Pediatric Endocrinology

FIFTH EDITION

Volume 1

Pediatric Endocrinology

FIFTH EDITION

Volume 1
Obesity, Diabetes Mellitus, Insulin Resistance, and Hypoglycemia

EDITED BY

Fima Lifshitz

Pediatric Sunshine Academics, Inc. and
Sansum Medical Research Institute
Santa Barbara, California, U.S.A.

University of Miami
Miami, Florida, U.S.A.

Health Science Center, State University of New York
Brooklyn, New York, U.S.A.

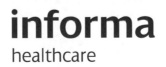

New York   London

Informa Healthcare USA, Inc.
270 Madison Avenue
New York, NY 10016

© 2007 by Informa Healthcare USA, Inc.
Informa Healthcare is an Informa business

No claim to original U.S. Government works
Printed in the United States of America on acid-free paper
10 9 8 7 6 5 4 3 2 1

International Standard Book Number-10: 0-8493-4068-3 (Hardcover)
International Standard Book Number-13: 978-0-8493-4068-0 (Hardcover)

Visit the Informa Web site at
www.informa.com

and the Informa Healthcare Web site at
www.informahealthcare.com

"Gracias a la vida que me ha dado tanto"
and has given me health to enjoy my life
and wisdom to do right.

Fima Lifshitz, M.D.

As Osler once said, "Read with two objects: first, to acquaint yourself with the current knowledge on a subject and the steps by which it has been reached; and second and more important, read to understand and analyze your cases." The fifth edition of the textbook of *Pediatric Endocrinology* provides the reader with an opportunity to meet both objectives, combining an update on the latest developments in the field of pediatric endocrinology with providing practical information on how this knowledge can be applied to patient care.

Books are a reflection of their times. It is not surprising, therefore, that the evolution of pediatric endocrinology over the past two decades is reflected by the changes that have occurred in this textbook since its initial printing in 1985. The first edition of *Pediatric Endocrinology* consisted of 27 chapters with 668 pages; the current edition consists of two volumes containing 53 chapters with a total of more than 1300 pages. The expansion in the size of the book reflects the rapid expansion of knowledge that has occurred in the field over the last 22 years. In 1985, only three chapters with 60 pages were devoted to the diagnosis and treatment of Type 1 diabetes mellitus and ketoacidosis, while Type 2 diabetes and obesity were not addressed. The current edition has been split into two separate but complementary volumes; the first volume covering disorders of carbohydrate metabolism (obesity, T1DM, T2DM, insulin resistance, and hypoglycemia) in 20 chapters with 510 pages and the second volume dealing with "traditional" endocrinology (growth, adrenal, sexual, thyroid, calcium, and fluid balance) in 33 chapters with 768 pages. The increase in the number of chapters and pages devoted to obesity and diabetes reflects the increased prevalence of these disorders in the pediatric population and is concordant with the patient distribution in many pediatric endocrine practices.

This book, therefore, provides an in-depth coverage of the disease states seen in the early 21st century. It provides the readership with an opportunity to explore the wonders of the science and the clinical breadth of pediatric endocrinology by just turning the pages. Osler wisely said, "To study the phenomena of disease without books is to sail an uncharted sea, while to study books without patients is to not go to sea at all." This book provides the sail, the boat, and the rudder; the clinicians must determine how to apply it to their patients.

Janet H. Silverstein, M.D.
Professor of Pediatrics
University of Florida
Gainesville, Florida, U.S.A.

The previous four editions of *Pediatric Endocrinology*, progressively, have been a dominating educational tool for subspecialists in pediatric endocrinology, genetics, nutrition, etc., and for pediatric generalists. The fifth edition exceeds my expectations and will exceed yours. The expansion of the text into two volumes could be discouraging to the prospective owner. It should not be. The educational leadership and organizational talent of Dr. Lifshitz have provided us with a text that now has necessarily expanded into two volumes as the scope of the specialty expanded. The new organization enhances the use of this textbook, permitting the reader initially to be very focused in obtaining the information he/she seeks, but it subsequently supplements that information as time permits by going to other chapters, each written by different well-known authors. Examination of Dr. Lifshitz's preface of this text and the indexed outline of chapters permits confirmation of my conclusion.

The multiple contributing authors also deserve strong commendations for the excellent content of this two volume text. The collaboration of multiple authors for each subsection permits the presentation of broader perspectives than if a single author had been responsible.

I have considered the presence of each of the previous four editions of *Pediatric Endocrinology* a necessity on my shelf because of their high quality as a diagnostic and therapeutic tool in the practice of pediatrics and pediatric endocrinology. The fifth edition similarly will be a necessary and welcomed addition on the shelf reserved for my favorite textbooks. I personally extend my thanks and congratulations to Dr. Lifshitz and to each of his contributors in producing this excellent and timely textbook.

Robert M. Blizzard, M.D.
Department of Pediatrics and
Children's Medical Center
University of Virginia
Charlottesville, Virginia, U.S.A.

Foreword

Dr. Fima Lifshitz's expansive view of the scope of pediatric endocrinology is reflected in the fifth edition of his classic textbook *Pediatric Endocrinology*, first published in 1985. Each edition has improved upon its predecessor by adding new chapters on topics relevant to the rapidly developing science and changing the practice of pediatric endocrinology. Unlike other textbooks of pediatric endocrinology, which tend to be largely devoted to classical pediatric endocrine subjects, Lifshitz's *Pediatric Endocrinology* has an expanded scope as it covers not only these subjects but is equally devoted to what might be referred to as Metabolic Endocrinology thereby reflecting the true practice of the specialty. The latter includes the various forms of diabetes mellitus, hypoglycemia, obesity and its related disorders, insulin resistance, lipid disorders and various genetic disorders of metabolism.

With 53 fully inclusive chapters, the fifth edition of *Pediatric Endocrinology* has expanded to two volumes. A substantial portion of volume one is devoted to metabolic endocrinology, whereas volume two contains chapters on all the classical topics in pediatric endocrinology including growth, adrenal, sexual, thyroid, calcium, and fluid balance disorders as well as other miscellaneous endocrine alterations. This textbook also provides valuable information on a variety of topics relevant to pediatricians, pediatric endocrinologists and academic clinicians throughout the world.

The two volumes complement each other and together provide comprehensive coverage of the contemporary practice of the expanded scope of pediatric endocrinology and metabolism.

Dr. Lifshitz has carefully selected pertinent topics and superb authors, all experts in their respective fields, who are both investigators and clinicians. As a result, *Pediatric Endocrinology* is characterized by an exceptional blend of rigorous scholarship and pragmatism, which undoubtedly contributes to its broad appeal and will ensure its continued success.

I congratulate Dr. Lifshitz on admirably accomplishing the monumental task of editing, unassisted, a textbook of this magnitude and complexity and ensuring that each chapter meets his exacting standards of scholarship, clinical relevance and clarity of exposition. It has been an honor and a privilege to serve as a contributor to *Pediatric Endocrinology* and to write this Foreword.

Joseph I. Wolfsdorf, M.B., B.Ch.
Children's Hospital and
Harvard Medical School
Boston, Massachusetts, U.S.A.

In this age of molecular science, our knowledge of the genetic basis of endocrine disorders is rapidly expanding. As we come to understand the etiology of the disease with pinpoint accuracy, our treatments become more effective and tailored to our patients' needs. Current molecular research impacts treatment when clinicians can use such findings to guide their therapies. This textbook serves as a crucial bridge between the molecular laboratory and the clinical practice, encouraging translational research.

Dr. Fima Lifshitz has again put together an authoritative, current and important text to serve the burgeoning field of pediatric endocrinology. I know that it will continue to be an invaluable tool for both clinicians and researchers.

Maria I. New, M.D.
Professor of Pediatrics
Director, Adrenal Steroid Disorders Program
Mount Sinai School of Medicine
New York, New York, U.S.A.

The good life is one inspired by love and guided by knowledge. —Bertrand Russell

The fifth edition of *Pediatric Endocrinology* marks the 22nd anniversary of this textbook. This edition has built upon the accumulated experience of the previous versions and every one of the chapters has been thoroughly updated; thereby its content enhances the reputation that *Pediatric Endocrinology* has enjoyed as "the classic book in the field." Each of the topics of the chapters of the fifth edition of this book addresses one of the many potential alterations of patients referred to the pediatric endocrinologist for evaluation and treatment. Together, they provide the most updated information needed by the physician caring for these children, yet written with the detail required by the subspecialist in academic settings. The chapters are written in a didactic manner, containing practical information, with comprehensive discussions that address all clinical situations. Thereby, the book serves to increase the knowledge of both the practitioner and the subspecialist. The fifth edition of *Pediatric Endocrinology* constitutes a state-of-the art textbook, written by mature, well-established contributors who transmit their knowledge in an erudite manner, covering the theoretical and the clinical considerations of each entity.

Since the first edition of *Pediatric Endocrinology* published in 1985, the field has grown and has evolved. The state of knowledge and the scientific basis of the practice of the specialty are markedly different from that of two decades ago. This edition encompasses the current status of the specialty and the care of patients with pediatric endocrine diseases. The ever-increasing scope of the science of endocrinology and the rapid acquisition of new knowledge are captured and synthesized in each chapter by experts in all aspects of the specialty. The clinical care and practical aspects of pediatric endocrinology are written by those who are committed to the practice of the specialty.

The fifth edition of *Pediatric Endocrinology* comprises two volumes—each one dealing with major areas in the field. The expanded version of the textbook allows a comprehensive review of the multiple advances and provides the reader the factual information to address all the concerns that arise when caring for children with endocrine-related alterations. Each one of these two books contains comprehensive chapters of specific entities that contain sufficient detailed information to cover the topic in its entirety. Thereby, each volume constitutes a book in its own right, yet both complement each other and together they form the resource in the field in an integrated easy-to-read and clearly written manner.

Volume 1 of *Pediatric Endocrinology* is devoted to obesity, diabetes mellitus, insulin resistance and hypoglycemia, with a special section on private practice and clinical research. Currently, caring for patients with these diseases constitutes a major part of the pediatric endocrinologist's time and effort. Thus, the expanded review of these topics reflects the true state of the specialty. Whereas previous editions of this book already contained chapters dealing with obesity and diabetes in children, long before these entities attracted the full attention of pediatric endocrinologists; other texts in the field have barely addressed these topics. However in this fifth edition of *Pediatric Endocrinology*, these entities are fully expanded to provide the reader with a substantive appraisal of the subjects and of the current issues. The major public health problem of obesity is most blatantly visible; yet it is often a neglected disease. In this book, obesity is discussed from a pediatric endocrinologist's perspective, with attention given to all aspects of the disease; including the epidemic and the mechanisms of the illness. The genetics and the single gene disorders that are manifested with obesity are reviewed as are the prevention and treatment of this disorder and the comorbidities. Included are also the chapters that address the current state of knowledge of the insulin resistance/metabolic syndrome and the diseases that often result from insulin resistance, such as hypertension and hyperlipidemia. The long-term endocrine alterations that follow the birth of a small-for-gestational-age infant are reviewed, with particular detail to the development of the insulin resistance syndrome, appearing later on in the life of such children.

There was a time when pediatric endocrinologists were not involved with the care of children with diabetes or with the teaching and research of this disorder; that was the past. Currently, the care for such patients demands the attention of the specialist; pediatric endocrinologists are now intimately involved in providing care and advancing the knowledge of the disease through clinical and basic science research. This is evident in each of the chapters of this book, which pertain to all aspects of diabetes mellitus. Included in the book is an update of the new clinical multicenter research programs designed to address the causes of Type 1 diabetes and chapters dealing with the theoretical and practical aspects of the care of such patients. Also, there is an expanded chapter dealing with Type 2 diabetes mellitus because this disease has become a more prominent area for the pediatric endocrinology specialty. In the section on hypoglycemia, the disorders that produce this alteration are reviewed with attention paid to the pathophysiology, its causes and the treatment, both in children and in neonates. The emergencies that pediatric endocrinologists deal when consulted for patients with inborn errors of metabolism are thoroughly addressed and the norms for the assessment of newborn screening alterations are provided. Finally, there are new chapters dealing with the current realities in the field, namely the private practice of the subspecialty and the performance of clinical trials by both the academic pediatric endocrinologist and the physician committed to patient care. There is also a comprehensive reference resource containing frequently used charts and tables needed for the assessment of endocrine patients.

Volume 2 of *Pediatric Endocrinology* is devoted to growth, adrenal, sexual, thyroid, calcium and fluid balance disorders, with a special section on radiation terrorism. The web resources available to the pediatric endocrinologist and the dynamic and genetic tests utilized in the care of patients with endocrine diseases are also contained therein. The diseases reviewed in this volume have been traditionally included within the realm of the pediatric endocrinology specialty and were included in previous editions of the book. However in the fifth edition of *Pediatric Endocrinology*, the specific chapters dealing with each of these entities are thoroughly reviewed and completely updated with attention given to the clinical and pathophysiological aspects of the disease. The book contains sections devoted to (i) growth and growth disorders, (ii) adrenal disorders, (iii) sexual development abnormalities, (iv) thyroid disorders, (v) calcium and mineral metabolism disorders, (vi) miscellaneous endocrine entities and (vii) endocrine testing protocols. In these sections, the diseases that afflict children cared for in a pediatric endocrine service are discussed. In the fifth edition of *Pediatric Endocrinology*, there are new chapters dealing with specific advances in the field of growth hormone insufficiency, the molecular basis of growth disorders and the integrity of the IGF system for appropriate growth. Also, there is a chapter on the transition from adolescence to adulthood of the growth hormone–deficient patient and the deficiency of this hormone in adults. The skeletal dysplasias leading to short stature and the syndromes leading to overgrowth and tall short stature are thoroughly reviewed.

The neonatal screening program is now widely used for the diagnosis of multiple inborn errors of metabolism, hypothyroidism and congenital adrenal hyperplasia. Thus, a readily available resource of the standards and guidelines for the care of newborns with abnormal newborn screens is found in the book. The chapters on traditional diseases of the adrenal cortex and medulla, as well as the sexual differentiation disorders and thyroid and parathyroid alterations, provide great detail in comprehensive reviews of all the alterations of patients with diseases of these endocrine glands. Also, there are new chapters dealing with rickets and osteoporosis and brittle bone syndromes, as the scope of the specialty has demanded that pediatric endocrinologists deal with patients with these entities. A major source of concern to pediatricians in practice is also addressed in this book, namely the patient with nonendocrine diseases associated with abnormal endocrine tests, often causing referrals to the pediatric endocrinologist. In this era, a chapter of radiation terrorism was necessary to bring to the pediatric endocrinologist the necessary information "to be aware and prepared." Additionally, the chapter dealing with the use of the web provides an important practical update to the practicing physician for the recognition of genetic syndromes in pediatric endocrinology. Finally, all the chapters address the diagnostics of endocrine function and disease with algorithms and updated tables, special growth charts, dynamic endocrine testing protocols and interpretation of the data. Altogether, the book provides the necessary information to facilitate the care of the pediatric endocrine patient and the understanding of the diseases that they present.

Sophocles said it long ago: "Look and you will find it—what is unsought will go undetected."

Fima Lifshitz, M.D.

Acknowledgments

This book was supported in part by Pediatric Sunshine Academics, Inc. a nonprofit corporation which promotes pediatric endocrinology and nutrition research and education. The contributions of the authors of each chapter are greatly appreciated; without their cooperation, the book would not have been realized. All manuscripts were paperless, electronic versions and thus saved trees and tested and improved my computer skills. This task would not have been possible without the help of my wife, Jere, who was always there to solve and improve upon the intricacies of computing, and I thank her foremost for her encouragement with the editing of the book and her love.

Fima Lifshitz, M.D.

Contents

SECTION III: INSULIN RESISTANCE AND ITS COMPLICATIONS

SECTION IV: HYPOGLYCEMIA

SECTION V: SPECIAL CONSIDERATIONS AND RESOURCES

Jose E. Abdenur Division of Metabolism, PSF-Children's Hospital of Orange County, Orange, California, U.S.A.

Ramin Alemzadeh Department of Pediatrics, Medical College of Wisconsin, Milwaukee, Wisconsin, U.S.A.

David B. Allen Department of Pediatrics, University of Wisconsin Children's Hospital, University of Wisconsin School of Medicine, Madison, Wisconsin, U.S.A.

Henry Anhalt Division of Pediatric Endocrinology and Diabetes, Saint Barnabas Medical Center, Livingston, New Jersey, and Department of Pediatrics, State University of New York, Health Science Center, Brooklyn, New York, U.S.A.

Yong Bao Department of Pediatric Endocrinology, Mailman Center for Child Development and Department of Pediatrics, Miller Medical School, University of Miami, Miami, Florida, U.S.A.

Dorothy J. Becker Department of Pediatrics, Children's Hospital of Pittsburgh, University of Pittsburgh School of Medicine, Pittsburgh, Pennsylvania, U.S.A.

Gary Berkovitz Department of Pediatric Endocrinology, Mailman Center for Child Development and Department of Pediatrics, Miller Medical School, University of Miami, Miami, Florida, U.S.A.

Amrit Bhangoo Division of Pediatric Endocrinology, Infants and Children's Hospital of Brooklyn, Maimonides Medical Center, and Department of Pediatrics Health Science Center, State University of New York, Brooklyn, New York, U.S.A.

Diego Botero Department of Pediatrics, Children's Hospital Boston, Harvard Medical School, Boston, Massachusetts, U.S.A.

Adriana A. Carrillo Department of Pediatric Endocrinology, Mailman Center for Child Development and Department of Pediatrics, Miller Medical School, University of Miami, Miami, Florida, U.S.A.

Martin Charron Division of Nuclear Medicine, Research for Diagnostic Imaging, Hospital for Sick Children, University of Toronto, Toronto, Ontario, Canada

Hofit Cohen The Institute of Lipid and Atherosclerosis Research, The Chaim Sheba Medical Center, Tel-Hashomer and Sackler Faculty of Medicine, Tel Aviv University, Tel Aviv, Israel

Ellen Lancon Connor Department of Pediatrics, University of Wisconsin, Madison, Wisconsin, U.S.A.

Giulia Costi Universitá Degli Studi Di Parma, Parma, Italia

Richard M. Cowett CIGNA Insurance, Pittsburgh, Pennsylvania, U.S.A.

John S. Dallas Pediatric Endocrinology, Cook Children's Medical Center, Fort Worth, Texas, U.S.A.

Middey Damian Department of Pediatric Endocrinology, Mailman Center for Child Development and Department of

Pediatrics, Miller Medical School, University of Miami, Miami, Florida, U.S.A.

Frank B. Diamond, Jr. Division of Pediatric Endocrinology and Diabetes, All Children's Hospital, St. Petersburg, and Department of Pediatrics, University of South Florida School of Medicine, Tampa, Florida, U.S.A.

Ruben Diaz Division of Endocrinology, Children's Hospital Boston, Havard Medical School, Boston, Massachusetts, U.S.A. and Division of Endocrinology, Hospital Sant Joan de Deu, Barcelona, Spain

Allan L. Drash Department of Pediatrics, Children's Hospital of Pittsburgh, University of Pittsburgh School of Medicine, Pittsburgh, Pennsylvania, U.S.A.

Graeme Eisenhofer Clinical Neurocardiology Section, National Institute of Neurological Disorders and Stroke, National Institutes of Health, Bethesda, Maryland, U.S.A.

Berrin Ergun-Longmire Division of Pediatric Endocrinology, UMDNJ/Robert Wood Johnson Medical School, New Brunswick, New Jersey, U.S.A.

Oscar Escobar Department of Pediatrics, Children's Hospital of Pittsburgh, University of Pittsburgh School of Medicine, Pittsburgh, Pennsylvania, U.S.A.

Hussien M. Farrag Baystate Medical Center, Tufts University School of Medicine, Springfield, Massachusetts, U.S.A.

Patricia Y. Fechner Division of Pediatric Endocrinology and Diabetes, Stanford University, Stanford, California, U.S.A.

Amy Fleischman Division of Endocrinology, Children's Hospital Boston, Harvard Medical School, Boston, Massachusetts, U.S.A.

Thomas P. Foley, Jr. Departments of Pediatrics and Epidemiology, School of Medicine, Graduate School of Public Health, University of Pittsburgh, Children's Hospital of Pittsburgh, Pittsburgh, Pennsylvania, U.S.A.

Lucia Ghizzoni Università Degli Studi Di Parma, Facoltà Di Medicina E Chirurgia, Istituto Di Clinica Pediatrica, Parma, Italia

Catherine Gordon Divisions of Endocrinology and Adolescent/Young Adult Medicine, Children's Hospital Boston, Harvard Medical School, Boston, Massachusetts, U.S.A.

Adda Grimberg Department of Pediatrics, University of Pennsylvania School of Medicine, and Division of Pediatric Endocrinology and Diabetes, The Children's Hospital of Philadelphia, Philadelphia, Pennsylvania, U.S.A.

Isil Halac Division of Pediatric Endocrinology, Children's Memorial Hospital, Northwestern University, Chicago, Illinois, U.S.A.

Michael J. Haller Division of Pediatric Endocrinology, Department of Pediatrics, University of Florida, Gainesville, Florida, U.S.A.

Christopher P. Houk   Backus Children's Hospital, Mercer University School of Medicine, Savannah, Georgia, U.S.A.

Stephen A. Huang   Division of Endocrinology, Children's Hospital Boston, Harvard Medical School and Thyroid Section, Brigham and Women's Hospital, Boston, Massachusetts, U.S.A.

Julie R. Ingelfinger   Department of Pediatrics, Harvard Medical School and Pediatric Nephrology Unit, MassGeneral Hospital for Children at Massachusetts General Hospital, Boston, Massachusetts, U.S.A.

Muhammad A. Jabbar   Department of Pediatrics, Hurley Medical Center, Michigan State University School of Medicine, Flint, Michigan, U.S.A.

Winston W. K. Koo   Department of Pediatrics, Obstetrics and Gynecology, Hutzel Hospital and Children's Hospital of Michigan, Wayne State University, Detroit, Michigan, U.S.A.

Anna Kozupa   Reproductive Biology and Medicine Branch, National Institute of Child Health and Development, National Institutes of Health, Bethesda, Maryland, U.S.A.

Edward P. Krenzelok   Department of Pharmacy and Pediatrics, Pittsburgh Poison Center, Children's Hospital of Pittsburgh, University of Pittsburgh, Pittsburgh, Pennsylvania, U.S.A.

Roberto Lanes   Unidad de Endocrinologia Pediatrica, Hospital de Clinicas Caracas, Caracas, Venezuela

Peter A. Lee   Penn State College of Medicine, The Milton S. Hershey Medical Center, Hershey, Pennsylvania, and Indiana University School of Medicine, Indianapolis, Indiana, U.S.A.

Phillip D. K. Lee   Reproductive Medicine and Metabolism, Clinical Development, Serono, Inc., Rockland, Massachusetts, U.S.A.

Fima Lifshitz   Pediatric Sunshine Academics Inc. and Sansum Medical Research Institute, Santa Barbara, California, and Department of Pediatrics, University of Miami, Miami, Florida, and Department of Pediatrics, Health Science Center, State University of New York, Brooklyn, New York, U.S.A.

Karen Lin-Su   Department of Pediatrics, Mount Sinai School of Medicine, New York, New York, U.S.A.

Faina Linkov   Department of Epidemiology, Graduate School of Public Health, University of Pittsburgh, Pittsburgh, Pennsylvania, U.S.A.

Shannon P. Lyles   Division of Pediatric Endocrinology, Department of Pediatrics, University of Florida, Gainesville, Florida, U.S.A.

Noel K. Maclaren   Department of Pediatrics, New York-Presbyterian Hospital, Weill Medical College of Cornell University, and Bioseek Endocrine Clinics, New York, New York, U.S.A.

Joseph A. Majzoub   Department of Pediatrics, Division of Endocrinology, Children's Hospital Boston, Harvard Medical School, Boston, Massachusetts, U.S.A.

Richard Mauseth   Woodinville Pediatrics, Woodinville, Washington and Department of Pediatrics, University of Washington School of Medicine, Seattle, Washington, U.S.A.

Maria Verónica Mericq G.   Department of Medicine, Institute of Maternal and Child Research, University of Chile, Las Condes, Santiago, Chile

Claude J. Migeon   Department of Pediatrics, Johns Hopkins Hospital, Johns Hopkins University, School of Medicine, Baltimore, Maryland, U.S.A.

Jennifer Miller   Division of Pediatric Endocrinology, Department of Pediatrics, University of Florida, Gainesville, Florida, U.S.A.

Brandon M. Nathan   Pediatric Endocrinology and Metabolism, Rainbow Babies and Children's Hospital, Case Western Reserve University School of Medicine, Cleveland, Ohio, U.S.A.

E. Kirk Neely   Division of Pediatric Endocrinology and Diabetes, Stanford University, Stanford, California, U.S.A.

Maria I. New   Department of Pediatrics, Adrenal Steroid Disorders Program, Mount Sinai School of Medicine, New York, New York, U.S.A.

Karel Pacak   Reproductive Biology and Medicine Branch, National Institute of Child Health and Human Development, National Institutes of Health, Bethesda, Maryland, U.S.A.

John A. Phillips III   Departments of Pediatrics, Medicine, Biochemistry and Pathology, Vanderbilt University School of Medicine, Nashville, Tennessee, U.S.A.

Horacio Plotkin   Departments of Pediatrics and Orthopedic Surgery, University of Nebraska Medical Center and Children's Hospital, Omaha, Nebraska, U.S.A.

Michel Polak   Pediatric Endocrinology Unit, Hôpital Necker-Enfants Malades, Paris, France

Raphaël Rappaport   Pediatric Endocrinology and Gynecology, Hopital Necker-Enfants Maldes, Paris, France

David L. Rimoin   Medical Genetics Institute, Cedars-Sinai Medical Center and the David Geffen School of Medicine at UCLA, Los Angeles, California, U.S.A.

Russell Rising   EMTAC, Inc., Miami, Florida, U.S.A.

Allen W. Root   Division of Pediatric Endocrinology and Diabetes, All Children's Hospital, St. Petersburg, Florida and Departments of Pediatrics and Biochemistry and Molecular Biology, University of South Florida College of Medicine, Tampa, Florida, U.S.A.

Arlan L. Rosenbloom   Division of Pediatric Endocrinology, Department of Pediatrics, University of Florida, Gainesville, Florida, U.S.A.

Ron G. Rosenfeld   Lucile Packard Foundation for Children's Health, Palo Alto, California, and Departments of Pediatrics and of Cell and Developmental Biology, Oregon Health and Science University, Portland, Oregon, U.S.A.

Raanan Shamir   Division of Gastroenterology and Nutrition, Meyer Children's Hospital of Haifa, and Ruth and Bruce Rappaport Faculty of Medicine, Technion, Haifa, Israel

Mordechai Shohat   Department of Pediatrics and Genetics, Rabin Medical Center and Sackler School of Medicine, Tel Aviv University, Tel Aviv, Israel

Janet H. Silverstein Division of Pediatric Endocrinology, Department of Pediatrics, University of Florida, Gainesville, Florida, U.S.A.

Abhinash Srivatsa Department of Pediatrics, Division of Endocrinology, Children's Hospital Boston, Harvard Medical School, Boston, Massachusetts, U.S.A.

Ömer Tarim Division of Pediatric Endocrinology, Department of Pediatrics, Uludağ University Faculty of Medicine, Gorukle, Bursa, Turkey

Elisabeth Thibaud Pediatric Endocrinology and Gynecology, Hopital Necker-Enfants Maldes, Paris, France

Guy Van Vliet Department of Pediatrics, University of Montréal, Endocrinology Service, Sainte-Justine Hospital, Montréal, Québec, Canada

David A. Weinstein Glycogen Storage Disease Program, Department of Pediatrics, University of Florida, College of Medicine, Gainesville, Florida, U.S.A.

William E. Winter Department of Pathology, Immunology and Laboratory Medicine, University of Florida, Gainesville, Florida, U.S.A.

Selma Feldman Witchel Division of Pediatric Endocrinology, Children's Hospital of Pittsburgh, University of Pittsburgh, Pittsburgh, Pennsylvania, U.S.A.

Joseph I. Wolfsdorf Division of Endocrinology, Department of Medicine, Children's Hospital Boston, and Department of Pediatrics, Harvard Medical School, Boston, Massachusetts, U.S.A.

Donald Zimmerman Division of Pediatric Endocrinology, Children's Memorial Hospital, Northwestern University, Chicago, Illinois, U.S.A.

1

Obesity in Children

Ramin Alemzadeh
Department of Pediatrics, Medical College of Wisconsin, Milwaukee, Wisconsin, U.S.A.

Russell Rising
EMTAC, Inc., Miami, Florida, U.S.A.

Fima Lifshitz
*Pediatric Sunshine Academics Inc. and Sansum Medical Research Institute,
Santa Barbara, California, and Department of Pediatrics, University of Miami, Miami, Florida,
and Department of Pediatrics, Health Science Center, State University of New York,
Brooklyn, New York, U.S.A.*

PREVALENCE

Obesity is one of the most complex and poorly understood clinical syndromes affecting children and adults throughout the world. In the last decade the estimated number of adults with excess weight has increased dramatically, from 200 million to 300 million affected individuals (1). The current prevalence of this disorder ranges from 5% to 10% of the population in some African and Asian countries to over 75% in urban Samoa (2). Since 1980 obesity rates have risen threefold or more in some areas of North America, United Kingdom, Eastern Europe, Middle East, the Pacific Islands, and Australia. In Mexico the prevalence of obesity also exhibited a dramatic increase between 2000 and 2003, obesity now being present in 60% of women and 50% of men (3). Mendez et al. recently observed that, in most developing countries, prevalence rates of overweight in young women exceed prevalence rates of underweight in both urban and rural areas particularly in countries at higher levels of socioeconomic development where the rates of obesity exceed 60% (4).

The prevalence and trends of obesity among U.S. adults markedly increased in the last decade of the last century (5). Approximately 127 million adults in the United States were overweight, 60 million were obese and 9 million were extremely obese in 2004 (6). Among different immigrant subgroups, number of years of residence in the United States was associated with higher prevalence and degree of obesity beginning after 10 years. The prevalence of obesity among immigrants living in the United States for at least 15 years approached that of U.S.-born adults (7). The percentage of overweight children and adolescents has increased by almost 50% in the last two decades of the 20th century (8). The prevalence and trends of overweight among U.S. children and adolescents have continued to increase (9). Among 2- through 5-year old children, the prevalence in 1999–2000 was 10.4%; among 6 through 11 years—15.3%; and among the 12- through 19-year-old group—15.5%. Similar results were observed by other investigators, who also showed that 22.6% of 2- to 5-year-old and 30% of 6- to 19-year-old children were at risk for overweight, as defined by a body mass index (BMI) ≥85th percentile for age (10). In the United States, the increase in the incidence of overweight has been more significant among African-Americans and Hispanic children and adolescents (11). The overweight prevalence increased to 21.5% among African-Americans, 21.8% among Hispanics, and 12.3% among non-Hispanic whites.

Increases in maternal anthropometry have also been associated with higher birth weight of infants at or after term (12). But the rate of weight gain during the first year of life and not birth weight, predicted BMI in childhood (13,14) or adulthood (15). It has long been observed that about 40% of overweight children will continue to have increased weight during adolescence and 75% to 80% of obese adolescents will become obese adults (16). Moreover, more than one-third of overweight children will eventually become obese adults (17). A child with a high BMI percentile has a high risk of being overweight or obese at 35 years of life and this risk increases with age (18), and childhood BMI was associated with adult adiposity (19).

Obesity in children is expected to continue to increase in the 21st century, but the consequences of this disease may be more severe as the duration of obesity will be longer. It may therefore have a greater deleterious impact on health and the rate of morbidity and mortality than obesity starting in adulthood.

MORBIDITY

Obesity in childhood is a major public health problem as it increases the risks of developing a number of health conditions and diseases (Table 1). These comorbidities have been associated with the increased mortality rates attributed to obesity. The number of deaths associated with obesity in the United States has been reported to be as high as over 430,000 per annum, a number that exceeds that attributed to smoking (20), though others reported a lower death rate, 112,000 of obesity-attributable deaths (21). The actual death rate prevalence of obesity continues to be debated (22–24) though there is a general agreement that the impact of this disease is enormous. Recently, Olshansk et al. suggested that in the 21st century, American obese children may die before their parents due to a potential decline in life expectancy (22).

Obesity decreases longevity, a 7- to 8-year loss of lifespan in 40-year-old nonsmoker individuals and a 13- to 14-year less lifespan in smokers (25); when obesity occurred by 20 to 30 years of age there was a 22% reduction in longevity, 17 to 20 less lifespan (26). Thus it could be expected that the impact of obesity starting earlier in life, beginning during childhood, would be more dramatic and lifespan would be further impaired. In a study by Must et al., long-term morbidity and mortality of overweight adolescents were examined (27). They demonstrated that obesity in adolescent subjects was associated with an increased risk of mortality from all causes and disease-specific mortality among men, but not among women. The risk of morbidity from coronary heart disease and atherosclerosis was increased in both men and women who had been obese in adolescence. However, in a study by Freedman et al., childhood overweight was related to adverse risk factors among adults, but associations were weak and were attributable to the strong persistence of weight status between childhood and

Table 1 Comorbidities Associated with Obesity in Children

Insulin resistance syndrome
Type 2 diabetes mellitus
Hypertension
Dyslipidemia
Cardiovascular disease
Renal alterations and hyperuricemia
Early puberty
Polycystic ovary syndrome
Cholecystitis
Fatty liver disease
Sleep apnea
Respiratory infections and asthma
Orthopedic alterations
Dermatologic alteatios
Nutritional deficits
Birth defects in offsprings
Increased risk of cancer
Psychosocial problems
Eating disorders
Depression

adulthood (28). This suggested that body weight reduction in the young may decrease the risks for many of the obesity-related health disorders.

Medical Complications

The altered nutritional state in obesity results in several alterations that have been linked as comorbidities of the disease. Hyperinsulinemia is strongly linked with cardiovascular diseases, Type 2 diabetes mellitus, hyperlipidemia, and hypertension (29). Obesity is associated with hypertension in 10% to 30% of children (30) regardless of age, gender, and duration. Obese children and adolescents tend to have elevated levels of total serum cholesterol, triglycerides, and low-density lipoprotein, and decreased levels of high-density lipoproteins (30,31). They are also at increased risk for coronary heart disease (31–33). With few exceptions, the clinical features of cardiovascular heart disease are not apparent until the third or fourth decade of life. However, there is substantial evidence that the atherosclerotic process is initiated during childhood (32–34).

Sensitivity to insulin glucose-mediated disposal may be altered in obese children (35). When insulin secretion cannot maintain the degree of hyperinsulinemia needed to overcome the resistance, Type 2 diabetes mellitus develops. However even when individuals secrete enough insulin to remain nondiabetic, if they present an altered glucose-mediated disposal with hyperinsulinemia they remain at increased risk to develop a cluster of abnormalities that have been given various names, best described as insulin resistance syndrome (IRS) (Vol. 1; Chap. 11). IRS was first described by Reaven in 1988 (29) and has been referred as syndrome X, metabolic syndrome, and dysmetabolic syndrome, the latest being the term used for ICD-9 coding 277.9. However the primary reason to select the term IRS is that the term denotes the central role of hyperinsulinemia in the pathogenesis of the cluster of abnormalities which characterize the syndrome, namely a clinical quartet of hyperinsulinemia, hyperlipidemia, hypertension, and subsequent cardiovascular disease (35–38). Clustering features of the IRS are independent of gender and age in both black and white populations (39).

It should be kept in mind that IRS may occur in individuals who are not obese and that many obese may not present this syndrome. It is believed that obesity is a risk factor for the development of IRS and it is a component of this metabolic syndrome since it has been described in obese children (40) and adolescents (41). However, only one-third of obese children and adolescents have IRS (42), though it was present with increased frequency and severity with a prevalence of up to 50% in severely obese youngsters (35). IRS was more highly prevalent among U.S. adults (43). Fasting insulin levels can help identify children with hyperinsulinemia: normal: < 15 IU/mL; borderline: 15 to 20 IU/mL; and high: > 20 IU/mL (44). The characterization of IRS and the recommended intervention in the pediatric population was clearly defined (45). Hyperinsulinemia and insulin resistance account for the observed highly prevalent abnormalities in glucose tolerance in obese adolescents (46) and for the development of acanthosis nigricans, a hyperpigmentation of skin, which is commonly seen in the back of the neck, axillae, and other flexural areas (47). Hyperinsulinemia is usually accompanied by hyperandrogenism, which leads to hirsutism and polycystic ovary (PCO) syndrome (48). Amenorrhea, oligomenorrhea, and/or dysfunctional uterine bleeding are common among obese adolescent females. Some of these patients will also develop PCO (48–50). PCO is now recognized as a component of the IRS (Vol. 1; Chaps. 11 and 13). Insulin-lowering agents have become the norm in the management of PCO (51).

There is a large body of literature demonstrating that the lipotoxic fat is the visceral adipose tissue; this may account for the differences in the prevalence of insulin resistance in obese individuals (52,53). Chen et al. suggested that this syndrome is characterized by the linking of a metabolic entity (hyperinsulinemia/insulin resistance, hyperlipidemia, and obesity) to hemodynamic factors resulting in hypertension through a shared correlation with hyperinsulinemia/insulin resistance (54). Low-grade systemic inflammation, elevated leptin concentration, and low adiponectin level are described in very young obese children, correlating with a range of variables of metabolic syndrome. Inflammation and adipocytokines can play an important role in the etiopathogeny of metabolic syndrome (55).

Cardiorespiratory fitness or physical fitness of the individual is an attribute that determines the alterations in glucose-mediated transport by the muscle, thus inactivity and inaction play an important role in the clinical expression and complications of the syndrome (56,57). However, genetic components also play an important role as there may be mitochondrial activity alterations (58) and alterations in the retinoid X receptor heterodimers (59).

Individuals who present with insulin resistance may benefit from treatment aimed to reduce hyperinsulinemia independent of glycemia (60). The presence of hyperinsulinemia favors the maintenance of the obese state by stimulating lipogenesis via activation of lipoprotein lipase and by inhibiting lipolysis (61). It has also been known that the lipogenic action of insulin occurs at a lower insulin concentration than its glycoregulatory action (62). Additionally hyperinsulinemic obese children oxidized more fat and less glucose than their lean counterparts (63). This impairment of glucose metabolism may, in part, be caused by an excessive utilization of fatty substrate (64). The extent of the changes in insulin levels correlated with increasing fat cell size and degree of obesity particularly in individuals with central obesity (65,66).

Nonautoimmune forms of youth-onset diabetes have become increasingly prevalent as rates of obesity in children and adolescents accelerated (67). Health professionals have recognized an emerging epidemic

of Type 2 diabetes, mainly affecting minorities (68–70). Epidemiological data suggest an almost fourfold increase in the prevalence of Type 2 diabetes among minority groups such as Native, African, and Hispanic Americans aged 10 to 19 years over the past 10 years (67,71). Increasing prevalence of Type 2 diabetes in the youth is not limited to North America. For instance, among Japanese junior high school students, the incidence of Type 2 diabetes is almost seven times more than for Type 1 diabetes mellitus (72,73). Impaired glucose tolerance was highly prevalent among obese children irrespective of ethnicity and was associated with insulin resistance, while beta-cell function was still relatively preserved (46). Those with insulin resistance often developed Type 2 diabetes mellitus over a two-year follow-up (35). However an earlier onset of Type 1 diabetes mellitus in childhood has also been observed with increasing body weight patterns (74). Additional information on Type 2 diabetes mellitus in children is presented in Vol. 1; Chap. 9.

Renal sequelae of obesity have been identified as yet another obesity-related morbidity (75). Obese adolescents present proteinuria, which has distinct clinical and pathologic features and may be associated with significant renal complications. Such proteinuria may respond to weight reduction and/or treatment with angiotensin-converting enzyme inhibitors. Obesity-related glomerulopathy is distinct from idiopathic focal segmental glomerulosclerosis, with a lower incidence of nephrotic syndrome, more indolent course, consistent presence of glomerulomegaly, and milder foot process fusion or effacement (76). The 10-fold increase in incidence over 15 years suggests a newly emerging epidemic.

Increased cholesterol turnover and its concentration in the bile of obese individuals predispose them to a high incidence of nonalcoholic steatohepatitis (77). Nonalcoholic liver disease is a major cause of liver-related morbidity and is usually associated with the presence of insulin resistance in individuals with obesity (78,79). Gallbladder disease, cholelithiasis, has been reported to be three times more common in morbidly obese people than in normal subjects (80). Gallstones may also result while the obese person is on a hypocaloric diet. This may be due to mobilization of adipose tissue cholesterol during weight loss (81). Furthermore, the risk of colorectal cancer and gout was increased among women who had been obese in adolescence. Finally, obesity in adolescence was a more significant predictor of these risks than being overweight in adulthood (82).

Rapid weight gain or obesity during infancy and childhood are also risk factors for frequent respiratory infections (83). The work of breathing is increased in obese individuals and larger body mass places increased demands for oxygen consumption and carbon dioxide elimination. Many obese subjects suffer from chronic hypoxemia secondary to ventilation–perfusion mismatch. This is characterized by increased ventilation of upper lobes and increased perfusion of the lower lobes. Insufficient elimination of carbon dioxide, in some obese subjects, leads to hypo-ventilation (Pickwickian) syndrome (84), which is characterized by chronic hypoxemia and hypercapnia. These subjects have blunted respiratory drive to both hypoxemia and hypercapnia.

However, parents of obese children and adolescents usually report that their children snore loudly and sometimes appear to stop breathing during sleep. The apnea may be obstructive, central, or combined. In most patients, no anatomical abnormalities of the upper airway contribute to the development of obstructive sleep apnea (OSA) (85). It has been shown that the occurrence of OSA in obese subjects is related to the size of the region enclosed by the mandible (86,87) and sites and sizes of fat deposits around the pharynx, as well as the weight of the subjects. In patients with OSA, alveolar hypoventilation results from increased oxygen demand during the apnea episode. Coexistent cardiopulmonary or neuromuscular disease in subjects with OSA can play a role in the development of alveolar hypoventilation. During the apnea episodes, the systemic blood pressure increases whereas the heart rate and cardiac output decrease. Apnea-associated cardiac arrhythmias have been frequently observed in patients with OSA and increase their risk for cardiovascular mortality (88). Relief of respiratory obstruction alleviates OSA. This may be accomplished by weight loss and continuous positive airway pressure during sleep.

The prevalence of asthma and obesity has increased substantially in recent decades, leading to speculation that obese persons might be at increased risk of asthma development (89). In adults, cross-sectional, case–control, prospective, and weight-loss studies are cumulatively consistent with a role for obesity in the pathogenesis of asthma. However, a study has suggested that increased BMI is associated with asthma and atopy in women but not men. Population-attributable fraction calculations estimate that 28% of asthma developing in women after age 9 is due to overweight (90).

In children, a significant association between excess weight and asthma incidence has been observed (91). However, these findings remain controversial because of the methodological limitations of many studies (89). Population surveys do suggest that persons with asthma are disproportionately obese compared with persons who have never had asthma. Weight-loss studies on the basis of behavioral change and bariatric studies have shown substantial improvements in the clinical status of many obese patients with asthma who lost weight (92). Clarifying the nature of the relationship between obesity and asthma incidence and the role of weight management among patients with asthma are both critical areas with important implications for the prevention and treatment of asthma.

Orthopedic complications of obesity are believed to be largely of mechanical nature. During childhood, slipped capital femoral epiphysis, Legg-Calve-Perthes disease, and genu valgum tend to be more common in obese subjects. Orthopedic disorders such as Blount's disease (tibia vara) and slipped capital femoral epiphysis are frequently seen in obese adolescents (93,94). In addition, overweight children are more likely to have persistent symptoms six months after an acute ankle sprain suggesting increased risk of chronic orthopedic morbidity in obese following acute injury (95).

Obesity denotes ingestion of excess calories but it does not necessarily denote intake of excess micronutrients. These children are at risk for iron deficiency and have been shown to have this alteration frequently, though they may not present anemia (96). There has been increasing evidence that maternal obesity is associated with an increased risk of congenital malformations, particularly neural tube defects (97,98). Folic acid may not play a protective role in obese women (99). These findings add to the long list of obstetric morbidities among overweight pregnant women and point to the need to prevent excess weight gain in young women who may get pregnant.

Psychosocial Impact and Psychopathology
Psychosocial Impact
In addition to the medical complications associated with obesity, the juvenile-onset obese subject is also at risk for psychological morbidity (100). It has also been shown that obesity tends to confer disability greater than that associated with other forms of chronic illness (101). This disability seems to be linked to the public nature of obesity. Peer group discrimination prompts parents to seek treatment for their obese child. Even young school-aged children have been observed to view their overweight classmates as less desirable playmates (102). Overweight children are frequently teased on the playground and usually excluded from games. Obese children are under considerable psychological stress and are generally viewed by society as clumsy, unattractive, and overindulgent.

Overweight children, as young as five years of age associate their obesity with both lower body esteem and perceived cognitive ability (103). A parent's concern about obesity and restriction of food were associated with negative self-evaluations among girls (104). In one study a mother's own dietary restraint and concern about daughter's obesity predicted child-feeding practices. This suggests that a mother's control over her daughter's feeding practices and concern about the child's obesity may be an important influence on the daughter's eating habits and relative weight (105). Moreover, obese elementary school-aged girls were more likely to be dieting and express concern about their overweight than similarly aged boys (106). All of these results suggest that childhood obesity has an impact early in a child's life and on the whole family.

Lowered self-image, heightened self-consciousness, and impaired social functioning have been noted in individuals who either become or remain obese during adolescence (103). Studies of obese adolescents have demonstrated obsession with being overweight, passivity, and withdrawal from social contact (106). Some investigators have found similarities between the behavior of obese subjects and racial minorities expressing prejudice (107). In fact, it has been shown that the obese persons were less likely to get admitted to a college than their lean counterparts, although there were no significant differences in their application rates, academic standing, or economic background (108). Moreover, obese individuals are 20% less likely to marry and are of lower income status than normal-weight individuals with other chronic medical conditions.

Severely obese children and adolescents (aged 5–18 years) have lower health-related quality of life problems than children and adolescents who are healthy and living in a similar environment. This is also compared with those children diagnosed as having cancer (109). However, others have suggested that obese children tend to demonstrate only decreased physical and social functioning without significant reduction in emotional and school functioning compared with normal-weight children (110). Nevertheless, physicians, parents, and teachers need to be aware of the risk for impaired health-related quality of life among obese children and adolescents in order to target interventions that could improve present and future overall health.

Psychopathology

Although there have been many studies of psychopathology in obesity, whether obesity is associated with psychiatric disorders is controversial. Clinical studies generally suggest that obese persons seeking weight-loss treatment have elevated rates of mood and binge-eating disorders (BED) (111,112). Of people in weight-loss programs about 30% have a BED and these people have a higher prevalence of overweight categories than those who do not have BED (113,114). On the other hand, community studies suggested that obese persons did not have elevated rates of psychopathology, including depressive disorders (115). However, chronic obesity was associated with oppositional defiant disorders in boys and girls (116) and other studies found an association between obesity, depression, and BED in severely obese individuals (117).

Thus, in evaluating obese patients presenting for treatment a diagnosis of BED should be considered. The *Diagnosis and Statistical Manual of Mental Disorders* (DSM-IV-TR) defines an episode of binge eating by two features: eating in a discrete period of time (i.e., two hours) an amount of food that is definitely larger than most people would consume and by a sense of lack of control over eating during the episode and feeling that one cannot stop or control what one is eating. According to the DSM-IV BED and bulimia nervosa share the same core of recurrent binge eating; however, the bulimic patients present other inappropriate eating behaviors to compensate for the binges, such as self-induced vomiting, laxative misuse and excessive exercise, among other distinguishing features.

It should also be kept in mind that severe chronic mental illness is often complicated by obesity. In over 60% of patients with schizoaffective disorder and bipolar disorder psychotropic drugs were used (118,119). The choice of antipsychotic drugs used in children is particularly poignant in schizophrenia (120). Olanzapine is frequently used as it is effective in inducing remission of mental symptoms, but it is associated with marked weight gain leading to obesity. As the weight problem progresses adherence to the medication decreases, even with newer antipsychotic medications (121).

Depression during childhood is also positively associated with BMI during adulthood. This association cannot be explained by various potential confounding variables and may develop over time as children pass into their adult years (122). Depressed adolescents are also at increased risk for the development and persistence of obesity during adolescence. Understanding the shared biological and social determinants linking depressed mood and obesity may inform the prevention and treatment of both disorders (123). Additionally, the medications used to treat depressive disorders may also impact body weight gain (124). While a cross-sectional study observed that overeating among adolescents is associated with a number of adverse behaviors and negative psychological experiences (115), further research is needed to identify whether objective overeating is an early warning sign of additional psychological distress or is a potential consequence of compromised psychological health.

Dieting/Body Image Problem

There is a culture of body image in our society, thus it is important to pay close attention to the behavioral and mental health concerns for children and adolescents. The American Academy of Pediatrics *Diagnostic and Statistical Manual for Primary Care* (DSM-PC) distinguishes dieting/body image behaviors that were, in the past, difficult to categorize as eating disorders. Children and adolescents may exhibit behaviors that do not meet full DSM-IV criteria, yet still deserve attention. The two specific complexes in the DSM-PC–related diagnostic categories include dieting/body image behaviors and purging/binge-eating behaviors (125). There are two levels of pathology for both of these behavior patterns in children that do not fulfill DSM-IV criteria for an eating disorder. In DSM-PC, *variations* constitute minor deviations from normal that still might be of concern for a parent or clinician (125). An adolescent with a dieting/body image problem will be one who exhibits voluntary food limitation in a pursuit of thinness. If an adolescent experiences a systematic fear of gaining weight that extends beyond a simple dieting/body image variation with a more severe intensity and purging/binge-eating behaviors, a more severe problem needs to be appropriately diagnosed in accordance with DSM criteria.

Children want to be thin. They like to be slim and trim and they fear being even a bit overweight.

This fear is present among all individuals, even those who are not overweight, but who want to be thinner (126,127). Even children, by the time they reach the first grade of school, prefer other disabilities to obesity (128). The desire to be thin constitutes a problem that must be considered as a form of social obesity. This phenomenon often translates as a fear of obesity and may lead to both health-promoting and health-compromising eating behaviors (126,127). The appropriate health-promoting activities include exercising; eating healthy foods, limiting the amount of food eaten; and avoiding sweets. The health-compromising activities might be the same but of a more extreme degree and may also involve the use of diet pills, laxatives, or water pills; self-induced vomiting; skipping meals; dieting and fasting (129).

While children should be learning to enjoy food, it appears that they often diet without supervision. There is a high prevalence of extreme measures taken by high school students throughout the country to avoid obesity (130,131). They often diet and have inappropriate eating habits and purging behaviors. Young persons, even when they are not overweight, diet to avoid obesity at a time when they are still growing and developing (127,130,132). This can adversely affect their growth, resulting in nutritional growth retardation (133). Based on gender, weight control behaviors were found in 56.7% of adult women, 50.3% of adult men, 44.0% of adolescent girls, and 36.8% of adolescent boys (134). Moses et al. showed that high school adolescents in an affluent suburban location were dieting at a very high rate (127). Dieting occurred in normal-weight and underweight students. However, the proportion of the overweight students who were dieting was relatively low: 50% to 60%. A distorted perception of ideal body weight (below appropriate body weight for height) was very prevalent among high school students. Adolescents knew what their ideal weight should be, but preferred to be 10% less than their ideal weight for their height (127).

Dieting in childhood is a common habit even in young children (129). Abramovitz and Birch found that 34% to 64% of the girls had ideas about dieting and weight loss and understood the link between eating and body shape (135). They modified their eating behaviors, such as drinking diet shakes and sodas, and use of special diet foods, and had restrictive eating behaviors. Mothers played a very important role in modeling both health-promoting and health-compromising eating behaviors. Girls whose mothers reported current or recent food restriction were more than twice as likely to have ideas about dieting (135). Another factor found to influence children's ideas, concepts, and beliefs about dieting was a family history of overweight. The media was also mentioned by 55% of the children as a source of dieting ideas (136).

Children not only diet, but also worry about their body appearance, are concerned about and dissatisfied with their body image; 55% of girls and 35% of boys in grades 3 to 6 want to be thinner (136). Body image dissatisfaction is an important risk factor for eating disturbances, 4.8% of them had scores on the Children's Version of the Eating Attitudes Test suggestive of anorexia nervosa (137). Eating disturbances that emerged during childhood led to inhibited and secretive eating, overeating, and vomiting. Maternal body dissatisfaction, internalization of the thin ideal, dieting, bulimic symptoms, and maternal and paternal body mass prospectively predicted the emergence of childhood eating disturbances. Infant feeding behavior and body mass during the first month of life also predicted the emergence of eating disturbances (137).

Parents who worry about their children becoming overweight may set the stage for a vicious cycle. Maternal perceptions of weight status of children is often wrong (138). Those parents who control what and how much their children eat may impede energy self-regulation and put these children at higher risk for overweight (139). These findings suggest that the optimal environment for children's development of self-control of energy intake is that in which parents provide healthy food choices but allow children to assume control of how much they consume (139). The Framingham Children's Study showed that children whose parents had high degrees of dietary control had greater increases in body fatness than did children whose parents had the lowest levels of dietary restraint and disinhibition (140). The relationship between dieting and weight change is also important among children. Dieting to control weight is not only ineffective but may actually promote weight gain (141). Health-compromising behaviors and the fear of obesity may have detrimental consequences in children (134).

ECONOMIC IMPACT OF OBESITY

The increasing prevalence of obesity is associated with rising health care costs. The cost of treating obesity-related illnesses to the economy of the U.S. business sector has escalated in recent years. It has been estimated that over 9.0% of annual medical expenditures are related to obesity (142). Health insurance expenditures for treating obesity-related illnesses such as hypertension, Type 2 diabetes, and coronary artery disease amounted to 43% of the total amount. Additional costs include increased sick leave, and life and disability insurance payments. In 2003, annual U.S. obesity-attributable medical expenditures were estimated at $75 billion in 2003 dollars, and approximately one-half of these expenditures were financed by Medicare and Medicaid (143). Other countries have seen similar obesity-related increases in health care costs (144), and spend a considerable amount of available health care dollars for treating obesity-related comorbidities.

Most obesity-related expenditures relate to obese adults. There are few studies of the economic impact of childhood obesity (145). The medical expenditures of 6- to 17-year children quadrupled from

1979–1981 to 1997–1999. The cost of care for obese children will likely surpass the costs above mentioned statistics once they reach adulthood. They will like present earlier and more severe comorbidities as their obesity will be longer and perhaps worse than that of the current populations. Although, some managed care organizations are now beginning to offer benefits for the treatment of childhood obesity through better access to established community childhood obesity programs (146) their impact in reducing the prevalence and severity of obesity and its complications remains to be proven.

ASSESSMENT

The measurement of body weight, the parameter commonly used to assess adiposity, is not an optimal method to differentiate between being overweight and being obese. Indeed, individuals with larger than average body frames or excess muscle mass (athletes) may be mistakenly considered obese since they have excess body weight. However, obesity may also be prevalent among athletes, i.e., one-fourth of NFL football players had BMIs in the class 2 range, denoting a body weight that would not be due only to a healthy increase in lean body mass (147). Moreover, in a primary care setting, the excess body weight at the time of a visit to a pediatrician is not usually plotted on a growth chart and does not appear to be a concern as obese children are rarely referred to specialists, whereas underweight children usually get a work up and are often referred to a subspecialty (148). The referral of obese children to pediatric endocrinologists is usually late, occurring long after obesity onset, usually seeks an assessment of endocrine comorbidities and IRS, and is ineffective for the treatment of obesity (149).

Growth

Plotting the growth and weight of children in age-specific growth charts allows a precise assessment of a child's status. It helps the clinician to evaluate a child's weight and its relationship to height, and it provides a view of the growth pattern, which determine the gravity of the situation. The importance of growth charts in the evaluation of childhood obesity is illustrated in the example shown in Figure 1. Julie was a five-year-old girl with a pattern of morbid obesity. Review of her growth records revealed that Julie's rate of weight gain became excessive after three months of age and progressed at an accelerated pace after one year of age. This coincided with an acceleration of linear growth but of a lesser magnitude than that of weight gain. The final point on Julie's growth chart (weight: 50 kg; height: 116.5 cm) represents 249% of her ideal body weight for height. In contrast, in Figure 2, the growth chart of Michael with a pattern of constitutional overweight is shown. In this patient, body weight progression was constant

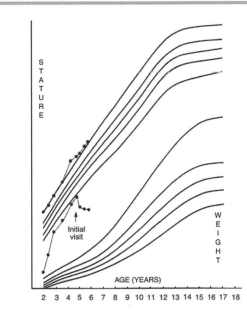

Figure 1 Growth chart of Jullie, a patient with obesity (see text).

throughout, being two major percentiles above that of height with an excess weight for height of 38% throughout his lifespan.

These two types of growth patterns provide clear evidence of two distinct clinical patterns of obesity necessitating different approaches. In Julie's case,

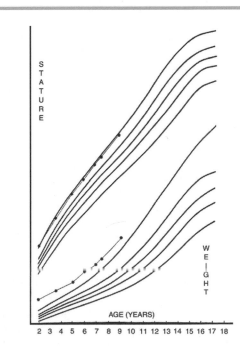

Figure 2 Growth chart of Michael, a patient with constitutional overweight (see text).

all efforts need to be made to stop the disproportionate body weight accretion including new patential therapies (150). In Michael's case, caution must be exercised not to interfere with the balance and adjustment already achieved by the patient in maintaining body weight. In a survey of high school children, Pugliese et al. showed that constitutional patterns of overweight are encountered in about 25% of high school students with excess body weight for height, remaining proportional throughout their school years (151). The morbid obesity pattern of growth was rare, observed in 0.8% of students. Therefore, the clinical assessment of an obese child must include measurements of height and weight progression for the proper assessment and recommendations for treatment.

Body Mass Index

BMI is a widely used method to define the relationship between weight and height (152). Charts of BMI relative to age are used to determine childhood obesity. BMI percentiles can be downloaded directly from the Centers for Disease Control (153). They are easy to use, nonintrusive, and have been validated against measures of body fat. The BMI is calculated as weight (kg)/height (m^2) and provides a practical clinical tool for classification of individuals with normal weight and those with various degrees of obesity. In the adult a grade I obesity is that with a BMI of 25 to 29; grade II is a BMI of 30 to 40; and grade III is one with a BMI of more than 40. The BMI system of classification of obesity is important because it denotes the risk for medical complications of obese patients, which increase at BMI levels above 25 (154). Individuals with a BMI above 27 have a markedly increased risk for hypertension, hypercholesterolemia, and diabetes mellitus. In contrast, when the BMI index is less than 25, there are no apparent physical effects of obesity on the individual, although there may be social and psychological concerns with body appearance. However, the use of BMI has limited applications in the assessment of overweight children since its calculation is based primarily on a stable height, which is not applicable to growing children. Also, the BMI can underestimate the percentage of lean body mass since it does not account for variations in musculature. This BMI paradox was clearly illustrated by Yajnik and Yudkin (155).

Children's BMIs at or above the 85th percentile are considered overweight and those above the 95th percentile are obese. Furthermore, no differences in the relationship between BMI and age exist among boys and girls up to age 20 in the United States, United Kingdom, Japan, and Singapore (156). The BMI charts clearly denote the usual percentiles and will distinguish a stage 1 obese child when the BMI is between the 85th and the 95th percentile for age. However, it will not determine the stage 2 or 3 of obesity as it does for the adult as the excess total BMI will vary with the age of the child. We have utilized an excess of >50% over the 50th percentile for age to define stage 2 obesity and an excess of >100% over the 50th percentile to define stage 3 obesity in children.

There are several potential errors associated with BMI as an indicator of obesity in children (157). The increasing height in children from birth until adulthood may cause a difference in the weight-for-height relationship assumed in current BMI-for-age charts. Gender and age also affect body weight and height. Furthermore, puberty may introduce another change in the weight-for-height relationship. Ethnic origin and social class may also affect both body weight and height. Nonetheless, BMI correlates (>0.8) with body fat as determined by both skinfold thickness measurements and by densitometry (158). This suggests that BMI is a reasonable criterion for determining obesity in children and adolescents. However in adults, these relations are simpler because adult height is assumed to be fixed. Therefore, body weight is adjusted for height only. However the progression of the BMI as the child grows will be a more appropriate longitudinal measurement, as it denotes the accumulation of excess fat over time and whether this is progressing in the same percentile or if it is crossing percentiles, as in the case of body weight progression mentioned above.

It should be kept in mind that the BMI adjustment for the age of the child may change over time. One study found that the power used to adjust height (Benn index) changed from 2.0 to 3.5 over the first 20 years of life in order to maintain the best relationship with skinfold thickness. The strongest relationships with skinfold thickness were obtained in children between 9 and 10 years old. Using only a Benn index of 2.0 may introduce subtle errors in BMI when used in younger children. Taller children will tend to have greater BMIs than shorter children. However, trying to correct for age with the Benn index will lead to more errors than if just one standard Benn index of 2.0 is used (159).

Skinfold

Skinfold thickness from several separate sites, including both trunk and extremities, provide a reliable estimate of obesity and regional fat distribution, if properly measured. The correlation of multiple skinfold measurements with total body adiposity is in the range of 0.7 to 0.8. One problem with skinfold measurements is that the equations used must be changed for age, gender, and ethnic background. Body fat increases with age, even though the sum of the skinfolds remains constant. This means that the fat deposition with age occurs in large part at sites other than subcutaneous ones (160). Also, triceps skinfold (TSF), which is typically the site of measurement, is often difficult to grasp and measurement reliability can be poor. It has been observed that there is a strong correlation between BMI and TSF among age- and gender-matched groups, suggesting that these measures are interchangeable for use in classifying individuals and in the evaluation of secular trends of obesity and morbid obesity (161). However, it should be noted that the clinician measuring skinfolds should be appropriately trained to be accurate.

Body Fat Measurement

Body composition tables for age and sex of children are in Vol. 1; Chap. 20. Additional information regarding body fat may be elicited from National Health and Nutrition Examination Survey (NHANES) measurements by participant age and gender—eight years and older (162).

Several methods are available for the estimation of body fat content. These include methods that measure body density: body weight in and out of the water. This process makes it possible to fractionate the body into its fat and lean components, assuming a density for fat of $0.91 \, g/cm^2$. The technique remains basically a research method. The recent availability of the BodPod Body Composition System allowed accurate determinations of body composition without the associated problems with hydrostatic weighting (163). The principle of the method is similar to hydrostatic weighting except that body volume is now obtained by air displacement. Subjects sit for two minutes in a 450 L chamber and a moving diaphragm determines the difference in air pressure between where the subject is sitting in the front chamber and a rear reference chamber. The pressure difference, along with the subject's body weight, is used to calculate body volume. From these results, body density is calculated and any of the standard equations for calculating fat-free mass (FFM) and fat mass can be used. The procedure is entirely safe and requires no special cooperation on the part of the subject and has been validated against hydrostatic weighting (164). Furthermore, the BodPod Body Composition System can accommodate adults up to 160 kg (350 lb). In children the BodPod Body Composition System may underestimate body fat up to 3% when compared with dual-energy X-ray absorptiometry measurements (165). Recently the same manufacturer produced a BodPod for infants (PEA POD), which has been validated and is now commercially available (166).

However, bioelectrical impedance analysis has been commonly used as a noninvasive and inexpensive method for estimation of body fat and lean mass (167). Bioelectrical impedance relies on the association between conductivity and tissue fluid and electrolyte content. It has proved to be fairly reliable in assessing total body water, but is less reliable in the estimation of body fat, especially in obese children (168,169).

Other noninvasive methods, such as the use of ultrasound waves applied to the skin, can provide a measure of fat depth (170). However, the data derived from the ultrasound method were 15% to 25% lower than that obtained by calipers. The authors concluded

that the ultrasound-derived body fat estimates represented only the subcutaneous body fat and not the whole-body adiposity (i.e., visceral fat). On the other hand, other studies have shown that sonography is a reliable tool in measuring small variations in quantities of intra-abdominal (visceral) fat and is superior to waist-to-hip ratio (WHR) in evaluating regional fat distribution and visceral adiposity (171).

Dual-energy X-ray absorptiometry has been shown to be a reliable method for estimating FFM and body fat. It has a unique ability to provide precise measures of regional fat mass, lean mass, and bone mineral content (172–174). Computerized axial tomography (CT) scan and magnetic resonance imaging (MRI) can also be used to quantitate lean and fat tissue. They provide accurate anatomical details and can reliably measure total and regional body adiposity (175). In a recent study, Ross et al. (176) demonstrated that MRI can provide a reliable measure of subcutaneous and visceral adipose tissue in obese subjects. A principal benefit of measuring adipose tissue by MRI or CT is the development of mathematical equations from external anthropometry that can predict MRI adipose tissue. However, the cost precludes the use of these methods for clinical purposes.

Validation for the use of total body electrical conductivity (TOBEC) for body composition measurements in children has allowed accurate determinations of FFM and fat mass without the assumptions associated with other methods. This method is appealing due to its ease of use, lack of radiation exposure, and the fact that little subject cooperation is required. The entire procedure takes only five minutes and does not require that infants or young children be sedated, though it does require the subject to remain still. The instrument registers the magnitude of the magnetic field disruption and provides a value referred to as the TOBEC number. The square root of the TOBEC number has been found to be directly correlated with FFM and fat mass (177).

There are multiple popular technologies to determine body fat: a Google search in October 2005 listed 15,700 sites. Some of the most frequently used ones are: (i) Body Fat Scales-Are they worth it? (178); (ii) Fat Track Pro Digital Body Fat Measurement System-Nutricraze (179); (iii) Equistat: Total body water and ECFV measured using bioelectrical impedance (180); (iv) Body Composition-Tanita Innerscan (181); (v) Balance Beam Scale-seca 700 (182); and (vi) DietMaster 2000 Software: Body Composition Screen (183). These technologies have not been standardized in children and have high replication errors.

Fat Distribution

It has long been known that there are major morphological and metabolic features that differentiate upper from lower body obesity (184–186). Body fat distribution is more important than percentage of body fat in predicting morbidity. Adults with a preponderance of abdominal fat (android) as measured by a WHR in excess of 0.8 have a higher frequency of hypertension, hyperinsulinemia, diabetes, and hyperlipidemia than equally obese individuals with predominantly pelvic (gynecoid) fat distribution (187,188). In children there is also an increased prevalence of obesity-related morbidities with increasing WHR (189) Thus, the evaluation of body fat distribution is an essential element in the assessment of obesity. However, it has been observed that WHR cannot predict visceral adiposity in obese individuals as accurately as other more sophisticated methods (170,173). CT scan, or MRI, measures of visceral-to-subcutaneous fat tissue ratio (VSR) has been shown to be a better index of regional fat distribution than WHR (190,191). Furthermore, VSR correlates more closely with metabolic variables such as levels of serum lipids, insulin, and glucose than WHR.

However, the clinical use of waist measurements to assess the presence of upper body obesity in obese children is of practical significance. It may be associated with development of acanthosis nigricans along the skin creases of posterior cervical, axillary, and other flexural areas. Waist circumference (WC) measurement is at least as strong as is BMI in predicting cardiovascular disease risk (192) and there was a correlation between the WC and the presence of risk obesity-related comorbidities. The WC of more than 102 cm in men and more than 88 cm in women have been recommended for determination of obesity-related comorbidities (193). Also, Wang et al. demonstrated that both overall and abdominal adiposity strongly and independently predict risk of Type 2 diabetes (194) and that WC is a better predictor than is WHR. However, these investigators suggested that the currently recommended cutoff for WC of 102 cm for men may need to be reevaluated; a lower cutoff may be more appropriate. Recently the percentiles of WC of children of various racial backgrounds were published (195). These tables are shown in Vol. 1; Chap. 20.

WHO IS AT RISK?

It has been shown that parental fatness is related to future obesity in their children. Obese parents impose a great risk that their children will be overweight. When both parents are overweight, about 80% of their children will be obese. When one parent is obese, this incidence decreases to 40%; and when both parents are lean, obesity prevalence drops to approximately 14% (191). There is more than a 75% chance that children aged 3 to 10 will be overweight if both parents were obese. This drops to a 25% to 50% chance with just one obese parent. These statistics suggest that lifestyle modification and treatment intervention at an early age may be important for preventing future adolescent and adulthood obesity (196). However, the reasons for these associations are not clear since most of the studies fail to separate the genetic and environmental influences in a critical way.

The susceptibility to obesity may begin in utero and in early life (Vol. 1; Chap. 12). Maternal-uterine restraint and rapid early catch-up growth are strong risk factors for the development of obesity and its complications (197). Roberts et al. (198) showed that excessive weight gain among a group of infants born to obese mothers was accompanied by reduced level of *energy expenditure for activity*. Furthermore, Ravussin et al. observed decreased levels of energy expenditure in obese compared with nonobese families (199). These findings are in accordance with the energy intake at six months, which predicted body fatness by one year of age (200). In contrast, several studies have found that energy intake in infants less than three months old is not a determinant of body fatness by two to three years of age (201,202).

The metabolic studies in infants cited above (199–202), which tried to identify alterations in metabolic rate that may contribute to future obesity, were inconclusive due to methodology limitations. Recent improvements in indirect calorimetry technology have enabled more accurate measurements of infant energy expenditure. With the new Enhanced Metabolic Testing Activity Chamber (EMTAC), validated for accurate measurements of the components of energy expenditure, such as resting and sleeping metabolic rates, along with physical activity, in infants (203,204), the relationship between maternal obesity and infant feeding-interactions was studied (205). Infants born to obese mothers consumed more energy more rapidly, and more energy as carbohydrate than normal-weight counterparts. Most of the increased intake was from complementary feedings. Furthermore, obese mothers spent less time interacting and feeding their infants who slept longer. However, there were no differences in total daily energy expenditures, resting metabolic rate, and sleeping metabolic rate between infants born to obese and normal-weight mothers. These variations in feeding-interacting practices appeared to be more important than the inborn metabolic parameters in predisposing them to obesity.

There is a strong influence of many environmental factors on the rate of weight gain, with or without a genetic susceptibility (206). Weight gain and adiposity in infancy and early childhood are influenced by several environmental factors (207). For instance, birth weight, duration of feeding, male gender, and age at the introduction of solid foods seem to affect the rate of weight gain during the first year of life. Maternal weight becomes a significant determinant for adiposity during the second year of life when the maternal environmental influences contribute to the development of obesity, since they determine the child's energy intake and expenditure (208). Vigorous feeding of infants and children may set the stage for the development of obesity (205,209,210). Overweight children have been observed to eat more rapidly and chew their food less than those of normal weight (209).

Body adiposity and growth of newborns are influenced by maternal weight and rate of weight gain during the prenatal period (211). Infants of diabetic mothers have increased body adiposity at birth and at one year of age (212) and macrosomic infants of mothers with gestational diabetes mellitus (GDM) have evidence of increasing body size and adiposity with increasing age and that maternal GDM and maternal prepregnant adiposity are predictors of such growth patterns (213).

GENETICS

It has long been known that obesity runs in families. The role of genetics in obesity was evaluated by Stunkard et al., who demonstrated no relationship between the body fat indices of adoptive parents and their adoptive children (214). They showed that BMI of biological parents was more closely correlated with the weight status of their offspring even when they did not live together. The importance of the genetic component was also confirmed by studies involving monozygotic twins (215). The BMIs of identical twins reared apart compared with those reared together were essentially the same. In addition, the correlation coefficients utilized to estimate the heritability of skinfold thickness in twins showed that there was a significant environmental component among children less than 10 years, whereas heritability estimated in twins more than 10 years of age was very high (216). The heritability of body fatness and of body fat distribution in adulthood was 65% to 80%, which is similar to the heritability of height.

In a study involving Swedish adult twins, Heitmann et al. (217) suggested that although food choices seemed to also play a role in the frequency of consumption of various foods, genetics also influenced the preference for several foods. However, there was no evidence that the consumption frequency of any of the foods was differentially associated with expression of genes responsible for weight gain. In a separate study, Faith et al. (218) showed that genetic influences played a role in percent body fat (PBF) in twins, including monozygotic and dizygotic pairs, from 3 to 17 years of age. The analyses indicated significant genetic influences on PBF, with genes estimated to account for 75% to 80% of the phenotypic variation. The remaining variation was attributable to nonshared environmental influences.

A poignant example of the role of genetics and environment in determining the development of obesity was clearly illustrated by the Pima Indian studies. Those living in the United States developed severe obesity whereas their counterparts living across the border in Sonora Mexico did not (219,220). Energy expenditures played a most important role in the same genetic component. Indeed, it is likely that the combination of continuous food abundance and physical inactivity eliminates the evolutionarily programmed biochemical cycles emanating from feast-famine and physical activity-rest cycles, which in turn abrogates the cycling of certain metabolic processes, ultimately resulting in metabolic derangements such as obesity and Type 2 diabetes (221). Perhaps a critical mechanism to break the stall of the metabolic processes would be through exercise or via the regulation of "physical activity genes," some of which may also be potential candidates for the "thrifty genes" of our hunter-gatherer ancestors (222).

Genes

The genetics of body weight regulation have been precisely documented (223). Several genome scans have been performed for adult obesity and obesity-related phenotypes in various ethnic groups (224–226). Different chromosomal regions have also been identified in these whole-genome scans including linkage to chromosomes 2p, 7q, 10p and q and 2p (227–230). Saar et al. performed a genome scan for childhood and adolescent obesity in German families (231). The chromosome 10p linkage can be considered one of the most consistent findings in obesity scans. Indeed, candidate genes localized within the chromosome 10 and 11 regions of interest including glutamic acid decarboxylase 2 (chromosome 10) and angiotensin receptor-like 1 (ciliary neurotrophic factor, galanin, and uncoupling proteins 2 and 3) show some potential. Further, these linkage studies in children and adolescents suggest that the genetic basis of childhood and adolescent obesity might not differ that much from adult obesity.

Essential maternal–placental factors that include maternal genetic material from the mother or from fetal placenta include the mitochondrial DNA 16189 variant and H19 (232). These maternal genetic factors may also play a role in the way the infant grows and in the development of obesity and comorbidities late in life. In particular these influence smaller, growth-restrained infants. Fetal genes include the insulin gene (INS) variable number of tandem repeat (VNTR), which is known to be associated with birth size and cord blood insulin-like growth factor (IGF) -2 levels (233). These fetal gene effects are more evident in the absence of maternal-uterine growth restraint. During postnatal life, the INS VNTR III/III genotype remains associated with body size, including BMI and WC, and also lower insulin sensitivity among girls.

However, there are significant gene–environment interactions that may determine the development of obesity. Rapid "catch-up" early postnatal weight gain, which follows maternal-uterine restraint, strongly predicts later childhood obesity and insulin resistance (197). Among these children, those with INS VNTR class I alleles are more obese. For further review of the endocrine/genetic adaptations present in growth-restricted infants see Vol. 1; Chap. 12. Genetic factors that influence early growth may have conferred some early survival advantage in human history during times of undernutrition. These genetic factors and their interactions with maternal and childhood environmental factors that influence childhood growth may now contribute to the early development of adult disease risk as there is abundant nutrition and rising obesity rates. Their identification may help the development of targeted early interventions to prevent the progression toward adult disease.

Human Single Gene Mutations

The most dramatic examples of the role of genetics in the control of body weight are evident by the existence of single gene mutations that result in marked obesity. Table 2 summarizes the mode of inheritance of these single genes and literature references (234–253). Additionally there are single gene mutations in rodents that are associated with obesity (254,255). Humans and rodents share some of these mutations. In monogenetic or dysmorphic forms of obesity, transmitted by both recessive and dominant modes of inheritance, there are also alterations in energy balance that result in obesity.

Patients with Prader-Willi syndrome are characterized by hyperphagia, hypotonia, developmental delay, hypogonadism, and short stature (234). In these children, obesity may start during the first year of life and becomes prominent by the second year, which in the presence of hyperphagia can result in morbid obesity. They show extreme elevations of Ghrelin, the hunger hormone (235). It was previously suggested that a low metabolic rate caused the obesity in these children (236). However, it has been demonstrated that a lower energy requirement of these children is due to less FFM and not to an unusually low metabolic rate (237). Translocation or deletion of chromosome 15 q11-q12 uniparental maternal disomy, has been reported in about 50% of these patients (238).

Lawrence-Moon-Bardet-Biedl syndrome is another dysmorphic form of obesity characterized by retinitis pigmentosa, hypogonadism, mental retardation, and polydactyly. It is inherited by an autosomal recessive gene located in chromosome 16q21 15q22-q23 (239). It is believed that excessive weight gain in these children is caused by disturbance of hypothalamic appetite center(s), which leads to increased food intake. Pseudohypoparathyroidism (Type 1A) (PHP) is also associated with obesity and short stature and is characterized by short fourth metacarpal, short thick neck, rounded facies, mental retardation, and hypocalcemia (240). It is commonly inherited as an autosomal dominant trait and may be accompanied by hypothyroidism and gonadal failure. The gene is located in chromosome 20q13.2. These patients present a germline loss of function mutations in the alpha subunit of the ubiquitously expressed G protein that couples many hormone receptors to the adenylate cyclase second messenger system. The hypothalamic GS protein-coupled melanocortin 4 (MC4) receptor in the hypothalamus, which mediates the effects of leptin on inhibition of satiety as described below. PHP patients present genetic mutations in GS alpha, which result in severe obesity and hyperphagia (241). Other genetic syndromes that include obesity are Alstrom, Carpenter, Cohen, and proopiomelanocortin (POMC). The mechanisms of excess weight gain in these patients have not been elucidated, but their gene mutations have been characterized (Table 2).

Obesity due to POMC deficiency is another example of a single gene mutation leading to obesity (250). The symptoms of severe early-onset obesity, adrenal insufficiency, and red hair that define POMC deficiency syndrome. This was described in children with complete loss-of-function mutations of the human POMC gene. In POMC deficiency, obesity reflects the lack of POMC-derived peptides as ligands at the MC4 and MC3 receptors, which are expressed in the hypothalamic leptin–melanocortin pathway of body weight regulation. Hypocortisolism and alteration of pigmentation are caused by the lack of POMC-derived peptides at the adrenal MC2 receptor and the skin MC1 receptor, respectively. These patients were

Table 2   Human Gene Mutations Associated with Obesity

Syndrome	Chromosome	Phenotype	References
Prader-Labhart-Willi	15q11-q12[a]	Mental retardation, short stature hypotonia cryptorchidism	234–238
Alstrom	2p14-p13[b]	Blindness, retinal degeneration, nerve deafness, nephropathy hypogonadism, Type 2 diabetes	255
Lawrence-Moon-Bardet-Biedl	16q21 and 15q22-q23[b]	Retinitis pigmentosa, mental retardation, polydactyly, hypogonadism	239
Carpenter	Unknown[b]	Mental retardation, acrocephaly poly- or syndactyly, hypogonadism	255
Cohen	8q22-q23[b]	Mental retardation, microcephaly, short stature	255
Pseudohypoparathyroidism (Type 1A)	20q13.2[c]	Mental retardation, short stature, subcutaneous calcifications, short metacarpals	240–241
Beckwith-Weidermann	11p15.5[b]	Hypoglycemia/hyperinsulinemia hemihypertrophy	255
Nesidioblastosis	11p15.1[bc]	Hypoglycemia/hyperinsulinemia	255
Prohormone convertase	5q15-q21[a]	Hypogonadotropic hypogonadism, hypocortisolism	255
Leptin deficiency	7q313[b]	Hyperphagia, delayed puberty, hypometabolic	242–244
Leptin receptor	1p31-p32[b]	Hyperphagia, delayed puberty, hypometabolic, altered leptin transduction	245–249
POMC	2p23.3[b]	Red hair, hyperphagia, adrenal insufficiency	250
MC4R deficiency	18q22[c]	Early-onset hyperphagia, binge eating, increased growth and bone density	251–253

[a]Uniparental maternal disomy.
[b]Recessive.
[c]Dominant.
Abbreviation: POMC, proopiomelanocortin.
Source: Adapted from Ref. 254.

diagnosed based on the clinical trials of red hair, adrenal insufficiency, and early-onset severe obesity. One previously described translation initiation mutation (C3804A) as well as one new nonsense (A6851T) and two new frame-shift mutations (6996del and 7100 + 2G) were found in homozygosity or compound heterozygosity. The heterozygous parents were found to have high normal or mildly elevated body weight, suggesting a dosage effect of the POMC gene product on weight regulation. To compensate for the lack of hypothalamic melanocortin function, two patients were treated with intranasal ACTH4-10, a melanocortin fragment for which an anorexic effect has been described recently. During three months with increasing doses of ACTH4-10, no change of body weight or metabolic rate was observed, suggesting that at least in these two POMC-deficient patients ACTH 4–10 is without any compensatory effect. In the same two patients, further investigation revealed a mildly elevated thyroid-stimulating hormone (TSH). However, a one-year treatment with thyroid hormone did not result in a significant reduction of body weight.

It is known that the loss of function mutations of the melanocortin 4 receptor (MC4R) gene lead to severe obesity in humans and in mice. These genetic mutations are the most common cause of monogenic human obesity since they disrupt the appetite control centers in the hypothalamus (251). In 2003, there were two papers published which clarified the clinical syndrome resulting from the mutations in the appetite controlling MC4R gene. In the first paper, Farooqi et al. (252) determined the nucleotide sequence of the MC4R gene, which is known to be a cause of a monogenic form of obesity. They studied 500 probands with severe obesity and examined the cosegregation of identified mutations in these families, and in the subjects who were found to have MC4R deficiency they performed a metabolic-endocrine evaluation and characterized their clinical phenotype. The results were correlated with the signaling properties of mutant receptors. Twenty-nine probands (5.8%) had mutations in MC4R; 23 were heterozygous and six were homozygous. Mutation carriers were severely obese; their mean percentage of body fat was 43% of their body composition. Excess body weight gain was evident since the first year of life. They also presented increased lean body mass, increased linear growth, hyperphagia, and severe hyperinsulinemia. However, serum leptin and lipid levels, metabolic rate, and thyroid, adrenal and reproduction function were normal. Homozygous individuals were more severely affected than the heterozygous ones. The subjects with mutations who retained some residual signaling capacity had a less severe phenotype than those with a totally absent signaling capacity. MC4R mutations resulted in a distinct obesity syndrome inherited in a co-dominant manner. The authors concluded that MC4R alterations play a key role in the development of a distinct form of severe obesity commencing in early childhood.

In the second paper, Branson et al. (253) studied the interactions of genetic and environmental factors, which may have a bearing on the development of obesity in MC4R-affected individuals. Four hundred sixty-nine severely obese white subjects with an average age of 42 years and with a mean body-mass index of 44, and 25 control subjects with normal weight and no history of obesity or dieting were included in this study. They sequenced (i) the complete MC4R coding region, (ii) the POMC gene region, which encodes the α-melanocyte-stimulating hormone (MSH), and (iii) the binding domain of the leptin receptor (LEPR) gene (245). They also obtained detailed data concerning phenotypes, resting energy expenditure, diet-induced thermogenesis, serum leptin levels, and eating behaviors. Twenty-four of the 469 obese subjects (5.1%) and one of the 25 controls (4%) had MC4R mutations, including five novel variants. All mutation carriers reported binge-eating behavior, defined as repeated rapid consumption at least twice per week of an unusually large amount of food in the absence of hunger, causing the subject to feel embarrassed, depressed or guilty and out of control. This 100% prevalence of binge eating in MC4R mutation patients was compared with a 14% frequency of such behavior in obese subjects without genetic mutations. The prevalence of binge eating was similar among carriers of mutations in the LEPR to that of noncarriers. No mutations were found in the region of POMC encoding an MSH. The authors concluded that binge eating is a major phenotypic characteristic of subjects with a mutation in MC4R, a candidate gene for the control of eating behavior.

These two papers simultaneously published in the *New England Journal of Medicine* are landmark studies. They contribute greatly to the understanding of the pathogenesis of obesity in humans. Farooqi et al. determined that the proportion of obesity attributed to a mutated gene of MC4R is as high as 6% of severely obese individuals who had obesity since early childhood. Thus, patients carrying MC4R mutations constituted an important subgroup of the severely overweight population. Given the high prevalence of observed MC4R deficiency, it appears that this condition represents the most common form of monogenic obesity in humans. Pediatricians and pediatric endocrinologists should be on the look out for this, especially in children who gain excess weight beginning in early childhood. Clinically, these patients differ from those with Prader-Willi syndrome, who also have another form of monogenic severe obesity, by the normal stature and muscle development, which are abnormal in Prader-Willi syndrome.

The second study showed that overweight people who are binge eaters are more likely to harbor genetic mutations of MC4R than overweight people who constantly overeat. Until now, binge eating was considered a psychological phenomenon or disorder as described above in the section of psychosocial alterations. For the first time a genetically driven characteristic was demonstrated. MC4R mutations appeared to disrupt brain signals governing satiety. Both studies clearly document that there are severely obese individuals who overeat, not because of lack of will power, but because they have a genetically determined pathological syndrome.

However, these data also demonstrate that there are some individuals who have genetically determined mutations, yet are not obese. The reverse also occurs; specifically, binge-eating behavior may occur and not be found to be associated with genetic mutations of MC4R. Thus, these two reports also support the thesis that the etiology of obesity is multifactorial, even in individuals who have a genetically determined alteration in the appetite control centers in the hypothalamus. In these patients, as well as in other obesities, excess energy intake over energy expenditures must occur for obesity to develop.

A major advance in understanding the pathogenesis of obesity was the discovery of the hormone leptin (246). It is produced by adipose tissue and has been found to modify feeding behavior in rodents by suppressing food intake and stimulating energy expenditure (247,248). The *ob/ob* and *db/db* mice have mutations in the genes encoding LEPR (249). These experimental animal models allowed for the evaluation of leptin metabolism in obese humans (256). Consequently, individuals with total or partial leptin deficiency and leptin resistance due to a defect in LEPR were rapidly recognized (242–244,256–261). These single gene anomalies are associated with hypogonadotropic hypogonadism (258), hyperphagia, and severe early-onset obesity (244,257). Congenital leptin deficiency was shown to be due to homozygocity of the delta 133G mutation (261). It has also been associated with missense mutations accompanied by multiple endocrine alterations, decreased sympathetic tone, and immune dysfunction (243). In these patients there was improvement as they got older. Additionally, leptin deficiency has been described in a group of individuals who were genetically partially deficient of this hormone (244). Leptin treatment has been shown to reverse this obesity phenotype (242,243). In these patients leptin induced decreased appetite and food intake and produced weight loss by decreasing fat mass without reducing lean body mass, which further supports the critical role of leptin in energy regulation and body weight maintenance (246,249). However, leptin treatment is not effective in patients with exogenous obesity (260) as they present a relative leptin-resistant state with elevated leptin levels. Indeed, obesity has been linked to leptin resistance and low levels of circulating leptin receptor, indicating that high levels of leptin cannot mediate its beneficial effects (261).

FOOD INTAKE REGULATION
Orexicans and Anorexicans

Recent evidence suggests a critical role for the brain in the regulation of food intake, body adiposity, and

Table 3 Food Intake Regulation

Hypothalamus (arcuate nucleus; MC4R)	
Orexicants	Anorexicants
Ghrelin	Leptin
CCK	α-MSH and POMC
Cortisol	Insulin
Agouti-related protein	Serotonin
Neuropeptide-Y	Dopamine
Orexin	PC-1
Melanin Con H	β-Adrenergic
GABA	PYY
α-Adrenergic	GLP-1
Endocannabinoids	GIP

Abbreviations: CCK, cholecystokinin; α-MSH, α-melanocyte-stimulating hormone; POMC, proopiomelanocortin; GABA, gamma-amino butyric acid; GLP-1, glucagon-like peptide 1; GIP, glucose dependent insulinotropic peptide.

gastrointestinal tract (Fig. 3) (262,263). The neuronal systems that regulate appetite and satiety, energy consumption, energy expenditure, and endogenous glucose production sense and modulate input from a variety of orexicans and anorexicans (Table 3) that play a role in food intake regulation. These include hormonal (i.e., insulin and leptin) and nutrient-related (i.e., glucose and free fatty acids) signals that transmit information about body energy stores and existing energy availability (264,265). Consequently, body weight is maintained in response to a variety of stimuli which increase or suppress energy intake, energy expenditure, and hepatic glucose homeostasis (266). Defects in the secretion or action of orexicans or anorexicans acting on the hypothalamic sensing of adiposity- or nutrient-related signals, or in the neuronal responsiveness to these inputs at the arcuate nucleus of the hypothalamus, predispose to both positive energy balance and increased glucose production (264). If these defects are sustained, pathological weight gain and insulin resistance will result.

List and Habener described the model of the homeostatic circuit regulating energy balance via the MC4 receptor located in the arcuate nucleus in the hypothalamus (267). These authors described the current knowledge of food intake regulation of the hormonal and neural influences on the appetite control centers in the hypothalamus (Fig. 4). They present an integrated circuit involving the adipose tissue, stomach, small intestine, and the large intestine which communicates through neural pathways with the appetite and satiety centers in the brain (Fig. 4). MC4R deficiency is clearly implicated in the etiopathogenic mechanisms in some cases of severe obesity and binge eating, through short-circuiting the regulation of appetite in the hypothalamus. MC4R deficiency decreases the signals of anorixegenic pathways, such as corticotropin-releasing hormone (CRH) and thyrotropin-releasing hormone (TRH); and prevents the inhibition of orexigenic pathways, such as MSH and orexin. The result is increased food intake. The melanocortin agonist α-MSH is a peptide that is produced by the POMC, and

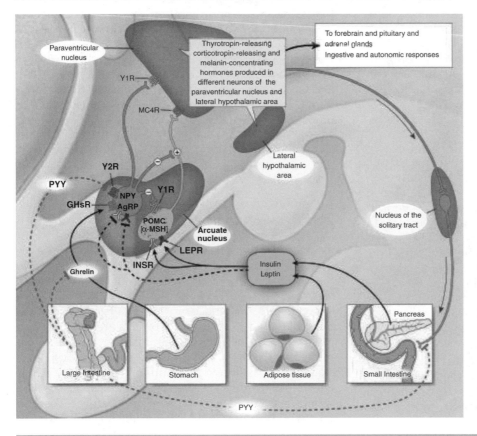

Figure 3 Interactions among hormonal and neural pathways that regulate food intake and body-fat mass. In this schematic diagram of the brain, the dashed lines indicate hormonal inhibitory effects, and the solid lines stimulatory effects. The paraventricular and arcuate nuclei each contain neurons that are capable of stimulating or inhibiting food intake. *Abbreviations*: Y1R and Y2R, Y1 and Y2 subtypes of the neuropeptide Y (NPY) receptor; MC4R, melanocortin 4 receptor; PYY, peptide YY3-36; GHsR, growth hormone secretagogue receptor; AgRP, agouti-related protein; POMC, proopiomelanocortin; α-MSH, α-melanocyte-stimulating protein; LEPR, leptin receptor; INSR, insulin receptor. *Source*: From Ref. 262.

is an agonist of MC4R. On the other hand, leptin reduces food intake through stimulation of the expression of POMC and the production of α-MSH, while inhibiting MC4R antagonists such as the agouti-related protein. The abnormal molecular physiology demonstrated in MC4R-deficient patients constitutes an important concept of a missing link between genes and behavior. However, there is a lot more to be uncovered before we fully understand satiety in individuals with MC4R gene mutations, as well as in other obesity syndromes, and in normal individuals (268).

Leptin

Increased adiposity leads to increased leptin production in fat tissue. Leptin decreases feeding behavior and encourages weight loss (246). Leptin stimulates neurons in the arcuate nucleus of the hypothalamus that coexpress the anorexigenic hormones such as α-MSH, a cleavage product of POMC and cocaine- and amphetamine-regulated transcript (246). Leptin also inhibits neurons in the arcuate nucleus that coexpress the orexigenic hormones, agouti-related protein, and neuropeptide Y (NPY). The neurons in the arcuate nucleus project to other regions of the hypothalamus (including the paraventricular nucleus and the lateral hypothalamic area–parafornical area), where α-MSH binds to its receptor, MC4R, resulting in an upregulation of anorexigenic effectors and a downregulation of orexigenic effectors.

Bouret et al. examined the effect of leptin deprivation and leptin administration upon the density of the neural projections between the arcuate nucleus and the paraventricular nucleus, dorsomedial hypothalamic nucleus, and lateral hypothalamic area in intact and leptin-deficient (*ob/ob*) mice (269). These observations showed that leptin is essential for the development of hypothalamic neural pathways that convey leptin downstream signals. This property was expressed in the neonatal period and was promoted by the neonatal surge in leptin secretion (270).

Ghrelin

Ghrelin, a 28-amino acid acylated hormone produced predominantly by the stomach (271), acts as a growth hormone secretagogue through its receptors located on hypothalamic neurons and in the brainstem. The main function of ghrelin is the regulation of pituitary growth hormone secretion independently of growth-hormone releasing hormone (GHRH) and somatostatin. It has been suggested that ghrelin is an endocrine link between the stomach, hypothalamus, and pituitary and it is important for the regulation of energy balance (272–274). In humans, ghrelin changes significantly throughout development, correlating with anthropometric and metabolic parameters during extrauterine life. The highest levels of ghrelin are found during early postnatal life, when growth hormone begins to exert its effects on growth and important changes in food intake occur (275). Plasma ghrelin concentrations are negatively correlated with body weight, percentage body fat, as well as plasma leptin and insulin, suggesting that plasma ghrelin is downregulated in obesity. This may result from increased concentrations of both leptin and insulin, and reduced plasma ghrelin concentrations may represent adaptation to a positive energy balance associated with obesity (276).

Peptide Tyrosine–Tyrosine

The gut hormone peptide tyrosine-tyrosine (PYY), which is released postprandially from the gastrointestinal tract, has recently been shown to be a physiological regulator of food intake (277). Peripheral administration of PYY reduces feeding in rodents via the Y2 receptor and is thought to primarily involve modulation of the hypothalamic arcuate nucleus circuitry. In humans a single 90-minute infusion of PYY has been shown to markedly reduce subsequent 24-hour caloric intake in lean, normal-weight and obese subjects (150). Moreover, obese subjects have been found to have low levels of fasting and postprandial PYY, suggesting a role for this hormone in the pathogenesis of obesity. Potential therapeutic manipulations based on the PYY system include development of Y2 agonists, exogenous administration of PYY or increased endogenous release from the gastrointestinal tract.

Endocannabinoids

This newly discovered system contributes to the physiological regulation of energy balance, food intake, and lipid and glucose metabolism through both central and peripheral effects (278). This system consists of endogenous ligands and two types of G-protein–coupled cannabinoid receptors: CB1 in the brain and peripheral organs including adipose tissue, gastrointestinal tract, adrenal and liver (279); and CB2 in the immune system (280). The endocannabinoid system is overactivated in genetic animal models of obesity (281) and in response to exogenous stimuli such as excessive food intake (282).

Miscellaneous

Alterations in dopamine systems and/or abnormalities of monoamines can cause various types of hyperphagia (283). Two main systems are implicated in food intake regulation: NPY and POMC. α-MSH is a tridecapeptide cleaved from POMC that acts to inhibit food intake. The predominant NPY orexigenic receptors are NPY-Y1 and NPY-Y5, and the two anorexigenic melanocortin receptors involved in hypothalamic food intake control are MC3-R and MC4-R. Both neuropeptides interact with monoamines in the hypothalamus to control physiologic states such as hunger, satiation, and satiety (284). On the other hand, serotonin is believed to act as a satiety factor and an inhibitor of feeding reward in the hypothalamus (285). Serotonin suppresses food intake and body weight, acting mainly through the serotonin 1B receptor. Also, dopamine regulates hunger and satiety by acting in specific hypothalamic areas, through the D1 and D2 receptors (284,285). In an experimental animal model of hyperphagia

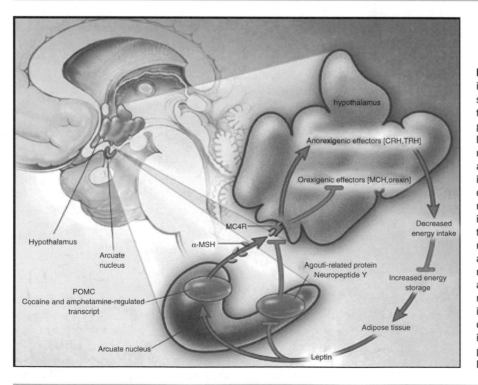

Figure 4 Increased adiposity leads to increased leptin production in fat tissue. Leptin stimulates neurons in the arcuate nucleus of the hypothalamus that coexpress the anorexigenic hormones: α-melanocyte-stimulating hormone [α-MSH, a cleavage product of proopiomelanocortin (POMC)] and cocaine- and amphetamine-regulated transcript. Leptin also inhibits neurons in the arcuate nucleus that coexpress the orexigenic hormones: agouti-related protein and neuropeptide Y. The neurons in the arcuate nucleus project to other regions of the hypothalamus (including the paraventricular nucleus and the lateral hypothalamic area–parafornical area), where α-MSH binds to its receptor, MC4R, resulting in an upregulation of anorexigenic effectors such as corticotropin-releasing hormone (CRH) and thyrotropin-releasing hormone (TRH) and a downregulation of orexigenic effectors such as melanin-concentrating hormone (MCH) and orexin. Agouti-related protein acts as an antagonist of MC4R. *Source*: From Ref. 267.

and obesity, venteromedial hypothalamic (VMH)-lesioned rat, a disturbance of norepinephrine (NE) and dopamine (DA) neurons in the hypothalamus is observed (286). It has been suggested that an increment of the activities of NE and DA systems in the central nervous system (CNS) as a whole and some irregularity in the sympatho-adrenal system might contribute to VMH obesity (286).

Finally, a number of gut hormones give feed back to appetite-controlling areas of the CNS in the regulation of meal size and frequency (287,288). Cholecystokinin (CCK), glucose-dependent insulinotropic peptide, and glucagon-like peptide 1 regulate satiety as enterogastrons and incretins. They also directly affect the satiety centers. Therefore, these peptides may participate in the pathogenesis of eating disorders (289). In mouse brainstem nucleus tractus solitarius POMC neurons are activated by CCK and feeding-induced satiety and that activation of the neuronal MC4-R is required for CCK-induced suppression of feeding. Thus, the melanocortin system provides a potential substrate for integration of long-term adipostatic and short-term satiety signals (290). Hirschberg et al. evaluated CCK levels in a group of obese women with polycystic ovary syndrome. They observed that women with PCO syndrome have reduced postprandial CCK secretion and deranged appetite regulation associated with increased levels of testosterone; implying that impaired CCK secretion may play a role in the greater frequency of binge eating and overweight in women with PCO syndrome (291). Further studies are needed to evaluate the role of CCK in long-term eating behavior in humans.

Adipose Tissue Endocrine Functions

Adipose tissue is comprised of lipid-filled cells surrounded by a matrix of collagen fibers, vessels, fibroblasts, and immune cells. Its main function is the storage of triglycerides for times of energy deprivation. However, it secretes hormones and other products and is involved in various aspects of metabolism that directly affect the onset of obesity. It metabolizes sex steroids and glucocorticoids. For example, 17-beta-hydroxysteroid oxidoreductase converts androstenedione to testosterone and estrone to estradiol. This may be important for fat distribution. Estrogens stimulate fat accumulation in the breast and subcutaneous tissue, while androgens promote central obesity. Alteration of these interconversions may predispose individuals to reproductive disorders and certain cancers (292,293).

Adipose tissue also produces and secretes certain inflammatory cytokines, for example, tumor necrosis factor alpha (TNF-α) and interleukin-6 (IL-6). It has been suggested that both of these cytokines help prevent obesity through inhibition of lipogenesis, increased lipolysis, and promotion of adipocyte death via apoptosis. However, TNF-α has been found to be a mediator of IRS in obesity (294,295). C-reactive protein, stimulated by elevated IL-6, has been found to be correlated with obesity, IRS, elevated TNF-α, and endothelial dysfunction (296).

Alteration of coagulation and complement factors may contribute to the obesity-associated cardiovascular disease. Fibrinogen and plasma activator inhibitor Type-1 (PAI-1) are altered in obesity and may be involved in myocardial infarction. Much of the PAI-1 is synthesized by adipose tissue and is increased in proportion to visceral adiposity. This may serve as a link between abdominal/central obesity and cardiovascular disease (297).

Adiponectin

Plasma concentrations of adiponectin, a novel adipose-specific protein with putative anti-athrogenic and anti-inflammatory effects, were recently found to be decreased in individuals with obesity, Type 2 diabetes, and cardiovascular disease conditions commonly associated with IRS (298). The degree of hypoadiponectinemia is more closely related to the degree of insulin resistance and hyperinsulinemia than the degree of adiposity and glucose intolerance. Ogawa et al. recently reported that hypoadiponectinemia was associated with visceral fat accumulation and IRS (299).

Resistin

Resistin, an adipocyte-derived cytokine, causes insulin resistance and glucose intolerance in mice (300). Resistin gene expression was reported to be similar in both the subcutaneous abdominal and omental depots (301). The abdominal depots showed a 418% increase in resistin mRNA expression compared with the thigh. Increased resistin expression in abdominal fat could explain the increased risk of Type 2 diabetes associated with central obesity. However, Bo et al. suggested that serum resistin is weakly associated with metabolic abnormalities in subjects with normal BMI, while in overweight/obese patients this correlation is not significant, perhaps due to their higher fat content (302). Serum resistin is directly correlated with markers of inflammation (C-reactive protein) and inversely with markers of oxidative stress (nytro-tirosine), suggesting that resistin has antioxidant properties and is secreted in response to a chronic low-grade inflammation. Finally, a recent study by Reinehr et al. showed that while girls demonstrated higher resistin concentrations than boys, there was no significant change in serum resistin despite weight reduction and improved insulin sensitivity, implying that there is no relationship between resistin, insulin resistance index, and weight status in childhood (303).

Visfatin

This newly identified adipocytikine is highly enriched in the visceral fat of both humans and mice and has been shown to have increasing expression levels during the development of obesity (304). Visfatin has insulin-mimetic effects by binding and activating the insulin receptor leading to lowered plasma glucose. Mice heterozygous for a targeted mutation in the visfatin gene had modestly higher levels of plasma glucose relative to wild-type littermates.

Acquired Hypothalamic Alterations

Lesions of the ventromedial area of the hypothalamus (VMH) may result form inflammatory processes such as encephalitis, arachnoiditis, tuberculosis, or trauma, or malignancy (Frohlich syndrome) (305,306). Children with hypothalamic obesity may present with a history of foraging and stealing foods. They have a voracious appetite and may display frequent tantrums if food is denied. In children, craniopharyngioma is the most common CNS tumor that leads to hypothalamic and pituitary dysfunction (307). Hypothalamic obesity is often coupled with other hypothalamic–pituitary disturbances, which may exacerbate the obesity (e.g., growth hormone deficiency or hypothyroidism), but the obesity resists treatment with hormonal replacement (308,309). It is believed that hypothalamic injury leads to alterations in the appetite center, which can cause hyperphagia and obesity (310). However, there is increasing evidence that the hyperinsulinemia seen in this disorder plays a role in the development of obesity. An animal model of VMH damage results in hyperphagia, obesity, hyperinsulinemia, and insulin resistance (311,312). It is believed that VMH damage causes a disinhibition of vagal tone (313) at the pancreatic beta cell, which leads to insulin hypersecretion and resultant obesity (314). Lustig et al. recently demonstrated that children with hypothalamic obesity have excessive insulin secretion during a standard oral glucose tolerance test (315) and treatment with octreotide, a long-acting somatostatin receptor agonist (316), attenuated hyperinsulinemia and promoted weight loss.

HORMONAL ALTERATIONS

Mild obesity may occur in adolescent patients with Klinefelter (317) and Turner syndromes (318). It is believed that hypogonadism results in excessive deposition of fat due to the deficiency of the sexual anabolic hormones, which are responsible for the growth of muscle. In Klinefelter syndrome, this effect is enhanced by the unopposed influence of estrogen, leading to further fat accumulation in the hips and buttocks to produce the characteristic eunuchoid appearance.

Adrenals

Adrenal glucocorticoid production is enhanced in obese children (319). They tend to maintain normal serum cortisol levels due to increased urinary clearance and a stimulatory effect on ACTH release with increased production of dehydroepiandrosterone and testosterone. Increased production of adrenal sex steroids leads to early adrenarche (pubarche), advanced skeletal maturity, and early onset of puberty in obese children (318,320).

Elevated plasma cortisol is related to the hyperinsulinemia of obesity and contributes to the characteristic body fat distribution and altered body composition (321). In obese children, serum levels of epinephrine and norepinephrine remain normal. Adrenal hypercorticolism (Cushing syndrome) is a rare cause of obesity, but the use of corticosteroid therapy for a variety of inflammatory and allergic conditions is associated with excess weight gain, which resolves once the treatment ceases. Patients with Cushing syndrome can be differentiated from those with exogenous obesity by the decreased growth that accompanies excess cortisol.

Growth

Reduced serum concentrations of GH are characteristically seen in obese children and adolescents and have been attributed to diminished GH secretion as well as accelerated GH clearance (322). Basal GH levels and GH release in response to pharmacologic stimuli namely arginine, insulin, l-dopa, clonidine, and GHRH are diminished in obese children and adults (322). However, the pituitary potential to secrete GH is conserved in obesity (323,324). The concentrations of IGF-1 tend to vary as it circulates bound to specific proteins called IGF-binding proteins (IGFBPs) with variable affinities (325,326). Obese children present normal growth in spite of reduced GH secretion, likely due to the combination of increased total growth hormone binding protein (GHBP) and normal GH–GHBP complex serum concentrations, which corresponds to increased GH receptor (GHR) numbers and normal serum GH stores (327). This allows for the achievement of normal levels of IGF-1 and IGFBP-3 levels. This is accompanied by reduced IGFBP-2 serum levels and a lower ratio of IGFBP-2/IGF-1 in obese children, which may suggest an increase of tissue IGF-1 bioavailability, thus promoting its action (327).

Increased adiposity appears to have profound effects on the complex interplay among GH, IGF-1, and IGFBPs during puberty. There is an increase in the ratio of free to total IGF-1, which may help to explain the lack of alterations of pubertal growth spurt in obese adolescents, even in the presence of lower GH levels. The discordance between the low GH and normal IGF-1 levels may be explained by increased hepatic sensitivity to GH stimulating a higher IGF-1 generation in response to a single dose of growth hormone when compared with lean individuals (328). However, in the absence of GH, sex hormones stimulate growth through a direct GH-independent effect on the bone growth centers. Leptin, insulin, and sex hormones locally activate the IGF system in the epiphyseal growth plate (329). Thus, the proposed mechanisms include hyperinsulinism-stimulated growth, decreased IGFBP-1 levels resulting in increased bioavailable (free) IGF-1, and enhanced growth plate stimulation by sex steroids (increased aromatization by the greater adipose mass) (330). Moderate caloric restriction (40%) in mice decreased circulating IGF-1 levels by 70% and tibial growth decreased by 5%. Subsequently, leptin treatment corrected the growth deficit despite further reductions in circulating IGF-I levels (331). Therefore, the growth-promoting consequences of obesity are multifactorial involving multiple factors including enhanced hepatic GH sensitivity.

The lean body mass is often increased in obese children (332). They are commonly tall for their age but there is a potential for reduced growth performance with obesity treatment. This is inherent to the reduction in nutrient intake of obesity treatment programs. For example, a reduction in height velocity was found in children undergoing an energy-restrictive 6-month obesity treatment protocol. However, those on a 12-month, less energy restrictive obesity treatment protocol, showed no reductions in height velocity. Furthermore, both groups had similar heights from baseline until 12 months, suggesting that the children given the restrictive 6-month protocol showed catch-up growth once this treatment was terminated (333). However, the more restrictive group had smaller increases in FFM after 12 months than the less restricted treatment groups.

Epstein et al.'s unique data on 10-year follow-up of children showed no significant changes in final adult height with obesity treatment (334). Furthermore, multiple regression analysis found that childhood percentage of overweight did not contribute to predicting height change. However, a reduction in the percentile for height did occur in children from baseline to 10 years after treatment. The mean height of the children was over the 70th percentile for age prior to, and it decreased to just over the 50th percentile after 10 years of obesity treatment. These studies suggest that children participating in comprehensive obesity treatment programs may attain an appropriate adult height for their parents (334). However, there is a potential for decreased growth even under the best treatment protocols and children who diet without appropriate supervision present growth failure (126).

Prolactin

Basal prolactin levels are normal or slightly elevated in obese children. However, the prolactin response to provocative stimuli is often diminished (335). Lala et al. suggested that decreased serotonin in the brain was a potential mechanism for the blunted prolactin response (336). Others have hypothesized that this may be due to a hypothalamic defect that contributes to the abnormal prolactin response and aberrant appetite regulation, especially when prolactin response does not return to normal with weight loss in the same obese patients (337).

Thyroid

Thyroid function tests including serum levels of thyroxine (T4), free T4, and TSH levels are normal in obese individuals, but serum concentrations of triiodothyronine (T3) are elevated, likely due to increased peripheral conversion of T4 to T3 (338). Furthermore, TSH response to TRH stimulation has been reported to be variable (65,338). The blunted TSH response to TRH stimulation in obesity is believed to be due to increased somatostatinonergic tone because somatostatin inhibition by pyridostigmine pretreatment significantly enhances the TSH response in obese adults but not in obese children (339). Hypothyroidism is not a common cause of obesity. However it has long been shown that excessive weight gain, secondary to an underactive thyroid gland, is due to a combination of decreased metabolic rate and enhanced fluid retention (340). In children, hypothyroidism is associated with poor linear growth. Therefore, a normally growing overweight child is not likely to be hypothyroid.

Reproductive Hormones

Puberty may begin early in tall overweight children with advanced skeletal age (320). Pubertal elevations of follicular-stimulating hormone have been observed in the 7- to 9-year-old girls, without any changes in luteinizing hormone levels (320). This is compounded by an adiposity-related decrease in circulating concentrations of sex hormone-binding globulin (SHBG). This results in a higher fraction of free or unbound serum sex steroids that are more bioactive than the ones in lean subjects. In general, the SHBG abnormalities correlate with the degree of obesity, which are reversed with weight loss. Low serum estradiol levels and elevated progesterone levels have been observed in young prepubertal and early pubertal obese girls compared with age-matched lean girls (320).

As discussed above hyperinsulinemia is usually accompanied by hyperandrogenism, which leads to hirsutism and PCO (48). Amenorrhea, oligomenorrhea, and/or dysfunctional uterine bleeding are common among obese adolescent females. Some of these patients will also develop PCO syndrome (48–50). PCO is now recognized as a component of the IRS (Vol. 1; Chaps. 11 and 13). Insulin-lowering agents have become the norm in the management of PCO (51).

Obese adolescent boys appear to have an attenuated testicular response to human chorionic gonadotropin, This is probably an artifact of decreased SHBG. Indeed, Glass (65) demonstrated that despite a decrease in SHBG levels, free testosterone levels and dihydrotestosterone levels remain normal in obese subjects. Aromatization of androgens to estrogens by adipose tissue, in males, appears to be enhanced without clinical feminization (65). However, free and total testosterone levels may be diminished in morbidly obese males. This is commonly associated with decreased gonadotropin levels, suggesting some degree of hypogonadotropic hypogonadism (248). These alterations in pituitary and gonadal hormones return to normal range with weight loss (341). Indeed, since circulating leptin correlates directly with fat mass and serves as a permissive signal for stimulation of reproductive system, its rising serum concentrations in obesity may alter reproductive function in obese individuals (342).

Conversely, precocious puberty may lead to obesity. Children with idiopathic precocious puberty prior to treatment show no differences in regard to lean or fat mass. However, during long-term treatment with gonadotropin-releasing hormone (GnRH) children present a reduction of lean mass and increased fat mass which may lead to obesity (343). This may be due to a shortening of the prepubertal growing period and by the so-called menopausal effect of the treatment. In another study, both boys and girls with precocious puberty had BMI scores above the 85th percentile prior to and during treatment with GnRH. After treatment the scores still remained above the 85th percentile suggesting that children with precocious puberty are prone to obesity though treatment of precocious puberty itself did contribute to obesity (344).

Parathyroid Hormone

Serum parathyroid hormone (PTH), adjusted for age, physical activity, and serum calcium, were positively associated with BMI in both sexes, and serum PTH was an independent predictor of obesity (345). It has been hypothesized that increased free intracellular calcium in adipocytes blunts the lipolytic response to catecholamines by activating phosphodiesterase 3B—the same enzyme that mediates the antilipolytic effect of insulin—while also compromising the efficiency of insulin-stimulated glucose uptake (346). Physiological increases in PTH have been shown to increase fat cell calcium content, implying that high dietary intake of calcium and/or dairy products may reduce the risk for obesity, diabetes, and IRS. Other dietary measures, which downregulate PTH—such as vitamin D and phosphate and salt intakes—may similarly affect these. It has been shown that body weight is elevated in elderly subjects with both primary and secondary hyperparathyroidism and that insulin resistance is associated with both forms of hyperparathyroidism (347). However, the relationship between PTH level and body adiposity has not been evaluated in children and adolescents. Furthermore, it is unlikely that downregulation of PTH would promote significant weight reduction, but it may diminish risk for weight gain and diabetes, and plausibly may potentiate attainable fat loss with caloric restriction and/or increased physical activity.

Dietary calcium plays a pivotal role in the regulation of energy metabolism; high calcium diets attenuate adipocyte lipid accretion and weight gain during periods of overconsumption of an energy-dense diet and increase lipolysis and preserve thermogenesis during caloric restriction, thereby markedly accelerating weight loss (348). Intracellular calcium has a key role in regulating adipocyte lipid metabolism and triglyceride storage, with increased intracellular calcium resulting in stimulation of lipogenic gene expression and lipogenesis, suppression of lipolysis, and increased lipid filling and adiposity (349). Increased calcitriol released in response to low calcium diets stimulates calcium influx in human fat cells and thereby promotes adiposity. Accordingly, suppressing calcitriol levels by increasing dietary calcium has been postulated as an attractive target for the prevention and management of obesity (350). Clinical and epidemiological data demonstrate a reduction in the odds of being obese with increasing dietary calcium intake (351). Particularly, dairy sources of calcium have been shown to exert a greater anti-obesity effect than supplemental sources of this mineral on adipocyte metabolism, possibly due to the effects of other bioactive compounds, such as the angiotensin-converting enzyme inhibitor found in milk (352). Dietary patterns characterized by increased dairy consumption have a strong inverse association with IRS among overweight adults and may reduce risk of Type 2 diabetes and cardiovascular disease (353). Currently, issues involving low consumption of dairy products and calcium are the focus of much debate and discussion among scientists and lay community. Nevertheless, it has been shown that calcium intake and dairy product intake have beneficial roles in a variety of chronic diseases (354). Also, dairy products provide a rich source of vitamins and minerals; calcium intakes of children have increased over time, yet intakes are not meeting the current adequate intake calcium recommendations; dairy intake has decreased, and soft drink consumption and, possibly, consumption of calcium-fortified products have increased (355). Intake of dairy products have a positive nutritional influence on diets of children and adolescents, particularly from school meals, and there are many factors which influence children's milk consumption, all of which need to be considered to promote adequate calcium intakes by children (356).

ENERGY BALANCE

A body weight setpoint is believed to exist for maintenance of energy balance (357). This biological setpoint for body adiposity functions as a point of stable equilibrium. In a malnourished state with resultant weight loss, the body will decrease the relative energy expenditure by metabolic adaption, which reduces the rate of weight loss (357). The setpoint model has been proposed to quantify this biological process and is unique in predicting energy expenditure during weight loss as a function of the setpoint FFM ratio and setpoint energy expenditure, eliminating the various controlling characteristics such as age, gender, and heredity. This setpoint can permanently and pathologically be displaced by extreme stress situations such as chronic metabolic and psychological stress, trauma, starvation, exercise, infections, hormones, drugs, and/or chemicals disrupting the endocrine system (358).

Obesity is a heterogenous group of disorders that result from an energy imbalance over an extended period of time in which energy intake exceeds expenditure. It is superficially apparent that obese subjects ingest more food relative to their needs. However, it has long been debated if calorie intake differs between overweight and normal-weight individuals (359,360), suggesting that obese subjects have "increased metabolic efficiency." They may expend relatively fewer calories to maintain body weight due to loss of lean body mass (361,362) resulting from repeated weight reduction attempts that lead to alterations in body composition and decreased FFM. However, there have been multiple attempts to elucidate if there is an intrinsic alteration in metabolic rates that sets the stage for the development of obesity (363).

The main determinant of basal metabolic rate (BMR) is FFM and the main determinant of energy expenditure is physical activity. It is believed that minor alterations in any of these could result in positive energy balance and lead to obesity over time. For example, obligatory energy expenditure, reflected by a decreased resting metabolic rate (RMR), could be the consequence of an increased metabolic efficiency in obese persons. On the other hand, a reduced level of energy expenditures due to a reduced activity could also lead to an increased energy balance and weight gain. The resting energy expenditure and the baseline activity levels are thought to be genetically determined. There are data among obese Pima Indians showing low BMR values and, therefore, enhanced metabolic efficiency of energy consumption among some families with obesity (364,365). Ravussin et al. demonstrated a reduced rate of energy expenditures to be a risk for the development of obesity (363). These investigators showed that energy expenditure correlated with the rate of change in body weight over a two-year follow-up period. In 95 Pima Indian adults, the estimated risk of gaining more than 7.5 kg in body weight was increased fourfold in persons with a low adjusted 24-hour energy expenditure (200 kcal/day below predicted values) when compared with persons with a high 24-hour energy expenditure (200 kcal/day above predicted values). In another 126 subjects, the adjusted metabolic rate at rest at the initial visit was also found to predict the gain in body weight over a 4-year follow-up period. When the 15 subjects who gained more than 10 kg were compared with the remaining 111 subjects, the initial mean adjusted metabolic rate at rest was lower in those who gained weight and increased after a mean weight gain of 15.7 kg. In a group of 94 siblings from 36 families, values for adjusted 24-hour energy expenditure aggregated in families. Indeed, Rising et al. showed that in Pima Indians, despite a higher body fat content, older individuals utilize less fat than their younger counterparts (365) and that reduced fat utilization and decreased BMR with age may both contribute to increasing obesity in older individuals.

However, other studies demonstrated that BMR values, corrected for FFM, among obese subjects were relatively higher than those in nonobese subjects (366), suggesting that attainment of energy balance and weight maintenance in obese individuals requires a larger energy intake than in nonobese individuals. Failure of some obese subjects to lose weight while eating a diet reported as low in calories is due to an energy intake that is higher than required for the energy expenditures of the individuals, not to an abnormality in thermogenesis (367).

Finally, maintenance of a reduced or elevated body weight is associated with compensatory changes in energy expenditures while the patient diets (368). These oppose the dietary intake to allow the maintenance of body weight. Leibel et al. repeatedly measured 24-hour total energy expenditure, resting and nonresting energy expenditure, and the thermic effect of feeding in 18 obese subjects and 23 subjects who had never been obese (368). The subjects were studied at their usual body weight and after losing 10% to 20% of their body weight by underfeeding or gaining 10% by overfeeding. Maintenance of a body weight at a level 10% or more below the initial weight was accompanied by a mean reduction in total energy expenditure of 6 kcal/kg of FFM per day in the subjects who had never been obese and 8 kcal/kg/day in the obese subjects. Resting energy expenditure and nonresting energy expenditure each decreased 3 to 4 kcal/kg of FFM per day in both groups of subjects. Maintenance of body weight at a level 10% above the usual weight was associated with an increase in mean total energy expenditure of 9 kcal/kg of FFM per day in the subjects who had never been obese and 8 kcal/kg/day in the obese subjects. The thermic effect of feeding and nonresting energy expenditure increased by approximately 1 to 2 and 8 to 9 kcal/kg of FFM per day, respectively, after weight gain. These changes in energy expenditure were not related to the degree of adiposity or the sex of the subjects. These compensatory changes may account for the poor long-term efficacy of treatments for obesity (368).

Further, humans expend energy through nonpurposeful exercise and through changes in posture and movement that are associated with the routines of daily life [nonexercise activity thermogenesis (NEAT)] (369). Levine et al. demonstrated that obese individuals were seated, on average, two hours longer per day than lean individuals (370). However, posture allocation did not change when the obese individuals lost weight or when lean individuals gained weight, suggesting that it is biologically determined. Levine et al. suggested that if obese individuals adopted the NEAT-enhanced behaviors of their lean counterparts, they might expend an additional 350 calories/day. The RMR represents 50% to 70% of daily energy expenditure and covers the energy necessary for body maintenance, including cellular metabolism and whole-body functions such as ventilation, circulation, and tissue oxygen uptake. RMR seems to be present for a given person, although it does decline with age. Because humans have evolved behavioral strategies (clothing) to maintain body temperature in cold environments, thermogenesis accounts for only 10% of daily energy expenditure and includes the energy required to digest, absorb, transport, and store ingested food. This leaves 20% to 40% of daily energy expenditure for the most variable component, physical activity. The energy cost of physical activity can be divided into planned physical activity, such as sport and exercise, and spontaneous physical activity or NEAT, which includes all involuntary muscle activities such as fidgeting, muscle tone, and maintenance of posture. When people decide to enhance energy expenditure to control body weight, only structured exercise is usually included in their calculations. It is likely that focusing on modifying NEAT behaviors (standing instead of sitting, fidgeting instead of keeping still, or simply walking) can burn the necessary extra calories to control body weight (370).

Differences of up to 500 calories/day in energy expenditures as a result of spontaneous physical activity (i.e., fidgeting) were observed among obese children compared with normal-weight children (371). Differences in BMR and physical activity were found in three- to five-year-old offspring of obese parents. BMR of children with at least one obese parent was 10% lower than that of children with lean parents (372). Children of lean parents had about twice the energy expenditure for physical activities of children with at least one obese parent, suggesting that children of obese parents are less physically active.

Some of the physiological energy balance components of obesity described in adults may also apply to children from the time of birth. For example, a change in the utilization of nutrients as determined by the RQ (373), a lower than average body temperature (374) and sleeping body core temperature (364) may contribute to additional positive energy balance, thus leading to body weight gain. Microneurographic recordings of sympathetic nervous system activity showed lower sympathetic nervous system activity occurs in obese adults (375). However, these potential causes of childhood obesity have not been studied in children.

PHYSICAL ACTIVITY AND FITNESS

While it is generally believed that a sedentary lifestyle increases the risk for obesity, others suggest that decreased physical activity level (PAL) is a consequence of obesity (376). For instance, in Pima Indians: at age five years, obesity is associated with decreased participation in sports and increased television viewing but not with a decreased PAL, whereas, at age 10 years, obesity is associated with decreased participation in sports, increased television viewing, and a decreased PAL, suggesting that a decrease in PAL in free-living conditions seems to follow, not precede, the development of obesity.

Physical activity in children has declined over recent decades implying an increasingly sedentary lifestyle in Western industrialized countries. Reports have indicated that physical activity declines almost 50% during adolescence, with girls becoming increasingly more sedentary than boys (377). A recent observation is that this pattern is due to a gender dimorphism in the developmental changes in energy expenditure before adolescence, independent of body composition, with a conservation of energy use in girls achieved through an appreciable reduction in physical activity (378).

Social and environmental influences are also believed to have major roles in the gender and developmental variation in physical activity (379). Understanding the psychosocial determinants of physical activity in children is critical for the treatment and prevention of childhood obesity. Strauss et al. suggested that children and adolescents are largely sedentary and that correlates of high- and low-level physical activity are different. For instance, time spent on sedentary activities is inversely correlated with moderate-level activity, while self-efficacy and social influences are positively correlated with more intense physical activity. In addition, increased high-level physical activity is an important component in the development of self-esteem in children (380).

Obese individuals have often been described as sluggish or lazy. A study of children and adolescents by Bullen et al. (381) indicated that obese youngsters were less active than their peers. However, an earlier study, which measured caloric expenditure by measuring oxygen consumption, found that obese individuals actually expended more calories through activity than did normal-weight individuals (382). Maffeis et al. (383) recently demonstrated that walking and running are energetically more expensive for obese children than for nonobese children.

Child obesity experts have suggested that the relationship between television and obesity may be the consequence of decreased energy expenditures and enhanced food consumption during viewing. This may be due to the influence of food advertisements (384,385). Experimental studies have demonstrated that a causal relationship exists between specific televised messages and children's eating behavior (386) and between television viewing and participation in sports (387). Earlier studies among children and adolescents found an association between hours of television viewing and the development of obesity (388). Indeed, this association was further supported by a recent observation that the levels of physical activity and hours of television viewing tend to have a strong relationship with body weight and degree of obesity among children (389). It is also possible that the way a child watches television and the content of the television programs may be more important than the number of viewing hours. However, it has been recently shown that television viewing has a fairly profound lowering effect on metabolic rate in both lean and obese individuals. Also, a TV in the child's bedroom is an even stronger marker of increased risk of being overweight especially in preschool children (390). This may be an important factor in susceptible children who are at risk for weight gain and potentially lead to obesity (385).

The estimates of energy requirements for children were derived in a time when more physical exertion was needed for daily living; therefore, energy requirements for children may be overestimated for today's sedentary lifestyle. Prentice et al. (391) measured energy expenditure in children aged 0 to 3 years by the doubly labeled water method and found that energy needs were overestimated by 15% as originally recommended by the World Health Organization (WHO) (392). Goran et al. (393) likewise showed that energy requirements were 25% overestimated for four- to six-year-old children. Fontvieille et al. (394) found that energy requirements for five- to six-year-old children were overestimated by 24% in comparison with that calculated according to the WHO. The sedentary lifestyles of today's children may easily account for consistent overestimates of childhood energy requirements. Indeed, children living a sedentary lifestyle with unlimited access to food are prone to consuming more energy than they expend, and therefore are at increased risk of obesity.

Furthermore, low cardiorespiratory fitness is an independent predictor of cardiovascular disease in obese adult men. This is comparable with diabetes mellitus, high blood pressure, and smoking (395). Myers et al. studied exercise capacity as a predictor of mortality in adults (396). He demonstrated that after adjustment for age, the peak exercise capacity measured in metabolic equivalents (MET) was the strongest predictor of the risk of death among both normal subjects and those with cardiovascular disease. Absolute peak exercise capacity was a stronger predictor of the risk of death than the percentage of the age-predicted value achieved, and there was no interaction between the use or nonuse of beta-blockade and the predictive power of exercise capacity. Each 1-MET increase in exercise capacity conferred a 12% improvement in survival. Mayer et al. suggested that exercise capacity is a more powerful predictor of mortality among men than other established risk factors for cardiovascular disease (397,398).

NUTRITIONAL CONSIDERATIONS

The role of dietary intake in obesity remains controversial, although new data have shed more light on this subject. Obese patients often claim that they do not ingest excess food (399). These patients often seek medical evaluation for failure to lose weight despite a history of severe caloric restriction. They are fre-

quently thought to be hypometabolic and are often treated with thyroid or other hormones to facilitate weight loss. This is neither safe nor necessary; moreover, the observed minus the total predicted energy expenditure varies in relation to weight progression (368). Patients who gain weight increase their metabolic rate whereas those who are on diets and are losing weight may reduce their energy expenditure by 10% to 20%. Thus the results of dietary efforts can only be successful if the reduced intakes are accompanied by increased energy expenditures to overcome the metabolic adaptations that occur with dieting.

A number of studies have demonstrated that obese individuals tend to underreport food intake compared with normal-weight subjects (367,400,401). Indeed, careful metabolic balance studies in some obese adults have shown a failure to lose weight despite self-reported low caloric intakes. This may be due to substantial misreporting of food intake and physical activity and not to an abnormality in thermogenesis (366). However, the problem is often confounded in the clinical setting by the difficulties in assessing food intake and food efficiency.

A high susceptibility to obesity may also be the result of unlimited availability of palatable and high-calorie-density foods. Laboratory adult rats fed a "supermarket diet" consisting of high-carbohydrate/high-fat foods (i.e., chocolate chip cookies, marshmallows, peanut butter, etc.), gained 2.5 times more weight than normal controls (402). In some animals, the weight gain was not reversed after the rat was switched back to chow. It is believed that supermarket diets increase the number and size of fat cells. In children the portion size offered and the type of food given also play a role. Repeated exposure to a larger portion size of macaroni and cheese resulted in 25% more calorie intake when compared with feedings of an age-appropriate serving size, particularly in older children (403). Therefore, while younger children may be better at regulating the amount of food consumed they may lose this ability as they grow older if exposed to large portion sizes (404).

Dietary composition and different rates of nutrient utilization of ingested diets can influence body weight maintenance. Using indirect calorimetric technique in nonobese males, Flatt et al. (405) demonstrated that under sedentary conditions, ingested carbohydrates are quickly metabolized while the rate of fat oxidation remains unchanged. Moreover, it has been suggested that the body tightly regulates carbohydrate balance for up to 36 hours after ingestion and is not affected by alteration in the body's fat balance (405). On the other hand, fat balance is believed to be regulated over a varying long term and it may take several days before the fat balance adjusts to new levels of fat ingestion. Thus, it is believed that excessive fat consumption over a long period of time will result in a positive fat balance and weight gain (406,407).

Therefore, a number of medical organizations including the American Heart Association (408) and the American Diabetes Association (409) recommend consumption of low-fat diets in the prevention and treatment of obesity. However, the relationship between the dietary fat and obesity has recently been questioned (410–412), since both cross-sectional and longitudinal analyses have failed to show a consistent association between dietary fat and body fat (413,414). Furthermore, recent studies indicate that weight loss on low-fat diets is usually modest and transient (410,415). It is also noteworthy that the rate of obesity has continued to rise in the United States despite reported reduction in mean fat intake over the past 30 years, from 42% to about 34% of dietary calories (412,413,416–418).

Glycemic index (GI) is another dietary factor that may influence body weight. GI is a property of carbohydrate-containing food that describes the rise of blood-glucose after a meal (419). The GI of a meal is determined mainly by the amount of carbohydrate content and by other dietary factors affecting food digestibility, gastrointestinal motility, or insulin secretion (including carbohydrate type, food structure, fiber, protein, and fat) (419–422). The average American diet contains starchy foods that are primarily refined grain products, cereals, and potatoes and have a high GI. In contrast, vegetables, legumes, and fruits generally have a low GI (423). It has been suggested that a potential adverse consequence of the decrease observed in mean fat intake in recent years is a concomitant increase in dietary GI. A reduction of dietary fat tends to cause a compensatory increase in sugar and starch intake (424–426). In fact, a rise in total carbohydrate consumption and GI of American diets over the past two decades has been reported (413,424,426). Since fat slows gastric emptying (420), carbohydrate absorption from low-fat meals may be accelerated.

According to food supply data, U.S. consumption of added sugars increased 23% from 1970 to 1996 (427). Nine specific foods and beverages accounted for 73% of all the added sugars in the American diet. Soft drinks, carbonated sodas, and fruit drinks provided 43%, while candy, cakes, ice cream, ready-to-eat cereal, sugar and honey, cookies and brownies, and syrups and toppings each accounted for 4% to 5% of the added sugars. As the intake of soft drinks, carbonated sodas, and fruit-flavored drinks has increased, the consumption of milk and pure fruit juice has decreased and the quality of nutrient-rich foods containing Vitamins A, C, D, riboflavin and folate, and the minerals calcium, magnesium and phosphorous diminished (428). Diets high in added sugar have been associated with several health problems, including obesity, bone loss and fractures, dyslipidemia, cardiovascular disease, and dental caries. However, no single factor, including added sugar consumption, can be linked to their etiology. Indeed, the intake of non-nutritive sweeteners

has increased significantly, while the prevalence of obesity continues to rise. Similarly, caries occurrence is compounded by frequency of meals and snacks, oral hygiene, fluoride supplementation and fluoride toothpaste. Although added sugar consumption has increased, the prevalence of caries has declined, probably due to fluoride supplementation and improved dental care. Similarly, the consequences of dyslipidemia (i.e., coronary artery disease and its complications) also have declined. Heart disease mortality has steadily declined for the past 30 years, and death rates were reduced independently of dietary intake. Although it is widely agreed that milk and soft drink intake are inversely related, it remains to be determined whether this is a cause and effect phenomenon. Ingestion of a variety of all foods in moderation is essential. Added sugars belong to the same biochemical class as other carbohydrates, and as such are processed in predictable metabolic pathways (428). Their intake, however, is best limited to the recommended modest amounts as part of a well-balanced diet over time (429).

High-carbohydrate diets have been demonstrated to increase basal plasma insulin levels in animals and humans (430,431). Dennison et al. suggested that consumption of "fruit drinks" equal to or greater than 12 fl oz/day by young children was associated with short stature and with obesity (432). Indeed, marked obesity has been associated with elevated basal plasma insulin secretory response to glucose and protein (433,434). The hyperinsulinemia of obesity has been regarded as a compensatory adaptation to the peripheral insulin resistance characteristics of the obese state (435). Since the diets of moderately obese individuals are excessive in both total calories and in the quantity of carbohydrate ingested, the hyperinsulinemia of obesity may also be a consequence of these dietary factors rather than merely a secondary response to insulin resistance. Indeed, it has recently been shown that voluntary intake after a high-GI meal was 53% greater than that after a medium-GI meal, and 81% greater than that after a low-GI meal. In addition, compared with the low-GI meal, the high-GI meal resulted in higher serum insulin levels, plasma glucagon levels, postabsorptive plasma glucose, and serum fatty acids levels, along with an elevation in plasma epinephrine (436). It is, therefore, likely that the slower absorption of glucose after ingestion of high-GI meals induces a sequence of hormonal and metabolic changes that promote excessive food intake in obese adolescents. Recently, Spieth et al. suggested that a low-GI diet in the treatment of childhood obesity resulted in greater weight loss than a standard reduced-fat diet (437).

Reduced meal frequency, or gorging (i.e., one to two meals daily), has been associated with an increased risk of obesity (438,439). This is also associated with high fasting serum lipid and insulin levels. Insulin stimulates hepatic synthesis of cholesterol and tissue lipogenesis (440,441). Increasing meal frequency or nibbling has been shown to significantly lower serum cholesterol and insulin levels (442). This is thought to have a beneficial effect in decreasing triglyceride synthesis in adipose tissue through a reduction in postprandial glucose and insulin levels. However, this effect may be significantly minimized by a parallel reduction in the postprandial thermogenesis stimulated by insulin and glucose (443).

FINAL CONSIDERATIONS

Obesity and significant comorbidities are reaching epidemic proportions among children. A variety of genetic, environmental, and other factors accounts for the development of obesity. Understanding the role of leptin in regulating food intake and energy expenditure is an important discovery. It has been identified as a component of the pathophysiological alterations in this entity, including hyperinsulinemia and its complications. Inborn alterations of leptin have also been identified in individuals with severe morbid obesity. However, most obese populations exhibit various degrees of leptin desensitization. Early recognition of excessive weight gain in relation to linear growth is important and should be closely monitored by pediatricians and health care providers. The use of BMI percentiles may also help to identify children at risk and quantify the severity of obesity. A recent study by Quattrin et al. demonstrated that in the majority of referred samples of obese children to pediatric endocrinologists, overweight started in the preschool years (149). The referral to the endocrinologist, occurring after a prolonged interval from the obesity onset, was ineffective in treating obesity. Hyperinsulinemia and hypercholesterolemia are often present also at a young age. These obesity comorbidities in association with high prevalence of parental obesity and Type 2 diabetes expose these youths to high risk for developing Type 2 diabetes and coronary heart disease. These data underscore the need for early family-based behavioral-lifestyle intervention programs to be made available to pediatricians, enabling them to target the "at risk for overweight" preschool children and their likely overweight parents.

Prevention is critical, since effective treatment of this disease is limited. Food management and increased physical activity must be encouraged, promoted, and prioritized to protect children. Dietary practices must foster moderation and variety, with a goal of setting the appropriate eating habits for life. Advocacy is needed to elicit insurance coverage of the disease.

ACKNOWLEDGMENTS

This work was supported in part by NIH grant (#2R44HD038180–04) and by Pediatric Sunshine Academics Inc.

REFERENCES

1. Controlling the Global Obesity Epidemic. World Health Organization Obesity and Overweight Fact Sheet, 2003 (http://www.who.int/nut/obs.htm).
2. Hodge AM, Dowse GK, Zimmet PZ, Collins VR. Prevalence and secular trends in obesity in Pacific and Indian Ocean island populations. Obes Res 1995; 2: 77S–87S.
3. Fernald LC, Gutierrez JP, Neufeld LM, et al. High prevalence of obesity among the poor in Mexico. JAMA 2004; 291:2544–2545.
4. Mendez MA, Monteiro CA, Popkin BM. Overweight exceeds underweight among women in most developing countries. Am J Clin Nutr 2005; 81:714–721.
5. Flegal KM, Carroll MD, Ogden CL, Johnson CL. Prevalence and trends in obesity among US adults, 1999–2000. JAMA 2002; 288:1723–1727.
6. American Obesity Association. AOAFact Sheets Obesity in the US, 2004, http://www.obesity.org/subs/fastfacts/obesity_youth.shtml.
7. Goel MS, McCarty EP, Phillips RS, Wee CC. Obesity among US immigrant subgroups by duration of residence. JAMA 2004; 292:2860–2867.
8. Troiano RP, Flegal KM. Overweight children and adolescents: description, epidemiology, and demographics. Pediatrics 1998; 101:497–504.
9. Ogden CL, Flegal KM, Carroll MD, Johnson CL. Prevalence and trends in overweight among US children and adolescents, 1999–2000. JAMA 2002; 288:1728–1732.
10. Hedley AA, Ogden CL, Johnson CL, Carroll MD, Curtin LR, Flegal KM. Prevalence of overweight and obesity among US children, adolescents, and adults, 1999–2002. JAMA 2004; 291:2847–2850.
11. Strauss RS, Pollack HA. Epidemic increase in childhood overweight, 1986–1998. JAMA 2001; 286:2845–2848.
12. Kramer MS, Morin I, Yang H, et al. Why are babies getting bigger? Temporal trends in fetal growth and its determinants. J Pediatr 2002; 141:538–542.
13. Stettler N, Zemel BS, Kumanyika S, Stallings VA. Infant weight gain and childhood overweight status in a multi-center, cohort study. Pediatrics 2002; 109:194–199.
14. Ong KK, Ahmed ML, Emmett PM, Preece MA, Dunger DB. Association between postnatal catch-up growth and obesity in childhood: prospective cohort study. BMJ 2000; 320: 967–971.
15. Gasser T, Ziegler P, Seifert P, Molinari L, Largo RH, Prader A. Prediction of adult skinfolds and body mass from infancy through adolescence. Ann Hum Biol 1995; 22:217–233.
16. Merritt RJ. Obesity. Curr Probl Pediatr 1982; 12:1–58.
17. Stark O, Atkins E, Wolff OH, Douglas JW. Longitudinal study of obesity in the National Survey of Health and Development. Br Med J 1981; 283:13–17.
18. Sun SS, Wu W, Chumlea WC, Roche AF. Predicting overweight and obesity in adulthood from body mass index values in childhood and adolescence. Am J Clin Nutr 2002; 76:1650–1650.
19. Freedman DS, Khan LK, Serdula MK, Dietz WH, Srinivasan SR, Berenson GS. The relation of childhood BMI to adult adiposity: the Bogalusa Heart Study. Pediatrics 2005; 115:22–27.
20. Mokdad AH, Marks JS, Stroup DF, Gerberding JL. Actual causes of death in the United States, 2000. JAMA 2004; 291:1238–1245.
21. Flegal KM, Graubard BI, Williamson DF, Gail MH. Excess deaths associated with underweight, overweight, and obesity. JAMA 2005; 293:1861–1867.

22. Olshansk SJ, Passaro DJ, Hershow RC, et al. A potential decline in life expectancy in the United States in the 21st century. N Engl J Med 2005; 352:1138–1145.

23. Mokdad AH, Marks JS, Stroup DF, Gerberding JL. Correction: actual causes of death in the United States, 2000. JAMA 2005; 293:293–294.

24. Jemal A, Ward E, Hao Y, Thun M. Trends in the leading causes of death in the United States, 1970–2002. JAMA 2005; 294:1255–1259.

25. Peeters A, Barendregt JJ, Willekens F, Mackenbach JP, Al Mamun A, Bonneux L. Obesity in adulthood and its consequences for life expectancy: a life-table analysis. Ann Intern Med 2003; 138:24–32.

26. Fontaine KR, Redden DT, Wang C, Westfall AO, Allison DB. Years of life lost due to obesity. JAMA 2003; 289:187–193.

27. Must A, Jacques PF, Dallal GE, Bajema CJ, Dietz WH. Long-term morbidity and mortality of overweight adolescents. A follow-up of the Harvard Growth Study of 1922 to 1935. N Engl J Med 1992; 327:1350–1355.

28. Freedman DS, Khan LK, Dietz WH, Srinivasan SR, Berenson GS. Relationship of childhood obesity to coronary heart disease risk factors in adulthood: the Bogalusa Heart Study. Pediatrics 2001; 108:712–718.

29. Reaven GM. Role of insulin resistance in human disease. Diabetes 1988; 37:1595–1607.

30. Williams DP, Going SB, Lohman TG, et al. Body fatness and risk for elevated blood pressure, total cholesterol, and serum lipoprotein ratios in children and adolescents. Am J Public Health 1992; 82:358–363.

31. Webber LS, Srinivasan SR, Wattigney WA, Berenson GS. Tracking of serum lipids and lipoproteins from childhood to adulthood: the Bogalusa heart study. Am J Epidemiol 1991; 133:884–899.

32. Webber LS, Cresanta JL, Voors AW, Berenson GS. Tracking of cardiovascular disease risk factor variables in school-age children. J Chron Dis 1983; 36:647–660.

33. Stary HC. Evolution and progression of atherosclerotic lesions in coronary arteries of children and young adults. Arteriosclerosis 1989; 9(suppl 1):I19–I32.

34. Berenson GS, Wattigney WA, Tracy RE, Newman WP 3rd, Srinivasan Dalferes ER Jr., Strong JP. Atherosclerosis of the aorta and coronary arteries and cardiovascular risk factors in persons aged 6 to 30 years and studied at necropsy (The Bogalusa Heart Study). Am J Cardiol 1992; 70:851–858.

35. Weiss R, Dziura J, Burgert TS, et al. Obesity and the metabolic syndrome in children and adolescents. N Engl J Med 2004; 350:2362–2374.

36. Williams B. Insulin resistance and syndrome X. Lancet 1994; 344:521–524.

37. McLaughlin TL. Insulin resistance syndrome and obesity. Endocr Pract 2003; 9:58–62.

38. Landsberg L. Hypertension and insulin resistance syndrome. Endocr Pract 2003; 9:63–66.

39. Chen W, Srinivasan SR, Elkasababny A, Berenson GS. Cardiovascular risk factor clustering features of insulin resistance syndrome (syndrome X) in a biracial (black-white) population of children, adolescents, and young adults. Am J Epidemiol 1999; 150:666–674.

40. Arsalanian S, Suprasongsin C. Insulin sensitivity, lipids, and body composition in childhood: is "syndrome X" present? J Clin Endocrinol Metab 1996; 81:1058–1062.

41. Steinberger J, Moorehead C, Katch V, Rochini AP. Relationship between insulin resistance and abnormal lipid profile in obese adolescents. J Pediatr 1995; 126: 690–695.

42. Viner RM, Segal TY, Lichtarowicz-Krynska E, Hindmarsh P. Prevalence of the insulin resistance syndrome in obesity. Arch Dis Child 2005; 90:10–14.

43. Ford ES, Giles WH, Dietz WH. Prevalence of the metabolic syndrome among US adults: findings from the third National Health and Nutrition Examination Survey. JAMA 2002; 287:356–359.

44. William CL, Hayman LL, Daniels SR, et al. Cardiovascular health in childhood: a statement for health professionals from the Committee on Atherosclerosis, Hypertension, and Obesity in the Young (AHOY) of the Council on Cardiovascular Disease in the Young, American Heart Association. Circulation 2002; 106:143–160.

45. Cruz ML, Goram MI. The metabolic syndrome in children and adolescents. Curr Diab Rep 2004; 4:53–62.

46. Sinha R, Fisch G, Teague B, et al. Prevalence of impaired glucose tolerance among children and adolescents with marked obesity. N Engl J Med 2002; 346:802–810.

47. Flier JS. Metabolic importance of acanthosis nigricans. Arch Dermatol 1985; 121:193–194.

48. Ehrmann DA. Polycystic ovary syndrome. N Engl J Med 2005; 352:1223–1236.

49. Ciampelii M, Fulghesu AM, Cucinelli F, et al. Impact of insulin and body mass index on metabolic and endocrine variables in polycystic ovary syndrome. Metabolism 1999; 48:167–172.

50. Nestler JE. Insulin resistance syndrome and polycystic ovary syndrome. Endocr Pract 2003; 9:86–89.

51. De Leo V, la Marca A, Petraglia F. Insulin-lowering agents in the management of polycystic ovary syndrome. Endocr Rev 2003; 24:633–667.

52. Janssen I. Combined influence of body mass index and waist circumference on coronary artery disease risk factors among children and adolescents. Pediatrics 2005; 115:1623–1630.

53. Zhu S, Wang Z, Heshka S, Heo M, Faith MS, Heymsfiled SB. Waist circumference and obesity-associated risk factors among whites in the third National Health and Nutrition Examination Survey: clinical action thresholds. Am J Clin Nutr 2002; 76:743–749.

54. Chen W, Srinivasan SR, Li S, Xu J, Berenson GS. Metabolic syndrome variables at low levels in childhood are beneficially associated with adulthood cardiovascular risk: the Bogalusa Heart Study. Diabetes Care 2005; 28:126–131.

55. Valle M, Martos R, Gascon F, Canete R, Zafra MA, Morales R. Low-grade systemic inflammation, hypoadiponectinemia and a high concentration of leptin are present in very young obese children, and correlate with metabolic syndrome. Diabetes Metab 2005; 31:55–62.

56. Balady GJ. Survival of the fittest—more evidence. N Engl J Med 2002; 346:852–854.

57. Chakravarthy MV, Booth FW. Inactivity and inaction: we can't afford either. Arch Pediatr Adolesc Med 2003; 157:731–732.

58. Petersen KF, Dufour S, Befroy D, Garcia R, Shulman GI. Impaired mitochondrial activity in the insulin-resistant offspring of patients with type 2 diabetes. N Engl J Med 2004; 350:664–671.

59. Shulman AI, Mangelsdorf DJ. Retinoid' receptor heterodimers in the metabolic syndrome. N Engl J Med 2005; 353:604–615.

60. Davidson MB. Is treatment of insulin resistance beneficial independent of glycemia? Diabetes Care 2003; 26: 3184–3186.

61. Caro JF, Dohm LG, Pories WJ, Sinha MK. Cellular alterations in liver, skeletal muscle, and adipose tissue responsible for insulin resistance in obesity and type II diabetes. Diabetes Metab Rev 1989; 5:665–689.

62. Schade DS, Eaton RP. Dose response to insulin in man: differential effects on glucose and ketone body regulation. J Clin Endocrinol Metab 1977; 44:1038–1053.

63. Le Stunff C, Bougneres PF. Time course of increased lipid and decreased glucose oxidation during early phase of childhood obesity. Diabetes 1993; 42:1010–1016.

64. Randle PJ, Garland PB, Hales CN, Newsholme EA. The glucose fatty-acid cycle: its role in insulin sensitivity and the metabolic disturbance of diabetes mellitus. Lancet 1963; 1:758–789.

65. Glass AR. Endocrine aspects of obesity. Med Clin North Am 1989; 73:139–160.

66. Rosenbaum M, Leibel RL. Pathophysiology of childhood obesity. Adv Pediatr 1988; 35:73–137.

67. Pontiroli AE. Type 2 diabetes mellitus is becoming the most common type of diabetes in school children. Acta Diabetol 2004; 41:85–90.

68. Glaser NS. Non-insulin-dependent diabetes mellitus in childhood and adolescence. Pediatr Clin North Am 1997; 44:307–337.

69. Dean HE, Mundy RLL, Moffatt M. Non-insulin-dependent diabetes mellitus in Indian children in Mannitoba. Can Med Assoc J 1992; 147:52–57.

70. Dean H. NIDDM-Y in First Nation children in Canada. Clin Pediatr 1998; 37:89–96.

71. Pinhas-Hamiel O, Dolan LM, Daniels SR, Standiford D, Khoury PR, Zeitler P. Increased incidence of non-insulin-dependent diabetes among adolescents. J Pediatr 1996; 128:608–615.

72. Kitagawa T, Owada M, Urakami T, Tajima N. Epidemiology of type 1 (insulin-dependent) and type 2 (non-insulin-dependent) diabetes mellitus in Japanese children. Diabetes Res Clin Pract 1994; 24(suppl):S7–S13.

73. Kitagawa T, Owada M, Urakami T, Yamauchi K. Increased incidence of non-insulin-dependent diabetes mellitus among Japanese school children correlates with an increased intake of animal protein and fat. Clin Pediatr 1998; 37:111–115.

74. Betts P, Mulligan J, Ward P, Smith B, Wilkin T. Increasing body weight predicts the earlier onset of insulin dependent diabetes in childhood. The accelerator hypothesis. Diabet Med 2005; 22:144–151.

75. Adelman RD, Restaino IG, Alon US, Blowey DL. Proteinuria and focal segmental glomerulosclerosis in severely obese adolescents. J Pediatr 2001; 138:481–485.

76. Kambham N, Markowitz GS, Valeri AM, Lin J, L'Agati VD. Obesity-related glomerulopathy: an emerging epidemic. Kidney Int 2001; 59:1498–1509.

77. Nanda K. Non-alcoholic steatohepatitis in children. Pediatr Transplant 2004; 8:613–618.

78. Matteoni CA, Younossi, Gramlich T, Boparai N, Liu YC, McCallough AJ. Nonalcoholic fatty liver disease: a spectrum of clinical and pathological severity. Gastroenterology 1999; 116:1413–1419.

79. Sanyal AJ, Campbell-Sargent C, Mirshahi F, et al. Non-alcoholic steatohepatitis: association of insulin resistance and mitochondrial abnormalities. Gastroenterology 2001; 120:1183–1192.

80. Bennion LJ, Knowler WC, Mott DM, Spagnola AM, Bennett PH. Development of lithogenic bile during puberty in Pima Indians. N Engl J Med 1979; 300: 873–876.

81. Liddle RA, Goldstein RB, Saxton J. Gallstone formation during weight-reduction dieting. Arch Intern Med 1989; 149:1750–1753.

82. Dietz WH Jr. Obesity in infants, children and adolescents in the United States. I. Identification, natural history and aftereffects. Nutr Res 1981; 1:117–137.

83. Tracey VV, De NC, Harper JR. Obesity in respiratory infection in infants and young children. Br Med J 1971; 1:16–18.

84. Mallory GB Jr., Fiser DH, Jackson R. Sleep-associated breathing disorders in morbidly obese children and adolescents. J Pediatr 1989; 115:892–897.

85. Strollo PJ Jr., Rogers RM. Obstructive sleep apnea. N Engl J Med 1996; 271:99–104.

86. Shelton KE, Gay SB, Hollowell DE, Woodson H, Suratt PM. Mandible enclosure of upper airway and weight in obstructive sleep apnea. Am Rev Respir Dis 1993; 148: 195–200.

87. Horner RL, Mohiaddin RH, Lowell DG, et al. Sites and sizes of fat deposits around the pharynx in obese patients with obstructive sleep apnea and weight matched controls. Eur Respir J 1989; 2:613–622.

88. Shepard JW Jr. Cardiopulmonary consequences of obstructive sleep apnea. Mayo Clin Proc 1990; 65:1250–1259.

89. Ford ES. The epidemiology of obesity and asthma. J Allergy Clin Immunol 2005; 115:897–909.

90. Hancox RJ, Milne BJ, Poulton R, et al. Sex differences in the relation between body mass index and asthma and atopy in a birth cohort. Am J Respir Crit Care Med 2005; 171:440–445.

91. Bibi H, Shoseyov D, Feigenbaum D, et al. The relationship between asthma and obesity in children: is it real or a case of over diagnosis? J Asthma 2004; 41:403–410.

92. Spivak H, Hewitt MF, Onn A, Half EE. Weight loss and improvement of obesity-related illness in 500 U.S. patients following laparoscopic adjustable gastric banding procedure. Am J Surg 2005; 189:27–32.

93. Kelsey JL, Acheson RM, Keggi KJ. The body build of patients with slipped capital femoral epiphysis. Am J Dis Child 1972; 124:276–281.

94. Kling TF Jr. Angular deformities of the lower limbs in insulin-dependent diabetes mellitus among adolescents. J Pediatr Children Orthop Clin North Am 1987; 18:513–527.

95. Timm NL, Grupp-Phelan J, Ho ML. Chronic ankle morbidity in obese children following an acute ankle injury. Arch Pediatr Adolesc Med 2005; 159:33–36.

96. Nead KG, Halterman JS, Kaczorowski JM, Auinger P, Weitzman M. Overweight children and adolescents: a risk group for iron deficiency. Pediatrics 2004; 114:104–108.

97. Neaye RL. Maternal body weight and pregnancy outcome. Am J Clin Nutr 1990; 52:273–279.

98. Shaw GM, Velie EM, Schaffer D. Risk of neural tube defect-affected pregnancies among obese women. JAMA 1996; 275:1093–1096.

99. Werler MM, Louik C, Shapiro S, Mitchell AA. Prepregnant weight in relation to risk of neural tube defects. JAMA 1996; 275:1089–1092.

100. Wadden TA, Stunkard AJ. Psychopathology and obesity. Ann N Y Acad Sci 1987; 499:55–56.

101. Gortmaker SL, Must A, Perrin JM, Sobol AM, Dietz WH. Social and economic consequences of overweight in adolescence and young adulthood. N Engl J Med 1993; 329: 1008–1012.

102. Staffieri JR. A study of social stereotype of body image in children. J Pers Soc Psychol 1967; 7:101–104.

103. Stunkard A, Burt V. Obesity and the body image. II. Age at onset of disturbances in body image. Am J Psychiatry 1967; 123:1443–1447.

104. Davison KK, Birch LL. Weight status, parent reaction, and self-concept in five-year-old girls. Pediatrics 2001; 107:46–53.

105. Birch LL, Fisher JO. Mothers' child-feeding practices influence daughters' eating and weight. Am J Clin Nutr 2000; 71:1054–1061.

106. Vander Wall JS, Thelen MH. Eating and body image concerns among obese and average weight children. Addit Behav 2000; 25:775–778.

107. Monello LF, Mayer F. Obese adolescent girls: a unrecognized "minority" group? Am J Clin Nutr 1963; 13:35–39.

108. Canning H, Mayer J. Obesity: its possible effect on college acceptance. N Engl J Med 1996; 275:1172–1174.

109. Schwimmer JB, Burwinkle TM, Varni JW. Health-related quality of life of severely obese children and adolescents. JAMA 2003; 289:1813–1819.

110. Williams J, Wake M, Hesketh K, Maher E, Waters E. Health-related quality of life of overweight and obese children. JAMA 2005; 293:70–76.

111. Cugini P, Cilli M, Salandri A, et al. Anxiety, depression, hunger and body composition: III. Their relationships in obese patients. Eat Weight Disord 1999; 4:115–120.

112. Decaluwe V, Braet C. Prevalence of binge-eating disorder in obese children and adolescents seeking weight-loss treatment. Int J Obes Relat Metab Disord 2003; 27:404–409.

113. Telch CF, Pratt EM, Niego SH. Obese women with binge eating disorder define the term binge. Int J Eat Disord 1998; 7:115–117.

114. deZwaan M. Binge eating disorder and obesity. Int J Obes Relat Metab Disord 2001; 25(suppl 1):S51–S55.

115. Ackard DM, Neumark-Sztainer D, Story M, Perry C. Overeating among adolescents: prevalence and associations with weight-related characteristics and psychological health. Pediatrics 2003; 111:67–74.

116. Mustillo S, Worthman C, Erkanli A, Keeler G, Angold A, Costello EJ. Obesity and psychiatric disorder: developmental trajectories. Pediatrics 2003; 111:851–859.

117. Carpenter KM, Hasin DS, Allison DB, Faith MS. Relationships between obesity and DSM-IV major depressive disorder, suicide ideation, and suicide attempts: results from a general population study. Am J Public Health 2000; 90:251–257.

118. Allison DB, Fontaine KR, Heo M, et al. The distribution of body mass index among individuals with and without schizophrenia. J Clin Psychiatry 1999; 60; 215–220.

119. Allison DB, Casey DE. Antipsychotic-induced weight gain: a review of the literature. J Clin Psychiatry 2001; 62(suppl 7): 22–31.

120. Schaeffer JL, Ross RG J. Childhood-onset schizophrenia: premorbid and prodromal diagnostic and treatment histories. Am Acad Child Adolesc Psychiatry 2002; 41: 538–545.

121. Lieberman JA, Stroup TS, McEvoy JP, et al. Effectiveness of antipsychotic drugs in patients with chronic schizophrenia. N Engl J Med 2005; 353:1209–1223.

122. Pine DS, Goldstein RB, Wolk S, Weissman MM. The association between childhood depression and adulthood body mass index. Pediatrics 2001; 107:1049–1056.

123. Goodman E, Whitaker RC. A prospective study of the role of depression in the development and persistence of adolescent obesity. Pediatrics 2002; 110:497–504.

124. Schwartz TL, Nihalani L, Virk S, Jindal S, Chilton M. Psychiatric medication-induced obesity: treatment options. Obes Rev 2004; 5:233–238.

125. Kreipe RE. Eating disorders in adolescents and older children. Pediatr Rev 1999; 12:410–421.

126. Pugliese MT, Lifshitz F, Grad G, Fort P, Marks-Katz M. Fear of obesity: a cause of short stature and delayed puberty. N Engl J Med 1983; 309:513–518.

127. Moses N, Banilvy M, Lifshitz F. Fear of obesity among adolescent girls. Pediatrics 1989; 83:393–398.

128. Richardson SA, Goodman N, Hastorf H, et al. Cultural uniformity in reaction to physical disabilities. Am Sociol Rev 1961; 26:241–247.

129. Neumark-Sztainer D, Hannan P. Weight-related behaviors among adolescent girls and boys: results from a national survey. Arch Pediatr Adolesc Med 2000; 154:569–577.

130. Lifshitz F. Fear of obesity in childhood. Ann N Y Acad Sci 1993; 699:230–236.

131. Lifshitz F, Tarim O, Smith MM. Nutrition in adolescence. Review. Endocrinol Metab Clin North Am 1993; 22: 673–683.

132. Pugliese M, Lifshitz F, Fort P, Recker B, Ginsberg L. Pituitary–hypothalamic response in adolescents with growth failure due to fear of obesity. J Am Coll Nutr 1987; 6:113–120.

133. Lifshitz F, Moses N, Cervantes C, Ginsberg L. Nutritional dwarfing in adolescents. Semin Adolesc Med 1987; 3: 255–266.

134. Neumark-Sztainer D, Rock CL, Thornquist MD, Cheskin LJ, Neuhouser ML, Barnett MJ. Weight-control behaviors among adults and adolescents: associations with dietary intake. Prev Med 2000; 5:381–391.

135. Abramovitz B, Birch L. Five-year-old girls' ideas about dieting are predicted by their mothers' dieting. J Am Diet Assoc 2000; 100:1157–1163.

136. Schur E, Sanders M, Steiner H. Body dissatisfaction and dieting in young children. Int J Eat Disord 2000; 27:74–82.

137. Stice E, Agras W, Hammer L. Risk factors for the emergence of childhood eating disturbances: a five-year prospective study. Int J Eat Disord 1999; 25:375–387.

138. Maynard LM, Galuska DA, Blanck HM, Serdula MK. Maternal perceptions of weight status of children. Pediatrics 2003; 111:1226–1231.

139. Johnson S, Birch L. Parents' and children's adiposity and eating style. Pediatrics 1994; 94:653–661.

140. Hood MY, Moore LL, Sundarajan-Ramamurti A, Singer M, Cupples LA, Ellison RC. Parental eating attitudes and the development of obesity in children. The Framingham Children's Study. Int J Obes 2000; 24:1319–1325.

141. Field AE, Austin SB, Taylor CB, et al. Relation between dieting and weight change among preadolescents and adolescents. Pediatrics 2003; 112:900–906.

142. http://www.healthaffairs.org.

143. Finkelstein EA, Fiebelkorn IC, Wang G. State-level estimates of annual medical expenditures attributable to obesity. Obes Res 2004; 12:18–24.

144. Birmingham CL, Muller JL, Palepu A, Spinelli JJ, Anis AH. The cost of obesity in Canada. Can Med Assoc J 1999; 160:483–488.

145. Wang G, Dietz WH. Economic burden of obesity in youths aged 6 to 17 years: 1979–1999. Pediatrics 2002; 109(5):e81–e91.

146. Pronk NP, Boucher J. Systems approach to childhood and adolescent obesity prevention and treatment in a managed care organization. Int J Obes Rel Metab Disord 1999; 2:S38–S42.

147. Harp JB, Hecht L. Obesity in the national football league. JAMA 2005; 293:1061–1062.

148. Miller LA, Grunwald GK, Johnson SL, Krebs NF. Disease severity at time of referral for pediatric failure to thrive and obesity: time for a paradigm shift? J Pediatr 2002; 141:121–124.

149. Quattrin T, Liu E, Shaw N, Shine B, Chiang E. Obese children who are referred to the pediatric endocrinologist: characteristics and outcome. Pediatrics 2005; 115:348–351.

150. Batterham RL, Cohen MA, Ellis SM, et al. Inhibition of food intake in obese subjects by peptide YY3-36 N Engl J Med 2003; 349:941–948.

151. Pugliese MT, Recker B, Lifshitz F. A Survey to determine the prevalence of abnormal growth patterns in a suburban school district. J Adolesc Health Care 1988; 9: 181–182.

152. Hammer LD, Kraemer HC, Wilson DM, Ritter PL, Dornbusch SM. Standardized percentile curves of body-mass

index for children and adolescents. Am J Dis Child 1991; 145:259–263.

153. http://www.cdc.gov/nchs/data/ad/ad314.pdf.

154. National Center for Health Statistics, U.S. Department of Health, Education and Welfare. NCHS Growth Curves for Children: Birth to 18 years. Series H, No. 165, DHEW Publication No. (PHS) 78–1650, 1977.

155. Yajnik CS, Yudkin JS. The Y–Y paradox. Lancet 2004; 363:163.

156. Franklin MF. Comparison of weight and height relations in boys from 4 countries. Am J Clin Nutr 1999; 70:157S–162S.

157. Bellizzi MC, Dietz WH. Workshop on childhood obesity: summary of the discussion. Am J Clin Nutr 1999; 70:173S–175S.

158. Malina RM, Katzmarzyk PT. Validity of the body mass index as indicator of the risk and presence of overweight in adolescents. Am J Clin Nutr 1999; 70:131S–136S.

159. Dietz WH, Bellizzi MC. Introduction: the use of body mass index to assess obesity in children. Am J Clin Nutr 1999; 70:123S–125S.

160. Durnin JV, Womersley J. Body fat assessed from total body density and its estimation from skinfold thickness: measurements on 481 men and women aged from 16 to 72 years. Br J Nutr 1974; 32:77–97.

161. Must A, Dallal GE, Dietz WH. Reference data for obesity: 85th and 95th percentiles of body mass index (wt/ht2) and triceps skinfold thickness. Am J Clin Nutr 1991; 53:839–846.

162. http://www.cdc.gov/nchs/about/major/nhanes/test-comp.

163. Megan AM, Gomez TG, Bernauer EM, Mole PM. Evaluation of a new air displacement plethysmograph for measuring human body composition. Med Sci Sport Exerc 1995; 27:1686–1691.

164. de Ridder CM, de Boer RW, Seidell JC, et al. Body fat distribution in pubertal girls quantified by magnetic resonance imaging. Int J Obes Relat Metab Disord 1992; 16:443–449.

165. Lockner DW, Heyward VH, Baumgartner RN, Jenkins KA. Comparison of air-displacement plethysmography, hydrodensitometry, and dual X-ray absorptiometry for assessing body composition of children 10 to 18 years of age. Ann N Y Acad Sci 2000; 904:72–78.

166. Ma G, Yao M, Liu Y, et al. Validation of a new pediatric air-displacement plethysmograph for assessing body composition in infants. Am J Clin Nutr 2004; 79:653–660.

167. Guo SM, Roche AF, Houtkooper L. Fat-free mass in children and young adults predicted from bioelectric impedance and anthropometric variables. Am J Clin Nutr 1989; 50:435–443.

168. Houtkooper LB, Going BS, Lohman TG, Roche AF, Van Loan M. Bioelectrical impedance estimation of fat-free mass in children and youth: a cross-validation study. J Appl Physiol 1992; 72:366–373.

169. Wells JC, Fuller NJ, Dewit O, Fewtrell MS, Elia M, Cole TJ. Four-component model of body composition in children: density and hydration of fat-free mass and comparison with simpler models. Am J Clin Nutr 1999; 69:904–912.

170. Czinner A, Varady M. Quantitative determination of fatty tissue on body surface in obese children by ultrasound method. Pediatr Pathol 1992; 27:7–10.

171. Armellini F, Zamboni M, Rigo L, et al. Sonography detection of small intra-abdominal fat variations. Int J Obes 1991; 15:847–852.

172. Ellis KJ. Measuring body fatness in children and young adults: comparison of bioelectric impedance analysis, total body electrical conductivity, and dual-energy X-ray absorptiometry. Int J Obes Relat Metab Disord 1996; 20:866–873.

173. Kohrt WM. Preliminary evidence that DEXA provides an accurate assessment of body composition. J Appl Physiol 1998; 84:372–377.

174. Paradisi G, Smith L, Burtner C, et al.. Dual energy X-ray absorptiometry assessment of fat mass distribution and its association with the insulin resistance syndrome. Diabetes Care 1999; 22:1310–1317.

175. Kvist H, Chowdhury B, Grangard U, Tylen U, Sjostrom L. Total and visceral adipose-tissue volumes derived from measurements with computed tomography in adult men and women: predictive equations. Am J Clin Nutr 1988; 48:1351–1361.

176. Ross R, Shaw KD, Martel Y, de Guise J, Avruch L. Adipose tissue distribution measured by magnetic resonance imaging in obese women. Am J Clin Nutr 1993; 57:470–475.

177. Fiorotto ML, Cochran WJ, Klish WJ. Fat-free mass and total body water of infants estimated from total body electrical conductivity measurements. Pediatr Res 1987; 22:417–421.

178. www.forum.lowcarber.org/archive/index.php/t-48103.html.

179. www.nutricraze.com/health_talk/Fat-Track-Pro-Digital-Body-Fat-Measurement-System-to-424.html.

180. www.equistat.co.uk/research.htm.

181. www.scales-r-us.com/scales.php/Scales/146.

182. www.medicalscales.com/seca/adult/700.html.

183. www.nutrition-software-review.toptenreviews.com/diet-master-2000-software.html.

184. Kissebah AH, Vydelingum N, Murray R, et al. Relation of body fat distribution to metabolic complications of obesity. J Clin Endocrinol Metab 1982; 54:254–260.

185. Evans DJ, Hoffmann RG, Kalkhoff RK, Kissebah AH. Relationship of body fat topography to insulin sensitivity and metabolic profiles in premenopausal women. Metabolism 1984; 33:48–75.

186. Kalkhoff RK, Hartz AH, Rupley D, Kissebah AH, Kelber W. Relationship of body fat distribution to blood pressure, carbohydrate tolerance, and plasma lipids in healthy obese women. J Lab Clin Med 1983; 102:621–627.

187. Peiris AN, Hennes MI, Evans DJ, Wilson CR, Lee MB, Kissebah AH. Relationship of anthropometric measurements of body fat distribution to metabolic profile in premenopausal women. Acta Med Scand Suppl 1988; 723:179–188.

188. Peiris AN, Struve MF, Mueller RA, Lee MB, Kissebah AH. Glucose metabolism in obesity: influence of body fat distribution. J Clin Endocrinol Metab 1988; 67:760–767.

189. Hirschler C, Aranda V, Calcagno MdeL, Maccalini G, Jadzinsky M. Can waist circumference identify children with the metabolic syndrome? Arch Pediatr Adolesc Med 2005; 159:740–744.

190. Zamboni M, Armellini F, Milani MP, et al. Evaluation of regional body fat distribution: comparison between W/H ratio and computed tomography in obese women. J Intern Med 1992; 232:341–347.

191. Garn SM, Sullivan TV, Hawthorne VM. Fatness and obesity of the parents of obese individuals. Am J Clin Nutr 1989; 50:1308–1313.

192. Reeder BA, Senthilselvan A, Despres J, et al. The association of cardiovascular disease risk factors with abdominal obesity in Canada. Canadian Heart Health Surveys Research Group. CMAJ 1997; 157(suppl 17):S39–S45.

193. Okosun IS, Choi S, Dent MM, Jobin T, Dever GE. Abdominal obesity defined as a larger than expected waist girth is

associated with racial/ethnic differences in risk of hypertension. J Hum Hypertens 2001; 15:307–312.

194. Wang Y, Rimm EB, Stampfer MJ, Willett WC, Hu FB. Comparison of abdominal adiposity and overall obesity in predicting risk of type 2 diabetes among men. Am J Clin Nutr 2005; 81:555–563.

195. Fernandez JR, Redden DT, Pietrobelli A, Allison DB. Waist circumference percentiles in nationally representative samples of African-American, European-American, and Mexican-American children and adolescents. J Pediatr 2004; 145:439–444.

196. Gray GA. Contemporary Diagnosis and Management of Obesity. Newtown, PA: Handbooks in Health Care, 1998:120.

197. Ong KK, Dunger DB. Birth weight, infant growth and insulin resistance. Eur J Endocrinol 2004; 151(suppl 3): U131–U139.

198. Roberts SB, Savage J, Coward WA, Chew B, Lucas A. Energy expenditure and intake in infants born to lean and overweight mothers. N Engl J Med 1988; 318:461–466.

199. Ravussin E, Burnand B, Schutz Y, Jequier E. Twenty-four-hour energy expenditure and resting metabolic rate in obese, moderately obese, and control subjects. Am J Clin Nutr 1982; 35:566–573.

200. Dewey KG, Heinig MJ, Nommsen LA, Peerson JM, Lonnerdal B. Breast-fed infants are leaner than formula-fed infants at 1y of age: the DARLING study. Am J Clin Nutr 1993; 57:140–145.

201. Wells JC, Stanley M, Laidlaw AS, Day JM, Davies PS. Energy intake in early infancy and childhood fatness. Int J Obes Relat Metab Disord 1998; 22:387–392.

202. Davis PS, Wells JC, Fieldhouse CA, Day JM, Lucas A. Parental body composition and infant energy expenditure. Am J Clin Nutr 1995; 61:1026–1029.

203. Cole CR, Rising R, Hakim A, et al. Comprehensive assessment of the components of energy expenditure in 97 infants using a new infant respiratory chamber. J Am Coll Nutr 1999; 18:233–241.

204. Rising R, Duro D, Cedillo M, et al. Daily metabolic rate in healthy infants. J Pediatr 2003; 143:180–185.

205. Rising R, Lifshitz F. Relationship between maternal obesity and infant feeding-interactions. Nutr J 2005; 4:17.

206. Hill JO, Peters JC. Environmental contributions to the obesity epidemic. Science 1998; 280:1371–1374.

207. Kramer MS, Barr RG, Leduc DG, Boisjoly C, McVey-White L, Pless IB. Determinants of weight and adiposity in the first year of life. J Pediatr 1985; 106:10–14.

208. Cutting TM, Fisher JO, Grimm-Thomas K, Birch LL. Like mother, like daughter: familial patterns of overweight are mediated by mothers' dietary disinhibition. Am J Clin Nutr 1999; 69:608–613.

209. Drabmam RS, Cordua GD, Hammer D, Jarvie GJ, Horton S. Developmental trends in eating rates of normal and overweight preschool children. Child Dev 1979; 50:211–216.

210. Agras WS, Kraemer HC, Berkowitz RI, Korner AF, Hammer LD. Does a vigorous feeding style influence early development of adiposity? J Pediatr 1987; 110: 799–804.

211. Udal JN, Harrison GG, Vaucher Y, Walson PD, Morrow G III. Interaction of maternal and neonatal obesity. Pediatrics 1978; 62:17–21.

212. Vohr BR, McGarvey ST. Growth patterns of large-for-gestational-age and appropriate-for-gestational-age infants of gestational diabetic mothers and control mothers at age 1 year. Diabetes Care 1997; 20:1066–1072.

213. Vohr BR, McGarvey ST, Tucker R. Effects of maternal gestational diabetes on offspring adiposity at 4–7 years of age. Diabetes Care 1999; 22:1284–1291.

214. Stunkard AJ, Srensen TI, Hanis C, et al. An adoption study of human obesity. N Engl J Med 1986; 314:193–198.

215. Stunkard AJ, Harris JR, Pedersen NL, McClearn GE. The body-mass index of twins who have been reared apart. N Engl J Med 1990; 322:1483–1487.

216. Bray GA. The inheritance of corpulence. In: Cioffi LA, James WPT, Van Itallie TB, eds. The Body Weight Regulatory System: Normal and Disturbed Mechanisms. New York: Raven Press, 1981:61–64.

217. Heitmann BL, Harris JR, Lissner L, Pedersen NL. Genetic effects on weight change and food intake in Swedish adult twins. Am J Clin Nutr 1999; 69:597–602.

218. Faith MS, Pietrobelli A, Nunez C, Heo M, Heymsfield SB, Allison DB. Evidence for independent genetic influences on fat mass and body mass index in a pediatric twin sample. Pediatrics 1999; 104:61–67.

219. Valencia ME, Bennett PH, Ravussin E, Esparza J, Fox C, Schultz LO. The Pima Indians in Sonora, Mexico. Nutr Rev 1999; 57:S55–S57.

220. Esparza J, Fox C, Harper IT, Bennett PH, Schultz LO, Valencia ME, Ravussin E. Daily energy expenditure in Mexican and USA Pima Indians: low physical activity as a possible cause of obesity. Int J Obes Relat Metab Disord 2000; 24:55–59.

221. Ravussin E, Bogardus C. Energy expenditure in the obese: is there a thrifty gene? Infusionstherapie 1990; 17:108–112.

222. Chakavarthy MV, Booth FW. Eating, exercise, and "thrifty" genotypes: connecting the dots toward an evolutionary understanding of modern chronic diseases. J Appl Physiol 2004; 96:3–10.

223. Barsh GS, Farooqi IS, O'Rahilly S. Genetics of body-weight regulation. Nature 2000; 404:644–651.

224. Walder K, Hanson RL, Kobes S, Knowler WC, Ravussin E. An autosomal genomic scan for loci linked to plasma leptin concentration in Pima Indians. Int J Obes Relat Metab Disord 2000; 24:559–565.

225. Duggirala R, Blangero J, Almasy L, et al. A major locus for fasting insulin concentrations and insulin resistance on chromosome 6q with strong pleiotropic effects on obesity-related phenotypes in nondiabetic Mexican Americans. Am J Hum Genet 2001; 68:1149–1164.

226. Zhu X, Cooper RS, Luke A, et al. A genome-wide scan for obesity in African-Americans. Diabetes 2002; 51: 541–544.

227. Perusse L, Rice T, Chagnon YC, et al. A genome-wide scan for abdominal fat assessed by computed tomography in the Quebec Family Study. Diabetes 2001; 50:614–621.

228. Comuzzie AG. A major quantitative trait locus determining serum leptin levels and fat mass is located on human chromosome 2. Nat Genet 1997; 15:273–276.

229. Lee JH, Reed DR, Li WD, et al. Genome scan for human obesity and linkage to markers in 20q13. Am J Hum Genet 1999; 64:196–209.

230. Feitosa MF, Borecki IB, Rich SS, et al. Quantitative-trait loci influencing body-mass index reside on chromosomes 7 and 13: the National Heart, Lung, and Blood Institute Family Heart Study. Am J Hum Genet 2002; 70:72–82.

231. Saar K, Geller F, Ruschendorf F, et al. Genome scan for childhood and adolescent obesity in German families. Pediatrics 2003; 111:321–327.

232. Petry CJ, Ong KK, Barratt BJ, et al. ALSPCA Study Team. Common polymorphism in H19 associated with birth-weight and cord blood IGF-II levels in humans. BMC Genet 2005; 6:22.

233. Bazaes RA, PetryCJ, OngKK, et al. Insulin gene VNTR genotype is associated with insulin sensitivity and secretion in infancy. Clin Endocrinol (Oxf) 2003; 59: 599–603.

234. Bray GA, Dahms WT, Swerdloff RS, et al. The Prader-Willi syndrome: a study of 40 patients and a review of the literature. Medicine (Baltimore) 1983; 62:59–80.

235. DelParigi A, Teschop M, Heiman ML, et al. High circulating ghrelin: a potential cause for hyperphagia and obesity in Prader-Willi syndrome. J Clin Endocrinol Metab 2002; 87:5461–5464.

236. Bekx MD, Carrel AA, Shriver TC, Li Z, Allen DB. Decreased energy expenditure is caused by abnormal body composition in infants with Prader-Willi syndrome. J Pediatr 2003; 143:372–376.

237. Schoeller DA, Levitksy LL, Bandini LG, Dietz WW, Walczak A. Energy expenditure and body composition in Prader-Willi syndrome. Metabolism 1988; 37:115–120.

238. Ledbetter DH, Riccardi VM, Airhart SD, Strobel RJ, Keenan BS, Crawford JD. Deletions of chromosome 15 as a cause of the Prader-Willi syndrome. N Engl J Med 1981; 304:325–329.

239. Bauman ML, Hogan GR. Laurence-Moon-Biedl syndrome. Report of two unrelated children less than 3 years of age. Am J Dis Child 1973; 126:119–126.

240. Spiegel AM. Pseudohypoparathyroidism. In: Scriver CR, Beaudet AL, Sly WS, Valle D, eds. The Metabolic Basis of Inherited Disease. New York: McGraw-Hill, 1989: 2013–2027.

241. Ong KK, Amin R, Dunger DB. Pseudohypoparathyroidism—another monogenic obesity syndrome. Clin Endocrinol 2000; 52:389–391.

242. Farooqi IS, Jebb SA, Langmack G, et al. Effects of recombinant leptin therapy in a child with congenital leptin deficiency. N Engl J Med 1999; 341:879–884.

243. Ozata M, Ozdemir IC, Licinio J. Human leptin deficiency caused by a missense mutation: multiple endocrine defects, decreased sympathetic tone, and immune system dysfunction indicate new targets for leptin action, greater central than peripheral resistance to the effects of leptin, and spontaneous correction of leptin-mediated defects. J Clin Endocrinol Metab 1999; 84:3686–3695.

244. Farooqi IS, Keogh JM, Kamath S, et al. Partial leptin deficiency and human adiposity. Nature 2001; 414:34–35.

245. Zhang Y, Proenca R, Maffei M, Barone M, Leopold L, Friedman JM. Positional cloning of the mouse obese gene and its human homologue. Nature 1994; 372:425–432.

246. Diamond F. The endocrine function of adipose tissue. Growth Genetics Horm 2002; 18:17–23.

247. Flier JS. Leptin expression and action: new experimental paradigms. Proc Natl Acad Sci U S A 1997; 94:4242–4245.

248. Flier JS. Clinical review 94: what's in a name? In search of leptin's physiologic role. J Clin Endocrinol Metab 1998; 83:1407–1413.

249. Campfiled LA, Smith FJ, Guisez Y, Devos R, Burn P. Recombinant mouse OB protein: evidence for a peripheral signal linking adiposity and central neural networks. Science 1995; 269:546–549.

250. Krude H, Biebermann H, Schnabel D, et al. Obesity due to proopiomelanocortin deficiency: three new cases and treatment trials with thyroid hormone and ACTH4-10. J Clin Endocrinol Metab 2003; 88:4633–4640.

251. Mergen M, Mergon H, Ozata M, Oner R, Oner C. A novel melanocortin 4 receptor (MC4R) gene mutation associated with morbid obesity. J Clin Endocrinol Metab 2001; 86:3448.

252. Farooqi IS, Keogh JM, Yeo GS, Lank EJ, Cheetham T, O'Rahilly S. Clinical spectrum of obesity and mutations in the melanocortin 4 receptor gene. N Engl J Med 2003; 348:1085–1095.

253. Branson R, Potoczna N, Kral JG, Lentes KU, Hoehe MR, Horber FF. Binge eating as a major phenotype of melanocortin 4 receptor gene mutations. N Engl J Med 2003; 348:1096–1103.

254. Kleinman RE, ed. Pediatric Obesity in Pediatric Nutrition Handbook. American Academy of Pediatrics, 2004:565.

255. Leibel RL, Chua SC, Rosenbaum M. Obesity: the molecular physiology of weight regulation. In: Scriver CR, Beaudet AL, Sly WS, Valle D, eds. The Metabolic Basis of Inherited Disease. 8th ed. New York: McGraw-Hill, 2001:3965–4028.

256. Chu NF, Wang DJ, Shieh SM, Rimm EB. Plasma leptin concentrations and obesity in relation to insulin resistance syndrome components among school children in Taiwan—The Taipei Children Heart Study. Int J Obes Relat Metab Disord 2000; 24:1265–1271.

257. Montague CT, Farooqi IS, Whitehead JP, Soos MA, Rau H, Wareham NJ, et al. Congenital leptin deficiency is associated with severe early-onset obesity in humans. Nature 1997; 387:903–908.

258. Strobel A, Issad T, Camoin L, Ozata M, Strosberg AD. A leptin missense mutation associated with hypogonadism and morbid obesity. Nat Genet 1998; 18:213–215.

259. Mergen M, Mergen H, Ozata M, Oner R, Oner C. A novel melanocortin 4 receptor (MC4R) gene mutation associated with morbid obesity. J Clin Endocrinol Metab 2001; 86:3448.

260. Heymsfield SB, Greenberg AS, Fujioka K, et al. Recombinant leptin for weight loss in obese and lean adults: a randomized, controlled, dose-escalation trial JAMA 1999; 282:1568–1575.

261. Gibson WT, Farooqi IS, Moreau M, et al. Congenital leptin deficiency due to homozygosity for the Delta133G mutation: report of another case and evaluation of response to four years of leptin therapy. J Clin Endocrinol Metab 2004; 89:4821–4826.

262. Korner J, Leibel RL. To eat or not to eat? How the gut talks to the brain. N Engl J Med 2003; 349:926–928.

263. Seeley RJ, Woods SC. Monitoring of stored and available fuel by the CNS: implications for obesity. Nat Rev Neurosci 2003; 4:901–909.

264. Schwartz MW, Porte D Jr. Diabetes, obesity, and the brain. Science 2005; 307:375–379.

265. Obici S, Feng Z, Arduini A, Conti R, Rossetti L. Inhibition of hypothalamic carnitine palmitoyltransferase-1 decreases food intake and glucose production. Nat Med 2003; 9:756–761.

266. Obici S, Zhang BB, Karkanis G, Rossetti L. Hypothalamic insulin signaling is required for inhibition of glucose production. Nat Med 2002; 8:1376–1382.

267. List JF, Habener JF. Defective melanocortin 4 receptor in hyperphagia and morbid obesity. N Engl J Med 2003; 348: 1160–1163.

268. Gotoda T. Binge eating as a phenotype of melanocortin 4 receptor gene mutations. N Engl J Med 2003; 349:606–609.

269. Bouret SG, Draper SJ, Simerly RB. Trophic action of leptin on hypothalamic neurons that regulate feeding. Science 2004; 304:108–110.

270. Pinto S, Roseberry AG, Liu H, et al. Rapid rewiring of arcuate nucleus feeding circuits by leptin. Science 2004; 304:110–115.

271. Broglio F, Arvat E, Benso A, et al. Ghrelin: endocrine and non-endocrine actions. J Pediatr Endocrinol Metab 2002; 15:1219–1227.

272. Kojima M, Hosoda H, Date Y, Nakazato M, Matsuo H, Kangawa K. Ghrelin is a growth-hormone-releasing acylated peptide from stomach. Nature 1999; 402:656–660.

273. Nakazato M, Murakami N, Date Y, et al. A role for ghrelin in the central regulation of feeding. Nature 2001; 409: 194–198.

274. Tschop M, Smiley DL, Heiman ML. Ghrelin induces adiposity in rodents. Nature 2000; 407:908–913.

275. Soriano-Guillen L, Barrios V, Chowen JA, et al. Ghrelin levels from fetal life through early adulthood: relationship with endocrine and metabolic and anthropometric measures. J Pediatr 2004; 144:30–35.

276. Tschop M, Weyer C, Tataranni PA, Devanarayan V, Ravussin E, Heiman ML. Circulating ghrelin levels are decreased in human obesity. Diabetes 2001; 50:707–709.

277. Renshaw D, Batterham RL. Peptide YY: a potential therapy for obesity. Curr Drug Targets 2005; 6:171–179.

278. Di Marzo V, Goparaju SK, Wang L, et al. Leptin-regulated endocannabinoids are involved in maintaining food intake. Nature 2001; 410:822–825.

279. Bensaid M, Gary-Bobo M, Escalngo A, et al. The cannabinoid CB1 receptor antagonist SR141716 increases Acrp30 mRNA expression in adipose tissue of obese fa/fa rats and in cultured adipocyte cells. Mol Pharmacol 2003; 63:908–914.

280. Howlett AC, Breivogal CS, Childers SR, Deadwyler SA, Hampson RE, Porrino LJ. Cannabinoid physiology and pharmacology: 30 years of progress. Neuropharmacology 2004; 47(suppl 1):345–358.

281. Di Marzo V, Bifulco M, De Petrocellis. The endocannabinoid system and its therapeutic applications. Nat Rev Drug Discov 2004; 3:771–784.

282. Ravinet Trillou C, Arnon M, Delgorge C, et al. Anti-obesity effect of SR141716, a CB1 receptor antagonist, in diet-induced obese mice. Am J Physiol Regul Integr Comp Physiol 2003; 284:345–353.

283. Cabeza de Vaca S, Hao J, Afroz T, Krahne LL, Carr KD. Feeding, body weight, and sensitivity to non-ingestive reward stimuli during and after 12-day continuous central infusions of melanocortin receptor ligands. Peptides 2005; 26:2314–2321.

284. Ramos EJ, Meguid MM, Campos AC, Coelho JC. Neuropeptide Y, alpha-melanocyte-stimulating hormone, and monoamines in food intake regulation. Nutrition 2005; 21:269–279.

285. Brunetti L, Di Nisio C, Orlando G, Ferrante C, Vacca M. The regulation of feeding: a cross talk between peripheral and central signalling. Int J Immunopathol Pharmacol 2005; 18:201–212.

286. Takahashi A, Ishimru H, Ikarashi Y, Maruyama Y. Aspects of hypothalamic neuronal systems in VMH lesion-induced obese rats. J Auton Nerv Syst 1994; 48:213–219.

287. Beglinger C. Overview. Cholecystokinin and eating. Curr Opin Investig Drugs 2002; 3:587–588.

288. Nauck MA, Meier JJ, Creutzfeldt W. Incretins and their analogues as new antidiabetic drugs. Drug News Perspect 2003; 16:413–422.

289. Tomasik PJ, Sztefko K, Starzyk J. Cholecystokinin, glucose dependent insulinotropic peptide and glucagon-like peptide 1 secretion in children with anorexia nervosa and simple obesity. J Pediatr Endocrinol Metab 2004; 17: 1623–1631.

290. Fan W, Ellacott KL, Halatchev IG, Takahashi K, Yu P, Cone RD. Cholecystokinin-mediated suppression of feeding involves the brainstem melanocortin system. Nat Neurosci 2004; 7:335–336.

291. Hirschberg AL, Naessen S, Stridsberg M, Bystrom B, Holtet J. Impaired cholecystokinin secretion and disturbed appetite regulation in women with polycystic ovary syndrome. Gynecol Endocrinol 2004; 19:79–87.

292. Siiteri PK. Adipose tissue as a source of hormones. Am J Clin Nutr 1987; 45:277S–282S.

293. Bjorntorp P. The regulation of adipose tissue distribution in humans. Int J Obes Rel Metab Disord 1996; 20:291–302.

294. Sethi J, Hotamisligil GS. The role of TNFa in adipocyte metabolism. Semin Cell Dev Biol 1999; 10:19–29.

295. Hotamisligil GS, Arner P, Caro JF, Atkinson RL, Spiegelman BM. Increased adipose tissue expression of tumor necrosis factor-alpha in human obesity and insulin resistance. J Clin Invest 1995; 95:2409–2415.

296. Yudkin JS, Stehouwer CD, Emeis JJ, Coppack SW. C-reactive protein in healthy subjects: associations with obesity, insulin resistance, and endothelial dysfunction: a potential role for cystokines originating from adipose tissue? Arteriorcler Thromb Vasc Biol 1999; 19:972–978.

297. Shimomura I, Funahashi T, Takahashi M, et al. Enhanced expression of PAI-1 in visceral fat: possible contributor to vascular disease in obesity. Nat Med 1996; 2:800–803.

298. Weyer C, Funahashi T, Tanaka S, et al. Hypoadiponectinemia in obesity and type 2 diabetes: close association with insulin resistance and hyperinsulinemia. J Clin Endocrinol Metab 2001; 86:1930–1935.

299. Ogawa Y, Kikuchi T, Nagasaki K, et al. Usefulness of serum adiponectin level as a diagnostic marker of metabolic syndrome in obese Japanese children. Hypertens Res 2005; 28:51–57.

300. Steppam CM, Lazar AM. Resistin and obesity-associated insulin resistance. Trends Endocrinol Metab 2002; 13:18–23.

301. McTernan CL, McTernan PG, Harte AL, Levick PL, Barnet AH, Kumar S. Resistin, central obesity, and type 2 diabetes. Lancet 2002; 359:46–47.

302. Bo S, Gambino R, Pagani A, Guidi S, Gentile L, Cassader M, Pagano GF. Relationships between human serum resistin, inflammatory markers and insulin resistance. Int J Obes Relat Metab Disord 2005; xx:xx–xx.

303. Reinehr T, Roth CL, Menke T, Andler W. Resistin concentrations before and after weight loss in obese children. Int J Obes (Lond) 2005; 90:6386–6391.

304. Fukuhara A, Matsuda M, Nishizawa M, Segawa K, Tanaka M, Kishimoto K, et al. Visfatin: a protein secreted by visceral fat that mimics the effects of insulin. Science 2005; 307:426–430.

305. Bray G, Gallagher TF Jr. Manifestations of hypothalamic obesity in man: a comprehensive investigation of eight patients and a review of the literature. Medicine (Baltimore) 1975; 54:301–330.

306. Didi M, Didock E, Davies HA, Oligvy-Stuart AL, Wales JKH, Shalet SM. High incidence of obesity in young adults after treatment of acute lymphoblastic leukemia of childhood. J Pediatr 1995; 127:63–67.

307. Ullrich NJ, Scott RM, Pomeroy SL. Craniopharyngioma therapy. Long-term effects on hypothalamic function. Neurologist 2005; 11:55–60.

308. Thomsett MJ, Conte FA, Kaplan SL, et al.. Endocrine and neurologic outcome in childhood craniopharyngioma: review of effect of treatment in 42 patients. J Pediatr 1980; 97:728–735.

309. Sorva R. Children with craniopharyngioma: early growth failure and rapid postoperative weight gain. Acta Paediatr Scand 1988; 77:587–592.

310. Sklar CA. Craniopharyngioma: endocrine sequalae of treatment. Pediatr Neurosurg 1994; 21:120–123.

311. Jeanrenaud B. A hypothesis on the aetiology of obesity: dysfunction of the central nervous system as a primary cause. Diabetologia 1985; 28:502–513.

312. Powley TL, Laughton W. Neural pathways involved in the hypothalamic integration of autonomic responses. Diabetologia 1981; 20:378–387.

313. Ionescu E, Rohner-Jeanrenaud F, Berthoud HR, Jeanrenaud B. Increases in plasma insulin levels in response to electrical stimulation of the dorsal motor nucleus of the vagus nerve. Endocrinology 1983; 112:904–910.

314. Rohner-Jeanrenaud F, Jeanrenaud B. Involvement of the cholinergic system in insulin and glucagon oversecretion of genetic preobesity. Endocrinology 1985; 116:830–834.

315. Lustig RH, Rose SR, Burghen GA, et al. Hypothalamic obesity caused by cranial insult in children: altered glucose and insulin dynamics and reversal by somatostatin agonist. J Pediatr 1999; 135:162–168.

316. Koontz AJ, MacDonald LM, Schade DS. Octreotide: a long-acting inhibitor of endogenous hormone secretion for human metabolic investigations. Metabolism 1994; 43:24–31.

317. Ratcliffe SG, Bancroft J, Axworthy D, McLaren W. Klinefelter's syndrome in adolescence. Arch Dis Child 1982; 57:6–12.

318. Polychronakos C, Letarte J, Collu R, Ducharme JR. Carbohydrate intolerance in children and adolescents with Turner syndrome. J Pediatr 1980; 96:1009–1014.

319. Jabbar M, Pugliese M, Fort P, Recker B, Lifshitz F. Excess weight and precocious pubarche in children: altera-somatostation-like immunoreactivity in obese children. Eur J Pediatr 1987; 146:48–50.

320. Kaplowitz PB, Slora EJ, Wasserman RC, Podlow SE, Herman-Giddens ME. Earlier onset of puberty in girls: relation to increased body mass index and race. Pediatrics 2001; 108:347–353.

321. Freedman DS, Srinivasan SR, Burke GL, et al. Relation of body fat distribution to hyperinsulinemia in children and adolescents: the Bogalusa Heart Study. Am J Clin Nutr 1987; 46:403–410.

322. Vanderschueren-Lodeweyckx M. The effect of single obesity on growth and growth hormone. Horm Res 1993; 40:23–30.

323. Bowers CY. A new dimension on the induced release of growth hormone in obese subjects. J Clin Endocrinol Metab 1993; 76:817–818.

324. Cordido F, Penalua A, Dieguez C, Casanueva FF. Massive growth hormone (GH) discharge in obese subjects after the combined administration of GH-releasing hormone and GHRP-6: evidence for a marked somatotroph secretory capability in obesity. J Clin Endocrinol Metab 1993; 76:819–823.

325. Leroith D. Insulin-like growth factors. N Engl J Med 1997; 336:633–637.

326. Attia N, Tamborlane WV, Heptulla R, et al. The metabolic syndrome and insulin-like growth factor I regulation in adolescent obesity. J Clin Endocrinol Metab 1998; 83:1467–1471.

327. Ballerini MG, Ropelato MG, Domene HM, Pennisi P, Heinrich JJ, Jasper HG. Differential impact of simple childhood obesity on the components of the growth hormone-insulin-like growth factor (IGF)-IGF binding proteins axis. J Pediatr Endocrinol Metab 2004; 17:749–757.

328. Phillip M, Moran O, Lazar L. Growth without growth hormone. J Pediatr Endocrinol Metab 2002; 15(suppl 5):1267–1272.

329. Gleeson HK, Lissett CA, Shalet SM. Insulin-like growth factor-I response to a single bolus of growth hormone is increased in obesity. J Clin Endocrinol Metab 2005; 90:1061–1067.

330. Maor G, Rochwerger M, Segev Y, Phillip M. Leptin acts as a growth factor on the chondrocytes of skeletal growth centers. J Bone Miner Res 2002; 17:1034–1043.

331. Gat-Yablonski G, Ben-Ari T, Shtaif B, et al. Leptin reverses the inhibitory effect of caloric restriction on longitudinal growth. Endocrinology 2004; 145:343–350.

332. Forbes GB. Influence of nutrition. In: Forbes GB, ed. Human Body Composition: Growth, Aging, Nutrition and Activity. New York: Springer-Verlag, 1987:209–247.

333. Amador M, Ramos LT, Morono M, Hermelo MP. Growth rate reduction during energy restriction in obese adolescents. Exp Clin Endocrinol 1990; 96:73–82.

334. Epstein LH, Valoski A, McCurley J. Effect of weight loss by obese children on long-term growth. Am J Dis Child 1993; 147:1076–1080.

335. AvRuskin TW, Pillai S, Kasi K, Juan C, Kleinberg DL. Decreased prolactin secretion in childhood obesity. J Pediatr 1985; 106:373–378.

336. Lala VR, Ray A, Jamias P, et al. Prolactin and thyroid status in prepubertal children with mild to moderate obesity. J Am Coll Nutr 1988; 7:361–366.

337. Kopelman PG, Pilkington TR, Jeffcoate SL, White N. Persistence of defective hypothalamic control of prolactin secretion in some obese women after weight reduction. Br Med J 1980; 281:358–359.

338. Danforth E Jr. Adaptive thermogenesis and thyroid hormones. In: Bjorntorp P, Cairella M, Howard A, eds. Recent Advances in Obesity Research III. London: John Libbey, 1980:228–235.

339. Mancini A, Fiumara C, Conte G, et al. Pyridostigmine effects on TSH response to TRH in adult and children obese subjects. Horm Metab Res 1993; 25:309–311.

340. Kyle LH, Ball MF, Doolan PD. Effect of thyroid hormone on body composition in myxedema and obesity. N Engl J Med 1966; 275:12–17.

341. Clement K, Vaisse C, Lahlou N, et al. A mutation in the human leptin receptor gene causes obesity and pituitary dysfunction. Nature 1998; 392:398–401.

342. Bajari TM, Nimpf J, Schneider WJ. Role of leptin in reproduction. Curr Opin Lipidol 2004; 15:315–319.

343. Chiumello G, Brambilla P, Guarneri MP, Russo G, Manzoni P, Sgaramella P. Precocious puberty and body composition: effects of GnRH analog treatment. J Pediatr Endocrinol Metab 2000; 13:S791–S794.

344. Palmert MR, Mansfield MJ, Crowley WF Jr. Crigler JF Jr., Crawford JD, Boepple PA. Is obesity an outcome of gonadotropin-releasing hormone agonist administration? Analysis of growth and body composition in 110 patients with central precocious puberty. J Clin Endocrinol Metab 1999; 12:4480–4488.

345. Kamycheva E, Sundsfjord J, Jorde R. Serum parathyroid hormone level is associated with body mass index. The 5th Tromso study. Eur J Endocrinol 2004; 151(2):167–172.

346. McCarty MF, Thomas CA. PTH excess may promote weight gain by impeding catecholamine-induced lipolysis—implications for the impact of calcium, vitamin D, and alcohol on body weight. Med Hypotheses 2003; 61:535–542.

347. Bolland MJ, Grey AB, Gamble GD, Reid IR. Association between primary hyperparathyroidism and increased body weight: a meta-analysis. J Clin Endocrinol Metab 2005; 90:1525–1530.

348. Shi H, Dirienzo D, Zemel MB. Effects of dietary calcium on adipocyte lipid metabolism and body weight regulation in energy-restricted aP2-agouti transgenic mice. FASEB J 2001; 15:291–293.

349. Zemel MB. Regulation of adiposity and obesity risk by dietary calcium: mechanisms and implications. J Am Coll Nutr 2002; 21(2):146S–151S.

350. Shi H, Norma AW, Okamura WH, Sen A, Zemal MB. 1alpha, 25-dihydroxyvitamin D3 inhibits uncoupling protein 2 expression in human adipocytes. FASEB J 2002; 16(13):1808–1810.

351. Zemel MB, Richards J, Mathis S, Milstead A, Gebhardt L, Silva E. Dairy augmentation of total and central fat loss in obese subjects. Int J Obes Relat Metab Disord 2005; 29:391–397.

352. Zemela MB, Miller SL. Dietary calcium and dairy modulation of adiposity and obesity risk. Nutr Rev 2004; 62:125–131.

353. Pereira MA, Jacobs DR Jr., Van Horn L, Slattery ML, Kartashov AI, Ludwig DS. Dairy consumption, obesity, and the insulin resistance syndrome in young adults: the CARDIA study. JAMA 2002; 287:2081–2089.

354. Niklas TA. Calcium intake trends and health consequences from childhood through adulthood. J Am Coll Nutr 2003; 22:340–356.

355. Veug3lers PJ , Fitzgerald AL, Johnston E. Dietary intake and risk factors for poor diet quality among children in Nova Scotia. Can J Public Health 2005; 96:212–216.

356. Niklas TA, Demory-Luce D, Yang SJ, Baranowski T, Zakeri I, Berenson G. Children's food consumption patterns have changed over two decades (1973–1994): the Bogalusa heart study. J Am Diet Assoc 2004; 104: 1127–1140.

357. Kozusko FP. Body weight setpoint, metabolic adaption and human starvation. Bull Math Biol 2001; 63:393–403.

358. Peters A, Schweiger U, Pellerin L, et al. The selfish brain: competition for energy resources. Neurosci Biobehav Rev 2004; 28:143–180.

359. Maxfield E, Konishi F. Patterns of food intake and physical activity in obesity. J Am Diet Assoc 1966; 49:406–408.

360. Dwyer JT, Feldman JJ, Mayer JK. Adolescent dieters: who are they? Physical characteristics, attitudes and dieting practices of adolescent girls. Am J Clin Nutr 1967; 20:1045–1056.

361. Rossner S. Weight cycling a "new" risk factor? J Intern Med 1989; 226:209–211.

362. Steen SN, Oppliger RA, Brownell KD. Metabolic effects of repeated weight loss and regain in adolescent wrestlers. JAMA 1988; 260:47–50.

363. Ravussin E, Lillioja S, Knowler WC, et al. Reduced rate of energy expenditure as a risk factor for body-weight gain. N Engl J Med 1988; 318:467–472.

364. Rising R, Fontvieille AM, Larson DE. Racial difference in body core temperature between Pima Indian and Caucasian men. Int J Obes Rel Metab Disord 1995; 19:1–5.

365. Rising R, Tataranni PA, Snitker S, Ravussin E. Decreased ratio of fat to carbohydrate oxidation with increasing age in Pima Indians. J Am Coll Nutr 1996; 15:309–312.

366. Bandini LG, Schoeller DA, Dietz WH. Energy expenditure in obese and nonobese adolescents. Pediatr Res 1990; 27:198–203.

367. Lichtman SW, Pisarska K, Berman ER, et al. Discrepancy between self-reported and actual caloric intake and exercise in obese subjects. N Engl J Med 1992; 327:1893–1898.

368. Leibel RL, Rosenbaum M, Hirsch J. Changes in energy expenditure resulting from altered body weight. N Engl J Med 1995; 332:621–628.

369. Ravussin E. Physiology. A NEAT way to control weight? Science 2005; 307:530–531.

370. Levine JA, Lanningham-Foster LA, McCrady SK, et al. Interindividual variation in posture allocation: possible role in human obesity. Science 2005; 307:584–586.

371. Ravussin E, Lillioja S, Anderson TE, Christin L, Bogardus C. Determinants of 24-hour energy expenditure in man. Methods and results using a respiratory chamber. J Clin Invest 1986; 78:1568–1578.

372. Griffiths M, Payne PR. Energy expenditure in small children of obese and nonobese parents. Nature 1976; 260:698–700.

373. Zurlo F, Lillioja S, Puente AED, et al. Low ratio of fat to carbohydrate oxidation as a predictor of weight gain: study of 24-h RQ. Am J Physiol 1990; 259:E650–E657.

374. Rising R, Keys A, Ravussin E, Bogardus C. Concomitant interindividual variation in the body temperature and metabolic rate. Am J Physiol 1992; 263:E730–E734.

375. Spraul M, Ravussin E, Fontvieille AM, Rising R, Larson DE, Anderson EA. Reduced sympathetic nervous activity. A potential mechanism predisposing to body weight gain. J Clin Invest 1993; 92:1730–1735.

376. Salbe AD, Weyer C, Harper I, Lindsay RS, Ravussin E, Tataranni PA. Assessing risk factors for obesity between childhood and adolescence: II. Energy metabolism and physical activity. Pediatrics 2002; 110:307–314.

377. Rowland TW. Exercise and Children's Health. Champaign, IL: Human Kinetics Books, 1990:356.

378. Goran MI, Gower BA, Nagy TR, Johnson RK. Developmental changes in energy expenditure and physical activity in children: evidence for a decline in physical activity in girls before puberty. Pediatrics 1998; 101:887–891.

379. Garcia AW, Broda MA, Frenn M, Coviak C, Pender NJ, Ronis DL. Gender and developmental differences in exercise beliefs among youth and prediction of their exercise behavior. J School Health 1995; 65:213–219.

380. Strauss RS, Rodzilsky D, Burack G, Colin M. Psychosocial correlates of physical activity in healthy children. Arch Pediatr Adolesc Med 2001; 155:897–902.

381. Bullen BA, Reed RB, Mayer J. Physical activity of obese and nonobese adolescent girls appraised by motion picture sampling. Am J Clin Nutr 1964; 14:211–223.

382. Waxman M, Stunkard AJ. Caloric intake and expenditure of obese boys. J Pediatr 1980; 96:187–193.

383. Maffeis C, Schutz Y, Schena F, Zaffanello M, Pinelli L. Energy expenditure during walking and running in obese and nonobese prepubertal children. J Pediatr 1993; 123: 193–199.

384. Gorn GJ, Goldberg ME. Behavioral evidence for the effects of televised food messages on children. J Consumer Res 1982; 9:200–205.

385. Klesges RC, Shelton ML, Klesges LM. Effects of television on metabolic rate: potential implications for childhood obesity. Pediatrics 1993; 91:281–286.

386. Jeffrey DB, McLellarn RW, Fox DT. The development of children's eating habits: the role of television commercials. Health Educ Q 1982; 9:174–189.

387. Williams TM, Handford AG. Television and other leisure activities. In: Williams TM, ed. The Impact of Television: A Natural Experiment in Three Communities. Orlando, FL: Academic Press, 1986:143–213.

388. Dietz WH Jr., Gortmaker SL. Do we fatten our children at the television set? Obesity and television viewing in children and adolescents. Pediatrics 1985; 75:807–812.

389. Andersen RE, Crespo CJ, Bartlett SJ, Cheskin LJ, Pratt M. Relationship of physical activity and television watching with body weight and level of fatness among children: results from the Third National Health and Nutrition Examination Survey. JAMA 1998; 279:938–942.

390. Dennison BA, Erb TA, Jenkins PL. Television viewing and television in bedroom associated with overweight risk among low-income preschool children. Pediatrics 2002; 109:1028–1035.

391. Prentice AM, Lucas A, Vasquez-Velaquez L, Davies PS, Whitehead RG. Are current dietary guidelines for young children a prescription for overfeeding? Lancet 1988; 2:1066–1069.

392. Energy and protein requirements. Report of a joint FAO/ WHO ad hoc expert committee, Rome, March 22 to April 2, 1971. FAO Nutr Meet Rep Ser 1973; 52:1–118.

393. Goran MI, Carpenter WH, Poehlman ET. Total energy expenditure in 4-to-6-yr-old children. Am J Physiol 1993; 264:E706–E711.

394. Fontvieille AM, Harper IT, Ferraro RT, Spraul M, Ravussin E. Daily energy expenditure by five-year-old children measured by doubly labeled water. J Pediatr 1993; 123:200–207.

395. Wei M, Kampert JB, Barlow CE, et al. Relationship between low cardiorespiratory fitness and mortality in normal-weight, overweight, and obese men. JAMA 1999; 282:1547–1553.

396. Myers J, Prakash M, Froelicher V, Do D, Partington S, Atwood JE. Exercise capacity and mortality among men referred for exercise testing. N Engl J Med 2002; 346:793–801.

397. Katzmarzyck PT, Church TS, Janssen I, Ross R, Blair SN. Metabolic syndrome, obesity, and mortality: impact of cardiorespiratory fitness. Diabetes Care 2005; 28: 391–397.

398. Lee S, Kuk JL, Katzmarzyck PT, Blair SN, Church TS, Ross R. Cardiorespiratory fitness attenuates metabolic risk independent of abdominal subcutaneous and visceral fat in men. Diabetes Care 2005; 28:895–901.

399. Schoeller DA. How accurate is self-reported dietary energy intake? Nutr Rev 1990; 48:373–379.

400. Mertz W, Tsui JC, Judd JT, et al. What are people really eating? The relation between energy intake derived from estimated diet records and intake determined to maintain body weight. Am J Clin Nutr 1991; 54:291–295.

401. Bandini LG, Schoeller DA, Cyr HN, Dietz WH. Validity of reported energy intake in obese and nonobese adolescents. Am J Clin Nutr 1990; 52:421–425.

402. Sclafani A, Springer D. Dietary obesity in adult rats: similarities in hypothalamic and human obesity syndromes. Physiol Behav 1976; 17:461–471.

403. Fisher JQ, Rolls BJ, Birch LL. Children's bite size and intake of an entrée are greater with large portions than with age appropriate or self selected portions. Am J Clin Nutr 2003; 77:1170–1184.

404. Rolls BJ, Engell D, Birch LL. Serving portion size influences 5 year old but not 3 year old children's food intake. J Am Diet Assoc 2000; 100:232–234.

405. Flatt JP, Ravussin E, Acheson KJ, Jequier E. Effects of dietary fat on postprandial substrate oxidation and on carbohydrate and fat balances. J Clin Invest 1985; 76: 1019–1024.

406. Schutz Y, Flatt JP, Jequier E. Failure of dietary fat intake to promote fat oxidation: a factor favoring the development of obesity. Am J Clin Nutr 1989; 50:307–314.

407. Golay A, Bobbioni E. The role of dietary fat in obesity. Int J Obes Rel Metab Disord 1997; 21:S2–S11.

408. Rolls BJ, Shide DJ. The influence of dietary fat on food intake and body weight. Nutr Rev 1992; 50:283–290.

409. America Heart Association. Dietary guidelines for healthy American adults: a statement for health professionals from the nutrition committee. Circulation 1996; 94:1795–1800.

410. American Diabetes Association. Nutrition recommendations and principles for people with diabetes mellitus. Diabetes Care 2000; 23:S43–S46.

411. Katan MB, Grundy SM, Willott WC. Should a low fat, high-carbohydrate diet be recommended for everyone? Beyond low-fat diets. N Engl J Med 1997; 337:563–566.

412. Larson DE, Hunter GR, Williams MJ, Kekes-Szabo T, Nyikos I, Goran MI. Dietary fat in relation to body fat and intraabdominal adipose tissue: a cross-sectional analysis. Am J Clin Nutr 1996; 64:787–788.

413. Allred JB. Too much of a good thing? An overemphasis on eating low-fat foods may be contributing to the alarming increase in overweight among US adults. J Am Diet Assoc 1995; 95:417–418.

414. Nicklas TA. Dietary studies of children: the Bogalusa Heart Study experience. J Am Diet Assoc 1995; 95: 1127–1133.

415. Kant AK, Graubard BI, Schatzkin A, Ballard-Barbash R. Proportions of energy intake from fat and subsequent weight change in the NHANES 1 epidemiologic follow-up study. Am J Clin Nutr 1995; 61:11–17.

416. Lissner L, Heitman BL. Dietary fat and obesity: evidence from epidemiology. Eur J Clin Nutr 1995; 49:79–90.

417. Lenfant C, Ernst N. Daily dietary fat and total energy hyperinsulinemia of obesity. N Engl J Med 1971; 285: 827–831.

418. Stephen AM, Wald NJ. Trends in individual consumption of dietary fat in the United States, 1920–1984. Am J Clin Nutr 1990; 52:457–469.

419. Wolever TM, Jenkins DJ, Jenkins AL, Josse RG. The glycemic index: methodology and clinical implications. Am J Clin Nutr 1991; 54:846–854.

420. Bjork I, Granfeldt Y, Liljeberg H, Tovar J, Asp N-G. Food properties affecting the digestion and absorption of carbohydrates. Am J Clin Nutr 1994; 59:699S–705S.

421. Granfeldt Y, Hagander B, Bjork I. Metabolic responses to starch in oat and wheat products. On the importance of food structure, incomplete gelatinization or presence of viscous dietary fiber. Eur J Clin Nutr 1995; 49:189–199.

422. Welch IM, Bruce C, Hill SE, Read NW. Duodenal and ileal lipid suppresses postprandial blood glucose and insulin responses in man: possible implications for dietary management of diabetes mellitus. Clin Sci 1987; 72:209–216.

423. Trout DL, Behall KM, Osilesi O. Prediction of glycemic index for starchy foods. Am J Clin Nutr 1993; 58:873–878.

424. Foster-Powell K, Miller JB. International tables of glycemic index. Am J Clin Nutr 1995; 62:871S–890S.

425. Stephen AM, Sieber GM, Gerster YA, Morgan DR. Intake of carbohydrate and its component-international comparisons, trends overtime, and effects of changing to low fat diet. Am J Clin Nutr 1995; 62:851S–867S.

426. Nicklas TA, Webber LS, Koschak ML, Berenson GS. Nutrient adequacy of low fat intakes for children: the Bogalusa Heart Study. Pediatrics 1992; 89:221–228.

427. Popkin BM, Haines PS, Patterson RE. Dietary changes in older Americans 1977–1987. Am J Clin Nutr 1992; 55: 823–830.

428. Harnack LJ, Jeffery RW, Boutelle KN. Temporal trends in energy intake in the United States: an ecologic perspective. Am J Clin Nutr 2000; 71:1478–1484.

429. Lifshitz F. Commentary: Soft drinks replacing healthier alternatives in American diet. AAP News 2002; 20:36–37.

430. Grey NJ, Goldring S, Kipnis DM. The effect of fasting, diet, and actinomycin D on insulin secretion in the rat. J Clin Invest 1970; 49:881–889.

431. Grey NJ, Kipnis DM. Effect of diet composition on the hyperinsulinemia of obesity. N Engl J Med 1971; 285: 827–831.

432. Dennison BA, Rockwell HL, Baker SL. Excess fruit juice consumption by preschool-aged children is associated with short stature and obesity. Pediatrics 1997; 99:15–22.

433. Bagdade JD, Bierman EL, Porte D Jr. The significance of basal insulin levels in the evaluation of the insulin response to glucose in diabetic and nondiabetic subjects. J Clin Invest 1967; 46:1549–1557.

434. Floyd JC Jr., Fajans SS, Conn JW, Khoph RF, Rull J. Stimulation of insulin secretion by amino acids. J Clin Invest 1966; 1487–1502.

435. Rabinowitz D, Zierler KL. Forearm metabolism in obesity and its response to intra-arterial insulin. Characterization of insulin resistance and evidence for adaptive hyperinsulinism. J Clin Invest 1962; 41:2173–2181.

436. Ludwig DS, Majzoub JA, Al-Zahrani A, Dallal GE, Blanco I, Roberts SB. High glycemic index foods, overeating, and obesity. Pediatrics 1999; 103:E26.

437. Spieth LE, Harnish JD, Lenders CM, et al. A low-glycemic index diet in the treatment of pediatric obesity. Arch Pediatr Adolesc Med 2000; 154:947–951.

438. Bray GA. Lipogenesis in human adipose tissue: some effects of nibbling and gorging. J Clin Invest 1972; 51:537–548.

439. Fabry P, Tepperman J. Meal frequency a possible factor in human pathology. Am J Clin Nutr 1970; 23:1059–1068.

440. Dietschy JM, Brown MS. Effect of alterations of the specific activity of the intracellular acetyl CoA pool on apparent rates of hepatic cholesterogenesis. J Lipid Res 1974; 15:508–516.

441. Lakshmanan MR, Nepokroeff CM, Ness GC, Dugan RE, Porter JW. Stimulation by insulin of rat liver β-hydroxy-β-methylglutaryl coenzyme A reductase and cholesterol-synthesizing activities. Biochem Biophys Res Commun 1973; 50:704–710.

442. Jenkins DJ, Wolever TM, Vuksan V, et al. Nibbling verses gorging: metabolic advantages of increased meal frequency. N Engl J Med 1989; 321:929–934.

443. Acheson K, Jequier E, Wahren J. Influence of β-adrenergic blockade on glucose-induced thermogenesis in man. J Clin Invest 1983; 72:981–986.

2

Treatment of Pediatric Obesity

Diego Botero
*Department of Pediatrics, Children's Hospital Boston, Harvard Medical School,
Boston, Massachusetts, U.S.A.*

Fima Lifshitz
*Pediatric Sunshine Academics Inc. and Sansum Medical Research Institute,
Santa Barbara, California, and Department of Pediatrics, University of Miami, Miami, Florida,
and Department of Pediatrics, Health Science Center, State University of New York,
Brooklyn, New York, U.S.A.*

INTRODUCTION

The main goal of therapy in childhood obesity should be to achieve lifelong weight control. Therefore, it is important to assess the child and the family in order to plan an appropriate therapeutic approach. It is essential to know the child's pattern of growth and weight gain (Vol. 1; Chap. 1). Children who are gaining excess weight and present upward crossing of percentiles require a more intensive therapeutic strategy than those who are overweight, but are maintaining a pattern of weight progression and follow the same percentile, as they grow older. In general, any treatment plan for children with obesity should aim to induce decreased energy intake and increased energy expenditure, while maintaining normal growth. Intervention to induce weight loss must consider all the factors believed to play a role in the obesity of a particular child.

In a clinical setting, only proven effective treatment modalities should be utilized for the treatment of children. A study reported medical complications in up to 80% of children who were on unsupervised diets (1). In addition, medically supervised diets may not be effective and may actually promote weight gain (2). However, most of our present experience in the treatment of obesity centers on environmental and behavioral factors; these represent the primary areas of intervention. Thus, the cornerstone of the treatment for childhood obesity includes dietary intake, physical activity, and behavior modification. However, genetic influences are also very significant in the development of obesity as well as in the response to treatment, and these need be considered in the plan. Genetics also help to identify the child at risk; early intervention for the child predisposed to obesity is needed, before obesity reaches severe proportions. Furthermore, any form

of treatment for obesity should take into account potential underlying medical conditions (i.e., hypotonia, mental retardation, medications, etc.) that may frustrate or render it ineffective. The presence of obesity-related comorbidities in children warrant early medical intervention and/or preventive measures implemented as soon as recognized. Therefore, an individualized therapeutic plan with specific desired goals should be established.

Prior to the initiation of any form of therapy, a comprehensive medical evaluation is necessary. This should comprise the assessment of the rate of growth and weight gain, medical conditions, developmental milestones, and family history. The latter is essential to identify children at risk for the type of obesity and/or the risk factors present in the family, i.e., hypertension, diabetes mellitus, and hyperlipidemia. Furthermore, the assessment should also include nutritional, psychological, and physical fitness evaluations. Obese children are not usually "overnourished" in all aspects. Indeed, the reverse may be true, because excess calorie intake may increase the requirements of essential nutrients that may not be provided by the diet that leads to excess weight gain. For example, obesity is often associated with mineral and vitamin deficits (3). In addition, obese adolescents and adults may engage in binge eating (4) and may be under tremendous psychological stress. These individuals have a higher dropout rate from weight reduction programs than those who do not binge. Additionally, the obese child must be assessed for comorbidities associated with obesity (Vol. 1; Chaps. 1 and 11).

However, the usual medical evaluation of the overweight child leaves much to be desired; it often falls short of the recommended practices (5). In addition, obese children are not referred for treatment on a timely basis, whereas children who fail to gain weight are usually promptly assessed (6). The majority of obese patients referred to a pediatric endocrinologist arrive after a prolonged interval from the onset of obesity (7). The use of popular diets without medical supervision may be detrimental.

The treatment of pediatric obesity may be successful with dietary intake, physical activity, and lifestyle changes (8). One-third of the children initially treated in a multidisciplinary program maintained their reduced weight after 5 and 10 years. Furthermore, preadolescent children showed better responses to initial treatment and maintenance of long-term weight loss. These data are encouraging, but more research needs to be done to determine compliance with treatment and maintenance of weight loss into adulthood, particularly in a clinical setting. Intensive therapies such as pharmacotherapy with antiobesity medications or bariatric surgery should be reserved for the treatment of morbidly obese adolescents who present with severe obesity related comorbidities. Regardless of the treatment strategy, close monitoring of growth and pubertal development is a top priority, because growth and pubertal development may be compromised with severe caloric restriction.

This chapter provides an action-oriented approach for pediatricians and pediatric endocrinologists. In this chapter, we begin with a broad overview of pediatrician involvement in prevention strategies, including public health initiatives. We then describe lifestyle-based treatments of pediatric obesity, followed by a discussion of intensive therapies.

PREVENTION

The prevention of obesity in children may be a cost-effective approach to combating the obesity epidemic and its comorbidities in adults, with pediatricians playing a role not only in clinic settings but also through public health initiatives. A policy statement on prevention of pediatric overweight and obesity was issued by the American Academy of Pediatrics (AAP) (9). It encouraged pediatricians to advocate for policies and programs that allow changes in the "obesogenic" environment, in addition to screening for overweight and associated comorbidities and offering clinical advice for prompt interventions.

Recommendations for preventing childhood obesity should be applied from prenatal life onward. Low birth weight due to maternal undernutrition, smoking, or placental insufficiency or large size at birth attributable most often to gestational diabetes mellitus, may be associated with obesity later in life (10). Obese parents impose a great risk for their children to be overweight (11). Although still controversial, breastfeeding has been considered to be a protecting factor for future obesity (12). Although recently, the differences in body mass index (BMI) later in life, between breastfed and nonbreastfed subjects in a

systematic review of published studies were very small (13). These factors suggest that lifestyle modification and early intervention may be important to prevent future adolescent and adult obesity (14). One of the most effective strategies for implementation of an active lifestyle early in life is the reduction in sedentary activities. This can be achieved by simple measures, such as by limiting television viewing (15).

Preventive measures implemented in schools may have a significant impact in the epidemic of overweight children. School cafeterias should provide a healthful diet including fresh fruits, salads, and vegetables. Sugary drinks and foods with a high content of simple carbohydrates should be banned (16,17). Physical activity should be mandatory at all ages. Guided exercise and after-school programs for physical education should be part of a health curriculum. Table 1 depicts the most effective prevention strategies to accomplish these goals.

Long-term follow up of children treated with diet, exercise, and behavior modification attained lower weights 5 to 10 years later than those children treated in other ways (18–20). However, not all obese children who were initially successful in reducing their body weight with a treatment program were able to maintain their reduced relative body weight later on in life. Nevertheless, these studies were not made to be compared with each other, and did not have similar designs and/or control populations. In addition, the increasing prevalence of childhood and adolescent obesity (21) suggests that even the most successful treatment program may be of limited benefit if it relies on the traditional doctor/patient interaction model. Furthermore, the frequent presence of the metabolic syndrome among obese individuals (i.e., hyperinsulinemia) and family history of Type 2 diabetes, hypertension and/or hyperlipidemia, may play a major role in patient's response to conventional weight management strategies (22). Insulin resistance and obesity are more resistant to weight loss than that observed in normoinsulinemic obese children (23) (Vol. 1; Chaps. 1 and 11).

Therefore, the development of effective methods for weight reduction should be encouraged and multidisciplinary research implemented to identify factors that prevent relapses. However, the pediatrician should always exercise simple methods to assess body weight progression by plotting height and weight on the growth chart of their patients and discussing the patterns with the families. This clinical practice standard is recommended by the AAP, but is often not being done (24). There are other methods for the rapid assessment of the nutritional status of patients that should be routinely used, even in a busy practice, because the identification of the problem of obesity and discussing it with the family may be a good first start (25).

Children should be encouraged to develop healthy eating habits and exercise patterns that prevent excessive weight gain. This is especially

Table 1 Strategies to Be Implemented in Prevention of Childhood Obesity

Pregnancy
  Normalize body mass index prior to pregnancy
  Do not smoke
  Maintain moderate exercise as tolerated
  Meticulous glucose control, in gestational diabetics
Postpartum and infancy
  Breast-feeding is preferred for a minimum of three months
  Postpone introduction of solid foods and sweet liquids
Families
  Eat meals as a family in a fixed place and time
  Do not skip meals, especially breakfast
  No TV during meals
  Use small plates and keep serving dishes away from the table
  Avoid unnecessary sweet or fatty foods and soft drinks
  Remove televisions from children's bedrooms; restrict times for TV viewing
    and video games
Schools
  Eliminate fundraisers with candy and cookie sales
  Review contents of vending machines for healthier choices
  Install water fountains
  Educate teachers, especially physical education and science faculty,
    about basic nutrition and benefits of physical activity
  Educate children from preschool through high school on appropriate diet
    and lifestyle
  Mandate minimum standards for physical education, including
    30–45 minutes of strenuous exercise two to three times weekly
  Encourage the "walking school bus"
Communities
  Increase family-friendly exercise/play facilities for all age children
  Discourage the use of elevators and moving walkways
  Provide information on how to shop and prepare healthier versions of
    cultural-specific foods
Healthcare providers
  Explain biological and genetic noncontrollable contributions to obesity
  Give age-appropriate expectations for body weight in children
  Work toward classifying obesity as a disease to promote recognition,
    reimbursement for care, and willingness and ability to
    provide treatment
Industry
  Mandate age-appropriate nutrition labeling for products aimed at
    children (e.g., red-light/green-light foods with portion sizes)
  Encourage marketing of interactive video games in which children must
    exercise in order to play
  Use celebrity advertising directed at children for healthful foods to
    promote breakfast and regular meals
Government and regulatory agencies
  Classify obesity as a legitimate disease
  Find novel ways to fund healthy lifestyle programs, i.e., with revenues
    from food/drink taxes
  Subsidize government-sponsored programs to promote consumption of
    fresh fruits and vegetables
  Provide financial incentives to industry to develop more healthful
    products and to educate the consumer on product content
  Provide financial incentives to schools that initiate innovative physical
    activity and nutrition programs
  Allow tax deductions for the cost of weight loss and exercise programs
  Provide urban planners with funding to establish bicycle, jogging, and
    walking paths
  Ban advertising of fast foods directed at preschool children, and restrict
    advertising to school-age children

Source: From Ref. 5.

important for children in high-risk groups, for instance, those with obese parents (11) and those who are overweight by the time they enter school (26).

Health professionals should inform parents of the potential risks and provide instructions on preventive measures at an early age. The introduction of a variety of nutritious foods to children's diets will lead to the development of healthy eating practices that may last a lifetime. Relatively free access to the popular servings of large-portion meal sizes results in increased calorie intake (27). This increases the chances of overeating and may encourage the development of obesity over time in predisposed children. A high susceptibility to obesity may also be the result of unlimited availability of palatable and high-calorie-dense foods. Laboratory adult rats fed a "supermarket diet" consisting of high-carbohydrate/high-fat foods (i.e., chocolate chip cookies, marshmallows, peanut butter, etc.), gained 2.5 times more weight than normal controls (28). In some animals, the weight gain was not reversed after the rat was switched back to chow. The intake of high-calorie-dense food diets may lead to increase the number and size of fat cells. Additionally, diets that are high-calorie-dense may result in overweight and iron deficiency (3).

Other lifestyle changes may be important in addressing the prevention of obesity. A desirable approach should include reduction of sedentary activities, such as television viewing and computer and video game use. In a comprehensive study of 198 third- and fourth-grade students who participated in a six-month course geared toward reduction in television viewing, videotape, and game use, the children in the intervention group reduced their BMI, triceps skinfold thickness, waist circumference, and waist-to-hip ratio as compared with the control group of children, who did not change their television-viewing habits (15). Moreover, children in the intervention group self-reported fewer hours watching television and consuming fewer meals in front of the television. However, no changes were detected between the two groups about high-fat food intake, physical activity, and cardiorespiratory fitness. These results suggest that just reducing television viewing and video game use contribute to positive changes in obesity indices in children.

Primary public health measures are critical to formulate a sound approach to the prevention of obesity in children, and the pediatrician and pediatric endocrinologist need to play an advocacy role to achieve these goals. Schools and government agencies, as well as food industries, have responsibility to support measures that can improve the food habits and exercise patterns of children and adults. The schools should play an active role in providing healthy food choices in the cafeteria and provide appropriate exercise programs for normal-weight and obese children separate from competitive athletics. Government and local authorities can insist that schools implement and promote physical fitness programs and provide easy access to exercise facilities in the community. The media must also assume a responsible position with regard to idealized concepts of beauty by appropriate programming and feeding of messages to children and to society.

LIFESTYLE-BASED TREATMENTS
Dietary Approaches

The role of dietary intake in obesity remains controversial, although new data have shed more light on this subject (29). Obese individuals often claim that they do not ingest excess food (30). These patients often seek medical evaluation for failure to lose weight despite a history of severe caloric restriction. There are no differences in resting energy expenditure (REE) or in metabolic rates between diet-sensitive and diet-resistant obese individuals (31). The differences in lean body mass account for the variations in weight reduction induced by diet restrictions in obese individuals. They are not "hypometabolic," they ingest excess calories for their energy expenditures. Patients who gain weight increase their metabolic rate, whereas those who are on restrictive diets and are losing weight may reduce their energy expenditure by 10% to 20%. Thus, the results of dietary efforts can only be successful if the reduced energy intake is accompanied by increased energy expenditures to overcome the metabolic adaptations that occur with dieting. A number of studies have demonstrated that obese individuals tend to underreport food intake as compared with normal-weight subjects (32–34). Indeed, careful metabolic balance studies in obese adults showed that failure to lose weight, despite self-reported low caloric intakes, was due to substantial misreporting of food intake and physical activity, not to an abnormality in thermogenesis. However, the problem is often confounded in the clinical setting by the difficulties in assessing food intake and food efficiency.

Dietary composition and different rates of nutrient utilization of ingested diets may influence body weight. Using indirect calorimetric technique in nonobese males, Flatt et al. (35) demonstrated that under sedentary conditions, ingested carbohydrates were metabolized quickly, while the rate of fat oxidation remained unchanged. Moreover, it appears that the body tightly regulates carbohydrate balance for up to 36 hours after ingestion and it does not alter the body's fat balance (36). On the other hand, fat balance is regulated over the long term, and it may take several days before the fat balance adjusts to new levels of fat ingestion. Thus, excessive fat consumption over a prolonged period will result in a positive fat balance and weight gain (37,38). Therefore, a number of medical organizations including the American Heart Association (39) and the American Diabetes Association (40) currently recommend consumption of low-fat (LF) diets in the prevention and treatment of obesity.

However, the relationship between the dietary fat and obesity has been questioned (41–43) because both cross-sectional and longitudinal analyses have failed to show a consistent association between dietary fat and body fat (44,45). Furthermore, recent studies indicate that weight loss with LF diets is usually modest and transient (42,46). It is also noteworthy that the rate of obesity has continued to rise in the United States, despite reported reduction in mean fat intake over the past 30 years, from 42% to about 34% of dietary calories (43,44,47,48).

Similarly, in a randomized trial of low-carbohydrate (LC) diets used for the treatment of obesity, there was modest weight loss for the first six months of therapy, but there was poor long-term adherence and the body weight loss was no longer significant after 12 months (49). In addition, in a recent study, the effectiveness of various popular diets in adults was tested. It was clearly shown that the diets work as long as the individuals adhere to the diet (50). Obese adults were given one of the following diets: Atkins, Ornish, Weight Watchers, or Zone. The study was carried out in a single center as a randomized trial of 160 patients, 40 in each diet. They all modestly reduced weight and improved cardiovascular risk factors, but there was poor adherence to all diets. The better outcomes occurred in the patients who adhered to the diets, though the Weight Watchers had better adherence rates. Therefore, a calorie is a calorie no matter how it is ingested, though a well-balanced diet may be easier to consume for prolonged periods.

In children short-term weight loss was attained in randomized, controlled trials of dietary interventions, ranging from LF to LC prescriptions (Table 2) (51).

However, due to the lack of controlled studies in children, no definitive conclusions can be derived regarding the long-term effects of these diets in youth. Although energy restricted, LF diets were endorsed by the AAP (52) and the U.S. Department of Agriculture (53) among others, no long-term clinical data are available to support implementation of this specific dietary approach as the most effective therapy. A systematic review of 22 randomized-controlled trials with greater than or equal to six months duration in overweight children could not achieve any conclusions about the effectiveness of the different interventions, due to the absence of large long-term randomized studies (54).

The glycemic index (GI) is another dietary factor that may influence body weight. GI is a property of carbohydrate-containing food that describes the rise of blood-glucose after a meal (55). The GI of a meal is determined mainly by the amount of carbohydrate content and by other dietary factors affecting food digestibility, gastrointestinal motility, or insulin secretion (including carbohydrate type, food structure, fiber, protein, and fat) (56–59). The average American diet contains starchy foods that are primarily refined grain products, cereals, and potatoes and have a high GI. In contrast, vegetables, legumes, and fruits have generally a low GI (60). The potential adverse consequence of the decreased, observed fat

Table 2 Dietary Approaches Currently Available

Type of diet	Carbohydrate/fat (%)	Example
Very low fat	70–75/≤10	Ornish diet
Low fat	45–65/<35	Dictary Guidelines for Americans 2005
Low energy density	Variable	Volumetricss
Low carbohydrate	≤10/60	Atkins diet
Low-glycemic load	Variable	South Beach diet

Source: Adapted from Ref. 51.

intake might be related to a concomitant increase in dietary GI. A reduction of dietary fat tends to cause a compensatory increase in sugar and starch intake (61–63). In fact, a rise in total carbohydrate consumption and GI of American diets, over the past two decades, has been reported (61,63). Because fat slows gastric emptying (59), carbohydrate absorption from LF meals is accelerated, and results in faster, higher blood-glucose concentrations.

Diets that include a low GI/load approach have received increased attention and are currently under investigation. GI is defined as the area under the glucose curve after ingesting a 50 g carbohydrate meal, divided by the glucose area under the curve that results after consuming a standard reference food (glucose or bread) containing 50 g carbohydrate, multiplied by 100 (55). Glycemic load (GL) on the other hand is the arithmetic product of the amount of carbohydrate consumed and the GI. Thus, while the GI refers to the effect on postprandial glycemia by the specific source of carbohydrate, the GL accounts for not only the source, but also the quantity of carbohydrate (64). Most refined grain products have a high GI. On the other hand, nonstarchy vegetables, legumes, nontropical fruits, and whole grains have a low GI (65). Table 3 depicts the GI and GL of some representative food items. The reader is referred to the International table of GI and GL values of over 13,000 data entries representing over 750 types of food (60). That paper also lists the GL associated with the consumption of specified serving sizes of different foods.

Figure 1 depicts the low GI food pyramid (66). Several studies relating GI to hunger have demonstrated beneficial effects of low GI compared with high-GI meals (66). The rapid absorption of glucose after consumption of high-GI foods induces a sequence of hormonal and metabolic changes that promote excessive food intake. Figure 2 shows the acute metabolic response to three different breakfasts (low, medium, and high GI) in a group of pubertal adolescent boys.

The high-GI breakfast induced higher glycemic and insulin responses compared to the medium and low-GI meals. Similarly, plasma glucagon level and free fatty acid concentrations were suppressed to a greater degree after the high-GI meal compared the low-GI meal. Higher concentration of counter regulatory hormones correlated with the high-GI meal versus

Table 3 Glycemic Index and Glycemic Load of Representative Foods

Food	Glycemic index[a]	Glycemic load[b]
Instant rice	91	24.8 (110 g)
Baked potato	85	20.3 (110 g)
Corn flakes	84	21.0 (225 mL)
Carrot	71	3.8 (55 g)
White bread	70	21.0 (2 slices)
Rye bread	65	19.5 (2 slices)
Muesli	56	16.8 (110 mL)
Banana	53	13.3 (170 g)
Spaghetti	41	16.4 (55 g)
Apple	36	8.1 (170 g)
Lentil beans	29	5.7 (110 mL)
Milk	27	3.2 (225 mL)
Peanuts	27	3.2 (225 mL)
Broccoli	14	0.7 (30 g)

Note: To determine the glycemic index of a specific food, subjects are given a test food and a control food on separate days, each food containing 50 g of available carbohydrate, and changes in blood glucose concentration are measured. Glycemic index is calculated with the trapezoidal rule as the increment area under the blood glucose curve for 2 hours after the test food is eaten divided by the corresponding area after the control food is eaten, multiplied by 100%. Values for the most commonly consumed carbohydrate-containing foods have been determined and can be obtained from published lists. Ellipses indicate value not computed; the values for most nonstarchy vegetables are too low to measure.
[a]Glycemic index values are taken from Foster-Powell and Miller (16) and expressed as a percentage of the value for glucose.
[b]Glycemic load is calculated as the glycemic index multiplied by grams of carbohydrate per serving size (15), indicated in parentheses, divided by 100%.
Source: From Ref. 65.

the low-GI meal. Similarly, greater ratings of hunger occurred after consuming the high-GI breakfast compared to the medium- and low-GI meals.

A 12-month randomized control trial (68) comparing the effects of a low GI/load diet versus

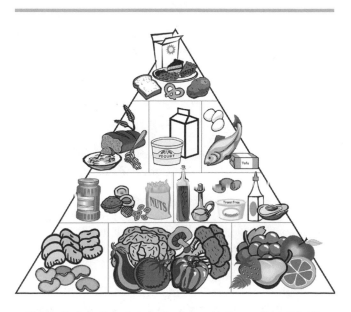

Figure 1 Low glycemic index food pyramid. *Source*: From Ref. 66.

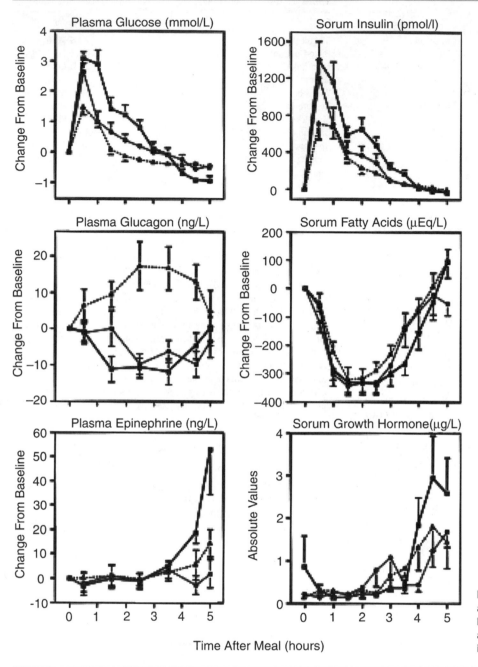

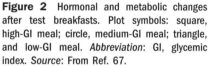

Figure 2 Hormonal and metabolic changes after test breakfasts. Plot symbols: square, high-GI meal; circle, medium-GI meal; triangle, and low-GI meal. *Abbreviation*: GI, glycemic index. *Source*: From Ref. 67.

conventional LF diet in 14 obese adolescents showed a reduction of BMI at 12 months of -1.3 ± 0.7 units in the low-GI group versus 0.7 ± 0.5 units in the LF group ($p = 0.02$). Similarly, fat mass decreased more in the experimental group (-3.0 ± 1.6 kg) compared to the conventional group (1.8 ± 1.0 kg, $p = 0.1$). Insulin resistance assessed by the homeostasis model assessment also increased less in the experimental group. A randomized-controlled 12-week trial compared the effects of a LC diet with self-selected energy intake to a LF diet with self-selected energy intake on weight loss in overweight adolescents (69). Adolescents in the LC group lost 9.9 ± 9.3 kg

compared with 4.1 ± 4.9 kg for teens in the LF group ($p < 0.04$). Eight of 16 subjects in the LC group lost more than 1 kg/wk compared with 4 of 14 in the LF group ($p < 0.05$).

Spieth et al. suggested that a low-glycemic-index diet in the treatment of childhood obesity resulted in greater weight loss than a standard reduced-fat diet (70). It has been shown that voluntary intake after a high-GI meal was 53% greater than after a medium-GI meal, and was 81% greater than after a low-GI meal. In addition, compared with the low-GI meal, the high-GI meal resulted in higher serum insulin levels, plasma glucagon levels, postabsorptive plasma glucose, and serum fatty acids levels, along with an elevation in plasma epinephrine (68). It is, therefore, likely that the rapid absorption of glucose after ingestion of high-GI meals induces a sequence of hormonal and metabolic changes that promote excessive food intake in obese adolescents.

When comparing the standard low-calorie, LF diet versus the LC diet, the LC diet resulted in greater high-density lipoprotein-cholesterol (HDL-C) and lower triglyceride (TG) levels compared to the LF diet. A randomized study by Samaha et al. (71), conducted in 132 obese adults for six months comparing a carbohydrate-restricted diet with a LF diet revealed greater weight loss (–5.8 vs. –1.9 kg), better insulin sensitivity, and lower TG levels in those that received the LC diet. A one-year study by Foster et al. (49) on 63 obese adults reported a more favorable lipid profile at one year of dietary treatment with the LC diet.

High-carbohydrate diets increase basal plasma insulin levels in animals and humans (72,73). Obesity is associated with elevated basal plasma insulin secretory response to glucose and protein (74,75). The hyperinsulinemia of obesity appears to be a compensatory adaptation to the peripheral insulin resistance that characterizes the obese state (76) (Vol. 1; Chap. 11). Because the diets of moderately obese individuals are usually excessive in both total calories and in the quantity of carbohydrate ingested, the hyperinsulinemia of obesity may also be a consequence of these dietary factors.

The traffic-light diet is another approach that may be suitable for preschool and preadolescent children. This consists of a 900 to 1300 kcal/day diet of "tagged" foods designed to meet the age recommendations for appropriate nutrient intake using the basic four food groups outlined in the food guide pyramid. These diet groups fit food into three categories: Green foods (go) can be consumed in unlimited amounts; yellow foods (caution) have average nutritional values within their group, and red foods (stop) provide less-nutrient density per calorie because of high-fat or simple carbohydrate content (77,78). Combined with a comprehensive treatment protocol, this diet was effective in obesity and changed eating habits in preadolescent children (78–81). Furthermore, weight loss up to 10 years was maintained when the traffic-light diet was combined with behavioral, exercise, and familial components of a comprehensive treatment program (18,19,82).

In summary, despite the controversy and lack of conclusive data on the most effective dietary approach to treat obesity, specific recommendations for a healthy diet along with physical activity can help most people to prevent, manage, and maintain weight loss. Long-term effects and safety of low-glycemic diets need to be evaluated in children. Although low-GI or GL diets appear to be promising in the management of obesity, large-scale long-term randomized-controlled trials are required before definitive conclusions can be drawn.

A healthful diet should include fruits, vegetables, legumes, and whole grains, and should restrict the intake of processed foods, sugary drinks, and foods with a high content of fat. Eating satisfying portions of low-energy-dense foods can help enhance satiety and control hunger while restricting energy intake for weight management (83). Providing older children and adults with larger portion sizes can lead to increased energy intake. One study showed that children ate 25% more when served a large entrée as compared with the amount ingested when they decided themselves (27).

Any dietary intervention in overweight children should provide a physiologic nutritional balance for growth and development. Severe caloric restriction may produce macro- and micronutrient deficits, electrolyte imbalances, and may compromise linear growth velocity. As discussed below, behavioral modification and family participation are critical components of any dietary intervention (77,82).

Food Management

Diets are most likely to succeed if individualized according to eating patterns, degree of motivation, intellect, amount of family support, and financial considerations. Therefore, a management approach to food intake is preferable to a diet prescription. A well-balanced calorie restrictive intake that provides all the necessary nutrients is the most effective and safest treatment for obesity (29). The reduction in caloric intake should consider the weight and weight history of the child. In addition, the usual calorie intake and the type of food consumed should be considered. In a study of lean and overweight adolescents, over consumption of fast food was prevalent among adolescents, though the obese individuals were less likely to compensate for the energy in fast food, by adjusting energy intake throughout the day, than the lean counterparts (84). Body size, rate of growth, degree of adiposity, desired weight, and estimated daily activity level must also be considered for the therapy plan. As a rule, moderately obese children should be placed on an energy intake and exercise level that will slow weight gain appropriate for their age and growth. In specific instances, to allow for parental or patient desires, it may be appropriate to design a nutrient intake to induce a slight weight loss. To accomplish this goal, for practical purposes it can be assumed that one pound of fat represents 3500 kcal.

The food choices must be individualized in accordance with the taste and preferences of the family and the patient, with an aim of meeting all the appropriate dietary requirements. This should be achieved gradually to ensure compliance, while appropriate eating patterns are established. It is important to correct all potential nutritional deficits at the beginning of the treatment and to assess for the frequent comorbidities associated with the disease. Initially, a 10% calorie reduction with the usual nutrient intake should be prescribed, and when to eat and how often should also be recommended. There are potential benefits from nibbling and avoiding gorging, thus consumption of multiple small meals is preferable to one large meal, though ultimately the amount consumed is most important (85). While on treatment it is important to monitor any alteration that may develop throughout the follow-up period.

The following is an example of an initial approach to the treatment of an obese adolescent: a 14-year-old boy with a weight of 72 kg and a BMI of 28% was examined because of obesity. The initial nutritional evaluation documented that he was ingesting the diet shown in Table 4. This diet is typical of this age group (86). Analysis of the diet revealed that he was ingesting 3200 kcal (44.5 kcal/kg/day), plus 28% of that recommended for his age/size. He was also ingesting 44% of the total calories from fat; 14.6% of the total calories from saturated fat with 723 mg cholesterol, all being very high. He also had a high sodium intake of 4739 mg, almost double than that recommended for his age (87).

Although his intake was very inappropriate, treatment was started with a slight modification to improve compliance. By eliminating one doughnut and switching from regular soda to diet soda, the energy intake was reduced to a level sufficient to avoid weight gain and maintain his current weight (38.5 kcal/kg/day). By simply eliminating those two items from the diet, there was a drop in calorie intake of 433 kcal/day. Other inappropriate dietary habits were not corrected, although the cholesterol intake also dropped by 19 mg/day. Once the patient adjusted to these simple changes, further work was necessary to improve upon the excess fat intake and reduce the amount of saturated fat from the diet. Patients who do not comply with simple measures

might not be sufficiently motivated or learn to improve their nutritional habits for life.

Another example is a 50 kg five-year-old patient with a BMI of 37% who was gaining weight rapidly and had biochemical abnormalities detected in the work up (i.e., hyperinsulinemia and hyperlipidemia). The patient and the family were highly motivated. Her caloric intake was 1400 to 1500 kcal/day. This level of energy intake was not excessive for maintenance of body weight (30 kcal/kg/day). However, it contained a high proportion of dietary fats. A realistic goal for her was set at 10% of body weight loss and then weight maintenance, until her weight would catch up with her height and normalize the height-to-weight ratio. This was a long-term plan that would require a successful attempt with three years of body maintenance.

Food management was initiated without reducing the total calories, because her total daily caloric intake did not appear to be excessive for weight. Her food choices were modified to reduce the fat intake. She was placed on a 1500 kcal meal plan with decreased fat content (30%), while increasing complex-carbohydrates (low GI). This included increasing vegetables in her diet and substituting low-calorie snacks for high-fat foods. She was given three meals and three snacks daily. It is recognized that frequent meals are more effective for weight control than one large meal, if reduced energy intake is accomplished (85). Therefore, her usual intake that consisted of one or two large meals per day was discouraged.

Day-to-day variations in caloric consumption are characteristic of normal eating patterns and thus they should be allowed as long as they not are excessive. For example, it would be appropriate for a girl on a 1500 kcal-meal plan to have a range of intakes from approximately 1200 to 1800 kcal/day. While assessment of the rate of weight loss and growth is important, periodic assessment of nutrient composition of the diet is essential. This is particularly important for such micronutrients as calcium, iron, magnesium, copper, zinc, folacin, and vitamins, because these are very likely to be deficient on a restricted dietary intake (44). However, it is important to reiterate that total energy intake, more than the type of energy consumption or distribution of calories, determines weight loss (29). Therefore, a balanced diet that provides a reduced intake is preferable because it achieves long-term weight control with healthier eating behaviors as described below.

Behavior Modification

Behavior intervention and lifestyle modification are essential components of a multidisciplinary obesity program (88). Behavioral treatment helps the overweight person develop skills to cope with an environment that promotes overeating and inactivity, whether implemented on an individual basis or in a

Table 4 Typical Intake of an Adolescent Evaluated for Obesity

	Energy (kcal)
Breakfast	
Two sausages and two eggs	300
Coffee (1 cup)	0
Whole milk (1 cup)	150
Fruit juice (1 cup)	110
Lunch	
McDonald's Quarter Pounder	525
French fries (10 strips)	160
Soda (1 can)	148
Dinner	
Half chicken breast	220
Baked potato (1)	220
Salad with dressing (8 oz)	85
Daily snack	
Donuts (2)	570
Chocolate chip cookies (3)	185
Ice cream (1 cup)	270
Potato chips (10 pieces)	105
Total	3207

Source: From Ref. 87.

group setting. The effects of an eight-month family-based behavioral intervention study reported by Epstein et al. (18) in a group of 6- to 11-year-old overweight children showed greater decreases in percent overweight compared to the control group 10 years after finishing the intervention.

The goal of behavioral treatment is to help overweight individuals to identify and modify conditions associated with sedentary lifestyle and maladaptive eating habits by using different strategies applied in a family-based context (77,84). Relevant behaviors should be identified and positive changes should be reinforced. For the behavioral approach to be effective, it must define reasonable, clear goals and must help the overweight patient to find not only what needs to be changed but also how to do so. Limitation in the intake of sugary beverages, reduction of television viewing, and increase in physical activity are the bases of behavioral modification. Most of the techniques of behavioral modification are based on the principles of classic behavioral conditioning techniques. The selection of the appropriate strategy should be based on the specific characteristics and needs of the patient. Table 5 depicts several strategies commonly used.

Of these strategies, monitoring has been considered as one of the most important techniques of behavior modification (89) because it appears to be crucial for long-term maintenance of weight loss. Patients or parents are encouraged to continually assess eating and exercise behaviors by keeping food and activity diaries.

Stimulus control is a technique used to create an environment with fewer opportunities to encourage a sedentary lifestyle or excessive caloric intake. Cognitive restructuring and goal specificity will provide the appropriate skills to counter unrealistic expectations and irrational attitudes regarding weight loss and body image. By increasing motivation, social support plays an important role in weight management. A family-based strategy is essential in the assessment and treatment of pediatric obesity.

Limitation of sedentary behaviors (television viewing, computer use, and video games) by positive reinforcement appears to be as effective as increasing physical activity (90). The reduction of sedentary behaviors in obese children results in lower intake of high-energy-density foods, increased energy expenditures, and indirectly promotes a more active lifestyle (90,91).

Exercise

Dietary treatment in childhood obesity should be combined with exercise to promote long-term weight loss. The metabolic response to caloric restriction is characterized by a reduction of the REE with subsequent decrease in caloric utilization (92,93). Exercise will improve health in general and will contribute to the maintenance of weight loss. By reducing visceral and total fat mass and increasing muscle mass, exercise enhances basal metabolic rate, which will contribute in maintaining a negative caloric balance (94).

In addition to weight control, physical activity has other health benefits including improvement of body composition and several obesity-related comorbidities such as dyslipidemia, i.e., reduction in low-density lipoprotein-cholesterol (LDL-C) and TG, increase in HDL-C, lower blood pressure, improvement in insulin sensitivity and endothelial function, and psychological well-being (95,96). Ferguson et al. (97) reported in a randomized crossover study, improvement of several components of the metabolic syndrome in a group of 70 children who underwent four months of intense exercise training. Improvements of plasma TG, insulin sensitivity, and reduction in total body fat occurred during the exercise-training period.

While programmed exercise typically includes aerobic sessions, lifestyle activity integrates exercise into daily routines and appears to be more successful, enjoyable, and sustainable. Increasing parents' physical activity should also be part of the intervention. Table 6 depicts some of the lifestyle activities that can be recommended as part of the behavior intervention.

The American Heart Association recommends that all children aged two and older should participate in at least 30 minutes of enjoyable, moderate-intensity activities every day. They should also perform at least 30 minutes of vigorous exercise at least three to four days each week to achieve and maintain a good level of cardiorespiratory fitness (98). The use of

Table 5 Common Strategies Used in Behavior Modification

Contingent reinforcement/incentives
Stimulus control
Parental monitoring/self-monitoring
Goal specificity
Planning ahead
Parental modeling
Problem solving
Cognitive restructuring
Social support
Stress management

Table 6 Practical Recommendations to Implement an Active Lifestyle

Promote reducing the time spent in sedentary behaviors such as television watching, video games, telephone, and computer use
Promote daily moderate to vigorous physical activity as part of the child's family's lifestyle by:
- Using active transportation (walking and biking)
- Walking to school if possible
- Avoid using elevators
- Planning summer day camps
- Increasing outdoor activities
- Participating in after-school programs of physical education

Note: Any exercise plan should be enjoyable, sustainable, and age appropriate.

pedometers, in combination with recordkeeping, may be an effective way of implementing an active lifestyle (99).

However, exercise should be prescribed on an individual basis with an exercise program based upon the initial fitness level (100). A slow progression of the intensity, frequency, and duration is required to achieve the goal of weight control. For instance, obese children may achieve maximal energy expenditure during a brisk walk, because prescriptions for more demanding physical activities like jogging are likely to be impossible at the start. Resistance training may also be a suitable component of a structured obesity-treatment program. One study found that weight loss was maintained for up to one year in obese preadolescents after completing a 10-week program that included resistance training combined with a low-calorie diet, behavior modification, and aerobic and flexibility exercises. Furthermore, compliance with the exercise regimen was 100% (101).

The amount and the density of physical activity have a direct influence on the energy expenditures. However, energy cost for most activities is generally greater for heavier people. There is also some evidence that increased activity in the obese individual may decrease appetite while increasing metabolic rate. Both obese and lean individuals experience a 19% to 30% decrease in resting metabolic rate within 24 to 48 hours following caloric restriction (31,102). Thus, caloric restriction without an increase in physical activity may not result in continued weight loss. Regular aerobic exercise combined with energy restriction will result in greater reductions in body weight than dieting alone. It should be kept in mind that energy expenditures are also significant through nonpurposeful exercise through daily activities (103).

Intermittent exercise and use of home exercise equipment are effective in inducing and maintaining weight loss in adults (104). Individuals who used the equipment longer were those who lost more weight and sustained their weight loss for longer periods of time. The type of exercise is also important: Long bouts of exercise of greater intensity were more beneficial. The benefits transcend those of body weight. The relationship between cardiorespiratory fitness and mortality in normal-weight, overweight, and obese men was clear (105). Fitness is an independent predictor of health, comparable to diabetes mellitus, cholesterol levels, hypertension, and smoking. However, the use of home devices to increase energy expenditures in children has not been scientifically evaluated.

Major benefits may be attained by simply engaging in leisure-time physical activity. This is often not achieved, because most persons trying to lose weight are not accomplishing the recommended combination of reducing calorie intake and engaging in leisure-time physical activity (150 minutes/week) (106). If the two patients mentioned above are given dietary treatment added to their treatment regimen

a habit of walking 20 minutes/day, they would enhance their energy expenditure by 5.8 kcal/minute. In other words, they would increase their energy expenditures by 116 kcal/day. This will enhance the reductions in energy intake induced by the dietary restriction, therefore increasing weight loss and enhancing their health. The amount of energy necessary for various physical activities is shown in Table 7.

Energy expenditure is related to the size of the individual and should, therefore, be related to body weight. The usual dietary energy allowance for children 4 to 18 years varies between 34 and 82 kcal/kg/day. For competitive and long-endurance exercises in children, energy expenditure should be increased by 17.6 to 52.8 kcal/kg/day above usual.

Family Involvement

Supportive counseling and reinforcement can help set the goals for health professionals, patient, and parent. This may allow for long-lasting results and avoidance of failure and frustration. Refusal to adhere to a weight-reduction plan may be due to lack of family support, insufficient motivation, or other psychological stresses. For instance, it was demonstrated that children of married parents lose weight at higher rates than those of divorced parents (77). When a weight-reduction plan is recommended,

Table 7 Energy Expenditure in Occupational, Recreational, and Sports Activities (kcal/minute) for a 50 kg Individual

Activity	Calories expended per 50 kg (110 lb)
Basketball	6.9
Cycling	
Leisure	5.9
Racing	8.5
Computer typing	1.4
Dancing	
Ballroom	2.6
Vigorous	8.4
Eating (sitting)	1.2
Football	6.6
Gymnastics	3.3
Swimming	
Backstroke	8.5
Breaststroke	8.1
Crawl, fast	7.8
Crawl, slow	6.4
Tennis	5.5
Volleyball	2.5
Fishing	3.1
Gardening: mowing	5.6
Marching	7.1
Running: 8 min/mile	10.8
Sitting quietly	1.1
Skiing (hard snow): moderate speed	6.0
Walking (comfortable pace)	
Fields and hillsides	4.1
Grass track	4.1
Writing (sitting)	1.5

Source: From Ref. 87.

conflicts frequently arise between the patient and nondieting family members, regarding the degree of dietary restriction and who is permitted to eat different foods.

Dietary restriction should not be introduced in a punitive fashion. In some cases, the obese child and the entire family may benefit and adhere to a diet similar in composition, if not quantity. Participation of the entire family should help minimize the feelings of isolation of the overweight child. Family involvement is essential for the success of any obesity treatment plan. Children whose families are involved in their treatment protocol lose more weight and maintain it for more prolonged periods that those whose families are not participatory. Eating patterns, food choices, and other behavioral factors of importance in obesity are family characteristics.

Food management and physical exercise are essential components for the development of effective treatment. The area of greatest concern for psychologists is how to get children to alter food intake and activity behaviors. Because the primary focus is on changing the child's behavior, parenting skills represent an integral component of the intervention. Stimulus-control procedures for the behavioral control of overeating have led to the development of several behavioral techniques for the treatment of obesity. These include self-monitoring of body weight and/or food intake, goal setting, reward and punishment, aversion therapy, social reinforcement, and stimulus control. Several of these modifications have been found to be effective with children (18,19,78–80,107). The interventions assume that the obese child is an overeater who is hypersensitive to food stimuli and can be trained to behave like a nonobese person and subsequently lose weight. Moreover, positive family support improved the degree of immediate and long-term weight loss in children and adolescents (18,79,80).

Any program designed specifically for treating obese children must include a group format with individualized counseling, parent participation, frequent sessions over a long period of time, appropriate exercise, and changes in the home environment to reinforce changes in the child's lifestyle. The behavior modification sessions should include the family self-monitoring, goal setting and contracting, parenting skills training, skills for managing the high-risk situation, and skills for maintenance and relapse prevention (80).

THERAPEUTIC GOALS

Initial therapeutic goals to treat obesity should be determined taking into account age, BMI percentile, the pattern of weight progression, and the presence of comorbidities. Children and adolescents with a BMI greater than or equal to 95th percentile and those who are overweight (85th–95th percentile) who

present with significant comorbidities, should be treated. Obese children age two to six and those older than six years need a program implemented for weight maintenance or weight loss, respectively (108). Excessive caloric restriction is contraindicated in children as it may compromise growth and development. An overweight child should have a well-balanced diet with sufficient calories to promote growth, but with an intake restricted enough to produce weight loss. The normalization of the body weight and BMI, although a theoretical long-term goal, may not be a realistic expectation in many patients.

In obese adults, significant improvement in obesity-related metabolic, orthopedic, and cardiopulmonary comorbidities occurs after modest weight loss of 5% to 10% of body weight (109). However, the most important problem remains—the poor maintenance of treatment induced weight loss and relapse prevention in both adult and pediatric obese patients. An extended treatment intervention program based on a problem-solving model therapy appears to be effective in long-term management of obesity (110).

Yo-Yo Weight Cycling

A very important therapeutic goal is to avoid weight cycling; it has a profound effect on body composition and its metabolic efficiency (102). Weight loss followed by weight gain results in loss of muscle; increased fat; greater risk of heart disease; and frustration (111,112). Chronic dieters learn to cope with dieting. They develop a very efficient mechanism to maintain their weight with fewer and fewer calories, with each attempt to lose weight. There is loss of muscle mass and an increased fat mass. These body composition changes during weight cycling decrease metabolic expenditures and lead to an elevation of basal insulin and lipoprotein lipase levels (113), resulting in more fat deposition. In addition to changes in the body composition, the patient becomes psychologically frustrated because of failure to achieve the desired weight loss. The outcome is a patient who ingests very few calories and yet cannot lose weight.

Chronic dieters may also increase their risk for heart disease more than if excess weight remained at a stable level. Dieting leads to fat mobilization and during the regaining phase there is increased abdominal adiposity. The regained weight is more likely to be distributed into the upper body, where it is potentially more harmful (114) and associated with a higher incidence of heart disease and glucose intolerance (115). Appropriate strategies to avoid weight cycling should be considered at the beginning of a child's weight-reduction program; those who are not fully committed or motivated should not start. When a child is ready to participate in a weight reduction program, it should represent a serious commitment of all involved.

Fat and Sugar Substitutes

Bulking agents and nonprescription diet aids, such as methylcellulose and other noncaloric bulk materials, have been used in experimental and clinical attempts to inhibit food intake. The rationale for the use of such agents is that they swell in the stomach and supposedly give a feeling of satiety. Indeed, several lines of evidence suggest that dietary fiber may play a key role in the regulation of circulating insulin levels. Dietary fiber reduces insulin secretion by slowing the rate of nutrient absorption following a meal (56,116). In the experimental setting, insulin sensitivity increases (57) and body weight decreases (58) in animals fed high-fiber diets. In addition, fiber consumption predicted insulin levels, weight gain, and other cardiovascular heart disease (CVD) risk factors more strongly than total or saturated fat consumption. Therefore, high-fiber diets (10–15 g/day) may protect against obesity and CVD by lowering insulin levels (59).

There are many misconceptions about the benefit of the use of nonnutritive sugar substitutes and the consumption of foods containing nonnutritive sweeteners. Currently, nonnutritive sweeteners approved for use in the United States include saccharin, aspartame, acesulfame K, and sucralose. Other sweeteners include sorbitol, mannitol, and xylitol. Many obese individuals consume foods containing these sweeteners, thinking they are reducing their caloric intake. However, many of these foods contain either the same amount of or more calories than their regular sweetened counterparts. For example, dietetic chocolate contains 168 calories per 2 oz serving. Regular sweetened chocolate contains only 150 calories for a similar-sized serving (117). Therefore, without proper advice from a dietician, many obese individuals may be over consuming calories by including dietetic foods in their diets. These foods also tend to be more expensive.

INTENSIVE THERAPIES

Very low-calorie diets (VLCD), pharmacotherapy, and bariatric surgery have been recommended for morbidly obese adults; however, they are still considered as experimental approaches for treating obese children. Although there are no clear guidelines to define what pediatric population should be offered these interventions, emerging data suggests that intensive therapy may be beneficial for severely obese adolescents or severe obesity-related comorbidities. Long-term clinical trials are warranted to assess the risks and benefits of intensive therapies on growth, puberty, and psychological development in children and adolescents.

Very Low-Calorie Diets

The national task force on the prevention and treatment of obesity published a report on the efficacy of VLCD on weight reduction in adults (118). Although rapid weight loss could be achieved, the long-term evolution of obese patients on these diets was disappointing. Slowly but surely they regained their weight and within one to five years they were of the same weight as before the treatment, regardless of the diet given.

There are few studies documenting the success of structured programs for treating childhood obesity that encompass the use of VLCD. LC diets are usually high in protein and fat. They involve intake of large amounts of meat and restrict carbohydrate-containing foods such as fruits, vegetables, and grain products. The high intake of fat in such diets can increase the risk of coronary heart disease and other problems such as gallstones and high cholesterol. The body depends heavily on its fat stores for energy, while on a LC diet. This can lead to ketosis. The rapid weight loss on these diets is composed of 60% to 70% water and the dieters often regain weight rapidly, once normal eating is resumed (119,120). Very low-calorie restriction using a protein-sparing, modified fast (PSMF) diets (400–800 kcal/day) is designed to produce rapid weight loss of up to 2.3 kg/week (5 lb), while preserving vital lean body mass. The protein is provided as lean meat or fish, or in a milk or egg-based liquid formula. It has been suggested that these diets spare body protein by decreasing insulin levels and enhancing fat breakdown (121), while inhibiting the release of amino acids from muscle (122). However, in the past, several deaths have been associated with the use of these formulas (35). Moreover, these quick-fix weight-loss schemes may be unsafe for use in children and do not promote healthy eating behavior for long-lasting weight control.

Nutritionally balanced VLCD, combined with exercise, may improve the outcomes in structured obesity treatment programs for children (81,123). Obese individuals who entered a structured 10-week program that included exercise and behavior modification, along with a VLCD showed good response. After 10 weeks, BMI decreased from 33.8 to 29.6. Fat mass was reduced without decrements in both lean body mass or energy expenditure (29). These results suggest that a multidisciplinary structured program for treating severely obese children that is maintained for long periods of time may yield positive results. However, the metabolic adaptations during energy restriction and the implications to the different diets that may affect the fuel regulatory system (121) need be kept in mind, particularly in growing children.

Pharmacological Treatment

The administration of weight-loss medications in children and adolescents must be conducted under medical supervision and as part of a clinical trial. Only antiobesity medications that are proven safe and effective in this age group should be prescribed. Pharmacological treatment should never replace diet and lifestyle changes and it should be implemented only as a supplement to standard treatment. Behavioral and pharmacological treatments appear to be additive in adult studies. Thus, the amount of weight loss depends on the intensity of behavioral approach.

Pharmacological treatment of obesity is still controversial. Long-term use of medications to suppress appetite or antiobesity pills is not indicated for the treatment of pediatric obesity unless dealing with a morbidly obese adolescent (124). Studies involving the use of anorectic drugs alone or in combination with behavior therapy have demonstrated that weight loss is no greater than when behavior therapy was used alone. When the drugs were stopped, the weight was regained more rapidly. However, the combination of medication and group lifestyle modification resulted in more weight loss than either medication or lifestyle modification alone (125). Furthermore, the effectiveness of appetite-suppressant drugs (i.e., amphetamines) appears to decrease with time and there may be side effects. The addictive potential of amphetamines and the risk of depression associated with fenfluramine have resulted in the minimal use of these agents in children and adolescents. The use of serotonin agonists such as fluoxetine and fenfluramine in the short term may be useful as an adjunct in weight-loss programs for children and adolescents (124,126). These drugs seem to decrease appetite and carbohydrate craving. Although they are by no means the solution to weight loss, they may help individuals at the beginning of a weight loss program by suppressing appetite. They must be used with caution and for a very limited time (127). In fact, serious side effects such as pulmonary hypertension and valvular heart lesions have been associated with the use of fenfluramine and its derivative, dexfenfluramine, in combination with another appetite suppressant (i.e., phentermine) (128). Recently rimonabant, a selective cannabinoid 1-receptor blocker, was shown to reduce body weight and waist circumference and improved the profile of several metabolic risk factors in obese adults (129).

Another potential antiobesity medication is metformin, an antihyperglycemic drug, which has been reported to enhance insulin sensitivity leading to reduced appetite and body weight in obese children and adults (130). Fremark et al. recently demonstrated that a six-month trial of metformin treatment (500 mg twice daily) in a group of obese adolescents caused significant reductions in BMI, fasting glucose, and insulin compared to a placebo group. In a two-month study, Metformin (850 mg twice daily) in a group of adolescents on a hypocaloric diet caused significant reductions in weight, fasting insulin, leptin, and lipids compared to a placebo group (131). The use of diazoxide, an inhibitor of glucose-mediated insulin secretion, in a group of hyperinsulinemic obese adults was effective in short-term weight reduction with few adverse effects (132). Daily subcutaneous administration of octreotide (somatostatin analogue), an inhibitor of pancreatic insulin secretion, to a group of children and adolescents with hypothalamic obesity secondary to cancer therapy likewise resulted in significant reduction in body weight over a six-month period (133). The results of these studies imply that attenuation of hyperinsulinemia of obesity may be of therapeutic benefit in the management of this disorder. However, long-term efficacy and safety of these agents have yet to be evaluated in children.

The administration of exogenous leptin has been shown to result in loss of body fat in animals with elevated leptin levels (134), as well as in humans with leptin deficiency, by reducing food intake (Vol. 1; Chap. 1). However, in the ordinary obese patient, Heymsfield et al. demonstrated that a six-month administration of subcutaneous recombinant leptin in high dosages induced mild weight loss in some obese adults with elevated endogenous leptin concentrations if maintained on a diet and exercise regimen (135). Additional research into the potential role for leptin and other related hormones for the treatment of human obesity is needed, though these do not appear to provide the magic bullet for most obese patients.

At the present time, orlistat and sibutramine are the only antiobesity drugs approved by the FDA for long-term use in adults. Orlistat has also been approved by the FDA for the treatment of obesity in children older than 12 years and sibutramine for use in adolescents over 16 years of age (136). Orlistat, an inhibitor of gastrointestinal lipases, blocks the absorption of up to one-third of fat intake. It has no systemic activity. Most of its side effects are related to fat malabsorption. Abdominal pain, flatulence, diarrhea, steatorrhea, increased defecation, and fecal urgency and incontinence are the most common side effects. These side effects can be ameliorated by reducing the intake of fat. Supplementation with vitamins A, D, E, and K is recommended as the long-term use of orlistat may compromise the absorption fat-soluble vitamins. The recommended dose is 120 mg three times a day with meals. The use of inhibitors of digestive enzymes, such as intestinal lipase, in obese and diabetic adult patients has been shown to be beneficial for weight reduction and improved glycemic control (137,138).

The study by McDuffie et al. (139), determined the safety and efficacy of orlistat plus behavior intervention among overweight African-American and Caucasian adolescents. Patients received six months of treatment with orlistat (120 mg three times daily) as well as a six-month comprehensive behavior intervention. The study participants showed decrease in weight, BMI, total cholesterol, LDL-C, fasting insulin, and fasting glucose. The mean weight loss over six months was 3.75 kg. A multicenter 54-week randomized, double-blind study (140) in 539 obese adolescents of age 12 to 16 years compared the effect of orlistat versus placebo The orlistat group showed a 0.55 units decrease in BMI, while the placebo group experienced an increment of 0.31 units. Up to 50% of patients taking orlistat experienced mild to moderate GI side effects compared with 13% in the placebo group. No significant differences between both groups with respect to lipids, glucose, and insulin were reported.

Sibutramine, an anorectic agent that inhibits neuronal reuptake of serotonin, norepinephrine, and dopamine (141) has also been used in overweight adolescents. Its main side effects are mild hypertension and tachycardia (which improved with weight loss), insomnia, anxiety, headaches, and depression. The medication is contraindicated in hypertension, cardiovascular disease, or in combination with monoamin oxidase inhibitors, selective serotonin reuptake inhibitors, erythromycin, and ketoconazole. The safety and efficacy of sibutramine have not been established in pediatric patients under the age of 16 years. Although several studies in adults have shown modest weight reduction (2–10 kg) (125,142) only a few trials have been conducted in children (142,143). In a six-month randomized, double-blind placebo-control-study (143) in 82 obese adolescents aged 13 to 17 years, there was a 7.8 kg weight loss in the sibutramine group compared with 3.2 kg in the placebo group six months after discontinuation of the drug. Forty-four percent of sibutramine patients developed tachycardia and mild hypertension. The starting dose of sibutramine was 5 mg/day. Patients were titrated to 10 mg/day at week 3 and 15 mg/day at week 7. Another recent six-month placebo-control study (23) in 60 obese adolescents aged 14 to 17 years showed a decrease of 3.56 BMI units compared with 0.9 units in the placebo group. No differences in blood pressure or heart rate were reported.

In summary, weight loss associated with both orlistat and sibutramine are additive to behavior modification and lifestyle changes. True benefit versus conventional therapy remains to be determined in additional large long-term placebo-controlled trials.

Bariatric Surgery

Bariatric surgery is a therapeutic option in patients with extreme obesity and significant comorbidities. A systematic review and meta-analysis of bariatric surgery in adults concluded that it is an effective weight loss method for morbidly obese adults resulting in improvement of significant comorbidities (144). Despite the phenomenal growth in the use of this procedure, research on this intervention continues to be reported primarily as case series, and substantial gaps in bariatric surgery research need be filled (145). The procedure use, type, recurrences, readmissions rates, and mortality—all need to be fully studied (146).

Four types of surgical procedures have been used to change eating behavior: Jejunoileal and gastric bypass, gastric plication, and jaw wiring. The jejunoileal bypass procedures are usually followed by a large weight loss. However, significant complications

including diarrhea, vitamin D deficiency with osteomalacia, vitamin B12 and folate deficiencies, renal (oxalate) calculi, hyperuricemia, and liver disease follow these procedures (147). A second procedure is the gastric bypass, which appears to be effective in producing weight loss without serious late complications seen with the jejunoileal procedure (148). Gastric plication (gastroplasty), involving a stapling procedure, is also widely used. Following the gastric bypass or gastroplasty procedure, patient's food intake is decreased by the sensation of fullness. They also show less anxiety, depression, irritability, and preoccupation with food during weight loss compared with their weight-reduction attempts before the surgical procedure (149). In controlled studies, gastric bypass appears slightly more effective than gastroplasty. Although successful initially in almost all patients, the failure rate for both procedures is high (up to 50%) (150). The laparoscopic adjustable gastric banding in the treatment of obesity in adults appears to be more benign in terms of morbidity and mortality rates. It is as effective, at least for four years, as other procedures (151).

Clinical data show significant long-lasting weight loss in severely overweight adults in addition to improvement of other comorbidities including dyslipidemia, Type 2 diabetes mellitus, obstructive sleep apnea (OSA), and better psychological status. The few studies done in children (152,153) show results very close to the ones reported in adults.

Guidelines for bariatric surgery in obese adolescents were proposed by an expert panel on child and adolescent obesity in July 2004 shown in Table 8 (154).

The two current procedures done in adolescents are the roux-en-y gastric bypass and the adjustable gastric banding. At the present time, this last procedure does not have FDA approval for patients less than 18 years of age. Complications of bariatric surgery include: macro and micronutrient malabsorption, iron-deficiency anemia, variable degree of diarrhea, gastrointestinal leakage, stomach and small bowel obstruction, dumping syndrome, cholecystitis, pulmonary emboli and bleeding, atelectasis, and

Table 8 Guidelines and Recommendations for Bariatric Surgery in Adolescents

Have failed greater than or equal to six months of organized attempts at weight management, as determined by their primary care provider
Have attained or nearly attained physiologic maturity
Be very severely obese (BMI≥40) with serious obesity-related comorbidities or have a BMI of greater than or equal to 50 with less severe comorbidities
Demonstrate commitment to comprehensive medical and psychological evaluations both before and after surgery
Agree to avoid pregnancy for at least one year postoperatively
Be capable of and willing to adhere to nutritional guidelines postoperatively
Provide informed assent to surgical treatment
Demonstrate decisional capacity
Have a supportive family environment

Source: From Ref. 154.

pneumonia. Weight regain has been reported in up to 15% of patients. A meta-analysis of bariatric surgery in adults has reported an operative mortality of 1.1% (144). The laparoscopic technique has less mortality and complications compared to the open laparotomy surgery.

A report on bariatric surgery in 13 obese adolescents by Inge at al (155), showed significant weight loss by 12 months postoperatively with a reduction in BMI from 59 to 38 kg/m² (143–103 kg) and in body fat content from 47% to 36% by three months. A review on a 20-year data base on bariatric surgery in 33 adolescent's aged 12 to 18 years revealed a significant weight loss and improvement of most of the obesity-associated comorbidities one year after the surgery (153). Several complications were reported in this study, including pulmonary embolism, wound infection, stomal stenoses, marginal ulcers, small bowel obstruction, incisional hernias, and micronutrient deficiencies. Five patients regained most of the lost weight from 5 to 10 years postoperatively.

In summary, although short-term results of bariatric surgery in adolescents appear to be positive, there is a need for further research to determine the long-term effects of this procedure in this population. Surgical procedures of this type in this specific population need to be done as part of clinical trials lead by a multidisciplinary team including surgeons with expertise and experience. The development of other less-aggressive techniques is being actively investigated in adults, such as an implantable pacemaker that may signal the brain that the stomach is full. However, in all instances bariatric surgery should always be part of an obesity treatment program with dietary, physical activity, and behavior modification.

Treatment of Comorbidities

Obesity is one of the most common chronic disorders in childhood and there is increasing awareness of the long-term health complications of this disease. Yet many pediatricians do not offer treatment to obese children in the absence of comorbid conditions (156). Additionally, health insurance organizations are unlikely to reimburse for treatment of obesity, unless medical comorbidities are documented. However, the most widely spread consequences of childhood obesity may be psychological, social, including lower perceived competences and self-worth (157,158). Obese children and adolescents have impaired lower health-related quality of life than lean counterparts, and their quality of life may be as bad as that of newly diagnosed cancer patients (158). Most often, either obesity-related comorbidities or psychiatric conditions are readily apparent or are responsible for the differences in health-related quality of life. Thus even in the absence of comorbid disease, obese children need to have targeted interventions to improve their health-related quality of life, before, during, and after other medical interventions.

Obesity often presents multiple medical comorbidities, which are reviewed in Vol. 1; Chap. 1. These need to be addressed and treated accordingly. Often the therapy is primarily directed to improve the excess weight and physical fitness of the patient through lifestyle and behavior modification. These treatment interventions may reduce the risk of developing complications such as diabetes mellitus (159). The amount of weight loss and improved fitness need not be marked to improve obesity-related comorbidities (108). The specific treatment modalities of the frequent comorbid conditions of obesity are reviewed in other chapters of the book, including diabetes (Vol. 1; Chaps. 5 and 8), insulin resistance/dysmetabolic syndrome (Vol. 1; Chap. 11), hyperlipidemia (Vol. 1; Chap. 14), hypertension (Vol. 1; Chap. 13), and polycystic ovary disease (Vol. 2; Chap. 13). Orthopedic complications, including slipped capital femoral epiphysis, and Legg-Perthes disease need to be kept in mind (160,161).

Sleep apnea, brief periods of breathing cessation or hypopnea, and marked reduction in tidal volume, are common during sleep in obese patients (162). The prevalence of OSA in children has been estimated to be between 1% and 3% in preschool and school age children (163). The occurrence is higher in obese subjects and is related to the size of the region enclosed by the mandible, sites of fat deposits around the pharynx as well as the subject's body weight (164,165). The clinical presentation of OSA may include simple snoring and daytime sleepiness and narcolepsy. The severity of these symptoms is what usually determines decisions about diagnostic testing and management (166). Only a small proportion of cases are accurately assessed and/or diagnosed; this is due to insufficient awareness of the sleep disturbances among physicians and families, though the risk of this comorbidity is enormous (167–170). The gold standard diagnostic test, polysomnography, requires considerable expertise and is labor intensive and time consuming, particularly in children. A positive clinical assessment of OSA may be associated with negative polysomnography and may improve with tonsillectomy and adenoidectomy (171). Once OSA is diagnosed, continuous positive airway pressure treatment may be required, though there other methods that may be used if this treatment is not tolerated, i.e., mandibular-advancement appliance and uvulopalatopharyngoplasty (172). However, weight loss should be pursued; if this is accomplished the need for these therapies may cease.

CONCLUSION AND FINAL CONSIDERATIONS

Obesity and the multiple comorbidities associated with this disease have reached epidemic proportions among children and adolescents. The development of obesity depends on a variety of genetic, environmental, and sociocultural factors. The elucidation of the role of leptin and multiple other hypothalamic mechanisms involved in the regulation of food intake and energy expenditure constitutes important discoveries that may affect the treatment of obesity in the future. The pathophysiological role of hyperinsulinimia and its role in the development of the long-term complications associated with the disease may also have an impact in the early intervention of obese children. Early recognition of excessive weight gain in relation to linear growth is important and should be closely monitored by pediatricians and health care providers. The use of BMI percentiles may also help to identify children at risk and quantify the severity of obesity. Prevention is critical, because effective treatment of this disease is limited. Food management and increased physical activity must be encouraged, promoted, and prioritized to protect children. Dietary practices must foster moderation and variety, with a goal of setting the appropriate eating habits for life. Advocacy is also needed to elicit insurance coverage for the treatment of the disease.

A multidisciplinary approach to pediatric obesity should include diet, exercise, and behavior therapy. The modification of population lifestyle conditions that support an obesogenic environment is crucial in order to ameliorate the epidemic of pediatric obesity. The advocacy of healthy eating habits and active lifestyle by primary care providers is essential in the prevention and treatment of pediatric overweight. Intensive therapies such as VLCD, pharmacotherapy or bariatric surgery are an option in selected patients but only after documented failure of structured interventions. Long-term placebo control studies to assess the risk and benefits of intensive therapies in children and adolescents are still unavailable.

However, there is ample evidence that diet and lifestyle play important roles in the development of obesity, though the understanding of the inter-relationship regarding health outcomes continues to evolve. Lifestyle factors and dietary intake may be amenable to modification as shown by the decrease of cigarette smoking and the reduction of high fat dietary intake over the past decades. The effectiveness of the interventions to prevent and to treat obesity vary, but it is clear that those who practice one or more healthy behaviors such as increased physical activity may make healthier choices in other healthier behaviors. Walking may improve health outcomes beyond weight control, it may also reduce the risk of dementia and improve cognitive skills in later life (173). Additionally, the concept of the "healthy" obesity in a physically fit individual who exercises regularly and eats a healthful diet needs to be kept in mind. Obese individuals may enjoy psychosocial quality of life (174) and may enjoy health with morbidity and mortality rates similar to the nonobese individual (175).

The reader is also referred to the strategic plan for the National Institute of Health Obesity Research and the science-based solutions to obesity that need be considered (176), including the role of academia, government, and industry (177). Many consumers desire alternative treatment programs (178). Of interest and worthy of consideration may be the Internet behavioral and weight loss-related programs that are now readily available. These need to be appropriately tested and their effectiveness and efficacy proven, though there are reports that adding e-mail counseling to a basic Internet weight-loss intervention results in significant benefits (179). As we move into the 21st century, with increased availability of Internet facilities and with more expertise in handling such resources by children, there may be a role for web-based treatment programs.

ACKNOWLEDGMENTS

This work was supported in part by Pediatric Sunshine Academics, Inc. and NIH grant 2R-44–HD0381080 04.

REFERENCES

1. Lifshitz F, Tarim O, Smith MM. Nutrition in adolescents—review. Endocrinol Metab Clin North Am 1993; 22:673–683.
2. Field AE, Austin SB, Taylor CB, et al. Relation between dieting and weight change among preadolescents and adolescents. Pediatrics 2003; 112:900–906.
3. Nead KG, Halterman JS, Kaczorowski JM, Auinger P, Weitzman M. Overweight children and adolescents: risk group for iron deficiency. Pediatrics 2004; 114:104–105.
4. Lowe MR, Caputo GC. Binge eating in obesity. Toward the specification of predictors. Int J Eating Disord 1991; 10:49–55.
5. Barlow SE, Dietz WH, Klish WJ, Trowbridge FL. Medical evaluation of overweight children and adolescents: reports from pediatricians, pediatric nurse practitioners, and registered dieticians. Pediatrics 2002; 110:222–228.
6. Miller LA, Grunwald GK, Johnson SL, Krebs NF. Disease severity at time of referral for pediatric failure to thrive and obesity: time for a paradigm shift? J Pediatr 2002; 141:121–124.
7. QuattrinT, Liu E, Shaw N, Shine B, Chiang E. Obese children who are referred to the pediatric endocrinologist: characteristics and outcome. Pediatrics 2005; 115:348–351.
8. Epstein LH, Valoski AM, Kalarchian MA, McCurley J. Do children lose and maintain weight easier than adults: a comparison of child and parent weight changes from six months to ten years. Obes Res 1995; 3:411–417.
9. Krebs NF, Jacobson MS. American Academy of Pediatrics Committee on Nutrition. Prevention of pediatric overweight and obesity. Pediatrics 2003; 112:424–430.
10. Bhargava SK, Sachdev HS, Fall CH, et al. Relation of serial changes in childhood body-mass index to impaired glucose tolerance in young adulthood. N Engl J Med 2004; 350:856–975.
11. Garn SM, Sullivan TV, Hawthorne VM. Fatness and obesity of parents of obese individuals. Am J Clin Nutr 1989; 50:1308–1313.
12. Hediger ML, Overpeck MD, Kuczmarski RJ, Ruan WJ. Association between infant breastfeeding and overweight in young children. JAMA 2001; 285:2453–2460.
13. Owen CG, Martin RM, Whincup PH, Davey-Smith G, Gillman MW, Cook DG. The effect of breastfeeding on

mean body mass index throughout life: a quantitative review of published and unpublished observational evidence. Am J Clin Nutr 2005; 82:1298–1307.

14. Gray GA. Contemporary Diagnosis and Management of Obesity. In: Handbooks in Healthcare. Pennsylvania: Newton, 1998:120.

15. Robinson TN. Reducing children's television viewing to prevent obesity: a randomized controlled trial. JAMA 1999; 282:1561–1567.

16. Speiser PW, Rudolf MC, Anhalt H, et al. Childhood obesity. J Clin Endo Metab 2005; 90:1871–1887.

17. Ludwig DS, Peterson KE, Gortmaker S. Relation between consumption of sugar-sweetened drinks and childhood obesity: a prospective, observational analysis. Lancet 2001; 357:505–508.

18. Epstein LH, Valoski A, Wing RR, McCurley J. Ten-year follow-up of behavioral family-based treatment for obese children. JAMA 1990; 264:2519–2523.

19. Epstein LH, Valoski AM, Wing RR, McCurley J. Ten year outcomes of behavioral family-based treatment for child hood obesity. Health Psychol 1994; 13:373–383.

20. Nuutinen O, Knip M. Long-term weight control in obese children: persistence of treatment outcome and metabolic changes. Int J Obes 1992; 16:279–287.

21. Troiano RP, Flegal KM. Overweight children and adolescents: description, epidemiology and demographics. Pediatrics 1998; 101:497–504.

22. Sigal RJ, El-Hashimy M, Martin BC, Soeldner JS, Krolewski AS, Warram JH. Acute postchallenge hyperinsulinemia predicts weight gain: a prospective study. Diabetes 1997; 46:1025–1029.

23. Godoy-Matos A, Carraro L, Vieira A, et al. Treatment of obese adolescents with sibutramine: a randomized, double-blind, controlled study. J Clin Endocrinol Metab 2005; 90: 1460–1465.

24. Committee on Practice and Ambulatory Medicine. American Academy of Pediatrics Policy Statement. Recommendations for Preventive Health Care. Pediatrics 2000; 105:645–646.

25. Gans KM, Ross E, Barner CW, Wylie-Rosett J, McMurray J, Eaton C. REAP and WAVE: new tools to rapidly assess/discuss nutrition with patients. J Nutr 2003; 132:556S–562S.

26. Black O, James WPT, Besser CM. A report of the Royal College of Physicians. J R Coll Physicians Long 1983; 17:5–65.

27. Orlet Fisher J, Rolls BJ, Birch LL. Children's bite size and intake of an entree are greater with large portions than with age-appropriate or self-selected portions. Am J Clin Nutr 2003; 77:1164–1170.

28. Sclafani A, Springer D. Dietary obesity in adult rats: similarities in hypothalamic and human obesity syndromes. Physiol Behav 1976; 17:461–471.

29. Golay A, Allaz AF, Ybarra J, et al. Similar weight loss with low-energy food combining or balanced diets. Int J Obes Relat Metab Disord 2000; 24:492–496.

30. Schoeller DA. How accurate is self-reported dietary energy intake? Nutr Rev 1990; 48:373–379.

31. Leibel RL, Rosenbaum M, Hirsch J. Changes in energy expenditure resulting from altered body weight. N Engl J Med 1995; 332:621–628.

32. Mertz W, Tsui JC, Judd JT, Reiser S, et al. What are people really eating? The relation between energy intake derived from estimated diet records and intake determined to maintain body weight. Am J Clin Nutr 1991; 54:291–295.

33. Bandini LG, Schoeller DA, Cyr HN, Dietz WH. Validity of reported energy intake in obese and nonobese adolescents. Am J Clin Nutr 1990; 52:421–425.

34. Lichtman SW, Pisarska K, Berman ER, et al. Discrepancy between self-reported and actual caloric intake and exercise in obese subjects. N Engl J Med 1992; 327:1893–1898.

35. Flatt JP, Ravussin E, Acheson KJ, Jequier E. Effects of dietary fat on postprandial substrate oxidation and on carbohydrate and fat balances. J Clin Invest 1985; 76:1019–1024.

36. Schutz Y, Flatt JP, Jequier E. Failure of dietary fat intake to promote fat oxidation: a factor favoring the development of obesity. Am J Clin Nutr 1989; 50:307–314.

37. Golay A, Bobbioni E. The role of dietary fat in obesity. Int J Obes Relat Metab Disord 1997; 21:S2–S11.

38. Rolls BJ, Shide DJ. The influence of dietary fat on food intake and body weight. Nutr Rev 1992; 50:283–290.

39. Krauss RM, Deckelbaum RJ, et al. Dietary guidelines for healthy American adults. A statement for health professionals from the nutrition committee, American Heart Association. Circulation 1996; 94:1795–1800.

40. American Diabetes Association. Nutrition recommendations and principles for people with diabetes mellitus. Diabetes Care 2000; 23(S1):S43–S46.

41. Katan MB, Grundy SM, Willett WC. Should a low-fat, high-carbohydrate diet be recommended for everyone? Beyond low-fat diets. N Engl J Med 1997; 337:563–566.

42. Larson DE, Hunter GR, Williams MJ, Kekes-Szabo T, Nyikos I, Goran MI. Dietary fat in relation to body fat and intraabdominal adipose tissue: a cross-sectional analysis. Am J Clin Nutr 1996; 64:687–684.

43. Allred JB. Too much of a good thing? An overemphasis on eating low-fat foods may be contributing to the alarming increase in overweight among US adults. J Am Diet Assoc 1995; 95:417–418.

44. Nicklas TA. Dietary studies of children: The Bogalusa Heart Study experience. J Am Diet Assoc 1995; 95:1127–1133.

45. Kant AK, Graubard BI, Schatzkin A, Ballard-Barbash R. Proportions of energy intake from fat and subsequent weight change in the NHANES 1 epidemiologic follow-up study. Am J Clin Nutr 1995; 61:11–17.

46. Lissner L, Heitman BL. Dietary fat and obesity: evidence from epidemiology. Eur J Clin Nutr 1995; 49:79–90.

47. Lenfant C, Ernst N. Daily dietary fat and total energy hyperinsulinemia of obesity. N Engl J Med 1971; 285: 827–831.

48. Stephen AM, Wald NJ. Trends in individual consumption of dietary fat in the United States, 1920–1984. Am J Clin Nutr 1990; 52:457–469.

49. Foster GD, Wyatt HR, Hill JO, et al. A randomized trial of low-carbohydrate diet for obesity. N Engl J Med 2003; 348:2082–2090.

50. Dansinger ML, Gleason JA, Griffith JL, Selker HP, Schaefer EJ. Comparison of the atkins, ornish, weight watchers, and zone diets for weight loss and heart disease risk reduction: a randomized trial. JAMA 2005; 293:43–53.

51. Ebbeling C. Dietary approaches for obesity treatment and prevention in children and adolescents. In: Handbook of Pediatric Obesity: Epidemiology Etiology and Prevention.

52. Committee on Nutrition. American Academy of Pediatrics. Obesity in children. In: Pediatric Nutrition. Elk Grove, Il: American Academy of Pediatrics, 1998:423–458.

53. US Department of Health and Human Services, Public Health Service. The Surgeon General's Report on Nutrition and Health. Washington, DC: DHHS (PHS), 1998.

54. Summerbell CD, Ashton V, Campbell KJ, Edmunds L, Kelly S, Waters E. Interventions for treating obesity in children. Cochrane Database Syst Rev 2003; 3:CD001872.

55. Wolever TM, Jenkins DJ, Jenkins AL, Josse RG. The glycemic index: methodology and clinical implications. Am J Clin Nutr 1991; 54:846–854.

56. Bjorck I, Granfeldt Y, Liljeberg H, Tovar J, Asp NG. Food properties affecting the digestion and absorption of carbohydrates. Am J Clin Nutr 1994; 59:699S–705S.

57. Granfeldt Y, Hagander B, Bjorck I. Metabolic responses to starch in oat and wheat products. On the importance of food structure, incomplete gelatinization or presence of viscous dietary fiber. Eur J Clin Nutr 1995; 49:189–199.

58. Welch IM, Bruce C, Hill SE, Read NW. Duodenal and ileal lipid suppresses postprandial blood glucose and insulin responses in man: possible implications for dietary management of diabetes mellitus. Clin Sci 1987; 72:209–216.

59. Trout DL, Behall KM, Osilesi O. Prediction of glycemic index for starchy foods. Am J Clin Nutr 1993; 58:873–878.

60. Foster-Powell K, Miller JB. International tables of glycemic index. Am J Clin Nutr 1995; 62:871S–890S.

61. Stephen AM, Sieber GM, Gerster YA, Morgan DR. Intake of carbohydrate and its components—international comparisons, trends overtime, and effects of changing to low-fat diets. Am J Clin Nutr 1995; 62:851S–867S.

62. Nicklas TA, Webber LS, Koschak ML, Berenson GS. Nutrient adequacy of low fat intakes for children: the Bogalusa Heart Study. Pediatrics 1992; 89:221–228.

63. Popkin BM, Haines PS, Patterson RE. Dietary changes in older Americans 1977–1987. Am J Clin Nutr 1992; 55: 823–830.

64. Salmeron J, Manson JE, Stampfer MJ, Colditz GA, Wing AL, Willett WC. Dietary fiber, glycemic load, and risk of non–insulin-dependent diabetes mellitus in women. JAMA 1997; 277:472–477.

65. Ludwig DS. The glycemic index. JAMA 2002; 287:2414–2423.

66. Ebbeling CB, Ludwig DS. Dietary approaches for obesity treatment and prevention in children and adolescents. In Doran MI, Sothern MS, eds. Handbook of Pediatric Obesity: Etiology, Pathophysiology, and Prevention. CRC Press, 2006:311–312.

67. Ludwig DS, Majzoub JA, Al-Zahrani A, Dallal GE, Blanco I, Roberts SB. High glycemic index foods, overeating, and obesity. Pediatrics 1999; 103:E26.

68. Ebbeling CB, Leidig MM, Sinclair KB, Hangen JP, Ludwig DS. A reduced-glycemic load diet in the treatment of adolescent obesity. Arch Pediatr Adolesc Med 2003; 157: 773–779.

69. Sondike SB, Copperman N, Jacobson MS. Effects of a low-carbohydrate diet on weight loss and cardiovascular risk factor in overweight adolescents. J Pediatr 2003; 142: 253–258.

70. Spieth LE, Harnish JD, Lenders CM, et al. A low-glycemic index diet in the treatment of pediatric obesity. Arch Pediatr Adolesc Med 2000; 154:947–951.

71. Samaha FF, Iqbal N, Seshadri P, et al. A low-carbohydrate as compared with a low-fat diet in severe obesity. N Engl J Med 2003; 348:2074–2081.

72. Grey NJ, Goldring S, Kipnis DM. The effect of fasting, diet, and actinomycin D on insulin secretion in the rat. J Clin Invest 1970; 49:881–889.

73. Grey N, Kipnis DM. Effect of diet composition on the hyperinsulinemia of obesity. N Engl J Med 1971; 285:827–831.

74. Bagdade JD, Bierman EL, Porte D Jr. The significance of basal insulin levels in the evaluation of the insulin response to glucose in diabetic and nondiabetic subjects. J Clin Invest 1967; 46:1549–1557.

75. Floyd JC Jr., Fajans SS, Conn JW, Knopf RF, Rull J. Stimulation of insulin secretion by amino acids. J Clin Invest 1966; 45:1487–1502.

76. Rabinowitz D, Zierler KL. Forearm metabolism in obesity and its response to intra-arterial insulin. Characterization of insulin resistance and evidence for adaptive hyperinsulinism. J Clin Invest 1962; 41:2173–2181.

77. Epstein LH, Valoski A, Koeske R, Wing RR. Family-based behavioral weight control in obese young children. J Am Diet Assoc 1986; 86:481–484.

78. Valoski A, Epstein LH. Nutrient intake of obese children in a family-based behavioral weight control program. Int J Obes 1990; 14:667–677.

79. Epstein LH, Wing RR, Steranchak L, Dickson B, Michelson J. Comparison of family based behavior modification and nutrition education for childhood obesity. J Pediatr Psychol 1980; 5:25–36.

80. Epstein LH, Valoski AM, Vara LS, et al. Effects of decreasing sedentary behavior and increasing activity on weight change in obese children. Health Psychol 1995; 14:109–115.

81. Robinson TN. Behavioural treatment of childhood and adolescent obesity. Int J Obes Rel Metab Disord 1999; 23(S2): S52–S57.

82. Epstein LH, Wing RR. Behavioral treatment of childhood obesity. Psychol Bull 1987; 101:331–342.

83. Ello-Martin JA, Ledikwe JH, Rolls B. The influence of food portion size and energy intake: implications for weight management. Am J Clin Nutr 2005; 82(S1):236S–2341S.

84. Ebbeling CB, Sinclair KB, Pereira MA, Garcia-Lago E, Feldman HA, Ludwig DS. Compensation for energy intake from fast food among overweight adolescents. JAMA 2004; 291:2828–2833.

85. Parks EJ, McCrory MA. When to eat and how often? Am J Clin Nutr 2005; 81:3–4.

86. Mahan K, Escott-Stump S. Krauses's Food Nutrition and Diet Therapy. Philadelphia: WB Saunders, 1996:463–469.

87. Alemzadeh R, Rising R, Cedillo M, Lifshitz F. Obesity in children. In: Lifshitz F, ed. Pediatric Endocrinology. 4th ed. New York: Marcel Dekker, 2003:823–828.

88. Haddock CK, Shadish WR, Klesges RC, Stein RJ. Treatments for childhood and adolescent obesity. Ann Behav Med 1994; 16:235–244.

89. Wadden TA, Sarwer DB. Behavioral treatment of obesity: new approaches to an old disorder. In: Goldstein D, ed. The Management of Eating Disorders. Totowa NJ: Humana Press, 1999:173–199.

90. Epstein LH, Paluch RA Gordy CC, Dorn J. Decreasing sedentary behaviors in treating pediatric obesity. Arch Pediatr Adolecs Med 2000; 154:220–226.

91. Epstein LH, Paluch RA, Kilanowski CK, Raynor HA. The effect of reinforcement or stimulus control to reduce sedentary behavior in the treatment of pediatric obesity. Health Psychol 2004; 23:371–380.

92. Apfelbaum M, Bostsarron J, Lacatis D. Effect of caloric restriction and excessive caloric intake on energy expenditure. Am J Clin Nutr 1971; 24:1405–1409.

93. Doucet E, St-Pierre S, Alméras N, Després JP, Bouchard C, Tremblay A. Evidence for the existence of adaptive thermogenesis during weight loss. Br J Nutr 2001; 85:715–723.

94. Grundy SM, Blackburn G, Higgins M, Lauer R, Perri MG, Ryan D. Physical activity in the prevention and treatment of obesity and its comorbidities: evidence report of independent panel to assess the role of physical activity in the treatment of obesity and its comorbidities. Med Sci Sports Exerc 1999; 31:1493–1500.

95. Goodpaster BH, Katsiaras A, Kelley DE. Enhanced fat oxidation through physical activity is associated with improvements in insulin sensitivity and diabetes. Diabetes 2003; 52:2191–2197.

96. Gutin B, Barbeau P, Owens S, et al. Effects of exercise intensity on cardiovascular fitness, total body composition, and visceral adiposity of obese adolescents. Am J Clin Nutr 2002; 75:818–826.

97. Ferguson MA, Gutin B, Le NA, et al. Effects of exercise training and its cessation on components of the insulin resistance syndrome in obese children. Int J Obes Relat Metab Disord 1999; 23:889–895.

98. Williams CL, Hayman LL, Daniels SR, et al. Cardiovascular healthy in childhood. A statement for health professionals from the committee on atherosclerosis, hypertension, and obesity in the young (AHOY) of the council on cardiovascular disease in the young, American Heart Association. Circulation 2002; 106:143–160.

99. Tudor-Locke CE, Myers AM. Methodological considerations for researchers and practitioners using pedometers to measure physical (ambulatory) activity. Res Q Exerc Sport 2001; 72:1–12.

100. Hagan RD, Upton SJ, Wong L, Whittam J. The effects of aerobic conditioning and/or caloric restriction in overweight men and women. Med Sci Sports Exerc 1986; 18:87–94.

101. Sothern MS, Hunter S, Suskind RM, Brown R, Udall JN Jr., Blecker U. Motivating the obese child to move: the role of structured exercise in pediatric weight management. South Med J 1999; 92:577–584.

102. Ravussin E, Burnand B, Schutz Y, Jequier E. Energy expenditure before and during energy restriction in obese patients. Am J Clin Nutr 1985; 41:753–759.

103. Ravussin E. A NEAT way to control weight. Science 2005; 307:530–531.

104. Jakicic JM, Winters C, Lang W, Wing RR. Effects of intermittent exercise and use of home exercise equipment on adherence, weight loss, and fitness in overweight women: a randomized trial. JAMA 1999; 282:1554–1560.

105. Wei M, Kampert JB, Barlow CE, et al. Relationship between low cardiorespiratory fitness and mortality in normal-weight, overweight, and obese men. JAMA 1999; 282:1547–1553.

106. Serdula MK, Mokdad AH, Williamson DF, Galuska DA, Mendlein JM, Heath GW. Prevalence of attempting weight loss and strategies for controlling weight. JAMA 1999; 282:1353–1358.

107. Sothern MS, von Almen TK, Schumacher HD, Suskind RM, Blecker U. A multidisciplinary approach to the treatment of childhood obesity. Del Med J 1999; 71:255–261.

108. Barlow SE, Dietz WH. Obesity evaluation and treatment: expert committee recommendations. Pediatrics 1998; 102: e29–e29.

109. Goldstein DJ. Beneficial health effects of modest weight loss. Int J Obesity 1991; 397:397–415.

110. Perri M, McKelvey D, Renjilian D, Nezu A, Shermer R, Viegener B. Relapse prevention training and problem solving therapy in the long-term management of obesity. J Consult Clin Psych 2001; 69:722–726.

111. Rossner S. Weight cycling a "new" risk factor? J Intern Med 1989; 226:209–211.

112. Steen SN, Oppliger RA, Brownell KD. Metabolic effects of repeated weight loss and regain in adolescent wrestlers. JAMA 1988; 260:47–50.

113. Brownell KD, Greenwood MR, Stellar E, Sharager EE. The effects of repeated cycles of weight loss and regain in rats. Physiol Behav 1986; 30.459–464.

114. Ross R, Shaw KD, Martel Y, de Guise J, Avruch L. Adipose tissue distribution measured by magnetic resonance imaging in obese women. Am J Clin Nutr 1993; 57: 470–475.

115. Peiris AN, Hennes MI, Evans DJ, Wilson CR, Lee MB, Kissebah AH. Relationship of anthropometric measurements of body fat distribution to metabolic profile in premenopausal women. Acta Med Scand 1988; 723(suppl):179–188.

116. Wolver TM, Jenkins DJ, Jenkins AL, Josse RG. The glycemic index: methodology and clinical implications. Am J Clin Nutr 1991; 54:846–854.

117. Wunschel IM, Sheikholislam BM. Is there a role for dietetic foods in the management of diabetes and/or obesity? Diabetes Care 1978; 1:247–249.

118. National Task Force on the Prevention and Treatment of Obesity, National Institutes of Health. Very low-calorie diets. A review. JAMA 1993; 270:967–974.

119. Andersen T, Backer OG, Stokholm KH, Quaade F. Randomized trial of diet and gastroplasty compared with diet alone in morbid obesity. N Engl J Med 1984; 310:352–356.

120. Wadden TA, Stunkard AJ. Controlled trial of very low calorie diet, behavior therapy, and their combination in of carbohydrate and its components—international com- the treatment of obesity. J Consult Clin Psychol 1986; 54:482–488.

121. Flatt JP, Blackburn GL. The metabolic fuel regulatory system: implications for protein-sparing therapies during caloric deprivation and disease. Am J Clin Nutr 1974; 27:175–187.

122. Sherwin RS, Hendler RG, Felig P. Effect of ketone infusion on amino acid and nitrogen metabolism in man. J Clin Invest 1975; 55:132–139.

123. Sothern MS, Loftin M, Suskind RM, Udall JN Jr., Blecker U. The impact of significant weight loss on resting energy expenditure in obese youth. J Invest Med 1999; 47: 222–226.

124. Boeck MA. Safety and efficiency of fiuoxetine in morbidly obese adolescent females. Int J Obes 1991; 15(S3):60.

125. Wadden TA, Berkowitz RI, Womble LG, et al. Randomized trial of lifestyle modification and pharmacotherapy for obesity. New Eng J Med 2005; 353:2111–2120.

126. Selikowitz M, Sunman, Pendegast A, Wright S. Fenfiuramine in Prader-Willi syndrome: a double blind, placebo controlled trail. Arch Dis Child 1990; 65:112–114.

127. Oleandri SE, Maccario M, Rossetto R, et al. Three-month treatment with metformin or dexfenfiuramine does not modify the effects of diet on anthropometric and endocrine-metabolic parameters in abdominal obesity. J Endocrinol Invest 1999; 22:134–140.

128. Abenhaim L, Moride Y, Brenot F, et al. Appetite-suppressant drugs and the risk of primary pulmonary hypertension. N Engl J Med 1996; 335:609–616.

129. Despres JP. Golay A, Sjostrom L. Effects of rimonabant on metabolic risk factors in overweight patients with dyslipidemia. N Engl J Med 2005; 353:2121–2134.

130. Freemark M, Bursey D. The effect of metformin on body mass index and glucose tolerance in obese adolescents and fasting hyperinsulinemia and a family history of type 2 diabetes. Pediatrics 2001; 107:E55.

131. Kay JP, Alemzadeh R, Langley G, D'Angelo L, Smith P, Holshouser S. Beneficial effects of metformin in normoglycemic morbidly obese adolescents. Metabolism 2001; 50: 1457–1461.

132. Alemzadeh R, Langley G, Upchurch L, Smith P, Slonim AE. Beneficial effect of diazoxide in obese hyperinsulinemic adults. J Endocrinol Metab 1998; 83:1911–1915.

133. Lustig RH, Rose SR, Burghen GA, et al. Hypothalamic obesity caused by cranial insult in children: altered glucose and insulin dynamics and reversal by somatostatin agonist. J Pediatr 1999; 135:162–168.

134. Pelleymounter MA, Cullen MJ, Baker MB, et al. Effects of the obese gene product on body weight regulation in ob/ob mice. Science 1995; 269:540–543.

135. Heymsfield SB, Greenberg AS, Fujioka K, et al. Recombinant leptin for weight loss in obese and lean adults. JAMA 1999; 282:1568–1575.

136. Joffe A. Pharmacotherapy for adolescent obesity. JAMA 2005; 293:2932–2934.

137. Matsuo T, Odaka H, Ikeda HE. Effect of an intestinal disccharidase inhibitor (AO-128) on obesity and diabetes. Am J Clin Nutr 1992; 55:314S–317S.

138. James WP, Avenell A, Broom J, Whitehead J. A one-year trial to assess the value of orlistat in the management of obesity. Int J Obes Rel Metab Disord 1997; 21:S24–S30.

139. McDuffie JR, Calis KA, Uwaifo GI, et al. Efficacy of orlistat as an adjunct to behavioral treatment in overweight African American and Caucasian adolescents with obesity-related co-morbid conditions. J Pediatr Endocrinol Metab 2004; 17:307–319.

140. Chanoine JP, Hampl S, Jensen C, Boldrin M, Hauptman J. Effects of orlistat on weight and body composition in obese adolescents. JAMA 2005; 293:2873–2883.

141. Halpern A, Mancini MC. Treatment of obesity: an update on anti-obesity medications. Obesity Reviews 2003; 4:25–43.

142. Ioannides-Demos LL, Proietto J, McNeil JJ. Pharmacotherapy for obesity. Drugs 2005; 65:1391–1418.

143. Berkowitz RI, Wadden TA, Tershakovec AM, Cronquist JL. Behavior therapy and sibutramine for the treatment of adolescent obesity. JAMA 2003; 289:1805–1812.

144. Buchwald H, Avidor Y, Braunwald E, et al. Bariatric Surgery a systematic review and meta-analysis JAMA; 292:1724–1737.

145. Courcoulas AP, Flum DR. Filling the gaps in bariatric surgical research. JAMA 2005; 294:1957–1960.

146. Wolfe BM, Morton JM. Weighing in on bariatric surgery: procedure use, readmission rates, and mortality. JAMA 2005; 294:1960–1963.

147. O'Leary JP. Gastrointestinal malabsorptive procedures. Am J Clin Nutr 1992; 55:567S–570S.

148. Alden JF. Gastric and jejunoileal bypass: a comparison in the treatment of morbid obesity. Arch Surg 1997; 112:799–806.

149. Saltzstein EC, Gutmann MC. Gastric bypass for morbid obesity; preoperative and postoperative psychological evaluation of patients. Arch Surg 1980; 115:21–23.

150. Freeman JB, Burchett H. Failure rate with gastric partitioning for morbid obesity. Am J Surg 1977; 112:799–806.

151. Chapman AE, Kiroff G, Game P, et al. Laparoscopic adjustable gastric banding in the treatment of obesity: a systematic literature review. Surgery 2004; 135:326–351.

152. Inge TH, Garcia V, Daniels S, et al. A multidisciplinary approach to the adolescent bariatric surgical patient. J Pediatr Surg 2004; 39:442–447.

153. Sugerman HJ, Sugerman EL, DeMaria EJ, et al. Bariatric surgery for severely obese adolescents. J Gastrointest Surg 2003; 7:102–107.

154. Inge TH, Krebs NF, Garcia VF, et al. Bariatric surgery for severely overweight adolescents: concerns and recommendations. Pediatrics 2004; 114:217–223.

155. Inge TH, Lawson ML, Garcia VF, Kirk S, Daniels S. Body composition changes after gastric bypass in morbidly obese adolescents. Obes Res 2004; 12:A53.

156. Jonides L, Buschbacher V, Barlow SE. Management of child and adolescent obesity: psychological, emotional, and behavioral assessment. Pediatrics 2000; 110:215–221.

157. Dietz WH. Health consequences of obesity in youth: childhood predictors of adult disease. Pediatrics 1998; 101:518–525.

158. Schwimmr JB, Burwinkle TM, Varni JW. Health related quality of life of severely obese children and adolescents. JAMA 2003; 289:1813–1819.

159. Tuomilehto J, Lindstrom J, Eriksson JG, et al. Prevention of type 2 diabetes mellitus by changes in lifestyle among subjects with impaired glucose tolerance. N Engl J Med 2001; 344:1343–1350.

160. Kelsey JL, Acheson RM, Keggi KJ. The body build of patients with slipped capital femoral epiphysis. Am J Dis Child 1972; 124:276–281.

161. Kling TF Jr. Angular deformities of the lower limbs in children. Orthop Clin North Am 1987; 18:513–527.

162. Young T, Palta M, Dempsey J, Skatrud J, Weber S, Badr S. The occurrence of sleep-disordered breathing among middle-aged adults. N Engl J Med 1999; 328:1230–1235.

163. Gislason GO, Benediktsdot B. Snoring, apneic episodes, and nocturnal hypoxemia among children 6 months to 6 years old. Chest 1955; 107:53–966.

164. Horner RL, Mohiaddin RH, Lowell DG, et al. Sites and sizes of fat deposits around the pharynx in obese patients with obstructive sleep apnea and weight matched controls. Eur Respir J 1989; 2:613–622.

165. Shelton KE, Gay SB, Hollowell DE, Woodson H, Suratt PM. Mandible enclosure of upper airway and weight in obstructive sleep apnea. Am Rev Respir Dis 1993; 148:195–200.

166. Felmons WW. Obstructive sleep apnea. N Engl J Med 2002; 347:498–504.

167. Rosen RC, Rosekind M, Rosevear C, Cole WE, Dement WC. Physicians education in sleep and sleep disorders: a national survey of US medical schools. Sleep 1993; 338:1230–1235.

168. He J, Kryger MH, Zirick FJ, Conway W, Roth T. Mortality and apnea index in obstructive sleep apnea: experience in 385 male patients. Chest 1988; 94:9–14.

169. Partinen M, Guilleminault C, Quera-Silva MA, Jamieson A. Obstructive sleep apnea and cephalometric roentgenogram: The role of anatomic upper airway abnormalities in the definition of abnormal breathing during sleep. Chest 1988; 93:1199–1205.

170. Hla KM, Young TB, Bidwell T, Palta M, Skatrud JB, Dempsy J. Sleep apnea and hypertension: a population based study. Ann Intern Med 1994; 120:118–128.

171. Goldstein NA, Pugazhendhi V, Rao SM, et al. Clinical assessment of pediatric obstructive sleep apnea. Pediatrics 2004; 114:33–43.

172. Strollo PJ, Rogers RM. Obstructive sleep apnea. N Engl J Med 1996; 334:99–104.

173. Abbott RD, White LR, Ross GW, Masaki KH, Curb JD, Petrovitch H. Walking and dementia in physically capable elderly men. JAMA 2004; 292:1447–1453.

174. Sarlio-Lahteenkorva S, Stunkard A, Rissanen A. Psychosocial factors and quality of life in obesity. Int J Obes Relat Metab Disord 1995; 19(S6):S1–S5.

175. Barlow CE, Kohl HW, Gibbons LW, Blair SN. Physical fitness, mortality and obesity. Int J Obes Relat Metab Disord 1995; 19(S4):S41–S44.

176. Spiegel AM, Alving BM. Executive summary of the strategic plan for National Institutes of Health Obesity Research. Am J Clin Nutr 2005; 82(S1):211S–214S.

177. Blackburn GL, Walker WA. Science-based solutions to obesity: what are the roles of academia, government, industry and health care? Am J Clin Nutr 2005; 82(S1):207S–2010S.

178. Sherwood NE, Morton N, Jeffery RW, French SA, Neumark-Sztainer D, Falkner NH. Consumer preferences in format and type of community weight control programs. Am J Health Promot 1998; 13:1343–1350.

179. Tate DF, Jackvony EH, Wing RR. Effects of Internet behavioral counseling on weight loss in adults at risk for type 2 diabetes: a randomized trial. JAMA 2003; 289:291.

180. Tate DF, Jackvony EH, Wing RR. Effects of internet behavioral counseling on weight loss in adults at risk for type 2 diabetes: a randomized trial. JAMA 2003; 289:1833–1836.

3

Diabetes in the Child and Adolescent: Diagnosis and Classification

Arlan L. Rosenbloom

Division of Pediatric Endocrinology, Department of Pediatrics, University of Florida,
Gainesville, Florida, U.S.A.

INTRODUCTION

Until the 1970s, the care and investigation of childhood diabetes was pursued by internists, pediatricians, nephrologists, and general physicians. In 1971, it was estimated that visits for diabetes by those 0 to 15 years of age were equally divided among internists, general physicians, and general pediatricians (1). At that time, there were few pediatric endocrinologists, virtually none in private practice, and most of them did not consider diabetes to be an endocrine disorder. The third, 1965, edition of what was then the only textbook of pediatric endocrinology devotes a short paragraph to diabetes mellitus as one of half a dozen causes of hyperglycemia (2). By 1993, pediatric endocrinologists accounted for 35% of all visits of 0 to 21-year-old diabetes patients and nearly half of these were to private practicing pediatric endocrinologists; the remainder were 37% to internists (most likely the older adolescents and young adults) and 28% to general pediatricians (3). In pediatric endocrinology practice, diabetes now accounts for 50% to 60% of the workload (3). The movement of diabetology into mainstream pediatric endocrinology has multiple causes beyond the clinical importance and challenge of the problem, including the scientific excitement about diabetes research (and its funding!), the extensive endocrine physiology that diabetes affects, and the inclusion of diabetes in the accreditation requirements of training programs and board certification for pediatric endocrinology.

This history deserves consideration and reflection because pediatric endocrinologists are presently engaged in a comparable revolution in what is considered to be within the purview of pediatric endocrinology. The contemporary epidemic of Type 2 diabetes (T2DM) in youth has confronted pediatric diabetes specialists with a major responsibility for a condition that was previously rare in the pediatric age group. Furthermore, pediatric endocrinologists have had to reconsider the associated problem of obesity, which has long been a frequent reason for referral to the endocrine clinic, but rarely dealt with after ruling out unusual syndromic or medical causes. This obesity epidemic has had pediatric endocrinologists dealing with various comorbidities of insulin resistance that were formerly the exclusive domain of physicians treating adults. As they earlier did for Type 1 diabetes (T1DM), pediatric diabetologists are becoming involved in developing teams to deal with this difficult and growing clinical challenge of obesity and T2DM.

DIAGNOSIS

The diagnosis of diabetes includes a wide variety of diseases characterized by hyperglycemia. Because insulin is the only physiologically important hypoglycemic hormone, hyperglycemia is the result of either impaired secretion of insulin from the beta cells of the pancreas (T1DM) or resistance to the effect of insulin in the liver, muscle, and fat cells exceeding a limited capacity of the pancreas to compensate (T2DM). Criteria for the diagnosis of diabetes have recently been revised and categories of impaired glucose tolerance and impaired fasting glucose added, reflecting the recognition that these preclinical glucose intolerance states are associated with increased cardiovascular morbidity (4). The information in Table 1 is based on the current recommendations of the American Diabetes Association (ADA) (4). There is no reason to apply different criteria with children and adolescents.

ETIOLOGIC CLASSIFICATION OF DIABETES

In 1997, the American Diabetes Association published revisions of the classification of diabetes based on etiology and these were modified in 1999 (4). Early taxonomy had the common forms of diabetes separated by age of onset (juvenile and maturity or adult), which a 1979 report of the U.S. National Diabetes Data

Table 1 Criteria for the Diagnosis of Diabetes

Symptoms plus casual[a] plasma glucose concentration $\geq$200 mg/dL (11 mmol/L), or

Fasting plasma glucose $\geq$126 mg/dL (7 mmol/L), or

Two-hour plasma glucose $\geq$200 mg/dL (11 mmol/L) during an OGTT. The test should be performed using a glucose load containing the equivalent of 75 g anhydrous glucose dissolved in water for those weighing >43 kg and 1.75 g/kg for those weighing <43 kg[a]

[a]Casual is defined as any time of day without regard to the time of the last meal. The OGTT should be done following 2–3 days of a high carbohydrate diet. In practice, however, obtaining a plasma glucose two hours after a high carbohydrate breakfast may be more practical and as informative. We only use OGTT for research purposes.

Note: In the absence of marked hyperglycemia with decompensation, these criteria should be confirmed by repeat testing on a different day. OGTT is not recommended for routine clinical use.

Impaired glucose tolerance = two-hour plasma glucose 140–200 mg/dL.

Impaired fasting glucose = 100–125 mg/dL.

Abbreviation: OGTT, oral glucose tolerance test.

Group revised to emphasize treatment, using the terms insulin-dependent and noninsulin-dependent diabetes for the principal forms (5). Contemporary understanding of the pathogenesis of various forms of diabetes has made this classification based on treatment inappropriate. Table 2 is adapted from the classification published by the ADA expert committee (4).

Type 1 Diabetes

Diabetes occurring in childhood remains predominantly immune-mediated T1DM associated with histocompatibility locus (HLA) specificities. Idiopathic T1DM may be difficult to distinguish from the immune-mediated form. Many, if not most, African-American patients who have T1DM without evidence of autoimmunity have what has been termed atypical diabetes mellitus (ADM) or "flatbush" diabetes (6,7). This condition has its onset throughout childhood and rarely past age 40, and is not associated with HLA specificities. Further characteristics are described in Table 3. T1DM is discussed in Vol. 1; Chaps. 4, 5, and 6.

Type 2 Diabetes

T2DM in childhood and adolescence now accounts for 10% to 50% or more of new patients with diabetes in the 10 to 19-year age group, depending on the ethnic/racial mix of the population served (9). For the population as a whole, adults and children, T2DM accounts for 90% to 95% of all diabetes (4). For further information, refer to Vol. 1; Chap. 9.

Maturity Onset Diabetes of the Young

This is a stable form of youth onset (under 25 years of age) diabetes inherited in an autosomal dominant fashion and affecting almost exclusively Caucasians (Table 3). Six molecular defects have been identified, affecting beta cell function. Its frequency among

Table 2 Etiologic Classification of Diabetes Mellitus

Type 1 diabetes[a] (β-cell destruction), usually leading to absolute insulin deficiency
  Immune mediated
  Idiopathic
Type 2 diabetes[a] (may range from predominantly insulin resistance with relative insulin deficiency to a predominantly secretory defect with insulin resistance)
Other specific types
  Genetic defects of β-cell function
    Maturity onset diabetes of the young
    Mitochondrial defects
  Genetic defects in insulin action
    Type A insulin resistance
    Leprechaunism
    Rabson-Mendenhall syndrome
    Lipoatrophic diabetes
  Diseases of the exocrine pancreas
    Pancreatitis
    Trauma/pancreatectomy
    Neoplasia
    Cystic fibrosis
    Hemochromatosis
    Fibrocalculous pancreatopathy
  Endocrinopathies
    Acromegaly
    Cushing's syndrome
    Glucagonoma
    Pheochromocytoma
    Hyperthyroidism
    Somatostatinoma
    Aldosteronoma
  Drug- or chemical-induced
    Vacor
    Pentamidine
    Nicotinic acid
    Glucocorticoids
    Thyroid hormone
    Diazoxide
    β-adrenergic agonists
    Thiazides
    Dilantin
    α-interferon
    Atypical antipsychotics
  Infections
    Congenital rubella
    Cytomegalovirus
  Uncommon forms of immune-mediated diabetes
    "Stiff-man" syndrome
    Anti-insulin receptor antibodies
  Other genetic syndromes sometimes associated with diabetes
    Down syndrome
    Klinefelter syndrome
    Turner syndrome
    Wolfram syndrome
    Friedreich ataxia
    Huntington chorea
    Laurence-Moon-Biedl syndrome
    Myotonic dystrophy
    Porphyria
    Prader-Willi syndrome
Gestational diabetes mellitus

[a]Patients with any form of diabetes may require insulin treatment at some stage of their disease. Such use of insulin does not, of itself, classify the patient.

Table 3 Classification of the Types of Diabetes Seen in Children

	Type 1	ADM	Maturity onset diabetes of the young	Type 2
Age at onset	Throughout childhood	Pubertal	Pubertal	Pubertal
Predominant race or ethnic distribution	All (low frequency in Asians)	African-American	Caucasian	Hispanic, African-American, Native-American
Onset	Acute, severe	Acute, severe	Subtle	Subtle to severe
Islet autoimmunity	Present	Absent	Absent	Unusual
Insulin secretion	Very low	Moderately low	Variable	Variable
Insulin sensitivity	Normal (with blood glucose control)	Normal	Normal	Decreased
Ketosis, DKA at onset	Up to 40%	Common	Rare	Up to 33%
Obesity	As in population	As in population	Uncommon	>90%[a]
Proportion of diabetes	−70–80%[a]	<10%	<5%	20–25%[a]
Percentage of probands with affected 1° relative	5–10%	>75%	100%	~80%
Mode of inheritance	Non-Mendelian, generally sporadic	Autosomal dominant	Autosomal, dominant	Non-Mendelian, strongly familial

[a]The proportion of pediatric diabetes patients having Type 2 diabetes will vary with racial/ethnic mix of the population and it is increasing.
Abbreviation: ADM, atypical diabetes mellitus.
Source: From Ref. 8.

diabetes patients is reported to vary from <0.2% to 5% in various populations (10). The genetic forms of diabetes are reviewed in Vol. 1; Chap. 10.

Mitochondrial Mutations

Diabetes and deafness may be associated as a result of mutations in mitochondrial DNA (11–13).

Genetic Defects in Insulin Action

Genetically determined abnormalities of insulin action are very rare as a cause of diabetes, ranging from mild hyperinsulinemia with modest hyperglycemia to severe diabetes (14). The structure and function of the insulin receptor are intact in the insulin resistance of lipoatrophic diabetes, indicating that the defect lies in postreceptor transduction (15).

Diseases of the Exocrine Pancreas

Diffuse injury to the pancreas needs to be relatively extensive to result in diabetes because of the small volume occupied by the beta cells, with the exception of carcinoma involving the pancreas, a problem not seen in pediatrics. With improved survival, increasing numbers of patients with cystic fibrosis are developing diabetes (16).

Endocrinopathies

Diabetes has been described in adults with hormone excess syndromes including acromegaly, Cushing syndrome, glucagonoma, and pheochromocytoma (17). There has been recent concern about the use of pharmacologic doses of growth hormone in children who do not have growth hormone deficiency, which may be increasing the risk for Type 2 diabetes (18,19).

Drug or Chemical-Induced Diabetes

A large number of drugs used in pediatric care can impair insulin secretion, increase gluconeogenesis, or increase insulin resistance, resulting in hyperglycemia or the precipitation of diabetes in a susceptible individual (20,21). The rat poison, Vacor, and pentamidine given intravenously, can permanently destroy beta cells (22–25). The class of atypical antipsychotic drugs (clozapine, olanzapine, quetiapine, and risperidone) has been associated with precipitation of diabetes and ketoacidosis, often with clearing of the diabetes on cessation of the drug (26). Exact mechanisms are uncertain, but beta cell toxicity and weight gain with insulin resistance have been implicated. Other drugs can impair insulin action, probably the most common being glucocorticoids (20,21).

Infections

Numerous viruses have been implicated in the induction of diabetes, but the strongest evidence of a direct causation comes from the experience with congenital rubella (27), fortunately now rarely seen.

CLASSIFICATION OF DIABETES IN CHILDHOOD

Table 3 describes the characteristic features of the common types of diabetes seen in childhood and Table 4 summarizes clinical characteristics helpful in distinguishing T1DM and T2DM in children and adolescents.

In those with acute onset who are not obese and not African-Americans, T1DM is highly likely and further testing is not necessary. Nonobese African-American youngsters with acute onset diabetes who have a three-generation family history of diabetes indicative of autosomal dominant transmission and do not have islet autoimmunity markers are very likely to have ADM. Islet cell autoimmunity testing should be considered in obese patients having acute onset; if this is not practical or if the patient has acanthosis nigricans, the ability to reduce and stop

Table 4 Differentiating Type 1 from Type 2 Diabetes in Children and Adolescents

Demographics	Type I	Type 2	Comment
Family history	3–5%	74–100%	Extensive family history suggests T2; T2 affects minorities disproportionately
Age or pubertal status	Variable	> 10 or pubertal[a]	Type 1 can occur at any age; only 10% of Type 2 children are younger than 10 or prepubertal
Gender	Female = male	Female > male	Some gender difference in T2 may reflect differences in use of medical care
Presentation			
Asymptomatic	Rare	Common	Type 2 often detected incidentally on routine physical examination
Symptom duration	Days or weeks	Weeks or months	Predominant symptoms are polyuria, polydipsia, polyphagia, and nocturia
Weight loss	Common	Common	Type 2 children lose more pounds; Type 1 usually lose greater % body weight
HHS[b]	Very rare	Occurs	Type 2 can develop severe, fatal dehydration and electrolyte disturbance
Physical findings			
Body mass index (BMI) at diagnosis	≤75 percentile	≥85 percentile	Those with BMI 75–85th percentile often present greatest diagnostic challenge
Acanthosis	No	Common	Useful marker in hyperglycemic child
Biochemistry at diagnosis			
Hyperglycemia	Variable	Variable	Degree of hyperglycemia at diagnosis is not useful in delineating diabetes type
Ketosis and ketonuria	Common	Common	Not useful for diagnosis of diabetes type
Acidosis	Common	Moderately common	Not useful for diagnosis of diabetes type
Other markers			
HbA	Elevated	Elevated	Not useful for diagnosis of diabetes type
Insulin or C-peptide/serum	Low (may be normal early)	Normal-high	Hyperinsulinism reflects insulin resistance Low levels may be found in T2 at diagnosis; repeat 3–6 mo after diagnosis may be elevated
Autoimmune markers	Common	Uncommon	Includes anti-islet cell and anti-GAD Antibodies; absence does not rule out T1

[a]Occasionally in 8–10-year-old group and as young as 4 yr.
Abbreviation: HHS, hyperglycemic hyperosmolar state.
Source: Adapted from Hale DE: Type 2 diabetes: an increasing pediatric problem (unpublished).

the acutely required insulin over the first several months with weight reduction, exercise, and oral hypoglycemic therapy as necessary, will clarify the diagnosis.

With insidious onset, obese individuals can be considered to have T2DM. If the patient is lean, islet autoantibody testing will be helpful and, if positive, indicate early detection of T1DM. Absence of islet cell autoimmunity in the lean individual may indicate MODY, in which case testing of family members will be productive; the pattern of autosomal dominant transmission may not emerge unless apparently unaffected family members are tested. Fasting C-peptide or insulin measurements may be of value, with elevated levels indicative of T2DM; repeated testing after one year or more may be needed for those who have normal results. One can assume that an individual with persistent normal C-peptide levels can be treated as T2DM, regardless of the presence or absence of diabetes-related autoimmunity.

A study of 700 newly diagnosed 5 to 19-year-old patients from three university centers in Florida over a five-year period indicated that 3% of those initially classified as T1DM (17 out of 605) were later classified as T2DM and that 8% of those initially diagnosed as T2DM were subsequently reclassified as having

T1DM (6 out of 77) (28). Most of the 17 originally considered to have T1DM and later determined to have T2DM were diagnosed with ketosis or in ketoacidosis. Those six individuals with an initial diagnosis of T2DM who were subsequently considered to have T1DM were, typically, overweight youngsters without diabetes-related antibodies; however, over the next few years they had a clinical course most consistent with T1DM. In this relatively sophisticated clinical setting, the proportion of patients in whom classification may be problematic was less than 5% of newly diagnosed children and youth.

The distinctions indicated by the typical features in Tables 3 and 4 are not always as certain as one would like. There are a number of reasons for classification difficulty. With the increased frequency of obesity in childhood, a substantial number of newly diagnosed T1DM and ADM patients will be obese, suggesting the possibility of T2DM. Insulin or C-peptide measurements at the onset of diabetes may not be helpful because there may be reasonable beta cell function during the recovery phase ("honeymoon") of autoimmune diabetes and, conversely, glucose toxicity/lipotoxicity in nonautoimmune diabetes will impair insulin secretion at the time of testing. Because some T2DM patients and almost all ADM have ketoacidosis, this feature is not helpful to distinguish non-T1DM from T1DM.

There are also some classification difficulties that suggest that there will be further refinement of diabetes classification in years to come and that the contemporary distinction between two major forms of diabetes, T1DM and T2DM, will come to be seen as simplistic. Challenges to the concept of two main and distinct forms of diabetes have accumulated for the last 40 years. There was little diabetes among Yemenite immigrants to Israel, but 25 years later they had a 40-fold increase in the frequency of diabetes with proportions of insulin dependency similar to that among Israelis of European origin, suggesting common environmental influences, most likely nutritional, for both T1DM and T2DM (29). The specificity of a family history of T2DM is low because of the high frequency of this disorder in the general population, particularly in minority populations. Furthermore, a family history of T2DM is three times as common with T1DM as in the general population and, conversely, T1DM is more frequent in the relatives of patients with T2DM (30,31). Genetic interaction between T1DM and T2DM is further suggested by HLA haplotype interaction in families with both T1DM and T2DM (32). The finding of islet autoimmunity markers at onset in substantial percentages of children with typical T2DM unrelated to degree of obesity or treatment requirement has been a further assault on the notion of immune-mediated diabetes as a distinct and uniform clinical and pathologic entity (33–35).

While the investigators sort out the uncertainties in our classification of diabetes, the clinician has the advantage of dealing with the individual patient whose treatment should always be determined by individual characteristics, rather than absolute diagnostic classification.

REFERENCES

1. Rosenbloom AL, Ongley JP. Who provides what services to children in private medical practice? Am J Dis Child 1974; 127:357–361.
2. Wilkins L. The Diagnosis and Treatment of Endocrine Disorders in Childhood and Adolescence. 3rd ed. Springfield, IL: Charles C. Thomas, 1965:542.
3. Rosenbloom AL, Deeb LC, Allen L, Pollock BH. Characteristics of pediatric endocrinology practice: a workforce study. Endocrinologist 1998; 8:213–218.
4. American Diabetes Association. Position statement: diagnosis and classification of diabetes mellitus. Report of the expert committee on the diagnosis and classification of diabetes mellitus. Diabetes Care 2005; 28:S37–S42.
5. National Diabetes Data Group. Classification and diagnosis of diabetes mellitus and other categories of glucose intolerance. Diabetes 1979; 28:1039–1057.
6. Winter WE, Maclaren NK, Riley WJ, Clarke DW, Kappy MS, Spillar RP. Maturity-onset diabetes of youth in black Americans. N Engl J Med 1987; 316:285–291.
7. Banerji MA, Chaiken RL, Juey H, et al. GAD antibody negative NIDDM in adult with black subjects with diabetic ketoacidosis and increased frequency of human leukocyte antigen DR3 and DR4: flatbush diabetes. Diabetes 1994; 43:741–745.
8. Rosenbloom AL. Type 2 diabetes in children. American Association for Clinical Chemistry. Diagn Endocrinol, Immunol Metabolism 2000; 18:143–153.
9. American Diabetes Association. Type 2 diabetes in children and adolescents: consensus conference report. Diabetes Care 2000; 23:381–389.
10. Winter WE. Molecular and biochemical analysis of the MODY syndromes. Pediatric Diabetes 2000; 1:88–117.
11. Reardon W, Ross RJM, Sweeney MG, et al. Diabetes mellitus associated with a pathogenic point mutation in mitochondrial DNA. Lancet 1992; 340:1376–1379.
12. van den Ouwenland JMW, Lemkes HHPJ, Ruitenbeek W, et al. Mutation in mitochondrial tRNA (Leu(URR) gene in a large pedigree with maternally transmitted type II diabetes mellitus and deafness. Nature Genet 1992; 1:368–371.
13. Kadowaki T, Kadowaki H, Mori Y, et al. A subtype of diabetes mellitus associated with a mutation of mitochondrial DNA. N Engl J Med 1994; 330:962–968.
14. Taylor SI. Lilly lecture: molecular mechanisms of insulin resistance: lessons from patients with mutations in the insulin-receptor gene. Diabetes 1992; 41:1473–1490.
15. Rosenbloom AL, Goldstein S, Yip CC. Normal insulin binding to cultured fibroblasts from patients with lipoatrophic diabetes. J Clin Endocrinol Metab 1977; 44:803–806.
16. Moran A, Doherty L, Wang X, Thomas W. Abnormal glucose metabolism in cystic fibrosis. J Pediatr 1998; 133:10–17.
17. Berelowitz M, Eugene HG. Non-insulin-dependent diabetes mellitus secondary to other endocrine disorders. In: LeRoith D, Taylor SI, Olefsky JM, eds. Diabetes Mellitus. New York: Lippincott-Raven, 1996:496–502.
18. WS Cutfield, P Wilton, H Bennmarker, et al. Incidence of diabetes mellitus and impaired glucose tolerance in children and adolescents receiving growth hormone treatment. Lancet 2000; 355:610–613.
19. Rosenbloom AL. Hot topic. Fetal growth, adrenocortical function, and the risk for type 2 diabetes. Pediatric Diabetes 2000; 1:150–154.
20. Pandit MK, Burke J, Gustafson AB, Minocha A, Peiris AN. Drug-induced disorders of glucose tolerance. Ann Int Med 1993; 118:529–540.
21. O'Byrne S, Feely J. Effects of drugs on glucose tolerance in non-insulin-dependent diabetes (parts I and II). Drugs 1990; 40:203–219.
22. Bouchard P, Sai P, Reach G, Caubarrere I, Ganeval D, Assan R. Diabetes mellitus following pentamidine-induced hypoglycemia in humans. Diabetes 1982; 31:40–45.
23. Assan R, Perronne C, Assan D, Chotard L, Mayaud C, Matheron S, Zucman D. Pentamidine-induced derangements of glucose homeostasis. Diabetes Care 1995; 18:47–55.
24. Gallanosa AG, Spyker DA, Curnow RT. Diabetes mellitus associated with autonomic and peripheral neuropathy after Vacor poisoning: a review. Clin Toxicol 1981; 18:441–449.
25. Esposti MD, Ngo A, Myers MA. Inhibition of mitochondrial complex I may account for IDDM induced by intoxication with rodenticide Vacor. Diabetes 1996; 45:1531–1534.
26. Rettenbacher MA. Disturbances of glucose and lipid metabolism during treatment with new generation antipsychotics. Curr Opin Psychiatry 2005; 18(2):175–179.
27. Forrest JA, Menser MA, Burgess JA. High frequency of diabetes mellitus in young patients with congenital rubella. Lancet 1971; 2:332–334.

28. Macaluso CJ, Bauer UE, Deeb LC, et al. Type 2 diabetes mellitus among Florida children and adolescents, 1994 through 1998. Public Health Rep 2002; 117:373–379.

29. Keen H, Jarrett RJ. Environmental factors and genetic interactions. In: Creutzfeld W, Kobberling J, Neel JV, eds. The Genetics of Diabetes Mellitus. Berlin: Springer-Verlag, 1976:203–214.

30. Gottlieb MS. Diabetes in offspring and siblings of juvenile- and maturity-onset-type diabetics. J Chronic Dis 1980; 33: 331–339.

31. Dahlquist G, Blom L, Tuvemo T, Nystrom L, Sandstrom A, Wall S. The Swedish childhood diabetes study—results from a nine year case register and a one year case-referent study indicating that type 1 (insulin-dependent) diabetes mellitus is associated with both type 2 (non-insulin-dependent) diabetes mellitus and auto-immune disorders. Diabetologia 1989; 32:2–6.

32. Li H, Lindholm E, Almgren P, et al. Possible human leukocyte antigen-mediated genetic interaction between type 1 and type 2 diabetes. J Clin Endocrinol Metab 2001; 86:574–582.

33. Hathout EH, Thomas W, El-Shahawy, Nabab F, Mace JW. Diabetic autoimmune markers in children and adolescents with type 2 diabetes. Pediatrics (http://www.pediatrics.org/cgi/content/full/107/6/e102), 2001.

34. Umpaichitra V, Banerji MA, Castells S. Autoantibodies in children with type 2 diabetes mellitus. J Pediatr Endocrinol Metab 2002; 15:525–530.

35. Rosenbloom AL. Obesity, insulin resistance, beta cell autoimmunity, and the changing clinical epidemiology of childhood diabetes. Diabetes Care 2003; 26:2954–2956.

4

Type 1 Diabetes in the Child and Adolescent

Michael J. Haller, Janet H. Silverstein, and Arlan L. Rosenbloom

Division of Pediatric Endocrinology, Department of Pediatrics, University of Florida, Gainesville, Florida, U.S.A.

TYPE 1 DIABETES MELLITUS

Type 1 diabetes mellitus (T1DM) is a heterogeneous disorder characterized by autoimmune-mediated destruction of pancreatic beta cells culminating in absolute insulin deficiency. T1DM is most commonly diagnosed in children and adolescents and requires exogenous insulin replacement. Terms such as "juvenile diabetes" and "insulin-dependent diabetes" have been replaced as they no longer adequately reflect our understanding of the natural history and pathophysiology of T1DM. This chapter provides a review of our current understanding of the epidemiology, etiology, presentation, and complications of T1DM.

EPIDEMIOLOGY

The past 30 years have seen a rapid increase in knowledge of the epidemiologic patterns and natural history of T1DM, knowledge that was anticipated to provide insight into the critical environmental contribution to the development of this disease and direction for potential cure (1). While this information has heightened understanding of T1DM, we have yet to develop an intervention to prevent T1DM or to identify the environmental triggers.

The Multi-National Project for Childhood Diabetes (Diabetes Mondiale) study was initiated by the World Health Organization in 1990 to investigate and monitor the patterns of incidence of T1DM (2). This remarkable study encompassed surveillance of 4.5% of the world's population 14 years of age and under, representing probably the largest standardized survey for any disease (3). From 1990 to 1994, nearly 20,000 cases of T1DM in children less than or equal to 14 years were diagnosed in the 75 million sample population and annual incidence rates were calculated per 100,000. The terminology used in discussing the epidemiology of T1DM includes the standard definitions of incidence, prevalence, frequency, and epidemic (4). There was greater than a 350-fold variation in incidence among the 100 populations studied, from 0.1/100,000 per year in China and Venezuela to 36.8 in Sardinia and 36.5 in Finland. Very high incidence, considered equal to or greater than 20, was also found in Sweden, Norway, Portugal, United Kingdom, Canada, and New Zealand (Fig. 1).

Wide variation in incidence has been seen between neighboring areas in Europe and North America. For example, across the eastern border of Finland and Russia there is a sixfold gradient in the incidence of T1DM between areas in geographic proximity despite equal frequencies of high-risk and low-risk genotypes (5). In the Americas, Alberta and Prince Edward Island, across the continent from each other, have comparable annual incidence rates of 24 and 24.5, whereas U.S. rates vary from 11.7 in Chicago to 17.8 in Pennsylvania. While the rate in Puerto Rico, 17.4, is virtually identical to that in Pennsylvania, the rate in neighboring and ethnically similar Cuba is only 2.9 (3). The overall incidence of T1DM in the United States is estimated to be between 15 and 17 while the prevalence in U.S. children is 1.7 to 2.5/1000 (3). More than 13,000 U.S. children are diagnosed with T1DM each year (6).

Migrant populations provide an interesting perspective on environmental contributions to the development of T1DM. A number of observations have indicated that susceptibility is affected by environmental change. Israeli children living in Canada have a fourfold greater incidence than those in Israel (3). Where T1DM in the Indian population is very low, Indian children migrating to England from South Africa developed incidence rates comparable with those of English children in the community (7). Japanese living in Hawaii are five times more likely to have T1DM than those in Japan, a country with a very low incidence of T1DM. Ethnic French and Italian children in Montreal have twice the incidence of diabetes as those in their native lands (8–10).

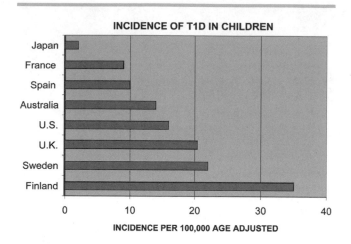

INCIDENCE OF T1D IN CHILDREN

INCIDENCE PER 100,000 AGE ADJUSTED

Figure 1 Incidence of Type 1 diabetes mellitus in children. Incidence per 100,000 age-adjusted varies greatly from country to country even in the same geographic region.

There is considerable evidence for an increasing frequency of T1DM, a further profound argument for environmental influences. While many autoimmune diseases disproportionately affect women, T1DM generally affects males and females equally, although some reports indicate a slight male excess among those younger than 20 years (11,12). The temporal trend has been noted in steadily increasing incidence rates in European countries since the 1950s (13–15). France saw a 4.9% rise in incidence between 1980 and 1998 (16). From 1983 through 2000 Sweden reported a 2.2% annual increase in incidence while Lithuania reported a 2.3% annual rise in incidence (17).

Epidemics have been described outside Europe, one striking report being a single year nearly sixfold increase in the Virgin Islands in 1984 (18). There is also evidence that the average age of onset of diabetes is decreasing (19,20). Consistent with the occasional observation of an epidemic increase in T1DM, modest seasonality has been documented, with a peak in winter months and a summertime dip (14,21,22).

ETIOLOGY AND PREVENTION

Over the past 30 years, the combined use of genetic, autoimmune, and metabolic markers has dramatically improved the ability to predict the development of T1DM. Current understanding of T1DM pathogenesis is that T1DM develops in genetically predisposed individuals who are exposed to an environmental trigger which initiates autoimmune destruction of beta cells via autoreactive T cells (1). Beta-cell injury results in the release of antigens not previously seen by the immune system resulting in production of antibodies to these antigens. Autoantibodies are not themselves pathogenic but instead indicate altered cellular proteins resulting from the inflammatory

process of autoimmunity. The appearance of insulin autoantibodies (IAA), islet cell antibodies (ICA), glutamic acid decarboxylase (GAD_{65}) antibodies, and antibodies to tyrosine phosphatase (IA-2 or ICA512) indicate ongoing autoimmune disease and these antibodies may be present in the serum for many years before the development of overt diabetes. GAD_{65} antibodies are present in 75% of newly diagnosed diabetes patients (23) and IA-2 are present in 50% to 60% of patients at diabetes onset (24). The number of types of autoantibodies and their titers are independent predictors of T1DM risk. ICA titers of greater than 40 Juvenile Diabetes Foundation units convey a 60% to 70% risk of developing diabetes over five to seven years (25). ICA at a young age denote a much greater risk than in older subjects. The presence of ICA in the first few years of life conveys a 10-year risk of developing diabetes of nearly 90%, whereas a 40-year-old found to be ICA positive has a 30% 10-year risk. After 10 years of overt diabetes, fewer than 5% of patients have detectable ICA. Although IAA may be the first autoantibodies to appear in the development of T1DM, they are not by themselves strong predictors of developing T1DM. When IAA are found in combination with other autoantibodies, however, the risk for T1DM increases significantly. In the large NIH funded Diabetes Prevention Trial-Type 1 (DPT-1) five-year risk of T1DM was 20% to 25% for subjects with one autoantibody marker, 50% to 60% for subjects with two markers, nearly 70% for those with three markers, and almost 80% for those with four autoantibody markers (Table 1) (26). As the autoimmune process continues, there is gradual loss of beta-cell mass with the first demonstrable abnormality being loss of first-phase insulin response (FPIR) during intravenous glucose tolerance testing (IVGTT). This is followed by abnormal oral glucose tolerance testing and finally, overt diabetes (Fig. 2) (1,24,27).

The presence of immune markers before the onset of diabetes has permitted development of prediction models to determine who is at risk for developing disease. The immunoassays (GAD_{65}, IA-2) are more easily applied for large-scale use than previous assays for islet-cell autoimmunity, have a high predictive value for T1DM, and are more reproducible than ICA assays. Using models based on antibody characteristics, autoantibody-positive relatives of T1DM subjects can be classified into groups with risks of diabetes ranging from 5% to 90% within five years (28). Other risk factors include young age, absolute number of autoantibodies,

Table 1 Autoantibody Number and Five-Year Risk of Diabetes

Number of autoantibodies	Five-year risk of developing diabetes (%)
0	0.2
1	20
2	50
3	70
4	80

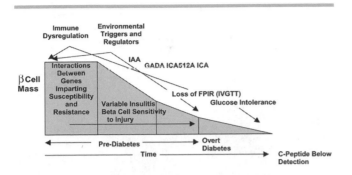

Figure 2 Modern model of the pathogenesis and natural history of Type 1 diabetes. The modern model expands and updates the traditional model by inclusion of information gained through an improved understanding of the roles for genetics, immunology, and environment in the natural history of Type 1 diabetes. *Abbreviations*: FPIR, first-phase insulin response; IVGTT, intravenous glucose tolerance test, IAA, insulin autoantibodies; ICA, islet cell autoantibodies; ICA 512, autoantibodies against the islet tyrosine phosphatase; GAD, glutamic acid decarboxylase. *Source*: Adapted from Ref. 27.

high titer antibodies, low FPIR to IVGTT, and high-risk human leukocyte antigen (HLA) genotypes (DR3/4, DQB0302/DQB0201) (Table 2) (29,30). The persistent loss of FPIR to IVGTT predicts progression to overt diabetes over the next five years in greater than 85% (31).

While autoantibody testing has fostered the development of accurate T1DM prediction models, standard autoantibody testing of all newly diagnosed patients is not recommended, except when there is difficulty differentiating new onset T1DM from Type 2 diabetes or when patients are being screened for enrollment in intervention studies. For patients not being seen at a research institution, we recommend having diabetes-related autoantibody studies sent to an experienced reference laboratory.

Environmental Triggers

The importance of environmental factors in the initiation of the autoimmune response that ultimately results in diabetes is suggested by the observations that only 30% of identical monozygotic twins are concordant for T1DM (32) and that the incidence of diabetes is rising, with a decrease in mean age of onset, despite a stable genetic pool (3,17,20). Many factors have been linked to increased risk of diabetes, including congenital rubella infection (33), enteroviral infection (34,35), lack of exposure to early infection

(the "farm" hypothesis) (36), and even vitamin D deficiency (37). In addition, some environmental factors, such as vaccination, have been implicated by concerned parents despite the overwhelming evidence that standard vaccination does not increase risk for T1DM (38). Many other agents have been implicated, but only those figuring in preventive trials will be discussed in detail.

Cow's Milk

A triggering effect of cow's milk has been proposed, based on molecular mimicry due to the structural similarity of a 17-amino acid fragment (ABBOS) of bovine serum albumin to an islet antigen (ICA 69). Although Karjalainen et al. found antibodies to bovine serum albumin in children with new-onset diabetes, but not controls (39), the Diabetes Auto-immunity Study of the Young (DAISY) found no association between islet autoimmunity and early cow's milk exposure (40). The Trial to Reduce Type 1 diabetes mellitus in the Genetically at Risk (TRIGR) was designed to test the hypothesis that avoidance of nutritional cow's milk proteins for at least the first six months of life would reduce diabetes in the high-risk population. Smaller pilot studies in Finland have demonstrated significant decreases in islet autoimmunity in those children who avoided cow's milk (41). Nearly 2400 infants will be enrolled in TRIGR. Infants with high-risk HLA genotypes DQB10302 and/or DQB10201 and who are negative for the protective genotypes DQB10602, 0603, or 030 are eligible. Mothers are encouraged to breast feed. The intervention group receives a casein hydrolysate formula after full breast feeding, whereas the control group receives a cow's milk-containing formula. The intervention group is advised to avoid beef and cow's milk products in the diet. At the two-year observation point, IA-2, GAD_{65}, and ICA titers were measured in 173 children. Three of 84 children (3.6%) in the casein hydrolysate intervention group developed at least one autoimmune marker compared with 10 of 89 (11.2%) in the control group ($p = 0.056$) (42). TRIGR's 10-year prospective trial is not yet complete. As the final analysis of the cow's milk hypothesis remains incomplete, we do not advise parents to make any dietary changes in attempts to decrease diabetes risk. Because of the many other well demonstrated benefits of breast feeding, we advise all new mothers to breast feed, as recommended by the American Academy of Pediatrics.

Viral Agents/Vaccines

Studies from Sweden and Finland found more frequent immunoglobulin (Ig)M antibodies to enterovirus in pregnant women whose children subsequently developed diabetes than in control women (43,44). Molecular mimicry between the P2-D protein of coxsackie virus and the GAD protein make this an

Table 2 Absolute Risk for Type 1 Diabetes Mellitus According to DR/DQ Genotypes

DR/DQ	Risk	First-degree relative	Population
DR 3/4, DQ 0201/0302	Very high	1/4–5	1/15
DR 4/4, DQ 0300/0302	High	1/6	1/20
DR 3/3, DQ 0201/0201	High	1/10	1/45
DR4/x, DQ 0302/x (x≠0602)	Moderate	1/15	1/60
X/X	Low	1/125	1/600
DR0403 or DQ0602	Protected	1/15,000	1/15,000

attractive hypothesis. Other viruses implicated have been chickenpox, mumps, measles, enteric cytopathic human orphan, rotavirus, and rubella (in utero infection) (43,45). In fact, nearly 20% of children with congenital rubella infection are ICA-positive (33). Immunization, specifically for diptheria-pertussis-tetanus and hemophilus influenza, has also been implicated in the increased incidence of T1DM (46). Such a relationship has not been substantiated in recent large studies (38,47).

PANDA and TEDDY

Despite growing understanding of the natural history of T1DM, knowledge of the complex interplay between environment and genetics is limited. The Pediatric Assessment of Newborns for Diabetes Autoimmunity (PANDA) study is a pilot effort in which HLA typing is done from filter paper blood spots along with the neonatal screening laboratory work (48). Those babies with high-risk HLA haplotypes (DR3 and DR4, DQA0302/501, and DQB0301,0201) have blood specimens taken for ICA studies. Families keep records of foods eaten, immunizations, and illnesses, and the subjects are tested for islet autoantibodies every six months in the initial couple of years and then annually. Correlations of the appearance of islet autoimmunity with history of environmental exposure may help identify the environmental factors that trigger the autoimmune cascade and permit specific preventive intervention.

On a larger scale, The Environmental Determinants of Diabetes in Youth (TEDDY) consortium of six international centers (four in the United States and two in Europe) seeks to identify the infectious agents, dietary factors, and other environmental factors associated with T1DM in genetically susceptible people (49,50). We strongly encourage all pregnant women to have their newborns screened for participation in studies such as TEDDY. The ability of observational studies to provide new information on the pathogenesis of T1DM depends on the continued involvement of dedicated study participants.

Intervention Trials

As the ability to predict diabetes has increased, intervention trials have moved from treating new-onset patients to targeting those at high risk of developing T1DM. One of the major impediments to effective intervention trials has been that as prediction accuracy improves the potential for effective intervention declines (Fig. 3). Early studies were aimed at treatment of newly diagnosed patients with immunosuppressive agents, while more recent studies attempted to prevent the disease in high-risk individuals. Because of the lack of adequate efficacy to justify the potential toxicities of the immunosuppressive agents used, efforts were made to design trials using safer agents and to initiate treatment at an earlier stage of the disease.

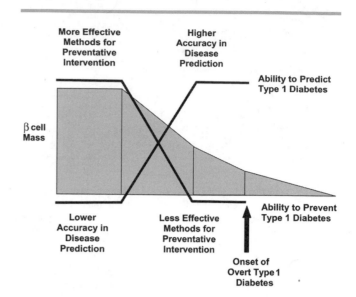

Figure 3 The "treatment dilemma" for Type 1 diabetes. Many studies from animal models of Type 1 diabetes in combination with a much more limited series of investigations in human beings suggest that early intervention not only is more effective in terms of disease prevention, but also often requires more benign forms of therapy. In contrast, the ability to identify an individual who will truly develop Type 1 diabetes (among an at-risk population) increases as the individual approaches onset of overt disease. *Source:* Adapted from Ref. 27.

Cyclosporine

In the 1980s, cyclosporine administration to newly diagnosed patients increased the frequency and duration of clinical remission, as determined by residual C-peptide secretion. Unfortunately, the remission was not long-lived and the effect was lost when the cyclosporine was stopped (51). Reports of cyclosporine-induced nephrotoxicity led to cessation of its use (52).

Azathioprine

Azathioprine given to newly diagnosed patients resulted in increases in C-peptide levels that were short-lived despite continued use of the immunosuppressive agent. Predictors of success with these agents were older age, lack of ketoacidosis at diagnosis, early initiation of treatment, and higher C-peptide levels at diabetes onset (53).

High-Dose Insulin

Treatment of new-onset patients with high-dose insulin using the Biostator, a device which measured venous blood-glucose every few minutes and provided intravenous insulin to maintain normoglycemia, proved as effective as azathioprine in preserving beta-cell function. Nevertheless, as with the immunosuppressive agents, the results were transient (54).

Nicotinamide

Nicotinamide is a free radical scavenger that interferes with the autoimmune destruction of beta cells primarily by acting as an antioxidant. Nicotinamide therapy restores cellular NAD+ levels, helps to prevent damage from inflammatory macrophages, and promotes increased beta-cell regenerative capacity (55,56). Nicotinamide prevented diabetes in animal models. Because nicotinamide is a safe drug, the initial positive results in animal models and population-based studies made it an attractive candidate for DPTs.

Nicotinamide decreased the incidence of T1DM by 41% in a study done in 80,000 five- to seven-year-old New Zealand school children (57,58). Among the 20,000 children who were tested for ICA, 185 were positive and 173 of them accepted treatment with nicotinamide for upwards of seven years; the incidence of T1DM in the treated group was approximately 7/100,000, significantly lower than the 16 to 18/100,000 per year incidence in the background population. These findings led to the initiation of a large European multicenter study, the *European Nicotinamide Diabetes Intervention Trial*. This trial was a double-blind placebo-controlled study enrolling first-degree relatives who were ICA-positive. Enrollment began in 1994 and was completed in 1998. Among 50,000 first-degree relatives of children with T1DM, 552 had ICA with normal oral glucose testing. The final analysis showed that nicotinamide was ineffective in decreasing the incidence of T1DM (59).

Oral and Subcutaneous Insulin—DPT-1

Initiated in 1994, the DPT-1 was designed to determine if antigen-based therapy could prevent diabetes in at-risk individuals. Insulin was used as the antigen, based on studies showing that low-dose parenteral insulin given to ICA-positive relatives with low FPIR resulted in reduced development of diabetes compared with controls who refused insulin prophylaxis (60). In the DPT-1, patients with ICA were considered high risk if they had low FPIR to IVGTT (>50% risk of developing diabetes over five years) and were randomized to receive low-dose subcutaneous insulin or to receive no intervention. Subjects with ICA and normal FPIR were assigned to the intermediate risk group (25–50% chance of developing diabetes over five years) and were randomly assigned to receive oral insulin or placebo. Unfortunately, the study revealed no differences in development of diabetes between the high-risk insulin-treated group and controls (61). Although DPT-1 was unsuccessful in preventing T1DM, the undertaking resulted in the formation of an integrated network with core laboratories providing standardized testing and a centralized data/statistical center, which has provided the framework for future multicenter intervention trials.

TrialNet

The most recent prevention/intervention development is the creation of the multicenter cooperative group known as TrialNet. This collaborative network is similar to the childhood cancer cooperative groups and will enable the undertaking of multiple pilot studies involving primary and secondary prevention strategies in different population groups at different stages of the disease process. These studies will not only ascertain the efficacy of intervention, but also should lead to greater insight into the pathogenesis of the disease. For example, while DPT-1 was not powered to perform certain subgroup analyzes, there was a suggestion that subjects in the oral insulin arm with the highest IAA titers benefited from therapy (62). Through TrialNet a new adequately powered study is being initiated to determine if the original observation from DPT-1 is valid. We recommend considering all eligible patients for participation in TrialNet sponsored studies. However, careful consideration must be given to the patient's likelihood to complete the study and comply with the study requirements. Patients with a history of poor compliance or in unstable social situations often are unwilling or unable to fully participate in intervention studies.

Trial to Reduce Insulin-Dependent Diabetes Mellitus in the Genetically at Risk

As previously discussed, the TRIGR study seeks to determine whether genetically at-risk infants who are not exposed to cow's milk for the first six months of life will be protected from the subsequent development of diabetes (63).

CLINICAL PICTURE

T1DM is usually diagnosed in a child with polydipsia and polyuria. In children, the third member of the classic diabetes triad, polyphagia, is often absent because ketosis can cause anorexia. The symptoms of diabetes are related to prolonged hyperglycemia. When blood-glucose concentrations exceed the renal threshold for reabsorption (~180 mg/dL), there is osmotic diuresis and glycosuria. Decreasing glucose uptake, hepatic gluconegenesis from muscle proteolysis, lipolysis, and chronic glycosuria result in weight loss and dehydration. Eventually, insulin deficiency, dehydration, and ketosis will progress to diabetic ketoacidosis (DKA) which is the manner of presentation for 20% to 40% of all newly diagnosed T1DM (64). Clinical features of DKA are listed in Chapter 8. Asymptomatic diabetes may be diagnosed by families or physicians if the children are involved in diabetes research studies or have other family members with T1DM.

T1DM is usually diagnosed in the outpatient setting when a slightly ill-appearing child is brought to the pediatrician for evaluation of weight loss and other nonspecific symptoms. The dehydration associated with polyuria may result in nonspecific symptoms of constipation, headache, and abdominal pain, often interpreted as a viral syndrome, or gastro-enteritis if there is vomiting. Children who are vomiting but do not have diarrhea and are maintaining high urine output despite dehydration may have T1DM. Other causes for this combination of symptoms are rare (adrenal insufficiency, renal disease). In addition, enuresis in a previously toilet-trained child, nocturia, pyogenic skin infections, recurrent Candida diaper rash in babies and toddlers, and monilial vaginitis in teen-age girls also require consideration of diabetes.

Children in whom diabetes must be considered may, for practical purposes, be divided into three general categories: (i) those who have typical signs and symptoms of diabetes—polyuria, polydipsia, and weight loss; (ii) those who have glycosuria, without hyperglycemia, and (iii) those with transient hyperglycemia.

Renal glycosuria may be an isolated congenital disorder, a feature of the Fanconi syndrome and other renal tubular disorders, due to severe heavy metal intoxication, ingestion of certain drugs (e.g., outdated tetracycline), or result from inborn errors of metabolism such as cystinosis. When vomiting, diarrhea, or inadequate intake of food occurs in any of these conditions, starvation ketosis may ensue and simulate DKA. The absence of hyperglycemia eliminates the possibility of diabetes. Stress of illness, especially in the toddler age group, may be associated with glycosuria and moderate hyperglycemia. Blood glucose levels usually do not exceed 300–400 mg/dL (17–20 mmol/L), but values over 500 mg/dL (>27 mmol/L) have been reported (65). This usually occurs in the context of acute asthma exacerbation or during a hospital admission for severe infection or other serious illness. The hyperglycemia is usually transient and blood glucose levels normalize with resolution of illness. A similar clinical picture can be seen with glucocorticoid administration (66,67). The presence of ICA, IA-2, IAA, or GAD antibodies in those with stress or glucocorticoid-induced hyperglycemia may indicate limited beta-cell reserve and risk for future development of diabetes (24). Thus, autoantibodies against islet antigens should be measured in all instances of stress hyperglycemia. For a complete discussion of T1DM management in children, see Chapter 6.

COMPLICATIONS

The Diabetes Care and Complications Trial (DCCT) and the longitudinal follow-up of DCCT patients, the Epidemiology of Diabetes Interventions and Complications (EDIC) study, unequivocally demonstrated that tight glycemic control is critical in reducing both microvascular and macrovascular complications of diabetes (68). Insulin replacement makes it possible for the child with diabetes to attain a level of metabolic control that permits normal day-to-day functioning in school, play, and at home, with only occasional episodes of mild to moderate hypoglycemia and avoidance of ketoacidosis, despite high average

blood sugar concentrations. Awareness that this was the typical situation was limited until the development of self-monitoring of blood-glucose (SBGM) and measurement of glycohemoglobin (69,70). SBMG, HbA1c measurements, and the improvement in insulins and delivery systems have made it possible to attain a level of glucose control that will reduce the risk of long-term complications. The ability to normalize blood-glucose is now limited only by the frequency and severity of hypoglycemia (71). The contemporary goals of treatment of T1DM in children, therefore, include the traditional maintenance of a reasonably normal lifestyle and avoidance of the acute complications (see Chapter 6), but with the addition of the attainment of near-normal glycemia to reduce the risk of the long-term complications involving both microvascular and macrovascular disease. Microvascular disease is responsible for retinopathy, nephropathy, and neuropathy. Macrovascular complications affecting coronary, carotid, and other major vessels are increasingly recognized as beginning during childhood. Of particular interest in children have been joint and skin complications, and the effects on growth and development.

Joint Problems

Limited joint mobility (LJM) is one of the earliest clinically apparent long-term complications of T1DM in childhood and, following its initial description in 1974, was recognized to be a common feature of both Type 1 and Type 2 diabetes (72,73). LJM was described as bilateral painless, but obvious, contracture of the finger joints and large joints, with thick tight waxy skin, and short stature in three older teenagers with long-standing diabetes and early microvascular complications (72). Milder expression was subsequently recognized as affecting approximately 30% of youngsters with diabetes, a third of whom had involvement of more than two fingers or one finger and one large joint bilaterally (74). Variation in prevalence among various reports is related to the examination technique, the criteria, the age of the patients, and duration of diabetes. In older adult patients, examination is confounded by the presence of finger contracture related to age, occupation, and other problems affecting the joints more commonly in those with diabetes, such as Dupuytren disease, flexor tenosynovitis, or carpal tunnel syndrome (71).

The limitation in LJM is painless and only mildly disabling when severe. A simple examination method is to have the patient attempt to approximate palmar surfaces of the interphalangeal joints (Fig. 4). Passive examination is essential to confirm that inability to do so is due to LJM. Attained age seems more important than duration of diabetes or age of onset of diabetes in the evolution of LJM. With rare exception, LJM appears after the age of 10 years. The biochemical basis for LJM is likely glycation of protein with the formation of advanced glycation end products

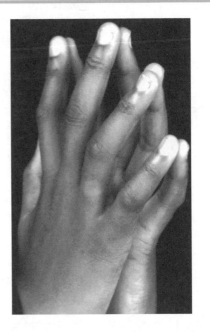

Figure 4 Inability to approximate the palmar surfaces of the fingers in a 14-year-old girl with diabetes for seven years.

(AGE). This results in increased stiffness of the periarticular and skin collagen with decreased range of motion.

As might be expected, the presence of LJM is associated with increased risk for the development of microvascular disease. The initial report of the prevalence of LJM included seven patients with severe changes, of whom five had clinically apparent retinopathy before the age of 18 years (73). In a longitudinal study of 169 patients with diabetes duration greater than 4.5 years, which was the shortest duration at which complications were noted, LJM was associated with an 83% risk for retinopathy, while the absence of LJM was associated with a 25% risk after 16 years of diabetes. The severity of microvascular changes also corresponded to the severity of LJM (75).

Both the prevalence and severity of LJM have decreased since the initial recognition in the 1970s, most likely the result of improved glucose control during this era (76). These study results are pertinent to the question of the importance of prepubertal duration and control of diabetes for the development of long-term microvascular complications. Even for the youngest age group studied or those with the shortest duration of diabetes, there was a marked decrease in the prevalence of LJM between the two eras, suggesting that improved control from the first years of childhood diabetes will reduce long-term complication risks.

Skin Problems

Necrobiosis lipoidica diabeticorum is a rarely seen pretibial lesion that is characterized by round or oval indurated plaques, with central atrophy and eventual ulceration. Unless they become infected, the lesions are painless. Relationship to diabetes control is uncertain, but there is an association with smoking, proteinuria, and retinopathy (77,78). Because these lesions do not heal well, trauma should be avoided and infection vigorously treated.

Lipoatrophy, indentation or atrophy of the subcutaneous tissue resulting from insulin injection, has become uncommon with the generalized use of recombinant-derived human insulin. It is presumed that the impurities in animal extract insulin or the foreign nature of that insulins led to the problem. It was thought to be immune-mediated, frequently following dermatomes and occurring symmetrically, distal from the actual injection sites. The lesions tended to resolve after a few years and were thought to be IgE-mediated. Mild atrophy is still seen occasionally with the contemporary insulins, affecting approximately 3% of patients 1 to 19 years old in one study (79). Lipoatrophy has even been reported with the use of insulin analogues (80,81). Injection site rotation may help decrease the risk of developing lipoatrophy.

When lipoatrophy develops, giving insulin injections around the edges of atrophic areas or using an alternative insulin analogue may be helpful.

Lipohypertrophy, which always occurs at the site of injection, is a local reaction to repeated injection trauma, usually from inadequate site rotation, with scarring and decreased sensitivity to pain. The lesion can occur quite early, however, and may not be abolished by site rotation (82). Unlike lipoatrophy, lipohypertrophy continues to be a frequent problem with improved insulin forms, present to some degree in as many as half of patients under 20 years of age (83). Both lipoatrophy and lipohypertrophy are associated with greater insulin antibody concentrations (79). The cosmetic effect is problematic, but most important is the possibility of varying absorption of insulin from areas of hypertrophy resulting in erratic glycemic control (84). Site rotation is also important in reducing the risk of developing lipohypertrophy. Once lipohypertrophy develops, injections into the area of induration should be discouraged. Most areas of lipohypertrophy will resolve within six to eight weeks if injections to the area are avoided. However, some areas of lipohypertrophy become permanent even with dedicated avoidance of injections to the area.

Cataracts

Cataracts occur rarely during recovery from ketoacidosis, typically in the newly diagnosed patient; they usually disappear rapidly but may persist, requiring surgical removal (85). In contrast to these "sugar" cataracts, subcapsular juvenile cataracts, associated with chronic hyperglycemia and caused by sorbitol accumulation, do not regress and always require removal.

Growth Failure and Delayed Sexual Maturation

Insulin has important influence on normal growth and development. Before the contemporary era of diabetes management, growth retardation and delayed puberty were frequently seen in pediatric diabetes clinics. In twin pairs discordant for diabetes, the development of diabetes before the onset of puberty was associated with invariably shorter stature than that of the nonaffected twin (86). Nonetheless, despite the generally nonphysiologic traditional means of treating diabetes, most children with diabetes did not have serious growth or maturational delay problems. With the significant advances in diabetes management over the last 30 years, with rate exception children with diabetes now experience normal timing of puberty, with normal growth and adult heights (87,88).

The effects of insulin on normal growth and development are largely mediated through the anabolic pathway and the growth hormone–insulin-like growth factor I (GH–IGF-I) axis. Deficiency of portal insulin delivery to the liver results in reduced circulating GH binding protein (GHBP) reflecting reduction in the cell surface receptor for GH, GH resistance, and diminished IGF-I production (89,90). The GH resistance also results in decreased production of IGFBP-3, the principal binding protein for circulating IGF-I, and increased production of IGFBP-1 and IGFBP-2 (91). These latter BPs, unlike IGFBP-3, do not deliver their bound IGF-I to tissues. Furthermore, there is increased proteolysis of IGFBP-3, decreasing its viability in the circulation. In addition to the GH resistance, reflected in the lower concentrations of circulating GHBP, there may be postreceptor defects in GH action mediated by the insulin deficiency. Diminished circulating total and free IGF-I levels are associated with GH hypersecretion because of the absence of negative feedback from IGF-I. This hypersomatotropism increases glycemia and decreases insulin sensitivity, but is reversible with adequate insulin replacement (92).

Growth failure and maturational delay with hepatomegaly and abdominal distention in insulin treated children was first described by Mauriac in 1930 (93). The regression of hepatomegaly in 13 such patients, following transfer from regular insulin to protamine zinc insulin, was noted in 1936 (94). Hepatomegaly was apparently a common complication in children in the era when only short-acting insulin was available and aglycosuria was the objective. This was exemplified in a series from the Joslin clinic in the late 1930s of 60 youngsters with hepatomegaly, growth failure, delayed sexual maturation, and severe uncontrollable diabetes with frequent hypoglycemia and ketoacidosis (95). Improvement was associated with the change to long-acting protamine zinc insulin.

There appear to be two forms of the Mauriac syndrome. In one form there is associated Cushingoid obesity and documented wide fluctuation between hyperglycemia and hypoglycemia, suggestive of a pattern of over- and under-insulinization, which would be expected with treatment using only soluble insulin, with secondary hyperadrenalism. Periods of over insulinization would appear to be essential for the development of obesity in this form of the syndrome, and for the induction of hyperadrenalism. More recent reports are of patients with Mauriac syndrome who do not have obesity, and are without a history of alternating hypoglycemia and ketoacidosis; these patients are unmistakably inadequately insulinized continuously (96,97).

In addition to insulin deficiency, associated autoimmune problems, such as hypothyroidism and celiac disease, can result in growth failure in children with T1DM. Approximately 20% of children with T1DM have evidence of autoimmune thyroid disease, determined by the presence of thyroid autoantibodies (98). Such autoantibodies should be tested for in all youngsters with T1DM at diagnosis and those who are positive should have annual determination of TSH levels. In addition, all children with T1DM should have TSH screening every one to two years and any time thyromegaly is noted or clinical thyroid dysfunction is suspected (99). If TSH is abnormal, free T4 and, if indicated, total T3 should be measured.

Celiac disease has been described in 5% to 8% of children with T1DM; tissue transglutaminase (tTG) antibodies should be sought in children with growth failure without obvious cause, even in the absence of diarrhea (100). Patients with T1DM should be tested soon after diagnosis for celiac disease, using tTG antibodies and serum IgA levels. Retesting should occur if growth failure, failure to gain weight, weight loss, or gastrointestinal symptoms occurs. Positive antibody tests should be confirmed and patients with confirmed positive tTG require small-bowel biopsy to definitively diagnose celiac disease. Individuals with confirmed celiac disease should follow a gluten-free diet. Consultation with a registered dietician is often helpful in teaching families how to manage both celiac disease and T1DM (99).

Eating disorders are also more common in children with diabetes than in the general population and should be considered in the assessment of any child who is not gaining weight or growing normally (101). Adolescent females with diabetes are 2.4 times more likely than those without diabetes to have clinical eating disorders and 1.9 times more likely to have a subclinical eating disorder. Mean HbA1c levels were higher in adolescents with diabetes who had an eating disorder than in those who did not (102).

Pathogenesis of Microvascular Complications

The hallmark of microvascular disease is thickened capillary basement membrane with alterations in membrane permeability and occlusion of small blood vessels. While many pathways explain some of the pathophysiology of diabetic complications, the single unifying mechanism for all hyperglycemia-induced tissue damage appears to be the increased production of reactive oxygen species (ROS) (103). The following pathways have all been used to explain the pathogenesis of microvascular complications:

Protein glycation. It has been well documented that improved glycemic control is associated with decrease in microvascular disease and its progression (104). This suggests that excess glucose per se has deleterious effects on tissues. Some of these effects appear to be through binding to collagen by posttranslational nonenzymatic means. The amidori glycation products undergo slow (nonenzymatic) chemical rearrangements to form irreversible AGE. These AGE accumulate in the extracellular matrix and vascular intracellular proteins to cause structural tissue alterations with progressive occlusion of blood vessels. This glycation may alter the charge of the proteoglycan component of the basement membrane, resulting in leakage of negatively charged proteins from the plasma. The pores in glomeruli may also undergo alterations in size resulting in protein leakage. The basement membrane thickening found in microvascular disease may be due to this glycation process, with accumulation of proteins that are not degradable. The nonenzymatic glycation of hemoglobin is an example of protein glycation and has been used as an indicator of glycemic control since the late 1970s.

Amidori products may be involved in induction of strand breakage in DNA by interfering with gene transcription. This may explain the "metabolic memory" observed in the EDIC study seven years after the conclusion of the DCCT. Although the mean HbA1c levels one year after conclusion of the DCCT were nearly identical between the former intensive and former conventional groups, the rate of worsening of retinopathy by three steps or more was significantly lower in the former intensive therapy group than in the former conventional group after seven years of follow-up (68). Similarly, the prevalence of micro-albuminuria (defined below) was 13.6% for the former conventional treatment group compared with 8.1% in the former intensive treatment group at study close-out; 15.8% of the former conventional group had albuminuria at seven years compared with only 6.8% of patients in the former intensive group (105).

Polyol pathway. Sorbitol (glucose alcohol) is enzymatically formed from glucose by aldose reductase. The higher the blood sugar concentration the more the sorbitol accumulation in a number of tissues, including lens and nerve. This influx of glucose into the polyol pathway is associated with decreased myoinositol uptake and decreased sodium/potassium/ATPase activity. These changes have been related to increased permeability and increased pressure and leakage in blood vessels, which may be related to the increased release of vasoconstrictive prostaglandins and decreased release of nitric oxide which mediates endothelium relaxation. The overall effect of these metabolic abnormalities is decreased vessel wall elasticity and microvascular hypertension (106).

PKC activation. Intracellular hyperglycemia increases the synthesis of diacylglycerol, a key activator of protein kinase C (PKC). The activation of PKC has multiple effects on gene expression which result in inflammation, increased ROS, and vascular dysfunction (103).

Hexosamine pathway. Hyperglycemia also increases the movement of glucose through the hexosamine pathway. Excess fructose-6-phosphate bypasses the glycolytic pathway and gets converted to N-acetyl glucosamine. Binding of N-acetyl glucosamine to transcription factors results in further pathologic changes in gene expression (103).

Abnormalities in the coagulation system. Elevated fibrinogen levels and other antithrombotic factors may result in increased platelet stickiness. In addition, increased prostaglandin metabolism induces coagulopathy, resulting in increased red blood cell aggregation and blockage of small capillaries (107).

Nephropathy

Micro-albuminuria, defined as urinary albumin excretion rates of 20–200 mcg/min or 30–300 mg/24 hr, is predictive of renal and cardiovascular disease (108). Concentration above 300 mg/24 hr is indicative of overt diabetic nephropathy. HbA1c level, low-density lipoprotein cholesterol (LDL-C) concentration, and body mass index (BMI) were all risk factors for the development of micro-albuminuria in 12.6% of 1134 men and women with T1DM aged 15 to 60 years during seven years follow-up in the EURO DIAB Prospective Complications Study (109).

Predictors of Nephropathy

Micro-albuminuria is rare before adolescence, as noted in a study of the prevalence and progression of micro-albuminuria and clinical proteinuria in 361 children with T1DM over the course of 12 years. While the incidence of any single episode of micro-albuminuria increased between the ages of 10 and 18 years (30.9% of males and 40.4% of females), persistent micro-albuminuria and progression from micro-albuminuria to macro-albuminuria was rare (110).

Persistently elevated levels of serum vascular endothelial growth factor may help to identify patients who are predisposed to develop persistent albuminuria (111). Eleven percent of 101 children and adolescents with diabetes who initially had normal urine albumin excretion developed persistent micro-albuminuria during eight years of follow-up with an odds ratio of 4.1 for the occurrence of micro-albuminuria if vascular endothelial growth factor serum levels were elevated.

Other predictors of persistent albuminuria are high HbA1c and high baseline albumin excretion rates, occurring in 12.8% of 339 Danish children and adolescents with T1DM over a six-year period (112).

This was a higher incidence than in a large American cross-sectional survey of 702 children and adolescents with average diabetes duration of 7.6 years. In this study, micro-albuminuria, defined as an albumin excretion rate greater than or equal to 15 mcg/min measured on at least two of three urine collections, increased from 5.1% to 11.6% after 10 years of diabetes duration and completion of puberty; maternal hypertension was a significant risk factor, but patients' blood pressure was not, and HbA1c had a borderline effect (113). These findings contrast with other studies in which there is strong association between development of micro-albuminuria and HbA1c values. A four-year follow-up of 279 patients with T1DM found that the rate of development of micro-albuminuria was 1.3/100 person-years in those with HbA1c levels less than 8%, whereas it was 5.1/100 person-years with HbA1c levels between 8% and 9%, 4.2 between 9% and 10%, and 6.7/100 person-years if HbA1c was greater than 10%. The risk of development of micro-albuminuria rose steeply between HbA1c values of 7.5% and 8.5%, emphasizing the importance of improved glycemic control (114).

The Pittsburgh Epidemiology of Diabetes Complications (EDC) study is an observational prospective study of 589 patients with onset of T1DM before the age of 17 years. Baseline LDL levels greater than or equal to 130, triglycerides greater than or equal to 150, systolic blood pressure greater than or equal to 130, and diastolic blood pressure greater than or equal to 85, conferred relative risks (RRs) of 2.2, 3.2, 2.3, and 2.5 for developing nephropathy over 10 years (115).

Homocysteine elevation has been considered a risk factor for premature cardiovascular disease. Young patients with T1DM diagnosed before the age of 12 years and with duration of disease longer than seven years who had albumin excretion rates of greater than 70 mcg/min had elevated homocysteine levels, indicating an association of diabetic nephropathy with premature cardiovascular disease (116). Fortunately, over the last 30 years, modern diabetes management has markedly decreased the incidence of severe nephropathy in adults who were diagnosed with T1DM as children (117,118).

Treatment of Nephropathy

Annual testing of the urine for albumin is recommended for children from 10 years of age and with five years of diabetes (99). The most convenient way to assess albuminuria is measurement of the urinary albumin to creatinine ratio obtained on a spot urine sample. Micro-albuminuria in a single specimen may not indicate fixed disease. Repeat testing is required to confirm persistent micro-albuminuria. It is also important to distinguish between orthostatic proteinuria and that due to diabetic renal disease. With orthostatic proteinuria a first void morning urine should not contain abnormal concentration of albumin while a late afternoon urine specimen often will.

The DCCT demonstrated that micro-albuminuria and overt nephropathy can be delayed or prevented by intensive diabetes treatment (105). However, the United Kingdom Prospective Diabetes Study (UKPDS) and other studies have shown that blood pressure control is at least as important as glycemic control in prevention of nephropathy and in decreasing the rate of decline of GFR in established disease in adults with Type 2 diabetes (119). Because of this increased risk for development of nephropathy, it is essential to pay close attention to maintaining blood pressure at normal values. Loss of nocturnal dip in blood pressure is often the first sign of hypertension, making ambulatory blood pressure monitoring a useful adjunct in evaluating children with borderline hypertension.

Persistent micro-albuminuria should be treated with an angiotensin-converting enzyme (ACE) inhibitor titrated to maintain normal albumin excretion. ACE inhibitors increase afferent vessel dilatation and decrease elevated intraglomerular pressures resulting in decreased albumin excretion. Although children and adolescents with micro-albuminuria have higher blood pressures than those with normal albuminuria (120–123), the beneficial effects of ACE inhibitors are observed whether or not the patient has hypertension (124). We recommend starting therapy with enalapril 5–10 mg daily and titrating upwards to achieve normal albuminuria and blood pressure.

The role of low protein diets in treatment of micro-albuminuria has been debated for several years; there are no long-term studies in children. Studies have shown protein restriction to slow the rate of decline of glomerular filtration rate (125) and decrease albumin excretion rates in adults with micro-albuminuria (126). Thus, a low protein diet of 0.6–0.8 g/kg of body weight may be helpful in decreasing albuminuria and slowing the decline in renal function in patients with persistent micro-albuminuria (126). High protein intake should be avoided in children with micro-albuminuria. Because of the importance of adequate dietary protein in the growing child, however, protein restriction below 15% of total daily calories is not justified.

Adolescents should be counseled to avoid smoking, because nicotine has profound vasoconstrictive effects which have been associated with progression of nephropathy in adults with T1DM (127).

Retinopathy

Retinopathy is the most common microvascular disease seen in children and adolescents with T1DM. Retinopathy is broadly defined as (i) background retinopathy, with the presence of microaneurysms only or microaneurysms and occasional dot-blot hemorrhages, and (ii) proliferative retinopathy, with growth of new vessels, glia, and fibrous tissue. Fluorescein angiography is used to document severity of retinopathy by showing areas of retinal ischemia, proliferation of new blood vessels, and permeability of the retinal vessels.

At diabetes diagnosis, there is increased blood flow through the retina. Initially, poor metabolic control may be associated with leakage of injected fluorescein into the vitreous (128), which is reversed by improved metabolic control. In addition, rapidly improving metabolic control may be associated with an initial worsening of diabetic retinopathy with subsequent long-term improvement (99). Anatomic disease results from increased vascular permeability and capillary and arteriolar occlusion within the retina. The increased permeability results in edema and the formation of hard exudates, whereas the occlusion results in the formation of microaneurysms, hemorrhages, soft exudates, and capillary dropout. The growth of new blood vessels, glia, and fibrous tissue in front of the retina can result in vitreous hemorrhage and retinal detachment from shrinkage of the proliferating tissue.

Although retinopathy has been reported to be present at onset of diabetes (129), it usually is not recognized before 5 to 10 years' duration and after the onset of puberty. By that time, 20% to 30% of patients will have background retinopathy, 30% to 50% after 10 to 15 years' diabetes duration, and 70% to 80% after 15 years of diabetes (130).

Predictors of Retinopathy

The incidence of retinopathy in 764 patients greater than 15 years of age in the European Diabetes (EURODIAB) prospective complications study was 56% after seven years of follow-up. Risk factors for development of retinopathy included high albumin excretion rate, elevated cholesterol and triglyceride levels, and increased waist to hip ratio. In contrast to other studies, there was no association between retinopathy and blood pressure, cardiovascular disease, or smoking in this study (131).

In a cross-sectional study of 725 African-Americans with T1DM in New Jersey, 3% had macular edema and 20.6% had retinal hard exudates. The severity of retinopathy correlated with the presence of proteinuria, higher LDL-C levels, systolic hypertension, poor glycemic control, and longer duration of disease. Hyperglycemia was strongly associated with retinopathy, with those patients whose HbA1c values were in the highest quartile being three times more likely to have retinopathy than those in the lowest quartile. Patients with renal disease were three times more likely to have retinopathy and 10 times more likely to have proliferative retinopathy than those without renal disease, and patients in the highest quartile of systolic blood pressure were three times more likely to have proliferative retinopathy than patients in the lowest quartile. Importantly, a large proportion of African-Americans with T1DM do not receive adequate eye care (132–134). Systolic

blood pressures above 120 mmHg conferred increased risk of proliferative retinopathy.

The Pittsburgh EDC found that systolic blood pressure greater than or equal to 120 mmHg conferred an RR of 1.6 for the development of proliferative retinopathy and the RR was 2.7 if systolic blood pressure was greater than or equal to 130 mmHg; diastolic blood pressure greater than 79 mmHg conferred an RR of 1.8; if diastolic blood pressure was greater than or equal to 85 mmHg, RR was 2.4, and if diastolic blood pressure was greater than or equal to 90 mmHg, the RR of proliferative retinopathy was 4.6 (115).

Homocysteine concentrations, which, as noted above, are elevated with cardiovascular disease, were higher in adolescents with proliferative retinopathy, further indicating a link between presence of microvascular complications and later onset of macrovascular disease and implicating a common pathologic mechanism in large and small vessels (116).

Treatment of Retinopathy

Because retinopathy is rare before puberty, many recommend a baseline screening at diabetes diagnosis to determine if preexisting eye disease is present. Otherwise, children with T1DM should begin regular ophthalmologic evaluation at the age of 10 years and following three to five years of diabetes (99). Once criteria for ophthalmologic evaluation have been met, current recommendations are that children with diabetes should be followed annually by an ophthalmologist. Recent studies indicate, however, that biennial screening may be adequate in well controlled children (135). ACE inhibitors have been shown to slow the progression of retinopathy in patients with and without hypertension; thus, the presence of retinopathy is an indication for initiation of such therapy (136). We recommend beginning enalapril 5–10 mg daily and closely monitoring the progression of retinopathy. Care must be taken to remind adolescent females that ACE inhibitors are contraindicated in pregnancy.

The use of retinal photocoagulation has markedly improved the prognosis for vision in patients with proliferative retinopathy (137). Although the mechanism of action is uncertain, it is thought that the photocoagulation destroys ischemic retinal tissue, thus removing the stimulus for neovascularization. Laser therapy is also used for macular edema by destroying leaking microaneurysms and dilated capillaries. In cases of proliferative retinopathy, panretinal photocoagulation will destroy retinal tissue outside the macula and optic nerve so that the remaining retina is not ischemic and will, therefore, not produce the growth factors that result in proliferative diabetic retinopathy. The panretinal photocoagulation has the adverse effects of compromising color discrimination, visual fields, and night vision. In the case of vitreous hemorrhage or detached retina, vitrectomy can be used to remove the blood from the vitreous or to reattach a retina that is in the process of detaching. Laser photocoagulation should be considered immediately upon diagnosis of proliferative retinopathy to prevent additional visual loss and prolong the period of useful vision (99).

Neuropathy

Although symptomatic neuropathy is uncommonly seen in children and adolescents with diabetes, sensory and autonomic motor nerve impairment can be demonstrated in young people. Peripheral neuropathy, including motor and sensory disturbances, as well as autonomic neuropathies, including gastrointestinal, cardiovascular, vasomotor instability, and hypoglycemia unawareness, have been described in childhood and adolescence. Evaluation of peripheral sensory function should be performed at each clinic visit by gently bending a 10 g monofilament against the great toe. Failure to feel the 10 g monofilament requires further evaluation for neuropathy.

The pathogenesis of neuropathy in diabetes is likely multifactorial. The aldose reductase system is present in the lens and peripheral nerves and is responsible for metabolism of glucose to sorbitol. High glucose levels will accelerate the synthesis of sorbitol, which is not freely diffusible. The sorbitol thus remains as an osmolar force within the nerve, causing swelling and possible destruction. Myoinositol, a component of neuronal cell membranes, and therefore involved in the control of neural transmission, has been found to be decreased in animals and humans with diabetes. In addition, the basement membrane of the Schwann cell is thickened and the vasa nervorum has capillary and arteriolar wall thickening by basement membrane accumulation, as part of the generalized microvascular disease of diabetes. Biopsy of affected nerves has shown numerous thrombosed vessels, axonal loss, and a characteristic segmental demyelination.

Peripheral Neuropathy

Clinical symptoms of peripheral neuropathy include bilateral numbness and paresthesias, especially pain and burning in the lower extremities, which is much worse at night. A decrease in the laboratory sense is usually the first clinical sign of neuropathy, followed by loss of ankle jerks and later by loss of pin prick sensation in a stocking distribution (138). The Pittsburgh EDC study found that 3% of 65 children under 18 years of age had neuropathy based on history and physical examination (139). Subclinical neuropathy, assessed by decreased motor nerve conduction velocities and sensory changes, is much more common, however, occurring in as many as 50% to 72% of adolescents (140).

Predictors of Neuropathy

Neuropathy has been correlated with hyperlipidemia, smoking (140), LJM (141), and albuminuria (138). A recent study of 1172 patients followed for an average of 7.3 years found that neuropathy, determined by clinical evaluation, quantitative sensory testing, and autonomic-function tests, developed in 23.5% of patients. Risk markers were HbA1c, duration of diabetes and, importantly, modifiable cardiovascular risk factors such as LDL-C, triglycerides, BMI, smoking, and blood pressure (138).

The Pittsburgh EDC study found the RR of developing peripheral neuropathy to be 2.2 if LDL-C was greater than 129 mg/dL and 1.5 if LDL-C was greater than 99 mg/dL but less than 130 mg/dL. Similarly, triglyceride levels greater than 140 mg/dL conferred a 1.5 RR. A systolic blood pressure greater than 130 mmHg was associated with an RR of 4.0 and a diastolic blood pressure greater than 85 mmHg with a 2.0 RR (115).

Improved metabolic control may result in resolution of sensory and motor nerve dysfunction as well as autonomic symptoms. The DCCT showed that intensive diabetes therapy decreased clinical neuropathy by 35% to 90% (68). Peripheral motor and sensory nerve conduction velocities were significantly faster after five years of intensive therapy compared with conventional treatment in the adolescent cohort (142).

Autonomic Neuropathy

Autonomic neuropathy most commonly results in gastroparesis, cardiovascular reflex loss, and hypoglycemic unawareness. Diabetic gastroparesis is associated with decreased gastric motility and delayed emptying time. Affected patients often complain of bloating and feelings of satiety following intake of small amounts of food and they often have anorexia and weight loss. There are some reports of resolution of gastroparesis with improved metabolic control (143,144). Diagnosis can be made by gastric emptying study. Use of metoclopramide or erythromycin may result in increased motility with resolution of symptoms. For patients with documented gastroparesis we recommend starting 5 mg metoclopramide and 5 mg/kg erythromycin before meals.

Autonomic neuropathy of the cardiovascular system results in heart rate abnormalities, especially fixed heart rate, and defects in central and peripheral vascular dynamics. Because of this, there is hyposensitivity to catecholamines and an inability to increase cardiac output resulting in hypotension with standing or exercise. Patients with autonomic neuropathy will frequently have a lower blood pressure when sitting or standing than when supine. Cardiovascular autonomic neuropathy is also a risk factor for painless myocardial ischemia and mortality (145).

Macrovascular Disease and Hyperlipidemia

Diabetes mellitus is a strong risk factor for cardiovascular disease conferring a two- to fourfold increased risk and considered to be equivalent to a previous cardiovascular event for predicting future events (146–149). Risk factors that independently increase cardiovascular risk in people with diabetes include smoking, hypertension, dyslipidemia, renal dysfunction, and hyperglycemia (150).

The Pathological Determinants of Atherosclerosis in Youth study involved more than 3000 young people who died between the ages of 15 and 34, evaluating risk factors for coronary heart disease by correlating pathologic findings of fatty streaks and lipid-laden plaques to blood lipid values, smoking, hypertension, and diabetes. There was a strong association of extent of disease with smoking, as measured by serum thiocyanate concentrations. All the aortas and about half of the right coronary arteries in the 15- to 19-year age group already had lesions, with 7% of the aortas and 12% of the right coronary arteries having raised lesions or advanced lesions of atherosclerosis. The percentage of intimal surface involved with lesions in both the aorta and right coronary artery was positively associated with very low density dipoprotien (VLDL) and LDL-C, with a 5% increase in surface involvement with each 1 standard deviation increase of LDL and VLDL cholesterol levels. Conversely, a 1 standard deviation increase in HDL cholesterol was associated with a 3% decrease in intimal surface involvement. HbA1c concentration was associated with more extensive and more advanced atherosclerosis in the aorta and right coronary artery, primarily in people between the ages of 25 and 34 years of age. The prevalence of raised lesions involving 5% or more of the intimal surface was twice as great in both the aorta and right coronary artery of people with hypertension throughout the entire 15- to 34-year age span (151).

The Bogalusa heart study reported the autopsy findings of 43 people aged 2 to 39 years who died from accidents or homicide and in whom antemortem data were available; 50% of children 2 to 15 years of age had fatty streak lesions in the coronary arteries and 8% had fibrous plaques in their coronary arteries. These atherosclerotic lesions correlated with BMI, systolic and diastolic blood pressure, total and LDL-C, and triglyceride levels (152). This indicates that the atherosclerotic process occurs early and underscores the importance of monitoring and treating, where appropriate, each of the risk factors for cardiovascular disease.

The increased cardiovascular risk in T1DM may be due to a number of factors, including endothelial dysfunction, increased arterial stiffness (148,153), and loss of endothelial integrity. One of the most important roles of the endothelium is the control of vascular tone through the production of nitric oxide. Hyperglycemia increases ROS, which directly reduce the bioavailability of nitric oxide, resulting in endothelial dysfunction (154). Endothelial dysfunction precedes atherosclerosis and can be used to predict cardiovascular events.

Predictors of Cardiovascular Disease

Recent studies have found higher levels of endothelin-1 (an indicator of endothelial damage) in patients with diabetes and hyperlipidemia than in controls; those patients with diabetes who had vascular complications had significantly higher endothelin-1 levels than did patients without complications (155). The patients with diabetes complications also had significantly higher apolipoprotein B levels compared with healthy controls. Patients without microvascular or macrovascular disease had levels similar to those of controls. Thus, it is possible that the susceptibility to the development of atherosclerosis might be attributed to the relationship between elevated lipid levels and endothelin-1 (155).

The Heart Outcome Prevention Evaluation Trial (156) was a cohort study of 5545 individuals aged 55 years or more with a history of cardiovascular disease or with diabetes mellitus and at least one cardiovascular risk factor. Of the 3498 subjects who fell into the latter category, micro-albuminuria increased the RR of major cardiovascular events (RR 1.83), all-cause death (RR 2.09), and hospitalization for congestive heart failure (RR 3.23). Any degree of albuminuria was a risk factor for cardiovascular disease, the risk increasing as the albumin to creatinine ratio increased. The use of the ACE inhibitor ramipril resulted in significant risk reduction of 25% for myocardial infarction, 37% for cardiovascular deaths, 33% for stroke, and 24% for all causes of mortality. ACE inhibition also reduced the risk of overt nephropathy by 22% and dialysis by 15%. The ramipril not only decreases blood pressure, but also has antithrombotic effects, reducing collagen-induced platelet aggregation by 18% and adenosine diphosphate-induced platelet aggregation by 39% (189). In addition, ACE inhibitors have effects on endothelium and fibrinolysis that are beneficial in preventing plaque rupture and subsequent thrombosis, two key events in the acute formation and progression of atherosclerotic disease (157).

As previously discussed, the Pittsburgh EDC found a strong correlation between lipid levels, blood pressure and risk of cardiovascular disease in their 10-year study of patients with diabetes diagnosed before the age of 18. Perhaps most importantly, tight glycemic control may decrease cardiovascular event rates in patients with T1DM and may demonstrate the same "metabolic memory" seen with microvascular complications. Mean HbA1c levels one year after conclusion of the DCCT were nearly identical between the former intensive and former conventional groups. While the EDIC cohort is still relatively young and the total event rates are still quite small, the intensive insulin therapy group demonstrated lower cardiovascular event rates than the conventional therapy group (158).

Treatment of Hyperlipidemia

The recommendation for adults with diabetes is to maintain LDL-C less than 100 mg/dL, triglycerides less than 150 mg/dL, and HDL greater than 40 mg/dL (159). Evidence continues to mount that even lower LDL levels result in decreased cardiovascular disease in high-risk patients (160). The 2005 ADA clinical practice recommendations now suggest that an LDL goal of less than 70 mg/dL should be used in high-risk patients with diabetes and cardiovascular disease (159). The data indicating that fatty streaks and atherosclerotic plaques are present during childhood show that the process begins early. Treatment goals in children are based on data obtained in adults and guidelines are similar; intervention should begin early.

Children with LDL-C levels greater than 160 mg/dL require pharmacologic intervention and treatment should be considered in children with LDL-C levels 130–159 mg/dL with a family history of CVD or additional CVD risk factors who cannot reach goal (LDL-C < 130 mg/dL) with lifestyle modification (99). Initial efforts to improve metabolic control with recommendations for diet and exercise should always be initiated when lipid levels exceed target. If fasting lipid profiles are not decreasing after three months, pharmacologic therapy should be initiated. Statins are now considered first-line therapy for hyperlipidemia and can be used in children 10 years and older (99,161). After confirming normal aspartate aminotransferase and alanine aminotransferase, we usually begin atorvastatin 10 mg daily. Fasting lipid levels should be rechecked six weeks after initiating therapy and the dose should be titrated upwards at 10 mg increments to achieve the target level of LDL-C. Adolescent females should be warned of the teratogenic potential of statins. In addition, we have begun to use cholesterol absorption inhibitors (ezetemibe) as adjunct therapy. We consider adding ezetemibe 10 mg daily if the LDL-C goal cannot be reached with 20 mg atorvastatin. Triglyceride elevation, too, should be vigorously treated. In some patients optimal blood-glucose levels will not be achieved despite intensive effort, resulting in isolated hypertriglyceridemia. In those instances, agents directed at lowering triglyceride levels, such as fibrates, should be considered. We recommend using fenofibrate 48 mg daily. Triglycerides should also be rechecked six weeks after initiating therapy and dose should be titrated upwards to achieve normal triglyceridemia.

Hypertension

The UKPDS showed that above a baseline systolic blood pressure of 110 mmHg, the higher the blood pressure, the greater the risk of cardiovascular disease (162). The Hypertension Optimal Therapy study compared the outcomes of maintaining diastolic blood pressure to goals of less than or equal to 90 mmHg, less than or equal to 85 mmHg, or less than or equal to 80 mmHg. In the 15,001 patients with diabetes mellitus at baseline, the rate of major cardiovascular events, defined as myocardial infarction, stroke, or death due to any cardiovascular event, revealed that the group randomized to maintain a diastolic blood pressure less than or equal to 80 mmHg had half the risk of major cardiovascular events compared with the group randomized to a blood pressure less than or equal to 90 mmHg. This differs from the results in the group without diabetes, in which the risk reduction was only 10% for the lower compared with the higher blood pressure readings (163), indicating that diabetes conferred an additional risk for cardiovascular disease.

Treatment of Hypertension

Children with high–normal blood pressure, defined as average systolic or diastolic blood pressure greater than the 90th percentile for age, sex, and height, should be given dietary (reduce salt intake) and exercise (30–60 minutes of daily exercise that raises heart rate) recommendations. If normalization of blood pressures is not reached within three to six months of lifestyle interventions, pharmacologic treatment should be initiated. Hypertension, defined as average systolic or diastolic blood pressure consistently greater than the 95th percentile for age, sex, and height on three separate occasions, should be treated with ACE inhibitors (159). As discussed above, we recommend starting with 5–10 mg enalapril daily and titrating upwards until blood pressure is normalized.

CONCLUSION

Since the discovery of insulin by Banting, Best, Collip, and McCleod in 1921, our understanding and management of T1DM have rapidly advanced. As we approach the 100-year anniversary of the discovery of insulin, we have an impressive armamentarium of insulins, delivery devices, and blood-glucose monitoring systems that allow us to provide excellent care for our patients. Nevertheless, the healthcare and quality of life costs of living with diabetes remain daunting. In addition, while our knowledge of T1DM has continued to grow, we still know relatively little about the true cause of pancreatic autoimmunity and how it relates to genetic and environmental risk. As we all hope for a day when patients will not be burdened with the difficulties of living with diabetes, we continue to explore the potential of environmental and pharmacological immune modification, islet cell transplantation, and stem cell regeneration to provide a gateway to the prevention and cure of T1DM.

REFERENCES

1. Atkinson MA. Thirty years of investigating the autoimmune basis for type 1 diabetes: why can't we prevent or reverse this disease. Diabetes 2005; 54(5):1253–1263.
2. WHO Multinational Project for Childhood Diabetes. WHO Diamond Project Group. Diabetes Care 1990; 13(10):1062–1068.
3. Karvonen M, Viik-Kajander M, Moltchanova E, Libman I, LaPorte R, Tuomilehto J. Incidence of childhood type 1 diabetes worldwide. Diabetes Mondiale (DiaMond) Project Group. Diabetes Care 2000; 23(10):1516–1526.
4. Fletcher R, Fletcher SW, Wagner EH. Clinical Epidemiology, the Essentials. 2nd ed. Baltimore: Williams and Wilkins, 1988.
5. Kondrashova A, Reunanen A, Romanov A, et al. A six-fold gradient in the incidence of type 1 diabetes at the eastern border of Finland. Ann Med 2005; 37(1):67–72.
6. http://www.cdc.gov/diabetes/projects/cda2.htm.
7. LaPorte R, Matsushima M, Chang Y-F. Prevalence and incidence of insulin-dependent diabetes. In: National Diabetes Data Group: Diabetes in America. 2nd ed. National Institutes of Health, National Institute of Diabetes and Digestive and Kidney Diseases, 1995:37–46.
8. Mimura G. Present status and future view of the genetics of diabetes in Japan. In: Mimura G, Baba S, Goto W, Kobberling J, eds. Clinical Genetics of Diabetes Mellitus, International Congress Series 597. Amsterdam: Excerpta Medica, 1982:13–18.
9. Kitagawa T, Fugita H, Hibi I. A comparative study of the epidemiology of IDDM in between Japan, Norway, Israel, and the United States. Acta Paediatr Jpn 1984; 26:275–281.
10. Siemiatycki J, Colle E, Campbell S, Dewar R, Aubert D, Belmonte MM. Incidence of IDDM in Montreal by ethnic group and by social class and comparisons with ethnic groups living elsewhere. Diabetes 1988; 37(8):1096–1102.
11. Krischer JP, Cuthbertson DD, Greenbaum C. Male sex increases the risk of autoimmunity but not type 1 diabetes. Diabetes Care 2004; 27(8):1985–1990.
12. Weets I, Van Autreve J, Van der Auwera BJ, et al. Male-to-female excess in diabetes diagnosed in early adulthood is not specific for the immune-mediated form nor is it HLA-DQ restricted: possible relation to increased body mass index. Diabetologia 2001; 44(1):40–47.
13. Gale EA. The rise of childhood type 1 diabetes in the 20th century. Diabetes 2002; 51(12):3353–3361.
14. Karvonen M, Tuomilehto J, Libman I, LaPorte R. A review of the recent epidemiological data on the worldwide incidence of type 1 (insulin-dependent) diabetes mellitus. World Health Organization DIAMOND Project Group. Diabetologia 1993; 36(10):883–892.
15. Diabetes Epidemiology Research International Group. Secular trends in incidence of childhood IDDM in 10 countries. Diabetes 1990; 39(7):858–864.
16. Mauny F, Grandmottet M, Lestradet C, et al. Increasing trend of childhood type 1 diabetes in Franche-Comte (France): analysis of age and period effects from 1980 to 1998. Eur J Epidemiol 2005; 20(4):325–329.
17. Pundziute-Lycka A, Dahlquist G, Urbonaite B, Zalinkevicius R. Time trend of childhood type 1 diabetes incidence in Lithuania and Sweden, 1983–2000. Acta Paediatr 2004; 93(11):1519–1524.
18. Tull ES, Roseman JM, Christian CL. Epidemiology of childhood IDDM in U.S. Virgin Islands from 1979 to 1988. Evidence of an epidemic in early 1980s and variation by degree of racial admixture. Diabetes Care 1991; 14(7):558–564.
19. Charkaluk ML, Czernichow P, Levy-Marchal C. Incidence data of childhood-onset type I diabetes in France during 1988–1997: the case for a shift toward younger age at onset. Pediatr Res 2002; 52(6):859–862.
20. Feltbower RG, McKinney PA, Parslow RC, Stephenson CR, Bodansky HJ. Type 1 diabetes in Yorkshire, UK: time trends in 0–14 and 15–29-year-olds, age at onset and age-period-cohort modelling. Diabet Med 2003; 20(6):437–441.
21. Weets I, Kaufman L, Van der Auwera B, et al. Seasonality in clinical onset of type 1 diabetes in Belgian patients above the age of 10 is restricted to HLA-DQ2/DQ8-negative males, which explains the male to female excess in incidence. Diabetologia 2004; 47(4):614–621.
22. Fleeger F, Rogers KD, Drash A, Rosenbloom AL. Age, sex, and season of onset of childhood diabetes in different geographic areas. Pediatrics 1979; 63:374–379.
23. Falorni A, Ackefors M, Carlberg C, et al. Diagnostic sensitivity of immunodominant epitopes of glutamic acid decarboxylase (GAD65) autoantibodies in childhood IDDM. Diabetologia 1996; 39(9):1091–1098.
24. Atkinson MA, Maclaren NK. The pathogenesis of insulin-dependent diabetes mellitus. N Engl J Med 1994; 331(21):1428–1436.
25. Schatz D, Krischer J, Horne G, et al. Islet cell antibodies predict insulin-dependent diabetes in United States school age children as powerfully as in unaffected relatives. J Clin Invest 1994; 93(6):2403–2407.
26. Winter WE, Harris N, Schatz D. Immunological markers in the diagnosis and prediction of autoimmune type 1a diabetes. Clin Diabetes 2002; 20(4):183–191.
27. Atkinson MA, Eisenbarth GS. Type 1 diabetes: new perspectives on disease pathogenesis and treatment. Lancet 2001; 358(9277):221–229.
28. Achenbach P, Warncke K, Reiter J, et al. Stratification of type 1 diabetes risk on the basis of islet autoantibody characteristics. Diabetes 2004; 53(2):384–392.
29. Krischer JP, Schatz D, Riley WJ, et al. Insulin and islet cell autoantibodies as time-dependent covariates in the development of insulin-dependent diabetes: a prospective study in relatives. J Clin Endocrinol Metab 1993; 77(3):743–749.
30. Riley WJ, Maclaren NK, Krischer J, et al. A prospective study of the development of diabetes in relatives of patients with insulin-dependent diabetes. N Engl J Med 1990; 323(17):1167–1172.
31. Group D-S. The Diabetes Prevention Trial Type 1 Diabetes (DPT-1). Diabetes 1994; 43(suppl):159A.
32. Hyttinen V, Kaprio J, Kinnunen L, Koskenvuo M, Tuomilehto J. Genetic liability of type 1 diabetes and the onset age among 22,650 young Finnish twin pairs: a nationwide follow-up study. Diabetes 2003; 52(4):1052–1055.
33. Ginsberg-Fellner F, Witt ME, Fedun B, et al. Diabetes mellitus and autoimmunity in patients with the congenital rubella syndrome. Rev Infect Dis 1985; 7(suppl 1):S170–S176.
34. Salminen K, Sadeharju K, Lonnrot M, et al. Enterovirus infections are associated with the induction of beta-cell autoimmunity in a prospective birth cohort study. J Med Virol 2003; 69(1):91–98.
35. Salminen KK, Vuorinen T, Oikarinen S, et al. Isolation of enterovirus strains from children with preclinical Type 1 diabetes. Diabet Med 2004; 21(2):156–164.
36. McKinney PA, Okasha M, Parslow RC, et al. Early social mixing and childhood Type 1 diabetes mellitus: a case–control study in Yorkshire, UK. Diabet Med 2000; 17(3):236–242.

37. Hypponen E, Laara E, Reunanen A, Jarvelin MR, Virtanen SM. Intake of vitamin D and risk of type 1 diabetes: a birth-cohort study. Lancet 2001; 358(9292): 1500–1503.

38. Hviid A, Stellfeld M, Wohlfahrt J, Melbye M. Childhood vaccination and type 1 diabetes. N Engl J Med 2004; 350(14):1398–1404.

39. Karjalainen J, Martin JM, Knip M, et al. A bovine albumin peptide as a possible trigger of insulin-dependent diabetes mellitus. N Engl J Med 1992; 327(5):302–307.

40. Norris JM, Beaty B, Klingensmith G, et al. Lack of association between early exposure to cow's milk protein and beta-cell autoimmunity. Diabetes Autoimmunity Study in the Young (DAISY). JAMA 1996; 276(8):609–614.

41. Akerblom HK, Virtanen SM, Ilonen J, et al. Dietary manipulation of beta cell autoimmunity in infants at increased risk of type 1 diabetes: a pilot study. Diabetologia 2005; 48(5):829–837.

42. Wilson DM, Buckingham B. Prevention of type 1a diabetes mellitus. Pediatr Diabetes 2001; 2(1):17–24.

43. Hyoty H, Taylor KW. The role of viruses in human diabetes. Diabetologia 2002; 45(10):1353–1361.

44. Dahlquist GG, Ivarsson S, Lindberg B, Forsgren M. Maternal enteroviral infection during pregnancy as a risk factor for childhood IDDM. A population-based case–control study. Diabetes 1995; 44(4):408–413.

45. Honeyman MC, Coulson BS, Stone NL, et al. Association between rotavirus infection and pancreatic islet autoimmunity in children at risk of developing type 1 diabetes. Diabetes 2000; 49(8):1319–1324.

46. Helmke K, Otten A, Willems WR, et al. Islet cell antibodies and the development of diabetes mellitus in relation to mumps infection and mumps vaccination. Diabetologia 1986; 29(1):30–33.

47. Hummel M, Fuchtenbusch M, Schenker M, Ziegler AG. No major association of breast-feeding, vaccinations, and childhood viral diseases with early islet autoimmunity in the German BABYDIAB Study. Diabetes Care 2000; 23(7):969–974.

48. Silverstein JH, Rosenbloom AL. New developments in type 1 (insulin-dependent) diabetes. Clin Pediatr (Phila) 2000; 39(5):257–266.

49. http://www.niddk.nih.gov/patient/TEDDY/TEDDY.htm.

50. http://www.teddystudy.org/.

51. Bougneres PF, Carel JC, Castano L, et al. Factors associated with early remission of type I diabetes in children treated with cyclosporine. N Engl J Med 1988; 318(11): 663–670.

52. Lipton R, LaPorte RE, Becker DJ, et al. Cyclosporin therapy for prevention and cure of IDDM. Epidemiological perspective of benefits and risks. Diabetes Care 1990; 13(7):776–784.

53. Silverstein J, Maclaren N, Riley W, Spillar R, Radjenovic D, Johnson S. Immunosuppression with azathioprine and prednisone in recent-onset insulin-dependent diabetes mellitus. N Engl J Med 1988; 319(10):599–604.

54. Shah SC, Malone JI, Simpson NE. A randomized trial of intensive insulin therapy in newly diagnosed insulin-dependent diabetes mellitus. N Engl J Med 1989; 320(9): 550–554.

55. Pozzilli P, Andreani D. The potential role of nicotinamide in the secondary prevention of IDDM. Diabetes Metab Rev 1993; 9(3):219–230.

56. Kolb H, Burkart V. Nicotinamide in type 1 diabetes. Mechanism of action revisited. Diabetes Care 1999; 22(suppl 2):B16–B20.

57. Elliott RB, Pilcher CC, Fergusson DM, Stewart AW. A population based strategy to prevent insulin-dependent diabetes using nicotinamide. J Pediatr Endocrinol Metab 1996; 9(5): 501–509.

58. Elliott RB, Chase HP. Prevention or delay of type 1 (insulin-dependent) diabetes mellitus in children using nicotinamide. Diabetologia 1991; 34(5):362–365.

59. Gale EA, Bingley PJ, Emmett CL, Collier T. European Nicotinamide Diabetes Intervention Trial (ENDIT): a randomised controlled trial of intervention before the onset of type 1 diabetes. Lancet 2004; 363(9413):925–931.

60. Keller RJ, Eisenbarth GS, Jackson RA. Insulin prophylaxis in individuals at high risk of type I diabetes. Lancet 1993; 341(8850):927–928.

61. Diabetes Prevention Trial–Type 1 Diabetes Study Group. Effects of insulin in relatives of patients with type 1 diabetes mellitus. N Engl J Med 2002; 346(22):1685–1691.

62. Skyler JS, Krischer JP, Wolfsdorf J, et al. Effects of oral insulin in relatives of patients with type 1 diabetes: The Diabetes Prevention Trial-Type 1. Diabetes Care 2005; 28(5):1068–1076.

63. Julius MC, Schatz DA, Silverstein JH. The prevention of type I diabetes mellitus. Pediatr Ann 1999; 28(9):585–588.

64. Mallare JT, Cordice CC, Ryan BA, Carey DE, Kreitzer PM, Frank GR. Identifying risk factors for the development of diabetic ketoacidosis in new onset type 1 diabetes mellitus. Clin Pediatr (Phila) 2003; 42(7):591–597.

65. Chernow B, Rainey TG, Heller R, Clapper M, Labow J. Marked stress hyperglycemia in a child. Crit Care Med 1982; 10(10):696–697.

66. Pandit MK, Burke J, Gustafson AB, Minocha A, Peiris AN. Drug-induced disorders of glucose tolerance. Ann Intern Med 1993; 118(7):529–539.

67. Henriksen JE, Alford F, Ward GM, Beck-Nielsen H. Risk and mechanism of dexamethasone-induced deterioration of glucose tolerance in non-diabetic first-degree relatives of NIDDM patients. Diabetologia 1997; 40(12):1439–1448.

68. Writing Team for the Diabetes Control and Complications Trial/Epidemiology of Diabetes Interventions and Complications Research Group. Effect of intensive therapy on the microvascular complications of type 1 diabetes mellitus. JAMA 2002; 287(19):2563–2569.

69. Sonksen PH, Judd SL, Lowy C. Home monitoring of blood-glucose. Method for improving diabetic control. Lancet 1978; 1(8067):729–732.

70. Rosenbloom A, Silverstein JH, Riley WJ, et al. Total glycosylated hemoglobin estimation in the management of children and youth with diabetes. Bull Int Study Group Diabetes Child Adolesc 1980; 4:24–25.

71. Davis S, Alonso MD. Hypoglycemia as a barrier to glycemic control. J Diabetes Complications 2004; 18(1):60–68.

72. Rosenbloom A, Frias, JL. Diabetes mellitus, short stature, and joint stiffness—a new syndrome. Clin Res 1974; 22:92A.

73. Grgic A, Rosenbloom AL, Weber FT, Giordano B, Malone JI, Shuster JJ. Joint contracture—common manifestation of childhood diabetes mellitus. J Pediatr 1976; 88(4 Pt 1): 584–588.

74. Rosenbloom AL. Limited joint mobility in insulin dependent childhood diabetes. Eur J Pediatr 1990; 149(6): 380–388.

75. Rosenbloom AL, Silverstein JH, Lezotte DC, Richardson K, McCallum M. Limited joint mobility in childhood diabetes mellitus indicates increased risk for microvascular disease. N Engl J Med 1981; 305(4):191–194.

76. Infante JR, Rosenbloom AL, Silverstein JH, Garzarella L, Pollock BH. Changes in frequency and severity of limited joint mobility in children with type 1 diabetes mellitus between 1976–78 and 1998. J Pediatr 2001; 138(1):33–37.

77. Verrotti A, Chiarelli F, Amerio P, Morgese G. Necrobiosis lipoidica diabeticorum in children and adolescents: a clue

for underlying renal and retinal disease. Pediatr Dermatol 1995; 12(3):220–223.

78. Kelly WF, Nicholas J, Adams J, Mahmood R. Necrobiosis lipoidica diabeticorum: association with background retinopathy, smoking, and proteinuria. A case controlled study. Diabet Med 1993; 10(8):725–728.

79. Raile K, Noelle V, Landgraf R, Schwarz HP. Insulin antibodies are associated with lipoatrophy but also with lipohypertrophy in children and adolescents with type 1 diabetes. Exp Clin Endocrinol Diabetes 2001; 109(8): 393–396.

80. Arranz A, Andia V, Lopez-Guzman A. A case of lipoatrophy with Lispro insulin without insulin pump therapy. Diabetes Care 2004; 27(2):625–626.

81. Griffin ME, Feder A, Tamborlane WV. Lipoatrophy associated with lispro insulin in insulin pump therapy: an old complication, a new cause. Diabetes Care 2001; 24(1):174.

82. Roper NA, Bilous RW. Resolution of lipohypertrophy following change of short-acting insulin to insulin lispro (Humalog). Diabet Med 1998; 15(12):1063–1064.

83. Kordonouri O, Lauterborn R, Deiss D. Lipohypertrophy in young patients with type 1 diabetes. Diabetes Care 2002; 25(3):634.

84. Young RJ, Hannan WJ, Frier BM, Steel JM, Duncan LJ. Diabetic lipohypertrophy delays insulin absorption. Diabetes Care 1984; 7(5):479–480.

85. Lang-Muritano M, La Roche GR, Stevens JL, Gloor BR, Schoenle EJ. Acute cataracts in newly diagnosed IDDM in five children and adolescents. Diabetes Care 1995; 18(10):1395–1396.

86. Tattersall RB, Pyke DA. Growth in diabetic children. Studies in identical twins. Lancet 1973; 2(7838):1105–1109.

87. Kanumakala S, Dabadghao P, Carlin JB, Vidmar S, Cameron FJ. Linear growth and height outcomes in children with early onset type 1 diabetes mellitus—a 10-yr longitudinal study. Pediatr Diabetes 2002; 3(4):189–193.

88. Lebl J, Schober E, Zidek T, et al. Growth data in large series of 587 children and adolescents with type 1 diabetes mellitus. Endocr Regul 2003; 37(3):153–161.

89. Menon RK, Arslanian S, May B, Cutfield WS, Sperling MA. Diminished growth hormone-binding protein in children with insulin-dependent diabetes mellitus. J Clin Endocrinol Metab 1992; 74(4):934–938.

90. Massa G, Dooms L, Bouillon R, Vanderschueren-Lodeweyckx M. Serum levels of growth hormone-binding protein and insulin-like growth factor I in children and adolescents with type 1 (insulin-dependent) diabetes mellitus. Diabetologia 1993; 36(3):239–243.

91. Munoz MT, Barrios V, Pozo J, Argente J. Insulin-like growth factor I, its binding proteins 1 and 3, and growth hormone-binding protein in children and adolescents with insulin-dependent diabetes mellitus: clinical implications. Pediatr Res 1996; 39(6):992–998.

92. Bereket A, Lang CH, Wilson TA. Alterations in the growth hormone-insulin-like growth factor axis in insulin dependent diabetes mellitus. Horm Metab Res 1999; 31(2–3): 172–181.

93. Mauriac P. Gros ventre, hepatomegalie, troubles de croissance chez les enfants diabetiques traites depuis plusiers annee par l'insuline. Gaz Hebd Med Bordeaux 1930; 26:402–410.

94. Rosenbloom A, Clark DW. Excessive insulin treatments and the Somogyi effect. In: Pickup J, ed. Difficult Diabetes. Oxford: Blackwell, 1985:103–131.

95. Marble A, White P, Bogan I, Smith R. Enlargement of the liver in diabetic children: I. Its incidence etiology and nature. Arch Intern Med 1938; 62:740–750.

96. Dorchy H, van Vliet G, Toussaint D, Ketelbant-Balasse P, Loeb H. Mauriac syndrome: three cases with retinal angiofluorescein study. Diabetes Metab 1979; 5(3): 195–200.

97. Winter RJ, Phillips LS, Green OC, Traisman HS. Somatomedin activity in the Mauriac syndrome. J Pediatr 1980; 97(4):598–600.

98. Kordonouri O, Klinghammer A, Lang EB, Gruters-Kieslich A, Grabert M, Holl RW. Thyroid autoimmunity in children and adolescents with type 1 diabetes: a multicenter survey. Diabetes Care 2002; 25(8):1346–1350.

99. Silverstein J, Klingensmith G, Copeland K, et al. Care of children and adolescents with type 1 diabetes: a statement of the American Diabetes Association. Diabetes Care 2005; 28(1):186–212.

100. Freemark M, Levitsky LL. Screening for celiac disease in children with type 1 diabetes: two views of the controversy. Diabetes Care 2003; 26(6):1932–1939.

101. Colton P, Olmsted M, Daneman D, Rydall A, Rodin G. Disturbed eating behavior and eating disorders in preteen and early teenage girls with type 1 diabetes: a case-controlled study. Diabetes Care 2004; 27(7):1654–1659.

102. Affenito SG, Adams CH. Are eating disorders more prevalent in females with type 1 diabetes mellitus when the impact of insulin omission is considered? Nutr Rev 2001; 59(6):179–182.

103. Brownlee M. The pathobiology of diabetic complications: a unifying mechanism. Diabetes 2005; 54(6):1615–1625.

104. The Diabetes Control and Complications Trial Research Group. The effect of intensive treatment of diabetes on the development and progression of long-term complications in insulin-dependent diabetes mellitus. N Engl J Med 1993; 329(14):977–986.

105. Writing Team for the Diabetes Control and Complications Trial/Epidemiology of Diabetes Interventions and Complications Research Group. Sustained effect of intensive treatment of type 1 diabetes mellitus on development and progression of diabetic nephropathy: the Epidemiology of Diabetes Interventions and Complications (EDIC) study. JAMA 2003; 290(16):2159–2167.

106. Greene DA, Lattimer SA, Sima AA. Sorbitol, phosphoinositides, and sodium-potassium-ATPase in the pathogenesis of diabetic complications. N Engl J Med 1987; 316(10): 599–606.

107. Lee P, Jenkins A, Bourke C, et al. Prothrombotic and antithrombotic factors are elevated in patients with type 1 diabetes complicated by microalbuminuria. Diabet Med 1993; 10(2):122–128.

108. Viberti GC, Hill RD, Jarrett RJ, Argyropoulos A, Mahmud U, Keen H. Microalbuminuria as a predictor of clinical nephropathy in insulin-dependent diabetes mellitus. Lancet 1982; 1(8287):1430–1432.

109. Chaturvedi N, Bandinelli S, Mangili R, Penno G, Rottiers RE, Fuller JH. Microalbuminuria in type 1 diabetes: rates, risk factors and glycemic threshold. Kidney Int 2001; 60(1):219–227.

110. Twyman S, Rowe D, Mansell P, Schapira D, Betts P, Leatherdale B. Longitudinal study of urinary albumin excretion in young diabetic patients—Wessex Diabetic Nephropathy Project. Diabet Med 2001; 18(5):402–408.

111. Santilli F, Spagnoli A, Mohn A, et al. Increased vascular endothelial growth factor serum concentrations may help to identify patients with onset of type 1 diabetes during childhood at risk for developing persistent microalbuminuria. J Clin Endocrinol Metab 2001; 86(8):3871–3876.

112. Olsen BS, Sjolie A, Hougaard P, et al. A 6-year nationwide cohort study of glycaemic control in young people with type 1 diabetes. Risk markers for the development of

retinopathy, nephropathy and neuropathy. Danish Study Group of Diabetes in Childhood. J Diabetes Complications 2000; 14(6):295–300.

113. Levy-Marchal C, Sahler C, Cahane M, Czernichow P. Risk factors for microalbuminuria in children and adolescents with type 1 diabetes. J Pediatr Endocrinol Metab 2000; 13(6):613–620.

114. Warram JH, Scott LJ, Hanna LS, et al. Progression of microalbuminuria to proteinuria in type 1 diabetes: non-linear relationship with hyperglycemia. Diabetes 2000; 49(1):94–100.

115. Orchard TJ, Forrest KY, Kuller LH, Becker DJ. Lipid and blood pressure treatment goals for type 1 diabetes: 10-year incidence data from the Pittsburgh Epidemiology of Diabetes Complications Study. Diabetes Care 2001; 24(6):1053–1059.

116. Chiarelli F, Pomilio M, Mohn A, et al. Homocysteine levels during fasting and after methionine loading in adolescents with diabetic retinopathy and nephropathy. J Pediatr 2000; 137(3):386–392.

117. Kong A, Donath S, Harper CA, Werther GA, Cameron FJ. Rates of diabetes mellitus-related complications in a contemporary adolescent cohort. J Pediatr Endocrinol Metab 2005; 18(3):247–255.

118. Nordwall M, Bojestig M, Arnqvist HJ, Ludvigsson J. Declining incidence of severe retinopathy and persisting decrease of nephropathy in an unselected population of Type 1 diabetes—the Linkoping Diabetes Complications Study. Diabetologia 2004; 47(7):1266–1272.

119. UK Prospective Diabetes Study Group. Tight blood pressure control and risk of macrovascular and microvascular complications in type 2 diabetes: UKPDS 38. BMJ 1998; 317(7160):703–713.

120. Dahlquist G, Rudberg S. The prevalence of microalbuminuria in diabetic children and adolescents and its relation to puberty. Acta Paediatr Scand 1987; 76(5):795–800.

121. Joner G, Brinchmann-Hansen O, Torres CG, Hanssen KF. A nationwide cross-sectional study of retinopathy and microalbuminuria in young Norwegian type 1 (insulin-dependent) diabetic patients. Diabetologia 1992; 35(11): 1049–1054.

122. Mortensen HB, Marinelli K, Norgaard K, et al. A nation-wide cross-sectional study of urinary albumin excretion rate, arterial blood pressure and blood glucose control in Danish children with type 1 diabetes mellitus. Danish Study Group of Diabetes in Childhood. Diabet Med 1990; 7(10):887–897.

123. Mathiesen ER, Ronn B, Jensen T, Storm B, Deckert T. Relationship between blood pressure and urinary albumin excretion in development of microalbuminuria. Diabetes 1990; 39(2):245–249.

124. Mathiesen ER, Hommel E, Giese J, Parving HH. Efficacy of captopril in postponing nephropathy in normotensive insulin dependent diabetic patients with microalbuminuria. BMJ 1991; 303(6794):81–87.

125. Walker JD, Bending JJ, Dodds RA, et al. Restriction of dietary protein and progression of renal failure in diabetic nephropathy. Lancet 1989; 2(8677):1411–1415.

126. Pedrini MT, Levey AS, Lau J, Chalmers TC, Wang PH. The effect of dietary protein restriction on the progression of diabetic and nondiabetic renal diseases: a meta-analysis. Ann Intern Med 1996; 124(7):627–632.

127. Sawicki PT, Didjurgeit U, Muhlhauser I, Bender R, Heinemann L, Berger M. Smoking is associated with progression of diabetic nephropathy. Diabetes Care 1994; 17(2):126–131.

128. Kohner EM, Hamilton AM, Saunders SJ, Sutcliffe BA, Bulpitt CJ. The retinal blood flow in diabetes. Diabetologia 1975; 11(1):27–33.

129. Rosenbloom AL, Malone JI, Yucha J, Van Cader TC. Limited joint mobility and diabetic retinopathy demonstrated by fluorescein angiography. Eur J Pediatr 1984; 141(3):163–164.

130. Lovestam-Adrian M, Agardh CD, Torffvit O, Agardh E. Diabetic retinopathy, visual acuity, and medical risk indicators: a continuous 10-year follow-up study in Type 1 diabetic patients under routine care. J Diabetes Complications 2001; 15(6):287–294.

131. Chaturvedi N, Sjoelie AK, Porta M, et al. Markers of insulin resistance are strong risk factors for retinopathy incidence in type 1 diabetes. Diabetes Care 2001; 24(2): 284–289.

132. Roy MS, Sponer R, Fjeldsa J. Molecular systematics and evolutionary history of kalats (genus *Sheppardia*): a pre-Pleistocene radiation in a group of African forest birds. Mol Phylogenet Evol 2001; 18(1):74–83.

133. Roy MS. Diabetic retinopathy in African Americans with type 1 diabetes: The New Jersey 725: I. Methodology, population, frequency of retinopathy, and visual impairment. Arch Ophthalmol 2000; 118(1):97–104.

134. Roy MS. Eye care in African Americans with type 1 diabetes: the New Jersey 725. Ophthalmology 2004; 111(5): 914–920.

135. Maguire A, Chan A, Cusumano J, et al. The case for biennial retinopathy screening in children and adolescents. Diabetes Care 2005; 28(3):509–513.

136. Chaturvedi N, Sjolie AK, Stephenson JM, et al. Effect of lisinopril on progression of retinopathy in normotensive people with type 1 diabetes. The EUCLID Study Group. EURODIAB Controlled Trial of Lisinopril in Insulin-Dependent Diabetes Mellitus. Lancet 1998; 351(9095): 28–31.

137. The Diabetic Retinopathy Study Research Group. Photocoagulation treatment of proliferative diabetic retinopathy: the second report of diabetic retinopathy study findings. Ophthalmology 1978; 85(1):82–106.

138. Tesfaye S, Chaturvedi N, Eaton SE, et al. Vascular risk factors and diabetic neuropathy. N Engl J Med 2005; 352(4): 341–350.

139. Maser RE, Steenkiste AR, Dorman JS, et al. Epidemiological correlates of diabetic neuropathy. Report from Pittsburgh Epidemiology of Diabetes Complications Study. Diabetes 1989; 38(11):1456–1461.

140. Kaar ML, Saukkonen AL, Pitkanen M, Akerblom HK. Peripheral neuropathy in diabetic children and adolescents. A cross-sectional study. Acta Paediatr Scand 1983; 72(3):373–378.

141. Starkman HS, Gleason RE, Rand LI, Miller DE, Soeldner JS. Limited joint mobility (LJM) of the hand in patients with diabetes mellitus: relation to chronic complications. Ann Rheum Dis 1986; 45(2):130–135.

142. White NH, Cleary PA, Dahms W, Goldstein D, Malone J, Tamborlane WV. Beneficial effects of intensive therapy of diabetes during adolescence: outcomes after the conclusion of the Diabetes Control and Complications Trial (DCCT). J Pediatr 2001; 139(6):804–812.

143. Reid B, DiLorenzo C, Travis L, Flores AF, Grill BB, Hyman PE. Diabetic gastroparesis due to postprandial antral hypomotility in childhood. Pediatrics 1992; 90 (1 Pt 1): 43–46.

144. White NH, Waltman SR, Krupin T, Santiago JV. Reversal of neuropathic and gastrointestinal complications related to diabetes mellitus in adolescents with improved metabolic control. J Pediatr 1981; 99(1):41–45.

145. Maser RE, Lenhard MJ. Cardiovascular autonomic neuropathy due to diabetes mellitus: clinical manifestations, consequences, and treatment. J Clin Endocrinol Metab 2005.

146. Laing SP, Swerdlow AJ, Slater SD, et al. Mortality from heart disease in a cohort of 23,000 patients with insulin-treated diabetes. Diabetologia 2003; 46(6): 760–765.

147. Laing SP, Swerdlow AJ, Slater SD, et al. The British Diabetic Association Cohort Study, I: all-cause mortality in patients with insulin-treated diabetes mellitus. Diabet Med 1999; 16(6):459–465.

148. Jarvisalo MJ, Raitakari M, Toikka JO, et al. Endothelial dysfunction and increased arterial intima-media thickness in children with type 1 diabetes. Circulation 2004; 109(14): 1750–1755.

149. Krolewski AS, Kosinski EJ, Warram JH, et al. Magnitude and determinants of coronary artery disease in juvenile-onset, insulin-dependent diabetes mellitus. Am J Cardiol 1987; 59(8):750–755.

150. Dahl-Jorgensen K, Larsen JR, Hanssen KF. Atherosclerosis in childhood and adolescent type 1 diabetes: early disease, early treatment? Diabetologia 2005.

151. McGill HC Jr., McMahan CA. Determinants of atherosclerosis in the young. Pathobiological Determinants of Atherosclerosis in Youth (PDAY) Research Group. Am J Cardiol 1998; 82(10B):30T–36T.

152. Berenson GS, Srinivasan SR, Bao W, Newman WP III, Tracy RE, Wattigney WA. Association between multiple cardiovascular risk factors and atherosclerosis in children and young adults. The Bogalusa Heart Study. N Engl J Med 1998; 338(23):1650–1656.

153. Haller MJ, Samyn M, Nichols WW, et al. Radial artery tonometry demonstrates arterial stiffness in children with type 1 diabetes. Diabetes Care 2004; 27(12):2911–2917.

154. Ceriello A. Endothelial cell dysfunction. Int Diabetes Monit 2005; 17(3):8–15.

155. Sarman B, Farkas K, Toth M, Somogyi A, Tulassay Z. Circulating plasma endothelin-1, plasma lipids and complications in Type 1 diabetes mellitus. Diabetes Nutr Metab 2000; 13(3):142–148.

156. Hope SA, Tay DB, Meredith IT, Cameron JD. Use of arterial transfer functions for the derivation of central aortic waveform characteristics in subjects with type 2 diabetes and cardiovascular disease. Diabetes Care 2004; 27(3):746–751.

157. Bauriedel G, Skowasch D, Schneider M, Andrie R, Jabs A, Luderitz B. Antiplatelet effects of angiotensin-converting enzyme inhibitors compared with aspirin and clopidogrel: a pilot study with whole-blood aggregometry. Am Heart J 2003; 145(2):343–348.

158. Nathan D. Effects of intensive diabetes management on cardiovascular events in DCCT/EPIC. In: 65th Annual American Diabetes Association Meeting, San Diego, CA, 2005.

159. Standards of Medical Care in Diabetes. Diabetes Care 2005; 28(suppl 1):S4–S36.

160. Ong HT. The statin studies: from targeting hypercholesterolaemia to targeting the high-risk patient. QJM 2005; 98(8):599–614.

161. McCrindle BW, Helden E, Cullen-Dean G, Conner WT. A randomized crossover trial of combination pharmacologic therapy in children with familial hyperlipidemia. Pediatr Res 2002; 51(6):715–721.

162. Adler AI, Stratton IM, Neil HA, et al. Association of systolic blood pressure with macrovascular and microvascular complications of type 2 diabetes (UKPDS 36): prospective observational study. BMJ 2000; 321(7258): 412–419.

163. Hansson L, Zanchetti A, Carruthers SG, et al. Effects of intensive blood-pressure lowering and low-dose aspirin in patients with hypertension: principal results of the Hypertension Optimal Treatment (HOT) randomised trial. HOT Study Group. Lancet 1998; 351(9118):1755–1762.

5

Diabetes Autoimmunity

William E. Winter

Department of Pathology, Immunology and Laboratory Medicine, University of Florida, Gainesville, Florida, U.S.A.

AUTOIMMUNITY TO THE PANCREATIC ISLETS
T1DM Classification of Diabetes Mellitus

In 1997, the American Diabetes Association (1) reclassified diabetes mellitus according to etiology into four major forms: Type 1, Type 2, other specific type of diabetes, and gestational diabetes mellitus (GDM). Therefore, the term Type 1 diabetes mellitus (T1DM) replaced the term insulin-dependent diabetes mellitus. Type 1 diabetes is insulinopenic diabetes that results from autoimmune beta cell destruction (Type 1A diabetes) or whose cause is unknown, but is believed most often to result from viral infection of the beta cells (Type 1B diabetes). In the remainder of this chapter, Type 1A diabetes will be referred to simply as Type 1 diabetes. Type 1 diabetes is an element of two immunoendocrinopathy syndromes: autoimmune polyglandular syndrome Type 2 (Vol. 1; Chap. 9) and the immunodysregulation, polyendocrinopathy, enteropathy, X-linked (IPEX) syndrome. Besides early-onset T1DM, disorders in the IPEX syndrome include severe enteropathy, eczema, anemia, thrombocytopenia, and hypothyroidism. The condition is usually lethal in infancy or childhood. Forkhead box P3 mutations (FoxP3) cause IPEX (2).

Non-insulin-dependent diabetes mellitus was reclassified in 1997 as Type 2 diabetes that results from insulin resistance in combination with relative insulinopenic beta cell failure. Other specific types of diabetes are forms of diabetes previously classified as secondary. These disorders include genetic defects of the beta cell (3–5), genetic defects in insulin action, diseases of the exocrine pancreas (6,7), endocrinopathies, drug- or chemical-induced diabetes (8,9), infections (10–12), uncommon forms of immune-mediated diabetes (13,14) and other genetic syndromes sometimes associated with diabetes. GDM is defined as diabetes that is first detected during pregnancy. The pathophysiology of GDM is similar to that of Type 2 diabetes. GDM usually resolves following delivery; however, women with GDM are at high risk of developing Type 2 diabetes later in life.

Clinical Impact of Type 1 Diabetes

Type 1 diabetes is a major clinical problem in both children and adults. Approximately 1:500 Caucasian people in Europe and North America are affected with Type 1 diabetes (15). Because of its high morbidity and mortality, it can be argued that jointly, Types 1 and 2 diabetes are the most significant endocrine disorders affecting Westernized populations. A variety of other disorders of carbohydrate metabolism result from autoimmune perturbations (Table 1). Type B insulin resistance, hypoglycemia resulting from insulinomimetic autoantibodies, and autoimmune hypoglycemia are discussed in Vol. 1; Chap. 15. These conditions singly and even collectively are all far less common than Type 1 diabetes.

Before the introduction of rigorous glycemic control as the standard-of-care as determined from the results of the Diabetes Control and Complications Trial (DCCT) (16), the expected lifespan from the time of diagnosis of Type 1 diabetes was otherwise reduced by one-third. For example if the normal life expectancy of a 10-year child was to age 70 with 60 more years of life expected, in Type 1 diabetes the expected lifespan would be reduced to age 50. Microvascular complications (retinopathy and nephropathy) are major causes of morbidity and mortality in Type 1 diabetes. Premature macrovascular disease (coronary artery, carotid artery, and peripheral vascular disease) and neuropathy are also major contributors to morbidity and mortality (Vol. 1; Chaps. 4, 6, and 11). The leading causes of premature death in Type 1 diabetes are coronary artery disease followed by renal failure. Hopefully with better diabetes management, these grim statistics can be avoided and revised. Tight glycemic control is also important in Type 2 diabetes for the avoidance of microvascular complications as illustrated by the results of the United Kingdom Prospective Diabetes Study (17). Follow up of the DCCT tight-control participants demonstrates continued benefit in the avoidance of microvascular and neuropathic complications (18) and lower rates of macrovascular disease (19).

Table 1 Autoimmune Disorders Involving Carbohydrate Metabolism

Type 1 diabetes
Type B insulin resistance
Hypoglycemia resulting from insulinomimetic autoantibodies
Autoimmune hypoglycemia

ETIOPATHOGENESIS

The majority of cases of Type 1 diabetes result from a cell-mediated autoimmune process that selectively destroys the pancreatic beta cells (e.g., Type 1A diabetes) (20–22). Both CD8 T cells and macrophages are believed to be responsible for beta cell necrosis. Islet cell autoimmunity can develop very early in life (23). It has been reported to develop prenatally (24) and is transferable by bone marrow transplantation (25). Roles for T helper Type 1 (Th1) and Th2 cells have been implicated (26).

Multiple lines of evidence support an autoimmune basis for Type 1 diabetes. In patients dying within six months of diagnosis of Type 1 diabetes, 60% to approximately 90% have pancreatic insulitis (27–29). Insulitis is the histological description of lymphocytic infiltration of the pancreatic islets with destruction of the beta cells and depletion in insulin content detected by immunohistochemistry. Both Biobreeding (BB) rats and nonobese diabetic (NOD) mice display insulitis (30). With increasing duration of the disease, there is progressive disappearance of pancreatic beta cells. Non-beta cells (alpha, gamma, and pancreatic polypeptide cells) are not subject to autoimmune targeting or permanent damage. Destroyed islets are depleted of beta cells yet alpha cells persist. The beta cell most likely carries antigens unique to insulin-producing cells not expressed in other islet cell types. Of the major antigens so far discovered that are targeted in Type 1 diabetes [e.g., glutamic acid decarboxylase (GAD), insulinoma-associated antigen 2 (IA-2), and islet sialoglycoconjugate], only insulin appears to be highly beta cell-specific (31).

In both animal models of Type 1 diabetes, the BB rat (32) and the NOD mouse (33,34), Type 1 diabetes can be transferred with lymphocytes from the spleens of acutely diabetic animals to nondiabetic animals. On the other hand, Type 1 diabetes cannot be transferred with serum. In NOD mice, CD4 T cells are specifically able to transfer Type 1 diabetes (35). NOD mice lacking B cells still develop Type 1 diabetes, further emphasizing the pivotal role of CD4 T cells in the pathogenesis of Type 1 diabetes (36). There is also a case report of Type 1 diabetes developing in a child with agammaglobulinemia, indicating that neither B cells nor antibody are necessary for the pathogenesis of Type 1 diabetes in humans (37). In pregnant women with Type 1 diabetes who express islet autoantibodies being of the immunoglobulin G (IgG) class (e.g., isotype), these autoantibodies do cross the placenta and are detectable in the blood stream but do not affect the carbohydrate metabolism in the newborn (38).

This provides in vivo human evidence that islet autoantibodies by themselves do not cause beta cell damage or destruction.

NATURAL HISTORY OF TYPE 1 DIABETES

The natural history of Type 1 diabetes can be schematized into a number of stages (Fig. 1). In Stage 1, where beta cell mass and function are normal, individuals who carry genetic susceptibility alleles to Type 1 diabetes suffer exposure to an environmental stimulus triggering islet inflammation (insulitis). The presumed release of sequestered or altered self-antigens explains, at least in part, the later development of islet autoantibodies that mark the recognition of Stage 2. In the absence of islet autoantibodies and any clinical evidence of beta cell dysfunction, insulitis is silent. Only a minority of genetically susceptible individuals develop islet autoantibodies and eventual T1DM. Thus in the natural history of Type 1 diabetes, a subset of autoantibody-positive individuals progress through varying stages of glucose intolerance to clinical diabetes (39).

In Stage 2, there is now serological evidence of humoral (and/or cell-mediated) autoimmunity [i.e., islet cell cytoplasmic autoantibodies (ICA), glutamic acid decarboxylase autoantibodies (GADA), insulinoma-2-associated autoantibodies (IA-2A), or

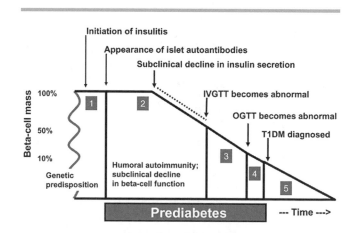

Figure 1 The natural history of Type 1 diabetes can be schematized into a number of stages. In Stage 1, where beta cell mass and function are normal, individuals who carry genetic susceptibility alleles to Type 1 diabetes suffer exposure to an environmental stimulus triggering islet inflammation (insulitis). The development of islet autoantibodies marks the recognition of Stage 2. During this stage, there is an approximate 50% decline in beta cell mass without detectable abnormalities by any form of glucose tolerance testing. The earliest functional beta cell abnormality that can be detected (Stage 3) is a decline in first-phase insulin response to intravenously administered glucose. Later intolerance to oral glucose challenges appears (Stage 4). After one to two years of glucose intolerance upon oral testing, a typical history of polyuria, polydipsia, and possible weight loss is identified heralding the diagnosis of diabetes (Stage 5). *Abbreviations*: IVGTT, intravenous glucose tolerance test; OGTT, oral glucose tolerance test; T1DM, Type 1 diabetes mellitus.

insulin autoantibodies (IAA)] without clinically detectable metabolic perturbations. However during this stage, there can be a 50% decline in beta cell mass without detectable abnormalities by any form of glucose tolerance testing. The earliest functional beta cell abnormality that can be detected (Stage 3) is a decline in first-phase insulin response to intravenously administered glucose at time 1 plus three minutes (40,41). Later, intolerance to oral glucose challenges appears. When there is glucose intolerance Stage 4 is reached. After one to two years of glucose intolerance upon oral testing, a typical history of polyuria, polydipsia, and possible weight loss is identified. Finally, with such frank hyperglycemia, diabetes is clinically diagnosed in Stage 5. Diabetic ketoacidosis may occur if the diagnosis of diabetes is delayed.

GENETICS OF TYPE 1 DIABETES

Susceptibility to Type 1 diabetes can be inherited although most cases (approximately 85%) of Type 1 diabetes occur sporadically (e.g., in the absence of an affected first-degree relative). Whereas the general population frequency of Type 1 diabetes in the United States is approximately 1:500 (0.2% of the population affected), siblings of Type 1 diabetes patients experience a 40-fold higher risk of developing Type 1 diabetes (e.g., 1:20 or 5% affected). Likewise offspring of a Type 1 diabetes father or mother are also at increased risk, respectively, 1 in 14 (7%; 35-fold increased risk) and 1 in 50 (2%; 10-fold increased risk). Ethnicity greatly influences risk for Type 1 diabetes. Finns experience the highest risk in the world (1:100) while peoples of China and Japan suffer the lowest risk for Type 1 diabetes worldwide (1:10,000) (42). Risks for Type 1 diabetes in Caucasian North Americans and Southern Europeans are lower than in Scandinavians being 1 in 500 as described above. Type 1 diabetes in African-Americans is approximately half as common as in Caucasians that is being approximately 1 in 1000.

HLA Susceptibility to Type 1 Diabetes

Inheritance of susceptibility to Type 1 diabetes is not Mendelian but instead is multifactorial and polygenic. Clearly no single gene allele is always associated with Type 1 diabetes nor are unique DNA sequences observed in Type 1 diabetes subjects (43). The association of specific human leukocyte antigen (HLA)-loci and Type 1 diabetes was first recognized in the 1970s for HLA-B alleles and then, more powerfully associated with DR alleles in the late 1970s and early 1980s. In the mid to late 1980s, the predominant role of HLA-DQB1 and A1 alleles was discovered in providing proclivity to Type 1 diabetes.

In studies from the University of Florida involving more than 1000 individuals with Type 1 diabetes, approximately 95% express at least one HLA-DR3 and/or DR4 allele. Compared with a general population frequency of approximately 3%, approximately 40% of Type 1 diabetes patients are heterozygous for HLA-DR3 and DR4. After DR3/DR4 heterozygotes, DR4 homozygosity is the next highest risk genotype followed by DR3 homozygotes and DR4/DRX heterozygotes (X = non-DR3/DR4 allele). Only 5% of Type 1 diabetes patients lack both HLA-DR3 and DR4. In individuals with HLA-DR3 or DR4, the second antigen excluding DR3 and DR4, is most commonly DR1. DR2 and DR5 are usually protective of Type 1 diabetes (44).

In contrast to the data in Caucasians, in African-Americans with Type 1 diabetes only 70% have a HLA-DR3 and/or DR4 allele suggesting greater heterogeneity of etiology of youth-onset diabetes in African-Americans than in Caucasians (45). In African-Americans, while HLA-DR4 is associated with Type 1 diabetes, DR3 is not. Thirty percent of African-Americans with youth-onset diabetes lack both DR3 and DR4 alleles. Islet cell cytoplasmic autoantibody frequencies at diabetes onset in African-Americans are also considerably lower than in Caucasians (40% in African-Americans vs. approximately 75% in Caucasian Americans) thus providing further evidence of etiological heterogeneity.

Using recombinant DNA methodologies, the serological DQw3 antigen associated with DR4 has been divided by analysis of DR4-related DQ beta genes (DQw3) into Type 1 diabetes-susceptible (DQB1*0302) and Type 1 diabetes-resistant or neutral (DQB1*0301 and DQB1*0303) Type 1-diabetes-risk subtypes (46). The susceptibility to Type 1 diabetes is inherited, at least in part, by way of inheritance of DQA1*0501–DQB1*0201 (associated with DR3) and DQA1*0301–DQB1*0302 (associated with DR4) or closely linked alleles (47). Individuals heterozygous for DQA1*0501–DQB1*0201/DQA1*0301–DQB1*0302 can have a 32-fold increased risk for Type 1 diabetes, which would be an absolute risk of approximately 6.4% risk based on a general population frequency of Type 1 diabetes of 1 in 500.

HLA-DQB1*0602 is highly protective of Type 1 diabetes with only 1 in 15,000 persons carrying this allele developing Type 1 diabetes (48). HLA-DQB1*0602 is also protective of Type 1 diabetes in subjects with autoimmune polyglandular syndrome Type 1 (49). The DR4 molecular split DR*0403 is also highly protective of the development of Type 1 diabetes.

For the DQB1 alleles associated with Type 1 diabetes at position 57 of the beta chain, there are nonaspartic acid residues (e.g., serine, valine, and alanine) as opposed to Type 1 diabetes-resistance alleles where aspartic acid is present (50). This amino acid difference alters the class II major histocompatibility complex (MHC) antigen-binding cleft and thus appears to influence which antigen-peptides are presented (51). Many studies have associated nonaspartic acid alleles with Type 1 diabetes susceptibility (52). Arginine at position 52 in the DQ alpha chain has also been related to Type 1 diabetes susceptibility (53). A combination of these DQA1 and DQB1 alleles (particularly in the *trans* configuration) further increases risk for Type 1 diabetes (54).

The DR2 and DR5 diabetes-resistance alleles associated DQA1–DQB1 haplotypes are, respectively, DQA1∗0102–DQB1∗0602 and DQA1∗0501–DQB1∗0301. As opposed to Caucasians and DQB1, in Japanese DQA1 alleles are the MHC susceptibility factors (55). However, Korean and Caucasian Type 1 diabetes subjects display similar HLA susceptibility patterns (56). It has been proposed that variations in population frequencies of DQB1 beta-chain nonaspartic acid alleles correlate with the population frequency of Type 1 diabetes (57). Several excellent overviews of the genetics of Type 1 diabetes have been published (58,59). The influences of various DQ loci are summarized in Table 2.

Studies of multiplex families show that the inheritance of Type 1 diabetes is associated with particular parental haplotypes. In sibling pairs with Type 1 diabetes, instead of the expected random haplotype distribution (25% HLA identical, 50% haploidentical, 25% nonidentical) a predominance of like-haplotypes is found (60% HLA identical, 35% haploidentical, < 5% nonidentical). There is an apparent transmission bias for Type 1 diabetes because approximately 7% of children fathered by Type 1 diabetes men develop Type 1 diabetes as opposed to 2% of the offspring of Type 1 diabetes mothers (60). This is due to the preferential inheritance of a DR4-bearing haplotype from the affected Type 1 diabetes father (70% transmission to offspring vs. expected 50% transmission) (61). In both Type 1 diabetes fathers and mothers, there is transmission bias of DR3 (60% transmission to offspring vs. expected 50% transmission).

Non-HLA Susceptibility to Type 1 Diabetes

Polygenic inheritance of susceptibility to Type 1 diabetes is certain (62). Polymorphisms in at least 14 different genetic loci have been associated with Type 1 diabetes in humans (63–67). The loci have been identified by population studies and sib-pair analysis.

Table 3 Confirmed Susceptibility Loci in Type 1 Diabetes

Locus	Location	Gene(s)
IDDM1	6p21	HLA-DR and DQ
IDDM2	11p15	Insulin
IDDM12	2q33	CTLA-4
	1p13	PTPN22

The loci can be classified according to the certainty with which the data supports a genetic association with Type 1 diabetes. Presently four loci have been confirmed as true susceptibility loci based upon adequately statistically powered studies, often in diverse populations (Table 3) (68). These loci are the MHC, the insulin gene, CTLA-4 (69) and PTPN22 (70). There are many unconfirmed loci: IDDM3 (15q26), IDDM4 (11q13), IDDM5 (6q25), IDDM6 (18q), IDDM7 (2q33), IDDM8 (6q2), IDDM9 (3q), IDDM10 (10p14-q11), IDDM11 (14q24-q31), IDDM13 (2q33), and IDDM15 (6q21). Data supporting IDDM7 (2q33), IDDM15 (6q21), IDDM10 (10p14-q11), and 16q22-q24 as significant diabetes susceptibility loci are increasing (71).

Despite this surfeit of potential loci, the MHC remains the most important susceptibility factor (Table 4) and provides 40% to 50% of genetic susceptibility to Type 1 diabetes as described above. The next most influential gene appears to be the insulin gene and its 5′ hypervariable region (HVR) (72). The insulin gene is located on chromosome 11p15. The gene has three exons separated by two introns: a 179-base pair (bp) intron within the 5′ untranslated region and a 786-bp intron within the coding region of the C-peptide. The order of the insulin chains encoded in the gene is beta chain: C-peptide:alpha chain. Three hundred and sixty-three base pairs upstream of the transcription start site is located the insulin-gene HVR which consists of 14- to 15-bp tandem repeats. This region has also been described as a region of variable numbers of tandem repeats (VNTR). While the number of repeats in HVR alleles in the human population varies greatly, the

Table 2 Relative Influence of HLA-DQ Alleles on Susceptibility to Type 1 Diabetes

DQ alleles				
DQB1	DQA1	Associated HLA-DR	T1DM influence	Relative influence[a]
0602	0102	DR15[b]	Protective	++++
0301	0501	DR5	Protective	+++
0302	0301	DR4	Susceptible	++
0201	0501	DR3	Susceptible	+

[a]Protective alleles are generally dominant over susceptibility alleles.
[b]DR15 is a split of DR2.
Abbreviations: HLA, human leukocyte antigen; T1DM, Type 1 diabetes mellitus.

Table 4 Risk Effect of Specific HLA Alleles for the Development of Type 1 Diabetes

HLA-DRB1	Absolute risk	Relative risk
Within families		
Random sibling risk	1:20	25
Sibling HLA identical to affected sibling	1:7	70
Sibling shares DR3/DR4 with affected sibling	1:4	125
Genetically identical to affected sibling (identical twin)	1:3–1:2	170–250
General population		
Random risk	1:500	1
DR3 (+)	1:400	1.25
DR4 (+)	1:400	1.25
DR3/DR4 (+)	1:40	12.5

Abbreviation: HLA, human leukocyte antigen.

alleles are usually described as class I alleles (approximately 40 repeats; < 600 bp in length; approximately two-thirds of the total allele population), class II alleles (approximately 95 repeats; 600–1600 bp in length; rare alleles), or class III alleles (approximately 170 repeats; > 1600 bp in length; approximately one-third of the total allele population). The class I alleles are associated with the Type 1 and Type 2 diabetes (73) and latent autoimmune diabetes in adults (74). The class I allele may not be expressed in the thymus abundantly, leading to impaired tolerance against insulin (75,76). Other researchers believe that the VNTR alleles may not be the primary susceptibility features of the insulin gene and may in turn be linked to another truly pathogenic focus (77). IDDM2 does not appear to influence susceptibility to other autoimmune disorders (78).

CTLA-4 is an abbreviation for cytotoxic lymphocyte-associated protein 4 or cytotoxic T-lymphocyte-associated serine esterase-4. The normal role of CTLA-4 is in downregulating the immune response. Unactivated T cells do not express CTLA-4 but with T-cell activation, CTLA-4 is expressed. CTLA-4 binds to B7 on antigen-presenting cells with 20 times higher affinity than the CD28:B7 interaction. The interaction of CTLA-4 with B7 impairs further T-cell activation serving to turn off the immune response. It is logical that a mutation or dysregulation of CTLA-4 could predispose to autoimmunity (79). For example, CTLA-4 or genes closely linked to CTLA-4 may influence the development of autoimmune thyroid disease such as Graves disease and Hashimoto thyroiditis (80–84).

The newest confirmed diabetes susceptibility locus is PTPN22 located on chromosome 1p13 that encodes a lymphoid protein tyrosine kinase (85–87). By dephosphorylating and inactivating T-cell receptor-associated Csk kinase, PTPN22 appears to be involved in preventing spontaneous T-cell activation (88). Like CTLA-4, PTPN22 may be involved in many forms of autoimmunity (89).

ENVIRONMENTAL TRIGGERS IN THE PATHOGENESIS OF TYPE 1 DIABETES

Because concordance for Type 1 diabetes in identical twins is only 33% to 50%, environmental factors are thought to play a significant role in triggering Type 1 diabetes (90). Environmental triggers of beta cell autoimmunity under investigation include diet/breast feeding (91), toxins, drugs, immunizations (92), viral infections (93–95), and stress. Suspected toxins include alloxan-like or streptozotocin-like agents that induce oxidant beta cell damage and smoked or cured mutton. Viral infections hypothesized to trigger Type 1 diabetes include coxsackie A, coxsackie B (96), cytomegalovirus, and ECHO virus (97), Epstein–Barr virus, rubella, mumps, and retroviruses. There is no unequivocal evidence to suggest that children should avoid cows' milk products to prevent Type 1 diabetes (98), although cow's milk bovine serum albumin, and

beta-lactoglobulin exposure have been found in various studies to act as diabetogenic influences (99). Immunizations are not associated with the development of Type 1 diabetes. The lay literature has often identified routine immunizations as the cause of many pediatric maladies, yet no proof of this can be found despite exhaustive searches.

Because of the inherent "plasticity" of the genome, especially with respect to T-cell receptor and immunoglobulin gene rearrangements, the supposition that monozygotic twins are immunogenetically identical can be seriously questioned (100). In persons who develop Type 1 diabetes, the relative contributions of genetic and interacting environmental factors appear to be highly variable. Genetic factors may predominate early in life whereas environmental "exposures" may become more important with advancing age. Presumably, once a person is predisposed to Type 1 diabetes by the possession of particular immune response genes (HLA-associated and those outside the MHC) and nonimmune response genes, the proper environmental exposure may trigger or foster the initiation of the autoimmune process. Unfortunately, the triggers to the development of Type 1 diabetes remain largely unknown (101–106).

ISLET AUTOANTIBODIES

In new-onset cases of Type 1 diabetes, 95% or more of individuals will exhibit at least one of the following autoantibodies: ICA, GADA (107), IA-2A (108,109), or IAA (Table 5) (110). The presence of any of these autoantibodies in the setting of diabetes establishes the diagnosis of Type 1 diabetes regardless of the phenotype of the diabetes: insulin-requiring or non-insulin requiring. The presence of the autoantibodies in nondiabetic individuals also predicts the development of Type 1 diabetes (111).

Islet Cell Cytoplasmic Autoantibodies

ICA are detected by indirect immunofluorescence using human blood group O pancreas as substrate. Because ICA react with intracellular antigens of all cells of the pancreatic islets, they are not involved in the pathogenesis of Type 1 diabetes. ICA was the first islet autoantibody assay developed and was first described in 1974 (112). ICA react with GAD, IA-2, and sialoglycoconjugate antigens in the pancreatic islets (113); non-GAD ICA have been reported (114). ICA are polyclonal including both kappa and lambda light chains and all four IgG subclasses (115). Standardization of ICA testing has been accomplished by workshops held under the aegis of the Juvenile

Table 5 Clinically Important Islet Autoantibodies in Type 1 Diabetes

Islet cell cytoplasmic autoantibodies
Glutamic acid decarboxylase autoantibodies
Insulinoma-2-associated autoantibodies
Insulin autoantibodies

Diabetes Foundation (JDF). This lead to the establishment of ICA titers being reported as JDF units.

At the time of diagnosis, 70% to 80% of Caucasian children with Type 1 diabetes have ICA; however, the frequency falls thereafter (116). By five years' duration of Type 1 diabetes, ICA frequency has declined to approximately 25%, and after 10 years, ICA persists in sera in less than 5%. First-degree relatives of Type 1 diabetes patients have a frequency of Type 1 diabetes similar to their ICA frequency (3–5%). In Pasco County, Florida in a study of approximately 10,000 normal school children, ICA were detected in 1 in approximately 250 children (117). The Type 1 Diabetes Prevention Trial (DPT-1) employed ICA testing for the identification of relatives of Type 1 diabetes subjects who were at risk of developing Type 1 diabetes (118,119).

In patients with clinically apparent Type 2 diabetes, some 5% to 15% are ICA-positive (120–122), and with time, these patients tend to progress to insulin dependence. These individuals also express higher frequencies of the Type 1 diabetes-associated HLA-DR alleles DR3 and DR4.

ICA and other islet autoantibodies usually predate the clinical presentation of Type 1 diabetes by months or years (123,124). ICA-positive, nondiabetic patients, evaluated serially by glucose tolerance testing, often show insulinopenia to intravenous glucose injection, while later, rises in fasting and stimulated glucose concentrations occur after oral glucose challenges (39–41,125). Higher titer ICA appear to predict an increased risk for the development of Type 1 diabetes in nondiabetic individuals. Furthermore, newly diagnosed individuals with Type 1 diabetes who have higher ICA titers are at higher risk to more rapidly lose endogenous C-peptide secretion (126). A similar claim has been made for higher titer GADA (127).

Glutamic Acid Decarboxylase Autoantibodies

In 1990, the M_r 64,000 (64 kDa) islet immunoprecipitable autoantigen was shown to be GAD (3). GADA are now detected predominantly by immunoprecipitation of radio-labeled antigen (e.g., a radio-binding assay).

GAD normally converts glutamate to gamma-amino butyric acid (GABA) in the nervous system. GABA is an inhibitory neurotransmitter. GAD is expressed predominantly in the central and peripheral nervous systems but is also expressed in testes, ovary, adrenal, pituitary, thyroid, islets, and kidney (128). Whereas the role of GAD in nervous tissue of converting glutamic acid to GABA is well recognized, the biologic role of GAD in the islets of Langerhans is unclear.

GAD comes in two molecular isoforms that are coded for by separate genes: GAD65 (chromosome 2), M_r approximately 65 kDa and GAD67 (chromosome 10), M_r approximately 67 kDa. GAD65 and GAD67 exhibit approximately 70% amino acid homology. GADA are most commonly directed against GAD65 (129–131).

Varying epitope reactivity for GADA among nondiabetic and diabetic individuals may explain why not all GADA in nondiabetic individuals predict Type 1 diabetes (132).

A primary sequence homology between portions of GAD and the P2-C protein expressed by coxsackie virus has been described (129). GAD cellular autoimmunity has been shown (133). In addition to GAD, cell-mediated immune responses to other islet antigens have been described, such as insulin secretory granule proteins and beta cell membrane antigens (134–136). One group of investigators propose that cellular and humoral GAD reactivity are inversely associated with Type 1 diabetes risk (137). Using the older immunoprecipitation assay, Atkinson et al. (138) showed that 64 kDa autoantibodies were highly predictive of Type 1 diabetes. Since of this initial report, many studies have confirmed that GADA in nondiabetic individuals predict the later development of Type 1 diabetes.

GADA in patients with clinical Type 2 diabetes correlates with insulin deficiency similar to ICA. Because of the attenuated pace of beta cell destruction and older-onset of disease, the term latent-autoimmune diabetes of adulthood (LADA) has been applied to such clinical circumstances (139–142).

Insulinoma-2-Associated Autoantibodies

The most recently identified autoantigen of great clinical importance is a member of the plasma membrane protein tyrosine phosphatase family: IA-2 (108,143,144). Besides the islets, IA-2 is found in other endocrine tissues such as the pituitary gland. Like GAD, the role of IA-2 in islets is controversial.

Similarly to GADA, IA-2A are detected predominantly by radio-immunoprecipitation. The immunoreactivity to the C-terminal portion of IA-2 is most highly associated with Type 1 diabetes. Whereas some IA-2 assays include the entire IA-2 molecule, many assays include only the C-terminal portion of the molecule, e.g., assays for ICA512 autoantibodies or IA-2c autoantibodies. A second transmembrane protein tyrosine phosphatase autoantigen (IA-2β) has been described (145). IA-2 and IA-2β share several common epitopes while other epitopes are unique to each molecule.

Insulin Autoantibodies

The only beta cell-specific autoantigen is insulin whose autoantibodies are detected in the IAA assay (110). IAA are determined by the immunoprecipitation of A-14 mono-iodinated insulin. The enzyme-linked immunosorbent method for the detection of IAA does not correlate with the development of Type 1 diabetes (146,147). Because the IAA assay requires several hundred microliters of serum, a micro-IAA assay has been developed. IAA are found in approximately 40% to 50% of newly diagnosed children with Type 1 diabetes (148). By themselves, IAA do not strongly predict the development of Type 1 diabetes in nondiabetic individuals. However, IAA together with ICA are highly predictive of insu-linopenia and the eventual development of Type 1 diabetes as demonstrated in DPT-1 (148).

Testing for IAA should be carried out before insulin administration is initiated. Insulin-treated patients frequently develop insulin antibodies that cannot be distinguished from IAA by the IAA assay. Insulin antibodies can arise even in individuals treated with human insulin. It is true that insulin antibodies take several days to a week or more to develop in response to exogenous insulin therapy; however in any one patient, the time at which insulin antibodies arise in response to insulin therapy is not known and thus blood for IAA should be drawn prior to the initiation of insulin injections.

Islet Autoantibody Testing

While autoantibodies to many other molecules have been described in Type 1 diabetes [e.g., anticarboxy-peptidase-H autoantibodies (149), 51 kDa aromatic-l-amino-acid decarboxylase autoantibodies (150), chymotrypsinogen-related 30 kDa pancreatic autoanti-bodies (151), DNA topoisomerase II autoantibodies (152), glima 38 autoantibodies (153), GLUT2 auto-antibodies (154), heat shock protein autoantibodies (155; controversial) ICA69 autoantibodies (156,157), insulin receptor autoantibodies (158), islet cell-specific 38 kDa autoantibodies (159,160), islet cell surface auto-antibodies (161,162), proinsulin autoantibodies (163), sex-determining region Y-related protein SOX13 auto-antibodies (164)], these assays are not sufficiently rigorous or the positivity rates sufficiently high to recommend that such assays be employed clinically in addition to ICA, GADA, IA-2A, or IAA.

While certain HLA types are more common in Type 1 diabetes than in controls, such as HLA-DR3, HLA-DR4, HLA-DQB1*0302 and HLA-DQB1*0201, HLA-typing is not diagnostic for Type 1 diabetes because these alleles do occur in the general population (165). As well, there are alleles protective of Type 1 diabetes such as HLA-DR2 and HLA-DQB1*0602; however, the presence of these alleles in any individual cannot be used to exclude Type 1 diabetes.

OTHER IMMUNE ABNORMALITIES IN TYPE 1 DIABETES

When ICA were first discovered, immunofluorescent staining of the islet limited to either glucagon-producing alpha cells or somatostatin-secreting delta cells was described in a minority of sera tested for ICA (166). ICA-positive sera react with all cells of the pancreatic islet. In a University of Florida study, the frequency of alpha-cell autoantibodies was found to be similar in controls and relatives of Type 1 diabetes patients (0.5% vs. 0.6%, respectively).

Subjects with alpha-cell autoantibodies did not display disturbed HLA-DR frequencies in contrast to nondiabetic individuals with ICA that exhibited increased frequencies of HLA-DR3 and DR4. Alpha-cell autoantibodies are apparently rare in Type 1 diabetes patients because alpha-cell autoantibodies were not found in any of 62 ICA-negative Type 1 diabetes patients studied. Biochemically, alpha-cell autoantibodies are not associated with any perturbations in glucagon secretion (167,168). Autoantibodies to the glucagon molecule have also been reported but do not cause disease (169,170).

Besides insulitis and islet autoantibodies (e.g., ICA, IAA, GADA, and IA-2A) a number of other immunological abnormalities have been described in Type 1 diabetes including: elevated levels of Ia (class II MHC) (171,172) and TAC (transferrin receptor)-positive T cells (activated T cells), increased K-cell levels, perturbed numbers or ratios of T-helper/inducer (CD4) and T-cytotoxic/suppressor (CD8) cells, lymphocytotoxic autoantibodies (173), circulating immune complexes (174), decreased IL-2 production by lymphocytes from Type 1 diabetes patients (175), impaired CD4-positive T-lymphocyte function (176), and decreased class I MHC expression (177). In vitro, lymphocytes from Type 1 diabetes patients have been shown to produce migration inhibition factor when exposed to xenogeneic islets or islet homogenates. Lymphocytes in vitro have produced islet adherence (178) and cytolysis and have inhibited insulin release. Variations in antigen-presenting cell function in Type 1 diabetes and prostaglandin synthase-2 expression have been described (179,180).

Further evidence of an autoimmune etiology for Type 1 diabetes is found in the association of Type 1 diabetes with other recognized autoimmune diseases [particularly Hashimoto thyroiditis (181,182) and atrophic gastritis (183,184)], and with disturbed frequencies of particular HLA-DR and DQ types (185). In contrast to many other autoimmune disorders, Type 1 diabetes is equal to or slightly more common in males than females and more commonly presents in childhood than in adult life. Other autoimmune diseases atypically more common in men than women include infantile polyarteritis nodosa and ankylosing spondylitis.

PREDICTION, IMMUNOTHERAPY, AND PREVENTION OF TYPE 1 DIABETES

In studies undertaken largely in the 1980s, immuno-suppression of newly diagnosed Type 1 diabetes patients with cyclosporin, or azathioprine and gluco-corticoids produced short-lived remissions (186–188). Because of the limited success of these trials and the intrinsic toxicities of such immunosuppressive agents, researchers have recently attempted to induce immunologic tolerance to beta cell antigens as a method of preventing Type 1 diabetes (189). The first beta cell antigen to be used in such trials was insulin by subcutaneous injection for high-risk individuals and oral insulin was administered to moderate-risk individuals (190). This was the basis for the DPT-1 study that started in 1993 and recently concluded (118,119). Unfortunately, neither approach was successful in abating the development of Type 1 diabetes. In another smaller study, oral insulin administration begun at disease onset was also ineffective in changing the disease course over the first 12 months following diagnosis (191).

Nasal insulin administration is being attempted in Finland in the Diabetes Prediction and Prevention trial (192,193). In New Zealand (194) and Canada, Texas and Europe (195), nicotinamide was studied as a beta cell selective antioxidant. Similar to the DPT-1 trial, nicotinamide was unfortunately ineffective in preventing diabetes (196). Several papers had previously disputed the concept that nicotinamide would be of benefit in preventing or treating Type I diabetes (197,198).

Recently, Herold and colleagues have had success in partially preserving insulin secretion in new-onset patients with Type 1 diabetes who were treated with an anti-CD3 monoclonal antibody (199,200). The monoclonal antibody is humanized to allow repeated use.

Eventual success in trials to prevent or treat new-onset Type 1 diabetes will revolutionize the management of autoimmune diabetes (201). However, at the present time, such intervention trials are to be considered strictly experimental (202). Islet beta cell and stem cell transplantation is a promising field in beta cell reconstitution (203–207).

PANCREAS, ISLET, AND STEM CELL TRANSPLANTATION

Since the time of the first pancreas transplant in December 1966, diabetologists have sought technologies aimed at restoring beta cell mass. Three general approaches exist: (i) whole or partial pancreas transplantation, (ii) islet transplantation, and (iii) cellular engineering to produce beta cell equivalents.

In certain circumstances pancreas transplantation is now an accepted modality for the treatment of Type 1 diabetes (208). Most pancreas transplants are performed at the time of kidney transplantation with both the kidney and the pancreas coming from the same cadaveric donor. Less commonly, pancreas transplantation is performed following an established kidney transplant. In such cases the kidney and pancreas come from different individuals. Isolated pancreas transplantation can be undertaken when a patient with Type 1 diabetes has frequent, severe hypoglycemia but adequate renal function. As of October 2002, almost 19,000 pancreas transplants had been carried out with about three quarters of these surgeries performed in the United States.

The issue of pancreatic exocrine drainage is significant: using various surgical techniques the exocrine secretions can be drained into the bladder or into the intestine. Technical failure rates vary between approximately 7% and approximately 15% with bladder drainage superior to enteric drainage. Other data favor enteric drainage over bladder drainage (209). The most common reported cause of graft failure is thrombosis. Other complications include pancreatitis and rejection. Whether bladder or enteric drainage is carried out, graft survival rates of 74% to 94% are reported with patient survival rates of 92% to 100%. Living donor pancreas transplants represent only 1 in 200 cases of transplanted individuals.

A successful simultaneous kidney–pancreas transplant improves 7- to 10-year patient survival compared with kidney transplantation alone, simultaneous kidney–pancreas transplant with subsequent pancreatic failure, and dialysis. With a successful pancreas transplant, normal glucose homeostasis can be achieved. Insulin levels are two- to threefold higher than normal when the venous drainage of the pancreas is routed systemically. However if the venous drainage of the pancreas enters the portal vein, insulin concentrations are as expected for glucocorticoid-treated renal transplant patients. Hypoglycemia becomes less pronounced and diminishes in frequency. In the nontransplanted kidney, after five years with a functioning pancreas transplant and reversal of diabetes for that length of time, the pathologic changes of diabetic nephropathy recede. Because diabetic retinopathy may worsen initially following pancreas transplantation, such patients require careful ophthalmologic follow-up. In patients without preexisting retinopathy, retinal surgery is less often needed three or more years after pancreas/kidney transplantation than after kidney transplantation alone. Sensory and autonomic neuropathies improve after pancreas transplantation. There is suggestive data that improvements in macrovascular disease also occur after pancreas transplantation. Quality of life is significantly improved in pancreas recipients.

Despite the many potential and real benefits of pancreas transplantation, this technique is available to, and appropriate for, only a very small fraction of the diabetic population. Overall there are currently approximately 500,000 people with Type 1 diabetes in the United States. The major challenges are the high cost of transplantation and the limited numbers of organs.

The promise of islet transplantation is that beta cell mass can be replenished without the surgical risks of pancreas transplantation and without the worries of vascular anastomoses or exocrine drainage. By infusing the islets into the liver via the portal system, the islets can seed a major target organ for insulin action. As well, if there is a recurrent need for additional islets, a relatively simple intravenous injection of islet cells can be carried out.

To perform islet transplantation, islets are isolated from the donor pancreas (210). Collagenase is infused intraductally. An automated digestion and purification technique allows released islets to be progressively collected. Separation of islets from nonislet tissue is accomplished by various ficoll centrifugations. Prior to transplant, the islets are incubated for 24 hours at 37°C.

Between 1983 and 2000, almost 500 islet transplants were attempted throughout the world. Transplanted islets must be protected from rejection similar to any other allogeneic tissue or organ that is transplanted. While being powerful immunosuppressive agents, glucocorticoids produce insulin resistance increasing the metabolic demand for insulin secretion by the beta cells. The calcineurin inhibitors are also directly toxic to beta cells. A glucocorticoid-free, sirolimus-based protocol developed at the University of Edmonton in Canada has produced the best islet transplant results (203). At two years post-transplant, 70% of patients maintained insulin independence. Transplanting sufficient numbers of islets is highly problematic. Recent trials have isolated islets from two pancreata prior to transplantation. This further complicates the limited availability of pancreata for pancreas or islet transplant. In contrast to pancreas transplantation which is an accepted medical therapy, islet transplantation is certainly still experimental.

Beta cell engineering has been studied in animal models of human diabetes but the field has not progressed to the point where trials in humans are being undertaken. Conceptually, beta cell-equivalent cells could be grown in vitro and would be available in unlimited quantities for transplantation. This is the single most important aspect of this research compared with pancreas or islet transplantation where a donor is always needed. It is highly unlikely that there will ever be sufficient pancreas donors to transplant every patient with Type 1 diabetes.

Many novel approaches are being studied that often involve stem cell technologies (211,212). Nonendocrine cells may be genetically modified to elaborate insulin in response to glucose (206). This could be carried out by gene therapy with an appropriate mix of transcription factor genes to turn on the correct genes for insulin production, glucose sensing, and insulin release (213). As well, nonendocrine stem, progenitor, or mature cells could be trans-differentiated into functional beta cells. Alternatively, islet stem or progenitor cells could be differentiated into beta cell equivalents. Embryonic stem cells are another potential cell source for differentiation into beta cells (214). Despite our optimism, the development of beta cells from stem cells is a daunting task (215). Some authors suggest that prevention of autoimmunity or interference in autoimmunity is a more reasonable short-term goal for abrogating Type 1 diabetes (216).

CLINICAL APPROACH TO THE DIAGNOSIS OF DIABETES

In lean children and adolescents that present with hyperglycemia, ketosis, polyuria, polydipsia, and weight loss, the diagnosis of Type 1 diabetes is usually not in doubt (Fig. 2). In such cases when the clinical diagnosis of Type 1 diabetes is certain, islet autoantibody testing does not add value to the management of the patient. While several studies have examined the role of islet autoantibodies in predicting the subsequent severity of hyperglycemia following diagnosis, such information is not sufficiently predictive to be of significant clinical use. Therefore, islet autoantibody testing is not justified to predict the clinical course of the disease.

There are situations where islet autoantibody testing can be very helpful. As obesity affects a greater and greater proportion of youth, it is possible to develop Type 1 diabetes and be obese. This could cause confusion with Type 2 diabetes. In such circumstances, any type of islet autoantibody positivity (ICA, GADA, IA-2A, IAA) establishes the diagnosis of Type 1 diabetes. Nevertheless, there may still be insulin resistance from the patient's obesity and a more complex picture of combined absolute insulinopenia and peripheral insulin resistance.

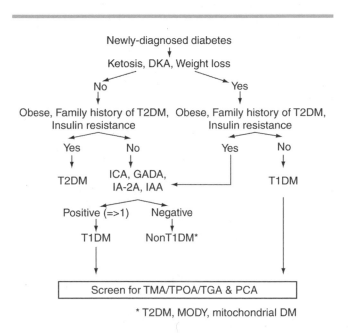

Figure 2 Children with newly diagnosed diabetes who are lean, insulin-sensitive and ketotic [or display diabetic ketoacidosis (DKA)] with weight loss are diagnosed with Type 1 diabetes. Ketotic children and adolescents with obesity, a family history of Type 2 diabetes mellitus (T2DM) and/or insulin resistance should undergo islet autoantibody testing. If ICA, GADA, IA-2A, or IAA are positive, Type 1 diabetes is present. If these markers are negative, some form of non-Type 1 diabetes (such as T2DM) is present. New-onset diabetes in children that do not display ketosis, DKA or weight loss who are obese, have a family history of T2DM and/or are insulin resistant have T2DM. Lean children with new-onset diabetes that are nonketotic should undergo islet autoantibody testing. If positive, Type 1 diabetes is present. If negative, some form of non-Type 1 diabetes (such as maturity-onset diabetes of youth) is present. *Abbreviations*: ICA, islet cell cytoplasmic autoantibodies; GADA, glutamic acid decarboxylase autoantibodies; IAA, insulin autoantibodies; IA-2A, insulinoma-2-associated autoantibodies, TMA, thyroid microsomal autoantibodies; TPOA, thyroperoxidase autoantibodies; TGA, thyroglobulin autoantibodies; PCA, parietal cell autoantibodies; T1DM, Type1 diabetes mellitus.

Another perplexing situation is the obese adolescent African-American who presents with diabetic ketoacidosis: is this Type 1 diabetes or Type 2 diabetes? There are reports in the literature of such adolescents being noninsulin-requiring after recovery from diabetic ketoacidosis (217) and possibly up to 25% of children with Type 2 diabetes present with diabetic ketoacidosis (218–221). Therefore, the lack of islet autoantibodies in such a circumstance supports the diagnosis of Type 2 diabetes.

Occasionally a lean youth presents with mild diabetes that is nonketotic and noninsulin-requiring for the control of hyperglycemia. The question arises if this is very early-onset Type 1 diabetes. The absence of any islet autoantibody suggests that a non-autoimmune etiology should be investigated such as maturity-onset diabetes of youth. Making the diagnosis of Type 1 diabetes is important: at the onset of Type 1 diabetes, rigorous early glycemic control has been shown to prolong beta cell function which makes the diabetes easier to control (222). If a youth does have Type 1 diabetes, immediate and aggressive insulin therapy should be instituted.

Because there are four main islet autoantibodies, a short discussion of their use is valuable. The most common islet autoantibodies are ICA and GADA, being present in 70% of more of new-onset Type 1 diabetes cases. IA-2A is less common with an approximate 60% frequency at onset. Least common of the islet autoantibodies is IAA. IAA are detected in approximately 50% or less of new-onset children. IAA are far less common in adults.

Based on the frequencies of the autoantibodies, it can be argued that if only one islet autoantibody is to be measured initially, it should be ICA or GADA (Fig. 3). If ICA is measured first and is positive, no further islet autoantibody testing is indicated to establish the diagnosis of Type 1 diabetes in a symptomatic

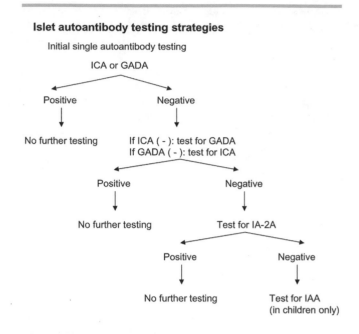

Figure 3 Based on the frequencies of the autoantibodies, it can be argued that if only one islet autoantibody is to be measured initially, it should be ICA or GADA. If ICA is measured first and is positive, no further islet autoantibody testing is indicated to establish the diagnosis of Type 1 diabetes in a symptomatic patient. On the other hand if GADA is measured first and is positive, no other testing is indicated. If both ICA and GADA are negative, IA-2A can be determined. If negative, IAA can be sought in children. *Abbreviations*: ICA, islet cell cytoplasmic autoantibodies; GADA, glutamic acid decarboxylase autoantibodies; IAA, insulin autoantibodies; IA-2A, insulinoma-2-associated autoantibodies.

patient. On the other hand if GADA is measured first and is positive, no other testing is indicated. If both ICA and GADA are negative, IA-2A can be determined. If negative, IAA can be sought in children.

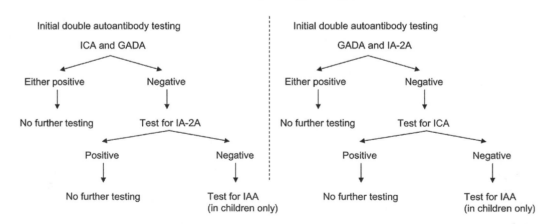

Figure 4 If two autoantibodies are to be ordered, then either ICA or GADA should be measured or GADA and IA-2A should be measured. *Abbreviations*: ICA, islet cell cytoplasmic autoantibodies; GADA, glutamic acid decarboxylase autoantibodies; IAA, insulin autoantibodies; IA-2A, insulinoma-2-associated autoantibodies.

Because IA-2A is not as common at the onset of Type 1 diabetes as either ICA or GADA, in single islet auto-antibody testing strategies, testing should not start with IA-2A.

If two autoantibodies are to be ordered, then either ICA or GADA should be measured or GADA and IA-2A should be measured (Fig. 4). Some reference laboratories do not offer ICA testing at their own facility because it requires human pancreatic substrate for indirect immunofluorescence. Nevertheless, there are university-based research laboratories that do offer ICA testing on a commercial basis. Thus those laboratories that do not offer ICA testing will begin with GADA and IA-2 measurements. However because ICA is more common at onset than IA-2A, the combination of initial testing for ICA and GADA would appear to have higher sensitivity than GADA and IA-2A.

Using a cascade strategy to detect islet autoantibodies in new-onset patients, one could test sequentially for GADA/ICA, IA-2A and then IAA and stop testing once one islet autoantibody was found to be positive. However if ICA, GADA, and IA-2A are all negative, the likelihood that IAA will be positive in isolation is very low. It can be questioned if IAA testing should be included in such a cascade scheme because of its rarity compared with the other islet autoantibodies. While the biochemical autoantibodies, GADA and IA-2A, provide many methodological advantages over ICA testing, ICA testing should not be abandoned because of its higher specificity than GAD or IA-2A and its ability to detect autoimmunity to several islet autoantigens not detected by the single GADA or IA-2A assays (223).

Whereas islet autoantibodies can be used to predict Type 1 diabetes, in the absence of effective preventative therapies, islet antibody screening outside of research settings is not indicated (224). Similarly while some success in preserving beta cell function has been demonstrated using an anti-CD3 monoclonal antibody in new-onset Type 1 diabetes (199), there is no routine recommendation to screen new-onset Type 1 diabetes patients for islet autoantibodies because the anti-CD3 therapy is experimental at this point.

In the prediction of Type 1 diabetes in nondiabetic individuals using islet autoantibody testing, it is now clear that the presence of a single autoantibody is not as powerful a predictor of the later development of Type 1 diabetes as positivity for multiple islet autoantibodies. Clearly when multiple islet autoantibodies are present, the risk for developing Type 1 diabetes rises substantially (225–228). Furthermore, in children when multiple-autoantibody-positivity-islet autoimmunity is coupled with depressed first-phase insulin response to intravenously administered glucose, risk for Type 1 diabetes can exceed 50% over five years' duration of follow-up and approaches 100% over 10 years.

REFERENCES

1. American Diabetes Association. Diagnosis and classification of diabetes mellitus. Diabetes Care 2005; 28(suppl 1): S37–S42.

2. Wildin RS, Smyk-Pearson S, Filipovich AH. Clinical and molecular features of the immunodysregulation, polyendocrinopathy, enteropathy, X linked (IPEX) syndrome. J Med Genet 2002; 39:537–545.

3. Taylor SI, Arioglu E. Genetically defined forms of diabetes in children. J Clin Endocrinol Metab 1999; 84: 4390–4396.

4. Winter WE, Nakamura M, House DV. Monogenic diabetes mellitus in youth: the MODY syndromes. Endocrinol Metab Clin North Am 1999; 28(4):765–785.

5. van den Ouweland JM, Lemkes HH, Trembath RC, et al. Maternally inherited diabetes and deafness is a distinct subtype of diabetes and associates with a single point mutation in the mitochondrial tRNA [Leu(UUR)] gene. Diabetes 1994; 43(6):746–751.

6. Moran A. Cystic fibrosis-related diabetes: an approach to diagnosis and management. Pediatr Diabetes 2000; 1: 41–48.

7. Marshall BC, Butler SM, Stoddard M, Moran AM, Liou TG, Morgan WJ. Epidemiology of cystic fibrosis-related diabetes. J Pediatr 2005; 146(5):681–687.

8. Karam JH, Lewitt PA, Young CW. Insulinopenic diabetes after rodenticide (Vacor) ingestion: a unique model of acquired diabetes in man. Diabetes 1980; 29:971–978.

9. Hauser L, Sheehan P, Simpkins H. Pancreatic pathology in pentamidine-induced diabetes in acquired immunodeficiency syndrome patients. Hum Pathol 1991; 229: 926–929.

10. Yoon JW, Austin M, Onodera T, Notkins AL. Virus-induced diabetes mellitus. N Engl J Med 1979; 300: 1173–1179.

11. Forrest JM, Menser MA, Burgess JA. High frequency of diabetes mellitus in young adults with congenital rubella. Lancet 1971; 2:332–334.

12. Cabrera-Rode E, Sarmiento L, Molina G, et al. Islet cell related antibodies and Type 1 diabetes associated with echovirus 30 epidemic: a case report. J Med Virol 2005; 76(3):373–377.

13. Elias D, Cohen IR, Schechter Y, Spirer Z, Golander A. Antibodies to insulin receptor followed by anti-idiotype antibodies to insulin in child with hypoglycemia. Diabetes 1987; 36:348–354.

14. Virally ML, Timsit J, Chanson P, Warnet A, Guillausseau PJ. Insulin autoimmune syndrome: a rare cause of hypoglycaemia not to be overlooked. Diabetes Metab 1999; 25(5): 429–431.

15. Winter WE, Signorino MR. Diabetes Mellitus: Pathophysiology, Etiologies, Complications, Management, and Laboratory Evaluation. Washington, DC: AACC Press, 2002:1–137.

16. The Diabetes Control and Complications Trial Research Group. The effect of intensive treatment of diabetes on the development and progression of long-term complications in insulin-dependent diabetes mellitus. N Engl J Med 1993; 329:977–986.

17. UKPDS Group. Intensive blood-glucose control with sulphonylureas or insulin compared with conventional treatment and risk of complications in patients with Type 2 diabetes (UKPDS 33). Lancet 1998; 352:837–853.

18. Diabetes Control and Complications Trial/Epidemiology of Diabetes Interventions and Complications Research Group. Retinopathy and nephropathy in patients with Type 1 diabetes four years after a trial of intensive

therapy. N Engl J Med 2000; 342:381–389 [Erratum: N Engl J Med 2000; 342:1376].

19. Nathan DM, Cleary PA, Backlund JY, et al. Diabetes Control and Complications Trial/Epidemiology of Diabetes Interventions and Complications (DCCT/EDIC) Study Research Group. Intensive diabetes treatment and cardiovascular disease in patients with Type 1 diabetes. N Engl J Med 2005; 353(25):2643–2653.

20. Kukreja A, Maclaren NK. Autoimmunity and diabetes. J Clin Endocrinol Metab 1999; 84(12):4371–4378.

21. Kawasaki E, Gill RG, Eisenbarth GS. Type 1 diabetes mellitus. In: Eisenbarth GS, ed. Endocrine and Organ Specific Autoimmunity. Austin, TX: RG Landes Company, 1999:149–182.

22. Badenhoop K, Boehm BO. Genetic susceptibility and immunological synapse in Type 1 diabetes and thyroid autoimmune disease. Exp Clin Endocrinol Diabetes 2004; 112(8):407–415.

23. Ziegler AG, Hummel M, Schenker M, Bonifacio E. Autoantibody appearance and risk for development of childhood diabetes in offspring of parents with Type 1 diabetes: the 2-year analysis of the German BABYDIAB Study. Diabetes 1999; 48(3):460–468.

24. Cilio CM, Bosco A, Moretti C, et al. Congenital autoimmune diabetes mellitus. N Engl J Med 2000; 342(20): 1529–1531.

25. Lampeter EF, Homberg M, Quabeck K, et al. Transfer of insulin-dependent diabetes between HLA-identical siblings by bone marrow transplantation. Lancet 1993; 341(8855):1243–1244.

26. Almawi WY, Tamim H, Azar ST. Clinical review 103: T helper Type 1 and 2 cytokines mediate the onset and progression of type I (insulin-dependent) diabetes. J Clin Endocrinol Metab 1999; 84(5):1497–1502.

27. Gepts W, Lecompte PM. The pancreatic islets in diabetes. Am J Med 1981; 70:105–115.

28. Foulis AK, Stewart JA. The pancreas in recent-onset type 1 (insulin-dependent) diabetes mellitus: insulin content of islets, insulitis and associated changes in the exocrine acinar tissue. Diabetologia 1984; 26:456–461.

29. Foulis AK, Liddle CN, Farquharson MA, Richmond JA, Weir RS. The histopathology of the pancreas in Type 1 (insulin-dependent) diabetes mellitus: a 25-year review of deaths in patients under 20 years of age in the United Kingdom. Diabetologia 1986; 29:267–274.

30. Logothetopoulos J, Valiquette N, Madura E, Cvet D. The onset and progression of pancreatic insulitis in the overt, spontaneously diabetic, young adult BB rat studied by pancreatic biopsy. Diabetes 1984; 33:33–36.

31. House DV, Nakamura M, Winter WE. Autoimmune markers of type I diabetes mellitus. In: Nakamura RM, Burek CL, Cook L, Folds JD, eds. Clinical Diagnostic Immunology: Protocols in Quality Assurance and Standardization. Cambridge, MA: Blackwell Science, 1998:234–249.

32. Crisa L, Mordes JP, Rossini AA. Autoimmune diabetes mellitus in the BB rat. Diabetes Metab Rev 1992; 8(1):4–37.

33. Tochino Y. The NOD mouse as a model of type I diabetes. Crit Rev Immunol 1987; 8:49–81.

34. Atkinson MA, Leiter EH. The NOD mouse model of Type 1 diabetes: as good as it gets? Nat Med 1999; 5:601–604.

35. Christianson SW, Shultz LD, Leiter EH. Adoptive transfer of diabetes into immunodeficient NOD-scid/scid mice. Relative contributions of CD4+ and CD8+ T-cells from diabetic versus prediabetic NOD. NON-Thy-1a donors. Diabetes 1993; 42(1):44–55.

36. Yang M, Charlton B, Gautam AM. Development of insulitis and diabetes in B cell-deficient NOD mice. J Autoimmun 1997; 10(3):257–260.

37. Martin S, Wolf-Eichbaum D, Duinkerken G, et al. Development of Type 1 diabetes despite severe hereditary B-lymphocyte deficiency. N Engl J Med 2001; 345(14): 1036–1040.

38. Ziegler AG, Hillebrand B, Rabl W, et al. On the appearance of islet associated autoimmunity in offspring of diabetic mothers: a prospective study from birth. Diabetologia 1993; 36(5):402–408.

39. Thai A-C, Eisenbarth GS. Natural history of IDDM. Diabetes Rev 1990; 1:1–14.

40. Srikanta S, Ganda OP, Jackson RA, et al. Pre-Type 1 (insulin-dependent) diabetes: common endocrinological course despite immunological and immunogenetic heterogeneity. Diabetologia 1984; 27:146–148.

41. Srikanta S, Ganda OP, Gleason RE, Jackson RA, Soeldner JS, Eisenbarth GS. Pre-Type 1 diabetes, linear loss of beta cell response to intravenous glucose. Diabetes 1984; 33:717–720.

42. Karvonen M, Viik-Kajander M, Moltchanova E, Libman I, LaPorte R, Tuomilehto J. Incidence of childhood Type 1 diabetes worldwide. Diabetes Mondiale (DiaMond) Project Group. Diabetes Care 2000; 23(10):1516–1526.

43. Becker KG. Comparative genetics of Type 1 diabetes and autoimmune disease, common loci, common pathways? Diabetes 1999; 48:1353–1358.

44. Maclaren N, Riley W, Skordis N, et al. Inherited susceptibility to insulin-dependent diabetes is associated with HLA-DR1, while DR5 is protective. Autoimmunity 1988; 1:197–205.

45. Winter WE, Maclaren NK, Riley WJ, Clarke DW, Kappy MS, Spillar RP. Maturity-onset diabetes of youth in Black Americans. N Engl J Med 1987; 316:285–291.

46. Khalil I, Deschamps I, Lepage V, al-Daccak R, Degos L, Hors J. Dose effect of cis- and trans-encoded HLA-DQ alpha beta heterodimers in IDDM susceptibility. Diabetes 1992; 41:378–384.

47. Ronningen KS. Genetics in the prediction of insulin-dependent diabetes mellitus: from theory to practice. Ann Med 1997; 29:387–392.

48. Greenbaum CJ, Schatz DA, Cuthbertson D, Zeidler A, Eisenbarth GS, Krischer JP. Islet cell antibody-positive relatives with human leukocyte antigen DQA1*0102, DQB1*0602: identification by the Diabetes Prevention Trial-Type 1. J Clin Endocrinol Metab 2000; 85(3):1255–1260.

49. Gylling M, Tuomi T, Bjorses P, et al. B-cell autoantibodies, human leukocyte antigen II alleles, and Type 1 diabetes in autoimmune polyendocrinopathy-candidiasis-ectodermal dystrophy. J Clin Endocrinol Metab 2000; 85(12):4434–4440.

50. Todd JA, Bell JI, McDevitt HO. HLA-DQ beta gene contributes to susceptibility and resistance to insulin-dependent diabetes mellitus. Nature 1987; 329:599–604.

51. Todd JA, Acha-Orbea H, Bell JI, et al. A molecular basis for MHC class II-associated autoimmunity. Science 1990; 240:1003–1008.

52. Baisch JM, Weeks T, Giles R, Hoover M, Stastny P, Capra JD. Analysis of HLA-DQ genotypes and susceptibility in insulin-dependent diabetes mellitus. N Engl J Med 1990; 322:1836–1841.

53. Owerbach D, Gunn S, Ty G, Wible L, Gabby KH. Oligonucleutide probes for HLA-DQA and DQB genes define susceptibility to Type 1 (insulin-dependent) diabetes mellitus. Diabetologia 1988; 31:751–757.

54. Gutierrez-Lopez MD, Bertera S, Chantres MT, et al. Susceptibility to Type 1 (insulin-dependent) diabetes mellitus in Spanish patients correlates quantitatively with expression of HLA-DQ alpha Arg 52 and HLA-DQ beta non-Asp 57 alleles. Diabetologia 1992; 35:583–588.

55. Ikegami H, Tahara Y, Topyon C, et al. Aspartic acid at position 57 of the HLA-DQ beta chain is not protective against insulin-dependent diabetes mellitus in Japanese people. J Autoimmunity 1990; 3:167–174.

56. Park Y, She JX, Wang CY, et al. Common susceptibility and transmission pattern of human leukocyte antigen DRB1-DQB1 haplotypes to Korean and Caucasian patients with Type 1 diabetes. J Clin Endocrinol Metab 2000; 85(12):4538–4542.

57. Dorman JS, LaPorte RE, Stone RA, Trucco M. Worldwide differences in the incidence of type I diabetes are associated with amino acid variation at position 57 of the HLA-DQ beta chain. Proc Natl Acad Sci USA 1990; 87:7370–7374.

58. She JX. Susceptibility to type I diabetes: HLA-DQ and DR revisited. Immunol Today 1996; 17(7):323–329.

59. Melanitou E, Fain P, Eisenbarth GS. Genetics of type 1A (immune mediated) diabetes. J Autoimmun 2003; 21(2): 93–98.

60. Warram JH, Krolewski AS, Gottlieb MS, Kahn CR. Differences in risk of insulin-dependent diabetes in offspring of diabetic mothers and diabetic fathers. N Engl J Med 1984; 311:149–152.

61. Vadheim CM, Rotter JI, Maclaren NK, Riley WJ, Anderson CE. Preferential transmission of diabetic alleles within the HLA gene complex. N Engl J Med 1986; 315: 1314–1318.

62. She JX, Marron MP. Genetic susceptibility factors in Type 1 diabetes: linkage, disequilibrium and functional analyses. Curr Opin Immunol 1998; 10(6):682–689.

63. Davies JL, Kawaguchi Y, Bennett ST, et al. A genome-wide search for human Type 1 diabetes susceptibility genes. Nature 1994; 371(6493):130–136.

64. Buzzetti R, Quattrocchi CC, Nistico L. Dissecting the genetics of Type 1 diabetes: relevance for familial clustering and differences in incidence. Diabetes Metab Rev 1998; 14(2):111–128.

65. Luo DF, Buzzetti R, Rotter JI, et al. Confirmation of three susceptibility genes to insulin-dependent diabetes mellitus: IDDM4, IDDM5 and IDDM8. Hum Mol Genet 1996; 5(5):693–698.

66. Pugliese A. Unraveling the genetics of insulin-dependent type 1A diabetes: the search must go on. Diabetes Rev 1999; 7:39–54.

67. Marron MP, Zeidler A, Raffel LJ, et al. Genetic and physical mapping of a Type 1 diabetes susceptibility gene (IDDM12) to a 100-kb phagemid artificial chromosome clone containing D2S72-TLA4-D2S105 on chromosome 2q33. Diabetes 2000; 49(3):492–499.

68. Maier LM, Wicker LS. Genetic susceptibility to Type 1 diabetes. Curr Opin Immunol 2005; 17(6):601–608.

69. Vaidya B, Pearce S. The emerging role of the CTLA-4 gene in autoimmune endocrinopathies. Eur J Endocrinol 2004; 150(5):619–626.

70. Kim MS, Polychronakos C. Immunogenetics of Type 1 diabetes. Horm Res 2005; 64(4):180–188.

71. Concannon P, Erlich HA, Julier C, et al. Type 1 Diabetes Genetics Consortium. Type 1 diabetes: evidence for susceptibility loci from four genome-wide linkage scans in 1,435 multiplex families. Diabetes 2005; 54(10):2995–3001.

72. She JX, Bui MM, Tian XH, et al. Additive susceptibility to insulin-dependent diabetes conferred by HLA-DQB1 and insulin genes. Autoimmunity 1994; 18(3):195–203.

73. Bell GI, Horita S, Karam JH. A polymorphic locus near the human insulin gene is associated with insulin-dependent diabetes mellitus. Diabetes 1984; 33(2):176–183.

74. Cerrone GE, Caputo M, Lopez AP, et al. Variable number of tandem repeats of the insulin gene determines susceptibility to latent autoimmune diabetes in adults. Mol Diagn 2004; 8(1):43–49.

75. Pugliese A, Zeller M, Fernandez A Jr. et al. The insulin gene is transcribed in the human thymus and transcription levels correlated with allelic variation at the INS VNTR-IDDM2 susceptibility locus for Type 1 diabetes. Nat Genet 1997; 15(3):293–297.

76. Vafiadis P, Bennett ST, Todd JA, et al. Insulin expression in human thymus is modulated by INS VNTR alleles at the IDDM2 locus. Nat Genet 1997; 15(3):289–292.

77. Barratt BJ, Payne F, Lowe CE, et al. Remapping the insulin gene/IDDM2 locus in Type 1 diabetes. Diabetes 2004; 53(7):1884–1889.

78. Tait KF, Collins JE, Heward JM, et al. Evidence for a Type 1 diabetes-specific mechanism for the insulin gene-associated IDDM2 locus rather than a general influence on autoimmunity. Diabet Med 2004; 21(3):267–270.

79. Ueda H, Howson JM, Esposito L, et al. Association of the T-cell regulatory gene CTLA4 with susceptibility to autoimmune disease. Nature 2003; 423(6939):506–511.

80. Barbesino G, Chiovato L. The genetics of Hashimoto's disease. Endocrinol Metab Clin North Am 2000; 29(2): 357–374.

81. Kotsa K, Watson PF, Weetman AP. A CTLA-4 gene polymorphism is associated with both Graves disease and autoimmune hypothyroidism. Clin Endocrinol (Oxf) 1997; 46(5):551–554.

82. Donner H, Braun J, Seidl C, et al. Codon 17 polymorphism of the cytotoxic T lymphocyte antigen 4 gene in Hashimoto's thyroiditis and Addison's disease. J Clin Endocrinol Metab 1997; 82(12):4130–4132.

83. Braun J, Donner H, Siegmund T, Walfish PG, Usadel KH, Badenhoop K. CTLA-4 promoter variants in patients with Graves' disease and Hashimoto's thyroiditis. Tissue Antigens 1998; 51(5):563–566.

84. Simmonds MJ, Gough SC. Unravelling the genetic complexity of autoimmune thyroid disease: HLA, CTLA-4 and beyond. Clin Exp Immunol 2004; 136(1):1–10.

85. Bottini N, Musumeci L, Alonso A, et al. A functional variant of lymphoid tyrosine phosphatase is associated with type I diabetes. Nat Genet 2004; 36(4):337–338.

86. Ladner MB, Bottini N, Valdes AM, Noble JA. Association of the single nucleotide polymorphism C1858T of the PTPN22 gene with Type 1 diabetes. Hum Immunol 2005; 66(1):60–64.

87. Vang T, Congia M, Macis MD, et al. Autoimmune-associated lymphoid tyrosine phosphatase is a gain-of-function variant. Nat Genet 2005; 37(12):1317–1319.

88. Zheng W, She JX. Genetic association between a lymphoid tyrosine phosphatase (PTPN22) and Type 1 diabetes. Diabetes 2005; 54(3):906–908.

89. Smyth D, Cooper JD, Collins JE, et al. Replication of an association between the lymphoid tyrosine phosphatase locus (LYP/PTPN22) with Type 1 diabetes, and evidence for its role as a general autoimmunity locus. Diabetes 2004; 53(11):3020–3023.

90. Akerblom HK, Knip M. Putative environmental factors in Type 1 diabetes. Diabetes Metab Rev 1998; 14:31–67.

91. Couper JJ, Steele C, Beresford S, et al. Lack of association between duration of breast-feeding or introduction of cow's milk and development of islet autoimmunity. Diabetes 1999; 48(11):2145–2149.

92. Graves PM, Barriga KJ, Norris JM, et al. Lack of association between early childhood immunizations and beta-cell autoimmunity. Diabetes Care 1999; 22(10):1694–1697.

93. Maclaren NK, Atkinson MA. Insulin-dependent diabetes mellitus: the hypothesis of molecular mimicry between

islet cell antigens and microorganisms. Mol Med Today 1997:76–83.

94. Law GR, McKinney PA, Staines A, et al. Clustering of childhood IDDM. Links with age and place of residence. Diabetes Care 1997; 20(5):753–756.

95. Honeyman MC, Coulson BS, Stone NL, et al. Association between rotavirus infection and pancreatic islet autoimmunity in children at risk of developing Type 1 diabetes. Diabetes 2000; 49(8):1319–1324.

96. Hyoty H, Hiltunen M, Knip M, et al. A prospective study of the role of coxsackie B and other enterovirus infections in the pathogenesis of IDDM. Childhood Diabetes in Finland (DiMe) Study Group. Diabetes 1995; 44(6):652–657.

97. Vreugdenhil GR, Schloot NC, Hoorens A, et al. Acute onset of type I diabetes mellitus after severe echovirus 9 infection: putative pathogenic pathways. Clin Infect Dis 2000; 31(4):1025–1031.

98. Maclaren NK, Atkinson MA. Is insulin-dependent diabetes mellitus environmentally induced? N Engl J Med 1992; 327:347–349.

99. Karjalainen J, Martin J, Knip M. A bovine albumin peptide as a possible trigger of insulin-dependent diabetes mellitus. N Engl J Med 1992; 327:302–307.

100. Verge CF, Gianani R, Yu L, et al. Late progression to diabetes and evidence for chronic beta-cell autoimmunity in identical twins of patients with type I diabetes. Diabetes 1995; 44(10):1176–1179.

101. Krokowski M, Caillat-Zucman S, Timsit J, et al. Anti-bovine serum albumin antibodies: genetic heterogeneity and clinical relevance in adult-onset IDDM. Diabetes Care 1995; 18(2):170–173.

102. Hummel M, Fuchtenbusch M, Schenker M, Ziegler AG. No major association of breast-feeding, vaccinations, and childhood viral diseases with early islet autoimmunity in the German BABYDIAB Study. Diabetes Care 2000; 23(7):969–974.

103. Cainelli F, Manzaroli D, Renzini C, Casali F, Concia E, Vento S. Coxsackie B virus-induced autoimmunity to GAD does not lead to Type 1 diabetes. Diabetes Care 2000; 23(7):1021–1022.

104. Casu A, Carlini M, Contu A, Bottazzo GF, Songini M. Type 1 diabetes in Sardinia is not linked to nitrate levels in drinking water. Diabetes Care 2000; 23(7):1043–1044.

105. Lonnrot M, Korpela K, Knip M, et al. Enterovirus infection as a risk factor for beta-cell autoimmunity in a prospectively observed birth cohort: the Finnish Diabetes Prediction and Prevention Study. Diabetes 2000; 49(8):1314–1318.

106. Juhela S, Hyoty H, Roivainen M, et al. T-cell responses to enterovirus antigens in children with Type 1 diabetes. Diabetes 2000; 49(8):1308–1313.

107. Baekkeskov S, Aanstoot HJ, Christgau S, et al. Identification of the 64K autoantigen in insulin-dependent diabetes as the GABA-synthesizing enzyme glutamic acid decarboxylase. Nature 1990; 34:151–156.

108. Rabin DU, Pleasic SM, Shapiro JA, et al. Islet cell antigen 512 is a diabetes-specific islet autoantigen related to protein tyrosine phosphatases. J Immunol 1994; 152(6):3183–3188.

109. Lan MS, Wasserfall C, Maclaren NK, Notkins AL. IA-2, a transmembrane protein of the protein tyrosine phosphatase family, is a major autoantigen in insulin-dependent diabetes mellitus. Proc Natl Acad Sci USA 1996; 93(13):6367–6370.

110. Palmer JP, Asplin CM, Clemons P, et al. Insulin antibodies in insulin-dependent diabetics before insulin treatment. Science 1983; 222(4630):133–139.

111. Winter WE. The use of islet autoantibody markers in the prediction of autoimmune Type 1 diabetes. Clin Immunol Newslett 1999; 19(3):25–39.

112. Bottazzo GF, Florin-Christensen A, Doniach D. Islet-cell autoantibodies in diabetes mellitus with autoimmune polyendocrine deficiencies. Lancet 1974; 2:1279–1283.

113. Nayak RC, Omar MAK, Rabizadeh A, Srikanta S, Eisenbarth GS. "Cytoplasmic" islet cell antibodies. Evidence that the target antigen is a sialoglycoconjugate. Diabetes 1985; 34:617–619.

114. Richter W, Seissler J, Northemann W, Wolfahrt S, Meinch H-M, Scherbaum WA. Cytoplasmic islet cell antibodies recognize distinct islet antigens in IDDM but not in stiff man syndrome. Diabetes 1993; 42:1642–1648.

115. Schatz DA, Barrett DJ, Maclaren NK, Riley WJ. Polyclonal nature of islet cell antibodies in insulin-dependent diabetes. Autoimmunity 1988; 1:45–50.

116. Neufeld M, Maclaren NK, Riley WJ, et al. Islet cell and other organ-specific antibodies in U.S. Caucasians and Blacks with insulin-dependent diabetes mellitus. Diabetes 1980; 29:589–592.

117. Schatz D, Krischer J, Horne G, et al. Islet cell antibodies predict insulin-dependent diabetes in United States school age children as powerfully as in unaffected relatives. J Clin Invest 1994; 93:2403–2407.

118. Diabetes Prevention Trial-Type 1 Diabetes Study Group. Effects of insulin in relatives of patients with Type 1 diabetes mellitus. N Engl J Med 2002; 346:1685–1691.

119. Skyler JS, Krischer JP, Wolfsdorf J, et al, Diabetes Prevention Trial-Type 1 Study Group. Effects of oral insulin in relatives of patients with Type 1 diabetes: The Diabetes Prevention Trial-Type 1. Diabetes Care 2005; 28(5):1068–1076.

120. Irvine WJ, McCallum CJ, Gray RS, Duncan LJP. Clinical and pathogenic significance of pancreatic islet-cell antibodies in diabetics treated with oral hypoglycemic agents. Lancet 1977; 1:1025–1027.

121. Di Mario U, Irvine WJ, Borsey DQ, Kyner JL, Weston J, Galfo C. Immune abnormalities in diabetic patients not requiring insulin at diagnosis. Diabetologia 1983; 25:392–395.

122. Niskanen L, Karjalaienen J, Sarlund H, Siitonen O, Uusitupa M. Five year follow-up of islet-cell antibodies in (non-insulin dependent) diabetes mellitus. Diabetologia 1991; 34:402–408.

123. Riley WJ, Maclaren NK, Krischer J, et al. A prospective study of the development of diabetes in relatives of patients with insulin-dependent diabetes. N Engl J Med 1990; 323:1167–1172.

124. Krischer JP, Cuthbertson DD, Yu L, et al. Screening strategies for the identification of multiple antibody-positive relatives of individuals with Type 1 diabetes. J Clin Endocrinol Metab 2003; 88(1):103–108.

125. Palmer JP. Predicting IDDM: use of humoral immune markers. Diabetes Rev 1993; 1:104–115.

126. Decochez K, Keymeulen B, Somers G, et al. Use of an islet cell antibody assay to identify Type 1 diabetic patients with rapid decrease in C-peptide levels after clinical onset. Belgian Diabetes Registry. Diabetes Care 2000; 23(8):1072–1078.

127. Torn C, Landin-Olsson M, Lernmark A, et al. Prognostic factors for the course of B cell function in autoimmune diabetes. J Clin Endocrinol Metab 2000; 85(12):4619–4623.

128. Vives-Pi M, Somoza N, Vargas F, et al. Expression of glutamic acid decarboxylase (GAD) in the alpha, beta and delta cells of normal and diabetic pancreas: implications for the pathogenesis of type I diabetes. Clin Exp Immunol 1993; 92(3):391–396.

129. Kaufman DL, Erlander MG, Clare-Salzler M, Atkinson MA, Maclaren NK, Tobin AJ. Autoimmunity to two forms of glutamate decarboxylase in insulin-dependent diabetes mellitus. J Clin Invest 1992; 89: 283–292.

130. Hagopian WA, Michelsen B, Karlsen AE, et al. Autoantibodies in IDDM primarily recognize the 65,000-M(r) rather than the 67,000-M(r) isoform of glutamic acid decarboxylase. Diabetes 1993; 42(4):631–636.

131. Luhder F, Schlosser M, Mauch L, et al. Autoantibodies against GAD65 rather than GAD67 precede the onset of Type 1 diabetes. Autoimmunity 1994; 19(2):71–80.

132. Hampe CS, Hammerle LP, Bekris L, et al. Recognition of glutamic acid decarboxylase (GAD) by autoantibodies from different gad antibody-positive phenotypes. J Clin Endocrinol Metab 2000; 85(12):4671–4679.

133. Atkinson MA, Kaufman DL, Campbell L. Response of peripheral blood mononuclear cells to glutamate decarboxylase in insulin-dependent diabetes. Lancet 1992; 339: 458–459.

134. Roep BO, Arden SD, de Vries RR, Hutton JC. T-cell clones from a type-1 diabetes patient respond to insulin secretory granule proteins. Nature 1990; 345:632–634.

135. Roep BO, Kallan AA, Duinkerken G, et al. T-cell reactivity to beta-cell membrane antigens associated with beta-cell destruction in IDDM. Diabetes 1995; 44:278–283.

136. Hummel M, Durinovic-Bello I, Ziegler A-G. Relation between cellular and humoral immunity to islet cell antigens in type I diabetes. J Autoimmun 1996; 9: 427–430.

137. Harrison LC, Honeyman MC, DeAizpurua HJ, et al. Inverse relation between humoral and cellular immunity to glutamic acid decarboxylase in subjects at risk of insulin-dependent diabetes. Lancet 1993; 341:1365–1369.

138. Atkinson MA, Maclaren NK, Scharp DW, Lacy PE, Riley WJ. 64 000 M$_r$ autoantibodies as predictors of insulin-dependent diabetes. Lancet 1990; 335:1357–1360.

139. Tuomi T, Groop LC, Zimmet PZ, Rowley MJ, Knowles W, Mackay IR. Antibodies to glutamic acid decarboxylase reveal latent autoimmune diabetes mellitus in adults with a non-insulin-dependent onset of disease. Diabetes 1993; 42:359–362.

140. Seissler J, de Sonnaville JJ, Morgenthaler NG, et al. Immunological heterogeneity in type I diabetes: presence of distinct autoantibody patterns in patients with acute onset and slowly progressive disease. Diabetologia 1998; 41(8): 891–897.

141. Carlsson A, Sundkvist G, Groop L, Tuomi T. Insulin and glucagon secretion in patients with slowly progressing autoimmune diabetes (LADA). J Clin Endocrinol Metab 2000; 85(1):76–80.

142. Pietropaolo M, Barinas-Mitchell E, Pietropaolo SL, Kuller LH, Trucco M. Evidence of islet cell autoimmunity in elderly patients with Type 2 diabetes. Diabetes 2000; 49(1):32–38.

143. Payton MA, Hawkes CJ, Christie MR. Relationship of the 37,000- and 40,000-M(r) tryptic fragments of islet antigens in insulin-dependent diabetes to the protein tyrosine phosphatase-like molecule IA-2 (ICA512). J Clin Invest 1995; 96(3):1506–1511.

144. Bonifacio E, Lampasona V, Genovese S, Ferrari M, Bosi E. Identification of protein tyrosine phosphatase-like IA2 (islet cell antigen 512) as the insulin-dependent diabetes-related 37/40K autoantigen and a target of islet-cell antibodies. J Immunol 1995; 155(11):5419–5426.

145. Lu J, Li Q, Xie H, et al. Identification of a second transmembrane protein tyrosine phosphatase, IA-2beta, as an autoantigen in insulin-dependent diabetes mellitus:

146. precursor of the 37-kDa tryptic fragment. Proc Natl Acad Sci USA 1996; 93(6):2307–2311.

146. Greenbaum CJ, Palmer JP, Kuglin B, Kolb H. Insulin autoantibodies measured by radioimmunoassay methodology are more related to insulin-dependent diabetes mellitus than those measured by enzyme-linked immunosorbent assay: results of the Fourth International Workshop on the Standardization of Insulin Autoantibody Measurement. J Clin Endocrinol Metab 1992; 74(5):1040–1044.

147. Levy-Marchal C, Bridel MP, Sodoyez-Goffaux F, et al. Superiority of radiobinding assay over ELISA for detection of IAAs in newly diagnosed type I diabetic children. Diabetes Care 1991; 14(1):61–63.

148. Atkinson MA, Maclaren NK, Riley WJ, Winter WE, Fisk DD, Spillar RP. Are insulin autoantibodies markers for insulin-dependent diabetes mellitus? Diabetes 1986; 35: 894–898.

149. Castano L, Russo E, Zhou L, Lipes MA, Eisenbarth GS. Identification and cloning of a granule autoantigen (carboxypeptidase-H) associated with type I diabetes. J Clin Endocrinol Metab 1991; 3:1197–1201.

150. Rorsman F, Husebye ES, Winqvist O, Bjork E, Karlsson FA, Kampe O. Aromatic-L-amino-acid decarboxylase, a pyridoxal phosphate-dependent enzyme, is a beta-cell autoantigen. Proc Natl Acad Sci USA 1995; 92(19): 8626–8629.

151. Kim YJ, Zhou Z, Hurtado J, et al. IDDM patients' sera recognize a novel 30-kD pancreatic autoantigen related to chymotrypsinogen. Immunol Invest 1993; 22(3):219–222.

152. Chang YH, Hwang J, Shang HF, Tsai ST. Characterization of human DNA topoisomerase II as an autoantigen recognized by patients with IDDM. Diabetes 1996; 45(4): 408–414.

153. Aanstoot HJ, Kang SM, Kim J, et al. Identification and characterization of glima 38, a glycosylated islet cell membrane antigen, which together with GAD65 and IA2 marks the early phases of autoimmune response in Type 1 diabetes. J Clin Invest 1996; 97(12):2772–2783.

154. Johnson JH, Crider BP, McCorkle K, Alford M, Unger RH. Inhibition of glucose transport into rat islet cells by immunoglobulins from patients with new-onset insulin-dependent diabetes mellitus. N Engl J Med 1990; 332:653–659.

155. Atkinson MA, Holmes LA, Scharp DW, Lacy PE, Maclaren NK. No evidence for serological autoimmunity to islet cell heat shock proteins in insulin dependent diabetes. J Clin Invest 1991; 8:21–24.

156. Pietropaolo M, Castaño L, Babu S, et al. Islet cell autoantigen 69 kD (ICA69): molecular cloning and characterization of a novel diabetes-associated autoantigen. J Clin Invest 1993; 92:359–371.

157. Lampasona V, Ferrari M, Bosi E, Pastore MR, Bingley PJ, Bonifacio E. Sera from patients with IDDM and healthy individuals have antibodies to ICA69 on western blots but do not immunoprecipitate liquid phase antigen. J Autoimmun 1994; (5):665–664.

158. Maron R, Elias D, DeJongh BM, et al. Autoantibodies to the insulin receptor in juvenile onset insulin dependent diabetes. Nature 1983; 303:81–88.

159. Pak CY, Cha CY, Rajotte RV, McArthur RG, Yoon JW. Human pancreatic islet cell specific 38 kilodalton autoantigen identified by cytomegalovirus-induced monoclonal islet cell autoantibody. Diabetologia 1990; 33(9):569–572.

160. Karounos DG, Thomas JW. Recognition of common islet antigen by autoantibodies from NOD mice and humans with IDDM. Diabetes 1990; 39(9):1085–1090.

161. Lernmark A, Freedman ZR, Hofmann C, et al. Islet-cell-surface antibodies in juvenile diabetes mellitus. N Engl J Med 1978; 299:375–380.

162. Maclaren NK, Huang S-W. Antibody to cultured human insulinoma cells in insulin-dependent diabetes. Lancet 1975; 1:997–999.

163. Bohmer K, Keilacker H, Kuglin B, et al. Proinsulin autoantibodies are more closely associated with type 1 (insulin-dependent) diabetes mellitus than insulin auto-antibodies. Diabetologia 1991; 34(11):830–834.

164. Kasimiotis H, Myers MA, Argentaro A, et al. Sex-determining region Y-related protein SOX13 is a diabetes autoantigen expressed in pancreatic islets. Diabetes 2000; 49(4):555–561.

165. Winter WE. Autoimmune disorders that influence carbohydrate metabolism. In: Nakamura RM, Keren DF, Bylund DJ, eds. Clinical and Laboratory Evaluation of Human Autoimmune Diseases. Chicago, IL: ASCP Press, 2002:345–372.

166. Bottazzo GF, Lendrum R. Separate autoantibodies to human pancreatic glucagon and somatostatin cells. Lancet 1976; 2:873–876.

167. Del Prete GF, Tiengo A, Nosadini R, Bottazzo GF, Betterle C, Bersani G. Glucagon secretion in two patients with autoantibodies to glucagon producing cells. Horm Metab Res 1978; 10:260–261.

168. Winter WE, Maclaren NK, Riley WJ, Unger, RH, Ozand P, Neufeld M. Pancreatic alpha cell autoantibodies and glucagon response to arginine. Diabetes 1984; 33: 435–437.

169. Baba S, Morita S, Mizuno N, Okada K. Autoimmunity to glucagon in a diabetic not on insulin. Lancet 1976; 12:585.

170. Sanke T, Kondo M, Moriyama Y, Nanjo K, Iwo K, Miyamura K. Glucagon binding autoantibodies in a patient with hyperthyroidism treated with methimazole. J Clin Endocrinol Metab 1983; 57:1140–1144.

171. Jackson RA, Haynes BF, Burch WM, Shimizu K, Bowring MA, Eisenbarth GS. Ia+ T cells in new onset Graves' disease. J Clin Endocrinol Metab 1984; 59:187–190.

172. Jackson RA, Morris MA, Haynes BF, Eisenbarth GS. Increased circulating Ia-antigen bearing T-cells in type I diabetes mellitus. N Engl J Med 1982; 306:785–788.

173. Serjeantson S, Theophilus J, Zimmet P, Court J, Corssley JR, Elliott RB. Lymphocytotoxic antibodies and histocompatibility antigens in juvenile-onset diabetes mellitus. Diabetes 1981; 30:26–29.

174. Virella G, Wohltmann H, Sagel J, et al. Soluble immune complexes in patients with diabetes mellitus: detection and pathological significance. Diabetologia 1981; 21: 184–191.

175. Zier KS, Keo MM, Speilman RS, Baker L. Decreased synthesis of interleukin-2 (IL-2) in insulin-dependent diabetes mellitus. Diabetes 1984; 33:552–555.

176. Schatz DA, Riley WJ, Maclaren NK, Barrett DJ. Defective inducer T-cell function before the onset of insulin-dependent diabetes mellitus. J Autoimmun 1991; 4:125–136.

177. Faustman D, Li XP, Lin HY, et al. Linkage of faulty major histocompatibility complex class I to autoimmune diabetes. Science 1991; 254(5039):1756–1761.

178. Lang F, Maugendre D, Houssaint E, Charbonnel B, Sai P. Cytoadherence of lymphocytes from type I diabetic subjects to insulin-secreting cells. Marker of anti-beta-cell cellular immunity. Diabetes 1987; 36(12):1356–1364.

179. Litherland SA, Xie XT, Hutson AD, et al. Aberrant prostaglandin synthase 2 expression defines an antigen-presenting cell defect for insulin-dependent diabetes mellitus. J Clin Invest 1999; 104(4):515–523.

180. Litherland SA, Xie TX, Grebe KM, Li Y, Moldawer LL, Clare-Salzler MJ. IL10 resistant PGS2 expression in at-risk/Type 1 diabetic human monocytes. J Autoimmun 2004; 22(3):227–233.

181. Riley WJ, Maclaren NK, Lezotte D, Spillar RP, Rosenbloom AL. Thyroid autoimmunity in insulin-dependent diabetes mellitus: the case for routine screening. J Pediatr 1981; 98:350–354.

182. McCanlies E, O'Leary LA, Foley TP, et al. Ashimoto's thyroiditis and insulin-dependent diabetes mellitus: differences among individuals with and without abnormal thyroid function. J Clin Endocrinol Metab 1998; 83(5): 1548–1551.

183. Riley WJ, Toskes PP, Maclaren NK, Silverstein JS. Predictive value of gastric parietal cell autoantibodies as a marker for gastric and hematological abnormalities associated with insulin-dependent diabetes. Diabetes 1982; 32:1051–1055.

184. Riley WJ, Winer A, Goldstein D. Coincident presence of thyrogastric autoimmunity at onset of Type 1 (insulin-dependent) diabetes. Diabetologia 1983; 24:418–421.

185. Nepom GT, Kwok WW. Molecular basis for HLA-DQ associations with IDDM. Diabetes 1998; 47(8):1177–1184.

186. Harrison LC, Colman PG, Dean B, Baxter R, Martin FI. Increase in remission rate in newly diagnosed type I diabetic subjects treated with azathioprine. Diabetes 1985; 34:1306–1308.

187. Silverstein J, Maclaren N, Riley W, Spillar R, Radjenovic D, Johnson S. Immunosuppression with azathioprine and prednisone in recent-onset insulin-dependent diabetes mellitus. N Engl J Med 1988; 319:599–604.

188. Martin S, Schernthaner G, Nerup J, et al. Follow-up of cyclosporin A treatment in Type 1 (insulin-dependent) diabetes mellitus: lack of long-term effects. Diabetologia 1991; 34(6):429–434.

189. Silverstein JH, Rosenbloom AL. New developments in Type 1 (insulin-dependent) diabetes. Clin Pediatr 2000; 39:257–266.

190. Fuchtenbusch M, Rabl W, Grassl B, Bachmann W, Standl E, Ziegler AG. Delay of type I diabetes in high risk, first degree relatives by parenteral antigen administration: the Schwabing Insulin Prophylaxis Pilot Trial. Diabetologia 1998; 41(5):536–541.

191. Pozzilli P, Pitocco D, Visalli N, et al. No effect of oral insulin on residual beta-cell function in recent-onset type I diabetes (the IMDIAB VII). IMDIAB Group. Diabetologia 2000; 43(8):1000–1004.

192. Hahl J, Simell T, Ilonen J, Knip M, Simell O. Costs of predicting IDDM. Diabetologia 1998; 41(1):79–85.

193. Kupila A, Sipila J, Keskinen P, et al. Intranasally administered insulin intended for prevention of Type 1 diabetes—a safety study in healthy adults. Diabetes Metab Res Rev 2003; 19(5):415–420.

194. Elliott RB, Chase HP. Prevention or delay of Type 1 (insulin-dependent) diabetes mellitus in children using nicotinamide. Diabetologia 1991; 34(5):362–365.

195. ENDIT Trial: European Nicotinamide Intervention Trial (Manna R, Migliore A, Martin LS, et al.). Nicotinamide treatment in subjects at high risk of developing IDDM improves insulin secretion. Br J Clin Pract 1992; 46(3):1–9.

196. Gale EA, Bingley PJ, Emmett CL, Collier T; European Nicotinamide Diabetes Intervention Trial (ENDIT) Group. European Nicotinamide Diabetes Intervention Trial (ENDIT): a randomised controlled trial of intervention before the onset of Type 1 diabetes. Lancet 2004; 363(9413):925–931.

197. Herskowitz RD, Jackson RA, Soeldner JS, Eisenbarth GS. Pilot trial to prevent type I diabetes: progression to overt IDDM despite oral nicotinamide. J Autoimmun 1989; 2(5): 733–737.

198. Vidal J, Fernandez-Balsells M, Sesmilo G, et al. Effects of nicotinamide and intravenous insulin therapy in newly

diagnosed Type 1 diabetes. Diabetes Care 2000; 23(3): 360–364.

199. Herold KC, Hagopian W, Auger JA, et al. Anti-CD3 monoclonal antibody in new-onset Type 1 diabetes mellitus. N Engl J Med 2002; 346(22):1692–1698.

200. Herold KC, Gitelman SE, Masharani U, et al. A single course of anti-CD3 monoclonal antibody hOKT3gamma1(Ala-Ala) results in improvement in C-peptide responses and clinical parameters for at least 2 years after onset of Type 1 diabetes. Diabetes 2005; 54(6): 1763–1769.

201. Pozzilli P. Prevention of insulin-dependent diabetes mellitus 1998. Diabetes Metab Rev 1998; 14(1):69–84.

202. Rosenbloom AL, Schatz DA, Krischer JP, et al. Therapeutic controversy: prevention and treatment of diabetes in children. J Clin Endocrinol Metab 2000; 85(2): 494–522.

203. Shapiro AM, Lakey JR, Ryan EA, et al. Islet transplantation in seven patients with Type 1 diabetes mellitus using a glucocorticoid-free immunosuppressive regimen. N Engl J Med 2000; 343(4):230–238.

204. Yang L, Li S, Hatch H, et al. In vitro trans-differentiation of adult hepatic stem cells into pancreatic endocrine hormone-producing cells. Proc Natl Acad Sci USA 2002; 99(12):8078–8083.

205. Chaudhari M, Cornelius JG, Schatz D, Peck AB, Ramiya VK. Pancreatic stem cells: a therapeutic agent that may offer the best approach for curing Type 1 diabetes. Pediatr Diabetes 2001; 2(4):195–202.

206. Peck AB, Ramiya V. In vitro-generation of surrogate islets from adult stem cells. Transpl Immunol 2004; 12(3–4): 259–272.

207. Peck AB, Yin L, Ramiya V. Animal models to study adult stem cell-derived, in vitro-generated islet implantation. ILAR J 2004; 45(3):259–267.

208. Larsen JL. Pancreas transplantation: indications and consequences. Endocr Rev 2004; 25(6):919–946.

209. Demartines N, Schiesser M, Clavien PA. An evidence-based analysis of simultaneous pancreas-kidney and pancreas transplantation alone. Am J Transplant 2005; 5(11):2688–2697.

210. Kim KW. Islet transplantation: a realistic alternative for the treatment of insulin deficient diabetes mellitus. Diabetes Res Clin Pract 2004; 66(suppl 1):S11–S117.

211. Yamada S, Kojima I. Regenerative medicine of the pancreatic beta cells. J Hepatobiliary Pancreat Surg 2005; 12(3):218–226.

212. Zhang YQ, Kritzik M, Sarvetnick N. Identification and expansion of pancreatic stem/progenitor cells. J Cell Mol Med 2005; 9(2):331–344.

213. Di Gioacchino G, Di Campli C, Zocco MA, et al. Transdifferentiation of stem cells in pancreatic cells: state of the art. Transplant Proc 2005; 37(6):2662–2663.

214. Calne R. Cell transplantation for diabetes. Philos Trans R Soc Lond B Biol Sci 2005; 360(1461):1769–1774.

215. Stainer D. No stem cell is an islet (yet). N Engl J Med 2006; 354(5):521–523.

216. Trucco M. Regeneration of the pancreatic beta cell. J Clin Invest 2005; 115(1):5–12.

217. Umpierrez G, Casals MMC, Gebhart SSP, et al. Diabetic ketoacidosis in obese African Americans. Diabetes 1995; 44(7):790–795.

218. Pinhas-Hamiel O, Dolan LM, Zeitler PS. Diabetic ketoacidosis among obese African-American adolescents with NIDDM. Diabetes Care 1997; 20(4):484–486.

219. Banerji MA. Impaired beta-cell and alpha-cell function in African-American children with Type 2 diabetes mellitus—"Flatbush diabetes". J Pediatr Endocrinol Metab 2002; 15(suppl 1):493–501.

220. Zdravkovic V, Daneman D, Hamilton J. Presentation and course of Type 2 diabetes in youth in a large multi-ethnic city. Diabet Med 2004; 21(10):1144–1148.

221. Sapru A, Gitelman SE, Bhatia S, Dubin RF, Newman TB, Flori H. Prevalence and characteristics of Type 2 diabetes mellitus in 9–18 year-old children with diabetic ketoacidosis. J Pediatr Endocrinol Metab 2005; 18(9):865–872.

222. Shah SC, Malone JI, Simpson NE. A randomized trial of intensive insulin therapy in newly diagnosed insulin-dependent diabetes mellitus. N Engl J Med 1989; 320(9): 550–554.

223. Dupre J, Mahon JL. Diabetes-related autoantibodies and the selection of subjects for trials of therapies to preserve pancreatic beta-cell function in recent-onset Type 1 diabetes. Diabetes Care 2000; 23(8):1057–1058.

224. Rabinovitch A, Skyler JS. Prevention of Type 1 diabetes. Med Clin North Am 1998; 82(4):739–755.

225. Bonifacio E, Genovese S, Braghi S, et al. Islet autoantibody markers in IDDM: risk assessment strategies yielding high sensitivity. Diabetologia 1995; 38(7):816–822.

226. Verge CF, Gianani R, Kawasaki E, et al. Prediction of type I diabetes in first-degree relatives using a combination of insulin, GAD, and ICA512bdc/IA-2 autoantibodies. Diabetes 1996; 45(7):926–933.

227. Maclaren N, Lan M, Coutant R, et al. Only multiple autoantibodies to islet cells (ICA), insulin, GAD65, IA-2 and IA-2beta predict immune-mediated (Type 1) diabetes in relatives. J Autoimmun 1999; 12(4):279–287.

228. Gardner SG, Gale EA, Williams AJ, et al. Progression to diabetes in relatives with islet autoantibodies. Is it inevitable? Diabetes Care 1999; 22(12):2049–2054.

6

Management of the Child with Type 1 Diabetes

Oscar Escobar, Allan L. Drash, and Dorothy J. Becker

*Department of Pediatrics, Children's Hospital of Pittsburgh, University of Pittsburgh
School of Medicine, Pittsburgh, Pennsylvania, U.S.A.*

INTRODUCTION

Four distinct aspects of diabetes management: the *control* of the disease, its *prevention*, the *prevention of complications*, and its *cure* have occupied the minds of physicians and researchers for decades. Since the first recognition of diabetes as a clinical entity, utmost attention has been paid to its control. Initial efforts were directed toward the amelioration of the symptoms of polyuria and polydipsia eventually leading to cachexia and ultimately to death within weeks or months. Severe dietary restriction, especially, in the intake of sugars and other carbohydrates, high fat diets, and even complete starvation were the only available strategies to achieve that goal prior to the discovery of insulin. These therapeutic approaches did not prevent but may have delayed death; however, it seems possible that the "ketogenic" type diet may have contributed to the progression of the final decompensation of the disease with ketosis and ketoacidosis.

The discovery of insulin in 1921–1922 by Paulesco in Romania and Banting and Best in Canada (1–3) divided the history of diabetes into two. When Banting and Best gave injections of pancreas extracts as management for this disease in humans, the expectations of the outcome changed drastically. Survival beyond the first months after diagnosis was now possible, starvation was not necessary, and patients could recover from their initial cachexia. Progressive refinement in the production of insulin by the pharmaceutical industry led to improved purification techniques, which helped circumvent initial problems with nonpurified pancreas extracts such as local and generalized reactions and immune-mediated inactivation of insulin. Years of research and sophistication of molecular engineering have led to the production of human insulin through recombinant DNA technology and the design of insulin analogs with specific pharmacokinetic profiles that allow extrarapid or protracted action of injected insulin.

Metabolic Disturbances as a Consequence of Insulin Deficiency

The hormone "insulin" has pervasive effects on overall energy homeostasis. The actions of insulin are multifold, with major effect on protein and fat metabolism in addition to its key role on carbohydrate metabolism. Insulin release is stimulated by dietary intake (glucose, amino acids, and, to a much lesser extent, fats and ketones). The body energy metabolism is alternatively under the direct control of insulin during the prandial and immediate postprandial periods, whereas it is probably under the control of glucagon and epinephrine in the distal postprandial periods, growth hormone and cortisol being added during intervals of fasting. The release of insulin from β-cells has been shown to occur in a pulsatile fashion. The frequency of the insulin secretory bursts varies among different species from every 4 to every 15 minutes. These bursts are thought to be the main mechanism for basal insulin secretion, which is regulated through neuronal, hormonal, and metabolic pathways. The postprandial increase in insulin secretion appears to be the result of an increase in both the mass and the frequency of the secretory insulin bursts. This has been equated to insulin bolus secretion (4). There has been a resurgence of interest of the role of incretins in the postprandial insulin secretory response. Recent studies have focused on glucagon-like peptide 1 and its analogs in the potentiation of insulin secretion in response to dietary carbohydrates and the possible therapeutic use especially in Type 2 diabetes (T2D) (5–7) but also on Type 1 diabetes (8). The overall effect in the normal healthy individual is very narrow variations in the concentration of all nutrients throughout the course of each day, despite feasting and fasting cycles. These well-regulated nutrient concentrations include glucose, amino acids, triglyceride, cholesterol, ketone bodies, and a number of energy intermediates such as lactate, pyruvate, and glycerol. The extremes of both hyper and hypoglycemia are avoided, as are significant variations in lipid and protein concentration. The failure of insulin secretion results in a disruption of the normal tight regulation of metabolism.

Hyperglycemia results as a consequence of impaired peripheral glucose uptake and increased hepatic glucose production, both from an increased rate of glycogenolysis and from an increased rate of gluconeogenesis. Hyperlipidemia results from a marked increase in the mobilization of preformed fat in adipose tissues, and ketonuria results if this process continues unabated, without intervention of insulin therapy. The concentration of several counter-regulatory hormones is increased, including growth hormone, adrenocorticotropic hormone (corticotropin), cortisol, glucagon, and, in extreme stress, the catecholamines. The combination of insulin deficiency and counter-regulatory hormone excess complicates the metabolic picture further, exacerbating hyperglycemia, hyperlipidemia, and ketogenesis, and leading to an increased rate of proteolysis and gluconeogenesis, placing the individual in negative nitrogen balance (9,10). Acidosis, an additional complicating factor, ensues as the result of direct and indirect effect of insulin deficiency. Increased serum ketone concentration is the main cause of acidosis in insulin deficiency. Buildup of excretable organic acids resulting from decreased renal clearance and accumulation of lactic acid resulting from anaerobic metabolism of peripheral tissues are two additional sources of acidosis occurring in the individual with moderate-to-severe fluid deficit.

COMPONENTS OF MANAGEMENT OF DIABETES IN CHILDREN

We are currently in the midst of a continuum of changes in the strategies, techniques, and objectives of Type 1 diabetes mellitus (T1DM) management. These include techniques for the assessment of metabolic control and new insulin formulations and delivery systems. Practical aspects of diabetic care are described in Vol. 1; Chap. 7.

Monitoring of Control
Blood Glucose Monitoring

The development of devices for self-monitoring of blood-glucose revolutionized the management of diabetes. The widespread utilization of these monitoring techniques has provided the patient as well as the therapeutic team quantitative means of assessing metabolic status over time. Reflectance photometry and electrochemistry are the most common technologies used in the home blood-glucose meters. Both technologies depend on an enzymatic reaction between the glucose present in the blood sample and glucose oxidase, glucose dehydrogenase, or hexokinase. The concentration of glucose is determined indirectly by quantification of the intensity of a colored product of such reaction in the reflectance meters and by the quantification of the number of electrons generated during the oxidation reaction in the electrochemistry meters. There have been steady improvements in the accuracy and simplicity in the home blood-glucose monitoring meters that use smaller amounts of blood and take shorter time to display results, thus making measurement of fingerprick glucoses much easier for patients. Some meters give results very close to standardized laboratory measurements (11). In general, the meters that use glucose oxidase methodology have received the widest acceptance, being the most specific for glucose measurements. Nevertheless, interference by medications may occur (12). The current excitement in glucose monitoring strategies has been the rapid advancement of continuous glucose monitoring sensing techniques by a number of manufacturing companies. These monitors are currently undergoing critical evaluation (13,14) with recent publications suggesting fairly good accuracy in the hyperglycemic range but insufficient sensitivity and specificity for accurate detection of hypoglycemia (15). A recent randomized clinical trial in insulin-requiring T1DM and in Type 2 diabetics supporting the utility of continuous monitoring in detecting both unsuspected hypoglycemia and hyperglycemia and allowing patients to make appropriate therapeutic adjustments remains to be confirmed in the pediatric population (16).

Glycosylated Hemoglobin

The advent of methodologies to measure glycosylation in 1979 revolutionized the assessment of metabolic control in diabetes, providing clinicians with "the test that does not lie"; however, its interpretation has often been hampered because of interlaboratory variations that preclude accurate comparisons for individuals as well as for clinical trials. Progress is being made toward international standardization of techniques (17,18). Because the Diabetes Control and Complications Trial (DCCT) used high-performance liquid chromatography for the measurement of glycosylated hemoglobin, this continues to be the gold standard. The advantage of refinements to this technique is the ability to detect abnormal hemoglobins that might interfere with the measurement of hemoglobin A_{1C}. In the presence of hemoglobinopathies, affinity chromatography is the methodology of choice (19) with measurements of total glycosylated hemoglobin (i.e., $HbA_{1A} + A_{1B} + A_{1C}$ and glycosylated abnormal hemoglobins such as HbC, HbS, or HbF). Most laboratories report the results as a calculated HbA_{1C}. Desktop devices for rapid measurements of HbA_{1C} (DCA 2000) are increasingly used with results available within minutes at the time of the patient–clinician interaction (20). The accuracy of those methodologies in the higher ranges is steadily improving. New single home-use, disposable technologies to measure HbA_{1C}

are being introduced. Currently, the correlation with gold standard methods is variable but improving, and the concept is very promising (21).

Insulin Therapy

The last 20 years have witnessed major changes in all aspects of insulin therapeutics. Improvement in manufacturing techniques has resulted in remarkably increased purity of commercially available insulin preparations. Mixed beef and pork insulin, formerly the standard of therapy, has been basically removed from the marketplace. Highly purified pork insulin is now withdrawn from the U.S. market after several years of availability. Human insulins produced by recombinant DNA technologies, which replaced the animal extracted insulin preparations, are now being displaced by new synthetic insulin analogs.

The use of insulin analogs has grown significantly and has the theoretical advantages over regular insulin as well as intermediate and long acting [Neutral Protamine Hagedorn (NPH), Lente, Ultralente], which have nonphysiologic peaks in their pharmacokinetic profile. Insulin analogs engineered to provide either extrarapid action or prolonged, peakless pharmacokinetics and thus more physiologic actions may allow much more precise "tailoring" of an individual patient's insulin therapeutic needs on the basis of the individual's personal lifestyle (22,23) with less risk of hypoglycemia. The improvement of insulin infusion devices, both external and implanted, also provides the potential for more physiologic insulin delivery (24). The prospect of ultrasonic enhanced transdermal delivery of insulin and oral insulin therapy has been considered as a potential way to treat diabetic patients. Trials of inhaled insulin are ongoing in adults and children (25–30).

With these methodological advances has come an increasing interest in attempting to normalize energy metabolism, with the anticipation that this will eliminate or reduce the serious vascular complications of diabetes. This therapeutic approach has been improperly referred to as "intensive insulin therapy" rather than the more appropriate intensive diabetes therapy (31). Unfortunately, many, both physicians and patients, have concluded that the way to improve diabetes management is simply to give insulin more often. This is a serious misconception. Intensive diabetes therapy also includes the need for intensive blood-glucose monitoring, frequent measurements of glycosylated hemoglobin, and close attention to lipid abnormalities, blood pressure, and dietary and activity regimens.

Successful therapeutic management of the child and adolescent with diabetes mellitus requires a highly integrated four-pronged approach: insulin administration, dietary management, physical activity, and education and emotional support (32–35).

Insulin Requirements

Initial insulin requirements during preadolescence are approximately 1.0 unit/kg/day. A partial remission, referred to as the "honeymoon period," is identified as a decline in insulin requirement below 0.5 units/kg/day associated with very good metabolic control as measured by near-normal glycosylated hemoglobin levels. This occurs with increasing frequency and duration in newly diagnosed patients after the first several weeks since diagnosis, with the nadir in insulin requirement reached on average between 12 and 16 weeks after diagnosis. During this period, insulin doses must be carefully adjusted downward to prevent hypoglycemia. In some cases, the evening dose needs to be entirely eliminated. This is particularly true in those children in the under six-year age group. It is our impression that the duration of this remission period is usually longer than experienced in the past and, in some cases, may last longer than two years before increasing insulin needs are again expressed. The maintenance of some residual C-peptide secretion by intensive therapy must be a goal of treatment in view of the beneficial effects on the prevention of microvascular complications seen in the DCCT (36). Eventually, in all patients, insulin requirements begin to climb after the nadir of remission and generally plateau at about 0.8 to 1.2 units/kg/day in the preadolescent and somewhat above this in the adolescent child. Pubertal development is associated with increased insulin requirements secondary to insulin resistance induced by changes in the hormonal milieu. It is not infrequent to find adolescent patients who require 1.5 to 1.8 units/kg/day in order to maintain target HbA_{1C} levels (37).

Available Insulin Preparations

Three major groups of insulin preparations have been available sequentially since the discovery of insulin: (i) insulin extracted from animal pancreases, specifically beef, beef–pork, and pork insulin, (ii) human insulin produced by recombinant DNA technology, and (iii) insulin analogs, also produced by recombinant DNA technology with the introduction of molecule modifications that change the pharmacokinetic profile (Table 1).

Highly purified pork insulin was the longest survivor of the first group; however, its production has been discontinued at the time of writing this chapter. The advent of recombinant human insulin led to the general wisdom that this should be the insulin of choice due to both theoretical and practical advantages. Immune alterations of the action of exogenous animal insulin were a main concern; however, insulin antibody formation was the same when using pure pork and human insulin. Severe hypoglycemia without the typical hypoglycemic symptoms was described more frequently in patients treated with human insulin preparations leading to the controversial suggestion that there is something

Table 1 Insulin Preparations in the United States

Insulin type	Brand name	Laboratory	Onset of action	Peak	Duration of action	pH	CSII	IV use
Nonhuman Insulins								
Pork Regular	Iletin II Regular	Lilly	0.5 to 1 hr	2 to 4 hr	6 to 12 hr	Neutral	No	Yes
Pork-NPH	Iletin II NPH	Lilly	1 to 2 hr	4 to 14 hr	10 to > 24 hr	Neutral	No	No
Pork Lente	Iletin II Lente	Lilly	1 to 3 hr	6 to 16 hr	12 to > 24 hr	Neutral	No	No
Human Insulins								
Human Regular	Humulin R	Lilly	0.5 hr	2.5 to 5 hr	5 to 8 hr	Neutral	No	Yes
	Novolin R	Novo-Nordisk	0.5 hr	2.5 to 5 hr	5 to 8 hr	Neutral	No	Yes
Human-NPH	Humulin N	Lilly	1 to 2 hr	4 to 14 hr	10 to > 24 hr	Neutral	No	No
	Novolin N	Novo-Nordisk	1 to 2 hr	4 to 14 hr	10 to > 24 hr	Neutral	No	No
Human Lente	Humulin L	Lilly	1 to 3 hr	6 to 16 hr	12 to > 24 hr	Neutral	No	No
Human Ultralente	Humulin U	Lilly	4 to 8 hr	10 to 30 hr	18 to > 36 hr	Neutral	No	No
Premixed insulins								
NPH + Regular	Humulin 70/30	Lilly	0.5 hr	4 to 8 hr	24 hr	Neutral	No	No
	Novolin 70/30	Novo-Nordisk	0.5 hr	4 to 8 hr	24 hr	Neutral	No	No
Lis-pro Protamin/ Lispro	Humalog Mix 75/25	Lilly	<0.5 hr	0.5 to 1.5 hr/2 to 4 hr	6 to 12 hr	Neutral	No	No
Aspart Protamine/ Aspart	Novolog Mix 70/30	Novo-Nordisk	<0.25 hr	1 to 4 hr	12 to 24 hr	Neutral	No	No
Rapid analogs								
Lis-Pro Insulin	Humalog	Lilly	<0.5 hr	0.5 to 1.5 hr	<6 hr	Neutral	Yes	No
Aspart Insulin	Novolog	Novo-Nordisk	<0.25 hr	40 to 50 min	3 to 5 hr	Neutral	Yes	No
Insulin glulisine	Apidra	Aventis	<0.25 hr	55 min	<6 hr	Neutral	Yes	No
Long-acting analogs								
Insulin Glargine	Lantus	Aventis	1 to 2 hr	No true peak	24 hr	Acid	No	No
Insulin Detemir	Levemir	Novo-Nordisk	1 to 2 hr	No true peak	24 hr	Neutral	No	No

Abbreviation: NPH, neutral protamine hagedorn.

uniquely different about the body's response to human insulin that increases the likelihood of hypoglycemia (38,39). Different human insulin formulations, each with its own pharmacokinetic profile, were produced by adding other compounds (such as protamine, Zinc, etc.) to the preparation without manipulating the insulin molecule itself. This led to the production of regular insulin, also called crystalline insulin (Fig. 1A), NPH, Lente, and Ultralente insulins. According to the experience of a multicenter study, one of the major disadvantages of human ultralente insulin in the pediatric population was its prolonged peak and increased frequency of hypoglycemia when compared to pork-NPH (Becker, unpublished). These preparations, particularly Lente and Ultralente, have been used less frequently over the last few years and have practically disappeared from the therapeutic armamentarium, which still includes regular and NPH insulin formulations. The latter have been increasingly replaced by the new insulin analogs with new preparations recently introduced. Key modifications to the insulin molecule are the basis for the design of insulin analogs. These modifications are responsible for a change in the pharmacokinetic profile by altering the speed of release of insulin from the subcutaneous tissue into the circulation, but do not affect the interaction of the insulin molecule with its receptors.

The introduction of insulin lispro, a rapid-acting insulin analog, in the last decade, has broadened the repertoire of therapeutic options. Insulin lispro is synthetically produced by recombinant DNA technology

introducing a reversal of the natural occurring sequence of proline and lysine in positions B-28 and B-29, respectively, to LysB28 and ProB29 (Fig. 1B). It is highly homologous with human insulin; yet, it does not self-associate into dimers as human insulin does. The stabilized hexamer complexes of insulin lispro immediately dissociate into monomeric subunits upon injection into the subcutaneous tissue. This characteristic confers insulin lispro at least three differences when compared to human regular insulin: the action starts earlier (5–15 minutes), the peak insulin concentration in plasma is higher (more than double), and the duration of action is shorter (less than four hours). Similar pharmacokinetic profiles are found in newer analogs, i.e., insulin aspart and insulin glulisine. Insulin aspart is also produced by recombinant DNA technology, substituting proline in position B28 by aspartic acid (Fig. 1C). This single substitution reduces the molecule's tendency to form hexamers and, like lispro, it is therefore more rapidly absorbed after subcutaneous injection than regular human insulin (40–42).

Insulin glulisine has been engineered so that the amino acid asparagine in position 3 of the β-chain has been replaced by lysine and the amino acid lysine in position 29 of the β-chain has been replaced by glutamic acid. Safety and efficacy studies in children have been recently published (Fig. 1D) (43). The replacement of human regular insulin by ultra–short-acting analogs has been shown to decrease the frequency of hypoglycemia in randomized trials in children (44–48).

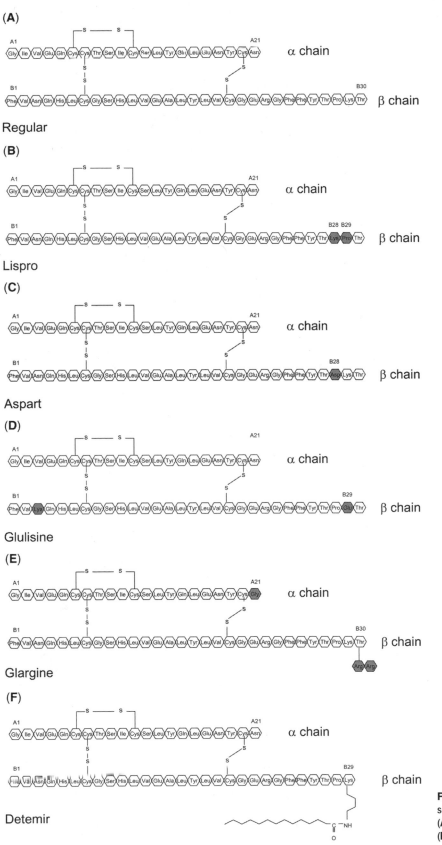

(A)

α chain

β chain

Regular

(B)

α chain

β chain

Lispro

(C)

α chain

β chain

Aspart

(D)

α chain

β chain

Glulisine

(E)

α chain

β chain

Glargine

(F)

α chain

β chain

Detemir

Figure 1 Schematic representation of the amino acid sequence of insulin and the currently available analogs: **(A)** regular insulin, **(B)** insulin lispro, **(C)** insulin aspart, **(D)** insulin glulisine, **(E)** insulin glargine, **(F)** insulin detemir.

More recently, long-acting insulin analogs have been synthesized with the idea of providing peak-less basal insulin concentrations. Also produced by recombinant DNA technology, these analogs are designed to have a longer duration of action by changing their isoelectric point (e.g., insulin glargine) or by promoting their binding to serum proteins such as albumin through the addition of fatty acids to the insulin molecule (e.g., insulin detemir) (40).

Insulin glargine has already been approved by the Food and Drug Administration (FDA) and is widely used in the United States. Two arginine molecules are added at the C-terminus of the β-chain. With these two extrapositive charges, the isoelectric point changes, rendering a molecule that is soluble at a more acidic pH and less soluble at the physiologic pH of the subcutaneous tissue. Another modification of the molecule, a substitution of asparagine in position 21 of the α-chain by glycine, is intended to protect it from deamidation and dimerization that would otherwise occur in the acidic solution in which it is formulated (Fig. 1E). The acidity of its formulation (pH: 4.0) allows insulin glargine to remain soluble. Once injected in the subcutaneous tissue, the solution is neutralized and forms microprecipitates from which insulin glargine is slowly released, providing virtually no peak concentrations and duration of action for at least 24 hours (49). Disadvantages of this type of insulin include the fact that it cannot be mixed with any other type of insulin, and, therefore, two separate injections must be given when the action of rapid insulin is needed at the same time. The acidic pH of the preparation seems to be responsible for a sensation of burning in the site of injection in some patients. Large multicenter trials of the effectiveness of these newer analogs in the pediatric population are being conducted in the United States. The use of insulin glargine has decreased the frequency of hypoglycemia in clinical trials (50).

Insulin detemir has just been approved in the United States in patients over six years at the time of writing this chapter. It has become popular in Europe. Insulin detemir is also considered a long-acting insulin analog providing "basal" insulin action with a duration of action for up to 24 hours. It is also produced by recombinant DNA technology. The amino acid threonine in position B29 is omitted, and a 14-carbon fatty acid (myristic acid) is attached to LysB29 (Fig. 1F). By virtue of this addition, insulin detemir increases its binding to serum proteins such as albumin. Slow release of insulin from albumin determines its pharmacokinetic profile characterized by the virtual absence of a peak and a prolonged duration of action (51) and has less variability in action than both NPH and glargine in adults (52). The pharmacokinetic profile of insulin detemir has been found to be consistent in children and adolescents (53).

It should be possible in the near future to tailor the individual patient's insulin management carefully to personal lifestyle and changing requirements. The availability of this new family of synthetic insulins will make the demise of animal insulin less painful for all of us.

Premixed insulins are an additional tool in the therapeutic repertoire. Highly popular for the management of insulin-requiring adults with T2D, their use in the treatment of T1DM in children and adolescents is less common in the United States and, in our experience, mostly restricted to adolescents who display poor compliance with their insulin administration, especially with regimens requiring multiple daily injections (MDI). The inability to adjust doses according to planned food intake, meal plans, or ambient blood sugars is the major drawback for the use of these combinations in children (54). Available premixed insulin preparations include combinations of NPH and regular insulin in a 70% to 30% ratio, lispro protamine and lispro insulin in a 75% to 25% ratio, and aspart protamine and aspart insulin in a 70% to 30% ratio.

Insulin Management Strategies

When insulin preparations with intermediate or prolonged duration of action such as protamin insulin (Hagedorn) and zinc protamin insulin (Scott and Fisher) in the mid-1930s, isophane insulin (Krayenbuhl and Rosenberg) in the mid-1940s and slow insulins (Hallas-Moller) in the early 1950s became available, insulin regimens were designed to provide insulin coverage for the 24-hour period with the minimum possible number of injections.

All these preparations were characterized by a distinct peak of action occurring several hours after being injected. The presence of such a peak was at the same time an advantage and a drawback. The advantage was the ability to provide robust insulin coverage for a meal taken several hours after the insulin injection, obviating the need for an additional shot at the time of that meal. The drawback was the increased risk of hypoglycemia at the time of that peak if not matched by timely food intake. One or two insulin doses per day given as combinations of "intermediate-" and "rapid"-acting insulin preparations became the standard of care. This strategy, later called "conventional insulin management" and popular for several decades, was challenged by the DCCT, which demonstrated that "intensive therapy," defined as the use of MDI (three or more) of insulin or continuous subcutaneous insulin infusion (CSII) via pump, along with more frequent blood-glucose monitoring, timely adjustment of insulin doses according to blood-glucose levels, dietary intake and anticipated exercise, and more frequent visits to the therapeutic team, was effective in delaying the onset and slowing down the progression of diabetic retinopathy, nephropathy, and neuropathy in adult and adolescent patients with T1DM (Table 2) (55).

There had already been a gradual movement toward intensification of diabetes management,

Table 2 Examples of Insulin Regimens

Regimen	Insulin preparations	Times
Two-shot-per day	Human NPH (N)	Breakfast: N + R/Log
	Regular (R) or rapid analog (Log)	Dinner: N + R/Log
Three-shot-per day	Human NPH (N)	Breakfast: N + Log
	Rapid analog (Log)	Dinner: Log
		Bedtime: N + Log
Basal-bolus	Insulin glargine (Glar)	Meals and snacks: Log
	Rapid analog (Log)	Breakfast or HS snack: Glar
Combination regimen	Insulin glargine (Glar)	Breakfast: N + Log
	Human NPH (N)	Lunch: no insulin
	Rapid analog (Log)	Dinner: Log
		HS snack: Glar + Log

Abbreviation: NPH, neutral protamine hagedorn.

climaxed by the results of the DCCT. The term "intensive insulin therapy" has unfortunately become embedded in our terminology and to the uninitiated may be interpreted to mean that overall diabetes management can be improved simply by increasing the frequency of insulin administration. The proper message, of course, is that improved results are accomplished in the great majority of patients only with intensification of all aspects of management. The "therapeutic set" of the diabetes team, with full cooperation of the patient and family, is directed toward achieving either optimal management utilizing whatever resources are available or something less. The concept of conventional versus intensive management must be set aside. We must undertake to do the very best we can with each patient, understanding that there are major differences in resources and abilities as well as many barriers to the achievement of near metabolic normality (56–59).

Fixed Meal-Insulin Regimens

Two-Shot-per-Day Regimen. While very young children could previously be reasonably managed using a two-shot-per-day split-dose regimen of pork-NPH insulin plus lispro insulin (or regular insulin) given before breakfast and before the evening meal, the same was not the case when using this schedule with human NPH insulin. The shorter time course of human NPH, particularly overnight (60), did not provide adequate glucose control, leading to morning hyperglycemia. Attempts to improve this by raising the dose increased the likelihood of nocturnal hypoglycemia. The recent complete withdrawal of pork insulin from the market has prompted an abandonment of this therapeutic strategy among most pediatric diabetologists.

Three-Shot-per-Day Regimen. Moving the evening dose of human NPH to bedtime was instituted to solve the above-mentioned difficulty; however,

short-acting insulin was still needed to cover the evening meal. This was the origin of the three-shot-per-day regimen consisting of a combination of human NPH and regular insulin, and later a rapid-acting analog at breakfast, a rapid-acting insulin at the evening meal and glargine or human NPH usually with a small dose of rapid-acting insulin given at the bedtime snack. This has been a widely used regimen in children, with the recent advantages of the short-acting analogs being lower post-prandial blood-glucose levels and less hypoglycemia, and thus theoretically better hypoglycemia awareness and counter-regulation in response to low blood sugars. An additional advantage of rapid-acting analogs in pediatric patients, especially in infants, whose food intake is often unpredictable, is the administration after eating due to their rapid onset of action, allowing for adjustments based on food intake.

Basal-Bolus Regimens

Multiple Daily Injections. The advent of long-acting, relatively peakless insulin analogs has allowed the design of insulin regimens, which more closely resemble the physiologic insulin secretion pattern, i.e., the basal insulin secretion and the meal-induced insulin bursts (bolus). The former is provided by the long-acting analogs, and the latter is provided as injections of short-acting analogs at the time of the meals. The same principle is used in CSII through insulin pumps. The basal-bolus regimen based on the use of insulin glargine, for instance, either one or twice daily at bedtime snack or at breakfast and the administration of a rapid analog with meals and snacks, provides great flexibility close to that of the insulin infusion pump, and increases the chances for good control in highly motivated patients.

Basal-bolus regimens have also prompted a change in the paradigm of insulin dose calculation. A transition is evolving from a "reactive" approach represented by the all so frequently used "sliding scales" designed to provide smaller doses of short-acting insulin when the blood sugar is lower and larger doses when the blood sugar is higher in a preset continuum of ranges, to a more "proactive" approach represented by a dual calculation of each dose of short-acting analog based on (i) the expected food intake and (ii) the current level of blood-glucose. The former calculation is, at the present time, based on the amount of carbohydrates contained in the meal to be ingested. Controversy exists as to how other macronutrients such as proteins and fats should also be taken into consideration. Nevertheless, for the sake of practicality and simplicity, using carbohydrates alone seems to be a reasonable practice if protein and fat are kept constant. Insulin to carbohydrate (I:CHO) ratios are initially estimated according to the patient's weight and modified thereafter depending on the need. Tables to calculate initial I:CHO ratios depending on body weight are available and typically range from 1 unit for every 5 g of carbohydrate in the heaviest individuals to 1 unit for every 50 to 100 g of carbohydrate in the smaller patients. It should be noted that these tables do not take into account the huge variability of insulin sensitivity in children related to pubertal status, physical fitness, etc. The second calculation frequently referred to as the "correction" is, in principle, the same as the previously used sliding scales. However, a mathematical calculation via a simple formula allows more precise computation of the insulin dose. The correction formula typically used is:

$$\text{Correction} = \frac{\text{MBG} - T}{\text{ISF}}$$

where MBG is the measured meter blood-glucose, T is the target blood-glucose, and ISF is the insulin-sensitivity factor. The target blood-glucose can be modified depending on the circumstances such as the age of the patient or the time of the day. Typically, higher targets are set for younger individuals and for the bedtime insulin dose calculation. The insulin sensitivity factor represents the theoretical number of points (mg/dL) of blood-glucose dropped by one unit of insulin and was devised in adults. Several ways of figuring out the initial calculation of ISF have been proposed. A common one is dividing 1800 (1900 in children younger than eight years of age) by the total daily dose of insulin required by a patient. These formulas also do not take into account individual variations in insulin sensitivity as described above and usually have to be adjusted.

Using a formula instead of a sliding scale is hoped to be useful in patients on CSII (see below). Current pumps have a computer where the parameters of the calculation (T,ISF) can be preentered and the MBG can be entered at the time of insulin dosing. The computer automatically calculates the correction dose. Current pumps can administer fractions of a unit of insulin, which is commonly the result of the calculation with the formula and may be important in small children; this is in contrast to injections when rounding down or rounding up becomes necessary in those circumstances. When the current MBG is lower than the target, a negative dosing is calculated and the pump's computer subtracts this amount from the dose calculated based on I:CHO ratio. Studies are currently being designed to critically assess what the best formulae are, and whether their introduction provides a real rather than a theoretical improvement in glycemic control.

Continuous Subcutaneous Insulin Infusion Therapy. In the early days of insulin pumps in the 1980s, we developed an extensive pump experience with our adolescent patients. Their initial metabolic response was gratifying in terms of decreasing glycosylated hemoglobin and blood-glucoses. As we followed these patients over time, however, the enthusiasm for living with a pump declined and their compliance with the intensive therapeutic regimen diminished. Thus, the early successes were lost. At that time, we concluded that the rigors of insulin pump therapy with the available pumps were such that few children or adolescents would adapt successfully to it and essentially discontinued pump use in our general clinic population (61). More recently, however, the advances in delivery systems have made pump therapy much easier for the patient with more reliable insulin delivery and less complications. The potential for success with pump therapy has been demonstrated in carefully selected patients who are either very mature and have made a clear commitment to improved health or have very dedicated families. Determining patient eligibility for CSII therapy has been a subject of controversy. Among the factors involved in this equation are the age of the patient, the degree of prior glycemic control, and multiple psychological, familial, cultural, and socioeconomic issues. The American Diabetes Association (ADA) suggests four basic conditions that should be met by the patient to increase the chances of obtaining benefit from CSII: (i) motivation, (ii) willingness to work in conjunction with the health care team, (iii) ability to demonstrate understanding of the technical aspects of correct use of the pump and, (iv) capacity of obtaining and interpreting the data to make decisions regarding pump programming (62,63).

Variations of the patient's age and the degree of prior glycemic control are major factors for the accounting heterogeneity of eligibility criteria for CSII in different centers. While some centers have been more liberal with the use of insulin pumps in younger patients including young children and even infants, others prefer to reserve this mode of therapy for older children, adolescents, and young adults capable of independent decision-making. The involvement of parents or caregivers is a *sine qua non* in the former group. The parental share of responsibility approaches 100% in the youngest patients, and should decrease in the older ones, although at least a certain degree of supervision continues to be highly recommended in the latter. It has been shown that improvement of glycemic control achieved by adolescent patients with the participation of their parents or responsible adults decreases significantly when these patients are left on their own (64), most probably reflecting a decrease in the frequency of blood-glucose monitoring and/or failure to give pre-meal insulin boluses. Poor judgment at the time of deciding on pump programming and bolus calculation according to the blood sugar level, the food to be eaten, and the amount of exercise predicted for the next minutes or hours would be additional concerns in some adolescents managed through CSII without parental involvement.

Our most recent experience with CSII showed that metabolic control improved in patients switched from MDI to CSII as manifested by a decrease of 0.5% of HbA_{1C} at three and six months after initiation. HbA_{1C} levels at 9 and 12 months after initiation of CSII was not significantly different from baseline. A similar difference in HbA_{1C} levels was observed between patients managed with MDI versus patients on CSII during the same observation period with lower HbA_{1C} levels in the latter. The patients who had a worsening of their diabetic control when switched to CSII were older than the patients who improved. They also had higher baseline levels of HbA_{1C}. Therefore, we found that the patients more likely to improve the metabolic control are those who have better control to begin with as compared to the patients with poorer control, who are older adolescents, and tend to worsen.

A beneficial effect of CSII found by others and us is the reduction in the frequency of severe hypoglycemia. We have not seen increase in body weight in patients managed with CSII as it occurred in the DCCT. Despite the lack of improvement in metabolic control in older adolescents with poorer control, reduction in the frequency of diabetic ketoacidosis (DKA) has been reported (65). However, in our clinic, this is frequently not achieved.

Approximately one-third of DCCT intensively managed patients were on an insulin infusion device. The general experience did not clearly document a benefit of either pump or multiple dose injection therapy. Since then, uncontrolled studies have suggested improved glycemic control and less hypoglycemia in children and adolescents in CSII (66), although similar results are not universal (67). Our own experience suggests that CSII does not improve glycemic control in those with high HbA_{1C} but can improve quality of life. The biggest risk is exaggerated expectations of pump therapy. Successful implementation of CSII therapy requires a dedicated, experienced team of diabetes caregivers available for very frequent telephone contact.

Insulin Dose Adjustments

By applying glucose goals derived from self-monitoring of blood-glucose, insulin adjustments are made as necessary to attempt continually to bring the patient's glucose variation into the target range. Of course, diet and exercise alterations are also considered and applied as necessary.

For the fixed insulin-meal regimens, we use a "10% rule" in terms of insulin changes. By summing the total insulin dose and dividing by 10, one obtains the number of units of insulin that is generally safe to increase or decrease in a patient who requires change. If the patient's blood-glucose levels are generally high throughout, then the distribution of the increase follows the current distribution, usually two-thirds added to the morning and one-third to the evening dosage. On the other hand, if the patient has a particular time point, for example before dinner, that is persistently out of range, then the dose modification applies only to the morning or lunch time insulin and the amount is determined by 10% of the morning dose. Again the distribution between NPH insulin and regular insulin or insulin lispro depends upon both pre- and postprandial blood-glucose levels. In the asymptomatic patient, we prefer to make insulin adjustments relatively slowly, after three to five days on a particular dose. On the other hand, if the patient is symptomatic and/or ketonuric, one must be more aggressive in moving toward a more acceptable blood-glucose excursion. Most patients are provided with insulin scales for their short-acting insulin doses. Additional modifications can be used in anticipation of planned activity, food intake, and to correct current hyperglycemia.

Insulin dose adjustments in the basal-bolus regimens should distinguish between these two components. In order to assess the dose of the basal insulin (i.e., the long-acting analog in the injection regimen or the basal rate in CSII), a meal and its associated bolus can be skipped. The blood sugar obtained prior to the following scheduled meal reflects the adequacy of the basal insulin dose during that period of the day. To assess the adequacy of the bolus calculation, a two-hour postprandial MBG should be obtained. As described above, formulas to assess boluses are a starting point and usually have to be adjusted up or down.

Somogyi Effect and Dawn Phenomenon

A very common management problem is illustrated by the child whose fasting blood-glucoses are consistently elevated. The usual strategy is to increase the evening intermediate-acting insulin (NPH) or the long-acting analog until fasting blood-glucoses are satisfactory. The common complication of this technique is that nocturnal hypoglycemia may be induced, with or without counter-regulatory hormone secretion recovery by the next morning. Nocturnal hypoglycemia is often masked by counter-regulation or waning of insulin action. This is particularly true with human insulin because of its shorter duration of action. The concept of the Somogyi phenomenon causing rebound hyperglycemia in the morning has been challenged although counter-regulation can account for post hypoglycemic euglycemia. Rebound hyperglycemia probably only occurs after active food therapy of low blood sugars (though this is not well reported in children).

If fasting glucose levels are elevated when a regimen with NPH or glargine given at bedtime is used, the addition of a short-acting analog at the bedtime dose may be beneficial, allowing a decrease of the dose of NPH or glargine to lower the risk of hypoglycemia in the middle of the night while controlling a hyperglycemic excursion as a result of the snack (68,69).

Elevated plasma glucose concentrations in the morning after 5 A.M. without preceding hypoglycemia characterize the "dawn" phenomenon. This occurs as a result of increased insulin requirements in the early morning, which could be related to either increased insulin clearance or decreased insulin action. An early morning surge of growth hormone, one of the insulin counter-regulatory hormones, has been hypothesized as a causal factor. Whether or not long-acting insulin analogs are able to avoid this morning rise in blood-glucose levels as a result of the dawn phenomenon in children and adolescents remains to be demonstrated in larger-scale pediatric trials. The use of CSII makes the management of the Somogyi and dawn phenomena much easier by manipulation of the basal rates.

Adjustments for Elective Surgery and Other Procedures

Children with diabetes undergoing elective surgery or other procedures which require fasting need to have appropriate insulin management before, during, and after the procedure. It is always a good idea to schedule these interventions all in the morning for several reasons: (i) the overnight natural fasting is usually adequate for anesthesia, (ii) the first scheduled procedure is less likely to be postponed, avoiding unnecessary prolongation of fasting with the concomitant risk for hypoglycemia, and (iii) insulin dose adjustments are easier and interfere less with the reinitiation of the home regimen. General guidelines may need modifications in certain circumstances. The recommendation in patients receiving a fixed meal-insulin regimen is to provide the usual doses of insulin the day before the intervention and to initiate fasting after midnight. One half to two-thirds of the intermediate insulin dose without fast acting insulin—unless the blood-glucose is high—is given in the morning prior to the procedure. The use of dextrose-containing intravenous fluids at maintenance rate is usually appropriate. The home insulin regimen can be restarted when the patient has finished the postoperatory recovery and is allowed to eat. In patients managed with a basal-bolus regimen, the recommendation is to keep the basal insulin (long-acting analog or basal rate through an insulin pump) unchanged and skip the breakfast bolus.

Adjustment for Exercise

Increased energy expenditure during exercise causing hypoglycemia is a well-known phenomenon requiring appropriate decreases in insulin doses or increased food intake. In contrast, acute stressful exercise can cause hyperglycemia due to release of hormones that antagonize insulin action (glucagon, growth hormone, epinephrine). The standard recommendation of providing 15 g of carbohydrate of rapid absorption may be insufficient to treat exercise-induced hypoglycemia in children and adolescents (70). Post-exercise hypoglycemia is often unrecognized and can occur hours later. Its prevention requires anticipation (71).

Adjustment for Intercurrent Illnesses

Intercurrent illnesses may have opposing effects in glycemic control in children. Common scenarios include viral or bacterial infections such as upper respiratory infections, gastroenteritis, acute pharyngitis, otitis media, and pneumonia among others. Decreased food intake is frequently seen in gastrointestinal and pharyngeal infections, and requires a decrease in insulin dosing. On the other hand, release of counter-regulatory hormones induced by fever and pain lead to hyperglycemia and increased ketogenesis. The balance between increased and decreased insulin requirements has to be addressed when managing diabetic children with intercurrent illnesses. "Sick day management" rules provide an initial guide for the parents but, not infrequently, professional assistance via telephone contact or direct visit to a medical facility is necessary to manage this delicate balance to avoid acute complications such as severe hypoglycemia or DKA. The appearance of urinary ketones in the face of hypoglycemia or normoglycemia in a child who has been refusing to eat is most probably the result of starvation ketogenesis. Attempts to provide calories should be made. In contrast, ketonuria in the presence of hyperglycemia, especially in a sick child, should alert the parents and the physician about impending ketoacidosis and should be managed promptly and aggressively.

Dietary Management

As stated above, the nutritional component is one of the cornerstones of diabetes management. The recommendations on nutritional intervention in diabetes have changed over the years. Before the discovery of insulin, the concept of dietary management relied on severe restriction of caloric intake leading to starvation diets. This was followed by low-carbohydrate high-fat diets and, most recently, higher-carbohydrate lower-fat diets (Table 3).

Our own recommendations since the early 70s have been 50% to 55% carbohydrate, 15% to 20% protein, and 30% fat with limitation of saturated fat and cholesterol to less than 10%. More recent recommendations suggest that 45% to 65% of the calories are derived from carbohydrates (73), making the now fashionable "low-carbohydrate diets" an inadequate alternative for diabetic individuals. On the other hand, the recommendation that 60% to 70% of the calories in the diet comes from a combination of carbohydrates and monounsaturated fat is supported in part by the finding that a high-carbohydrate diet leads to more hyperglycemia than a high monounsaturated-fat diet, while no differences were seen in the lipid profile between the two (74,75). The food

Table 3 Historical Perspective of Nutrition Recommendations

	Distribution of calories		
Year	Carbohydrate (%)	Protein (%)	Fat (%)
Before 1921	Starvation Diets		
1921	20	10	70
1950	40	20	40
1971	45	20	35
1986	Up to 60	12–20	<30
1994	a	10–20	a,b
2002	c	15–20	b,c

[a]Based on nutritional assessment and treatment goals.
[b]Approximately 10% from polyunsaturated fats and less than 10% from saturated fats.
[c]60–70% of the calories should come from carbohydrates and monounsaturated fat.
Note: Greater emphasis is placed on lifestyle changes.
Source: From Ref. 72.

intake of a diabetic child as well as that of any healthy child should be balanced; in other words, it should contain adequate amounts of carbohydrates, protein, fat, minerals, vitamins, fiber, and water.

The design of nutritional strategies for management of diabetes must be based on the procurement of basic goals, including: (i) the maintenance of near-normal glucose and lipid levels; (ii) the delivery of an adequate amount of calories to achieve normal growth and development in children and to avoid weight loss or excessive weight gain in all patients and, (iii) the prevention of nutrition-related complications such as hypoglycemia, renal disease, cardiovascular disease, hypertension, and autonomic neuropathy.

Therefore, diabetic patients should have meal plans designed for each individual, based on their needs and goals, taking into consideration age-related, cultural, as well as ethnic and financial issues. The concept of a unique "diabetic" or "ADA" diet should be replaced by a prudent meal plan. Furthermore, the term "diet" should be avoided given its connotation of imposed and "punitive" restriction. A newer term, "medical nutrition therapy," has been proposed by the ADA to replace others such as diet, dietary management, or diet therapy (76). Above all, healthy eating should be emphasized.

It is evident, from Table 3, that carbohydrate intake has become less restricted on recent recommendations. Carbohydrates are mainly of two kinds: complex carbohydrates or starches and simple sugars. Great emphasis has been given in the past to the avoidance of simple sugar intake in diabetic individuals. Although this continues to be truth, the restriction is less severe than originally proposed. Simple sugars naturally occurring in fruits (fructose) and milk (galactose), for instance, should be allowed within the meal plan. Fructose induces a smaller rise in blood sugar than isocaloric amounts of sucrose or other carbohydrates; however, in excess it may induce an undesirable increase in serum cholesterol and

low-density lipoprotein (LDL) cholesterol; therefore, fructose intake in diabetic individuals should be moderate and its use as a sweetener should be considered as not advantageous (77–79). Sucrose may also be component of the meal plan as long as it is not abused and is part of a meal rather than eaten alone. Glycemic excursions after ingestion of sucrose have been found to be of similar magnitude to those occurring after intake of white bread, refined rice, and cooked potatoes. Therefore, more attention has been paid to the total amount of carbohydrate and not the source of carbohydrate. Unfortunately, less attention has been paid to the factors that affect absorption of the carbohydrate, such as the rapid absorption in the liquid state or delayed absorption when eaten with fat or fiber.

Within the 30% of calories coming from fat, it is accepted that less than 10%, i.e., about one-third of those could come from saturated fat, another 10% from polyunsaturated fat, and yet another 10% or more from monounsaturated fat. Because LDL cholesterol is a major risk factor for both micro- and macrovascular disease in Type 1 diabetes (80,81), we advise that more attention be paid to the fat content of the diet. This is in addition to the importance of the role of fat in influencing glycemic excursions after a meal. The postprandial glucose excursion is determined by the rate of entry of glucose into the blood stream and the rate of disappearance of glucose, mainly the result if insulin-induced glucose cellular uptake. Absorption of carbohydrate from the gut is delayed by the presence of fat in the same meal, as it slows down the rate of gastric emptying (82). On the other hand, nutrients other than carbohydrates, mainly amino acids, also require insulin action. Hence, a protein meal increases glucose levels and requires insulin administration.

Limitations of protein content in the meals prior to the advent of albuminuria have been recommended because of the detrimental effect of protein excesses in animals (83). Though this effect has not yet been proven in children and adolescents, care to prevent protein overload to the kidneys appears to be prudent.

Food exchange lists have been created to help patients deal with the heterogeneity of nutrient composition of different foods with the purpose of providing some sort of standardization when designing a meal plan. These lists group certain foods together based on similarities in their composition. The carbohydrate group includes: starch, fruit, milk (skim, reduced fat, whole), other carbohydrates, and vegetables. The meat and meat-substitute group divides protein into: very lean, lean, medium fat, and high fat. Finally, the fat group includes lists of monounsaturated fats, polyunsaturated fats, and saturated fats. These lists are not a dietary formulation per se. The introduction of carbohydrate counting is an attempt to allow greater flexibility in meals, taking into account larger and smaller carbohydrate intake. This is a more realistic concept for daily living. The disadvantage is that all carbohydrates are treated as equal (e.g., complex and free sugars) and insulin needs for protein metabolism and effect of fat on absorption are ignored. It is recommended that a skilled dietician tailor the meal plan individually for each patient. It is clear that tailoring insulin needs according to carbohydrate counting or food exchanges and vice versa is not a straightforward task. "Carb counting" has risen in popularity as more than 90% of the calories coming from carbohydrates end up as glucose as compared to much less of the calories of protein and none from fat. The conclusion that carbohydrate is the only dietary source for blood-glucose is erroneous. Carbohydrate counting was originally initiated as a means to assist diabetic patients in designing their meal plan, especially for those with erratic meal planning. "Carb counting" offers the possibility of calculating by a rather simple mathematical formula, and involves initial training and attainment of skills to calculate the amount of insulin that should be given to cover the predicted blood-glucose rise after a certain food is eaten. This approach is usually used to calculate the insulin boluses to cover meals in patients receiving basal-bolus regimens of insulin including CSII. However, it should not be limited to this mode of insulin delivery. In addition, when teaching carbohydrate counting, the importance of stability of the other meal constituents should be emphasized.

The advent of basal-bolus regimens of insulin has greatly increased the flexibility of daily living, particularly in regard to the dietary intake. As the rigid, constant, and tightly scheduled meal plan to match the pharmacokinetic profiles of intermediate- and short-acting insulin preparations (as proposed in the fixed insulin-meal regimens) is no longer necessary, variation in timing and amount of meals and snacks, within certain limits, is now possible. Insulin boluses may vary in time and dose to match the food intake rather than vice versa. Skipping a meal or a snack does not pose the risk for hypoglycemia as in the fixed insulin-meal regimens. However, it has been our experience with some patients, especially teenagers, that this "freedom" is misunderstood and frequent snacks, not adequately covered with insulin, become the rule more than the exception, leading to significant hyperglycemia or, on the other hand, overbolusing for frequent snacks per day increases the risk of hypoglycemia. In those cases, reimplementation of a structured meal plan along with the basal-bolus regimen improves control in selected patients.

Exercise as a Therapeutic Modality

There is an increasing body of scientific data that suggests, but does not definitively prove, that physical fitness is a beneficial and highly desirable state for the patient with diabetes mellitus (84–88). Consequently, we recommend to our patients that they incorporate a regular exercise program into their daily lives. Exercise increases glucose utilization, and highly fit muscles have an increased sensitivity to insulin and, thus, glucose uptake. Our clinical observations include the following:

1. Highly fit children and adolescents with diabetes usually require less insulin per level of metabolic control.
2. These individuals are generally in better metabolic control than their relatively unfit diabetic peers.
3. The physically fit individual, particularly the competitive athlete, usually has a better self-image and a better appreciation of the importance of good diabetes management.
4. Episodic exercise, as opposed to regular exercise, which leads to an improved level of physical fitness, may result in either hypoglycemia or even the induction of DKA in very poorly controlled patients.
5. Our long-term diabetes complication studies indicate that those individuals who participated in competitive athletics during high school and college had a significant reduction in both diabetes-related morbidity and mortality when evaluated 10 to 30 years later.

Our recommendation to our patients—unfortunately rarely followed—is that they develop a daily exercise regimen (seven days per week) that involves a fairly vigorous level of exercise for approximately one hour each day. This could be most easily achieved by participating in competitive programs at the child's school, if available. If this is neither possible nor desirable, then other entirely satisfactory exercise activities can be substituted such as vigorous walking, jogging, swimming, aerobic dancing, tennis, and golf. The patients must understand the effects of exercise on blood-glucose and be ready to make necessary adjustments in insulin dose or diet. In general, we prefer to increase caloric intake before exercise rather than reduce insulin in the normal weight child, although either or both may be satisfactory solutions to problems of hypoglycemia associated with exercise. The very poorly controlled patient who desires to embark on an exercise program should be encouraged to improve overall metabolic control by increasing insulin dosage before embarking on an exercise regimen.

Education and Emotional Support

The importance of education as part of the integral management of diabetes cannot be overemphasized. Education should start at the very moment when the diagnosis of diabetes is made. However, the initial phase of shock experienced by parents in response to the new diagnosis in their child may interfere with the understanding of basic principles. That is why a well-balanced combination of emotional support and objective teaching is essential for the success of the initial education process. Previous misconceptions about diabetes that patients and their families may have when they are faced with this diagnosis for the first time should be clearly addressed at this point. When the child presents with severe DKA, the initiation of the education process should be deferred until the parents see signs of recovery and the child himself is able to participate in a teaching conversation, depending on age. However, the diabetes management team should be readily available to answer questions from the family members during this critical period to soothe their fears and to start building a nurturing relationship with them. That opportunity could be used to explain in very basic language the pathogenesis of diabetes and the pathophysiology of DKA as well as the reason for the clinical manifestations during the days prior to the diagnosis and at the time of presentation. This will help the family to recognize later on the signs of decompensation that need to be avoided (Table 4).

The education process should start immediately when the newly diagnosed child does not present in DKA or comes with a very mild DKA. The option of doing this initial education as an inpatient versus as an outpatient depends on several considerations including the resources available to the diabetes management team, third party reimbursement issues, and patient-related issues. Several investigators have addressed the question of differences in the outcome comparing inpatient versus outpatient education in the newly diagnosed patient. Initial retrospective studies suggested that the patients who received outpatient-based education at the time of diagnosis had lower rates of hospital readmission for diabetes-related problems than those who received inpatient education (89–91).

As very ill patients are always hospitalized initially, the problems with these studies are that they may be comparing outcomes in milder versus more-severe onset. In a prospective study comparing the outpatient education programs at Texas Children's Hospital in Houston, Texas, and Denver Children's Hospital in Denver, Colorado, with the inpatient education program at Children's Hospital of Pittsburgh in Pittsburgh, Pennsylvania, no significant differences were found in the outcome of multiple variables among the two approaches. The outcome measures considered in this study included: rates of hospital readmissions and/or emergency room visits, knowledge test scores, sharing of responsibilities, adherence to the diabetes regimen, family functioning scores, coping skills, and perceptions of quality of life (92–94).

Both inpatient and outpatient approaches have advantages and disadvantages as depicted on Table 4.

MANAGEMENT OF ACUTE COMPLICATIONS

The two major acute complications of T1DM in children are hypoglycemia and DKA. Preventing their occurrence is the first step in their management. The education provided by the therapeutic team and the compliance with the management plan exercised by the patients and their families are the mainstay for the prevention of such complications. Nevertheless, there may be circumstances that escape from the control of the therapeutic team or the patient that lead to the appearance of these complications. Managing them successfully will allow a smoother course of the disease with less interference in daily life and amelioration of the psychological burden that T1DM represents for the children and their caretakers.

Hypoglycemia

Once the diagnosis of T1DM has been made and the treatment with insulin has been instituted, the occurrence of hypoglycemia becomes a real possibility. In fact, this is the most common acute complication related to the management of T1DM in children (Vol. 1; Chap. 15). The pursuit of excellent metabolic control promoted by the results of the DCCT is associated with the cost of increased risk of moderate-to-severe hypoglycemia as seen in the patients receiving intensive therapy as compared to those receiving conventional treatment.

The definition of hypoglycemia has always been controversial. The severity of hypoglycemia has been linked to the need for assistance or the presence of changes in mental status. Children experiencing different degrees of hypoglycemia usually require assistance from a caretaker as compared to adults who can manage the situation on their own during less-severe episodes. Therefore, the definition used in the DCCT does not completely determine the severity of hypoglycemia in children. For this reason, an arbitrary cutoff in blood sugar level is used to define hypoglycemia in the pediatric age. We define mild

Table 4 Advantages and Disadvantages of Inpatient and Outpatient Diabetes Education

Inpatient setting
  Advantages
    Interaction between patient and family with the team in one place and during a few days
    Supervised environment, rapid response to possible complications
  Patients/family may feel safer
    Less trips of patient/family to medical facility
    Less difficulties in team member reimbursement
    Less reticence in early initiation of tight metabolic control
    Emphasis on the severity of the diagnosis
  Disadvantages
    Hospital stay increases general cost
    Less comfort for patient and family
    Removal of child from home environment
Outpatient setting
  Advantages
    Cost is reduced because hospital stay is avoided
    Family starts building self-confidence since early in the process
    Less disruption to the child
  Disadvantages
    Needs well-mounted and coordinated infrastructure of outpatient resources including sufficient well-trained personnel on 24-hr call
    If families cannot commute from home, housing at no cost to family must be available

hypoglycemia as a blood sugar level between 55 and 70 mg/dL, moderate hypoglycemia as a blood sugar level below 55 mg/dL without loss of consciousness, and severe hypoglycemia as any episode of hypoglycemia (blood sugar < 70 mg/dL) associated with loss of consciousness or seizures (95,96). In order to prevent hypoglycemia, every effort must be made to avoid a mismatch between the three major players in glycemic control, namely: insulin and exercise with their glucose-lowering effect versus food intake with its glucose-raising effect. Adequate insulin dose reductions in anticipation of decreased intake or increased physical activity are taught to patients and their families. Also, increases in carbohydrate intake are recommended in anticipation of and/or during prolonged exercise. When intermediate-action insulin preparations are used, the provision of a consistent bedtime snack, which includes protein and fat in addition to carbohydrate, has been, in our experience, a helpful practice to avoid overnight hypoglycemia induced by the prolonged peak of these insulins. Newer regimens using long-acting analogs are less likely to induce overnight hypoglycemia and the substitution of glargine for NPH at night has potential advantages.

Treatment of acute hypoglycemia depends on the severity of the episode. Parents should be taught about management of hypoglycemia from the time of diagnosis. Mild hypoglycemia can be treated by providing 15 g of carbohydrate of rapid absorption (three glucose tablets or 4 oz of orange juice) followed by a source of carbohydrate of slower absorption (six crackers). For moderate hypoglycemia, a larger initial load or rapid-absorption carbohydrate (four glucose tablets or 6–8 oz of orange juice) followed by crackers is recommended. Severe hypoglycemia requires the prompt use of subcutaneous glucagons injection (require training of parents or caretakers) or intravenous dextrose (0.1 mg/kg of dextrose 25%) if emergency medical services are available or the patient is in a medical facility (95). Frequent hypoglycemia, even if asymptomatic, causes hypoglycemia unawareness and failure of glucose counterregulation, placing patients at major risk for severe hypoglycemia. Death, while rare, is a constant fear. Thus avoidance of even mild hypoglycemia should be a therapeutic objective.

Diabetic Ketoacidosis

DKA is more frequently seen at presentation in newly diagnosed patients, although it also happens in individuals diagnosed previously. In the latter, physical stress, most frequently in the form of intercurrent infections, poor compliance with omission of insulin administration, or inadvertent interruption of insulin administration when using CSII, appear to be the main triggering events. The rate of DKA at onset of diabetes is variable, fluctuating between 15% and 67% in reports from Europe and the United States and probably higher in developing countries (97). The

pathophysiology and management of DKA are beyond the scope of this chapter and are covered in Vol. 1; Chap. 7.

THERAPEUTIC OBJECTIVES AND MONITORING REQUIREMENTS

The therapeutic goal for children with T1DM should be to provide comprehensive management striving for metabolic normalcy, physical and emotional health, and avoidance of diabetes-related complications, both acute and chronic, as they go through life. Unfortunately, even with the advances in intensive therapy, this is not now possible. Frequent therapeutic compromises are made between what the management team and the patients would like to achieve and what is reasonable within their personal life situations. In Table 5 are listed the principles of diabetes therapy as they have evolved over the last several years within the diabetes clinic at Children's Hospital of Pittsburgh.

Certainly a primary therapeutic objective is to eliminate the obvious symptoms of poorly controlled diabetes, including polyuria, polydipsia, and polyphagia. Conversely, both serious and frequent mild hypoglycemia should be avoided. Careful attention to physical growth and sexual maturation is important. Inadequate insulin therapy results in slow growth and delayed puberty. Unfortunately, the achievement of these important therapeutic goals is not enough. Many patients deny symptoms of either hyper- or hypoglycemia and are able to maintain normal growth and maturation while maintaining blood-glucose and glycosylated hemoglobin levels that are persistently too high.

Specific therapeutic objectives are presented in Table 6. Based on the DCCT results, primary therapeutic emphasis should be placed on achieving a metabolic status that is near normal while avoiding

Table 5 Principles of Diabetic Therapy

Elimination of the clinical features of inadequately controlled diabetes, including polyuria, polydipsia, and polyphagia
Prevention of diabetic ketoacidosis
Avoidance of hypoglycemia
Maintenance of normal growth and sexual maturation
Prevention of obesity
Early detection of associated diseases: a number of autoimmune diseases (such as Hashimoto's thyroiditis) and celiac disease, which occur with increased frequency in patients with IDDM; surveillance is important to detect these conditions in the early stages
Prevention and treatment of hyperlipidemia
Treatment of hypertension
Prevention of emotional disorders: the chronic and unrelenting demands of the disease and the therapeutic regimentation necessary to achieve reasonable control result in behavioral disability in a large number of families; the therapeutic program should be designed to prevent such problems or provide prompt and effective therapy as required
Early detection and treatment of eating disorders
Prevention of chronic vascular complications of diabetes

the known complications of this approach, including hypoglycemia and excessive weight gain. The primary biochemical guides to management include glycosylated hemoglobin obtained at least every three months and self-monitoring for blood-glucose carried out at least four times daily. A number of commercial techniques are available for determination of glycosylated hemoglobin. It is imperative that physicians be well acquainted with patients own laboratory assay, its normal range, and any special peculiarities of the assay. The currently used assays measure either glycosylated Hb or HbA$_{1C}$. The DCCT used a highly standardized method for measuring HbA$_{1C}$ that had an upper limit of normal of 6.05%, which remains the gold standard, though this is under discussion. The therapeutic goal of 6.5% in the intensively managed patients was achieved in only about 5%. At the close of the study, the mean HbA$_{1C}$ in the intensively managed adults was 7.1%, compared with 9% in the conventionally treated cohort. In those individuals who entered the study as adolescents, mean values were approximately 1% higher with the intensively treated adolescents with a mean of 8.1% and the conventional at 9.8%. Because the effectiveness of the

management appears to be comparable in both adults and adolescents in terms of minimizing rates of progression of vascular change, it seems reasonable to use the HbA$_{1C}$ value of 8% as a maximum therapeutic goal for adolescents participating in an optimized management program. It should be recognized that different assays have different normal ranges and may not read parallel to each other despite excellent statistical correlations.

There were no patients younger than 13 years of age on entry into the DCCT, and at the conclusion of the study, there were no individuals under 20 years of age. Consequently, one translates the conclusions of the DCCT to younger children with extreme caution. It is our view at this time that although the general principle of moving all patients toward physiologic homeostasis should be embraced, glycemic goals may have to be higher in the preadolescent, particularly the preschooler. It is important to focus on blood-glucose variation in these two younger groups, with very great emphasis on avoiding hypoglycemia in preschoolers (98). However, this should not be achieved at the expense of excessive hyperglycemia, which may also be a cause of cognitive dysfunction (95).

Traditionally, because of the impossibility of monitoring amino acid and lipid fluctuations on a day-to-day basis, blood-glucose measurements are the sole modality to assess and manipulate insulin and food therapies. It is important to recognize that although monitoring is "glucocentric," our therapy should be global in terms of insulin action. Routine frequent self-monitoring for blood-glucose is an essential component of good diabetes management. We recommend that at a minimum the patient carry out blood-glucose determinations before each meal and at bedtime. In addition, periodically, blood-glucose determination at 2 to 3 A.M. should be obtained to document whether hypoglycemia is occurring during sleep. Further, it is obvious that postprandial blood-glucose determinations should be obtained to assess the adequacy of insulin coverage for meals. Also, it is important to document symptomatic hypoglycemia by promptly doing a blood-glucose test. During illness, blood-glucose monitoring should be performed more frequently along with urine checks for ketones. Although there is a general correlation between the frequency of blood-glucose determinations and control, this is true only if the individual uses this information to make informed decisions regarding alteration in insulin dosage or other aspects of management. Here is where the recording of the blood-glucose levels on a log sheet or computer acquires its relevance. A single determination of blood-glucose at any one time gives valuable information that may lead to immediate therapeutic decisions. However, the other half of the information lies in the analysis of patterns appearing day to day when multiple measurements are reviewed as a whole. For instance, finding a significantly low blood

Table 6 Specific Monitoring and Objectives

Glycosylated hemoglobin (total HbA$_1$ or HbA$_{1c}$) should be obtained at least every 3 mo; the goal in patients participating in an optimized management program should be an HbA$_{1c}$ of less than 8% (the average of adolescents in the DCCT)

Self-monitoring for blood glucose should be carried out daily at least before each meal and at bedtime, and also at 3:00 A.M. 3–4 ×/mo and postprandially as indicated; the blood glucose goals in optimized patients should be in the range of 80–120 mg/dL before breakfast and 80–140 before meals and < 180 mg/dl postprandially (see text for goals for younger patients)

Urine testing: daily dipstick testing for glucose and ketones of the first voided urine in the morning unless blood sugar is measured more often at night; presence of ketonuria should lead to prompt consultation with the therapeutic team; minimal or no glycosuria or ketonuria is the goal

Urine testing for albumin: dipstick screening testing for albuminuria should be performed on a single voided specimen at each clinic visit; presence of albuminuria should promptly lead to assessment of an overnight or 24-hr urine collection; in the absence of postural proteinuria, overt proteinuria should result in a detailed renal evaluation and appropriate therapeutic intervention; microalbumin measurements are recommended for routine assessment. After 2–5 yr of Type 1 diabetes mellitus a timed overnight specimen is more convenient and avoids detection of postural proteinuria. Spot urine albumin/creatinine ratios are more costly and introduce two variables

Blood lipids: Blood should be obtained annually for determination of total cholesterol, high-density lipoprotein, low-density lipoprotein, very low-density lipoprotein, and triglycerides; the lipid fractions should be between the normal range for nondiabetic children and adolescents. If the triglycerides are above 120 mg/dL, a fasting level should be obtained and repeated. Increases may reflect inadequate diabetes management or genetic lipid alterations

Thyroid function should be assessed annually by determination of TSH; thyroid antibodies may be used as a screen.

Poor growth, erratic glycemic control or abdominal symptoms may be indicative of celiac disease and tissue transglutaminase antibodies should be measured along with IgA levels to decrease the risk of a false negative result. The need for routine screening remains controversial.

sugar in the mid-morning prompts immediate treatment of hypoglycemia with the use of a fast-acting carbohydrate such as glucose tablets or orange juice, but the recognition of a pattern of low blood sugars in the mid-morning over several consecutive days would call for its prevention by a decrease in the pre-breakfast fast-acting insulin, an adjustment in the content of breakfast, or both, to avoid this hypoglycemia on a continuous basis.

Although it is difficult for U.S. patients to obtain blood-glucose values at school before lunch, we insist that prelunch values be obtained routinely to assess properly the adequacy of the dose of short-acting insulin from the morning injection. Schools should make this as easy as possible for the patient. There are major advantages to the use of meters with extensive memory capacity, primarily to cross-check the patient's accuracy in the recording of blood-glucose results. However, the meter memory should not be used as an excuse for not recording the daily results in a format that is available for review by the parent as well as the team at and between outpatient visits. Some meters have the capability of downloading the blood-glucose records in a computer in different formats. When this feature is available and the patients can use it, they should be encouraged to perform the process of downloading on a frequent basis such as every few days, and not only every three months just prior to the follow-up visit in the diabetes clinic. Frequent downloading serves the same purpose as careful record keeping as it permits the review of blood-glucose trends and patterns, which are the basis for proactive adjustments in therapy.

The DCCT blood-glucose goals should be adopted for adolescent patients who have made a commitment to optimize management. The blood-glucose goals are directed toward achieving normal fasting blood-glucose in the range of 80 to 120 mg/dL (or 80–140 with meters calibrated to serum). Any other daytime determination should fall in the range of 80 to 140 mg/dL, with 3 A.M. values higher than 70 mg/dL. The DCCT results based on seven-point glucose profiles done once monthly gave a mean daily blood-glucose of 153 mg/dL in the intensively managed cohort compared with 230 mg/dL in the conventionally treated group. The results, although documenting the improved status of the intensively managed patients, further illustrates the difficulty in achieving blood-glucose goals close to the normal range.

Pediatric diabetologists are currently attempting to come to grips with the issues surrounding the general implementation of DCCT guidelines in the younger child. In the preadolescent (6–13 years of age), preprandial fasting levels should be moved as close as possible to adolescent blood-glucose goals: 80 to 140 mg/dL. This should be done as soon as patients can reliably detect and respond to hypoglycemic symptoms. Some preadolescent patients are stable and predictable enough in blood-glucose

excursions that careful management adjustments can be made to bring them in line with adolescent recommendations. For the preschool child, we continue to recommend that higher blood-glucose goals be implemented to minimize the danger of hypoglycemia. Our specific recommendations are for fasting blood-glucose to fall in the 100 to 160 mg/dL range and postprandial values in the 180 to 200 mg/dL range, while in toddlers, preprandial levels in the 80 to 180 range is the goal. Despite these higher goal ranges, HbA$_{1C}$ levels are usually lower in very young children than in adolescents.

With the widespread acceptance of routine self-monitoring of blood-glucose, urine glucose testing has largely been relegated to an assay of historical interest only. We think that this is a mistake, and the value of assessing nighttime control is major and can be assessed by routine daily testing for urine glucose and ketones in the first voided morning urine. A dipstick method is used to measure both glucose and ketones. The presence of ketonuria is always of importance. Ketonuria associated with negative or minimal glucose spill is suggestive of nighttime hypoglycemia. The combination of the high urinary glucose and ketones must be considered a strong indication of impending serious metabolic deterioration that requires careful follow-up. Under these circumstances, each successive voiding should be checked until ketonuria is clear. Communication with the therapeutic team is necessary to alter management as needed to prevent progression to DKA.

Urine protein determination is an essential component of routine management. In our clinic, a freshly voided specimen is checked at each visit using a microalbumin screening method. If positive, overt proteinuria should be assessed using a protein dipstick method that becomes positive with a urine albumin concentration of about 300 mg/L or total protein level of 500. More accurate methods for albumin determination are required to detect microalbuminuria (30–300 mg/24 hr), which may be indicative of impending, progressive renal disease. Proteinuria at this level or higher, if persistent, may be related to diabetes renal damage and is indicative of significant and serious pathology once infection is excluded. A carefully obtained 24-hour urine specimen or a timed overnight urine specimen obtained the morning before the clinic or office visit is possibly easier and more helpful in excluding orthostatic proteinuria. A spot urine albumin/creatinine ratio is the most convenient, but also the most costly and erratic assessment of microalbuminuria, and does not exclude orthostatic proteinuria.

Patients with poorly controlled diabetes mellitus frequently have elevations in several of the blood lipid fractions. As a component of assessment of control, we recommend that nonfasting lipids be screened annually for the determination of total cholesterol, LDL, high-density lipoproteins, and triglycerides. Total cholesterol values should be below 160 mg/dL,

LDL should be below 100 to 110 mg/dL, and triglycerides below 120 mg/dL. If triglycerides are elevated, a fasting specimen should be obtained. Elevated lipid values may be a result of either inadequate diabetes management or one of the forms of genetic hyperlipidemia. If the patient's diabetes control is unsatisfactory, the first objective should be to improve overall diabetes management and determine whether the elevated lipid fractions return toward the normal range. On the other hand, if persistent hyperlipidemia is identified in individuals with satisfactory diabetes control, then an evaluation for genetic hyperlipidemia should follow. Management should start with a strict diet. When this fails, pharmacologic therapy with lipid-lowering agents may become necessary.

Thyroid disease is commonly seen in association with IDDM. Hashimoto's thyroiditis, an autoimmune destructive process, appears to share many similarities with the mechanism of β-cell destruction leading to T1DM. In our experience, approximately 40% of our patients, particularly during the adolescent years, have evidence of Hashimoto's thyroiditis, including the presence of a goiter and/or elevations in thyroid antibodies. Approximately 10% of these patients develop hypothyroidism; a significantly smaller number develop hyperthyroidism. Timely diagnosis and appropriate management of these conditions are obviously important to the patient's well being. Careful examination of the patient's neck should be a part of each clinic visit, and assessment of thyroid function should occur as specifically indicated or on an annual basis. We recommend annual screening with measurement of thyroid-stimulating hormone (TSH). In the patient whose TSH is abnormally elevated or in whom a goiter or signs or symptoms of hypothyroidism are present, measurement of free thyroxine (free-T4) and thyroid antibodies, namely thyroglobulin antibodies (TG-Ab) and thyroid peroxidase antibodies (TPO-Ab), are also indicated. Thyrotropin receptor antibodies (TR-Ab) are indicated when a hyperthyroid state is suspected as a workup to rule out Graves' disease. Unexplained persistent hypoglycemia may be a subtle manifestation of hypothyroidism and, conversely, unexplained persistent hyperglycemia may be a subtle manifestation of a hyperthyroid state. Others suggest using TPO-Ab as the primary screen. This is more expensive in the United States, but their measurements every five years maybe adequate.

Another relatively common association has been documented between T1DM and celiac disease. The prevalence of celiac disease using screening tests among Type 1 diabetics has been calculated by different authors in Europe, Australia and the United States showing rates between 1.0% and 7.8% (99–101). Based on this, it has been suggested that all patients with Type 1 diabetes be screened for celiac disease. However, this recommendation remains controversial. The measurement of tissue transglutaminase antibodies is currently accepted as the most sensitive test to screen for celiac disease. The diagnosis, when suspected, is confirmed only with biopsy. We do not routinely perform "universal" screening for celiac disease in all our diabetic patients, but we certainly request transglutaminase antibodies in those patients who display poor linear growth, weight loss, or poor weight gain not clearly explainable by their degree of metabolic control, in patients with frequent hypoglycemia, and obviously in patients showing signs or symptoms of the disease. Investigations into the clinical significance of the presence of transglutaminase antibodies and the need for intestinal biopsy are under way. The unnecessary implementation of a burdensome gluten-free diet should be avoided. A similar genetic background, especially the high frequency of HLA-DR3 genotypes, has been postulated as the explanation for the simultaneous occurrence of T1DM and celiac disease (102). The proposition that gluten, the protein responsible for celiac disease, is a possible determinant for islet autoimmunity remains unconfirmed (103).

THE THERAPEUTIC TEAM

Medical care of the child with diabetes is quite different from that of most other diseases handled by the pediatrician. The primary focus is on education. A major responsibility for the physician is to ensure that the patient and family members are well educated about the diversity of problems associated with diabetes. This cannot be a one-time educational experience: it must be a constantly renewed and ongoing activity. However, the attainment of the knowledge is only half the battle. The knowledge gained about insulin administration, the utilization of monitoring information, dietary principles, and the incorporation of exercise into daily life, must be accepted by the patient, with adherence to the therapeutic regimen as a personal commitment for improved health. Each patient and family have their own unique barriers to full acceptance and incorporation of the recommended therapeutic regimen. Although most of these barriers are in the psychological sphere, other factors such as peer group pressures, financial problems, or unavailability of parents at appropriate times, may make the recommended therapeutic regimen difficult, if not impossible, to follow.

Although patients should take a leading role in the management of their diabetes, the physician diabetologist must serve as initial surrogate captain of the therapeutic team. It is the physician's responsibility to assess the unique characteristics of each patient and family and to determine the general therapeutic strategies to be used in an attempt to help the child achieve and maintain good health. Several other team members are essential for the development of an effective diabetes therapeutic program. The diabetes nurse educator plays a pivotal role. Although the experienced physician must always be involved in reinforcing the educational components of therapy, it is unlikely that the physician has sufficient time to carry out the primary educational activities. The nurse educator must become involved with the family as early as possible, usually during the time of initial diagnosis. It is clear from a number of studies that this is not an optimal time for teaching because of the family shock at the diagnosis of diabetes. However, we believe it is important to begin this process and ensure that the family has at least "survival skills," requiring three to five days of teaching. The educational process continues at each clinic visit and, if necessary, special educational sessions are set up with the diabetes educator outside the routine clinic schedule.

The dietitian assesses the family's knowledge of food and nutrition at the initial visit and begins constructing a meal plan appropriate to the particular child. At least an annual review by the dietitian of the patient's nutritional status is desirable. Specific issues about the appropriateness of particular food substances and insulin coverage can usually be handled by telephone consultation or at clinic visits. Label reading and carbohydrate counting are two concrete areas that need to be covered by the nutritionist at the initial education sessions at the time of diagnosis and need to be reinforced periodically during the outpatient follow-up visits. The assessment of the intake of protein and saturated fat is important.

The psychiatric social worker plays a special role within the diabetes therapeutic team. It is the social worker's responsibility to assess the strengths and weaknesses of the family as they relate to emotional issues, economic and community support, educational activities, etc. It is usually the social worker's assessment and recommendations that determine whether other professionals such as clinical psychologists and psychiatrists become promptly involved with the family. Prevention of severe problems is the goal. The development of psychiatric problems over time as a consequence of stresses of the disorder also calls for the social worker's reinvolvement. The social worker can be particularly useful in families with limited financial resources, helping them to obtain support for diabetes medications and supplies, and transportation to clinic appointments.

The core diabetes therapeutic team includes the physician diabetologist, diabetes nurse educator, dietitian, and psychiatric social worker. However, the central member of the team is the patient. The patient, when old enough to be involved in a meaningful way in decisions, or the parents of the younger child, must be incorporated from the beginning in the planning of the therapeutic strategies and in all other major decisions. It is not therapeutically meaningful to insist on an insulin therapy of three to four injections daily or using an insulin pump and a monitoring program of four glucose determinations daily when the patient frequently misses some injections of insulin and/or

refuses any monitoring. Although one continues to try to educate the patient and the family about the importance of a more comprehensive approach, at the same time it is essential to deal with reality. Most patients understand and appreciate the responsibility being placed upon them as part of the therapeutic team and respond maturely and appropriately to it. The need for the diabetes therapeutic team cannot be minimized. Creative new ways must be found to make these resources available to all children and adolescents with diabetes mellitus. University diabetes centers must provide the leadership and direction for the development of networks of diabetes therapeutic programs across geographic areas, involving small communities with apparently limited diabetes-related resources. The local family physician or pediatrician must be incorporated into the therapeutic team and given encouragement for periodic reeducation to function locally as the diabetes leader. In every community, it should be possible to identify nurses and dietitians who are willing to accept increased responsibility with appropriate, specifically pediatric, training to become the local diabetes educator or special diabetes dietitian. The university-based diabetes center or specialty clinic must be able to provide outreach to the local community diabetes program by providing periodic visiting specialists, local patient and professional teaching conferences, and referral services for especially difficult management problems.

Opportunities for educational renewal by the local team members must be available on a periodic basis. Such a networking program, once in place, should offer the benefits of diabetes team management to the great majority of children and adolescents with T1DM. Although the initial costs of such a program will clearly be in excess of current management activities, the long-term reduction in vascular complications will greatly reduce the health care costs associated with visual loss, end-stage renal disease, peripheral vascular disease, heart attacks, and strokes.

CLINICAL ASSESSMENT AND THERAPEUTIC DECISION MAKING

Children and adolescents with T1DM require regular ongoing physical, biochemical, and emotional assessment, and modification in all aspects of management to meet their changing needs and individual lifestyle requirements. Because of the complexity of this problem, we are convinced that this process should be carried out in a setting in which the talents of several diabetes therapeutic team members can be brought to bear on the situation of the patient and family.

We recommend that routine care involve a full clinic visit at a minimum of three-month intervals, with interim visits with the nurse educator or dietitian as required. The physician's routine evaluation should include a careful review of general health and diabetes management issues in the interval since the last examination. Frequency, severity, and management of hypoglycemia should be specifically investigated. Symptoms of hyperglycemia such as nocturia or urinary frequency should be documented. Dietary management should be reviewed by the physician, and specific dietary problems should be referred to the dietitian. An evaluation of physical activity should be obtained and the patient encouraged to participate in daily exercise to achieve superior physical fitness and assistance with dose adjustment made. Psychological issues should be reviewed, including how the patient is handling the personal problems of diabetes and its management, school performance, and interpersonal relationships at school and at home. Issues of sexuality and drug and alcohol abuse should be approached directly in a nonjudgmental fashion. The danger of conception without excellent glycemic control should be emphasized to sexually active girls who should be referred to a gynecologist or adolescent medicine specialist for additional counseling. All adolescent patients need to be made aware of emergency contraception methods (Vol. 2; Chap. 14).

Physical examination should be complete. Height and weight measurements should be transferred to a standard percentile growth grid in which assessment of growth parameters over time can be followed accurately. A declining growth rate or inadequate weight gain should result in careful review to determine whether this is a reflection of inadequate diabetes management or another problem. Excessive weight gain should also be addressed. In the adolescent patient, the physical examination should include determination of Tanner staging and information about menses in girls. Blood pressure should be carefully obtained with the patient in a relaxed state. Even moderate elevations above the appropriate blood pressure range for the age should lead to additional determinations during the visit and, if necessary, periodically by the school nurse or even with use of an ambulatory monitor. Persistent hypertension is a serious problem in the diabetic patient and must be aggressively evaluated and treated. The diabetologist should be comfortable and confident in carrying out a routine ophthalmologic examination looking for the early changes indicative of background retinopathy. Insulin injection sites should be carefully examined. Lipohypertrophy may result in impairment of insulin absorption and contribute to inadequate management. A complete neurological exam should also be performed.

A major portion of the routine visit is the review of the patient-generated blood-glucose records by the diabetologist. This is an opportunity to teach about diabetes therapeutics and encourage the patient's and parents' participation in the therapeutic decision-making. The individual's blood-glucose goals in the fasting and postprandial state are reviewed, and an assessment of the interim performance provided. The focus is on insulin adjustments, but the integration of diet and physical activity must also be emphasized in these discussions. Any therapeutic changes must be followed by a telephone conversation between the patient and the therapeutic team, which may include faxing the most recent blood-glucose results to a member of the therapeutic team. The results of the biochemical assessment are shared with the family and referring physician by letter within days of the clinic visit. Elevations in glycosylated hemoglobin levels, for example, may dictate more vigorous therapeutic changes than the initial review of the patient's blood-glucose record would suggest. When biochemical therapeutic goals are met, congratulations are due to the patient and family, with encouragement to keep up the good work. Lack of achievement of goals should not be presented in a negative or punitive fashion, but rather as encouragement to the patient and family to try even harder in the future with the assistance of the therapeutic team.

CONSULTATIONS AND REFERRALS

For the child and adolescent with diabetes mellitus, there may be several occasions on which the advice of physicians outside the therapeutic team is especially valuable. According to current guidelines, children with T1DM of at least five years' duration, as well as all patients during their adolescent years, undergo a thorough retinal exam through dilated pupils performed by an ophthalmologist or a trained optometrist on an annual basis. Many advocate waiting until eight years of diabetes duration in the prepubertal child in good control, but doing the exam after two years in poorly controlled patients. Ideally, the eye specialist should have experience in detecting early diabetic retinal changes. Fundus photography, either stereo color photography or fluorescein angiography, may be appropriate as a more sensitive assessment during the adolescent years. The detection of vascular changes in the eye by either the family physician or diabetologist should promptly result in a referral to an ophthalmologist. Although in most cases the ophthalmologist provides no therapeutic intervention at that time, the visit may provide an opportunity for the therapeutic team to reemphasize the importance of good diabetes management. Adolescent girls should be referred to a gynecologist or adolescent medicine clinic when sexually active.

The stress of diabetes and its management requirements exact a heavy toll in terms of behavioral problems and disabilities. In prospective studies carried out in our institution, nearly 50% of our patients experience significant psychopathology during adolescence (104). In most cases, this was pathological depression, requiring professional intervention. Other problems include antisocial acting-out behaviors, eating disorders, and adjustment problems. Eating disorders in patients with diabetes are much more common than in the general population and usually associated with poor control. These may include anorexia nervosa, bulimia, or omission of insulin delivery (105,106). It is essential for all therapeutic team members to be sensitive to behavioral issues and be prepared for referral to colleagues in psychiatry or psychology if necessary. There is a natural reticence on the part of most patients and families to accept psychiatric referrals. By including the behavioral scientist as an integral member of the therapeutic team from the beginning and emphasizing the importance of psychological well being as part of the management of the patient with diabetes, the likelihood of family cooperation, if active intervention therapy is needed, is increased.

Annual evaluation of possible renal involvement is also advised. Measurement of microalbuminuria is recommended on an annual basis in patients who have had diabetes for at least five years or those who are reaching puberty (107), and after two years if the disease is poorly controlled. Albumin excretion rate above 21 µg/min should be confirmed by repetition of the test within the following few weeks or months. A persistent overt proteinuria should ideally prompt the referral of the patient to the nephrologist. If the patient has not had poor glycemic control, causes other than diabetes should be excluded (108).

Eventually the patient followed by the pediatric diabetes specialist must be referred for adult care based on age. It is our preference to continue to work with these patients through adolescence; high school or college graduation is a natural time to terminate this therapeutic relationship and hand the patient over to an adult diabetologist. All too often, the young adult diabetic following high school graduation and either entry into the work force or departure from home for university is lost from the healthcare system and may not return for several years. Unfortunately, the return is frequently precipitated by an acute event such as retinal hemorrhage or other diabetic complications. It is not enough simply to refer the patient to the family doctor and assume that proper future management will be arranged locally. These patients deserve the opportunity to continue in a therapeutic environment characterized by the diabetes therapeutic team and led by a skilled internist or diabetologist. Assuring that this connection is made will go a long way toward minimizing serious complications during the patients' young adult years. The transition should be made in a well-planned and coordinated manner to avoid a series of difficulties associated with this change, which may have a negative impact on the glycemic control of the patient (109).

FUTURE DIRECTIONS
Inhaled Insulin

One of the major difficulties encountered by patients with diabetes is the need to inject insulin subcutaneously. The concept of using an alternate route for insulin administration was thought of even since the time of its discovery in the 1920s. Enteral administration of insulin is not feasible as this relatively large protein is readily digested in the gastrointestinal tract. The respiratory epithelium has been shown to be able to absorb insulin in a reproducible manner. Testing of inhaled insulin in humans was first performed in the 1990s. Two forms of inhaled insulin have been developed. One is a dry formulation of powdered insulin administered through a device in which a pulse of compressed air disperses the insulin into a chamber from which the patient inhales into the respiratory tract. The other one is an aqueous preparation delivered to the respiratory tract by inhalation after being aerosolized in a device equipped with a microprocessor (110–112). The absorption of insulin through the respiratory epithelium is faster than that from the subcutaneous tissue; however, the efficiency is lower because some of the insulin is lost within the delivery device or in the mouth. Therefore, higher doses are required when administering inhaled insulin as compared to subcutaneous injections. Some studies in adults have shown comparable glycemic control when compared to subcutaneous insulin injections (30). Increased compliance seems to be one of the advantages of this approach. One concern that has not been cleared is the long-term safety of inhaled insulin because of its repetitive interaction with the alveolar epithelium, given that insulin is an anabolic hormone with growth-promoting effects. Long-term safety has not been studied. The use in small children may be difficult because of the need for an appropriate inhalation technique. The inhaled insulin was approved by the FDA for use in adults for both Type 1 and T2D, mellitus and the cost is estimated to be $120 to $150 per month (113).

Amylin

The discovery in 1987 of amylin (114), a hormone produced in the β-cell and cosecreted with insulin, is now opening the possibilities for its clinical use. Amylin plays an important role in postprandial glucose regulation by suppressing postprandial glucagon secretion,(115) slowing the gastric emptying (116) and probably inducing an anorexigenic effect as shown in an animal model (117). Endogenous amylin production is impaired in individuals with β-cell failure seen in T1DM or later stages of T2DM. Administration by injection of pramlintide, an amylin analog along with insulin before meals to diabetic adults has been effective in decreasing postprandial hyperglycemia, decreasing appetite, and promoting weight loss or weight maintenance (118–120). Use of amylin analogs may prove useful as an adjunct therapy in children with T1DM to reduce the wide fluctuations in their blood-glucose, especially in the postprandial state (121). It requires additional injections because this polypeptide hormone cannot be given orally. This opens the potential for delivery through a continuous subcutaneous infusion pump with a mixture of insulin and "amylin" in the right proportion or with the development of pumps with dual cartridges to hold insulin and amylin separately.

Closing the Loop

The concept of an artificial pancreas has been proposed for decades. This "artificial pancreas" must have two major components: an afferent limb, represented by a real time continuous glucose sensing device, and an efferent limb, represented by an insulin delivery device with capability of delivery rate adjustments. A third element is the "communication" between these two components to close the loop. Current technology has provided all three elements: continuous real-time glucose sensing has been improved greatly, insulin infusion pumps have attained a significant degree of sophistication, and communication between these two via infrared signaling is available. However, the refinement is not yet such that allows the "artificial pancreas" to be a reality. The major setbacks are the limited time— usually three days—the currently available continuous glucose monitoring devices can work without interruption and the lag between insulin infusion in the subcutaneous tissue and actual insulin effect due to delayed absorption when compared to physiological insulin secretion into the portal system. The integration between glucose sensing and insulin delivery has to be coordinated through mathematical algorithms, which have been difficult to create given the complexity of insulin secretion regulation and the above-mentioned technical difficulties.

In the meanwhile, the constant improvements of continuous blood-glucose monitoring with real time display of results provide optimism in refining insulin delivery even without the closed loop. The lack of sensitivity and accuracy in detecting hypoglycemia in the currently available monitors is rapidly being corrected and new monitors are in the formal testing phases. Patient acceptability remains to be determined in large-scale trials such as those carried out by the DirecNet group.

REFERENCES

1. James T. History of medicine. Paulesco. S Afr Med J 1992; 82(2):123–125.
2. Murray I. Paulesco and the isolation of insulin. J Hist Med Allied Sci 1971; 26(2):150–157.
3. Bliss M. The discovery of insulin. McClelland, Stewart, eds. Chicago: University of Chicago Press, 1982.
4. Porksen N, Hollingdal M, Juhl C, et al. Pulsatile insulin secretion: detection, regulation, and role in diabetes. Diabetes 2002; 51(suppl 1):S245–S254.
5. Nauck MA. Glucagon-like peptide 1 (GLP-1) in the treatment of diabetes. Horm Metab Res 2004; 36(11–12):852–858.
6. Leon DD, Crutchlow MF, Ham JY, et al. Role of glucagon-like peptide-1 in the pathogenesis and treatment of diabetes mellitus. Int J Biochem Cell Biol 2005; 146(10): 4224–4233.
7. Fehse F, Trautmann M, Holst JJ, et al. Exenatide augments first and second phase insulin secretion in response to intravenous glucose in subjects with Type 2 diabetes. J Clin Endocrinol Metab 2005; 90(11):5991–5997.
8. Dupre J. Glycaemic effects of incretins in Type 1 diabetes mellitus: a concise review, with emphasis on studies in humans. Regul Pept 2005; 128(2):149–157.
9. Feldman JM. Pathophysiology of diabetes mellitus. In: Galloway JA, Potvin JH, Shuman CR, eds. Diabetes Mellitus. 9th. Indianapolis: Eli Lilly, 1988:28–44.
10. Gerich JA. Hormonal control of homeostasis. In: Galloway JA, Potvin JH, Shuman CR, eds. Diabetes Mellitus. 9th. Indianapolis: Eli Lilly, 1988:45–64.
11. Diabetes Research in Children Network (DirecNet) Study Group. A multi-center study of the accuracy of the one touch ultra home glucose meter in children with Type 1 diabetes. Diabetes Technol Ther 2003; 5(6):933–941.
12. Tang Z, Du X, Louie RF, et al. Effects of drugs on glucose measurements with handheld glucose meters and a portable glucose analyzer. Am J Clin Pathol 2000; 113(1): 75–86.
13. Diabetes Research in Children Network (DirecNet) Study Group. The accuracy of the CGMS in children with Type 1 diabetes: results of the diabetes research in children network (DirecNet) accuracy study. Diabetes Technol Ther 2003; 5:781–789.
14. Diabetes Research in Children Network (DirecNet) Study Group. Accuracy of the modified Continuous Glucose Monitoring System (CGMS) sensor in an outpatient setting: results from a diabetes research in children network (DirecNet) study. Diabetes Technol Ther 2005; 7:109–114.
15. Diabetes Research in Children Network (DirecNet) Study Group. Lack of accuracy of continuous glucose sensors in healthy, nondiabetic children: results of the Diabetes Research in Children Network (DirecNet) accuracy study. J Pediatr 2004; 144(6):770–775.
16. Garg S, Zisser H, Schwartz S, et al. Improvement in glycemic excursions with a transcutaneous, real-time continuous glucose sensor. A randomized trial. Diabetes Care 2006; 29(1):44–50.
17. Little RR, Wiedmeyer HM, England JD, et al. International standardization of glycohemoglobin measurements: practical application. Clin Chem 1993; 39(11 Pt 1):2356.
18. Little RR, Rohlfing CL, Wiedmeyer HM, et al., NGSP Steering Committee. The national glycohemoglobin standardization program: a five-year progress report. Clin Chem 2001; 47(11):1985–1992.
19. Schnedl WJ, Krause R, Halwachs-Baumann G, et al. Evaluation of HbA1c determination methods in patients with hemoglobinopathies. Diabetes Care 2000; 23(3): 339–344.
20. Diabetes Research in Children Network (DirecNet) Study Group. Comparison of fingerstick hemoglobin A1c levels assayed by DCA 2000 with the DCCT/EDIC central laboratory assay: results of a Diabetes Research in Children Network (DirecNet) study. Pediatr Diabetes 2005; 6(1):13–16.
21. Sicard DA, Taylor JR. Comparison of point-of-care HbA1c test versus standardized laboratory testing. Ann Pharmacother 2005; 39(6):1024–1028.
22. Galloway JA. New directions in drug development: mixtures, analogs, modeling. Diabetes care 1993; 16(3):16–23.
23. Chance RE, Frank BH. Research, development, production and safety of biosynthetic human insulin. Diabetes Care 1993; 16(3):133–142.

24. Saudek CD. Future developments in insulin delivery systems. Diabetes Care 1993; 16(3):122–132.

25. Laube BL. Treating diabetes with aerosolized insulin. Chest 2001; 120(suppl 3):99S–106S.

26. Tamborlane WV, Bonfig W, Boland E. Recent advances in treatment of youth with Type 1 diabetes: better care through technology. Diabet Med 2001; 18(11):864–870.

27. Steiner S, Pfutzner A, Wilson BRO, et al. TechnosphereTM/Insulin—proof of concept study with a new insulin formulation for pulmonary delivery. Exp Clin Endocrinol Diabetes 2002; 110(1):17–21.

28. Gerber RA, Cappelleri JC, Kourides IA, et al. Treatment satisfaction with inhaled insulin in patients with type 1 diabetes: a randomized controlled trial. Diabetes Care 2001; 24(9):1556–1559.

29. Skyler JS, Cefalu WT, Kourides IA, et al. Efficacy of inhaled human insulin in type 1 diabetes mellitus: a randomised proof-of-concept study. Lancet 2001; 357(9253):331–335.

30. Skyler JS, Weinstock RS, Raskin P, et al. Inhaled Insulin Phase III Type 1 Diabetes Study Group. Use of inhaled insulin in a basal/bolus insulin regimen in type 1 diabetic subjects: a 6-month, randomized, comparative trial. Diabetes Care 2005; 28(7):1630–1635.

31. Schade DS, Santiago JV, Skyler JS, et al. Intensive Insulin Therapy. Amsterdam: Excerpta Medica, 1983.

32. Drash AL. Clinical care of the diabetic child. Chicago: Year Book Medical Publishers, 1987.

33. Santiago JV. Insulin therapy in the last decade: a pediatric perspective. Diabetes Care 1993; 16(3):143–154.

34. Becker DJ. Management of insulin-dependent diabetes mellitus in children and adolescents. Curr Opin Pediatr 1991; 3:710–723.

35. Rother KT, Levitsky LL. Diabetes mellitus during adolescence. Adolescent endocrinology. Endocrinol Metab Clin North Am 1993; 22:553–572.

36. Effect of intensive therapy on residual beta-cell function in patients with type 1 diabetes in the diabetes control and complications trial. A randomized, controlled trial. The Diabetes Control and Complications Trial Research Group. Ann Intern Med 1998; 128(7):517–523.

37. Becker D. Individualized insulin therapy in children and adolescents with type 1 diabetes. Acta Pediatr 1998; 425(suppl):20–24.

38. Cryer P. Human insulin and hypoglycemia unawareness. Diabetes Care 1990; 13:536–538.

39. Orchard TJ, Maser RE, Becker DJ, et al. Human insulin use and hypoglycemia. Insights from the Pittsburgh Epidemiology Study. Diabetic Med 1991:469–471.

40. Bolli GB, Di Marchi RD, Park GD, et al. Insulin analogs and their potential in the management of diabetes mellitus. Diabetologia 1999; 42:1151–1167.

41. Brange J. The new era of biotech insulin analogues. Diabetologia 1997; 40:S48–S53.

42. Berger M, Heinemann L. Are presently available insulin analogues clinically beneficial? Diabetologia 1997; 40: S91–S96.

43. Danne T, Becker RHA, Heise T, Bittner C, Frick AD, Rave K. Pharmacokinetics, prandial glucose control, and safety of insulin glulisine in children and adolescents with type 1 diabetes. Diabetes Care 2005; 28:2100–2105.

44. Chase HP, Lockspeiser T, Perry B, et al. The impact of the diabetes control and complications trial and humalog insulin on glycohemoglobin levels and severe hypoglycemia in Type 1 diabetes. Diabetes Care 2001; 24:430–434.

45. Mohn A, Matyka KA, Harris DA, et al. Lispro or regular insulin for multiple injection therapy in adolescence. Differences in free insulin and glucose levels overnight. Diabetes Care 1999; 22:27–32.

46. Danne T, Deisst D, Hopfenmuller W, et al. Experience with insulin analogs in children. Horm Res 2002; 57:46–53.

47. Weinzimer SA, Doyle EA, Tamborlane WV. Disease management in the young diabetic patients: glucose monitoring, coping skills, and treatment strategies. Clin Pediatr 2005; 44:393–403.

48. Weinzimer SA, Ahern JH, Doyle EA, et al. Persistence of benefits of continuous subcutaneous insulin infusion in very young children with type 1 diabetes: a follow-up report. Pediatrics 2004; 114:1601–1605.

49. Ratner RE, Hirsch IB, Neifing JL, et al. Less hypoglycemia with insulin glargine in intensive therapy for type 1 diabetes. Diabetes Care 2000; 23(5):639–643.

50. Chase HP, Dixon B, Pearson JS, et al. Reduced hypoglycemic episodes and improved glycemic control in children with type 1 diabetes using insulin glargine and neutral protamine hagedorn insulin. J Pediatr 2003; 143:737–740.

51. Home P, Bartley P, Russell-Jones D, et al. Study to Evaluate the Administration of Detemir Insulin Efficacy, Safety and Suitability (STEADINESS) Study Group. Insulin detemir offers improved glycemic control compared with NPH insulin in people with type 1 diabetes: a randomized clinical trial. Diabetes Care 2004; 27(5):1081–1087.

52. Heise T, Nosek L, Ronn BB, et al. Lower within-subject variability of insulin detemir in comparison to NPH insulin and insulin glargine in people with type 1 diabetes. Diabetes 2004; 53(6):1614–1620.

53. Danne T, Lüpke K, Walte K, et al. Insulin detemir is characterized by a consistent pharmacokinetic profile across age-groups in children, adolescents, and adults with type 1 diabetes. Diabetes Care 2003; 26:3087–3092.

54. International Society for Pediatric And Adolescent Diabetes. Consensus Guidelines. The Netherlands: Medical forum International for the International society for Pediatric and Adolescent Pediatrics, 2000:1.

55. The Diabetes Control and Complications Trial Research Group. The effect of intensive treatment of diabetes on the development and progression of long-term complications in insulin dependent diabetes mellitus. N Engl J Med 1993; 329(14):977–986.

56. Rovet JF, Ehrlich RM. The effect of hypoglycemic seizures on cognitive function in children with diabetes: a 7-year prospective study. J Pediatr 1999; 134:503–506.

57. Becker D. Intensive diabetes therapy in childhood: is it achievable? Is it desirable? Is it safe? J Pediatr 1999; 134:392–394.

58. Ludvigsson J, Bolli GB. Intensive insulin treatment in diabetic children. Diabetes Nutr Metab 2001; 14(5): 292–304.

59. White NH, Cleary PA, Dahms W, et al. Beneficial effects of intensive therapy of diabetes during adolescence: outcomes after the conclusion of the Diabetes Control and Complications Trial (DCCT). J Pediatr 2001; 139(6): 804–812.

60. Heinemann L, Richter B. Clinical pharmacology of human insulin. Diabetes Care 1993; 16(3):90–100.

61. Becker DJ, Kerensky KM, Transue D, et al. Current status of pump therapy in childhood. Acta Pediatr Jpn 1984; 6:347–358.

62. American Diabetes Association Clinical Education Series: insulin infusion pump therapy. In: Intensive Diabetes Management. 2nd ed. Alexandria, Virginia: American Diabetes Association Inc, 1998:99–120.

63. Kaufman FR, Halvorson M, Fisher L, et al. Insulin pump therapy in Type 1 patients. J Pediatr Endocrinol Metab 1999; 12(3):759–764.

64. Anderson B, Ho J, Brackett J, et al. Parental involvement in diabetes management tasks: relationship to blood

glucose monitoring adherence and metabolic control in young adolescents with insulin dependent diabetes mellitus. J Pediatr 1997; 130:257–265.

65. Steindel BS, Roe TR, Costin G, Carlson M, Kaufman FR. Continuous subcutaneous insulin infusion (CSII) in children and adolescents with chronic poorly controlled type 1 diabetes mellitus. Diabetes Res Clin Pract 1995; 27(3):199–204.

66. Boland EA, Grey M, Oesterle A, et al. Continuous subcutaneous insulin infusion. A new way to lower risk of severe hypoglycemia, improve metabolic control, and enhance coping in adolescents with type 1 diabetes. Diabetes Care 1999; 22(11):1779–1784.

67. Maniatis AK, Klingensmith GJ, Slover RH. Continuous subcutaneous insulin infusion therapy for children and adolescents: an option for routine diabetes care. Pediatrics 2001; 107(2):351–356.

68. Zinman B. Insulin regimens and strategies for IDDM. Diabetes Care 1993; 16(3):24–28.

69. Bolli GB, Peniello G, Carmine G, et al. Nocturnal blood glucose control in Type 1 diabetes mellitus. Diabetes Care 1993; 16(3):71–89.

70. Tansey MJ, Tsalikian E, Beck RW, et al. The Diabetes Research in Children Network (DirecNet) Study Group. The effects of aerobic exercise on glucose and counterregulatory hormone concentrations in children with type 1 diabetes. Diabetes Care 2006; 29(1):20–25.

71. Tsalikian E, Mauras N, Beck RW, et al. Diabetes Research In Children Network Direcnet Study Group. Impact of exercise on overnight glycemic control in children with type 1 diabetes mellitus. J Pediatr 2005; 147(4):528–534.

72. Diabetes Care 1994; 17:519–522.

73. Institute of Medicine of the National Academies: Dietary Reference Intakes for Energy, Carbohydrate, Fiber, Fat, Fatty Acids, Cholesterol, Protein, and Amino Acids (Macronutrients). Washington, D.C: National Academy Press, 2002:1–8 http://www.iom.edu/Object.File/Master/4/154/0.pdf.

74. Perrotti N, Santoro D, Genovese S, et al. Effect of digestible carbohydrates on glucose control in insulin-dependent patients with diabetes. Diabetes Care 1984; 7:354–359.

75. Strychar IM, Blain E, Rivard M, et al. Association between dietary adherence measures and glycemic control in outpatients with type 1 diabetes mellitus and normal serum lipid levels. J Am Diet Assoc 1998; 98:76–79.

76. Franz MJ, Bantle JP, Beebe CA, et al. Evidence-based nutrition principles and recommendations for the treatment and prevention of diabetes and related complications. Diabetes Care 2002; 25:148–198.

77. Bantle JP, Laine DC, Thomas JW. Metabolic effects of dietary fructose and sucrose in types I and II diabetic subjects. JAMA 1986; 256:3241–3246.

78. Bantle JP, Swanson JE, Thomas W, et al. Metabolic effects of dietary fructose in diabetic subjects. Diabetes Care 1992; 15:1468–1476.

79. Bantle JP, Swanson JE, Thomas W, Laine DC. Metabolic effects of dietary sucrose in type II diabetic subjects. Diabetes Care 1993; 16:1301–1305.

80. Orchard TJ, Forrest KY, Kuller LH, et al. Lipid and blood pressure treatment goals for type 1 diabetes: 10-year incidence data from the Pittsburgh Epidemiology of Diabetes Complications Study. Diabetes Care 2001; 24(6):1053–1059.

81. Fried LF, Forrest KY, Ellis D, et al. Lipid modulation in insulin-dependent diabetes mellitus: effect on microvascular outcomes. J Diabetes Complications 2001; 15(3):113–119.

82. Collier G, McLean A, O'Dea K. Effect of co-ingestion of fat on the metabolic responses to slowly and rapidly absorbed carbohydrates. Diabetologia 1984; 26:50–54.

83. Toeller M, Buyken A, Heitkamp G, et al. The EURODIAB IDDM Complications Study. Protein intake and urinary albumin excretion rates in the EURODIAB IDDM Complications Study. Diabetologia 1999; 40:1219–1226.

84. LaPorte R, Dorman JS, Tajima N, et al. Pittsburgh insulin-dependent diabetes mellitus morbidity and mortality study: physical activity and diabetic complications. Pediatric 1986; 78:1027–1033.

85. Moy CS, LaPorte RE, Dorman J, et al. Physical activity, insulin dependent diabetes mellitus and death. Am J Epidemiol 1993; 137(1):74–81.

86. Zinman B. Exercise in the patient with diabetes mellitus. In: Galloway JA, Potvin JH, Schuman CR, eds. Diabetes Mellitus. 9th. Indianapolis: Eli Lilly, 1988:215–224.

87. Arslanian S, Nixon PA, Becker D, et al. Impact of physical fitness and glycemic control on in vivo insulin action in adolescents with IDDM. Diabetes Care 1990; 13:9–15.

88. Rigla M, Sanchez-Quesada JL, et al. Effect of physical exercise on lipoprotein(a) and low-density lipoprotein modifications in type 1 and type 2 diabetic patients. Metabolism 2000; 49(5):640–647.

89. Chase P, Crews K, Garg S. Outpatient management vs in-hospital management of children with new-onset diabetes. Clinical Pediatrics 1992; 31(8):450–456.

90. Swift P, Hearnshaw J, Botha J, et al. A decade of diabetes: keeping children out of hospital. Br J Med 1993; 307:96–98.

91. Lee P. An outpatient-focused program for childhood diabetes: design, implementation, and effectiveness. J Tex Med 1992; 88(7):64–68.

92. The Pennsylvania State University The Graduate School Department of health education comparing outpatient to inpatient diabetes education for newly diagnosed pediatric patients: an exploratory study. A Thesis in Health Education by Linda M. Siminerio Copyright 1998 Linda M. Siminerio Submitted in Partial Fulfillment of the Requirements for the Degree of Doctor of Philosophy May 1998.

93. Siminerio LM, Charron-Prochownik D, Banion C, et al. Comparing outpatient and inpatient diabetes education for newly diagnosed pediatric patients. Diabetes Educ 1999; 25(6):895–906.

94. Charron-Prochownik D, Maihle T, Siminerio L, et al. Outpatient versus inpatient care of children newly diagnosed with IDDM. Diabetes Care 1997; 20(4):657–660.

95. Ryan C, Gurtunca N, Becker D. Hypoglycemia: a complication of diabetes therapy in children. Pediatr Clin North Am 2005; 52:1705–1733.

96. American Diabetes Association Workgroup on Hypoglycemia. Defining and reporting hypoglycemia in diabetes: a report from the American Diabetes Association Workgroup on Hypoglycemia. Diabetes Care 2005; 28:1245–1249.

97. Dunger DB, Sperling MA, Acerini CL, et al. ESPE; LWPES. ESPE/LWPES consensus statement on diabetic ketoacidosis in children and adolescents. Arch Dis Child 2004; 89(2):188–194.

98. Ryan CM, Becker DJ. Hypoglycemia in children with type 1 diabetes mellitus. Risk factors, cognitive function, and management. Endocrinol Metab Clin North Am 1999; 28(4):883–900.

99. Cronin CC, Shanahan F. Insulin-dependent diabetes mellitus and coeliac disease. Lancet 1997; 349:1096–1097.

100. Hummel M, Ziegler AG, Bonifacio E. Type 1 diabetes mellitus, celiac disease and their association—lessons from antibodies. J Pediatr Endocrinol Metab 2001; 14(suppl 1):607–610.

101. Schuppan D, Hahn EG. Celiac disease and its link to type 1 diabetes mellitus. J Pediatr Endocrinol Metab 2001; 14(suppl 1):597–605.

102. Shanahan F, Mckenna R, McCarthy CF, et al. Coeliac disease and diabetes mellitus: a study of 24 patients with HLA typing. QJM 1982; 51:329–335.

103. Bonifacio E, Ziegler AG, Hummel M, et al. Gluten: is it also a determinant of islet autoimmunity? Diabetes Metab Rev 1998; 14(3):258–259.

104. Drash AL, Becker DJ. Behavioral issues in patients with diabetes mellitus, with special emphasis on the child and adolescent. In: Rifkin H, Porte D, eds. Ellenberg and Rifkin's Diabetes Mellitus Theory and Practice. 4th. New York: Elsevier, 1990:992–934.

105. Kelly SD, Howe CJ, Hendler JP, et al. Disordered eating behaviors in youth with type 1 diabetes. Diabetes Educ 2005; 31(4):572–583.

106. Mannucci E, Rotella F, Ricca V, et al. Eating disorders in patients with type 1 diabetes: a meta-analysis. J Endocrinol Invest 2005; 28(5):417–419.

107. Lane PH. Pediatric aspects of diabetic kidney disease. Adv Chronic Kidney Dis 2005; 12(2):230–235.

108. Chiarelli F, Trotta D, Verrotti A, et al. Treatment of hypertension and microalbuminuria in children and adolescents with type 1 diabetes mellitus. Pediatr Diabetes 2002; 3(2):113–124.

109. Tsamasiros J, Bartsocas CS. Transition of the adolescent from the children's to the adults' diabetes clinic. J Pediatr Endocrinol Metab 2002; 15(4):363–367.

110. Mandal TK. Inhaled insulin for diabetes mellitus. Am J Health Syst Pharm 2005; 62(13):1359–1364.

111. DeFronzo RA, Bergenstal RM, Cefalu WT, et al. Exubera Phase III Study Group. Efficacy of inhaled insulin in patients with type 2 diabetes not controlled with diet and exercise: a 12-week, randomized, comparative trial. Diabetes Care 2005; 28(8):1922–1928.

112. Harsch IA. Inhaled insulins: their potential in the treatment of diabetes mellitus. Treat Endocrinol 2005; 4(3):131–138.

113. New York Times January 28, 2006.

114. Cooper GJ, Willis AC, Clark A, et al. Purification and characterization of a peptide from amyloid-rich pancreases of Type 2 diabetic patients. Proc Natl Acad Sci USA 1987; 84:8628–8632.

115. Gedulin BR, Rink TJ, Young AA. Dose response for glucagonostatic effect of amylin in rats. Metabolism 1997; 46:67–70.

116. Sansom, M, Szarka LA, Camilleri M, et al. Pramlintide, an amylin analog selectively delays gastric emptying: potential role for vagal inhibition. Am J Physiol 2000; 278:G946–G951.

117. Bhavsar S, Watkins J, Young A. Synergy between amylin and cholecystokinin for inhibition of food intake in mice. Physiol Behav 1998; 64:557–561.

118. Hollander P, Maggs DG, Ruggles JA, et al. Effect of pramlintide on weight in overweight and obese insulin-treated type 2 diabetes patients. Obes Res 2004; 12(4):661–668.

119. Hollander PA, Levy P, Fineman MS, et al. Pramlintide as an adjunct to insulin therapy improves long-term glycemic and weight control in patients with type 2 diabetes: a 1-year randomized controlled trial. Diabetes Care 2003; 26(3):784–790.

120. Ratner R, Whitehouse F, Fineman MS, et al. Adjunctive therapy with pramlintide lowers HbA1c without concomitant weight gain and increased risk of severe hypoglycemia in patients with type 1 diabetes approaching glycemic targets. Exp Clin Endocrinol Diabetes 2005; 113(4):199–204.

121. Heptulla RA, Rodriguez LM, Bomgaars L, et al. The role of amylin and glucagon in the dampening of glycemic excursions in children with type 1 diabetes. Diabetes 2005; 54(4):1100–1107.

7

Practical Aspects of Diabetes Care

Shannon P. Lyles, Janet H. Silverstein, and Arlan L. Rosenbloom
*Division of Pediatric Endocrinology, Department of Pediatrics, University of Florida,
Gainesville, Florida, U.S.A.*

INTRODUCTION

Type 1 diabetes mellitus (T1DM) is a complex disease to manage, requiring a team effort in which the key player is the patient. Gone are the days of urine-glucose testing, boiling glass syringes, sharpening needles, and rigid diet restrictions. Technology and new medications continue to improve the lives of patients with this disease. Along with these new developments has come the need for increasing education and training of patients and health-care providers to effectively use these tools. This chapter will discuss technology and guidelines for blood glucose (BG) monitoring, continuous subcutaneous insulin infusion (CSII), and management of sick days, hypoglycemia, exercise, travel, and school days. While topics to be covered are directed to patients with T1DM, most of the information is applicable to children and youth with T2DM, as well.

BLOOD GLUCOSE MONITORING

Patients have a wide choice of meters to self-monitor their BG levels. BG levels should be tested at least four times per day, before breakfast, lunch, dinner, and at bedtime. Those on basal bolus regimens using multiple daily injections or pump therapy should additionally check before snacks so that appropriate doses of rapid-acting insulin can be taken. When initiating pump therapy or changing insulin regimens, more frequent monitoring is necessary throughout the day and night. In order to determine if the rapid-acting insulin dose is correct, two-hour postprandial BG levels are encouraged to assess the effectiveness of the insulin to carbohydrate ratio (I.C). If a patient is waking up with high BG levels, a 2 or 3 A.M. BG level should be obtained by the caregiver before adjusting the evening insulin dose upward, to ensure that the patient is not becoming hypoglycemic in the middle of the night and rebounding in the morning. If this were the case, the dose would need to be decreased instead of increased. It is also necessary to check the BG levels more frequently during illness (Table 1).

All of the meters listed in Table 1 can be downloaded to the computer with specific programs from each manufacturer. Some programs can be downloaded from the Internet for free while others must be purchased. Some meters are downloadable with an infrared port while others require a cable that hooks up to the meter. Even meters manufactured by the same company may require different cables for download. When downloading meters, a variety of reports may be generated including a logbook for a specified amount of time, data list with all results, statistics, averages, pie charts, line graphs, and highest and lowest readings. Most commonly, we view the 14-day logbook and statistics during clinic visits. The 14-day logbook also includes averages for each time of day. One of the most important pieces of information is the average number of BG tests per day. That information, in addition to the BG ranges and averages, is recorded in the clinic note (Table 2).

Patients and caregivers should be encouraged to keep a logbook with BG levels, insulin doses, and notes detailing events that may affect BG readings recorded, and bring both the logbook and the meter for download to the clinic visit. If a daily or weekly record is not kept, it is less likely that patients will recognize developing BG patterns. While a meter can record the date, time, blood glucose, and in some cases insulin dose, amount of carbohydrates eaten, or exercise done, that still does not provide as complete a picture as when the patient records these events in a logbook. Examples of extra information that can be recorded in a logbook might include whether the patient ate pizza and ice cream for dinner and ended up with hyperglycemia at bedtime, the patient went out to eat and miscalculated carbohydrates eaten and developed hypoglycemia one hour after finishing the meal, or the patient forgot to take a bolus for a mid-afternoon snack and had hyperglycemia pre-dinner. Logbooks can be obtained from the meter manufacturers.

We encourage patients to call for insulin dose adjustments if within one week, they have three BG readings less than 60 mg/dL or two less than

Table 1 BG Meter Comparison[a]

Manufacturer	Meter	Sample size (µL)	Result (sec)	Size (in.)	Weight (oz)	Number of results stored in memory	Alternate site testing approved
Lifescan	One Touch® Ultra®	1	5	3.12 × 2.25 × 0.85	1.5	150	Yes
	One Touch® Ultra Smart®	1	5	3.8 × 2.3 × 0.9	2.6	3000	Yes
	InDuo®	1	5	4.84 × 2.13 × 1.38	4.4	150	Yes
Roche	Accu-Chek® Advantage®	4	26	3.3 × 2.2 × 0.8	1.8	480	No
	Accu-Chek® Aviva®	0.6	5	3.7 × 2.0 × 0.9	2.1	500	Yes
	Accu-Chek® Active®	1	5 (in meter), 10 (out of meter)	4 × 1.7 × 0.9	2	200	Yes
	Accu-Chek® Compact®	1.5	8	4 × 2 × 1.2	4.2	100	Yes
Abbott Diabetes Care	FreeStyle®	0.3	7	2.03 × 3.82 × 0.98	2.04	250	Yes
	FreeStyle Flash™	0.3	7	1.6 × 3 × 0.8	1.4	250	Yes
	Precision Xtra®	1.5	10	2.9 × 2.1 × 0.6	1.48	450	Yes
Becton Dickinson	BD Logic®	0.3	5	3.6 × 2.2 × 0.9	2.65	250	Yes
Bayer	Ascensia Contour®	0.6	15	2.9 × 2.09 × 0.6	1.82	240	Yes

[a]While only 12 meters from 5 companies are highlighted, this list is not all-inclusive.
Abbreviation: BG, blood glucose.
Source: Adapted from Ref. 1.

50 mg/dL at the same time of day, or one unexplained reading less than 40 mg/dL.

Alternate Site Testing

Fingertips have been the traditional site for obtaining capillary blood for self-monitoring of glucose. However, there are various meters now on the market that are approved for alternate site testing (AST) in order to bypass the discomfort often associated with pricking the finger for a BG sample (13). AST can be done on the forearm, upper arm, palm of the hand, thigh, and calf. Patients need to refer to their BG meter manual to ensure that proper sites are being used because not all sites are approved for AST with each meter.

Several studies have compared AST with traditional finger stick BG monitoring. A study of 52 children and adolescents aged 6 to 17 years found preference for forearm testing; however, precision was less than with finger stick testing, BG readings were lower than with finger stick, and quick changes in postprandial glucose concentrations were picked up later (14). Another study with 29 subjects aged 5 to 17 years compared fingertip testing with palm or forearm testing. The recommendation from this study was that these two alternate sites are acceptable for use before and after meals, but the forearm should not be used during hypoglycemia, or if there is a risk of hypoglycemia, because of delay in detecting low BG levels. The palm is equivalent to the fingertip for detection of hypoglycemia (15).

We prefer that our patients use the traditional finger stick blood for glucose monitoring, especially at initiation of insulin therapy while insulin doses are being titrated. Later on, if the patient or caregiver asks if AST is acceptable, we tell them it is an alternative if they are fasting, or are not feeling hypoglycemic, or if the glucose concentration is not dropping quickly. If there is any doubt about the accuracy of an AST measurement, the BG result should be confirmed with a finger stick specimen.

Blood-Ketone Testing

The Precision Xtra BG meter is the only meter currently available to check for blood ketones. Blood-ketone testing differs from urinary ketones in that beta hydroxybutyrate (B-OHB) is measured instead of acetoacetate (AcAc) or acetone. This is primarily helpful in the diagnosis and monitoring of diabetic ketoacidosis (DKA) because treatment can begin sooner with the earlier detection of blood ketones. B-OHB is more elevated than AcAc in DKA and is a more accurate measure of recovery because it decreases in serum well ahead of urinary reduction of ketones. If a patient has large urinary ketones, the severity of ketosis can be determined by the blood–B-OHB level, and a more informed decision whether to treat at home or send the patient directly to the hospital can be made (16).

Serum levels of B-OHB less than 0.6 mmol/L are normal; so no adjustments are necessary. Supplemental insulin may be needed if the measurement is between 0.6 and 1.0 mmol/L. When levels reach 1.0 to 1.5 mmol/L, more insulin is needed along with supplemental fluids. Patients should call their diabetes care provider at this point if there is any doubt about treatment. We advise giving 10% of the total daily dose (TDD) of insulin as regular or rapid-acting analog and rechecking the B-OHB every four to six hours (regular), or every two to four hours for rapid-acting analog (lispro, aspart, or glulisine) until ketones clear or decrease. When B-OHB levels are greater than 1.5 to 3.0 mmol/L, the patient or caregiver should call the diabetes care provider immediately.

Table 2 Pros and Cons of Various BG Meters

Meter	Pros	Cons
One Touch® Ultra®	Small Ergonomic shape Result, in 5 sec Easy to set date and time Downloadable with One Touch® Diabetes Management Software	Must code test strips Date and time frequently reset by themselves
One Touch® UltraSmart®	Holds more results in memory than any other meter Has backlight 7, 14, 30, 60, and 90 day average all results, average by time of day, glucose range info, hypoglycemia info, daily food average Graphs results: all and time-specific Downloadable with One Touch® Diabetes Management Software Can input exercise and health checks such as HbA1C and blood pressure	Must code test strips Lots of bells and whistles Can be overwhelming to patients Must know keypad combinations to turn on backlight, reset date and time, etc.
InDuo®	Meter and insulin pen all in one for convenience Holds 3 mL insulin cartridge Downloadable with One Touch® Diabetes Management Software	Must code test strips Bulky Date and time frequently reset by themselves
Accu-Chek® Advantage®	Comfort curve test strip Large screen Ergonomic design Can be downloaded with Accu-Chek® Compass software	Must code test strips Results take 26 seconds Large sample size Being replaced by the Aviva®
Accu-Chek® Aviva®	7-, 14-, and 30-day averages Stores 500 BG results in memory Strip has wide mouth for easier sampling 150 automatic internal tests to ensure accuracy Small sample size Approved for all alternate site testing (AST) areas Ergonomic design Can be downloaded with Accu-Chek® Compass software	Must code test strips
Accu-Chek® Active®	Slender design 7- and 14-day averages Approved for all AST areas Cheaper test strips than other Accu-Chek® Meters Can be downloaded with Accu-Chek Compass Software	Must code test strips Hanging drop of blood must be applied to top of test strip Larger sample size
Accu-Chek® Compact®	Self-contained test strips No coding of test strips necessary Can be downloaded with Accu-Chek® Compass Software	Bulkier size Flip top often breaks off If test strip compartment opens test drum must reset to next available test strip
FreeStyle®	Smallest blood sample size (0.3 microliter) 14-day average Uses Coulometry Technology Downloadable with FreeStyle CoPilot™	Must code test strips
FreeStyle Flash™	Small size Smallest blood sample size Has backlight (screen and down strip) Uses Coulometry Technology 4 programmable alarms to remind patients when to test Downloadable with FreeStyle CoPilot™	Must code test strips
Precision Xtra®	Only meter to perform blood-ketone testing Can help diagnose diabetic ketoacidosis 7-, 14-, and 30-day averages Downloadable with Precision Link Software®	Must code test strips Separate test strips for BG– and blood-ketone-testing
BD Logic®	Holds 250 BG results in memory Shows 7- and 14-day averages Can record insulin type and doses Can "mark" specific insulin doses and BG results to indicate different times or doses Downloadable with the BD InterActiv™ Diabetes Software The Paradigm Link Version beams the blood glucose directly to the MiniMed insulin pump	Must code test strips Only holds up to 30 readings in memory without download Patient not keeping log book every day then will not be able to recall more than 30 readings "Marked" results are not averaged into the 7- or 14-day averages Not user-friendly

(Continued)

Table 2 Pros and Cons of Various BG Meters (*Continued*)

Meter	Pros	Cons
Ascensia Contour®	No coding of test strips necessary Control solution is marked with check mark Detects if strip does not have enough blood for sample Ergonomic design Downloadable with the Ascensia™ WIN Glucofacts™ Diabetes Management Software	

Abbreviation: BG, blood glucose.
Source: From Refs. 2–12.

The treatment is the same as for the levels of 1.0 to 1.5 mmol/L, except that 20% of the TDD may be needed instead of only 10%. If the blood-ketone test reveals levels in excess of 3 mmol/L, the patient should be sent immediately to the emergency department. Blood-ketone testing may facilitate earlier intervention and improved home management of impending ketoacidosis (16).

INSULIN INJECTIONS

The insulin regimen must be individualized to match the patient's physiology and lifestyle. Some things to consider when deciding which insulin regimen to assign a patient include:

- Compliance
- Education
- Supervision/support
- Math skills
- Problem solving skills

Types
Rapid-Acting Insulin Analogs
Humalog™ (insulin lispro):

- Onset: 15 to 30 minutes
- Peak: 0.5 to 2.5 hours
- Duration: 5 hours or less

Novolog™ (insulin aspart):

- Onset: 10 to 20 minutes
- Peak: 1 to 3 hours
- Duration: 3 to 5 hours

Apidra™ (insulin glulisine):

- Onset: 15 to 30 minutes
- Peak: 0.5 to 2.5 hours
- Duration: 5 hours or less

Short-Acting Insulin

Regular:

- Onset: 0.5 to 1 hour
- Peak: 2 to 5 hours
- Duration: 5 to 8 hours

Intermediate-Acting Insulin
NPH:

- Onset: 1 to 2 hours
- Peak: 2 to 12 hours
- Duration: 14 to 24 hours

Long-Acting Insulin Analogs

Lantus (insulin glargine):

- Onset: 1.5 hours
- Peak: small peak in the first three hours, then flattens out
- Duration: 20 to 24 hours

Levemir (insulin detemir):

- Onset: Steady state conditions after second injection
- Duration: dose-dependent, bid-dosing recommended (17,18)

Intermediate-/Rapid-Acting Insulin

Humalog Mix 75/25 (75% NPH/25% lispro):

- Onset: 15 to 30 minutes
- Peak: 0.5 to 2.5 hours
- Duration: up to 24 hours

Novolog Mix 70/30 (70% insulin aspart protamine suspension/30% aspart):

- Onset: 10 to 20 minutes
- Peak: 2.4 hours
- Duration: up to 24 hours

Intermediate-/Short-Acting Insulin

Humulin 70/30 (70% NPH/30% Regular):

- Onset: 30 to 60 minutes
- Peak: 0.5 to 2.5 hours
- Duration: up to 24 hours

Novolin 70/30 (70% NPH/30% Regular):

- Onset: 30 minutes
- Peak: 2 to 12 hours
- Duration: 24 hours (1)

Usage Guidelines

NPH/Rapid-Acting Insulin

We determine initial insulin dosages according to body weight, usually giving approximately one unit per kilogram per day. Once this dose is determined, we give approximately two-thirds of the TDD in the morning and one-third in the evening. The morning dose usually consists of two-thirds intermediate and one-third rapid-acting insulin, and the evening dose is broken down to 50% intermediate and 50% rapid-acting insulin. See Table 3 for sample calculations. We instruct patients to take their fixed-dose insulins, i.e., intermediate- or long-acting insulins within an hour before or after the scheduled time. This rule applies to patients on fixed doses of rapid-acting insulin analogs as well.

When patients and caregivers are not familiar with diabetes management but are able to mix insulins, it is easiest to begin insulin therapy with a combination of NPH and aspart/lispro/glulisine or, in some cases, regular. Initially, this minimizes the number of injections, often requiring only two to three per day. We do not start patients on regular insulin anymore unless they consume frequent snacks and the rapid-acting insulin does not provide adequate coverage. For the A.M. and P.M. injections, NPH and the rapid-acting insulin can be mixed. A variable dose of the rapid-acting insulin may be required with meals. If adjusting the morning NPH does not correct the high afternoon BG levels, an injection of rapid-acting insulin may be required at lunch. NPH taken at dinner, especially during adolescence, tends to run out before the morning, resulting in high level blood glucose even when the dose is increased. To deal with this phenomenon, NPH can be moved to bedtime, instead of before dinner. The rapid-acting insulin is then taken alone before dinner and the NPH alone before bedtime.

The principal drawback of this regimen is lack of flexibility. Patients are locked into rigid meal and snack times because the pharmacokinetics of insulin mandate that they eat to cover the peak concentrations of insulin. The daily schedule must include breakfast, lunch, mid-afternoon snack, dinner, bedtime snack, and possibly a mid-morning snack. While most patients using NPH and rapid-acting analog insulin do not count carbohydrates, the need to keep carbohydrate amounts consistent is necessary to maintain glycemic control with fixed dose regimens. Patients and caregivers need to understand that if more carbohydrates are consumed, larger amounts of insulin are necessary. Giving them guidelines such as adding one to two units of analog for every 15 g of carbohydrates consumed above their normal intake can help keep BG levels from increasing too much when extra carbohydrates are eaten.

If the patient or caregiver is unable to mix insulins together in a syringe because of low literacy or noncompliance, a premix of an intermediate plus rapid- or short-acting insulin can be used. While premixes are available in vials, dispensing them in pen form adds to the ease of use and may improve compliance. The patient simply has to dial the dose on the pen without having to worry about accurately reading lines on a syringe. The premix insulin is given as a standard dose for breakfast and dinner. The problems with the use of NPH are even greater for this regimen because it limits the ability to separately adjust the rapid- or the intermediate-acting insulin. Another disadvantage is that many patients on this regimen are less likely to use correction scales when BG levels are high, either because of inability to understand the concept or the need for an extra injection, which they are unwilling to take. The latter is especially true for those using insulin pens because that would require two injections at the same time.

Basal/Bolus Regimens

For patients and caregivers who are motivated, insulin glargine or detemir plus rapid-acting insulin allows the most flexibility of any multiple daily-injection regimen. Glargine and detemir are typically given initially as a single dose once daily. For young patients and those with nocturnal hypoglycemia, insulin glargine can be started in the morning. For patients who like to sleep in some days while waking up early on others, taking glargine or detemir at bedtime allows greater flexibility because they do not have to get up early to take their injection, eat, and then go back to bed, as recommended for patients on NPH regimens. While the most common times for administering insulin glargine are first thing in the morning or before bed, the injection can be given at any time because of its long duration of action and minimal variation in insulin concentration, so long as the time is consistent from day to day. For some patients, especially toddlers, glargine does not last a full 24 hours. Thus, if BG levels tend to be higher with increased duration following the injection, even after

Table 3 Initial Insulin Dose Calculations Based on Patient Weighing 48 kg

Type of insulin	Dose calculations
NPH + Aspart (A)/Lispro (L)/Glulisine (G)/Regular (R)	A.M.: 48 kg × 0.66 = 31.58 = 32 32 × 0.66 = 21.12 = 21 units NPH 32 × 0.33 = 10.56 = 11 units A/L/G/R P.M.: 48 kg × 0.33 = 15.84 = 16 16/2 = 8 so, 8 units NPH and 8 units A/L/G/R
Premixed insulins 70/30 or 75/25	A.M.: 48 kg × 0.66 = 31.58 = 32 units 70/30 or 75/25 P.M.: 48 kg × 0.33 = 15.84 = 16 units 70/30 or 75/25
Glargine (usually 60–70% of total NPH dose)	See above NPH calculation: A.M.= 21 units P.M.= 8 units, so 21 + 8 = 29 units NPH total daily 29 × 0.60 = 17.4 = 17 units Glargine or 29 × 0.70 = 20.3 = 20 units Glargine

increasing the dose, splitting the glargine dose should be considered. The way in which the dose is split must be individualized, though usual regimens are: 50/50, or two-thirds in the A.M. and one-third in P.M./hs, or two-thirds in the P.M./hs and one-third in the A.M.

The need to count carbohydrates for all meals and snacks and to give injections to cover carbohydrates eaten with these meals and snacks can lead to as many as 7 to 10 injections/day, depending on the frequency of snacking. Thus, the major disadvantage of glargine or detemir use is the number of injections of rapid-acting analog required, especially for patients who snack frequently. Patients tire of the frequent shots and may skip injections or snack without giving insulin coverage. The need to count carbohydrates for all food intake can also be overwhelming and requires support to patients, including nutrition counseling and telephone- or e-mail contact.

It is important to remember that patients may achieve better metabolic control if they change to a different regimen rather than attempting to adjust insulin within the current routine. If a more complex regimen worked for a while, but then circumstances change and that regimen no longer works, one can switch to a simpler regimen until the patient is ready to make changes. The same can happen for patients who had been placed on a regimen requiring minimal decision-making because of noncompliance, but are now able to take more responsibility for their diabetes management and can be prescribed a more complex regimen. The patient and caregiver must be aware of the pros and cons of each treatment program so they know what to expect from day to day.

CONTINUOUS SUBCUTANEOUS INSULIN INFUSION

Continuous subcutaneous insulin infusion or insulin pump therapy is the most intensive insulin management system currently in use, mimicking normal b-cell function in providing variable amounts of basal insulin throughout the day. The pump also allows delivery of a larger bolus dose of insulin to provide adequate insulin coverage for food intake.

The decision to initiate CSII must not be entered into without careful consideration of the following criteria for identifying appropriate candidates:

- Patients should have a history of keeping all clinic appointments. Patients who miss or cancel appointments are more likely to not adhere to the requirements of CSII treatment.
- A logbook should be kept for one month. This will be preparation for the detailed record keeping necessary for success on the pump.
- The patient or parent of the younger child must check blood glucose four to six times daily. For at least one week following initiation of CSII, pre– and two-hours-postprandial BG checks are needed.
- The patient or parent must be able to accurately count carbohydrates as evidenced by a satisfactory score on a carbohydrate counting test.

- The patient or parent must be able to appropriately calculate insulin dose for meal coverage using an insulin to carbohydrate ratio and correction factor.
- The patient or parent should contact the healthcare provider weekly to review BG levels. This will be preparatory for the frequent contact, which must be maintained with CSII.
- Hemoglobin A1C (HbA1C) level should be less than 9% or decreasing, indicating attention to diabetes management. This criterion can be negotiable under special circumstances (e.g., very young children).
- The most important criterion is that all members of the family, especially the child, must want the pump. The child will be the one wearing it, so the child's feelings must be considered.

After meeting these criteria, the patient and parents should attend an "Introduction to Insulin Pump" class. Often done in a group setting, this class should be maximally participatory, giving families the opportunity to pose questions about pump therapy. The interaction between families adds to the learning experience. Allowing the patient and parents to insert an infusion set in this controlled environment helps to dispel fear about the infusion set being painful.

It is a good idea for the child to wear a pump containing saline solution before beginning insulin treatment with the device. This gives the child a chance to see what it will be like to live with the pump continuously before making the final commitment to CSII. A saline delivering pump should be worn for three to seven days to allow the patient and parents the opportunity to manipulate the pump without fear of making a mistake that would have medical consequences. It also allows them to become comfortable with the different buttons and pump operations. It can be more beneficial for the parent of a young child, rather than the child, to wear the saline infusion pump because the parent will be the one manipulating the pump and doing the button pushing. Even elementary school-aged children, who are capable of button pushing, should have caregivers who are comfortable with all pump operations. As with conventional therapy, caregivers may relinquish responsibility to the child too quickly, without adequate supervision.

Another consideration is how soon after diagnosis, CSII should be considered. Some doctors offer it as initial treatment. This is based on the family's current understanding of diabetes management and ability to assimilate the basics of diabetes care. We have not yet done this. The time of diagnosis is highly stressful and educationally intense; teaching the requirements of pump therapy in addition to everything else that must be taught could be overwhelming for families. We have considered it best to wait until the family is comfortable with managing their child's diabetes and able to demonstrate the behaviors noted in the criteria above. After a month to several months, if the patient and caregivers meet the criteria and express interest in this therapy, they are eligible to go through pump class and proceed with initiation of CSII.

Once these eligibility requirements have been met and the patient or caregivers decide which pump they want, the insurance company must be contacted. Families should check with their health insurance carrier before initiating the pump preparation process to determine what their personal cost will be. The pump alone costs about $5000, with supplies exceeding $1500 per year. Coverage can vary from state to state, with some states requiring coverage for the pump and all associated supplies (Table 4) (19).

Infusion Site and Infusion Set

The insertion site for the infusion is the subcutaneous fat, as with traditional insulin injections. Appropriate loci for insertion are in the abdomen, arms, thighs, and buttocks. Site rotation is as important for CSII as for insulin injections. The site must be changed every two to three days or more frequently if problems occur with insulin delivery or site infections. Scar tissue or lipohypertrophy will develop with inadequate rotation and result in erratic insulin absorption. The new site must be at least a half inch from the old site. It is important to avoid areas of friction such as waistbands and clothing seams when deciding where to place the infusion set. The site should be at least two inches from a bone, a scar, or the umbilicus. The site should be changed in the morning, not at night, so that any problem with a new site will be detected early with BG monitoring throughout the day. Blood ketones can be checked in addition to urine ketones if the child is asleep, if urine cannot be obtained, or as clinically indicated. The blood glucose should be checked one to three hours after changing the site to ensure that the system is working. The site should be changed if two consecutive BG levels are above 240 mg/dL or moderate to large urine ketones are present (Fig. 1). Ketones are checked at a lower BG value with CSII because there is no long-acting insulin reserve; thus, if there is a problem with the system, the blood glucose and urine ketones or blood B-OHB levels are the first indicators of impaired insulin delivery. Indicators of site problems include redness, irritation, swelling, induration, discharge, or discomfort. Signs of infusion-set problems include air in the tubing, loose connection between cartridge and reservoir, insulin leakage at the infusion site, kinked cannula, air in the infusion set, blood in the infusion set, and loose adhesive backing caused by sweating or water activities.

Needle insertion discomfort can be alleviated by using an ice cube or analgesic cream such as ElaMax or Emla Cream, available at some pharmacies and medical supply stores. Standing up when inserting the needle/catheter into the abdomen, buttocks, or thighs can make the task easier. Facing a mirror can also be helpful.

Problems with nonadhesion of the infusion set can be alleviated by using an adhesive such as IV Prep™, Skin Prep, or Mastisol. Unisolve™ or Detachol™ can be used to remove adhesive agents. These are available at some pharmacies and medical supply stores, and online at Ferndale Laboratories. Some patients use Tegaderm™ to help with adhesion. Inserting through the Tegaderm works for some patients while others put it on top of the infusion set after needle insertion has been completed. Cutting a hole in the Tegaderm allows the infusion set to be disconnected from the cannula, if necessary.

The site should be checked by the patient or parent at least once a day and following vigorous activity as the catheter may become dislodged. A skin-protective agent such as IV Prep™ should be used before inserting the needle/catheter to avoid skin irritation. If a site becomes inflamed or irritated, a topical bacteriostatic agent such as Bactroban may be applied after removing the catheter. The patient or parent should be instructed to notify the health-care team immediately if there are any signs of infection, including fever, erythema, and pus or drainage from the site.

A variety of infusion sets are available with differing lengths of catheters and tubing. Age, size, and personal preference of the patient should all be taken into account. Some catheters are inserted perpendicular to the skin while others are inserted at an angle. There are inserters for some infusion sets, while others must be manually inserted. This is again a personal preference. Newer infusion sets include the inserter, set, and tubing as a disposable unit. With the exception of the MiniMed Paradigm model, pump infusion sets made by different companies are interchangeable among pump brands to allow patients more options. Younger patients and others with little subcutaneous fat may prefer infusion sets that are inserted perpendicular to the skin and have a shorter catheter. Patients who are very active or have more subcutaneous fat may benefit from angled sets, which have longer catheters. Occasionally, patients vary the type of set used depending on the insertion site.

Special Considerations

Teenage girls considering pump therapy may have body image concerns, making the realization that the pump will be attached at all times important. This offers the opportunity for creativity about how to wear the pump with various outfits. Toddlers and younger elementary school-age children are apt to experiment with pushing buttons on devices. To safeguard against accidental pushing of buttons with resultant insulin delivery, each pump has a block feature. When the block is turned on, no insulin bolus can be delivered. A special keypad combination must be pressed to unlock the pump and allow a bolus to be given. The buttocks are often the best insertion site in toddlers who might not have much subcutaneous fat on the arms, abdomen, or thighs. This site is an area

Table 4 Insulin Pump Comparison[a]

Manufacturer	Animas	Animas	Medtronic MiniMed	Medtronic MiniMed	Nipro Diabetes Systems	Sooil Development Co./DANA Diabecare	Smith's Medical/ Deltec
Model	IR-1250	IR-1000	Paradigm 515	Paradigm 715	Amigo	DANA Diabecare II	Cozmo
Size (in.)	2.9 × 2.0 × 0.76	3.5 × 2.2 × 0.71	3 × 2 × 0.8	3.6 × 2 × 0.8	3.28 × 2.18 × 0.93	2.95 × 1.77 × 0.74	3.2 × 1.8 × 0.90
Weight (oz)	3.13	3.5	3.8 (includes battery and reservoir filled to capacity)	3.8 (includes battery and reservoir filled to capacity)	3.1	1.8	3.3 (includes battery and reservoir filled to capacity)
Reservoir	Disposable plastic with 200 U	Disposable plastic with 300 U	Shock resistant disposable plastic with 176 U	Disposable plastic with 300 U	Disposable plastic with 300 U	Impact resistant disposable plastic	Disposable plastic with 300 U
Basal delivery (U)	0.025	0.05	0.05	0.05	0.05	0.1	0.05
Total number of basal patterns	4	4	3	3	1	1	4
Total number of basal rates per pattern	12	12	48	48	24	24	48
Temporary basal rate	Yes	Yes	Yes	Yes	Yes	Yes	Yes (8 customizable)
Temporary basal rate increase or decrease set as:	Percentage	Percentage	Percentage or units per hour	Percentage or units per hour	0–10 U/hr	0–32 U/hr	0–250% or U/hr
Temporary basal rate duration	30 min to 24 hr	30 min	30 min to 24 hr	30 min to 24 hr	15 min to 24 hr	Maximum is 12 hr	30 min to 72 hr
Maximum basal rate							
Bolus delivery in units including maximum bolus	0.05–25	0.1–25	0.1–25	0.1–25	0.1–25	0.1–87	0.05, 0.10, 0.50, 1.00, 2.00, or 5.00–75
Time it takes 1 U bolus to be delivered	Use selected	3 sec	40 sec	40 sec	3 or 15 sec	13 sec	1–5 min
Bolus types	Normal, carbohydrates, correction, combination, extended, audio, ezBolus	Normal, extended, combination, audio	Normal, square-wave, dual-wave, audio, carbohydrates, correction	Normal, square-wave, dual-wave, audio, carbohydrates, correction	Normal, extended	Normal, extended	Normal, carbohydrates, correction, combination, extended

Bolus calculator	Carb Smart Calculator	No	Bolus Wizard Calculator	Bolus Wizard Calculator	No	Dana Magic Bolus Calculator	Yes
Backlight	No	Yes	Yes	Yes	Yes	Yes	Yes
Type of battery	AA lithium or regular AA (shorter life)	Four 1.5 V model 357	One AAA alkaline	One AAA alkaline	One CR2 camera battery (3 V)	One 3.6 V DC	One AAA alkaline
Life of battery (wk)	6-8	8	2-3	2-3	4	8-12	4
Cost of battery per month (approximation)	<$2	$7	$2	$2	$8	$2.50	$1-2
Direct Communication with meter	No	No	Paradigm Link Blood Glucose Meter: BD Logic	Paradigm Link Blood Glucose Meter: BD Logic	No	No	Cozmonitor meter attaches directly to pump
Remote control	No	No	Yes (limited to suspend and bolus functions)	Yes (limited to suspend and bolus functions)	No	Yes (can perform all functions)	No
Computer program for download	ezManager Plus	ezManager Plus	Medtronic CareLink Therapy Management System (on web) and Paradigm PAL (pc based)	Medtronic CareLink Therapy Management System (on web) and Paradigm PAL (pc based)	Yes	Yes	CoZmanager PC Communications Software
Water rating	12 ft for 24 hr	12 ft for 24 hr	3 ft for 30 min (IPX7)	3 ft for 30 min (IPX8)	Water resistant	Water tight (IPX8)	Waterproof (IPX8): 8 ft for 30 min and 12 ft for 3 min
Optimal temperature range (°F)	41-104	41-104	34-108	34-108	41-104	32-104	35-104
Warranty (yr)	4	4	4	4	4	4	4
Special features	Has food database programmed into pump		Beams blood glucoses directly from Paradigm link meter to pump	Beams blood glucoses directly from Paradigm link meter to pump			Beams blood glucoses directly from Cozmonitor to pump
Customer support	(877)937-7867 24/7 Healthcare Professional Answers	(877)937-7867 24/7 Healthcare Professional Answers	(800)646-4633	(800)646-4633	(888)651-7867	(866)326-2832	(800)826-9703 24/7 RN/CDE Answers

aWhile 5 companies are highlighted, this list is not all-inclusive and new products are being developed continuously.

Source: Adapted from Ref. 1.

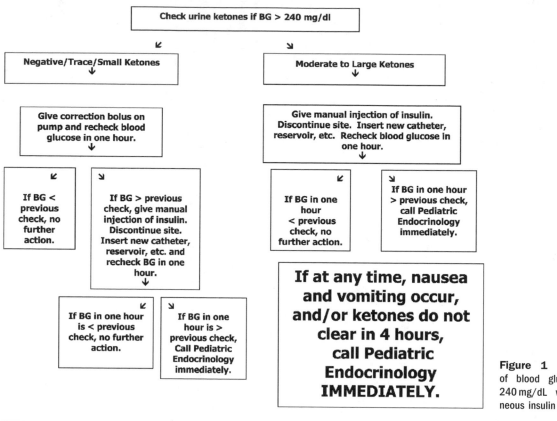

Figure 1 Guidelines for treatment of blood glucose (BG) greater than 240 mg/dL with continuous subcutaneous insulin infusion.

which the toddler cannot see, and would thus be less likely to pull out the catheter.

CSII Initiation

Insulin analogs are used in insulin pumps, including Aspart (Novolog), Lispro (Humalog), and Glulisine (Apidra). There are various ways to determine initial insulin dosages, which are dependent on the patient's previous insulin regimen. It is best to initiate CSII first thing in the morning so that any problems with insulin dose or insulin delivery will be recognized early (Table 5). If patients are started on the pump later in the day, slight adjustments for insulin given on the day of pump start may need to be made.

At initiation of CSII, the following instructions should be given to patients and their caregivers:

- BG levels should be checked before meals, two hours postprandial, bedtime, midnight, and 3 A.M.
- A correction dose of insulin should be given before breakfast, lunch, and dinner according to the prescribed correction factor.
- A correction dose should only be given two hours postprandial, bedtime, midnight, and 3 A.M. if the blood glucose is greater than 240 mg/dL. A correction dose of insulin should not be given for any BG value less than 240 mg/dL at these times because it will be impossible to determine if the correction dose or the basal rate is the cause of hypoglycemia following frequent insulin

correction boluses. In order to evaluate the appropriateness of the basal rates and bolus doses, patients should eat only breakfast, lunch, and dinner for the first week. This regimen obviously would require modification for the infant and toddler.

- It is recommended that patients or parents keep a detailed insulin pump log to keep track of BG levels, basal rates, boluses (food and correction), ketones, exercise, site changes, and food eaten. This will permit explanation of variations in BG levels more effectively to the healthcare provider (Fig. 2).

If BG levels are not in target range and it is not clear whether the basal rate or bolus dose needs to be adjusted, basal rate checks should be performed before making any adjustments. The criteria for checking basal rates include: no food for 4 to 5 hours, no bolus for 4 to 5 hours, and no exercise for 12 hours. Basal-rate checks can be performed for overnight, morning, afternoon, and evening time periods. The overnight basal-rate check should be performed first. If, at any time during a basal-rate check the patient experiences hypoglycemia, the patient should be treated and the basal-rate check repeated on another day.

Overnight Basal-Rate Check

- Check BG level, give bolus dose of insulin, and eat dinner by 7:00 P.M.

Table 5 How to Determine Initial Pump Doses

Type of insulin	Time of administration	Day before pump start	Day of pump start	Basal rate calculation
Glargine (Lantus)	q HS	Discontinue Glargine and give NPH at bedtime. Convert Glargine dose to NPH dose. TDD Glargine divided by 0.6 to 0.7 then multiply by 0.33	Patient to take analog only based on correction factor and insulin to carbohydrate ratio	TDD of Glargine divided by 24 for hourly rate
	q A.M.	Give usual Glargine dose	No Glargine the morning of pump start. Patient to take analog only based on correction factor and insulin to carbohydrate ratio	TDD of Glargine divided by 24 for hourly rate
	q A.M. and q P.M. or q A.M. and q HS (split dose)	Give usual Glargine doses	No Glargine the morning of pump start. Patient to take analog only based on correction factor and insulin to carbohydrate ratio	TDD of Glargine divided by 24 for hourly rate
NPH[a]	q A.M. and q P.M. or q A.M. and q HS	Give usual NPH doses	No NPH the morning of pump start. Patient to take analog only based on correction factor and insulin-to-carbohydrate ratio	TDD of NPH multiplied by 0.6–0.7 = Glargine dose. Divide Glargine dose by 24 for hourly rate

[a]For premixed 75/25 or 70/30 insulins, determine the equivalent NPH dose and follow above guidelines.
Abbreviation: TDD, total daily dose.

Insulin Pump Record

Name: <u>Brian Clark</u> Date of Pump Start: <u>9/10/96</u> Type of Insulin: <u>Novolog</u>

Insulin/Carbohydrate: <u>1:10</u> Correction Factor/Sensitivity: <u>BG-120÷50</u>

Basal Rate/s: <u>12am=1.0 4am=1.2 6am=1.1 12pm=1.0 7pm=1.1</u>

Date	12M	1A	2A	3A	4A	5A	6A	7A	8A	9A	10A	11A	12N	1P	2P	3P	4P	5P	6P	7P	8P	9P	10P	11P
BG				130					145		250			99		** 60		187				109		
Basal	1.0	1.0	1.0	1.0	1.2	1.2	1.1	1.1	1.1	1.1	1.1	1.1	1.0	1.0	1.0	1.0	1.0	1.0	1.0	1.1	1.1	1.1	1.1	1.1
Carb Grams				0					85		0			60		15		66				25		
Meal Bolus				0					8.5		0			6		0		6.6				2.5		
Correction Bolus				0					0.5		2.6			0		0		1.3				0		
Exercise															**									
Ketones											neg													
Site Change									*															

Breakfast	Snack	Comments
Milk=15 2 Large Biscuits=50 Apple=15 Low Carb Jelly=5	None	*Changed infusion site from abdomen to buttocks.
Lunch Ham Sandwich=15 Pear=15 Banana=30 Diet Cola=0	Snack Juice box to treat low BG	Comments **Played baseball from 1–3pm.
Dinner Spaghetti=40 Garlic Bread=20 Salad=6 Flavored Water=0	Snack Milk=15 ½ Granola Bar=10	Comments

Figure 2 Sample patient insulin pump log. *Abbreviation*: BG, blood glucose.

- Then, no food (unless low), insulin bolus, or exercise until the next morning.
- Check blood glucose at: 9:00 P.M., 12:00 A.M., 3:00 A.M., and 7 A.M.

Morning Basal-Rate Check

- Wake up and check blood glucose by 7:00 A.M.
- Skip breakfast.
- Then, no food (unless low), insulin bolus, or exercise until 11:00 A.M.
- Check blood glucose at: 7:00 A.M., 9:00 A.M., and 11:00 A.M.

Afternoon Basal-Rate Check

- Check blood glucose, give bolus dose of insulin, and eat breakfast by 7:00 A.M.
- Then, no food (unless low), insulin bolus, or exercise until 5:00 P.M.
- Check blood glucose at 12:00 P.M., 2:00 P.M., and 5:00 P.M.

Evening Basal-Rate Check

- Check blood glucose, give insulin bolus, and eat lunch by 12:00 P.M.
- Then, no food (unless low), insulin bolus, or exercise until 9:00 P.M.
- Check blood glucose at 5:00 P.M., 7:00 P.M., and 9:00 P.M.

The BG level should remain relatively constant if the basal dose is correct. It is important to review patterns of glycemia when making adjustments to basal rates or bolus algorithms. If basal-rate checks reveal patterns that need adjusting, the rate two hours before the abnormal pattern should be adjusted. It is ideal to get the overnight and fasting blood sugars under control first because they can affect the rest of the day's readings (Table 6).

In addition to setting basal rates for CSII, bolus doses must also be calculated, both for BG coverage and carbohydrate coverage. BG coverage is based upon each patient's individual insulin sensitivity factor (ISF). ISF is how much one unit of insulin will drop the blood glucose in mg/dL. To figure out the initial ISF, there are various rules to use, including the "Rule of 1800" or "Rule of 1500." Most commonly, we use the "Rule of 1500." We take the patient's TDD inclusive of long- and short-acting insulin, and divide 1500 by the TDD, rounding off to the nearest multiple of 5 or 10. These rules are a starting point, with adjustments made depending on the BG readings. Because insulin sensitivity increases at night and with increased exercise, patients often require less correction at these times. Therefore, we usually give half the usual dose to correct for hyperglycemia at bedtime (19).

Once the ISF is determined, the target BG level must be set. This will vary with age, with infants and toddlers having a higher BG target, from 100 to 180 mg/dL (110–200 at bedtime). School-age children usually have a target BG level of 90 to 180 mg/dL. At onset of puberty, the target range should be lowered to 90 to 130 mg/dL (20). Another option to

avoid nocturnal hypoglycemia is to increase the bedtime target blood glucose instead of increasing the bedtime ISF to account for increased insulin sensitivity. An example would be: if usual target blood glucose is 150 mg/dL, the bedtime target could be increased to 200 mg/dL. If changing the ISF or target blood glucose is too confusing for the patient, we advise using usual ISF and target, and dividing the correction in half.

For carbohydrate coverage, the I:C should be determined. Once again, there are algorithms for determining initial I:C. The most commonly used of these are the "Rule of 450" and the "Rule of 500" indicating the divisor for the patient's TDD. While some patients are on a consistent I:C for the entire day, many require a different I:C with each meal and snack. Patients who already have an I:C do not need to change the ratio initially when pump therapy is initiated, although adjustments may be required with CSII. The I:C can be determined for patients receiving a fixed dose of rapid-acting insulin before meals by determining how many carbohydrates are typically consumed and dividing that amount by the usual fixed insulin dose (19).

Once the ISF, target blood glucose, and I:C have been determined, the bolus dose of insulin can be calculated. The BG coverage (correction bolus) and carbohydrate coverage (carbohydrate bolus) must each be calculated and then added together to determine the mealtime bolus. To determine the coverage for hyperglycemia, the target BG level is subtracted from the current blood glucose and divided by the ISF. For the carbohydrate coverage, the total carbohydrates eaten are divided by the I:C. The two subtotals are combined for a complete bolus amount (Table 7). The ISF, target BG, and I:C can be preprogrammed into the newer "smart" pumps. When the patient or parent enters the BG reading and amount of carbohydrates eaten, the pump uses the settings to determine a bolus amount. This eliminates the need for the user to do the calculation. The bolus is not automatically delivered; each pump requires multiple button pushes before a bolus will be delivered. The patient or parent can choose to override or accept the suggested amount.

Typically, the carbohydrate and correction boluses are delivered as a standard bolus, whether delivered together or separately. This means the delivery occurs all at once as soon as the patient accepts and activates the dose. However, there are various types of advanced bolus features that can be performed with insulin pumps. A square wave or extended bolus is the entire calculated bolus extended over a specific period of time, usually two to three hours for high carbohydrate foods. A dual wave or combination bolus is used for high protein, high fat meals such as steak, pizza, or a bacon cheeseburger. Usually 20% to 30% of the total bolus is delivered initially, while 70% to 80% is then delivered over the next two to three hours. Some pumps also have audio

Table 6 Tips for Troubleshooting Hyperglycemia with Continuous Subcutaneous Insulin Infusion

Factors to consider when evaluating hyperglycemia	Possible cause/action
Infusion site	
Check infusion site for redness, swelling, hardness, drainage/discharge, and pain	Possible infection. Remove infusion set immediately. Check blood glucose and urine ketones. May need to give a manual injection and call Pediatric Endocrinology
	Refer to guidelines for blood glucose > 240
Lipohypertrophy (scar tissue or "puffy" areas)	Occurs when a site is used too often. Insulin absorption is erratic. Must rotate sites
Poor placement of infusion set	Site is in an area when constant friction occurs such as at the waistline or underwear seams or bands
Infusion set	
Air in tubing	Disconnect tubing from the site and prime until you have cleared the air in the tubing
Leakage at the site	Change infusion set and site immediately
Catheter dislodged or kinked	Change infusion set and site immediately. May need to use an adhesive to keep the infusion set adhered to the skin
Blood in infusion set	Change infusion set and site immediately
Set inserted at bedtime	Problems with the infusion set will not be detected because you are not checking your blood glucose during the night. Avoid nighttime changes unless you have problems. Perform site insertions in the morning
Omission of cannula bolus	Forgetting to fill the "dead space" in the cannula after inserting a new site will result in no insulin delivery for that amount (0.5, 0.7, etc.) and can result in high blood glucose because less basal is delivered
Insulin pump	
Time on pump is not correct	Basal rates will run according to the pump time and not the actual time. It can result in not enough or too much insulin delivered. Always review basal rate changes after entering them
Failure to activate bolus or basal rates	Look at the status screen or basal/bolus review to determine whether or not the desired delivery actually occurred
Placing the pump in suspend	Forgetting to resume delivery after suspending for exercise, etc.
Program/pump alarms	Refer to user manual and/or call 1–800 number
Incorrect clock time	Change clock to reflect present time
Low or dead battery	Change battery
Insulin	
Change in appearance, or exposure to high temperature or frozen	Exposure to extreme temperatures will damage insulin. It is possible to get a "bad" vial of insulin from the pharmacy or mail order supply company. Immediately change reservoir and insulin vial
Food	
Incorrect bolus or forgetting to bolus	Inaccurate carbohydrate estimation. Important to read labels and use resources to determine accurate carbohydrate counts
High protein or fat content in meal/snack	Protein and fat will delay the absorption of carbohydrate. High blood glucoses may occur later after eating larger quantities of protein or fat such as a 10 oz. steak, bacon cheeseburger, pizza, etc. Need to speak with your healthcare team about using an extended/square or dual wave bolus
Special occasions such as holiday meals, where a variety of foods are eaten over time	Same as for high fat or protein meals. Ask your healthcare team about using an extended/square or dual wave bolus
Poor timing of bolus	Forgetting a bolus and/or giving it late
Activity	
Decrease in activity or change in schedule	Decrease in normal activity such as long car rides or traveling, staying indoors during inclement weather, end of season for soccer, baseball, etc., may result in higher blood glucose levels
Blood glucose > 240 before exercise	Must check urine ketones if BG >240. If exercise occurs with moderate-to-large ketones, blood glucose will increase and nausea and vomiting may occur
	Do not exercise when urine ketones are moderate to large. Follow guidelines for blood glucose >240
Blood glucose (BG) monitoring	
Not enough BG checks	High blood glucoses are missed if not checking regularly before meals and at bedtime. Also, more frequent checks must be done during illness when blood glucoses tend to be higher
Persistent high blood glucose at particular times of the day	Changes in schedule, normal growth during childhood and adolescence, etc., hormonal changes during adolescence, menstrual cycles and pregnancy, will cause fluctuations in blood glucoses

(Continued)

Table 6   Tips for Troubleshooting Hyperglycemia with Continuous Subcutaneous Insulin Infusion (*Continued*)

Factors to consider when evaluating hyperglycemia	Possible cause/action
Incorrect sensitivity factor	Basal rate checks are performed to adjust for these situations
	May need to be changed due to an increase or decrease in total daily insulin usage due to a change in schedule, regular activity, growth, hormonal changes, etc.
Other	
Medication	Some medications will raise the blood glucose; steroids in particular, especially if taken for a period of time
Illness	Illness refers to any deviation from normal health such as a cold, sore throat, headache, recuperation from surgery and flu or virus. The stress of illness may result in high blood glucoses. Refer to Sick Day Guidelines
Hormonal	As previously noted, normal growth, adolescence, menses and pregnancy may result in higher blood glucoses

boluses, which means a specific button can be pushed without the patient looking at the pump and a preprogrammed increment bolus will be delivered, often with beeps played back for the patient to confirm the amount.

Insulin Pump Resources
Companies

Animas Corporation
200 Lawrence Drive
West Chester, PA 19389 USA
Tel: 610–644–8990 Fax: 610–644–8717
Info: 1–877–YES-PUMP (1-877–937–7867)
Service: 1–877–767–7373
www.animascorp.com

Disetronic Medical Systems, Inc.
11800 Exit 5 Parkway, Suite 120
Fishers, IN 46037
Tel: 866–703–3476 Fax: 888–810–0758
www.accu-chek.com

Medtronic MiniMed
18000 Devonshire Street
Northridge, CA 91325
1–800-MINIMED (1-800–646–4633)
www.minimed.com

Nipro Diabetes Systems

Tel: 888–651–7867 Fax: 954–435–9295
http://www.niprodiabetes.com

Smiths Medical MD, Inc. (formerly Deltec)
1265 Grey Fox Road
St. Paul, MN 55112 USA
1–800–826–9703
www.CozMore.com

Accessories

Diabetes Mall
http://www.diabetesnet.com

PumpPak.com
http://www.pumppack.com/

Pump Wear Inc.
http://www.pumpwearinc.com/

Unique Accessories Inc.
http://www.uniaccs.com/index.asp

Adhesives/Numbing Agents

Ferndale Laboratories:
Mastisol/Detachol
http://www.ferndalelabs.com

Emla Cream
http://www.emla-us.com/

Table 7   Sample Patient Calculation

Sample patient	ISF calculation using the "Rule of 1500"	I:C calculation using the "Rule of 500"	Bolus dose calculation for pump
Age = 10	TDD = 52 units	TDD = 52 units	BG = 225
Target BG = 150	1500/52 = 28.85 = 29, so round to nearest 5 or 10	500/52 = 9.6 = 10	Total Carbs = 75
Current BG = 225			
Current insulin dose	ISF = 30	I:C = 10	BG − target BG/ISF
Breakfast = 24 units NPH		So, 1 unit Aspart for every 10 carbohydrates consumed	225 − 150 = 75 ÷ 30 = 2.5 units
12 units Aspart			
			Total carbs 75 ÷ 10 = 7.5 units
Dinner = 8 units NPH			So, 2.5 + 7.5 = 10 units total bolus
8 units Aspart			
TDD = 52 units			

Abbreviations: TDD, total daily dose; BG, blood glucose.

SICK DAY MANAGEMENT

These guidelines for sick days are designed to help manage blood glucose and prevent or treat early ketoacidosis (DKA) during illness or stress. Insulin injections need to be continued even if the child refuses to eat or is vomiting. The notion of continuing to take insulin despite no food intake is counterintuitive for many parents, who need to appreciate the increased insulin requirements associated with stress of illness, resulting in counterregulatory hormone-induced gluconeogenesis and ketogenesis. BG levels should be checked more frequently than usual, at least every two to four hours. Urine or blood ketones should be checked often, as well. If the child is sick, ketones should be monitored even if the BG level is low or normal. If vomiting occurs, ketones should be checked each time the child urinates, with repeated testing at least every two to three hours. Sick-day management with use of serum B-OHB measurement was discussed in the monitoring section. Extra insulin may be necessary for the insulin resistance accompanying the illness or if ketones are present.

For negative, trace, or small ketonuria, increasing water intake, exercise, or insulin supplementation can be tried. For moderate or large ketonuria, extra insulin should be administered based on the TDD of insulin (Table 8).

For patients taking multiple daily injections, temporary adjustments may need to be made to I:C, target BG levels, and doses of the long-acting and/or rapid-acting insulins, even in the absence of ketonuria, if glucose levels remain elevated. Examples of adjustments to bring high BG levels down include: standard doses of intermediate or long acting insulin being increased, I:C being changed from 1:15 to 1:12 or 1:10, lowering target BG levels from 150 to 120 or 100, and adjusting the ISF because of insulin resistance associated with illness. More specifically, if the insulin sensitivity is normally 50, it may need to be changed to 30 or 25. All of these examples increase the insulin dosages to account for hyperglycemia accompanying illness.

Patients using CSII have another option for managing hyperglycemia on sick days. Pumps have a feature that allows a temporary basal rate to be programmed. The temporary rate can be set as units per hour or as a percentage of the usual rate. The percentage is most commonly used, leaving the pump to calculate the temporary rate. If the units per hour feature is used, the new basal rate per hour must be manually determined and entered into the pump. This feature may be useful if the patient is giving boluses and the BG remains high or if the patient is not eating and the BG remains high. It allows the basal rate to be temporarily increased and then decreased to usual rates when insulin sensitivity normalizes. A good starting place is a 20% to 30% increase for three to four hours. This period can be extended for as long as necessary to maintain BG levels in the target range. Sometimes temporary basal rates need to be set up to 50% more than regular basal rates for as long as 8 to 24 hours. This is a situation in which frequent BG checks are necessary. The usual rates can be restored when the patient's BG levels begin to normalize.

While most children become hyperglycemic with illness despite not eating, some will have a decrease in glycemia under these conditions. We provide the following guide to our patients for appropriate fluids for various BG ranges.

■ *If the blood glucose is below 120 mg/dL:*
FLUIDS: need to contain extra glucose such as soda or a sport drink with sugar added. The child should

Table 8 Ketone Management: How to Determine Supplemental Insulin Doses

Type of insulin	Moderate ketones	Large ketones
NPH + Lispro/Aspart/ Glulisine or NPH + Regular or 70/30 or 75/25	Add all doses and multiply the TDD by 15%. May give all as lispro/aspart/glulisine, all as Regular, or 50% as lispro/aspart/glulisine and 50% as Regular	Add all doses and multiply TDD by 20%. May give all as lispro/aspart/glulisine, all as Regular, or 50% as lispro/aspart/glulisine and 50% as Regular
Lantus + Lispro/Aspart/ Glulisine	Add Lantus dose to analog dose and multiply the TDD by 15%. Because patient's analog doses vary meal-to-meal and day-to-day estimate how much analog is taken on average with various meals and snacks. May give all as lispro/aspart/glulisine, all as Regular, or 50% as lispro/aspart/glulisine and 50% as Regular	Add lantus dose to analog dose and multiply the TDD by 20%. Because patient's analog doses vary meal to meal and day to day, estimate how much analog is taken on average with various meals and snacks. May give all as lispro/aspart/glulisine, all as Regular, or 50% as lispro/aspart/glulisine and 50% as Regular
Pump (Lispro/Aspart/ Glulisine)	Multiply the TDD, including the total basal rate and boluses, by 15%. Because bolus amounts vary from meal to meal and day to day estimate how much is taken on average with meals and snacks. Most pumps have a feature that shows Daily Totals. Access this feature and use the average. May give all as lispro/aspart/glulisine, all as Regular, or 50% as lispro/aspart/glulisine and 50% as Regular via a subcutaneous injection. Infusion set should be changed after the injection is given	Multiply the TDD, including the total basal rate and boluses, by 20%. Because bolus amounts vary from meal-to-meal and day-to-day, estimate how much is taken on average with meals and snacks. Most pumps have a feature that shows Daily Totals. Access this feature and use the average. May give all as lispro/aspart/glulisine, all as Regular, or 50% as lispro/aspart/glulisine and 50% as Regular via a subcutaneous injection. Infusion set should be changed after the injection is given

Abbreviation: TDD, total daily dose.

continue with glucose-containing drinks until the blood sugar is above 120 mg/dL.

- *If the blood glucose is between 120 and 180 mg/dL:*
  FLUIDS: need to contain approximately 15 g of carbohydrates such as half cup of ginger ale or cola, half cup of regular Jell-O®, half cup of juice, or half popsicle.
  FOODS: need to have at least 15 g of carbohydrates per serving. If the child cannot eat normal meals, possible "sick day" foods include: half cup of ice cream or sherbet, one slice of toast, or six saltines.
- *If blood glucose is above 180 mg/dL:*
  FLUIDS: need to have no calories such as diet soda, unsweetened tea, or water.
  FOODS: need to be small servings as tolerated.

If the child is nauseated or vomiting, give small sips of clear fluids (such as ice chips, popsicles, clear broth or bouillon, gelatin, water, or tea). Avoid orange juice, milk, or milk products. Speak with your diabetes team about fluid replacement and advancing to foods. Nutritional needs and insulin doses can change hour by hour depending on BG and urine ketone levels.

Some children and teens may benefit from an over-the-counter product to control nausea such as Emetrol®, which should be taken as directed on the bottle. Regular intake of cola, ginger ale, or other soda with the bubbles shaken out may also be helpful. If the child is vomiting, the diabetes team or primary physician needs to be involved. If the child has not been ill for more than a few hours and is not vomiting continuously, a Tigan or Phenergan suppository may control the vomiting and permit oral fluid intake, thus avoiding a visit to the emergency room for rehydration.

Elective Surgery

Elective surgery usually requires insulin dose adjustments, depending on the patient, the type of surgery, and time of surgery. Procedures should be scheduled as early in the morning as possible, with the first appointment of the day being ideal. Once parents are informed about any pre- or postsurgery dietary restrictions, they should contact their diabetes care provider. Sometimes, the surgeon prefers to talk to the diabetes care provider directly (21).

If local anesthesia is used, as in many dental procedures, there are no restrictions to meals before or after surgery. In these situations, small reductions in insulin dose may be made to account for decreased appetite such as from soreness of the mouth associated with dental surgery. If the patient does not eat before the procedure, the long-acting insulin may be administered before surgery, and the short-acting insulin after the procedure is done, but only if the patient eats. The easiest adjustments are made for patients on long-acting insulin analog or CSII. Long-acting analog treated patients often take their usual dose the night before or morning of surgery with supplemental bolus insulin as

needed for hyperglycemia (e.g., with the attendant anxiety) or when they eat. CSII patients can have their basal rates or bolus doses adjusted every hour as needed to keep up with their changing insulin needs (21).

General anesthesia places more restrictions on patients. Vomiting occurs more frequently after general anesthesia, which limits eating because of the risk of aspiration. This usually requires changing insulin doses. The dose of long-acting insulin can be decreased up to 50% with as needed coverage using short-acting insulin. Instead of using any long-acting insulin, supplemental doses of rapid-acting insulin can be given every two to three hours based on the BG levels, or if the procedure is long, the patient may be maintained with intravenous insulin, with dosage based on BG checks and determined by the doctor performing the procedure (21).

The most important consideration with elective surgery is frequent monitoring of BG levels before, during, and after surgery. While decreased eating may occur, which necessitates decreased insulin doses, the stress associated with the surgery could result in a need for increased insulin. Where the surgery is performed as well as its duration will determine who is responsible for monitoring BG levels during surgery. The anesthetist must check the glucose every one to two hours during the procedure. If the BG level begins to drop below 200 mg/dL, dextrose should be added to intravenous fluids (21).

HYPOGLYCEMIA

Causes of hypoglycemia include:

- Too much insulin
- Inadequate food intake
- Delayed meals or snacks
- Strenuous exercise (which can have an effect up to 24 hours later)

Hypoglycemia characteristics can vary greatly between patients and even from episode to episode in the same patient. It is important to stress to the patient and caregivers that they need to be familiar with the usual pattern for early recognition of hypoglycemia in future situations. Signs and symptoms of hypoglycemia include:

- Dizziness
- Shakiness
- Personality changes
- Irritability
- Sweating
- Changes in vision
- Weakness
- Headache
- Anxiety
- Inability to concentrate
- Tachycardia or palpitations

If any of these symptoms are present, the BG level should be checked. If less than 70 mg/dL, 15 grams of fast-acting carbohydrate should be given such as:

- Three to four glucose tablets
- Four ounces of juice
- One-third can of regular soda
- If the child is uncooperative, glucose gel may be used (1 tube = 15 g carbohydrate)
- Solid food should not be given until the BG level is greater than 70 mg/dL because the absorption rate is slowed if fat and protein are ingested before or simultaneously with fast-acting carbohydrate and the patient will have longer duration of hypoglycemia.

After 10 to 15 minutes, the BG level should be rechecked.

- If the BG level is still less than 70 mg/dL, treatment should be repeated with another 15 g of rapidly-acting carbohydrate the BG level checked every 10 minutes, and treatment repeated until the BG level is greater than 70 mg/dL.
- If the BG level is greater than 70 mg/dL and the time for the next snack or meal is more than 30 minutes, a snack should be given. It is safe to wait if the time for the next regular food intake is less than 30 minutes. For patients on long-acting insulin analog or CSII, an additional snack might not be necessary unless moderate to strenuous activity has been performed. Even then, bolus insulin for the additional snack may not be necessary.

In infants and toddlers, the following additional signs and symptoms of hypoglycemia may occur:

- Temper tantrums
- Falling asleep at unexpected times
- Uncontrollable crying
- Irritability
- Combativeness
- Pallor, shakiness, cold sweat
- Seizure

If any of these signs or symptoms is present in a conscious child, the BG level should be checked immediately. If less than 80 mg/dL, treatment is:

- To quickly give one to two ounces of sugar-containing liquid such as juice, regular soda, milk, or formula. This can be done by syringe if the child will not cooperate by drinking from a cup or bottle.
- If symptoms do not improve in 10 minutes, the above feeding should be repeated.
- If blood glucose is greater than 80 mg/dL after 10 to 15 minutes or when symptoms resolve, bottle-feeding or snack (e.g., cereal, crackers, sandwich, etc.) can be given.

If the child is already unconscious:

- Insta-glucose® (half a tube), cake icing, or honey should be placed between the gums and cheeks
- Glucagon 0.5 mg (0.5 cc) can be injected intramuscularly or subcutaneously

For patients using CSII, a special algorithm for treatment of BG readings less than 70 mg/dL should be followed (Fig. 3). Troubleshooting hypoglycemia in pump patients can be a challenge (Table 9).

If it is not possible to check the BG level and the patient is symptomatic, it is always prudent to treat it as a hypoglycemic episode. The goal is to prevent hypoglycemia, but if it occurs, to keep it from progressing to unconsciousness or seizure. Families, friends, coaches, and school personnel must be prepared for a hypoglycemic emergency.

The tight control associated with multiple daily injections and pump administration may increase the risk of hypoglycemia. We train our families in the use of glucagon emergency kits. Glucagon comes in 1 mg vials along with a syringe prefilled with diluent. For children less than eight years of age, 0.5 mg should be injected. For older children, 1 mg should be injected. In addition to the instructions for mixing, caregivers are taught that they can inject through the clothes, into the front of the leg or the upper arm; to turn the child onto one side because vomiting is not uncommon with glucagon injection; to check the blood glucose; and to call the physician. If the child is still unconscious after 10 minutes, the blood glucose should be rechecked. If the blood glucose is still below 80 mg/dL, they are instructed to repeat the injection of glucagon. There is no risk of overdosage with glucagon. As the child awakens and is able to swallow, give juice or regular soda and food such as crackers and cheese or a meat sandwich. If glucagon is administered, the caregiver should call the diabetes care provider after administration so that causes of the severe low can be ascertained and insulin dose adjustments made as necessary.

Fear of hypoglycemia is the major limiting factor to good diabetes control, both for caregivers and patients. This is especially true if the patient has ever experienced a severe hypoglycemic episode which has resulted in a seizure or unconsciousness, required glucagon administration, or required a call to emergency medical services. Patients do not like the way they feel when low, which can lead them to try to maintain higher BG levels. Caregivers who have had to deal with a severe hypoglycemic episode never forget the fear, anxiety, and guilt which can lead to underinsulinization of younger children. Depending on when and under what circumstances the hypoglycemic episode occurred, the patient or caregiver might try to avoid the same circumstances in the future, which can lead to withdrawal from important social, physical, or educational activities. If the low occurred during the night, caregivers often wake up frequently to check the child's blood glucose to prevent a recurrence. Even if the patient never actually had a severe low, the fear of one occurring can lead patients and caregivers to preoccupation with avoiding hypoglycemia.

Preparedness is the first step in dealing with hypoglycemia. Providing teenagers and caregivers of

```
┌─────────────────────────────────┐
│   Blood Glucose Less Than 70*   │
└─────────────────────────────────┘
                 ↓
┌─────────────────────────────────────────┐
│  Take 15 grams of fast-acting carbohydrate │
│     (each example is 15 grams)            │
│                                           │
│          3-4 glucose tablets              │
│                  or                       │
│             ½ cup juice                   │
│                  or                       │
│        1/3 can of regular soda            │
└─────────────────────────────────────────┘
                 ↓
┌─────────────────────────────────────────┐
│  Recheck Blood Glucose in 10-15 minutes  │
└─────────────────────────────────────────┘
         ↙                        ↘
```

| If blood glucose is greater than 80, no further action needed. May need a snack if activity is strenous. May not need to cover snack with insulin if it is less than 15 grams. | If blood glucose less than 80, repeat the fast-acting carbohydrate and recheck blood glucose in 10-15 minutes. |

```
                          ↙              ↘
```

| If blood glucose greater than 80, no further action. May need a snack if activity is strenous. May not need to cover snack with insulin if it is less than 15 grams. | If blood glucose is less than 80, eat a snack of complex carbohydrate and protein. May need to suspend pump if blood glucose is less than 60.* |

┌───┐
│ *If at any time, hypoglycemia results in unconsciousness or seizure, GIVE GLUCAGON IMMEDIATELY AND │
│ PLACE THE PUMP IN SUSPEND OR DISCONNECT. │
│ Remember to reconnect or resume pump operation once blood glucose is >80 and the │
│ child/adolescent/young adult is awake and able to eat. │
└───┘

Figure 3 Guidelines for treatment of blood glucose less than 70 mg/dL with continuous subcutaneous insulin infusion.

children with diabetes a list of "Don't Leave Home Without..." can be helpful and should include:

- Meter
- Strips
- Lancets
- Fast-acting carbohydrates (juice, glucose tabs, lifesavers)
- Insulin
- Syringes/pen needles
- Medic Alert or other emergency identification
- Glucagon kit

Because the risk of hypoglycemia is present with any insulin regimen, it is vital that patients and caregivers understand the importance of the child wearing a medical identification necklace or bracelet. Teenagers who begin to drive must also be taught to carry their BG meter with them at all times. They should check their BG level before driving. If they are to drive a long distance, the blood glucose should be monitored every hour or so. If the BG reading is less than 100 before driving, a 15 g carbohydrate snack should be ingested. If the patient begins to experience symptoms of hypoglycemia while driving, he/she should pull the car over, check the blood glucose, and if hypoglycemic, follow the above guidelines until the blood glucose is greater than 100 mg/dl. Along with their meter, a source of fast-acting carbohydrate such as juice, glucose tablets, or lifesavers should be kept in the car along with a more substantial snack such as a granola bar or cheese crackers. The fast-acting carbohydrate should not be kept in the locked glove compartment, but in a place that is easily accessible such as the visor or middle console of the car.

Prevention of hypoglycemia requires diligent BG monitoring and more frequent testing during illness, exercise, or when dose adjustments are being made. See the section on exercise for specific

Table 9 Tips for Troubleshooting Hypoglycemia with Continuous Subcutaneous Insulin Infusion

Factors to consider when evaluating hypoglycemia	Possible cause/action
Time of day	
Before breakfast	Check overnight basal rate, might be set too high
Before lunch	Check basal rate for the previous time period, might be set too high
	May represent overcorrection of a mid-A.M. snack
Before dinner	Check basal rate for the previous time period, might be set too high
	May represent overcorrection of a mid-afternoon snack
Before bed	Check basal rate for previous time period, might be set too high
	May represent overcorrection for dinner carbohydrates or over compensation for hyperglycemia
Nighttime	Check basal rate for previous time period, might be set too high
	May represent overcorrection for bedtime snack or over compensation for hyperglycemia
Food	
Two hours after a meal or snack	Review carbohydrate calculation and correction bolus if delivered. May have overestimated carbohydrates of correction. May need to change insulin/carbohydrate ratio or correction scale
Ingestion of alcohol	May cause hypoglycemia 6–8 hr after ingestion
	Eat while drinking alcohol. Always check blood glucose before driving, going to bed, and at 3:00 A.M.
	Advise friends of signs and symptoms of hypoglycemia
Timing of meal or correction bolus	Forgetting to perform the bolus (either before eating or to correct a high blood glucose) and then doing so later, without checking blood glucose
Activity	
Spontaneous or planned	Failure to check blood glucose before exercise, during exercise if longer than 1 hour and after exercise
	May need to snack before exercise
	Basal rate may need to be reduced or pump disconnected
	Basal rate may need to be reduced prior to or following activity (prolonged activity may result in hypoglycemia several hours later)
Blood glucose monitoring	
Failure to check blood glucose before a meal	May have low blood glucose already. Taking normal coverage for carbohydrates may prolong hypoglycemia
Failure to check blood glucose before bedtime	May be below target goal for blood glucose
Before, during, and after exercise, especially if a change in schedule has occurred, or a new activity is being introduced	Insulin sensitivity increases with regularly occurring physical activity. Insulin needs are different during the school year than on vacation or summer break
Must be performed more frequently if a child is too young to communicate symptoms or if there is hypoglycemia unawareness	May need to raise blood glucose goals and/or change insulin/carbohydrate ratio and/or correction scale (sensitivity)

guidelines on adjusting insulin dosages. Eating meals and snacks on time as well as understanding the timing of action of the insulin the patient is taking, including onset, peak, and duration, can help prevent lows. Knowing the individual's history and the pattern of response in the past to these variables can be helpful in determining therapy adjustments.

Resources for Medical Identification Accessories

American Medical Identifications, Inc.
PO Box 925617
Houston, TX 77292–5617
800–363–5985
Fax: 713–695–7358
www.americanmedical-id.com

Fifty50 Pharmacy
1420 Valwood Parkway, Suite 120
Carrollton, TX 75006

800–746–7505 or 972–243–2727
Fax: 800–769–6906 or 972–243–3111
www.FIFTY50.com

Lauren's Hope
1–800–360–8680
www.laurenshope.com

MedicAlert
2323 Colorado Ave
Turlock, CA 95382
1–800–ID-ALERT (1–800–432–5378)
www.medicalert.org

MediCharms
PO Box 558
Bryant, AR 72089
1–888–417–7591
www.MediCharms.com

Resources for Glucose Gel/Glucose Tablets

Insta-glucose
ICN Pharmaceuticals, Inc.

Costa Mesa, CA 92626 USA
www.instaglucose.com

Glutose-15
Paddock Laboratories, Inc.
3940 Quebec Avenue North
Minneapolis, Minnesota 55427
Phone: 763–546–4676 or 1–800–328–5113
Fax: 763–546–4842
http://www.paddocklabs.com/glutose.html

BD Glucose Tablets
Becton Dickinson
www.bddiabetes.com
(888) 232–2737

Dex 4 Glucose Tablets
Can-Am Care
(800) 461–7448

Resources for Glucagon Emergency Kits

Eli Lilly & Company
Indianapolis, IN 46285 USA
Glucagon Emergency Kit for Low Blood Glucose
http://www.lillydiabetes.com/about_diabetes/what_is_
    glucagon.jsp?reqNavId=1.6.6

Novo Nordisk
GlucaGen® Hypo Kit
1–800–727–6500
http://novonordisk.com/diabetes/public/hypokit/gluca
    genhypokit/default.asp

EXERCISE

Special instructions regarding insulin and carbo-hydrate adjustments to deal with exercise should be provided to patients and caregivers (Table 10).

Response to exercise is highly individual. While these guidelines provide a starting point, the exercise plan must be adapted to each patient. The first step is checking the BG level before, during, and after any exercise activity to see how the blood glucose responds. Keeping track of the adjustments made can help the individual create an exercise plan. By referring back to past exercise and what worked or did not work before, the patient should be able to avoid wide swings in BG levels with exercise. It is important for the family to know that the glucose levels may continue to fall for many hours after exercise.

Exercise may be planned or unplanned. If the patient knows that activity level will be increased the next day, long-acting insulin may be decreased by 10% to 20% the night before or the morning of increased activity. This might include the glargine dose before dinner or bedtime or the NPH dose before bedtime or breakfast. The rapid-acting insulin given on the day of increased activity may also need to be decreased by 10% to 20%. Some people may need a decrease in both the long-acting– and rapid-acting–insulin doses, whereas others may only need one of the insulins adjusted. This situation underscores the need to know what adjustment was made in the past and how it worked. The goal of therapy is to make insulin-dose adjustments that prevent hypoglcemia from occurring and thus avoiding the consumption of extra food. Eating to prevent hypoglycemia can be counterproductive and frustrating, especially for patients with weight control problems.

Some patients notice a spike in BG concentration after beginning exercise, especially in competitive sports activities, as the result of the surge of epineph-rine and, probably, cortisol. Often the blood glucose will come down on its own with no correction bolus of insulin. If a correction with rapid-acting insulin is given, the glucose may drop too low, but this is not a consistent finding. Thus, it is necessary to identify an individual's pattern.

The above general guidelines for mild, moder-ate, or strenuous activity may be used for patients using injections or CSII. However, patients using CSII may also program a temporary basal rate. The temporary basal rate can be set as units per hour or as a percentage of the usual basal rate as was

Table 10 Carbohydrate Adjustment for Varying Degrees of Activity[a]

Type of activity	Blood glucose reading (mg/dL) . . .	. . . Do this
Mild-to-moderate activity for 30 min or less (such as walking or biking leisurely)	< 100	Eat/drink 10–15 g carbohydrate
	100–240	No additional food needed
	> 240	No additional food needed
Moderate-to-strenuous activity (such as tennis, swimming, jogging, bicycling) or mild-to-moderate activity for more than 30 min (such as gardening, golfing, vacuuming)	< 100	Eat/drink 15 g carbohydrate before exercise, then 15 g/hr
	100–240	Eat/drink 10–15 g carbohydrate per hour
	> 240	Not necessary to increase food intake. If exercising for more than one hour—recheck blood glucose after an hour and make calorie adjustment at that time

[a]Some ketosis might occur as part of the physiologic response to exercise. Many years ago a study reported that intense physical activity in children with keto-nuria increased ketosis and blood glucose levels. However, the child with moderate-to-large ketonuria is not likely to pursue intensive exercise and we have never seen problems resulting from exercise in a child with ketonuria.

discussed in the sick-day management section. In order to properly use this feature with exercise, patients must know how their body responded in the past, whether, for example, the glucose dropped half an hour, one hour, two hours, or eight hours after exercise was begun.

The following recommendations provide beginning guidelines for temporary basal rates. If the blood glucose drops 30 minutes to an hour after beginning exercise, the basal rate should be decreased by 20% to 30% two hours before exercise through the end of exercise. If the BG levels normalize after finishing exercise, the usual basal rates can be resumed. However, if the patient continues to have decreasing BG levels for several hours after completion of exercise, the decreased basal rate should be continued for an additional one to three hours. Basal rates can be decreased by 20% to 30% for two to six hours after finishing exercise in those patients who develop hypoglycemia two to four hours after exercise. Some patients have to decrease basal rates by as much as 40% to 50% if the exercise is very strenuous. Patients with a very delayed hypoglycemic response, from 12 to 24 hours post exercise, may need a change in the next day's basal rates or insulin to carbohydrate ratios.

In addition to knowing how to program temporary basal rates, there are other considerations that must be taken into account when managing exercise in a child using CSII. First, patients can only be disconnected from the pump for one hour without rechecking the BG level. This applies to any type of exercise from swimming, to basketball, to gymnastics. The patient must check blood glucose before disconnecting. Table 9 can be followed for carbohydrate adjustment and exercise, but additional factors must be considered. A study of 10 children age 10 to 19 showed an increase in delayed hypoglycemia when the pump was worn during exercise, with nine patients experiencing lows afterward as opposed to only six having delayed lows when the pump was disconnected during exercise (22).

Some of the insulin pumps on the market are waterproof, while others are only watertight. We recommend that patients disconnect before engaging in any water sport regardless of the pump manufacturer's label regarding water activities. Reasons for this recommendation, besides the pump being such an expensive piece of equipment include: risk of leaking, pump becoming disconnected and getting lost in the water, dilemma of where to wear the pump, and tubing getting caught on something and yanking the infusion set out. Other sports or activities in which there is aggressive physical contact may require that the pump be removed, although some patients prefer to stay connected. If patients choose to stay connected, they may use special tapes or ace bandages to hold the pump closer to the body. Special cases and holders are also available.

TRAVEL
Supplies

When patients with diabetes are traveling, they need to be certain that they have all the necessary supplies to last the duration of their trip. A traditional rule is to take double the supplies thought to be necessary and to carry one complete set of supplies for the trip in the hand luggage. The following checklist outlines supplies that are essential for travel:

- Insulin vials and/or insulin pens
- Insulin syringes and/or insulin pen needles
- Ketone test strips
- BG meter and test strips
- Lancets/lancing device
- Fast-acting carbohydrates (juice box, glucose tablets, lifesavers, etc.)
- Glucagon Emergency Kit
- Snacks (in case of delayed meals, etc.)
- Alcohol Swabs
- Medical alert or other identification
- Travel letter from physician (see sample below)

For patients on CSII, additional supplies needed are:

- Reservoirs
- Infusion sets
- Batteries
- Prescription for long-acting insulin in case the pump fails

Box 1

Sample: "Insulin Injections Travel Letter"
Date: _____
To Whom It May Concern:
Re: (Patient's Name)
The above named child has Type 1 (insulin-dependent) diabetes. It is an imperative part of his/her care that this child be allowed to monitor his/her blood glucose at frequent intervals throughout the day. Injections of insulin may be required before meals, snacks, or to correct hyperglycemia (high blood glucose). A Glucagon Emergency Kit (containing a vial and syringe) may be needed to treat severe hypoglycemia (low blood glucose). Hyperglycemia and hypoglycemia are acute complications of diabetes management and must be treated in an expedient manner.
In order to perform the above mentioned functions, the following materials must be close at hand at all times: lancets to perform fingerstick blood glucose testing, blood glucose monitor, insulin, insulin syringes or pens with needles, alcohol swabs, snacks, and a Glucagon Emergency Kit.
If you should have any further questions, please feel free to contact us at (office phone #).
Sincerely,
Name of MD

Box 2

Sample: "Insulin Pump Travel Letter"
Date:_____
To Whom It May Concern:
Re: (Patient's Name)
The above named child has Type 1 (insulin-dependent) diabetes. It is
an imperative part of his/her care that this child be allowed to
monitor his/her blood glucose at frequent intervals throughout the
day. He/she is on an insulin pump, which delivers insulin
continuously over 24 hours. Injections of insulin may be required in
addition to the insulin he/she receives via the insulin pump. A
Glucagon Emergency Kit (containing a vial and syringe) may be
needed to treat severe hypoglycemia (low blood glucose).
Hyperglycemia and hypoglycemia are acute complications of
diabetes management and must be treated in an expedient manner.
In order to perform the above mentioned functions, the following
equipment and materials must be close at hand at all times: lancets to
perform fingerstick blood glucose testing, blood glucose monitor, test
strips for BS monitor, insulin, insulin syringes or pens with needles,
alcohol swabs, Glucagon Emergency Kit, snacks, and pump supplies
(insertion sites, insertion device, reservoirs, insulin pump, tubing).
If you should have any further questions, please feel free to contact us
at (office phone #).
Sincerely,
Name of MD

Box 1 and 2

The sample travel letters above should facilitate passing through airport security and customs. It is wise to keep all insulin and supplies in their original containers so that there is no question about the authenticity of the medications. Insulin pumps do not usually make metal detectors go off in airports. Most patients stay connected to their pump while passing through metal detectors. X-rays will not affect the pump settings or the insulin (23).

Insulin

Patients and caregivers should also know that in other countries insulin may come in different concentrations and that markings on syringes are made to correlate with the specific concentration. In the United States, all insulin is in U-100 (100 units/mL) concentration. If a patient were to get U-40 insulin and use it with a U-100 syringe, it would be less than half the correct dose. Names of insulins are also different in other countries (24).

Patients wonder about traveling with insulin when there is no refrigeration possible. As long as extreme cold (freezing) and warm temperatures above 86°F are avoided, insulin should stay viable for the duration of short trips. There are special travel cases that can be purchased to help keep insulin cool. While keeping insulin cool is usually the main concern, if the patient is traveling where the temperatures will reach freezing, patient should make sure to keep the insulin from freezing. Insulin that turns cloudy or has particles in it (clumping) should be exchanged for a new bottle to ensure proper dosing. Extreme temperatures can also affect BG monitor performance; the temperature range

for effective function of the individual's meter should either be in the manual or available online (24).

Insulin Adjustment

Travel often equates with long periods of decreased activity. This can lead to increased basal insulin needs. Frequent BG checks allow appropriate adjustments to be made to bolus doses. When crossing through time zones to the west, days are longer and to the east, days will be shorter. A good rule of thumb is to calculate the TDD and decrease or increase it by 2% to 4% for each hour of time change. When heading west, the patient should take extra rapid-acting insulin to cover extra meals because the day is longer, and take the normal dose of intermediate- or long-acting insulin at the new adjusted night time. When heading east, there may be fewer meals because of the shorter day. If the patient is taking a bedtime dose of intermediate- or long-acting insulin, it should be taken at the new adjusted nighttime. If heading east overnight, the patient should take the usual dinner dose and reduce the intermediate-acting insulin by 3% to 5% per hour of time change. If the overnight flight is less than four to five hours, supplementing rapid-acting insulin in place of intermediate bedtime insulin can be done as long as frequent BG monitoring is performed. If the flight is during the day, the patient can take the usual dose with breakfast and cut the intermediate-acting insulin by 3% to 5% at dinnertime for each hour of time change. Patients on CSII must remember to change their pump clock to the new time upon arrival at their destination (24).

Resources

Frio Cooling Wallet
Cooler Concept
337 Lake Hazelton Drive
Chaska, MN 55318
Phone: (952) 361–6683
Fax: (953) 361–6684
http://www.coolerconcept.com/

Diabetic Accessories
http://www.lifesolutionsplus.com/

Travel Tips

American Diabetes Association
Traveling with Diabetes Supplies
http://www.diabetes.org/advocacy-and-legalresources/
  discrimination/public_accommodation/travel.jsp

When You Travel
http://www.diabetes.org/pre-diabetes/travel/when-you-
  travel.jsp

NEW GADGETS
Continuous Glucose-Monitoring Systems

Continuous glucose monitoring provides a more in-depth picture of BG trends and excursions than

Table 11 Comparison: Self-monitoring Blood Glucose vs. CGMS

Type of monitoring	Pros	Cons
Self-monitoring blood glucose	Accurate, real time results May look at individual results for patterns Uses plasma or whole-blood sample	Intermittent Not predictive of future results Must operate each time test is performed
CGMS	Continuous Shows trends May predict future results Easy to operate once initialized algorithm to convert glucose concentration within interstitial fluid (ISF)	Multiple, fair accuracy results Too much data is generated. Can't look at each result = data overload Warm up and calibration required Calibration must be done with finger stick results Least accurate with hypoglycemia Skin irritation with some systems Rapidly changing glucose levels can have a lag between blood and ISF levels Limited reimbursement

Abbreviation: CGMS, continuous glucose-monitoring systems.

intermittent self-monitoring of blood glucose (Table 11). As postprandial glucose excursions are often missed with intermittent testing, continuous glucose-monitoring systems (CGMS) can provide information for dosage adjustments to minimize these excursions (25). CGMS does not eliminate the need for BG monitoring, which is required for calibration and for confirming BG values when intervention is required to treat hypoglycemia or hyperglycemia. Patients considering CGMS must be motivated and well trained in operating the equipment. Children with risk of hypoglycemia unawareness or who have a history of severe hypoglycemic episodes with consequent poor metabolic control because of parental fear of hypoglycemia are good candidates for CGMS.

Currently six continuous glucose-monitoring devices have received approval or are under consideration for approval by the U.S. Food and Drug Administration (FDA). All measure glucose concentration in tissue fluid, which is several magnitudes lower than in blood, requiring calibration against fingerstick BG measurements.

- GlucoWatch® G2™ Biographer by Cygnus
- Continuous Glucose-Monitoring System Gold by Medtronic MiniMed
- Guardian® Telemetered Glucose-Monitoring System by Medtronic MiniMed
- FreeStyle Navigator™ Continuous Glucose Monitor by Abbott Laboratories
- GlucoDay® by A. Menarinin Diagnostics
- Pendra® by Pendragon Medical
- Dexcom™ STS™ continous glucose monitoring system by Dexcom, Inc.

Some of these systems are discussed in greater detail below (25).

GlucoWatch® G2™ Biographer

The GlucoWatch consists of the G2 biographer and the AutoSensor. The G2 biographer looks like a watch and it calculates, stores, and displays glucose readings. Glucose is drawn from the skin by a process of reverse iontophoresis onto a pad in the AutoSensor, which then is analyzed and converted to a BG reading, which is displayed on the watch. The biographer gives glucose readings every 10 minutes, with up to 76 readings for 13 hours. A total of 8500 readings can be stored in its memory. The BG level shown is an average of the last two 10 minute readings. Each patient can set a high and low alarm, which will go off if the patient's BG reading goes outside the set limits. The GlucoWatch also shows trend arrows to let patients know if they are on the upward or downward swing. If the blood glucose shows a downward trend and will likely fall below the "low" preset value within the next 20 minutes, another alarm will sound. Finger stick BG values must be obtained to calibrate the AutoSensor, and if the glucose reading requires some type of intervention, either for a low or high blood glucose. Problems with the Glucowatch include the following:

- It takes two hours for the GlucoWatch to begin to display readings
- Perspiration can cause the Biographer to skip or quit monitoring
- It is not waterproof; so it cannot be worn during water activities
- Irritation frequently occurs at the site of the AutoSensor insertion (26)

In our patient population, the most common reason for using the Glucowatch was to monitor for nocturnal hypoglycemia, for the relief of caregivers who were not sleeping through the night. We found, however, that excitement over the device was short lived with the difficulty of the calibration process and skin irritation (26).

The results of a study evaluating youth and parental satisfaction with the GlucoWatch found that technical problems including site irritation, skipped readings, false alarms, and erroneous readings, were more frustrating than psychological aspects of wearing the device. This underscores the importance of overcoming these obstacles before the use of this device can become widespread (27).

Guardian® Telemetered Glucose-Monitoring System

The Medtronic Guardian has replaced the company's original CGMS, the CGMS System Gold. The CGMS System Gold was a three-day diagnostic tool that could only be downloaded at a clinic with the program software. Reports could be generated upon download to look at three-day patterns. We used this system when a patient came into clinic with unexplained erratic BG patterns or if we suspected high or low BG levels that were being missed with routine BG monitoring (28).

The new Guardian RT system shows real time BG values every five minutes and alarms to specified individual high and low BG settings. The system consists of a transmitter, a detached monitor, and a sensor, which is inserted subcutaneously. BG values should still be verified with a finger stick glucose value before management decisions are made. Because patients will be able to view glucose trends and excursions every five minutes, patterns will be picked up that would otherwise not be identified using traditional finger stick BG results. The Guardian can be downloaded so that therapy adjustments can be based on BG patterns (28).

FreeStyle Navigator™ Continuous Glucose Monitor

The Navigator is composed of a sensor, transmitter, and receiver. The sensor is inserted subcutaneously and attached to a sensor mount, which is patched onto the skin. The transmitter attaches to the sensor and receives the BG values with arrows indicating trends, and sends the values to the pager-sized receiver each minute. This is a wireless device and the receiver can be worn on a belt or carried in a purse, pocket, or briefcase up to 10 ft away from the transmitter. Like other continuous glucose monitors, high and low value alarms can be preset into the receiver. The information can be downloaded by the patient. While the sensor and transmitter are waterproof, the receiver is not (29).

Dexcom™ STS™ Continuous Glucose Monitoring System

The Dexcom™ STS™ system includes a glucose sensor, transmitter, and a monitor. The sensor is inserted into the abdomen where it can remain for up to 72 hours. There is a two hour calibration period in which two fingerstick blood glucose values must be obtained. Once calibration is complete glucose values and trends can be viewed on the monitor every five minutes. High and low values are preset into the monitor, so that alarms alert patients when blood glucose values are outside set ranges. Glucose trends for the previous one, three, or nine hours can be displayed. Transmitter batteries cannot be changed, so a new transmitter must be purchased for $250. At this time the life of the transmitter is unknown. Monitor batteries are rechargeable and must be charged for one hour every five days. Results from the Dexcom STS system are not meant to replace values from SMBG, but to enhance therapy adjustments. Calibration must be done every 12 hours to ensure accuracy (29a,29b).

Other BG Monitoring Possibilities

None of the following have been submitted to the FDA for approval. However, they present exciting possibilities.

Scanner

Pennsylvania State University researchers are developing a sensor that would be placed under the skin. The sensor is surrounded by glucose oxidase and a polymer that is responsive to changes in pH. Glucose oxidase becomes acidic when it comes in contact with glucose, causing changes in sensor vibrations, which are proportional to serum glucose concentrations and recorded by a scanner (30).

Light

University of Iowa researchers are investigating the use of light to measure interstitial fluid using the Sensys GTS by Sensys Medical (30). This is based on the finding that the amount of light that is absorbed or reflected when it passes through the skin is proportional to the glucose level of interstitial fluid. The Sensys GTS requires the arm to be placed in front of a computer like device and a light to shine on the arm, with the amount of light that is absorbed, measured, and recorded as a BG level.

Tattoo

Pennsylvania State and Texas A & M University researchers are developing a tattoo made out of small beads covered with fluorescent molecules, which become more fluorescent with hypoglycemia and less fluorescent with hyperglycemia. A device such as a watch would measure the fluorescence of the molecules to display a BG result (30).

Contact Lens

Researchers at the University of Pittsburgh are working on creating a material that would be a contact lens or put in the lower eyelid that would detect glucose levels in tears. The material would be visible to the naked eye and it would be compared to a color wheel to determine glucose levels. For example:

- Red = low
- Green = normal
- Violet = high

Some type of scanner that could be waved in front of the eye may be developed to quantitate glucose levels (30).

Insulin Pumps on the Horizon
Medtronic MiniMed
Implantable Pump

The Model 2007 implantable pump is already being distributed throughout Europe. Three hundred fifty subjects have been enrolled in studies designed to determine the effectiveness of this pump. The pump works by delivering bursts of insulin into the peritoneal cavity instead of the subcutaneous tissue, allowing quicker and more reliable absorption rates as the peritoneal venous circulation drains directly into the liver, mimicking physiologic insulin secretion into the portal vein.

Artificial Pancreas

Medtronic plans to develop a semiautomated closed-loop system as an artificial pancreas. This semiautomated system will consist of a sensor, which provides continuous glucose results that are converted to BG values using an algorithm that then suggests an insulin dose. The patient must choose to accept or reject the suggested dose before it is delivered through an external or implantable pump. Self-monitoring of BG levels via a finger stick must still be performed to calibrate the sensor. The main difference between the semiautomated and the closed-loop system is that the insulin dose is automatically delivered in the closed loop system once it is calculated via the algorithm (31).

Animas Corporation and Debiotech

Animas now has the rights to Debiotech's technology with regard to micropumps and microneedles for insulin administration and continuous glucose monitoring. Debiotech already has a micropump chip, the ChronoJet™; so Animas is working on developing an external insulin pump with this technology. The injection pump is tiny, lightweight, and can be taped right onto the skin. It is then controlled via a remote control device. The ChronoJet uses Micro-Electro-Mechanical System, which focuses on small size, safety, accuracy, and reliability. This technology is cheaper to manufacture while still maintaining accuracy, which should make it a viable option; either as a disposable device or as a device that can be used long-term.

OmniPod™ Insulin Management System by Insulet

The OmniPod™ is a device that is small and sticks to the skin like an infusion set. The tubing is enclosed in the OmniPod, thereby making it a wireless system. The OmniPod must be filled with insulin from a vial and has an automated insertion system in which the canula is inserted into the skin by pressing a button without use of an insertion device or manual insertion. Once these steps are performed, the Personal Diabetes Manager (PDM), a handheld device that has the insulin dose instructions preprogrammed into it, begins to deliver insulin. Different basal rates, bolus rates, safety features, and alarms can be set, and the PDM makes bolus suggestions. The PDM has no tubing attaching it to the OmniPod and can be carried in a pocket, purse, or briefcase. The PDM is also a BG monitor, thereby eliminating the need for a separate meter. The OmniPod should be changed at least every three days (33).

Insulin Pens

For convenience and ease of use, insulin pens are the preferred method of insulin administration for many patients and are now available for most types of insulin. Insulin pens can be prefilled with 3 mL of insulin and are fully disposable or have replaceable cartridges. Insulin pens should be considered for patients who are noncompliant with needles and syringes, for people who may have difficulty drawing up the correct dose in a syringe, for children and teens who require insulin at school, or children and teens "on the go." Because of the dead space in the pen needle, all insulin pens must be primed with at least two units of insulin every time a new pen needle is used until a drop of insulin appears at the needle tip. Most insulin pens dispense full units; however, the Novo-Pen® Junior comes in half unit increments, with each click being a half unit instead of a whole unit. Pen needles also come in different lengths and gauges to accommodate patient preference.

Syringes and Lancets
Syringes

Insulin syringes are manufactured in 3/10 cc, 1/2 cc, and 1 cc sizes, and insulin needles are of varying lengths and gauges. Choosing the right syringe for each patient should be according to age, size, and individual preference. Several companies are now making 3/10 cc syringes with half unit markings. This is especially useful for infants, toddlers, and children who require half unit dosing.

Lancets

We recommend that our patients use a single lancet for no more than one day. Although lancets have traditionally come singly, there is now an Accu-Chek® Multiclix lancet device which contains six lancets in one drum, which must be loaded into the device. This prevents the patient from having to carry around multiple lancets or handle the lancet, a useful feature for the school setting. The patient can decide when to rotate the drum to the next lancet. There are also 11 different depth settings to provide maximum comfort and adaptation to varying skin thickness (34). Another lancing device, the Pelikan Sun, has 50 self-contained lancets and 30 different depth settings. This electronic device releases each lancet using a Smart Lancing mechanism that is programmed for individualized speed and depth, thereby minimizing pain. As with the Accu-Chek device, individual lancets need not be handled (1). This device is still in development.

DIABETES EDUCATION
Survival Skills

The day a child is diagnosed with T1DM, the lives of the child and family are forever changed. Gone is the possibility of packing up and going somewhere on a moment's notice with minimal preparation. There are many new skills to acquire and information to learn. Not everything can be taught on the first day. Follow-up education the next day or within the next week should reinforce the topics taught initially, as well as go into more detail about each subject. The components of diabetes education can be found in Table 12 .

Each child's background and needs must be considered. Education must be individualized, depending on the child's age, family support, knowledge, and where the education is done. Some environments such as the emergency room or pediatric intensive care unit are less conducive to education than an outpatient clinic or even a private room on a pediatric ward of the hospital. The caregiver and patient responsiveness is also dependent on the child's medical condition at diagnosis, whether the child's diagnosis is based on symptoms alone or the child requires intensive care for ketoacidosis.

Continuous Education

Diabetes education is an ongoing process that should address issues that arise as the child ages and takes on more responsibilities. The child and family will require different levels of support through the years. For children who were diagnosed at a young age, caregivers receive all diabetes education. As these children grow up and tasks are transitioned from the caregiver to the child, they will require reinforcement of education related to all diabetes tasks. A specific example is the transition from the caregiver drawing up and giving the insulin injection to the child pushing the plunger, then drawing up the insulin, and eventually administering the injection. This transitioning of tasks can be difficult for the caregiver and patient alike, and must be individualized according to the child's developmental level and ability to accept the increased responsibility. If metabolic control worsens as more responsibility is handed to the child, the caregiver must reinstate close supervision (20).

Education must be geared toward different developmental levels, as outlined in the American Diabetes Association statement "Care of Children and Adolescents with Type 1 Diabetes" (20), with adolescence posing a particular challenge because of increasing independence and risk-taking behaviors. Topics to discuss include sex, alcohol, drug use, and smoking. Risks and consequences of these activities should be addressed. It is important to discuss birth control and the risk to the young woman and fetus if metabolic control is poor. Parents may need to be asked to leave the room so adolescents will be more open to discussions about their habits and concerns. For those old enough to drive, it is important to emphasize the importance of testing before driving, the need to wear a medical identification necklace or bracelet, and the need to carry juice or put glucose tablets on the windshield visor for easy access (20).

Education should not be done exclusively at each three-month clinic visit. While these regular visits are important to assess educational deficits, caregivers, and, eventually, patients themselves should be encouraged to call, e-mail, or fax BG values and insulin doses to the diabetes care provider regularly. This allows caregivers and patients to play an active role in problem solving, the best educational opportunity (20).

Self-Management

Diabetes self-management must address the different priorities and issues arising with each age throughout an individual's lifespan (Table 13) (20).

SCHOOL CARE

Sending a child with diabetes to school can often present added stressors to the child and parent alike. The amount of stress is often dependent on the child's age, duration of diabetes, as well as actual and perceived support at the school. Children with diabetes are covered under Section 504 of the Rehabilitation Act of 1973, the Individuals with Disabilities Education Act of 1991, and the Americans with

Table 12 Components of Diabetes Education

First day	Follow-up
Psychology 101: address guilt that the caregiver and/or child feels about diagnosis. They need to be assured they did nothing to cause it	Progression of hypoglycemia
What is diabetes?	Administration of Glucagon
How to check blood glucose levels	Specific meal plan: number of carbohydrates to eat with meals and snacks
How to draw up insulin in a syringe or insulin pen. If appropriate, how to mix different insulins in the same syringe	Ketone testing
How to give an insulin injection, including choosing and rotating injection sites	Sick day management
Basics about insulin regimen	Exercise
Signs/symptoms of hypoglycemia and hyperglycemia	School management plan
Treatment of hypoglycemia	Need for medic alert
Basic diabetes nutrition (general overview): When child should have meals and snacks and what child should or shouldn't eat—such as initially avoiding concentrated sweets	Answer any questions caregiver or patient may have
How to contact diabetes care provider in an emergency or if any questions arise	

Table 13 Self-Management Priorities and Issues by Age

Age (yr)	Priorities	Patient and family issues
0–1	Hypoglycemia: prevention, detection, treatment	Coping mechanisms: to deal with stress
	Trying to prevent wide swings in blood glucose (BG) levels	Burnout: primary caregivers need a break
1–3	Hypoglycemia: prevention, detection, and treatment	Adhering to a schedule
	Trying to prevent wide swings in BG levels secondary to erratic eating patterns	Dealing with erratic eating patterns: finicky eaters
		Burnout: primary caregivers need a break
		Testing of boundaries set by caregiver
		Lack of cooperation
3–7	Hypoglycemia: prevention, detection, and treatment	Appeasing guilt child may feel for diagnosis
	Erratic eating patterns and activities	Deciding who to involve in diabetes management and training them in what to do
	Praise for cooperation with diabetes tasks	
	Delegating diabetes tasks to other caregivers such as daycare and school personnel	
8–11	Flexibility for growing involvement in school and extracurricular activities	Continued delegation to other caregivers helping in diabetes management
	Education of patient to long- and short-term benefits of control	Primary caregivers stay involved while also allowing the child to have more independence occasionally
12–15	Puberty: growing insulin needs	Compromising between caregiver and teen on roles each is to have in diabetes care
	Maintaining good metabolic control is more of a challenge	Problem solving
	Peer pressure: weight and body image concerns increase	Minimizing and resolving issues related to diabetes management
		Be aware: risk behaviors (sex, driving, alcohol, drugs), depression, eating disorders
16–19	Begin transition from pediatric to adult endocrinologist	Independence: teens embracing it and caregivers allowing it
	Teen to take responsibility for care	Positive coping skills
		Minimizing and resolving issues related to diabetes management
		Be aware: risk behaviors (sex, driving, alcohol, drugs), depression, eating disorders

Source: Adapted from Ref. 20.

Disabilities Act. Public schools, day care centers, and all schools that receive federal funding fall under the jurisdiction of these Acts (35), requiring that the institutions provide adequate accommodation for children with diabetes. Parochial schools are exempt.

Before the school year begins, caregivers should set up a Diabetes Medical Management Plan meeting with school personnel in order to ensure that there is as little disruption to the child's day as possible. School nurses may be employed by the school full time, part time, or have only a very intermittent presence. There should be trained personnel, who are knowledgeable about diabetes designated to provide diabetes care and to act as the go to person for issues relating to diabetes that may arise during the day. When the caregivers meet with school personnel, at least two to three personnel should be appointed to learn how to care for the child with diabetes. At least one of the trained personnel should be available at school, for field trips, and other off-campus activities at all times. The school personnel should know how to:

- Check blood glucose
- Check urine or blood for ketones
- Recognize signs/symptoms of hypoglycemia and hyperglycemia
- Administer insulin injections
- Know the basics of insulin pump operation, if necessary (bolus, how to disconnect, etc.)

- Treat hypoglycemia
- Administer glucagon

While the child's primary teacher, coaches, and elective teachers do not have to be one of the trained personnel, all should be able to recognize symptoms of hypoglycemia and hyperglycemia and know what to do if the child were to experience very low BG levels while in their classroom (35).

In addition to appropriate supervision, the school must guarantee that, besides easy and quick access to supplies, the child must also be guaranteed privacy to check blood glucose levels and take insulin injections. The diabetes medical management plan should specify where the child should be able to test and perform these tasks. It is important to consider the age and responsibility level of the child when deciding on how much supervision, if any, is necessary. This should be specified in the individual health plan, which should be signed by the parents, health care team, and school nurse. Students should also be able to eat snacks and drink water whenever necessary during the school day. The child having symptoms indicative of hypoglycemia should never be sent alone to test for or treat low BG. All of these rules are also applicable to children while they ride the school bus to and from school (35).

The responsibilities of the caregiver include providing:

- Education of school personnel
- Supplies to school: insulin, insulin pens, syringes, pen needles, ketostix, glucagon, lancets, meter, test strips, sharps box, alcohol swabs, juice, crackers, glucose tablets, extra pump supplies, etc.
- Emergency contact information
- Specifications about meal and snack schedule for the child with diabetes
- Written medical management plan signed and dated by the child's diabetes care provider

Many schools prefer the use of insulin pens instead of vials and syringes because of ease of use. Especially if the trained personnel are nonmedical, they feel more comfortable dialing up an insulin dose in a pen rather than drawing it up in a syringe (35).

Resources

National Diabetes Education Program
http://www.ndep.nih.gov/

Helping the Student with Diabetes Succeed: A Guide for School Personnel
To receive first copy free and additional copies at $3/each:
Order Form http://www.childrenwithdiabetes.com/download/SGFlyerNDEP_April05.pdf
Direct Link http://www.ndep.nih.gov/diabetes/pubs/Youth_SchoolGuide.pdf
Call 1–800–438–5383, Fax (703) 738–4929, Mail National Diabetes Information Clearinghouse (NDIC) 1 Information Way Bethesda, MD 20892–3560

Diabetes Care Tasks at School: What Key Personnel Need to Know
American Diabetes Association
www.diabetes.org/schooltraining

Health in Action: Diabetes and the School Community, American School Health Association, American Diabetes Association, Aug/Sept. 2002, Vol 1, No. 1, 330–678–1601.

Your School & Your Rights: Protecting Children with Diabetes Against Discrimination in Schools and Day Care Centers (brochure)
American Diabetes Association 2001, Alexandria, VA
http://www.diabetes.org/type1/parents_kids/away/scrights.jsp

Fredrickson L, Griff M: *Pumper in the School, Insulin Pump guide for School Nurses, School Personnel and Parents. MiniMed Professional Education, Your Clinical Coach. First Edition*, May 2000. MiniMed, Inc., 1–800–440–7867.

Tappon D. Parker M, Bailey W: *Easy As ABC, What You Need to Know About Children Using Insulin Pumps in School.* Disetronic Medical Systems, Inc., 1–800–280–7801.

DIABETES CAMP

There is no other place quite like it. A place where a child with diabetes can go and feel like they are not the outsider, that they are not the only ones who must check their blood glucose and take insulin injections, a place where caregivers do not have to worry about who is taking care of their child's diabetes while they are not around. This place is diabetes camp. There are camps throughout the United States, whose main purpose and mission is to provide a safe environment for children with diabetes while challenging them in a fun environment, so that they learn how to take responsibility for their disease and do not feel limited by it. There are day camps, residential camps, camps for children of all ages, and camps for families.

Appropriate staff at camp includes doctors and nurses familiar with pediatric T1DM care, psychologists, registered dietitians, and volunteer staff for recreation and counselor positions. Oftentimes recreation staff and counselors are medical students, housestaff, pharmacy or nursing students, and many are ex-campers. Medical staff should have access to written policies, procedures, and diabetes management plans before and during camp. The counselors, recreational, and support staff should receive in depth training on diabetes management including insulin administration, treatment of hypoglycemia and hyperglycemia, ketone testing, emergency procedures, BG monitoring, etc. Support staff should have a clear picture of what to do in case of an emergency, whether diabetes related or not. There should not only be enough diabetes supplies to last the entire camp session, but also supplies for general first aid and general pediatric ailments (36).

Record keeping at camp for each individual camper is essential. A camper's daily record with BG levels, insulin doses, ketone testing results, activity level, and number of carbohydrates eaten can help medical staff determine what insulin dose adjustments are necessary. Regular BG checks should be performed before meals, snacks, activities, bedtime, and as needed throughout the day. Home insulin doses must often be decreased by 10% to 20% or more because of the increased activity level at camp, especially for children who are sedentary at home (36).

Regular meal and snack times should be available for food coverage of all insulin regimens. For campers on more flexible regimens such as insulin glargine or CSII, snacks consisting of low to no carbohydrates should be provided. A registered dietitian, if not available for the camp session, should look at the comprehensive menu for camp meals and snacks before the start of camp. The carbohydrate content and serving size should be displayed at meal times for campers and counselors alike. This provides an opportunity for campers to learn about carbohydrate counting while also assisting counselors in determining the correct insulin doses based on insulin to carbohydrate ratios (36).

Camp provides a structured environment that allows children with diabetes to learn how to manage their disease. Camp is often where a child first independently draws up his/her insulin or gives his/her first injection. Family weekend camps are also important in that they provide parents and children an opportunity to interact with others dealing with similar issues and allow parents and children close contact with diabetes health care providers who can provide education and answer questions in an informal atmosphere. The benefits of diabetes camp are enormous and all patients should be encouraged to attend them (36).

Resources

For a comprehensive list of diabetes camps:
http://www.childrenwithdiabetes.com/camps/

SUPPORT GROUPS

While diabetes camps are available at specified times throughout the year, many patients and caregivers need extra support throughout the entire year. Local support groups provide activities and support to patients and caregivers. Some support groups are geared to all families with a child with diabetes, while others target specific populations such as parents of preschoolers or teenagers on insulin pumps. Successful support groups need to:

■ Identify target population for support group
■ Identify a leader as well as support personnel to get the ball rolling
■ Identify resources for funding events (private donations/pharmaceutical sponsors/etc.)
■ Identify a location and time to meet
■ Identify frequency of meetings. Plan regular events. Participants should know how often to expect events or meetings.

Resources

For a list of support groups on Children with Diabetes Website: http://www.childrenwithdiabetes.com/support/

Juvenile Diabetes Research Foundation International
http://www.jdrf.org/

American Diabetes Association
http://www.diabetes.org

Medical Suppliers

Advanced Medical
1–866–716–9804
www.Advmedsolutions.com

CCS Medical
1–800–726–9811
www.ccsmed.com

Kelson Pharmacy: The Children's Pharmacy
1051 NW 14th Street Suite 160
Miami, FL 33136

866–796–2447
www.kelsonpharmacy.com

Liberty
1–800–288–6302
http://www.libertymedical.com

National Diabetic Pharmacies
2157 Apperson Drive
Salem, Virginia 24153
Tel: 1–877–637–8488 Fax: 1–888–268–6406
www.NationalDiabetic.com

CONCLUSION

While treatment principles and advances in technology are highlighted throughout this chapter, diabetes management depends on patient and caregiver ability to use the tools available to them. Encouraging patients and caregivers to ask questions about current treatment and imminent new therapies during clinic visits and visits between, via phone or email, helps them feel up to date and confident about how to better manage their disease. Patient oriented journals and reliable online resources should be suggested to foster further education and confidence, and an open door maintained for questions raised by these and less reliable sources. As investigators continue to develop improved ways of managing the disease, clinicians and educators must realize that diabetes affects every aspect of their patients' lives. The best technology cannot eliminate the increased psychological, emotional, financial, and social burden of diabetes. Patients with a positive attitude, however, can be empowered to effectively manage their diabetes without it ruling every aspect of their life, that is, living *with* their diabetes not *for* their diabetes.

REFERENCES

1. Diabetes Health Magazine. Spring 2005; 10–13, 17–20, 22–27, 36.
2. http://www.lifescan.com/products/meters/ultrasmart/fastfacts/ (accessed 10/18/05).
3. http://www.accu-chek.com/us/rewrite/content/en_US/2.1.2:20/article/ACCM_general_article_2502.htm(accessed 10/18/05).
4. http://www.accu-chek.com/us/rewrite/content/en_US/2.1.6:5/article/ACCM_general_article_2838.htm (accessed 10/18/05).
5. http://www.accu-chek.com/us/rewrite/content/en_US/2.1.1:10/article/ACCM_general_article_2354.htm(accessed 10/18/05).
6. http://www.accu-chek.com/us/rewrite/content/en_US/2.1.3:30/article/ACCM_general_article_2533.htm(accessed 10/18/05).
7. http://www.diabeteshealthconnection.com/products/monitors/freestyle/freestylemeter/facts.aspx (accessed 10/18/05).
8. http://www.diabeteshealthconnection.com/products/monitors/freestyle/freestyleflash/facts.aspx (accessed 10/18/05).

9. http://www.diabeteshealthconnection.com/products/monitors/precision/precisionxtra/facts.aspx (accessed 10/18/05).
10. http://www.bddiabetes.com/us/bgm/logic_product.asp (accessed 10/18/05).
11. http://www.bddiabetes.com/us/bgm/logic_memory.asp (accessed 10/18/05).
12. http://www.ascensia.ca/eng/prodserv/products/contour/index.asp (accessed 10/18/05).
13. http://www.childrenwithdiabetes.com/ast/ (accessed 10/21/05).
14. Greenhalgh S, Bradshaw S, Hall CM, et al. Forearm blood-glucose testing in diabetes mellitus. Archives of Disease in Childhood 2004; 89:516–518.
15. Lucidarme N, Alberti C, Zaccaria I, et al. Alternate-site testing is reliable in children and adolescents with type 1 diabetes, except at the forearm for hypoglycemia detection. Diabetes Care 2005; 28:710–711.
16. Burdick BS, Harris S, Chase HP. The importance of ketone testing. Pract Diabetol 2004; 23(2):3–11.
17. http://press.novonordisk-us.com/internal.aspx?rid=300 (accessed 12/6/05).
18. Bott S, Tusek C, Jacobsen LV, Kristensen A. Insulin detemir reaches steady-state after the first day of treatment and shows a peakless time-action profile with twice daily applications. Diabetologia 2003; 46(suppl 2):A271.
19. The pump advantage. In: Wolpert H, ed. Smart Pumping for People with Diabetes, Alexandria. Virginia: American Diabetes Association, 2002:10–11.
20. Silverstein J, Klingensmith G, Copeland K, et al. Care of children and adolescents with type 1 diabetes: a statement of the American Diabetes Association. Diabetes Care 2005; 28(1):186–212.
21. Chase HP. Sick Day and Surgery Management. In: Understanding Diabetes. 10th ed. University of Colorado Health Sciences Center, 2002:178–179.
22. Admon G, Weinstein Y, Falk B, et al. Exercise with and without an insulin pump among children and adolescents with type 1 diabetes mellitus. Pediatrics 2005; 116(3):e348–e355.
23. http://www.diabetes.org/advocacy-andlegalresources/discrimination/public_accommodation/travel.jsp (accessed 10/23/05).
24. Hanas R. Travel Tips. In: Type 1 Diabetes. New York: Marlowe and Company, 2005:294–299.
25. Klonoff DC. Continuous glucose monitoring: Roadmap for 21st century diabetes therapy. Diabetes Care 2005; 28(5):1231–1239.
26. http://www.glucowatch.com/us/pdfs/patient_brochure1.pdf (accessed 10/25/05).
27. The Diabetes Research in Children Network (DirecNet) Study Group. Youth and parent satisfaction with clinical use of the GlucoWatch G2 biographer in the management of pediatric type 1 diabetes. Diabetes Care 2005; 28(8):1929–1935.
28. http://www.minimed.com/professionals/guardianrt/index.html (accessed 10/24/05).
29. http://www.diabetesnet.com/diabetes_technology/therasense.php (accessed 10/25/05).
29a. http://www.fda.gov/cdrh/mda/docs/p050012.html (accessed 8\21\06).
29b. http://www.childrenwithdiabetes.com/continuous.html (accessed 8\21\06).
30. Kordella T. An "ouchless" future? Will the day come when you no longer have to prick, stick, jab or stab to check your glucose levels? Diabetes Forecast 2005; 58(4):51–53.
31. http://wwwp.medtronic.com/Newsroom/LinkedItemDetails.do?itemId=1101850830145&itemType= backgrounder& lang=en_US (accessed 10/24/05).
32. http://www.diabetesnet.com/diabetes_technology/insulin-pumps_future.php (accessed 10/25/05).
33. http://www.insulet.com/products/ (accessed 4/21/05).
34. http://www.accu-chek.com/us/rewrite/content/en_US/2.2.6:60/article/ACCM_general_article_2835.htm (accessed 10/17/05).
35. American Diabetes Association. Diabetes care in the school and day care setting. Diabetes Care 2005; 28(suppl 1):S43–S49.
36. American Diabetes Association. Diabetes care at diabetes camps. Diabetes Care 2005; 28(suppl 1):S50–S52.

8

Hyperglycemic Comas in Children

Arlan L. Rosenbloom
*Division of Pediatric Endocrinology, Department of Pediatrics, University of Florida,
Gainesville, Florida, U.S.A.*

INTRODUCTION

Diabetic ketoacidosis (DKA), occurring with both Type 1 (T1DM) and Type 2 diabetes (T2DM), and hyperglycemic hyperosmolar state (HHS), which occurs almost exclusively with T2DM, are associated with complications accounting for most of the diabetes-related morbidity and mortality in childhood (1). DKA is defined by venous pH less than 7.3 or serum bicarbonate concentration less than 15 mmol/L, with serum glucose concentration more than 200 mg/dL (11 mmol/L) (1). This is typically associated with glucosuria, ketonuria, and ketonemia. Near-normal circulating glucose concentrations may occur rarely in DKA with partial treatment or with pregnancy (2,3). HHS is the preferred nomenclature for what was long known as hyperglycemic hyperosmolar nonketotic state; the newer designation recognizes the frequent presence of mild ketosis. Hyperglycemic comas may be considered on a continuum from DKA with normal osmolality to HHS without ketosis (4). The emergence of T2DM in childhood (Vol. 1; Chap. 9), accounting for as much as 50% of newly diagnosed diabetes in the 10- to 19-year age group, depending on socioeconomic and ethnic composition of the population, has resulted in an appreciation of HHS as no longer a condition seen rarely outside of elderly populations (5–17). The criteria for HHS include plasma glucose concentration greater than 600 mg/dL (33.3 mmol/L), serum bicarbonate concentration greater than 15 mmol/L, no or small ketonuria, absent to small ketonemia, effective serum osmolality greater than 320 mOsm/kg, and stupor or coma (4).

FREQUENCY
Unset

DKA at onset of diabetes varies widely in frequency according to geographic region and correlates inversely with the regional incidence of T1DM; variation in the European diabetes study was from 11% to 67% (18). The frequency in Australia was 26% (19), and in New Zealand 63% in 1988/1989 and 42% in 1995/1996 (20). Children less than five years of age are more likely to have DKA at diagnosis as are children whose families do not have ready access to medical care for social or economic reasons (1,18–25). DKA at onset was seen in 28.4% of patients from Colorado, with the odds ratio for uninsured subjects compared to insured subjects being 6.2 and with significantly greater severity in the uninsured group (23). The only long-term reductions in frequency of DKA at onset in recent years have been reported where zealous efforts to educate the medical community have been made (19–21).

The frequencies of DKA at the onset of T2DM have been even more variable than those for T1DM. The American Diabetes Association consensus statement on T2DM in children estimated that 5% to 25% of new onset cases had DKA (26). Proportions as high as 52% are reported in populations of largely African-American youths, whereas lower proportions with DKA are seen among Hispanic, Caucasian, and Native American populations (27–31).

There is a single report on the frequency of HHS at the onset of T2DM in children, a review of 190 patients, of whom eight (4.2%) had HHS (16).

Recurrent

The risk of recurrent DKA among 1243 patients in Colorado was 8 episodes/100 patient years and 80% of episodes occurred among 20% of patients. Factors that increased the risk of recurrent DKA were poor metabolic control or previous episodes of DKA, female gender (peripubertal or adolescent), psychiatric disorders, including eating disorders, difficult or unstable family circumstances, limited access to medical services, and insulin pump therapy (as only rapid-acting or short-acting insulin is used in pumps, interruption of insulin delivery for any reason rapidly leads to insulin deficiency) (32). In the 1970s and 1980s, the establishment of treatment teams with intensive education of families on sick day management and 24-hour availability demonstrated profound reduction in recurrent DKA (33,34).

Recurrent DKA in T2DM is unusual, even in those who have had DKA at onset.

PATHOPHYSIOLOGY

DKA and HHS result from reduction in the net effective action of circulating insulin, producing intracellular starvation, which stimulates the release of the counter-regulatory hormones glucagon, catecholamines, cortisol, and growth hormone (Fig. 1).

These hormonal responses lead to accelerated hepatic and renal glucose production and impaired glucose utilization in insulin-dependent peripheral tissues (muscle, liver, and adipose), resulting in hyperglycemia, release of free fatty acids into the circulation from adipose tissue (lipolysis), and unrestrained hepatic fatty acid oxidation to ketone bodies (35). In HHS, plasma insulin concentrations may be inadequate to facilitate glucose utilization by insulin-sensitive tissues but adequate to prevent lipolysis and subsequent ketogenesis (4). Such an explanation would be consistent with the difference in the pathogenesis of T1DM and T2DM and the almost exclusive occurrence of HHS with T2DM. Both DKA and HHS are associated with glycosuria, leading to osmotic diuresis, with loss of water, sodium, potassium, and other electrolytes (4).

MORBIDITY AND MORTALITY

Mortality risks for each episode of DKA from national population-based studies are similar: 0.15% for the United States (36), 0.18% to 0.25% for Canada (37,38), and 0.31% for the United Kingdom (39). Cerebral edema accounts for 60% to 90% of this mortality (40–42). In a study of diabetes-related mortality over eight years

among insulin-treated patients under 25 years of age in Chicago, seven of the eight deaths at the onset of diabetes were in non-Hispanic African-Americans, who comprised less than half of the age specific population, and one death was in a Hispanic individual (28% of the population), with similar disproportion for all 30 deaths, emphasizing the sociodemographic specificity and preventability of such mortality (43). Other causes of death or disability with DKA or HHS in addition to cerebral edema include hypokalemia, hypophosphatemia, hypoglycemia, other intracerebral complications, peripheral venous thrombosis, mucormycosis, rhabdomyolysis, acute pancreatitis, acute renal failure, sepsis, aspiration pneumonia, and other pulmonary complications (1).

HYPERGLYCEMIC HYPEROSMOLAR STATE

Eight obese African-American youths thought to have died from DKA at onset of T1DM actually had previously unrecognized T2DM; seven of them met the criteria for HHS and not DKA (14,16). Hypokalemia resulting from failure to replace or from administration of bicarbonate was responsible for arrhythmia and cardiac arrest in three patients, and may have contributed, along with hypophosphatemia, in two others. One patient developed cerebral edema and another had pancreatitis and renal failure. Fourtner et al. (17) reported one death at onset of T2DM in their series, as a result of multisystem organ failure from HHS, while another patient survived rhabdomyolysis, acute renal failure, and pancreatitis. Another report described six male adolescent patients with hyperthermia and rhabdomyolysis at diabetes onset. Of the five who were obese, three met the criteria for HHS and two of these died, one with intractable arrhythmia and the other with multisystem failure (cardiac, pulmonary edema, and renal) (15).

Before these recent reports, HHS had been reported in few children and none had obesity, with the fatalities being only in those with mental retardation, which seemed to be a risk factor for the development of HHS (5–13). Three pubertal aged children, one with severe spastic quadriplegia, learning difficulties, and epilepsy, one with cystic fibrosis, and another without any premorbid condition, have recently been reported with HHS, and in two instances this was thought to be related to the ingestion of large volumes of high caloric fluids (44). Striking hyperosmolality and hypernatremia with DKA at onset have been described in five patients following ingestion of massive amounts of carbonated carbohydrate beverages and isotonic sports drinks; three of them required hemofiltration, but all survived without residual (45).

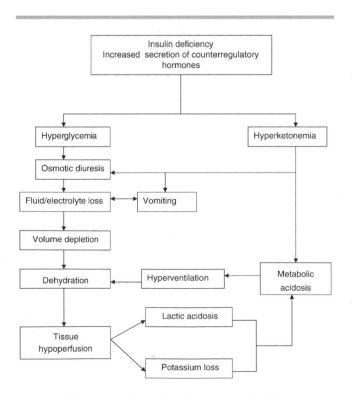

Figure 1 Pathogenesis of diabetic ketoacidosis.

RHABDOMYOLYSIS

This potentially lethal complication, already mentioned in relation to HHS, also occurs with DKA and is of uncertain etiology. Severe hyperglycemia and high osmolality, together with hypophosphatemia, are risk factors. A recent report in a 15-month old has added to the few pediatric cases reported (46). An early report in a 27-month-old boy led to a chart review of 133 children admitted with new onset diabetes, of whom 12 had significant orthotoluidine reactions in the urine; in only one case was urine myoglobin measured and it was extremely high. Another patient had an elevated serum CPK value three days after admission (47). Thus, mild rhabdomyolysis may be common in DKA, despite its infrequency as a clinical complication.

MUCORMYCOSIS

Mucormycosis is an acute, often rapidly fatal fungal infection that is an important cause of death in young patients with diabetes who have poor glycemic control and acute ketosis. Survival without disability is rare. Clinical features vary depending on the principal infection locus, which may be rhinocerebral, pulmonary, cutaneous, or gastrointestinal, or in the central nervous system (CNS) and may be disseminated. African-American race and history of poor compliance, as evidenced by poor clinic attendance, risk-taking behaviors, and high rate of hospital admission, were predictors of increased susceptibility to infection with mucormycosis in one study of five patients, which included only one survivor who had severe neurologic disability (48). Several systemic factors contribute to the predisposition to mucor infection in patients with diabetes. These include impaired neutrophil function, vascular insufficiency, and, in DKA, the acid environment and high blood-glucose concentration, which favor fungal growth.

PANCREATITIS

Acute pancreatitis is a well-recognized complication of DKA in adults, whereas it is unusual in children with T1DM. As noted above, however, pancreatitis may be a frequent and serious occurrence in children with HHS at onset of T2DM. Elevated amylase and lipase levels were common in children with T1DM and new onset DKA in a study of 50 patients, while only one individual with newly diagnosed diabetes without DKA had mildly elevated lipase. Lipase elevation was directly associated with degree of acidosis. One patient with persistent abdominal pain had abdominal computerized tomography (CT) scan confirmation of acute pancreatitis (49). Acute pancreatitis must be considered with abdominal pain that does not resolve with correction of acidosis.

PERIPHERAL VENOUS THROMBOSIS

A recent case series described deep venous thrombosis (DVT) in four of eight children with DKA who required femoral central venous catheter (CVC) placement (50), and three of six PICU patients with

DKA who required femoral CVC (out of 113 DKA/PICU patients) (51). All the latter patients were under 18 months of age and required long-term heparin therapy for persistent leg swelling; this frequency contrasted with complete absence of DVT in seven comparably aged patients with shock, who had femoral CVC for longer periods of time than did the DKA patients, suggesting a thrombotic diathesis in DKA beyond that which could be attributed to dehydration. In one of the patients, heterozygosity for factor V Leiden deficiency may have been contributory, but no other abnormalities were detected. While coagulation factor abnormalities have not been demonstrated in children with diabetes in the absence of DKA (52), von Willebrand factor activity has been noted to remain elevated at 120 hours following admission for DKA (53), suggesting that DKA and its treatment may result in a prothrombotic state and activation of vascular endothelium, predisposing to thrombosis.

INTRACEREBRAL COMPLICATIONS OTHER THAN IDIOPATHIC CEREBRAL EDEMA

Intracerebral complications, with or without associated edema, although by definition not idiopathic cerebral edema, account for an estimated 10% of all instances of neurologic collapse during ketoacidosis (1,40,54). Causes have included subarachnoid hemorrhage (40), basilar artery thrombosis (40), cerebral venous thrombosis (55,56), meningoencephalitis (57), and disseminated intravascular coagulation (58,59).

It is noteworthy that the five-year-old girl with established diabetes with mild ketoacidosis and microcytic anemia (a risk factor for thrombosis), who developed thrombosis in the straight sinus and the vein of Galen with ischemic changes in the thalamus, had a clinical picture indistinguishable from typical cerebral edema. She received anticoagulant therapy and made a full recovery with very mild learning disability as a residual (55). In contrast, the 11-year-old boy with DVT of the leg preceding admission for DKA at the onset of diabetes was found unconscious with fixed dilated pupils, but breathing. With cerebral edema, respiratory arrest would be expected with his unconsciousness and fixed dilated pupils as a reflection of brainstem herniation or compression from edema. Magnetic resonance imaging (MRI) two hours after his collapse showed acute infarction affecting multiple areas of the brain without hemorrhage or edema. He never recovered. His heterozygosity for factor V Leiden deficiency was thought to be responsible for the unusual occurrence of DVT in a child (56). Patients younger than 18 years of age with venous thrombosis are reported to have a greater than 50% likelihood of carrying a genetic thrombophilic defect, and two-thirds of such defects will be in factor V (60). Case series of cerebral venous thrombosis in children from various acute causes, including dehydration, indicate that thrombosis is unlikely to occur in the absence of background coagulopathy (61).

CEREBRAL EDEMA

The understanding of the epidemiology of cerebral edema, risk factors for its development, and intervention to minimize morbidity and mortality has greatly increased over the past decade. Recent exploration of pathogenesis using functional imaging methods promises new insight into this idiosyncratic and still enigmatic condition.

When two teenage patients with fatal cerebral edema were reported in 1967, there were only three others in the literature with a similar clinical history (62). By 1980, there were only 17 reported cases (63). By 1990, there were 40 reported cases, and an additional 29 were added in one report and 11 in another (40,64). Reports since 2000 have added another approximately 160 cases, collected over periods varying from 2 to 15 years. Most importantly, these reports have provided data on incidence, and within the limitations of retrospective analysis, added to the realization of the idiosyncratic nature of the occurrence of cerebral edema and the usual inability to assign iatrogenic causation (65,66).

Prevalence and Incidence

In 1990, Bello and Sotos (64) provided the first estimates of the incidence of cerebral edema in DKA based on their hospital experience with 1006 episodes in pediatric patients, of whom 11 had cerebral edema for an incidence of 1.1%. There was a striking difference between newly diagnosed patients who had a cerebral edema frequency of 3.3%, and established patients with frequency of 0.23%. This was, however, a biased population because more severely ill individuals would have been referred, reflected in the fact that some of those with cerebral edema arrived in advanced states of deterioration. The first population-based study, from a three-year U.K. experience involving nearly three times as many episodes, yielded a lower incidence of 0.7% overall, but also showed a marked discrepancy between the newly diagnosed, 1.2%, and established patients, 0.4% (41). Australian experience provides a higher incidence of 4.3% in newly diagnosed, 1.3% in established patients, and 2% overall (19). The North American multicenter study reported a cerebral edema incidence of 0.9% without differences between new onset and established patients (42). A prospective surveillance study in Canada of patients less than 16 years of age with DKA identified 13 verified cases of cerebral edema for a rate of 0.51% of episodes of DKA (38). Some of these frequency variations likely represent differences in case definition as well as referral patterns.

Morbidity and Mortality

Early case fatality and residual morbidity data based on case reports and litigated cases had an obvious ascertainment bias and also reflected later recognition of cerebral edema than with more recent population-based observations; in addition, appropriate intervention was less likely in these early or litigated cases. The most extensive series at the time (1990), analyzed 69 cases including 40 from the literature. The case fatality rate was 64% overall, with 14% surviving without disability, 9% with disability that did not preclude independence, and 13% with severe disability or vegetative state. In those who were treated before respiratory arrest, who would correspond more closely to subsequently reported instances, the case fatality was only 30%, with 30% surviving without disability, 26% with disability not precluding independence, and 13% with severe disability or vegetative state (24). Although the interventions in these cases were often after severe neurologic compromise and inadequate, the outcome with treatment is similar to contemporary population-based studies (Table 1).

Noteworthy in the most recent report, from Canada, 19% of cases of cerebral edema were present before treatment was undertaken, reinforcing previous observations of this phenomenon and the idiosyncratic, rather than iatrogenic, nature of this problem in most cases (38,40–42,66).

Risk Factors

As noted above, a number of reports suggest that young age, especially less than five years, carries an increased risk for the development of cerebral edema. While this may reflect the more rapid deterioration in this age group and greater delay in diagnosis because of nonspecificity of symptoms, it may also be due to greater susceptibility of the younger brain to metabolic and vascular changes associated with DKA. Greater severity of acidosis has been noted to be a risk factor, as have degree of hypocapnia and elevated serum urea nitrogen, all indicators of severity of ketoacidosis and dehydration (1). Treatment of acidosis with sodium bicarbonate infusion has been a significant association with the development of cerebral edema in one population-based case-control study (42). This association might reflect greater severity of ketoacidosis that is not adequately controlled for in the case-control design, rather than an effect of the bicarbonate itself (66).

Not only does younger age confer risk, but also the entire pediatric age group also carries a risk for cerebral edema associated with either DKA or HHS that is almost nonexistent in the adult population (67). In adult patients with HHS, this is true despite rapid rehydration and restoration of normal glycemia (68).

Table 1 Outcome with Cerebral Edema in Population-Based Studies

References	Glaser et al. (42)	Edge et al. (39)	Lawrence et al. (38)
Region	United States	United Kingdom	Canada
Death	21%	24%	22%
Permanent neurological sequela	21%	26%	8%
No permanent neurological sequela	57%	50%	70%

An inadequate increase in serum sodium concentration during treatment for DKA has been associated with increased risk for cerebral edema in several studies, which may reflect dysregulation of antidiuretic hormone secretion as a result of changes in the brain in those who are in the early, presymptomatic, stages of cerebral edema (42,69). That this might be the result of altered renal sodium handling due to cerebral injury, rather than the type or rate of fluid administration, is suggested by the absence of evidence of associations between volume or tonicity of fluids or the rate of change in serum glucose and risk of cerebral edema (1,38,40,42,65,70).

Poor outcome in the 61 children with cerebral edema from the North American multicenter study (42) was associated with greater neurologic depression at the time of diagnosis of their cerebral edema, and with initial serum urea nitrogen concentration. Importantly, intubation with hyperventilation to a pCO_2 less than 22 mmHg was also a risk factor, demanding caution in hyperventilating affected patients (71).

Mechanisms

Brain edema is a general term that refers to an increase of cerebral tissue water causing an increase of tissue volume (72). The prototypic forms are vasogenic, due to breakdown of the blood–brain barrier as around a tumor or with trauma; cytotoxic, from poisoning or metabolic derangement; and osmotic, as occurs with hyponatremia. While neither the cause nor the location of the fluid in the swollen brains of children with DKA- or HHS-related cerebral edema is known, the mechanism is likely to be complex, and it may not be the same in all affected individuals.

This complexity and variability is reflected in the time of onset and in the brain imaging findings. There is a bimodal distribution of the time of onset, with approximately two-thirds of patients developing signs and symptoms in the first six to seven hours and the rest from 10 to 24 hours after the start of treatment, with the early onset individuals tending to be younger (42,70). In an analysis of initial brain CT scans done 2 to 44 hours after establishment of the diagnosis of cerebral edema, 39% had no acute abnormalities visible, and this did not differ significantly between early and late onset subjects; 26% had diffuse edema, which was also similar between early and late onset. Three of the eight with diffuse edema also had hemorrhages and 17% of the entire group had only subarachnoid or intraventricular hemorrhage. Focal brain injury in the mesial basal ganglia and thalamus, the periaqueductal gray matter, and the dorsal pontine nuclei was seen in five subjects (22%), and these localized injuries occurred only in the early onset patients. These findings were not an artifact of the time that the studies were performed and thus truly reflect what appear to be widely varying pathology in the brain leading to the syndrome that falls under the rubric "cerebral edema" (70).

Functional brain imaging has permitted the beginning of understanding of the alterations in the brain with diabetes and with DKA. Single photon emission tomography using technetium with 31 10- to 18-year-old patients who were not affected with ketoacidosis and seven controls indicated significant brain hypoperfusion in those with diabetes mainly in the basal ganglia and frontal regions, suggesting underlying vascular changes that might be contributory to the risk for cerebral edema with the advent of DKA (73). Diffusion MRI, quantified as the apparent diffusion coefficient (ADC), is a technique that is highly sensitive for detecting edema. Conditions that expand the extracellular space, such as vasogenic edema, are characterized by increased ADC, while conditions that cause cellular swelling, such as hypoxic/ischemic injury or osmotic swelling, decrease the ADC. Perfusion MRI complements diffusion imaging by monitoring the first pass intravenously administered contrast agent (gadolinium) to assess relative cerebral blood flow (CBF) and cerebral blood volume. The prevailing hypothesis, despite the paucity of supporting data, has been that cerebral edema during treatment of DKA is the result of osmotic shifts resulting in cellular swelling. If this were the case, ADC should be decreased and cerebral perfusion diminished or unchanged. Fourteen children aged 3.5 to 15.5 years were studied during DKA treatment and after recovery, an appropriate approach because several studies have documented subtle cerebral edema changes on CT scan in children without significant neurologic symptoms during their treatment for DKA (74,75). ADC was significantly elevated during DKA treatment, which indicated increased water diffusion in all regions except the occipital gray matter, with reduction of ADC in the postrecovery MRI. Perfusion MRI during treatment showed significantly shorter mean transit times and higher peak tracer concentrations, suggesting increased CBF. These findings suggest that the predominant mechanism of edema formation is a vasogenic process rather than osmotic cellular swelling and further confirm the presence of subtle, asymptomatic cerebral edema during DKA treatment (76).

Patients with greater dehydration and those with more profound hypocapnia are at increased risk of symptomatic cerebral edema (42). Functional imaging studies (76) suggest that cerebral hypoperfusion before DKA treatment (73), followed by reperfusion, might lead to cerebral edema. Typically, ischemic brain injury is characterized in the acute-to-subacute phases by low ADC values (i.e., restricted diffusion), likely a result of both astrocytic swelling and diminished intracellular microcirculation. Elevated ADCs in DKA do not contradict a possible role for cerebral hypoperfusion in the pathogenesis of DKA-related cerebral edema. In fact, studies have demonstrated that the ADC may return to normal within one hour after reperfusion of ischemic tissue. The possibility remains that the initial and typical CNS response to DKA is vasogenic edema, while other insults leading to symptomatic cerebral edema might require prolonged hypoxia or further insult (inappropriate vasopressin release, fluid overload, and central hypoxia from rapid correction of peripheral acidosis with bicarbonate administration) leading to the superimposition of cellular edema (77).

Ketones have direct effects on brain microvascular endothelium and may alter permeability of the blood–brain barrier, and elevated levels may disrupt membrane structure by causing oxidative tissue damage through production of reactive oxygen species and by compromising free radical scavenging. These effects could contribute to cerebral edema. β-hydroxybutyrate was detected in brain by proton magnetic resonance (MR) spectroscopy in half of 25 children during or after treatment for DKA overall and in 90% of those tested within four hours of the start of treatment. Acetoacetate was detected in 60%, with greater frequency after four hours. This inverse relationship, as β-hydroxybutyrate is oxidized to acetoacetate, reflects changes in the serum concentrations of these substances with treatment. Ketones were detected in the brain more frequently in children with altered mental status during treatment (78).

Further insight into the background on which cerebral edema develops has been provided by MR imaging and MR spectroscopy of the brain in eight children with hyperglycemia with or without DKA, seven of whom were newly diagnosed. All had abnormal signal changes in the frontal region on fluid attenuated inversion recovery MR imaging, indicative of edema. Spectroscopic abnormalities were increased taurine, myoinositol, and glucose. The abnormalities varied in severity and did not correlate with any clinical or biochemical measures and were highly consistent between patients, thought to reflect homeostatic responses of the brain to prolonged hyperglycemia and associated osmotic pressure changes (79). Taurine has been considered important in neuroprotection and osmoregulation and has been implicated in animal models of cerebral edema.

Inflammatory mediators have also been implicated in the development of cerebral edema. Plasma cytokines, as markers of cellular activation, were elevated in six children and adolescents before treatment of severe DKA. There were significant decreases of some cytokines during treatment, while inflammatory cytokines increased, reaching a peak consistent with the peak time of cerebral edema development. Such elevation could have effects on capillary function that could contribute to the expression of clinical cerebral edema (80).

Monitoring

A model for early detection of cerebral edema has been developed based on the assumption that treatment modification has not prevented this complication and the strong evidence that early administration of mannitol prevents brain damage and death from cerebral edema (70). The model applied signs of neurologic impairment based on 26 case reviews, which were then

Table 2 Bedside Evaluation of Neurologic State of Children with Diabetic Ketoacidosis

Diagnostic criteria
Abnormal motor or verbal response to pain
Decorticate or decerebrate posture
Cranial nerve palsy (especially III, IV, VI)
Abnormal neurogenic respiratory pattern (e.g., grunting, tachypnea, Cheyne-Stokes, apneustic)
Major criteria
Altered mentation/fluctuating level of consciousness
Sustained heart rate deceleration (decline more than 20/min) not attributable to improved intravascular volume or sleep state
Age inappropriate incontinence
Minor criteria
Vomiting following initial treatment and its cessation, if present at admission
Headache (recurrent and more severe than on admission)
Lethargy or not easily aroused from sleep
Diastolic blood pressure greater than 90 mmHg
Age less than 5 yr old

tested with an independent sample of 17 patients who had previously been reported with symptomatic cerebral edema (40) for whom records were still available. The protocol allowed 92% sensitivity and 96% specificity for the recognition of cerebral edema early enough for intervention, using one diagnostic criterion, two major criteria, or one major plus two minor criteria (Table 2).

In effect this means that five youngsters will be treated for cerebral edema to prevent brain damage or death in one patient, a reasonable proposition considering the alternative of waiting for more stringent criteria to be met.

Treatment

The importance of early intervention, as soon as cerebral edema is suspected and especially before respiratory arrest, has been well documented (1,40,54,64). Intervention has included reduction in the rate of fluid administration, elevation of the head of the bed, and administration of intravenous (IV) mannitol in a dosage of 0.25 to 1.0 g/kg over 20 minutes with repeat as necessary in one to two hours. Although early intervention with mannitol has markedly improved outcome, the degree to which this has occurred is difficult to determine because increased recognition of the problem has undoubtedly led to less stringent case definition. In this context, it is interesting that the application of criteria developed from the most severe cases, when applied to a series of 69 consecutive cases thought to be uncomplicated, yielded three who met these criteria (4.3%) (70).

Mannitol has a variety of effects, which are not entirely understood, including lowering hematocrit and blood viscosity, which improves CBF and oxygenation, improvement in red cell deformability, vasoconstriction in areas of the brain with intact autoregulation or improved autoregulation from the effects of the mannitol on CBF and oxygenation, and direct osmotic effects with reduction in extracellular free water. Concerns about the risk of rebound edema and renal failure have not been borne out by any published reports. This is likely because these problems arise with long-term rather than acute use.

Hypertonic saline has been used in acute intracranial pressure reduction in head injury animal models and in patients undergoing surgical procedures in the supratentorial portion of the brain and has been considered at least as effective as mannitol (81–89). Its use in DKA-associated cerebral edema was initially described in a case report of a 13-year-old girl with relatively mild acidosis who developed a severe headache 20 minutes after the start of treatment and who had CT scan evidence of diffuse cerebral edema with transtentorial herniation. Deteriorating further despite infusion of mannitol, she was given 5 mL/kg of 3% saline rapidly and awoke with recovered neurologic function within five minutes (90). It seems reasonable to consider the use of 3% saline in patients who have not responded adequately to mannitol infusion of a dose of 1.0 g/kg.

Intubation is necessary for those who have progressed to respiratory compromise, an indicator of advanced neurologic deterioration. Aggressive hyperventilation was a significant risk factor for poor outcome in the study of Marcin et al. (71), similar to detrimental effects reported in head trauma and high-altitude exposure (1).

MANAGEMENT OF DIABETIC KETOACIDOSIS

The current consensus on management of DKA in children and adolescents has been developed from a conference of the European Society for Pediatric Endocrinology and the Lawson Wilkins Pediatric Endocrine Society (1). The management principles outlined should apply equally to pediatric HHS. Children with established diabetes, who are not vomiting or severely ill and whose caregiver has been trained in sick day management, can be managed at home or an outpatient facility, with appropriate supervision and follow-up (91–93). Children requiring IV rehydration over an extended period need to be admitted to a unit in which neurological status and vital signs can be monitored frequently and blood-glucose levels measured hourly (94). Nursing staff trained in monitoring and management of DKA should be available and there should be written guidelines (1). Those with severe DKA (long duration of symptoms, compromised circulation, and depressed level of consciousness) or with other factors increasing the risk for cerebral edema, i.e., age under five years, low pCO₂, and high serum urea nitrogen, should be in an intensive care unit, preferably pediatric, or an equivalent facility (1).

Evaluation

Differential diagnosis should include other causes of coma in children, which might be instead of or in addition to DKA (Table 3).

Table 3 Conditions Associated with Coma in Children

Metabolic derangements
Hyperglycemia (ketoacidosis, hyperosmolar state)
Hypoglycemia
Hepatic or uremic encephalopathy
Inborn errors of metabolism
Electrolyte imbalance (e.g., Addison disease, diabetes insipidus, water intoxication)
Lactic acidosis (salicylate poisoning)
Illicit substance or prescription drug
Hypoxia (CO, cyanide)
Postictal
Disturbances of the central nervous system
Meningitis
Encephalitis
Trauma/concussion
Hemorrhage (extradural, subdural, subarachnoid, intracerebral)
Brain tumor
Brain abscess
Cerebral thrombosis

Careful evaluation for infection is important; in one report approximately 30% of episodes were associated with infection, equally distributed between viral and bacterial (95). A weight should be obtained for calculation purposes.

The degree of dehydration can be estimated as 5% with reduced skin elasticity, dry mucous membranes, tachycardia, and deep breathing, up to 10% with capillary refill time greater than three seconds and sunken eyes. It is typical for calculations of fluid deficit to be based on 10% dehydration, which is a modest overestimate that does not appear to have clinical significance (96). The level of consciousness should be assessed using the Glasgow coma scale (GCS) (Table 4) (97). An initial blood sample should be tested for glucose, electrolytes, pH, urea nitrogen, creatinine, osmolality, ketones or β-hydroxybutyrate, hemoglobin and hematocrit, or complete blood count, keeping in mind that DKA is associated with leukocytosis that does not correlate with the presence or absence of infection (95). As a substitute for measured osmolality, calculated osmolality may be determined as: 2X(Na + K) + glucose in mmol/L + BUN/3. A urine specimen should be checked for ketones. Appropriate culture specimens should be obtained as indicated. If there is any possibility of delay in obtaining a serum potassium result, electrocardiographic monitoring should be done for potassium status (98,99). Continuous electrocardiographic monitoring using standard lead II should be done for severely ill patients or if the initial potassium level is less than 3 mEq/L or greater than 6 mEq/L; depressed T-waves indicate hypokalemia and peaked T-waves hyperkalemia (100).

Determination of glycohemoglobin (HbA1c) concentration will provide insight into the severity and duration of hyperglycemia in new patients and is useful for comparison to the previous determination in an established patient. It may also be useful to obtain a blood sample for measurement of free insulin before the administration of insulin to

Table 4 Glasgow Coma Scale or Score (GCS)

Best eye response	Best verbal response	Best verbal response (nonverbal children)	Best motor response
1. No eye opening	1. No verbal response	1. No response	1. No motor response
2. Eyes open to pain	2. No words, only incomprehensible sounds; moaning and groaning	2. Inconsolable, irritable, restless, cries	2. Extension to pain (decerebrate posture)
3. Eyes open to verbal command	3. Words, but incoherent[a]	3. Inconsistently consolable and moans; makes vocal sounds	3. Flexion to pain (decorticate posture)
4. Eyes open spontaneously	4. Confused, disoriented conversation[b]	4. Consolable when crying and interacts inappropriately	4. Withdrawal from pain
	5. Orientated, normal conversation	5. Smiles, oriented to sound, follows objects and interacts	5. Localizes pain
			6. Obeys commands

Note: The GCS consists of three parameters and is scored between 3 and 15; 3 being the worst and 15 the best. One of the components of the GCS is the best verbal response, which cannot be assessed in nonverbal young children. A modification of the GCS was created for children too young to talk.
[a]Inappropriate words, no sustained conversational exchange.
[b]Attention can be held; responds in a conversational manner, but shows some disorientation.
Source: From Ref. 97.

confirm an impression of failure to administer insulin as the cause of recurrent DKA (101).

The severely obtunded child will require continuous nasogastric suction for the prevention of pulmonary aspiration and may require oxygen. Bladder catheterization should be performed only in individuals who are unable to void on demand; older patients may have atonic bladder with urinary retention requiring initial catheterization, but not indwelling. Successful management and early intervention for complications require close monitoring. A flow chart should be maintained with as frequent entries as indicated by the patient's condition (Fig. 2) (101). Monitoring frequency recommendations are in Table 5 (102).

Fluid and Insulin Replacement

The goals of treatment with fluid and insulin are:

1. To restore perfusion, which will increase glucose use in the periphery, restore glomerular filtration, and reverse the progressive acidosis.
2. To arrest ketogenesis with insulin administration, reversing proteolysis and lipolysis while stimulating glucose uptake and processing, thereby normalizing blood-glucose concentration.
3. To replace electrolyte losses.
4. To avoid, insofar as possible, the complications of treatment or to intervene rapidly when they occur (102).

Fluid Therapy

- Dehydration can be assumed to be 5% to 10% (50–100 mL/kg). As noted above, clinical evaluation usually overestimates level of dehydration (96). Serum urea nitrogen and hematocrit may be useful for determining severity of extracellular fluid (ECF) contraction (92). Serum sodium concentration is not reliable for determining ECF deficit because of the osmotic effect of hyperglycemia-induced dilutional hyponatremia (103,104) and the low-sodium content of the elevated lipid fraction of the serum in DKA. Corrected sodium, i.e., for normal glucose level, can be estimated by adding 1.6 mEq to the measured value for each 100 mg/dL blood-glucose above normal (103).
- 20 mL/kg 0.9% NaCl should be provided in the first one to two hours to restore peripheral perfusion.

- Maintenance can be calculated as 1000 mL for the first 10 kg body weight + 500 mL for the next 10 kg + 20 mL/kg over 20 kg.
- The remainder of replacement after the loading dose based on 5% to 10% dehydration, and maintenance, can be distributed over the subsequent 22 to 23 hours. Some prefer to provide half of replacement in the first eight hours. It is important to consider fluids that have recently been administered orally at home (if not vomited) and parenteral fluids provided in the emergency room or referring institution.
- If osmolality (calculated or measured) is greater than 320 mosm/L, replacement can be calculated for correction in 36 hours and if greater than 340 mosm/L, in 48 hours. Except for severely ill and very young individuals, oral intake will begin before 24 hours.
- While urinary output should be carefully documented, urinary losses should not be added to fluid requirements (1).
- After initial 0.9% NaCl bolus, rehydration/maintenance should be continued with 0.45% NaCl. During rehydration, the measured Na can increase to the level of the corrected Na as glycemia declines and then decline to normal levels if the corrected level was elevated.
- The use of large amounts of 0.9% saline may result in hyperchloremic metabolic acidosis (105,106).
- To prevent unduly rapid decline in plasma glucose concentration and hypoglycemia, 5% glucose should be added to the IV fluid when the plasma glucose falls to 300 mg/dL (17 mmol/L). An efficient method of providing glucose as needed without long delays entailed by the changing of IV solutions is to have two IV fluid bags connected, one containing 10% dextrose and the appropriate sodium and potassium concentrations and the other with the same salt concentrations but no dextrose, the so-called "two bag system" (107).
- Potassium (20–40 mEq/L or up to 80 mEq/L as needed) can be provided as half KCL, half KPO_4 (to replenish low phosphate levels and to decrease the risk of hyperchloremia) or as half KPO_4 and half K acetate (which, like lactate, is converted to bicarbonate to help correct acidosis) after serum K reported as less than 6 mmol/L or urine flow is established. Serum potassium concentration increases by approximately 0.6 mEq/L for every 0.1 decrease in pH, so that the serum potassium level does not reflect the large deficit from diuresis and vomiting. Both potassium and phosphate shift markedly from

name _____ birthdate _____ admission date/time _____

weight _____ height _____ duration of diabetes _____

time								
hrs:min since admission								
Vital Signs								
temp								
pulse								
blood pressure								
respiratory rate								
GCS								
pupil size								
pupil reaction								
cap refill time								
Laboratory								
glucose								
pH								
sodium								
potassium								
chloride								
CO2								
HCO3								
BUN								
creatinine								
ketones serum								
ketones urine								
βOHbytyrate								
osmolality measured								
osmolality calculated								
calcium								
phosphorus								
magnesium								
Fluids and Insulin								
type								
potassium mEq/L								
rate								
intake								
urine output								
insulin units/hour								

Figure 2 Flow chart for monitoring the evolution of patients.

intracellular to extracellular compartments with acidosis and reenter cells rapidly with insulin-induced glucose uptake and rehydration (100,108).

■ Bicarbonate is very rarely indicated. There is no evidence that bicarbonate facilitates metabolic recovery. Restoring circulatory volume will improve tissue perfusion and renal function, increasing organic acid excretion and reversing lactic acidosis. The administration of insulin stops further synthesis of ketoacids and reactivates the Krebs cycle, permitting metabolism of them and regeneration of bicarbonate. Bicarbonate therapy may cause paradoxical CNS acidosis, rapid correction of acidosis can cause hypokalemia, the additional sodium can add to hyperosmolality, and

Table 5 Monitoring Treatment of Diabetic Ketoacidosis or Hyperglycemic Hyperosmolar State in Children

Measure	Interval
Clinical	
Vital signs	20–60 min[a]
Coma score	20–60 min[a]
Pupillary size and reaction	20–60 min[a]
Capillary refill time	30–60 min until < 3 sec
Laboratory	
Glucose	Hourly bedside; laboratory with electrolytes
Potassium	Hourly if < 3 or > 6 mmol/L
Sodium, potassium, CO2 or HCO3, venous pH, osmolality	Admission, 2, 6, 10, 24 hr
Serum urea nitrogen	Admission, 12, 24 hr
Calcium, phosphorus, magnesium	Admission, 12, 24 hr
β-hydroxybutyrate	Admission, 6, 12, 24 hr
Ketonuria	Admission, 4–6 hourly
Fluids	
Type and rate	
Potassium content and type	
Intravenous and oral intake	
Output (urine, gastrointestinal)	
Insulin	

[a] Depending on risk factors for cerebral edema.

alkali therapy can increase hepatic ketone production, potentially slowing recovery from ketosis (1). The extremely rare circumstance which may benefit from cautious alkali therapy is severe acidemia in which tachypnic response is inadequate or persistent compromised perfusion following initial fluid expansion suggests decreased cardiac contractility and peripheral vasodilatation (1). Safe administration to avoid risk of hypokalemia is to give 1 to 2 mEq/kg body weight or 80 mEq/m^2 body surface area over two hours (10). The NaCl concentration in the fluids should be reduced to allow for added Na ion.

Insulin

■ Insulin should be started after the initial fluid expansion is completed for a more realistic starting glucose level.
■ The most widely used system is 0.1 U/kg hourly as a continuous infusion, using a pump. 50 units of regular insulin is diluted in 50 mL normal saline to provide 1 U/mL.
■ A bolus dose is not necessary and may increase the risk of cerebral edema (109).
■ It may be more convenient in some settings to administer insulin subcutaneously. In adults, there did not seem to be any difference whether insulin was administered intravenously, intramuscularly, or subcutaneously after the first couple of hours of treatment (110–113). The first study of subcutaneous insulin in children with DKA using rapid-acting insulin analogue (lispro) provided a dose of 0.15 U/kg every two hours, finding no essential differences from children randomized to receive 0.1 U/kg/hr intravenously (114). The administration of 0.1 U/kg subcutaneously every hour may be preferable and can be adjusted to maintain blood-glucose concentration at approximately 250 mg/dL (11 mmol/L).

■ During initial fluid expansion, a high blood-glucose level may drop 200 to 300 mg/dL even without insulin infusion. High blood-glucose levels should drop 50 to 150 mg/dL/hr (but not more than 200 mg/dL/hr), and if they do not, the dose should be increased. This is rarely necessary.
■ If the blood-glucose level falls below 150 mg/dL with 10% dextrose solution running, the insulin dose should be reduced to 0.05 U/kg/hr.
■ Insulin should not be stopped or reduced below 0.05 U/kg/hr, because a continuous supply of insulin is needed to prevent ketosis and permit continued anabolism.
■ Persistent acidosis, defined as bicarbonate value less than 10 mmol/L after 8 to 10 hours of treatment, is usually caused by inadequate insulin effect, indicated by persistent hyperglycemia. Insulin dilution and rate of administration should be checked, and a fresh preparation made if older than six to eight hours. Too dilute a solution may enhance adsorption to the tubing. If insulin is being given by subcutaneous injection, inadequate absorption may be occurring or there may be resistance due to unusually high counter-regulatory hormones, as with concomitant febrile illness (102). Extremely rare causes of persistent acidosis are lactic acidosis due to an episode of hypotension, apnea, or inadequate renal competency in the handling of hydrogen ion as a result of an episode of renal hypoperfusion (102).

Transition

■ IV fluids can be stopped one to two hours after substantial consumption of oral fluids without vomiting.
■ Subcutaneous insulin injection can be started when the patient no longer needs IV fluids. It is most convenient to wait until the presupper or prebreakfast time to restart intermediate- or long-acting insulin. Until then, regular insulin 0.25 U/kg subcutaneously can be given every six hours approximately, and the insulin infusion stopped 60 to 120 minutes after the first subcutaneous dose of regular insulin or 15 to 30 minutes after rapid-acting insulin analogue.
■ Patients should not be kept in the hospital simply to adjust insulin dosage, because food, activity, and psychosocial environment in the hospital are not normal.

Prevention

The prevention of hyperglycemic coma in children and adolescents requires a diligent health-care system. The prevention of DKA at onset is possible when early diagnosis is made through genetic and immunologic screening of high-risk children (18,32). For the larger population, an example has been provided by the Italian school and physician awareness program directed at 6- to 14-year olds, which reduced the rates of DKA from 78% to near 0% over six years (21). The reports of death from HHS with undiagnosed T2DM emphasize the need to educate emergency physicians and others of the risk of this preventable mortality (16,17).

Recurrent DKA was demonstrated to be dramatically reduced 30 years ago by a comprehensive program involving outreach clinics, frequent routine and emergency telephone contact, and a camping program supported by a state program for children with special health-care needs. Private patients in the program had a reduction in hospital admission days from preintervention of 2.8 to 0.3/patient/yr and in the second year to 0/patient/year. The state program sponsored children had a reduction from 4.9 to 1.8/patient/yr and in the second year to 0.9/patient/yr (33). Guidelines for sick day management will vary depending on whether the child is being treated with multiple injections or uses a pump; recommendations are in Vol. 1; Chap. 7.

Patients with compliance problems resulting in recurrent DKA account for a disproportionate number of recurrent DKA episodes; in the U.K. surveillance study, 4.8% of patients accounted for 22.5% of all episodes (41). Insulin omission is the principal immediate reason for the development of DKA in children and adolescents, reflected in low or absent levels of free insulin (67). While psychosocial intervention is of importance, the necessity for assuring administration of insulin by responsible adults is paramount.

CONCLUSIONS

In addition to DKA, which occurs in T1DM and T2DM, HHS has been increasingly observed with the recent surge in incidence of T2DM. Frequency of DKA at onset of T1DM varies regionally and internationally from 10% to 70%, depending on availability of health care and frequency of diabetes. At the onset of T2DM, DKA occurs in 5% to 52%. One study suggests that approximately 4% of new T2DM presents with HHS. Variables of medical services and socioeconomic circumstances determine recurrent DKA rates, estimated to be 8 episodes/100 patient years, with 20% of patients accounting for 80% of the episodes. Mortality for each episode of DKA internationally varies from 0.15% to 0.31%, with idiopathic cerebral edema accounting for two-thirds or more of this mortality. Other causes of death or disability include untreated HHS, hypokalemia, hypophosphatemia, hypoglycemia, other intracerebral complications, peripheral venous thrombosis, mucormycosis, rhabdomyolysis, acute pancreatitis, acute renal failure, sepsis, aspiration pneumonia, and other pulmonary complications. Population-based studies from the United Kingdom, Australia, the United States, and Canada report cerebral edema incidence in DKA of 0.5% to 2.0%. As many as approximately 20% of occurrences of cerebral edema may be present before treatment is undertaken. Published information does not support the notion that treatment factors are causal in most cerebral edema. Younger age, greater severity of acidosis, degree of hypocapnia, and severity of dehydration have been suggested as risk factors in several studies. Bimodal distribution of the time of onset of cerebral edema and wide variation in brain imaging findings provide clues to the complexity and variability of this problem and the possibility of multiple causation of the clinical picture. Functional brain scanning has indicated that DKA is accompanied by increased CBF, suggesting that the predominant mechanism of edema formation

is a vasogenic process. A method of monitoring for diagnostic, major, and minor signs of cerebral edema has been proposed and tested, which indicates that intervention will be required in five individuals to provide early intervention for a single case of cerebral edema. The preferred intervention of mannitol infusion has typically been accompanied by intubation and hyperventilation, but recent evidence indicates outcome is adversely affected by aggressive hyperventilation.

The frequency of new onset DKA and its attendant morbidity and mortality cannot be reduced without a substantial investment in public, school, and physician education, for recognition of new onset diabetes before progression to acidosis. More focused investment in comprehensive supervision and 24-hour availability of knowledgeable health personnel are needed to prevent recurrent DKA. Studies of the efficacy and cost-effectiveness of such efforts are needed. The prevention of HHS and its attendant morbidity and mortality requires a high index of suspicion for the high-risk obese group who may not have typical signs and symptoms of diabetes and whose dehydration may be masked by their obesity. We are a long way from understanding enough about cerebral edema to know how to prevent it, but knowledgeable individuals treating DKA can prevent most of the devastating morbidity and mortality by early intervention. Increasingly sophisticated and perhaps bedside functional imaging techniques may be both informative and diagnostic. The recent observations of efficacy of hypertonic saline as an alternative to mannitol to treat cerebral edema suggest a need for further investigation.

REFERENCES

1. Dunger DB, Sperling MA, Acerini CL, et al. European society for paediatric endocrinology/Lawson Wilkins pediatric endocrine society consensus statement on diabetic ketoacidosis in children and adolescents. Pediatrics 2004; 113: e133–e140.
2. Burge MR, Hardy KJ, Schade DS. Short-term fasting is a mechanism for the development of euglycemic ketoacidosis during periods of insulin deficiency. J Clin Endocrinol Metab 1993; 76(5):1192–1198.
3. Pinkey JH, Bingley PJ, Sawtell PA, Dunger DB, Gale EA. Presentation and progress of childhood diabetes mellitus: a prospective population-based study. The Bart's-Oxford Study Group. Diabetologia 1994; 37(1):70–74.
4. American Diabetes Association. Position statement: hyperglycemic crises in patients with diabetes mellitus. Diabet Care 2001; 24(suppl):S83–S90.
5. Rubin HM, Kramer R, Drash A. Hyperosmolality complicating diabetes mellitus in childhood. J Pediat 1969; 74: 177–186.
6. Belmonte MM, Colle E, Murphy DA, Wiglesworth FW. Nonketotic hyperosmolar diabetic coma in Down's syndrome. J Pediat 1970; 77:879–881.
7. Ehrlich RM, Bain HW. Hyperglycemia and hyperosmolarity in an eighteen-month-old child. N Engl J Med 1967; 276:683–684.
8. Laugier J, Grenier B, Dupin M, Desbuquois G. Coma hyperosmolaire chez un enfant diabetique. Ann Pediat 1969; 16:604–607.

9. Thomsen K. Diabetic coma without ketonuria. Acta Paediat Scand 1971; 60:247–248.

10. Fernandez F, Hughes ER. Nonketotic hyperosmolar diabetic coma in an infant. J Pediat 1974; 84:606–614.

11. Dorchy H, Pardou A, Weemaes I, Loeb H. Coma hyperosmolaire acido-cetosique sans cetonurie initiale. Pediatrie 1975; 30:19–27.

12. Ginsberg-Fellner F, Primack WA. Recurrent hyperosmolar nonketotic episodes in a young diabetic. Am J Dis Child 1975; 129:240–243.

13. Vernon DD, Postellon DC. Nonketotic hyperosmolal diabetic coma in a child: management with low dose insulin infusion and intracranial pressure monitoring. Pediatrics 1986; 77:770–772.

14. Morales A, Rosenbloom AL. Death at the onset of type 2 diabetes (T2DM) in African-American youth. Pediatr Res 2002; 51:124A.

15. Hollander AS, Olney RC, Blackett PR, Marshall BA. Fatal malignant hyperthermia-like syndrome with rhabdomyolysis complicating the presentation of diabetes mellitus in adolescent males. Pediatrics 2003; 111:1447–1452.

16. Morales A, Rosenbloom AL. Death caused by hyperglycemic hyperosmolar state at the onset of type 2 diabetes. J Pediar 2004; 144:270–273.

17. Fourtner SH, Weinzimer SA, Katz LEL. Hyperglycemic hyperosmolar nonketotic syndrome in children with type 2 diabetes. Pediatr Diabet 2005; 6:129–135.

18. Lévy-Marchal C, Patterson CC, Green A, on behalf of the EURODIAB ACE study group. Geographical variation of presentation at diagnosis of type 1 diabetes in children: the EURODIAB Study. Diabetologia 2001; 44(Suppl 3):B75–B80.

19. Bui TP, Werther GA, Cameron EJ. Trends in diabetic ketoacidosis in childhood and adolescence: a 15-yr experience. Pediatr Diabet 2002; 3:82–88.

20. Jackson W, Hoffman PL, Robinson EM, Elliot RB, Pilcher CC, Cutfield WS. The changing presentation of children with newly diagnosed type 1 diabetes mellitus. Pediatr Diabet 2001; 2:154–159.

21. Vanelli M, Chiari G, Ghizzoni L, Costi G, Giacalone T, Chiarelli F. Effectiveness of a prevention program for diabetic ketoacidosis in children. An 8-year study in schools and private practices. Diabet Care 1999; 22:7–9.

22. Mallare JT, Cordice CC, Ryan BA, Carey DE, Kreitzer PM, Frank GR. Identifying risk factors for the development of diabetic ketoacidosis in new onset type 1 diabetes mellitus. Clin Pediatr 2003; 42:591–597.

23. Maniatis AK, Goehrig SH, Gao D, Rewers A, Walravens P, Klingensmith G. Increased incidence and severity of diabetic ketoacidosis among uninsured children with newly diagnosed type 1 diabetes mellitus. Pediatr Diabet 2005; 6:79–83.

24. Neu A, Willasch A, Ehehalt S, Hub R, Ranke MB, on behalf of the DIARY group Baden-Wuerttemberg. Ketoacidosis at onset of type 1 diabetes mellitus in children-frequency and clinical presentation. Pediatr Diabet 2003; 4:77–81.

25. Roche EF, Menon A, Gill D, Hoey H. Clinical presentation of type 1 diabetes. Pediatr Diabet 2005; 6:75–78.

26. American Diabetes Association. Type 2 diabetes in children and adolescents. Diabet Care 2000; 23:381–389.

27. Macaluso CJ, Bauer UE, Deeb LC, et al. Type 2 diabetes mellitus among Florida children and adolescents, 1994 through 1998. Public Health Rep 2002; 117:373–379.

28. Zdravkovic V, Daneman D, Hamilton J. Presentation and course of type 2 diabetes in youth in a large multi-ethnic city. Diabet Med 2004; 21:1144–1148.

29. Glaser NS, Jones KL. Non-insulin-dependent diabetes mellitus in Mexican-American children. West J Med 1998; 168:11–16.

30. Pinhas-Hamiel O, Dolan LM, Zeitler PS. Diabetic ketoacidosis among obese African-American adolescents with NIDDM. Diabet Care 1997; 20:484–486.

31. Scott CR, Smith JM, Cradock MM, Pihoker CI. Characteristics of youth-onset non-insulin dependent diabetes mellitus and insulin dependent diabetes mellitus at diagnosis. Pediatrics 1997; 100:84–91.

32. Predictors of acute complications in children with type 1 diabetes. JAMA 2002; 287:2511–2518.

33. Giordano B, Rosenbloom AL, Heller DR, Weber FT, Gonzales R, Grgic A. Regional services for children and youth with diabetes. Pediatrics 1977; 60:492–498.

34. Golden MP, Herrold AJ, Orr DP. An approach to prevention of recurrent diabetic ketoacidosis in the pediatric population. J Pediatr 1985; 107:195–200.

35. Foster DW, McGarry JD. The metabolic derangements and treatment of diabetic ketoacidosis. N Engl J Med 1983; 309(3):159–169.

36. Levitsky L, Ekwo E, Goselink CA, Solomon EL, Aceto T. Death from diabetes (DM) in hospitalized children (1970–1998) (abstract). Pediatr Res 1991; 29:A195.

37. Recent trends in hospitalization for diabetic ketoacidosis in Ontario children. Diabet Care 2002; 25:1591–1596.

38. Lawrence SE, Cummings EA, Gaboury I, Daneman D. Population-based study of incidence and risk factors for cerebral edema in pediatric diabetic ketoacidosis. J Pediatr 2005; 146:688–692.

39. Edge JA, Ford-Adams ME, Dunger DB. Causes of death in children with insulin-dependent diabetes 1990–96. Arch Dis Child 1999; 81:318–323.

40. Rosenbloom AL. Intracerebral crises during treatment of diabetic ketoacidosis. Diabet Care 1990; 13:22–33.

41. Edge JA, Hawkins MM, Winter DL, Dunger DB. The risk and outcome of cerebral oedema developing during diabetic ketoacidosis. Arch Dis Child 2001; 85:16–22.

42. Glaser N, Barnett P, McCaslin I, et al. Risk factors for cerebral edema in children with diabetic ketoacidosis. N Engl J Med 2001; 344:264–269.

43. Lipton R, Good G, Mikhailov T, Freels S, Donoghue E. Ethnic differences in mortality from insulin-dependent diabetes mellitus among people less than 25 years of age. Pediatrics 1999; 103:952–956.

44. Kershaw MJR, Newton TG, Barrett TG, Berry K, Kirk J. Childhood diabetes presenting with hyperosmolar dehydration but without ketoacidosis: a report of three cases. Diabet Med 2005; 22:645–647.

45. McDonnell CM, Pedreira CC, Vadamalayan B, Cameron FJ, Werther GA. Diabetic ketoacidosis, hyperosmolarity and hypernatremia: are high-carbohydrate drinks worsening initial presentation?. Pediatr Diabet 2005; 6:90–94.

46. Casteels, K, Beckers D, Wouters C, Van Geet C. Rhabdomyolysis in diabetic ketoacidosis. Pediatr Diabet 2003; 4:29–31.

47. Buckingham BA, Roe TF, Yoon J-W. Rhabdomyolysis in diabetic ketoacidosis. Am J Dis Child 1981; 135:352–354.

48. Moye J, Rosenbloom AL, Silverstein J. Clinical predictors of mucormycosis in type 1 diabetes in children. J Ped Endocrinol Metab 2002; 15:1001–1004.

49. Haddad NG, Croffie JM, Rugster EA. Pancreatic enzyme elevations in children with diabetic ketoacidosis. J Pediatr 2004; 145:122–124.

50. Gutierrez JA, Bagatell R, Samson MP, Theodorou AA, Berg RA. Femoral central venous catheter-associated deep venous thrombosis in children with diabetic ketoacidosis. Crit Care Med 2003; 31:80–83.

51. Worly JM, Fortenberry JD, Hansen I, Chambliss CR, Stockwell J. Deep venous thrombosis in children with diabetic ketoacidosis and femoral central venous catheters. Pediatrics 2004; 113:57–60.

52. Zeitler P, Thiede A, Muller HL. Prospective study on plasma clotting parameters in diabetic children—no evidence for specific changes in coagulation system. Exp Clin Endorinol Diabet 2001; 109:146–152.

53. Carl CF, Hoffman WH, Passmore GG, et al. Diabetic ketoacidosis promotes a prothrombotic state. Endo Res 2003; 29:73–82.

54. Roberts MD, Slover RH, Chase HP. Diabetic ketoacidosis with intracerebral complications. Pediatr Diabet 2001; 2: 109–114.

55. Keane S, Gallagher A, Aykroyd S, McShane MA, Edge JA. Cerebral venous thrombosis during diabetic ketoacidosis. Arch Dis Child 2002; 86:204–206.

56. Rosenbloom AL. Fatal cerebral infarctions in diabetic ketoacidosis in a child with previously unknown heterozygosity for factor V Leiden deficiency. J Pediatr 2004; 145:561–562.

57. Yoon J-W, Austin M, Onodera T, Notkins AL. Virus-induced diabetes mellitus. N Engl J Med 1979; 300: 1173–1179.

58. Cooper RM, Turner RA, Hutaff L, Prichard R. Diabetic keto-acidosis complicated by disseminated intravascular coagulation. South Med J 1973; 66:653–657.

59. Bonfanti R, Bognetti E, Meschi F, Medaglini S, D'Angelo A, Chiumello G. Disseminated intravascular coagulation and severe peripheral neuropathy complicating ketoacidosis in a newly diagnosed diabetic child. Acta Diabetol 1994; 31:173–174.

60. De Stefano V, Rossi E, Paciaroni K, Leone G. Screening for inherited thrombophilia: indications and therapeutic implications. Haematologica 2002; 87:1095–1108.

61. Carvalho KS, Bodensteiner JB, Connolly PJ, Garg BP. Cerebral venous thrombosis in children. J Child Neurol 2001; 16:574–580.

62. Young E, Bradley RF. Cerebral edema with irreversible coma in severe diabetic ketoacidosis. N Engl J Med 1967; 276:665–669.

63. Rosenbloom AL, Riley WJ, Weber FT, Malone JI, Donnelly WH. Cerebral edema complicating diabetic ketoacidosis in childhood. J Pediatr 1980; 96:357–361.

64. Bello FA, Sotos JF. Cerebral oedema in diabetic ketoacidosis in children (letter). Lancet 1990; 336:64.

65. Brown TB. Cerebral oedema in childhood diabetic ketoacidosis: Is treatment a factor?. Emerg Med J 2004; 21: 141–144.

66. Dunger DB, Edge JA. Predicting cerebral edema during diabetic ketoacidosis (editorial). N Engl J Med 2001; 344: 302–303.

67. Azzopardi J, Gatt A, Zammit A, Albert G. Lack of evidence of cerebral edema in adults treated for diabetic ketoacidosis with fluids of different tonicity. Diabetes Res Clin Practice 2002; 57:87–92.

68. Carroll P, Matz R. Uncontrolled diabetes mellitus in adults: experience in treating diabetic ketoacidosis and hyperosmolar nonketotic coma with low dose insulin and a uniform treatment regimen. Diabet Care 1983; 6:579–585.

69. Hale PM, Rezvani I, Braunstein AW, Lipman TH, Martinez N, Garibaldi L. Factors predicting cerebral edema in young children with diabetic ketoacidosis and new onset type I diabetes. Acta Paediatr 1997; 86: 626–631.

70. Muir AB, Quisling RG, Yang MCK, Rosenbloom AL. Cerebral edema in childhood diabetic ketoacidosis. Natural history, radiographic findings, and early identification. Diabet Care 2004; 27:1541–1546.

71. Marcin JP, Glaser N, Barnett P, et al. Factors associated with adverse outcomes in children with diabetic ketoacidosis-related cerebral edema. J Pediatr 2002; 141:793–797.

72. Pappius HM. Fundamental aspects of brain edema. In: Vinkin PJ, Bruyn GW, eds. Handbook of Clinical Neurology, Vol. 16. Part 1: Tumors of the Brain and Skull. Amsterdam: North Holland: Publishing Co., 1974: 167–185.

73. Salem MAK, Matta LF, Tantawy AAG, Hussein M, Gad GI. Single photon emission tomography (SPECT) study of regional cerebral blood flow in normoalbuminuric children and adolescents with type 1 diabetes. Pediatr Diabet 2002; 3:155–162.

74. Krane EJ, Rockoff MA, Wallman JK, Wolfsdorf JI. Subclinical brain swelling in children during treatment of diabetic ketoacidosis. N Engl J Med 1985; 312: 1147–1151.

75. Durr JA, Hoffman WH, Sklar AH, el Gammal T, Steinhart CM. Correlates of brain edema in uncontrolled IDDM. Diabetes 1992; 41:627–632.

76. Glaser N, Wooten-Gorges SL, Marcin JP, et al. Mechanism of cerebral edema in children with diabetic ketoacidosis. J Pediatr 2004; 145:164–171.

77. Levitsky LL. Symptomatic cerebral edema in diabetic ketoacidosis: the mechanism is clarified but still far from clear (editorial). J Pediatr 2004; 145:149–150.

78. Wooten-Gorges SL, Buonocore MH, Kuppermann N, et al. Detection of cerebral b-hydroxy butyrate, acetoacetate, and lactate on proton NMR spectroscopy in children with diabetic ketoacidosis. Am J Neuroradiol 2005; 26:1286–1291.

79. Cameron FJ, Kean MJ, Wellard RM, Werther GA, Neil JJ, Iner TE. Insights into the acute cerebral metabolic changes associated with childhood diabetes. Diabet Med 2005; 22: 648–653.

80. Hoffman WH, Burek CL, Waller JL, Fisher LE, Khichi M, Mellick LB. Cytokine response to diabetic ketoacidosis and its treatment. Clin Immunol 2003; 108:175–181.

81. Muizelaar JP, Marmarou A, Ward JD, et al. Adverse effects of prolonged hyperventilation in patients with severe head injury: a randomized clinical trial. J Neurosurg 1991; 75: 731–739.

82. Shapiro HM, Drummond JC. Neurosurgical anesthesia. In: Miller RD, ed. Anesthesia. 3rd. New York: Churchill Livingstone, 1990:1913–1914.

83. Zornow MH, Oh YS, Scheller MS. A comparison of the cerebral and haemodynamic effects of mannitol and hypertonic saline in an animal model of brain injury. Acta Neurochir Suppl 1990; 51:324–325.

84. Qureshi AI, Wilson DA, Traystman RJ. Treatment of elevated intracranial pressure in experimental intracerebral hemorrhage: comparison between mannitol and hypertonic saline. Neurosurgery 1999; 44:1055–1063.

85. Freshman SP, Battistella FD, Matteucci M, Wisner DH. Hypertonic saline (7.5%) versus mannitol: a comparison for treatment of acute head injuries. J Trauma 1993; 35: 344–348.

86. Berger S, Schurer L, Hartl R, Messmer K, Baethmann A. Reduction of post-traumatic intracranial hypertension by hypertonic/hyperoncotic saline/dextran and hypertonic mannitol. Neurosurgery 1995; 37:98–107.

87. Gemma M, Cozzi S, Tommasino C, et al. 7.5% hypertonic saline versus 20% mannitol during elective neurosurgical supratentorial procedures. J Neurosurg Anesthesiol 1997; 9:329–334.

88. Worthley LI, Cooper DJ, Jones N. Treatment of resistant intracranial hypertension with hypertonic saline. Report of two cases. J Neurosurg 1988; 68:478–481.

89. Qureshi AL, Suarez JI. Use of hypertonic saline solutions in treatment of cerebral edema and intracranial hypertension. Crit Care Med 2000; 28:3301–3313.

90. Curtis JR, Bohn D, Daneman D. Use of hypertonic saline in the treatment of cerebral edema in diabetic ketoacidosis (DKA). Pediatr Diabet 2001; 2:191–194.

91. Bonadio WA, Gutzeit MF, Losek JD, Smith DS. Outpatient management of diabetic ketoacidosis. Am J Dis Child 1988; 142(4):448–450.

92. Linares MY, Schunk JE, Lindsay R. Laboratory presentation in diabetic ketoacidosis and duration of therapy. Pediatr Emerg Care 1996; 12(5):347–351.

93. Chase HP, Garg SK, Jelley DH. Diabetic ketoacidosis in children and the role of outpatient management. Pediatr Rev 1990; 11(10):297–304.

94. Rosenbloom AL, Schatz DA. Diabetic ketoacidosis in childhood. Pediatr Ann 1994; 23:284–288.

95. Flood RG, Chiang VW. Rate and prediction of infection in children with diabetic ketoacidosis. Am J Emerg Med 2001; 19:270–273.

96. Koves IH, Neutze J, Donath S, et al. The accuracy of clinical assessment of dehydration during diabetic ketoacidosis in childhood. Diabet Care 2004; 27:2485–2487.

97. Teasdale G, Jennett B. Assessment of coma and impaired consciousness. A practical scale. Lancet 1974; 2(7872): 81–84.

98. Malone JI, Brodsky SJ. The value of electrocardiogram monitoring in diabetic ketoacidosis. Diabet Care 1980; 3(4):543–547.

99. Soler NG, Bennett MA, Fitzgerald MG, Malins JM. Electrocardiogram as a guide to potassium replacement in diabetic ketoacidosis. Diabetes 1974; 23(7):610–615.

100. Schatz DA, Rosenbloom AL. Diabetic ketoacidosis: management tactics in young patients. J Crit Illn 1988; 3:29–41.

101. Plasma free insulin concentrations: keystone to effective management of diabetes mellitus in children. J Pediatr 1981; 99:862–867.

102. Rosenbloom AL, Hanas R. Diabetic ketoacidosis (DKA): treatment guidelines. Clin Pediatr 1996; 35:261–266.

103. Katz MA. Hyperglycemia-induced hyponatremia—calculation of expected serum sodium depression. N Engl J Med 1973; 289(16):843–844.

104. Hillier TA, Abbott RD, Barrett EJ. Hyponatremia: evaluating the correction factor for hyperglycemia. Am J Med 1999; 106(4):399–403.

105. Adrogue HJ, Eknoyan G, Suki WK. Diabetic ketoacidosis: role of the kidney in the acid-base homeostasis re-evaluated. Kidney Int 1984; 25(4):591–598.

106. Oh MS, Carroll HJ, Uribarri J. Mechanism of normochloremic and hyperchloremic acidosis in diabetic ketoacidosis. Nephron 1990; 54(1):1–6.

107. Poirier MP, Greer D, Satin-Smith M. A prospective study of the "two bag system" in diabetic ketoacidosis management. Clin Pediatr 2004; 43:809–813.

108. Rosenbloom AL, Ongley JP. Serum calcium phosphorus and magnesium decrement during oral glucose tolerance testing: alteration in pre-clinical and overt diabetes mellitus in childhood. In: Catin M, Selig M, eds. Magnesium in Health and Disease. Jamaica, New York: Spectrum Publishers Inc, 1980:297–304.

109. Edge J, Jakes R, Roy Y, et al. The UK propsective study of cerebral oedema complicating diabetic ketoacidosis. Arch Dis Child 2005; 90(Suppl 11):A2–A3.

110. Fisher J, Shahshahani M, Kitabchi A. Diabetic ketoacidosis: low dose insulin therapy by various routes. N Engl J Med 1977; 297:238–243.

111. Sacks HS, Shahshahani M, Kitabchi AE, Fisher JN, Young RT. Similar responsiveness of diabetic ketoacidosis to low-dose insulin by intramuscular injection and albumin-free infusion. Ann Intern Med 1979; 90(1):36–42.

112. Umpierrez GE, Latif K, Stoever J, et al. Efficacy of subcutaneous insulin lispro versus continuous intravenous regular insulin for the treatment of patients with diabetic ketoacidosis. Am J Med 2004; 117(5):291–296.

113. Umpierrez GE, Cuervo R, Karabell A, Latif K, Freire AX, Kitabchi AE. Treatment of diabetic ketoacidosis with subcutaneous insulin aspart. Diabet Care 2004; 7(8):1873–1878.

114. Manna TD, Steinmetz L, Campos PR, et al. Subcutaneous use of a fast-acting insulin analog. An alternative treatment for pediatric patients with diabetic ketoacidosis. Diabet Care 2005; 28:1856–1861.

9

Type 2 Diabetes in the Child and Adolescent

Jennifer Miller, Janet H. Silverstein, and Arlan L. Rosenbloom

Division of Pediatric Endocrinology, Department of Pediatrics, University of Florida,
Gainesville, Florida, U.S.A.

INTRODUCTION

Type 2 diabetes mellitus (T2DM) in children and adolescents is becoming an increasingly important public health concern throughout the world. In North America, T2DM comprises 30% of all newly diagnosed diabetes in patients 10 to 20 years of age (1). Not surprisingly, this epidemic is closely associated with the increased prevalence of obesity among youth of all ethnic backgrounds (1,2), as increased visceral adipose tissue produces adipokines, which increase insulin resistance (3). There is a clear relationship between T2DM and the insulin resistance/metabolic syndrome, which includes abdominal obesity, disturbed glucose regulation, dyslipidemia, and hypertension (4). The contemporary epidemic of T2DM in youth has given pediatric diabetes specialists a major responsibility for a condition that was previously rare in the pediatric age group. As they earlier did for Type 1 diabetes mellitus (T1DM), pediatric diabetologists are developing teams to deal with this difficult and growing clinical challenge of obesity and T2DM.

Because of the relatively recent recognition of the problem in this age group, there may be many affected individuals who are undiagnosed, as well as many children who are misclassified as having T1DM. Risk factors for cardiovascular disease are already present at the time of diagnosis of T2DM, making immediate and continuing normalization of blood-glucose levels, blood pressure (BP), and lipids desirable.

EPIDEMIOLOGY

Beginning around 1990, pediatric endocrinologists, who had been aware for decades of a small proportion of their diabetes patients having Type 2 disease (5), noticed a sharp increase in the numbers of patients with T2DM (6). This was predominantly, but not exclusively, seen in the African-American and Mexican Hispanic-American population, indicating there may be ethnic differences in background insulin sensitivity. In studies from Cincinnati, Arkansas, and Texas, African-Americans accounted for 70% to 75% of pediatric T2DM (7,8). It is estimated that one-third of Mexican-American children and youth with diabetes in southern California and over two-thirds of those in South Texas have T2DM (9,10). Native Americans were the first to have been reported with a substantial number of children having T2DM, with a 1% prevalence noted as early as 1979 (11).

There is little argument that T2DM in children and adolescents has become an epidemic. The first recognition of a substantial prevalence was in 1977 among 15- to 24-year-old Pima Indians, with nine out of 1000 (0.9%) having diabetes associated with obesity and early onset of microvascular and cardiovascular complications (11). This was in a population in which 50% of adults have T2DM. Half of these youngsters had ketoacidosis. By the 1990s, 5% of 15- to 19-year-olds and 2.2% of 10- to 14-year-olds (previously 0%) had T2DM (12). Records from six Indian Health Service facilities in Montana and Wyoming showed that 53% of prevalent cases and 70% of incident cases were suspected to be T2DM, making the average annual incidence rate of T2DM for this population 23.3 per 100,000, four times higher than the incidence rate of T1DM in the same population (13). Among First Nations people in Canada, the frequency of T2DM in children and youth is comparable with that of T1DM in Caucasians (14).

Reports from throughout the United States show that the percentage of patients with new-onset diabetes diagnosed as having T2DM increased from 2% to 4% in 1994 to 20% to 50% by 2000 (15). The percentage of patients diagnosed with T2DM had previously been stable. Knowles reported approximately 3.5% of patients in a Cincinnati-based diabetes clinic having T2DM in 1971 (5); a similar proportion (2.4%) was noted from the same clinic between 1982 and 1992, with a sharp increase to 16% by 1994 (13). In Native North Americans, there have been four to six times as many females as males affected, but in the African-American and Mexican-American groups with T2DM, the sex ratio has been far less skewed, varying from 1.7 females for every male in African-Americans to nearly 1:1 in Mexican-Americans (16).

A study of 682 5- to 19-year-olds diagnosed between January 1, 1994 and December 31, 1998 at the three University-based diabetes centers in Florida found that 14% of the patients had T2DM. While 47% of T1DM patients were female, 63% of T2DM patients were female (17). In contrast to the studies from Arkansas and Cincinnati, African-Americans comprised only 46% of those with T2DM, while 22% were Hispanic, and the rest non-Hispanic whites. The risk for developing T2DM was three times greater for African-American youngsters and 3.5 times greater for Hispanics than for whites. During the initial year of the study, 8.7% of newly diagnosed patients were eventually classified as having T2DM, whereas in the last year of the study 19% were thus classified, indicating a twofold increase in the proportion of new diabetes patients in this age group having T2DM over the relatively brief period of five years (17).

The recognition of an epidemic of T2DM is not unique to North America. In Japan 80% of all new cases of diabetes in children and adolescents in 2000 were T2DM. Annual urine testing for glucose of schoolchildren in the Tokyo area has been carried out since 1975, followed by oral glucose tolerance testing for those who have glucosuria. In the primary school age group the incidence of T2DM increased from 0.2 per 100,000 in 1976 to 2 per 100,000 in 1995, while in the 12- to 15-year age group, there has been a doubling of incidence of T2DM from 7.2 to 13.9 per 100,000, paralleling increasing obesity rates (15). In contrast, the incidence of T1DM was 1.5 cases per 100,000 in 1976 and did not change appreciably over the next 20 years. Other reports indicate that increasing rates of T2DM with concurrent increases in obesity are also being observed in children in Thailand, China, India, New Zealand, Australia, and throughout Europe (15). The prevalence of T2DM in England is estimated at 0.2% and this problem is expected to be more prevalent with the epidemic of childhood obesity in that country (18).

A constant in the emergence of T2DM in young patients has been the association with obesity and increasing rates of that seminal condition. The U.S. National Health and Nutrition Examination Survey conducted between 1988 and 1994 found that 20% of children 12 to 17 years of age had body mass indexes (BMIs) above the 85th percentile for age, the definition of overweight, and that depending on ethnicity, 8% to 17% were obese, with a BMI greater than 95th percentile. Not only was there a doubling of the frequency of childhood obesity since 1980, but also the severity of obesity was greater (19).

In a 20-year study of 11,564 5- to 24-year-olds living in a biracial community in Louisiana (the Bogalusa Heart Study) from 1973 to 1994, there was a mean weight increase of 0.2 kg/yr and increased skinfold thickness. Overweight increased from 15% to 30%, and obesity from 5% to 11% in 5- to 14-year-olds and from 5% to 15% in 15- to 17-year-olds. The increases in the second 10 years of the study were 50% greater than those in the first 10 years (20). In the National Longitudinal Survey of Youth, a prospective cohort study of 8270 children aged 4 to 12 years, there was a significant increase in overweight and obesity between 1986 and 1998. The prevalence rates in 1998 for overweight were 38% for African-Americans and Hispanics and 26% for whites, while 22% of African-Americans and Hispanics and 12% of whites were obese (21).

Similar trends to those in the United States have been reported for Japan (22) and Western Europe (23). In Russia, 6% of approximately 7000 6- to 18-year-olds examined in 1992 were obese and 10% were overweight, using U.S. BMI reference data (24). Reports from 2003 from China indicated that 27.7% of boys and 14.1% of girls were overweight (25). In 1996 in the United Kingdom, 22% of 6-year-olds were overweight, and 10% were obese; by age 15, 31% were overweight and 17% obese (26). Numerous studies in Europe have indicated that the highest rates of childhood obesity occur in the eastern European countries, particularly Hungary, and in the southern European countries of Italy, Spain, and Greece (27).

ETIOLOGY

The question of nature versus nurture (genetics vs. environment) is raised frequently in discussions of the etiology of T2DM. The recent increase in T2DM prevalence in young patients has been so rapid that it can only be explained by changes in the environment. The most important of these is the increasing prevalence of obesity (28,29). Nonetheless, not all or even a majority of obese youngsters develop T2DM, emphasizing the importance of underlying genetic predisposition. The thrifty genotype hypothesis, advanced nearly 40 years ago and recently updated (30,31), explains the insulin resistance and relative beta-cell insufficiency that is associated with the development of obesity and T2DM as an adaptation for conserving energy and surviving famine. Until the modern era of ready availability of high calorie foods, such a genotype would have had great survival advantage. Numerous studies have demonstrated that both insulin resistance and limited pancreatic beta-cell capability to respond to the increased insulin requirements associated with obesity are the basic abnormalities in the development of T2DM (32–38) (Vol. 1; Chap. 11).

Insulin resistance affects glucose, lipid, and protein metabolism. Normal glycemic control requires the sensing of glucose concentration by the beta cells, the synthesis and release of insulin, the coupling of insulin to its receptors, and post-receptor insulin activation. This results in increased glucose uptake by muscles, fat, and liver tissue with decreased glucose production by the liver. In T2DM, there is peripheral insulin resistance in muscle and fat tissue, together with decreased pancreatic insulin secretion, and increased hepatic glucose output which results in hyperglycemia (Fig. 1) (39). Hyperglycemia can be promoted by protein tyrosine phophatases dephosphorylating the insulin receptor and its substrates

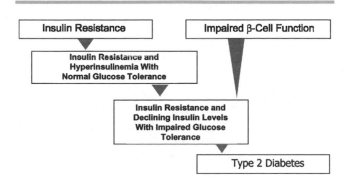

Figure 1   Development of T2DM. Peripheral insulin resistance in muscle and fat tissue, together with decreased pancreatic insulin secretion, and increased hepatic glucose output, results in hyperglycemia, which together with impaired beta-cell function results in T2DM. *Abbreviation*: T2DM, Type 2 diabetes mellitus. *Source*: Adapted from Ref. 39.

or by a protein called TRB3 blocking the actions of insulin in the liver (40).

The Role of Fetal and Childhood Nutrition

The association of lower birthweight, smaller head circumference, and thinness at birth with later development of insulin resistance and impaired glucose tolerance or T2DM suggested in utero programming that limited beta-cell capacity and induced insulin resistance in peripheral tissues (41,42). The maternal undernutrition that led to low birthweight was thought to impair development of the endocrine pancreas. The effect of fetal undernutrition on adult glucose tolerance has been confirmed in large studies in Sweden and the United States (43,44). Glucose intolerance was also found in adults who were the offspring of mothers who had starved during the last trimester of pregnancy during the Dutch famine at the end of World War II (45). Low birthweight has also been associated with increased cortisol axis activity in adults. South African non-obese 20-year-olds who had been underweight for gestational age had greater plasma cortisol response to adrenocorticotrophic hormone, higher BP, and more frequent impaired glucose tolerance compared with normal birthweight controls (46) (Vol. 1; Chap. 12).

Three studies of young subjects from high-risk populations substantiate the reports of the effect of fetal nutrition on the risk for development of the insulin resistance syndrome (IRS) (T2DM, hypertension, dyslipidemia) in adulthood. Current weight correlated with birthweight among 3061 Pima Indians aged 5 to 29 years, and two-hour glucose concentrations had a U-shaped relationship with birthweight in those greater than 10 years old, regardless of current weight. Thus, higher blood-glucose levels were present in those who had both high and low birthweights, irrespective of their current weight. The 2272 subjects without diabetes had negative correlations between birthweight and insulin resistance, determined by measurement of insulin concentrations at baseline and two hours following a glucose load. These findings support the hypothesis of a survival advantage for insulin resistance in low birthweight babies (47). These findings were confirmed in a study of 1492 individuals who were followed from birth through adulthood which found that thinness in infancy correlated with impaired glucose tolerance and T2DM in young adulthood (48).

In a study of 477 eight-year-old Indian children, insulin resistance variables and plasma total and low-density lipoprotein (LDL) cholesterol concentrations were strongly related to low birthweight but high-fat mass at eight years of age. Lower birthweight was associated with calculated insulin resistance, elevated systolic BP, fasting plasma insulin and 32 to 33 split proinsulin concentrations, plasma lipids, and glucose and insulin concentrations 30 minutes after glucose (49). Low birthweight Caucasian and African-American children ($n = 139$) studied when they were aged 4 to 14 years had significant differences between the two races in the effect of low birthweight on visceral fat mass as measured by dual-energy X-ray absorptiometry and computed tomography, fasting insulin, acute insulin response to intravenous glucose, beta-cell function, and high-density lipoprotein (HDL) cholesterol concentrations, indicative of the genetic differences suggested by the thrifty genotype hypothesis (50). These findings are consistent with the higher prevalence of T2DM in African-Americans.

Early childhood nutrition also is thought to play a role in the development of insulin resistance later in life. An association between high protein intake in infancy and later obesity has been suggested (51). Breast feeding results in a more appropriate caloric intake at a critical stage in development than bottle feeding, which is more likely to be associated with overfeeding and obesity. Glucose tolerance testing was carried out in 720 Pima Indians aged 10 to 39 years, including 325 who had been exclusively bottle-fed as infants, 144 who were exclusively breast-fed, and the rest partially breast-fed for the first two months of life. Those exclusively breast-fed had significantly lower rates of T2DM than those exclusively bottle-fed for each age decade, with an odds ratio for T2DM in exclusively breast-fed individuals of 0.41 (52). Furthermore, prolonged breast feeding markedly reduced the risk of overweight in nearly 10,000 five- to six-year-old German children; 3.8% of those exclusively breast-fed for two months were overweight versus 0.8% of those breast-fed for longer than 12 months (53). This finding may be due to the lower insulin responses and the lower energy and protein intake in breast-fed infants versus bottle-fed infants (51). The frequent overweight of the bottle-fed infant may contribute to insulin resistance and obesity in adolescence and young adulthood.

The thrifty phenotype hypothesis states that poor nutrition in fetal and early infant life would be detrimental to the development and function of the beta cells and insulin-sensitive tissues, primarily muscle, leading to insulin resistance. With obesity in later life, T2DM would develop. This hypothesis would explain the effect of fetal nutrition on later glucose tolerance and other manifestations of insulin insensitivity, such as hypertension and increased cardiovascular problems. These findings could also be interpreted as a reflection of the thrifty genotype hypothesis that defective insulin action in utero results in decreased fetal growth and obesity-induced impaired glucose tolerance in later childhood or adulthood (54). Genetic factors affecting birthweight and glucose metabolism are of interest in this regard. The polymorphism at the variable number of tandem repeats locus of the insulin chain is associated with decreased body length, weight, and head circumference at birth (55). Decreased birthweight has been associated with heterozygosity for a mutation in the glucokinase gene (56). Finally, the glucose transporter 4 expression is impaired in young adults with insulin resistance who had undernutrition in utero (57). These aspects are reviewed in greater detail in Vol. 1; Chap. 12.

The Role of Maternal Diabetes

The influence of the diabetic intrauterine environment on the risk of T2DM in children was first appreciated from studies in the Pima Indian population; the prevalence of diabetes in the offspring of Pima women with diabetes during pregnancy is significantly greater than in non-diabetic mothers or those who develop diabetes after delivery (58). In another study of the effect of maternal diabetes, fetal beta-cell function was assessed in 88 pregnancies with pregestational or gestational diabetes by measuring amniotic fluid insulin (AFI) concentration at 32 to 38 weeks of gestation and performing oral glucose tolerance tests annually in the offspring from 18 months of age. Only one of 27 adolescents with normal AFI had impaired glucose tolerance, in contrast to one-third of those with elevated AFI (59). These studies suggest a generation to generation accumulation of risk for T2DM that further increases the public health concern of the epidemic of this disease in young persons (60).

The Role of Puberty

In all reports of T2DM in childhood, the mean age at diagnosis is approximately 13.5 years, corresponding to the time of peak adolescent growth and development (7,9,10,13,14,16). Puberty is associated with relative insulin resistance, reflected in a two- to threefold increase in the peak insulin response to oral or intravenous glucose (61); insulin-mediated glucose disposal is approximately 30% lower in adolescents than in prepubertal children or young adults (62). The physiologic insulin resistance of puberty is of no consequence in the presence of adequate

beta-cell function. The cause of this physiologic resistance is likely the transitory increased activity of the growth hormone–insulin growth factor axis, which coincides with the physiologic insulin resistance of adolescence (1).

The Role of Obesity

The insulin resistance associated with obesity is the fundamental problem in T2DM in children and adolescents, as it is in adults. Total obesity is not as important as location of adipose tissue in causing insulin resistance (62). Visceral fat is more metabolically active than subcutaneous fat and produces adipokines that cause insulin resistance, thus predisposing to T2DM. The importance of location of excess adipose tissue in insulin resistance was validated by the finding that removal of subcutaneous adipose tissue with liposuction did not significantly alter levels of adipokines, insulin sensitivity, or other risk factors for coronary heart disease (BP, lipids) (63). That obese children have hyperinsulinism has been known for over 30 years (64,65). Obese children have approximately 40% lower insulin-stimulated glucose metabolism compared with the nonobese (62). African-American 5- to 10-year-olds, especially the girls, have reduced insulin sensitivity, and this correlates with increases in BP, triglycerides, subcutaneous fat, percentage of total body fat, and stage of sexual maturation (66). The amount of visceral fat in obese adolescents correlates directly with basal and glucose-stimulated insulin levels and inversely with insulin sensitivity (67). Insulin-stimulated glucose metabolism decreases while fasting insulinemia increases with increasing BMI (62).

The Role of Race, Gender, and Family History

There is a racial difference in the insulin responses to various stimuli that parallels the ethnic/racial differential in T2DM frequency. Greater insulin responses to oral glucose are seen in African-American children and adolescents than in European-American children after adjustments are made for weight, age, ponderal (obesity) index, and pubertal stage. This is indicative of compensated insulin resistance in the African-American youngsters (66,68,69). Both prepubertal and pubertal African-American children have higher fasting and stimulated insulin concentrations during glucose clamp studies than do European-American youngsters (70). Lipolysis is also significantly less in African-American children than in European-American children, suggesting an energy conservation phenotype that would have survival value in times of famine, but be detrimental with excess nutrition (thrifty genotype) (71).

A non-interventional cohort study showed that girls are more insulin resistant than boys as early as five years of age (72). The study also found that girls carry 26% more subcutaneous fat than boys, which

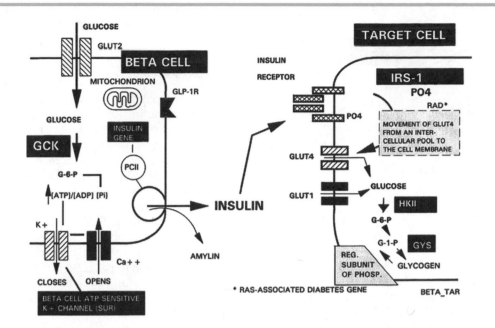

Figure 2 Beta-cell candidate genes in T2DM mellitus. Candidate genes include: GLUT2, which is responsible for the facilitative uptake of glucose by beta cells; GCK, which is the beta-cell glucose sensor; mitochondrial genes that provide power to the beta-cell (an increased ratio of ATP to ADP + Pi [(ATP)]/[(ADP) + (Pi)]); the ATP-sensitive potassium (K') channel (the SUR); GLP-1R that responds to GLP from the gastrointestinal tract; insulin; PCII (an example of an insulin-processing protein); and amylin, which is co-secreted with insulin. At the target cell (muscle, fat, or liver), candidate genes include: the insulin receptor; intracellular proteins that are phosphorylated (IRS1); GLUT1; hexokinase II, which catalyzes the conversion of glucose to glucose-6-phosphate; GYS, which regulates glycogen production; and the regulatory subunit of PHOSP that regulates glycogen breakdown. GLUT4 is also a candidate gene, but GLUT4 is expressed only in muscle and fat tissues and is not expressed in the liver. *Abbreviations*: T2DM, Type 2 diabetes mellitus; GLUT2, glucose transporter 2; GCK, glucokinase; SUR, sulfonylurea receptor; GLP-1R, beta-cell glucagon-like peptide-1 receptor; PCII, prohormone convertase II; IRS1, insulin receptor substrate-1; GYS, glycogen synthase; PHOSP, phosphorylase; ATP, adenosine triphosphate; ADP, adenosine diphosphate; *RAS-associated diabetes gene. *Source*: From Ref. 81.

may contribute to the development of insulin resistance in the female population. Therefore, sex-linked genes may contribute to the development of T2DM and the insulin resistance/metabolic syndrome in the current food-rich environment.

Prepubertal children who have a family history of T2DM have lower insulin-stimulated glucose disposal and non-oxidative glucose disposal than do those without such a family history, indicating that family history of T2DM is a risk factor for insulin resistance in children, as it is in adults (73).

Genetic Considerations

The evidence that T2DM is a genetic disease includes: the family clustering and segregation analyses that indicate that siblings of affected individuals have 3.5 times the general population risk of developing T2DM; studies of monozygotic twins that indicate a concordance of 80% to 100%, greater than twice the concordance for T1DM in dizygotic twins and in monozygotic twins; and the previously noted variations in insulin sensitivity and frequency of T2DM by ethnicity (74). With rare exception, T2DM in children and adolescents, as in adults, is polygenic.

The strategies for identification of T2DM susceptibility genes involve studying a candidate gene or scanning the human genome. With the candidate gene approach, there is a problem identifying or choosing an appropriate candidate, or the candidate may be unknown at the time of the study, as was the case with the MODY genes. With the genome scan approach, the entire genome is examined for linkages within families or associations within populations. In these analyses, micro-satellites are particularly useful and micro-assays of mRNA are able to identify gene patterns which are over- or underexpressed in specific disease states. Figure 2 illustrates possible candidate genes in the beta cell–target cell interaction.

Over 20 loci have been linked to or associated with T2DM in adults, the most important being non insulin dependent diabetes mellitus Type 1 (NIDDM1), described among Mexican-American siblings in Starr County Texas (75). This county, which is 97% Mexican-American, has the highest disease-specific diabetes mortality in Texas. The gene pool is 31% Native American. Four hundred seventy-four autosomal markers and 16 X-linked markers were examined in 170 affected siblings involving 300 affected siblings and 78 unaffected siblings. Identified as linked to T2DM was the NIDDM1 site on chromosome

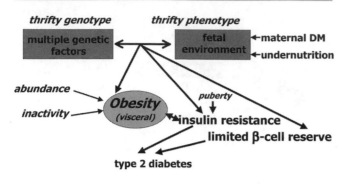

Figure 3 Factors implicated in the development of T2DM. *Abbreviation*: T2DM, Type 2 diabetes mellitus.

2, accounting for approximately 30% of family clustering, equal in importance, therefore, to the linkage with human leukocyte antigen in T1DM (76). This linkage was not identified in other populations, including non-Hispanic Caucasian, Japanese, French, Sardinian, and Finnish (74). The Calpain gene in the NIDDM1 region of chromosome 2 was subsequently found to be associated with T2DM in several of these populations, linked to different loci (77).

Calpains are calcium-activated neutral proteases that are ubiquitously expressed from fetal life through adulthood, functioning in signaling, proliferation, differentiation, and insulin-induced downregulation of IRS-1. Multiple polymorphisms of the gene encoding Calpain-10, encoded by the CAPN10 gene within the NIDDM1 region, have been found to be associated with T2DM. The highest risk combination of polymorphisms gives odds ratios of 2.8 to 3.6 in Mexican-Americans, 2.6 in Finns, and 5.0 in Germans (77). Non-diabetic Pima Indians who are homozygous for a common polymorphism of CAPN10 have reduced insulin-mediated glucose turnover as the result of decreased glucose oxidation

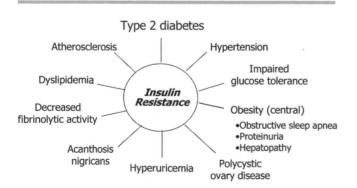

Figure 4 Comorbidities of insulin resistance. Comorbidities are often seen at the time of diagnosis in patients with T2DM. *Abbreviation*: T2DM, Type 2 diabetes mellitus. *Source*: Adapted from Ref. 1.

rates (78). Figure 3 summarizes the factors that have been discussed in the consideration of the development of T2DM.

CLINICAL PICTURE

The most striking difference between T1DM and T2DM is that in T2DM, hyperglycemia/diabetes is one of many manifestations of the IRS (a.k.a. the diabesity syndrome, syndrome X, or the metabolic syndrome), whereas T1DM is a disorder of insulin deficiency and is not usually associated with the comorbidities seen with insulin resistance early in the course of the disease (Fig. 4).

Distinguishing T1DM from T2DM at diagnosis is occasionally problematic (Vol. 1; Chap. 3). Most pediatric endocrinologists report that of the patients identified as having T2DM, 100% will have a BMI greater than 85% and 90% to 95% will have acanthosis nigricans (AN), a cutaneous manifestation of insulin resistance characterized by velvety, hyperpigmented skin, most often in intertriginous areas (79). However, with the epidemic of obesity in the United States, up to 24% of children with T1DM will be overweight at diagnosis, and non-Caucasian obese patients will often have AN. In contrast to T1DM, however, at presentation of T2DM, most children will have glycosuria, with mild or absent polyuria and polydipsia, and little to no recent weight loss. Although diabetic ketoacidosis (DKA) is not as common at presentation of T2DM as with T1DM, severe insulinopenia due to beta-cell dysfunction from glucose toxicity can result in DKA in patients with T2DM. The hyperglycemic hyperosmolar state (HHS) is a serious acute presentation that is almost exclusive to T2DM (80). While a family history of T2DM may be helpful in distinguishing T1DM from T2DM, as 74% to 100% of children with T2DM have a first- or second-degree relative with T2DM, T2DM is sufficiently frequent in the population, especially among ethnic minorities, that such a history will be frequently obtained among those with T1DM (81). Occasionally, diagnosis will only be clarified by observing the clinical course of the patient and may be helped by testing for the presence of diabetes-specific autoantibodies to islet cells (ICA), glutamic acid decarboxylase autoantibodies (GADA), insulin autoantibodies (IAA), and tyrosine dehydrogenase (IA-2). Diabetes-specific autoimmunity has been described with typical T2DM, however, was initially referred to as latent autoimmune diabetes of adults (LADA) (82,83). In the UK Prospective Diabetes Study, LADA was age-related, with 21% of T2DM patients 25 to 34 years old being ICA-positive, 34% GADA-positive, and 20% positive for both antibodies, decreasing to 4%, 7%, and 2%, respectively, in those 55 to 65 years of age. Antibody positivity was associated with significantly less overweight, higher HbA1c concentrations, and more rapid deterioration of beta-cell function (82). Among 764

Swedish patients aged 15 to 34 years with newly diagnosed diabetes, 76% were classified as T1DM, 14% as T2DM, and the rest unclassified. Forty-seven percent of T2DM patients and 59% of unclassified patients were positive for one or more diabetes-specific antibodies, with the antibody-positive T2DM or unclassified patients being significantly lighter, with lower C-peptide concentrations, than the antibody-negative patients (83). Two studies in children with T2DM have paralleled some, but not all of the findings in adults with T2DM. Among 48 children, 8% were positive for the ICA512 fragment, 30% were GADA-positive, and 35% IAA-positive; unlike in adults, there was no correlation between antibody positivity and degree of obesity (84). In a group of 37 African-American children and adolescents, 10.8% were positive for GADA, IA-2, or both, with no difference in treatment requirements (oral agent vs. insulin) related to the presence or absence of antibodies (85). Measurement of C-peptide levels to distinguish T1DM from T2DM may not be helpful because C-peptide levels may be low in children with T2DM at diagnosis due to the glucose toxicity to the beta cells, and in T1DM they may be adequate during the early recovery (honeymoon) phase.

Manifestations of the IRS include hypertension, endothelial dysfunction, atherosclerosis, dyslipidemia, a prothrombotic environment, impaired glucose tolerance, AN, hyperuricemia, polycystic ovary disease, and obesity, the core abnormality (Vol. 1; Chap. 11) (86). IRS increases the risk for development of cardiovascular disease. Individuals who have the components of IRS in youth track them into adulthood. The prevalence of IRS is 4% of all adolescents and 30% of overweight adolescents in the United States. The fact that IRS is being identified in younger individuals indicates that the development of cardiovascular disease will also occur earlier in adulthood.

Obesity itself has deleterious associations in childhood and adolescence that increase morbidity and contribute to cardiovascular risk. This increased risk of childhood obesity has been documented to be the result of the tracking of this obesity into adulthood, rather than specific effects during childhood (87,88). However, the clustering of risk factors (dyslipidemia, abdominal obesity, hypertension) in childhood causes adverse cardiovascular system changes beginning in childhood, which are predictive of adult-onset cardiovascular disease (89,90). Childhood obesity has been associated with elevated C-reactive protein and white blood cell counts, inflammatory indicators that have been implicated in adult cardiovascular disease (91), proteinuria and focal segmental glomerular sclerosis (92), obstructive sleep apnea and other respiratory problems (93), hepatic steatosis (94), and orthopedic problems (95) (Vol. 1; Chap. 1).

In adults, T2DM is strongly associated with increased risk factors for macrovascular disease. These risk factors include dyslipidemia, hypertension, oxidative stress, glycation of numerous vascular proteins, endothelial dysfunction, and abnormalities of platelet function and coagulation [increased fibrinogen, increased plasminogen activator inhibitor-1, decreased antithrombin III and other anticoagulant proteins, elevated factors VII and VIII, elevated vascular adhesion molecule 1, increased platelet adhesiveness and aggregation, decreased platelet nitric oxide (NO) production (NO mediates vasodilatation), decreased platelet prostacyclin production, and glycation of platelet proteins] (96).

Dyslipidemia

Lipoprotein abnormalities noted in T2DM are associated with increased cardiovascular disease and include hypertriglyceridemia, elevated very low-density lipoprotein, elevated LDL cholesterol, elevated lipoprotein (a), decreased HDL cholesterol, increased small dense LDL particles, decreased lipoprotein lipase activity, increased lipoprotein glycation, and increased lipoprotein oxidation (97).

This dyslipidemia reflects the reduction of insulin effect in adipose tissue, which is to store triglyceride and suppress hormone-sensitive lipase, the enzyme that breaks down triglycerides to release free fatty acids. Insulin also provides glucose to the fat cells for forming glycerol, the triglyceride backbone. With insulin resistance, there is abnormal breakdown of triglyceride and release of free fatty acids and glycerol, the latter contributing to gluconeogenesis. The free fatty acids cause insulin resistance in muscle tissue and, in the liver they are reconverted to triglyceride, driving the production of LDL, which is the lipoprotein carrier of triglycerides, and the other dyslipidemic changes follow. The reduction of insulin effect on lipoprotein lipase contributes to the elevated LDL levels. The hyperinsulinemia of the insulin resistance state further drives the synthesis of fatty acids from glucose in the liver (98).

Hypertension

Hypertension is estimated to account for 35% to 75% of diabetes complications involving both the microvasculature and the macrovasculature (99). Diabetes or impaired glucose tolerance doubles the risk of developing hypertension (100). There is emerging evidence of a genetic predisposition to hypertension and T2DM that is related to angiotensin-converting enzyme genotype (101). The hypertension in T2DM is multifactorial, due to volume expansion and increased vascular resistance, with reduced NO-mediated vasodilatation and increased activity of the renin–angiotensin system (96).

Endothelial Dysfunction

Endothelial dysfunction develops in the milieu of cardiovascular risk factors such as obesity, hypertension, dyslipidemia, insulin resistance, and T2DM. Endothelial dysfunction is one of the earliest signs of increased risk for cardiovascular disease, and has been shown to be predictive of cardiovascular events (102). Endothelial dysfunction is present in obese children, and is related to the amount of obesity as well as to the degree of insulin resistance (103).

Dysfunctional endothelium is associated with increased levels of cytokines and cellular adhesion molecules. The cytokines and cellular adhesion molecules mediate the recruitment of leukocytes, which then accumulate in the intima of the vessel wall, initiating atherosclerotic plaques (102). Activation of the endothelium leads to a proinflammatory, procoagulant, proadhesive surface. Additionally, the dysfunctional endothelium has reduced NO availability. NO-dependent processes, such as inhibition of platelet aggregation and coagulation and activation of fibrinolysis, are therefore decreased in the setting of endothelial dysfunction. Thus, the unopposed action of atherogenic factors that occurs as a result of endothelial dysfunction promotes atherogenesis and thrombosis (103).

Several cytokines produced by adipose tissue (adipokines) have been shown to be associated with endothelial dysfunction, including tumor necrosis factor alpha, interleukin-6, plasminogen activator inhibitor-1, leptin, and resistin (104). All of these adipokines are pro-inflammatory, and have been shown in in-vitro models to have activating effects on the endothelium and to contribute to the induction of thrombosis. On the other hand, the adipokine adiponectin, which is underexpressed in individuals with obesity or T2DM, decreases endothelial inflammation, inhibits vascular smooth muscle proliferation, and suppresses macrophage-to-foam cell transformation (105). Levels of adiponectin correlate inversely with other markers of inflammation, and low levels have been found to be associated with increased cardiovascular risk.

Acanthosis Nigricans

AN, an indicator of insulin resistance, is prominent in genetic IRS that are not associated with obesity. The frequency of AN in obese adolescents varies greatly by ethnicity, approximately 90% in Native Americans, approximately 50% in African-Americans, approximately 15% in Hispanic-Americans, and less than 5% in non-Hispanic Caucasians. As an indicator of hyperinsulinism, AN also varies by ethnicity inversely to its frequency of association with obesity (106). In a study of 139 overweight 6- to 10-year-olds, AN was present in 50% of African-Americans and 8.2% of whites. Half of those with fasting hyperinsulinemia did not have AN and AN was not considered a reliable marker for hyperinsulinemia in overweight children, despite its presence in a child with diabetes being an indicator of T2DM (107).

PREVENTION AND TREATMENT

The concept of prevention of T2DM arises naturally from the appreciation of its environmental causation.

Primary prevention would involve intervention to prevent the development of obesity or to correct obesity before the development of other features of IRS. Prevention of obesity is a societal challenge. The importance of primary prevention of obesity lies in the recognition that preclinical impairment of glucose tolerance as the result of obesity-induced insulin resistance conveys cardiovascular risk and that a substantial number of severely obese adolescents have impaired glucose tolerance (4).

From the individual physician standpoint, the major question is, "Who should be tested?" (1). Considerations of testing for T2DM in children began with the assumption that this will be done in obese individuals, making the determination of obesity the screening test. The testing for hyperglycemia then becomes a case finding exercise (108). The justifications for case finding include:

1. That the condition tested for is sufficiently common to provide a reasonable yield.
2. That the condition is serious in terms of morbidity and mortality.
3. That the condition has a prolonged latency without symptoms during which abnormality can be detected.
4. That a test is available which is sensitive, that is with few false negatives, and accurate with acceptable specificity, that is with a minimum number of false positives.
5. That an intervention is available which can prevent or delay disease onset or more effectively treat the condition if it is detected in the latency phase.

The first three conditions are unquestionably met by T2DM in children. The fourth criterion is met by plasma glucose measurement, with sensitivity and specificity dependent upon the circumstances of measurement. The last criterion, however, is extremely challenging, as will be discussed below. A consensus panel of the American Diabetes Association (1) answered the question posed above with the following recommendations:

Overweight defined as BMI greater than 85th percentile for age and sex, weight for height > 85th percentile, or weight > 120% of ideal for height, plus any two of the following risk factors:

- Family history of Type 2 diabetes in first- or second-degree relative
- Race/ethnicity (American-Indian, African-American, Hispanic, Asian/Pacific Islander)
- Signs of insulin resistance or conditions associated with insulin resistance (AN, hypertension, dyslipidemia, PCOS)

Age of initiation: age 10 or at onset of puberty, if puberty occurs at a younger age
Frequency: every two years
Test: Fasting plasma glucose preferred
These criteria were not databased, which is why the consensus panel provided a disclaimer that they should not replace individual clinical judgment. One might also take issue with the preference for the lower

cost and more convenient fasting plasma glucose, because two-hour postprandial plasma glucose increases earlier in the course of the development of T2DM, making it a more sensitive measure. Fasting hyperglycemia occurs later, and therefore is highly specific but relatively insensitive as a diagnostic test. However, higher fasting blood-glucose levels in the normoglycemic range [i.e. > 87 mg/dL (4.83 mmol/L)] have been shown to be a risk factor for T2DM in 26- to 45-year-old men (109). Random plasma glucose concentration can be measured in those with food intake shortly before testing, with a glucose concentration equal to 7.8 mmol/L or greater (140 mg/dL) serving as an indication for further testing.

Prevention of T2DM

Justification for primary prevention efforts in childhood has been the subject of wide publicity for the past several years, with recognition that obesity is associated with the rapid increase in incidence of T2DM in children (110–114). Obesity is associated with diminished school performance due to sleep apnea, torpor associated with physical inactivity, depression, and social stigmatization. Secondary prevention of obesity is rarely successful beyond the short-term and intervention in adult populations indicates enormous difficulty altering lifestyle and dietary habits.

The challenge for the pediatrician and for society is to counter eating and entertainment trends to provide popular social outlets that are highly attractive, heavily promoted, and readily available. Financially stressed school systems often sabotage community efforts by providing fast food concessions and vending machines containing soft drinks and high calorie snacks in exchange for financial support from the vendors. Food service in middle and high schools typically includes high fat, high calorie foods such as pizza and French fries. There are inadequate opportunities for non-competitive sports, such as aerobics and dance, permitting participation of all youngsters, and there has been a sharp reduction in compulsory physical education programs. For some minority youngsters, there is the additional problem of a lack of safe environments in which to be physically active, and lack of funding for after-school programs. Finally, school curricula have not effectively incorporated healthy lifestyle training.

A number of school-based and community-based programs have been developed targeting high-risk populations (14,113–118). School-based programs attempt modification of the food provided in school meals, incorporate healthy lifestyle training into classroom education, and create a school environment that promotes physical activity. Preschool and kindergarten through sixth-grade programs encourage family involvement, while high school-based programs focus on social networks and peer pressure in an effort to promote behavior change and reduce

risk factors. Short-term behavioral change has occurred with these programs, but long-term studies are needed to determine whether these changes persist and reduce the risk for Type 2 diabetes. A large NIH-funded longitudinal, multicenter randomized trial (STOPPT2DM) designed to assess the efficacy of a school-based intervention on obesity and T2DM prevention is currently underway.

Before the contemporary epidemic of T2DM, we had noted the occasional obese African-American teenager attending our diabetes adventure camp program and rapidly becoming normoglycemic with vigorous exercise, permitting withdrawal of insulin. This phenomenon has been documented in one week summer camp programs for North American Indian youth with T2DM, who are able to achieve normoglycemia after five days of increased physical activity. Unfortunately, the behaviors of camp are not maintained, with most of the youngsters reverting to poor glycemic control at home (116,119). Programs are in place that emphasize nutrition and exercise in schools, including those on Indian reservations throughout the United States, but their effectiveness has yet to be documented (118,120).

The cornerstone of prevention of T2DM is lifestyle modification. Both decreases in caloric intake and increased exercise are vital aspects of lifestyle modification for weight loss and prevention of T2DM. The benefits of exercise include improving the metabolic profile by improving insulin sensitivity, improving cardiovascular fitness, even without weight loss, and maintenance of weight loss (119,121). Several studies have shown improvements in endothelial function and inflammatory markers with exercise for just 30 minutes per day (122). Japanese researchers showed a halving of cardiovascular risk from just one hour of exercise per week (123). The Centers for Disease Control and Prevention recommends 30 minutes of moderate-intensity exercise seven days per week for every person in the United States (124). For those individuals attempting to achieve weight loss, the Institute of Medicine recommends 60 minutes of moderate-intensity exercise seven days per week (119). To achieve these recommendations, barriers to exercise, such as lack of motivation, lack of time, and lack of support, must be overcome (125).

The health-care system is increasing its appreciation of the magnitude of the problem of obesity/T2DM problem and all who have contact with at risk families need to emphasize the importance of early identification and intervention. Parent training by pediatricians, WIC nurses, and other health personnel should continue to promote prolonged breast feeding, which in addition to its many other benefits, reduces the risk of obesity in childhood (52,53). Parents also need to know that a fat baby is not a more healthy baby and that food should not be used as rewards (126). Because children with normal weight parents have a much lower risk of overweight (< 7% vs. 40%

with one overweight parent and 80% with two over-weight parents) lifestyle modification is important for the whole family and, of course, will not work for any one member by himself or herself (127). Physical activity must also be a family investment, with habits such as using stairs instead of elevators or escalators, walking or bicycling to school and to shop, and engaging in physically demanding chores, such as yardwork. The most effective single thing that can be done to increase children's physical activity is to turn off the television set and remove TVs from children's bedrooms (128). It is also important that meals be taken on schedule, in one place, with no other activity going on.

Studies in adults have shown improved glucose tolerance or reduction in the rate of development of T2DM for up to several years as a result of lifestyle interventions, including individualized counseling for weight reduction, reduced total and saturated fat intake, increased fiber intake, and exercise (129–131). Among the most sustained efforts was a 13-year project involving six communities, The Minnesota Heart Health Program. The project included adult education classes for weight control, exercise promotion, and cholesterol reduction, a worksite weight control program, a home correspondence course for weight loss, and a weight gain prevention program. Despite this intensive effort, there was a strong upward trend in weight, even when all potentially confounding variables were considered (132). Intervention with children, particularly preadolescents, should be more effective. In one study of family-based intervention involving 113 families, it was demonstrated that children had greater relative weight loss and better maintenance than the adults, with one-third of children remaining non-obese after 10 years (133). In another study of 24 families, including children 8 to 12 years old, two-thirds of the families completed the 10- to 12-session behavioral modification treatment program; those children who completed it lost weight. Weight loss was not maintained during 4 to 13 months of follow up, however (127). Even modest successes in the reported studies have to be interpreted with caution, because these are selected study populations, the numbers are small, and there is only short-term follow-up.

Diabetes prevention programs have to be designed with an understanding of the health beliefs and behaviors of the community. For example, one survey of American Indian youth with family members having diabetes did not relate the complications of retinopathy or amputation to the diabetes. Over half of the youth thought that diabetes was caused by bad blood, and greater than one-third attributed it to general weakness (134).

Unfortunately, less than 5% of people who attempt diet and exercise modifications to lose weight actually lose a significant amount of weight and maintain that weight loss for a long period of time, while greater than 90% regain their weight within one year

(135). Therefore, many patients and physicians seek pharmacologic intervention to achieve weight loss and prevent the onset of T2DM. Orlistat is currently approved for the reduction of body weight in children, but is associated with flatulence and fecal soilage, making it an unpopular choice (136). Those medications that have been effective in adults do not result in maintenance of weight loss when the drugs are stopped. Metformin has been studied in 29 black and white adolescents aged 12 to 19 years with BMI greater than $30 \, kg/m^2$, a family history of T2DM, elevated fasting insulin concentrations ($>15 \, \mu U/mL$), a family history of Type 2 diabetes, and normal fasting glucose and HbA1c levels (137). Subjects were randomized to receive metformin 500 mg twice daily or placebo for six months. Controls had an increase in BMI of 0.23 SD and metformin-treated subjects a decrease of 0.12 SD, a significant difference. There was also a significant decrease in fasting glucose concentrations and insulin levels in metformin-treated youngsters versus controls. Transient abdominal discomfort or diarrhea occurred in 40% of those taking metformin (137). This study, too, suffers from small numbers, short follow-up, and a select study population. In adults, lifestyle intervention was more effective than metformin in preventing progression from impaired glucose tolerance to T2DM (131).

The two most popular available medications for adults that promote weight loss are orlistat, an intestinal lipase inhibitor, and sibutramine, a central appetite regulator. Both of these medications result in a 5% to 10% loss of weight, with a concomitant decrease in insulin resistance and other cardiovascular risk factors (138). However, long-term studies have not yet been done evaluating the effects of these medications on mortality and cardiovascular morbidity.

Other potential pharmacologic therapies for obesity include topiramate, peptide YY3-36 (PYY), magnesium, and rimonabant (139). Topiramate is an anticonvulsant, which induces weight loss. While the effects of topiramate on weight loss are promising, the central nervous system-related side effect profile, which includes memory difficulty, concentration difficulty, and depression, precludes its use in children (140). PYY is a gut-derived peptide, which modulates appetite circuits in the hypothalamus. PYY concentrations are low in obese individuals, and the administration of this hormone reduces food intake in humans (141). Rimonabant is an endocannabinoid inhibitor, which has been shown to decrease appetite and weight in obese and overweight adults. One study showed that 39% of individuals treated with this medication lost 10% of their body weight at one year and 32% of those individuals were able to maintain their weight loss for two years (142). Pharmacologic manipulation of other gut-derived hormones and peptides related to hunger and satiety is being investigated. Magnesium deficiency has been associated with insulin resistance and increased risk for T2DM (143). Therefore, magnesium supplementation may be a potential tool in preventing the development of T2DM in obese children who are magnesium deficient.

Surgery is the last option for patients who have significant obesity-related morbidities and have failed lifestyle modification and medication. Bariatric surgery is being done for adolescents with obesity-related comorbidities in several centers (144). Gastric bypass, the traditional surgical procedure for weight loss, can have significant complications including nutrient malabsorption and even death. Newer techniques, which appear to be safer, include gastric banding and vagal nerve stimulators. However, the long-term safety and efficacy of these procedures have not been evaluated and the risks of doing the procedure must be weighed against the risks of not having the procedure done, thereby having to deal with the risks of obesity related comorbidities.

Treatment of T2DM

The treatment challenges of T2DM in children and adolescents differ greatly from those of T1DM, due largely to the nature of the disease and those most likely affected. While T1DM is distributed throughout the population, T2DM disproportionately affects families with fewer resources, paralleling the distribution of obesity in the population. Whereas T1DM occurs throughout childhood, predominantly during the time when parental influence predominates, T2DM affects mostly those in adolescence or beyond, when peer influence is most important. There is also a large difference in family experience, with only approximately 5% of families with a child with T1DM having affected family members, while 90% or more of youth with T2DM have family experience. These family members have typically failed to control their weight and glycemia, developing complications and creating an aura of despair and futility. Treatment priorities are also different between T1DM and T2DM. Extensive lifestyle modification, beyond insulin administration and glucose monitoring, is only required by those patients with T1DM who are overweight and inactive; however, the emphasis is on lifestyle modification in all those with T2DM and secondarily on glucose monitoring and hypoglycemic medication. Finally, technologic innovation has revolutionized management of T1DM with improved insulin purity and delivery, self-blood-glucose-monitoring, and the development of insulin analogues, with an artificial pancreas on the horizon along with the possibility of islet cell replacement. Technological developments have, however, been the underlying cause of the problem of T2DM, with advances in home entertainment systems, laborsaving devices, and transportation, and food preparation making calorically dense food increasingly available, desirable, and inexpensive.

Treatment Goals

The goals of treatment are to promote weight loss, normalize glycemia and HbA1c, control or prevent hypertension and hyperlipidemia, increase exercise capability, and reduce AN. Treatment is more important than might be indicated by the level of glycemia in some patients, because of the multitude of cardiovascular risk factors associated with insulin resistance. Just as in adults with newly diagnosed T2DM, young patients may already have evidence of complications reflecting a prolonged period of impaired glucose tolerance. Among 100 Pima Indian children and adolescents with T2DM, 7% had high cholesterol ($\geq$200 mg/dL), 18% had hypertension (BP $\geq$140/90, now considered far too high a cut off), and 22% had micro-albuminuria (albumin/creatinine $\geq$ 30) at the time of diagnosis. Ten years later, while still in their 20s, they had mean HbA1c of 12% indicative of poor control, 60% had micro-albuminuria and 17% macro-albuminuria (albumin/creatinine $\geq$ 300) (145). Japanese investigators have described a high risk of renal failure in those who developed T2DM under 30 years of age (146).

It is likely that reduction in the risk of complications may require more stringent glycemic control in the insulin resistance state of T2DM than is required in T1DM, with diligent attention to comorbidities. In the U.K. Prospective Diabetes Study there was a 25% decrease in the risk of microvascular complications when the average HbA1c decreased from 7.9% to 7.0% (147). Reduction in BP to below 144/82 resulted in a more dramatic decrease of 37% in the risk for microvascular disease, 44% decrease in stroke occurrence, and 36% decrease in heart failure (148).

Changing Behavior

The behavioral changes and motivation required are so extensive that the treatment team requires a psychologist or social worker. One of the simplest changes to make is to eliminate the frequent consumption of sugar-containing drinks, including high caloric soft drinks, sweetened tea, and juices, and substituting water, diet soft drinks, and artificial sweeteners for tea or Kool-Aid® (149). Consumption of sugar-sweetened beverages is strongly associated with an increased risk of childhood obesity and T2DM (150). Daily exercise should be documented in an attempt to break the vicious cycle of increased weight producing increased torpor, resulting in decreased activity and increased weight. As noted above, the most effective single method for doing this is turning off the TV. A relatively small reduction in weight, accomplished by an increase in activity, can restore euglycemia and decrease hyperinsulinemia, as in the camp experience.

The effectiveness of diet as a means of controlling T2DM in children was demonstrated in a short-term study of the use of a very low calorie ketogenic diet during which insulin or metformin treatment could be stopped with maintenance of normal blood-glucose concentrations (151).

The stages of behavioral change are outlined below (152):

Table 1 Hypoglycemic Agents

Drug type	Dosages (mg)	Action	Effect on BG	Risk of low BG	Weight increase	Lipid decrease
Biguanides [metformin, (Glucophage, Glucophage XR)]	500–2000	↓ Hepatic glucose output	++	0	0	+
Sulfonylureas [glipizide (Glucotrol, Glucotrol XL), glyburide (Micronase), Glimepiride (Amaryl)]	2.5–40	↑ Hepatic insulin sensitivity ↑ Insulin secretion and sensitivity	++	+	+	0
	2.5–20 1.25–2 1–8					
Meglitinide [repaglinide (Prandin)]	0.5–2	Short-term ↑ insulin secretion	++	+	+	0
Glucosidase inhibitors [acarbose (Precose), Miglitol (Glyset)]	25–100	Slow hydrolysis and absorption of complex CHO	+	0	0	+
Thiazolidinediones: [rosiglitazone (Avandia)]	4–8	↑ Insulin sensitivity in muscle and fat tissue	++	0	+/−	+
Thiazolidinediones: [pioglitazone (Actos)] Insulin	15–45	↓ Hepatic glucose output				
		↓ Hepatic glucose output; overcome insulin resistance	+++	+	++	+

Hypoglycemic Agents

Pharmacologic therapy either decreases insulin resistance, increases insulin secretion, slows postprandial glucose absorption, or, in the case of insulin injection, supplements inadequate secretion of insulin (Table 1).

Biguanides

The biguanides act on insulin receptors in the liver, reducing hepatic glucose production and in muscle and fat tissue enhancing insulin-stimulated glucose uptake. They have an anorexic effect, which can promote weight loss, and as noted above, metformin has been used for this purpose. It has also been used to reduce acanthosis and ovarian hyperandrogenism. Long-term use is associated with a 1% to 2% reduction in HbA1c, but a high rate of side effects, including transient abdominal pain, diarrhea, and nausea, limits compliance in adolescents (153). Metformin must not be given to patients with renal impairment, or who have hepatic disease, cardiac or respiratory insufficiency, or who are undergoing radiographic contrast studies because of the risk of lactic acidosis.

Metformin is the only oral hypoglycemic agent currently approved for use in children. FDA approval was based on a study of 80 previously untreated patients (aged 8–16 years) who were randomized to receive metformin or placebo in a multicenter study. Dosage began with 500 mg twice daily and increased to 2000 mg/day for over two weeks. Rescue criteria resulted in few placebo cases remaining by 16 weeks of the study. At four months or longer, the mean fasting glucose change from baseline was a decrease of 44 mg/dL with metformin and an increase of

20 mg/dL with placebo. The adjusted mean HbA1c with metformin was 7.5% and with placebo 8.6%. With metformin, there was no weight gain, and modest decrease in some patients, and lipid profiles improved. No serious adverse events were recorded (154). Review of 29 trials done using metformin compared with placebo, insulin, or other hypoglycemic agents in adults with T2DM showed that metformin not only normalizes blood sugars but also decreases cholesterol levels and lessens hypertension. Metformin may cause gastrointestinal upset, thus

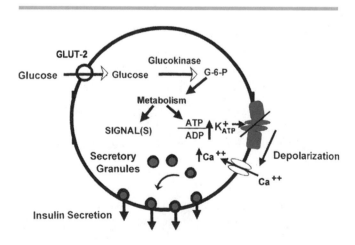

Figure 5 Binding sites for hypoglycemic agents. Sulfonylureas bind to specific receptors on the K+/ATP channel complex, while meglitinide and repaglinide bind to a separate site on the complex. *Abbreviation*: ATP, adenosine triphosphate.

decreasing compliance, but the extended-release formulation has less side effects, and tends to be better tolerated by patients (155). The extended-release formulation of metformin is given as a once-a-day dose usually in the evening. Dosing is begun at 500 mg/day and can be increased to a maximum of 2000 mg/day.

When metformin is not being effective, it is important to do an in-depth history of medication intake, including refill history from the pharmacy, which may demonstrate that the medication is not being taken. It must also be recognized that metformin may normalize ovulatory abnormalities in girls with PCOS or ovarian hyperandrogenism, increasing pregnancy risk.

Sulfonylurea and Meglitinide/Repaglinide

This group of drugs increases insulin secretion and is thus most useful when there is residual beta-cell function. The sulfonylureas bind to specific receptors on the K+/adenosine triphosphate (ATP) channel complex, while megilitinide and repaglinide bind to a separate site on the complex (Fig. 5). Activating ATP or binding by these drugs causes K+ channels to close, with resultant membrane depolarization, allowing calcium influx and insulin release. While ATP binding sites equilibrate rapidly, sulfonylurea sites do so slowly with prolongation of binding, explaining the sustained effects of traditional sulfonylureas. Meglitinide has an intermediate equilibration and binding duration, explaining its use for more rapid stimulation of insulin secretion, and need for pre-meal dosing (156). The major adverse effects of the sulfonylureas have been hypoglycemia, which, as noted above, can be prolonged, and weight gain, particularly troublesome for adolescent patients. Glimepramide, a third-generation sulfonylurea, has been compared with metformin in a pediatric T2DM trial, with comparable safety and efficacy (157).

Glucosidase Inhibitors

Alpha glucosidase inhibitors such as acarbose and miglitol reduce the absorption of carbohydrates in the upper small intestine by the inhibition of oligosaccharide breakdown, delaying absorption in the lower small intestine. This results in reduction in postprandial glycemia. Long-term use of glucosidase inhibitors is associated with a reduction in HbA1c of 0.5% to 1% (158). Flatulence associated with the use of these agents makes them unacceptable to young patients.

Thiazolidinediones

These drugs act directly on muscle, adipose tissue, and liver to increase insulin sensitivity, and are, therefore, considered specific agents for the manifold problems of the insulin sensitivity syndrome. They bind to nuclear proteins, activating peroxisome proliferator activator receptors (PPAR), orphan steroid receptors, which are particularly abundant in adipocytes, increasing formation of proteins involved in the nuclear-based actions of insulin. These include cell growth, adipose cell differentiation, regulation of insulin receptor activity, and glucose transport into cells. Long-term treatment with thiazolidinediones has been associated with a reduction in HbA1c of 0.5% to 1.3% (159). Side effects have included edema, weight gain, and anemia. The original member of this group of drugs, troglitazone, was associated with liver enzyme elevations in approximately 1% of those taking the drug, with mortality in some who had existing liver problems, resulting in its withdrawal from the market. The newer thiazolidinediones, rosiglitazone and pioglitazone, have not been shown to have significant hepatotoxicity.

The binding of thiazolidinediones to PPARγ receptors is ubiquitous and includes arterial walls, which contain muscle, affecting the growth of muscle cells and their migration in response to growth factors (160). These drugs also improve lipid profiles, decreasing LDL cholesterol and triglycerides, while increasing HDL cholesterol. These effects on vascular muscle and lipids could be important for the reduction of macrovascular disease associated with T2DM (161).

Rosiglitazone use in pediatric T2DM was compared with metformin in a 24-week double-blind study with 195 patients; reduction in HbA1c was comparable in both groups and there were no safety problems with the rosiglitazone. However, there was weight gain, as in adults taking thiazolidinediones (162).

Insulin

The development of T2DM is an indicator of limited beta-cell function, estimated to be approximately 50% by the time of diagnosis in adults, most of whom will be insulin-requiring by six or seven years later (163). Despite the insulin resistance, relatively small doses of supplemental insulin, a few units, may be sufficient to maintain euglycemia. Early normalization of blood sugars in patients with new-onset T2DM, using intensive insulin therapy, results in lower HbA1c and improvement of insulin area under the curve on oral glucose tolerance testing one year after diagnosis. Long-acting insulin analogues without peak effects, such as insulin glargine, may be especially useful for T2DM in combination with pre-meal meglitinide, particularly in those individuals who are unwilling to take metformin. Hypoglycemia has not been as common a side effect in T2DM as in T1DM, but weight gain is an important adverse effect. All patients with T2DM eventually require treatment with insulin because of ongoing loss of beta-cell function (147).

Incretins

Incretins are gut-derived factors that potentiate insulin secretion following the oral ingestion of nutrients. In the mid-1960s it was found that the insulin secretory response to oral glucose was stronger than the response to intravenous glucose, and, therefore, it was

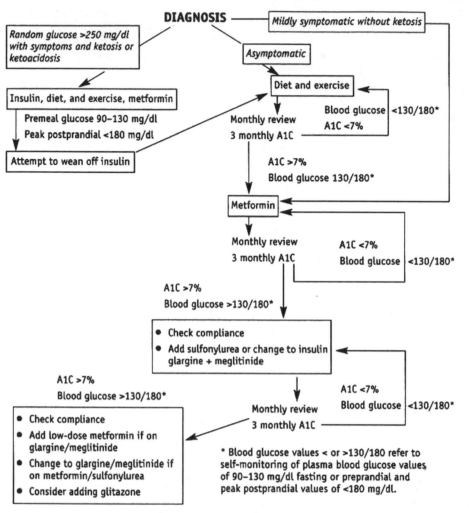

Figure 6   Decision tree for treatment of T2DM. *Blood glucose values < or >130/180 refer to self-monitoring of plasma blood-glucose values of 90–130 mg/dL fasting or preprandial and peak postprandial values of < 180 mg/dL. *Abbreviation*: T2DM, Type 2 diabetes mellitus.

recognized that gut-derived factors contribute to postprandial insulin response ("the incretin effect") (164). Glucagon-like peptide 1 (GLP-1) is a product of the glucagon gene and is secreted by the L-cells of the small and large intestine within 5 to 10 minutes following meal ingestion. GLP-1 exerts its effects by binding and activating receptors, which are found on the beta cells as well as many other tissues. GLP-1 enhances glucose-stimulated insulin release, is able to restore first-phase insulin release, decreases glucagons secretion, and slows gastric emptying (165). These effects of GLP-1 only occur when glucose levels rise above fasting concentrations. GLP-1 has been investigated as a treatment for obesity because of its effects on decreasing fluid and food intake. Additionally, GLP-1 has been shown in rodents to delay or prevent the loss of beta-cell mass, making it an important treatment consideration for the progressive disease of T2DM (166).

The two most well-studied incretins are GLP-1 and glucose-dependent insulinotropic polypeptide (also known as gastric inhibitory polypeptide). A GLP-1 mimetic (Exenatide; Byetta™) is being used

for the treatment of T2DM in adults (167). It is given as a twice daily injection. Side effects include nausea, vomiting, diarrhea, dyspepsia, jitteriness, dizziness, headache, and hypoglycemia, particularly when given with sulfonylurea. Safety and efficacy have not been established in pediatric patients, but it is likely that the need for twice daily injection and the side effect profile will make this an unacceptable treatment for children with T2DM.

Treatment Recommendations

Treatment decisions are based on symptoms, severity of hyperglycemia, the presence or absence of ketosis/ketoacidosis (DKA), or of dehydration. Signs of dehydration may be less obvious in the obese. Symptomatic youngsters with T2DM, in addition to frequently having ketoacidosis at diabetes onset, are at particular risk for the HHS, which carries a high mortality (80). DKA and HHS are discussed in Vol. 1; Chap. 8. A treatment decision tree for outpatient management is given in Figure 6 (168).

Metformin should be the first oral agent used, because it is associated with similar HbA1c reductions to sulfonylureas and thiazolidinediones, with minimal risk of hypoglycemia, and without weight gain. Furthermore, there may be greater effect on reducing LDL cholesterol and triglyceride levels than with a sulfonylurea. With failure of monotherapy using metformin over a three- to six-month period, sulfonylurea, meglitinide, or insulin can be added. Thiazolidinediones may be used in older adolescents. Combination formulations may result in better compliance (169).

It is important to counsel adolescents with T2DM about sexuality and pregnancy, and provide contraceptive advice as necessary, not only because metformin and thiazolidinediones may restore normal periods (170), but because oral agents should not be used during pregnancy.

Although routine self-monitoring of blood-glucose may not be needed as frequently as with T1DM, frequent monitoring is needed during periods of acute illness, during dosage adjustment, or with symptoms that indicate hyper- or hypoglycemia. It is also necessary to monitor for asymptomatic hypoglycemia in those individuals who are taking insulin or sulfonylureas. The frequency of routine self-monitoring of blood-glucose needs to be individualized, but include a combination of fasting in postprandial measurements.

Assessments of HbA1c concentration should be done at least twice a year and, if metabolic control is unsatisfactory and requires treatment adjustment, every three months. The involvement of a dietitian with skill in the management of nutritional problems in children with diabetes is essential; the dietary recommendations need to be culturally appropriate, sensitive to family style and resources, and need to be understood by all caregivers.

Treating Comorbidities

Hypertension is an independent risk factor for the development of albuminuria, retinopathy, and cardiovascular disease in T2DM in adults. Its importance is emphasized by the experience of the U.K. Prospective Diabetes Study, in which hypertension control was more important than blood-glucose control in reducing the risk of cardiovascular disease (148). BP should be measured at diagnosis and at least quarterly and compared with standards appropriate for age and height percentiles, as noted in the tables in Vol. 1; Chap. 13. Elevations must be treated aggressively if there is persistent elevation above the usual percentile for the child or above the 90th percentile for either systolic or diastolic pressure. Angiotensin-converting enzyme inhibitors (ACEI) are the initial drug of choice (172). As with T1DM, many physicians use ACEI prophylactically in patients with T2DM.

Lipid levels and urine albumin excretion should be measured shortly after diagnosis and annually, or more often if there is abnormality and treatment effects need monitoring. Exercise, weight loss, and glycemic control may be sufficient to correct hyperlipidemia. Dietary recommendations should be for the reduced fat diet consistent with step 2 American Heart Association guidelines. Lipid lowering medications should be added if lipids do not improve satisfactorily after three to six months of dietary and diabetes control efforts. HMG CoA reductase inhibitors (statins) are the most commonly used lipid lowering agents in pediatric patients; they are contraindicated in pregnancy or if there is risk of pregnancy (173).

Unlike the recommendations for T1DM, that regular monitoring for complications not begin until adolescence and three to five years of diabetes, monitoring lipids and urinary albumin excretion, and examining the retina in those with T2DM should begin at the time of diagnosis (1).

REFERENCES

1. American Diabetes Association. Type 2 diabetes in children and adolescents: consensus conference report. Diabetes Care 2000; 23:381–389.
2. Botero D, Woldsorf JI. Diabetes mellitus in children and adolescents. Arch Med Res 2005; 36:281–290.
3. Decsi T, Molnar D. Insulin resistance syndrome in children: pathophysiology and potential management strategies. Paediatr Drugs 2003; 5:291–299.
4. Weiss R, Dufour S, Taksali SE, et al. Prediabetes in obese youth: a syndrome of impaired glucose tolerance, severe insulin resistance, and altered myocellular and abdominal fat partitioning. Lancet 2003; 362:951–957.
5. Knowles HC. Diabetes mellitus in childhood and adolescence. Med Clin North Am 1971; 55:975–987.
6. Rosenbloom AL, Joe JR, Young RS, Winter WE. The emerging epidemic of type 2 diabetes mellitus in youth. Diabetes Care 1999; 22:345–354.
7. Pihoker C, Scott CR, Lensing SY, Cradock MM, Smith J. Non-insulin dependent diabetes mellitus in African-American youths of Arkansas. Clin Pediatr 1998; 37:97–102.
8. Upchurch SL, Brosnan CA, Meininger JC, et al. Characteristics of 98 children and adolescents diagnosed with type 2 diabetes by their health care provider at initial presentation. Diabetes Care 2003; 26:2209.
9. Glaser NS, Jones KL. Non-insulin-dependent diabetes mellitus in Mexican-American children. West J Med 1998; 168:11–16.
10. Neufeld ND, Raffal LF, Landon C, Chen Y-DI, Vadheim CM. Early presentation of type 2 diabetes in Mexican-American youth. Diabetes Care 1998; 21:80–86.
11. Savage PJ, Bennett PH, Senter RG, Miller M. High prevalence of diabetes in young Pima Indians. Diabetes 1979; 28:937–942.
12. Dabelea D, Hanson RL, Bennett PH, Roumain J, Knowler WC, Pettitt DJ. Increasing prevalence of type 2 diabetes in American Indian children. Diabetologia 1998; 41:904–910.
13. Pinhas-Hamiel O, Dolan LM, Daniels SR, Standiford D, Khoury PR, Zeitler P. Increased incidence of non-insulin dependent diabetes mellitus among adolescents. J Pediatr 1996; 128:608–615.
14. Dean HJ. NIDDM-Y in First Nation children in Canada. Clin Pediatr 1998; 39:89–96.

15. Pinhas-Hamiel O, Zeitler P. The global spread of type 2 diabetes mellitus in children and adolescents. J Pediatr 2005; 146:693–700.

16. Fagot-Campagna A, Pettitt DJ, Engelgau MM, et al. Type 2 diabetes among North American children and adolescents: an epidemiological review and a public health perspective. J Pediatr 2000; 136:664–672.

17. Macaluso CJ, Bauer UE, Deeb LC, et al. Type 2 diabetes mellitus among Florida children and adolescents, 1994 through 1998. Public Health Rep 2002; 117:373–379.

18. Drake AJ, Smith A, Betts PR, Crowne EC, Shield JP. Type 2 diabetes in obese white children. Arch Dis Child 2002; 86:207–208.

19. Troiano RP, Flegal KM. Overweight children and adolescents: description, epidemiology, and demographics. Pediatrics 1998; 101:497–504.

20. Freedman DS, Srinivasan SR, Valdez RA, Williamson DF, Berenson GS. Secular increases in relative weight and obesity among children over two decades: The Bogalusa Heart Study. Pediatrics 1997; 99:420–426.

21. Strauss RS, Pollack HA. Epidemic increase in childhood overweight, 1986–1998. JAMA 2001; 286:2845–2848.

22. Kitagawa T, Owada M, Urakami T, Yamauchi K. Increased incidence of non-insulin dependent diabetes mellitus among Japanese schoolchildren correlates with an increased intake of animal protein and fat. Clin Pediatr 1998; 37:111–115.

23. Sayeed MA, Hussain MZ, Banu A, Rumi MAK, Azad Khan AK. Prevalence of diabetes in a suburban population of Bangladesh. Diabetes Res Clin Pract 1997; 34:149–155.

24. Wang Y. Cross-national comparison of childhood obesity: the epidemic and the relationship between obesity and socioeconomic status. Int J Epidemiol 2001; 30:1129–1136.

25. Cheng TO. Childhood obesity in China. Health Place 2004; 10:395–396.

26. Ehtisham S, Barrett TG, Shawl NJ. Type 2 diabetes mellitus in UK children—an emerging problem. Diabetic Med 2000; 17:867–871.

27. Livingstone B. Epidemiology of childhood obesity in Europe. Eur J Pediatr 2000; 159(suppl 1):S14–S34.

28. Yanovski SZ, Yanovski JA. Obesity. N Engl J Med 2002; 346:591–602.

29. Blair SN, Nichaman MZ. The public health problem of increasing prevalence rates of obesity and what should be done about it. Mayo Clin Proc 2002; 77:109–113.

30. Neel JV. Diabetes mellitus: a "thrifty" genotype rendered detrimental by "progress"? Am J Hum Genet 1962; 14:353–362.

31. Lev-Ran A. Thrifty genotype: how applicable is it to obesity and type 2 diabetes? Diabetes Rev 1999; 7:1–22.

32. Lillioja S, Mott DM, Spraul M, et al. Insulin resistance and insulin secretory dysfunction as precursors of non-insulin-dependent diabetes mellitus: prospective studies of Pima Indians. N Engl J Med 1993; 329:1988–1992.

33. Haffner SM, Stern MP, Dunn J, Mobley M, Blackwell J, Bergman RN. Diminished insulin sensitivity and increased insulin response in non-obese, non-diabetic Mexican Americans. Metabolism 1990; 39:842–847.

34. Haffner SM, Miettinen H, Stern MP. Insulin secretion and resistance in non-diabetic Mexican Americans and non-Hispanic whites with a parental history of diabetes. J Clin Endocrinol Metab 1996; 81:1846–1851.

35. Groop L, Forsblom C, Lehtovirta M, et al. Metabolic consequences of a family history of NIDDM (the Botnia Study): evidence for sex specific parental effects. Diabetes 1996; 45:1585–1593.

36. Martin BC, Warram JH, Krolewski AS, Bergman RN, Soeldner JS, Kahn CR. Role of glucose and insulin resistance in development of type 2 diabetes mellitus: results of a 25 year follow-up study. Lancet 1992; 340:925–929.

37. Pigon J, Giacca A, Ostenson C-G, Lam L, Vranic M, Efendi S. Normal hepatic insulin sensitivity in lean, mild non-insulin-dependent diabetic patients. J Clin Endocrinol Metab 1996; 81:3702–3708.

38. O'Rahilly S, Turner RC, Matthew D. Impaired pulsatile secretion of insulin in relatives of patients with non-insulin-dependent diabetes. N Engl J Med 1988; 318:1225–1230.

39. Saltiel AR, Olefsky JM. Thiazolidinediones in the treatment of insulin resistance and type II diabetes. Diabetes 1994; 45:1661–1669.

40. Saltiel AR. Putting the brakes on insulin signaling. N Engl J Med 2003; 349:2560–2562.

41. Philipps K, Barker DJP. Fetal growth and impaired glucose tolerance in men and women. Diabetologia 1993; 36:225–228.

42. Phillips DIW, Barker DJP, Hales CN, Hirst S, Osmond C. Thinness at birth and insulin resistance in adult life. Diabetologia 1994; 37:150–154.

43. Lithell HO, McKeigue PM, Berglund L, Mohsen R, Lithell UB, Leon DA. Relation at birth to non-insulin-dependent diabetes and insulin concentrations in men aged 50–60 years. Br Med J 1996; 312:406–410.

44. Curhan GC, Willett WC, Rimm EB, Spiegelman D, Ascherio AL, Stampfer MJ. Birth weight and adult hypertension, diabetes mellitus, and obesity in US men. Circulation 1996; 94:3246–3250.

45. Ravelli AC, van der Meulen JH, Michels RP, et al. Glucose tolerance in adults after prenatal exposure to famine. Lancet 1998; 351:173–177.

46. Levitt NS, Lambert EV, Woods D, Hales CN, Andrew R, Seckl JR. Impaired glucose tolerance and elevated blood pressure in low birth weight, nonobese, young South African adults: early programming of cortisol axis. J Clin Endocrinol Metab 2000; 85:4611–4618.

47. Dabelea D, Pettitt DJ, Hanson RL, Imperatore G, Bennett PH, Knowler WC. Birthweight, type 2 diabetes, and insulin resistance in Pima Indian children and young adults. Diabetes Care 1999; 22:944–950.

48. Bhargava SK, Sachdev HS, Fall CHD, et al. Relation of serial changes in childhood body-mass index to impaired glucose tolerance in young adulthood. N Engl J Med 2004; 350:865–875.

49. Bavdekar A, Yajnik CS, Fall CHD, et al. Insulin resistance syndrome in 8-year old Indian children. Small at birth, big at 8 years, or both? Diabetes 1999; 48:2422–2429.

50. Li C, Johnson MS, Goran MI. Effects of low birth weight on insulin resistance syndrome in Caucasian and African-American children. Diabetes Care 2001; 24:2035–2042.

51. Koletzko B, Broekaert I, Demmelmair H, et al. Protein intake in the first year of life: a risk factor for later obesity? The E.U. childhood obesity project. Adv Exp Med Biol 2005; 569:69–79.

52. Pettitt DJ, Forman MR, Hanson RL, Knowler WC, Bennett PH. Breastfeeding and incidence of non-insulin-dependent diabetes mellitus in Pima Indians. Lancet 1997; 350:166–168.

53. Von Kries R, Koletzko R, Sauerwald T, et al. Breast feeding and obesity: cross-sectional study. BMJ 1999; 319:147–150.

54. Rosenbloom AL. Type 2 diabetes in children. American Association for Clinical Chemistry. Diagn Endocrinol Immunol Metabolism 2000; 18:143–153.

55. Dunger DB, Ong KK, Huxtable SJ, et al. Association of the INS VNTR with size at birth. ALSPAC study team. Avon longitudinal study of pregnancy and childhood. Nat Genet 1998; 19:98–100.

56. Hattersley AT, Beards F, Ballantyne E, Appleton M, Harvey R, Ellard S. Mutations in the glucokinase gene of the fetus result in reduced birthweight. Nat Genet 1998; xx:268–270.

57. Jaquet D, Vidal H, Hankard R, Czernichow P, Levy-Marchal C. Impaired regulation of glucose transporter 4 gene expression in insulin resistance associated with in utero undernutrition. J Clin Endocrinol Metab 2001; 86:3266–3267.

58. Pettitt DJ, Aleck KA, Baird HR, Carraher MJ, Bennett PH, Knowler WC. Congenital susceptibility to NIDDM: role of intrauterine environment. Diabetes 1988; 37:622–628.

59. Silverman BL, Metzger BE, Cho NH, Loeb CA. Impaired glucose tolerance in adolescent offspring of diabetic mothers. Relationship to fetal hyperinsulinism. Diabetes Care 1995; 18:611–617.

60. Dabelea D, Knowler WC, Pettitt DJ. Effect of diabetes in pregnancy on offspring: follow-up research in the Pima Indians. J Matern Fetal Med 2000; 9:83–88.

61. Rosenbloom AL, Wheeler L, Bianchi R, Chin FT, Tiwary CM, Grgic A. Age adjusted analysis of insulin responses during normal and abnormal oral glucose tolerance tests in children and adolescents. Diabetes 1975; 24:820–828.

62. Caprio S, Tamborlane WV. Metabolic impact of obesity in childhood. Endocrinol Metab Clin North Am 1999; 28:731–747.

63. Klein S, Fontana L, Young VL, et al. Absence of an effect of liposuction on insulin action and risk factors for coronary heart disease. N Engl J Med 2004; 350:2549–2557.

64. Drash AM. Relationship between diabetes mellitus and obesity in the child. Metabolism 1973; 22:337–344.

65. Martin MM, Martin AL. Obesity, hyperinsulinism, and diabetes mellitus in childhood. J Pediatr 1973; 82(2):192–201.

66. Young-Hyman D, Schlundt DG, Herman L, DeLuca F, Counts D. Evaluation of the insulin resistance syndrome and 5- to 10-year old overweight/obesity African-American children. Diabetes Care 2001; 24:1359–1364.

67. Caprio S. Relationship between abdominal visceral fat and metabolic risk factors in obese adolescents. Am J Hum Biol 1999; 11:259–266.

68. Svec F, Nastasi K, Hilton C, Bao W, Srinivasan SR, Berenson GS. Black-white contrasts and insulin levels during pubertal development: the Bogalusa Heart Study. Diabetes 1992; 41:313–317.

69. Jiang X, Srinivasan SR, Radhakrishnamurthy B, Dalferes ER, Berenson GS. Racial (black-white) differences in insulin secretion and clearance in adolescents: the Bogalusa heart study. Pediatrics 1996; 97:357–360.

70. Arslanian S. Insulin secretion and sensitivity in healthy African-American vs. American-white children. Clin Pediatr 1998; 37:81–88.

71. Danadian K, Lewy V, Janosky JJ, Arslanian S. Lipolysis in African-American children: is it a metabolic risk factor predisposing to obesity? J Clin Endocrinol Metab 2001; 86:3022–3026.

72. Webster-Gandy J, Warren J, Henry CJ. Sexual dimorphism in fat patterning in a sample of 5 to 7-year-old children in Oxford. Int J Food Sci Nutr 2003; 54:467–471.

73. Danadian K, Balasekaran G, Lewy V, Meza MP, Robertson R, Arslanian SA. Insulin sensitivity in African-American children with and without a family history of type 2 diabetes. Diabetes Care 1999; 22:1325–1329.

74. Lindgren CM, Hirschhorn JN. The genetics of type 2 diabetes. Endocrinologist 2001; 11:178–187.

75. Rosenbloom AL, House DV, Winter WE. Non-insulin dependent diabetes mellitus (NIDDM) in minority youth: research priorities and needs. Clin Pediatr 1998; 37:143–152.

76. Hanis CL, Boerwinkle E, Chakraborty R, et al. A genome-wide search for human non-insulin-dependent (type 2) diabetes genes reveals a major susceptibility locus on chromosome 2. Nat Genet 1996; 13:161–166.

77. Horikawa Y, Oda N, Cox NJ, et al. Genetic variation in the gene encoding calpain-IO is associated with type 2 diabetes mellitus. Nat Genet 2000; 26:163–175.

78. Baier LJ, Permana PA, Yang X, et al. A calpain 10 gene polymorphism is associated with reduced muscle mRNA levels and insulin resistance. J Clin Invest 2000; 106:R69–R73.

79. Zuhri-Yafi MI, Brosnan PG, Hardin DS. Treatment of type 2 diabetes mellitus in children and adolescents. J Pediatr Endocrinol Metab 2002; 15(suppl 1):541–546.

80. Morales A, Rosenbloom AL. Death at the onset of type 2 diabetes (T2DM) in African-American youth. J Pediatr 2004; 144:270–273.

81. Rosenbloom AL. Obesity, insulin resistance, beta cell autoimmunity, and the changing clinical epidemiology of childhood diabetes. Diabetes Care 2003; 26:2954–2956.

82. Turner R, Stratton I, Horton V, et al. for the UK Prospective Diabetes Study (UKPDS) Group. UKPDS 25: autoantibodies to islet cell cytoplasm and glutamic acid decarboxylase for prediction of insulin requirement in type 2 diabetes. Lancet 1997; 350:1288–1293.

83. Landin-Olsson M. Latent autoimmune diabetes in adults. Ann N Y Acad Sci 2002; 958:112–116.

84. Hathout EH, Thomas W, El-Shahawy, et al. Diabetic auto-immune markers in children and adolescents with type 2 diabetes. Pediatrics 2001; 107:e102.

85. Umpaichitra V, Banerji MA, Castells S. Autoantibodies in children with type 2 diabetes mellitus. J Pediatr Endocrinol Metab 2002; 15:525–530.

86. American Diabetes Association. Consensus development conference on insulin resistance. Diabetes Care 1998; 21:310–314.

87. Steinberger J, Moran A, Hong C-P, Jacobs DR, Sinaiko AR. Adiposity in childhood predicts obesity and insulin resistance in young adulthood. J Pediatr 2001; 138:469–473.

88. Freedman DS, Khan LK, Dietz WH, Srinivasan SR, Berenson GS. Relationship of childhood obesity to coronary heart disease risk factors in adulthood: the Bogalusa heart study. Pediatrics 2001; 108:712–718.

89. Berenson GS, Srnivasan SR. Cardiovascular risk factors in youth with implications for aging: the Bogalusa Heart Study. Neurobiol Aging 2005; 26:303–307.

90. Juonala M, Jarvisalo MJ, Maki-Torkko N, Kahonen M, Viikari JS, Raitakari OT. Risk factors identified in childhood and decreased carotid artery elasticity in adulthood: the Cardiovascular Risk in Young Finns Study. Circulation 2005; 112:1486–1493.

91. Visser M, Bouter LM, McQuillan GM, Wener MH, Harris TB. Low-grade systemic inflammation in overweight children. Pediatrics 2001; 107:e13.

92. Adelman RD, Restaino IG, Alon US, Blowey DL. Proteinuria and focal segmental glomerulosclerosis in severely obese adolescents. J Pediatr 2001; 138:481–485.

93. Smith JC, Field C, Braden DS, Gaymes CH, Kastner J. Coexisting health problems in obese children and adolescents that might require special treatment considerations. Clin Pediatr 1999; 38:305–307.

94. Strauss RS, Barlow SE, Dietz WH. Prevalence of abnormal serum aminotransferase values in overweight and obese adolescents. J Pediatr 2000; 136:727–733.

95. Kirpichnikov D, Sowers JR. Diabetes mellitus and diabetes-associated vascular disease. Trends Endocrinol Metab 2001; 12:225–230.

96. Laakso M. Lipids in type 2 diabetes. Semin Vasc Med 2002; 2:59–66.

97. Goldberg IJ. Diabetic dyslipidemia: causes and consequences. J Clin Endocrinol Metab 2001; 86:965–971.

98. Gress TW, Nieto FJ, Shahar E, Wofford MR, Brancati FL. Hypertension and antihypertensive therapy has risk factors for type 2 diabetes mellitus. Atherosclerosis Risk in Community Study. N Engl J Med 2000; 342: 905–912.

99. Salomaa VV, Strandberg TE, Vanhanen H, Naukkarinen V, Sarna S, Miettinen TA. Glucose tolerance and blood pressure: long-term follow-up in middle-age men. BMJ 1991; 302:493–496.

100. Wierzbicki AS, Nimmo L, Feher MD, Cox A, Foxton J, Lant AF. Association of angiotensin-converting enzyme DD genotype with hypertension in diabetes. J Hum Hypertens 1995; 9:671–673.

101. Poredos P. Endothelial dysfunction and cardiovascular disease. Pathophysiol Haemost Thromb 2002; 32:274–277.

102. Tounian P, Aggoun Y, Dubern B, et al. Presence of increased stiffness of the common carotid artery and endothelial dysfunction in severely obese children: a prospective study. Lancet 2001; 358:1400–1404.

103. Aldhahi W, Hamdy O. Adipokines, inflammation, and the endothelium in diabetes. Curr Diab Rep 2003; 3:293–298.

104. Shimabukuro M, Higa N, Asahi T, et al. Hypoadiponectinemia is closely linked to endothelial dysfunction in man. J Clin Endocrinol Metab 2003; 88:3236–3240.

105. Stuart CA, Gilkison CR, Smith MM, Bosma AM, Keenan BS, Nagamani M. Acanthosis nigricans as a risk factor for non-insulin dependent diabetes mellitus. Clin Pediatr 1998; 37:73–79.

106. Nguyen TT, Keil MF, Russell DL, et al. Relation of acanthosis nigricans to hyperinsulinemia and insulin sensitivity in overweight African-American and white children. J Pediatr 2001; 138:474–480.

107. Sackett DL, Holland WW. Controversy in detection of disease. Lancet 1975; 2:357–359.

108. Tirosh A, Shai I, Tekes-Manova D, et al.; Israeli Diabetes Research Group. Normal fasting plasma glucose levels and type 2 diabetes in young men. N Engl J Med 2005; 353(14):1454–1462.

109. Sokol RJ. The chronic disease of childhood obesity: the sleeping giant has awakened. J Pediatr 2000; 136:711–713.

110. Tersbakovec AM, Watson MH, Wenner WJ, Marx AL. Insurance reimbursement for treatment of obesity in children. J Pediatr 1999; 134:573–578.

111. Zwiaur KFM. Prevention and treatment of overweight and obesity in children and adolescents. Eur J Pediatr 2000; 159(suppl 1):S56–S68.

112. Segel DG, Sanchez JC. Childhood obesity in the year 2001. Endocrinologist 2001; 11:296–306.

113. Trevino RP, Pugh JA, Hernadez AE, Menchaca VD, Ramirez RR, Mendoza M. Bienestar: a diabetes risk factor prevention program. J School Health 1998; 68:62–66.

114. Epstein LH, Myers MD, Raynor HA, Saelens BE. Treatment of pediatric obesity. Pediatrics 1998; 101:554–570.

115. Cook VV, Hurley JS. Prevention of type 2 diabetes in childhood. Clin Pediatr 1998; 37:123–129.

116. Teufel NI, Ritenbaugh CK. Development of a primary prevention program: insight gained in the Zuni Diabetes Prevention Program. Clin Pediatr 1998; 37:131–141.

117. Gortmaker SL, Cheung LWY, Peterson KE, et al. Impact of a school-based interdisciplinary intervention on diet and physical activity among urban primary school children. Arch Pediatr Adolesc Med 1999; 153:975–983.

118. Macaulay AC, Paradis G, Potvin L, et al. The Kahnawake Schools Diabetes Prevention Project: intervention, evaluation and baseline results of a diabetes primary prevention program with a native community in Canada. Prev Med 1997; 26:779–790.

119. Jakicic JM. Exercise in the treatment of obesity. Endocrinol Metab Clin North Am 2003; 32:967–980.

120. Perry CL, Stone EJ, Parcel GS, et al. School-based cardiovascular health promotion: the child and adolescents trial for cardiovascular health (CATCH). J School Health 1998; 68:406–413.

121. Vestfold Heartcare Study Group. Influence on lifestyle measures and five-year coronary risk by a comprehensive lifestyle intervention programme in patients with coronary heart disease. J Cardiovasc Risk 2003; 10:429–437.

122. Moyna NM, Thompson PD. The effect of physical activity on endothelial function in man. Acta Physiol Scand 2004; 180:113–123.

123. Ishikawa-Takata K, Ohta T, Tanaka H. How much exercise is required to reduce blood pressure in essential hypertensives: a dose–response study. Am J Hypertens 2003; 16:629–633.

124. Cummings S, Parham ES, Strain GW. Position of the American Dietetic Association: weight management. J Am Diet Assoc 2002; 102:1145–1155.

125. Zabinski MF, Saelens BE, Stein RI, Hayden-Wade HA, Wilfley DE. Overweight children's barriers to and support for physical activity. Obes Res 2003; 11(2):238–246.

126. Baird J, Fisher D, Lucas P, Kleijnen J, Roberts H, Law C. Being big or growing fast: systematic review of size and growth in infancy and later obesity. BMJ 2005; 331(7522):929.

127. Levine MD, Ringham RM, Kalarchian MA, Wisniewski L, Marcus MD. Is family based behavioral weight control appropriate for severe pediatric obesity? Int J Eat Disord 2001; 30:318–328.

128. Robinson TM. Reducing children's television viewing to prevent obesity. A randomized controlled trial. JAMA 1999; 82:1561–1567.

129. Swinburn BA, Metcalf PA, Ley SJ. Long-term (five-year) effects of a reduced fat diet intervention in individuals with glucose intolerance. Diabetes Care 2001; 24:619–624.

130. Tuomilehto J, Lindstrom J, Eriksson JG, et al. Prevention of type 2 diabetes mellitus by changes in lifestyle among subjects with impaired glucose tolerance. N Engl J Med 2001; 344:1343–1350.

131. Diabetes Prevention Program Research Group. Reduction in the incidence of type 2 diabetes with lifestyle intervention or metformin. N Engl J Med 2002; 346: 393–403.

132. Jeffrey RW. Community programs for obesity prevention: the Minnesota Heart Health Program. Obesity Res 1995; 3(suppl 2):283S–288S.

133. Epstein LH, Valoski AM, Kalarchian MA, McCurley J. Do children lose and maintain weight easier than adults: a comparison of child and parent weight changes from six months to ten years. Obes Res 1995; 3:411–417.

134. Joe JR. Perceptions of diabetes by Indian adolescents. In: Joe JR, Young RS, eds. Diabetes as a Disease of Civilization: The Impact of Culture Change on Indigenous Peoples. Berlin: Mouton de Gruyter, 1994:329–356.

135. Miller WC. How effective are traditional dietary and exercise interventions for weight loss? Med Sci Sports Exerc 1999; 31:1129–1134.

136. Chanoine JP, Hampl S, Jensen C, Boldrin M, Hauptman J. Effect of orlistat on weight and body composition in obese adolescents: a randomized controlled trial. JAMA 2005; 293:2873–2883.
137. Freemark M, Bursey D. The effects of metformin on body mass index and glucose tolerance in obese adolescents with fasting hyperinsulinemia and a family history of type 2 diabetes. Pediatrics 2001; 107(4):E55.
138. Leung WY, Neil Thomas G, Chan JC, Tomlinson B. Weight management and current options in pharmacotherapy: orlistat and sibutramine. Clin Ther 2003; 25:58–80.
139. Thearle M, Aronne LJ. Obesity and pharmacologic therapy. Endocrinol Metab Clin North Am 2003; 32:1005–1024.
140. Bray GA, Hollander P, Klein S, et al. A 6-month randomized, placebo-controlled, dose-ranging trial of topiramate for weight loss in obesity. Obes Res 2003; 11:722–733.
141. Batterham RL, Cohen MA, Ellis SM, et al. Inhibition of food intake in obese subjects by peptide YY3-36. N Engl J Med 2003; 349:941–948.
142. Esposito K, Giugliano D. Effect of rimonabant on weight reduction and cardiovascular risk. Lancet 2005; 366:367–368 (author reply 369–370).
143. Huerta MG, Roemmich JN, Kington ML, et al. Magnesium deficiency is associated with insulin resistance in obese children. Diabetes Care 2005; 28:1175–1181.
144. Inge TH, Zeller M, Garcia VF, Daniels SR. Surgical approach to adolescent obesity. Adolesc Med Clin 2004; 15:429–453.
145. Fagot-Compagna A, Knowler WC, Pettitt DJ. Type 2 diabetes in Pima Indian Children: cardiovascular risk factors at diagnosis and 10 years later. Diabetes 1998(suppl 1):A155.
146. Yokoyama H, Okudaira M, Otani T, et al. High incidence of diabetic nephropathy in early-onset Japanese NIDDM patients. Risk analysis. Diabetes Care 1998; 21:1080–1085.
147. UKPDS Group. Intensive blood glucose control with sulphonylureas or insulin compared with conventional treatment and risk of complications in patients with type 2 diabetes (UKPDS 33) Lancet 1998; 352:837–853.
148. UKPDS Group. Tight blood pressure control and risk of macrovascular and microvascular complications in type 2 diabetes: UKPDS 38. Br Med J 1998; 317:703–713.
149. Ludwig DS, Peterson KE, Gortmaker SL. Relation between consumption of sugar sweetened drinks and childhood obesity: a prospective observational analysis. Lancet 2001; 357:505–508.
150. Apovian CM. Sugar-sweetened soft drinks, obesity, and type 2 diabetes. JAMA 2004; 292:927–934, 978–979.
151. Willi SM, Martin K, Datko FM, Brant BP. Treatment of type 2 diabetes in childhood using a very-low-calorie diet. Diabetes Care 2004; 227:348–353.
152. University of Texas Health Science Center at San Antonio/Department of Pediatrics and The Children's Center at the Texas Diabetes Institute. Kids, teens, and type 2 diabetes: what you need to know. An essential reference for school nurses, 2000.
153. DeFronzo RA, Goodman AM. Efficacy of metformin in patients with non-insulin dependent diabetes mellitus. The multicenter metformin study group. N Engl J Med 1995; 333:541–549.
154. Jones KL, Arslanian S, Peterokova VA, Park JS, Tomlinson MJ. Effect of metformin in pediatric patients with type 2 diabetes: a randomized controlled trial. Diabetes Care 2002; 25:89–94.
155. Timmins P, Donahue S, Meeker J, Marathe P. Steady-state pharmacokinetics of a novel extended-release metformin formulation. Clin Pharmacokinet 2005; 44:721–729.
156. Lebovitz HE. Insulin secretagogues, old and new. Diabetes Rev 1999; 7:139–152.
157. Gottschalk M, Danne T, Cara J, Vlajinic A, Izza M. Glimepramide (GLIM) vs metformin (MET) as monotherapy in pediatric subjects with T2DM: a single blind comparison study. Pediatr Diabetes 2005; 6(suppl 3):24–25 (abstract SP-18).
158. Chiasson J, Josse R, Hunt J, et al. The efficacy of acarbose in the treatment of patients with non-insulin-dependent diabetes mellitus. A multicenter controlled clinical trial. Ann Int Med 1994; 121:928–935.
159. Schwartz S, Raskin P, Fonseca V, Graveline JF. Effect of troglitazone in insulin treated patients with type 2 diabetes. N Engl J Med 1998; 338:861–866.
160. Law RE, Goetze S, Xi X-P, et al. Expression and function of PPARγ in rat and human vascular smooth muscle cells. Circulation 2000; 101:1311–1318.
161. Olefsky JM, Saltiel AR. PPARγ and the treatment of insulin resistance. Trends Endocrinol Metab 2000; 11:362–367.
162. Dabiri G, Jones K, Krebs J, et al. Benefits of rosiglitazone in children with T2DM. ADA Annual Meeting 2005 (abstract 1904-P).
163. Marble A, White P, Bogan I, Smith R. Enlargement of the liver in diabetic children: I. Its incidence etiology and nature. Arch Int Med 1938; 62:740–750.
164. Velasquez-Mieyer PA, Cowan PA, Umpierrez GE, Lustig RH, Cashion AK, Burghen GA. Racial differences in glucagon-like peptide-1 (GLP-1) concentrations and insulin dynamics during oral glucose tolerance test in obese subjects. Int J Obes Relat Metab Disord 2003; 27:1359–1364.
165. Leon DD, Crutchlow MF, Ham JY, Stoffers DA. Role of glucagon-like peptide-1 in the pathogenesis and treatment of diabetes mellitus. Int J Biochem Cell Biol 2005.
166. Aston-Mourney K, Proietto J, Andrikopoulos S. Investigational agents that protect pancreatic islet beta-cells from failure. Expert Opin Investig Drugs 2005; 14:1241–1250.
167. Summaries for patients. Exenatide or insulin glargine for suboptimally controlled diabetes? Ann Intern Med 2005; 143:I30.
168. Silverstein JH, Rosenbloom AL. Treatment of type 2 diabetes in children and adolescents. J Pediatr Endocrinol Metab 2000; 13(suppl 6):1403–1409.
169. Miller JL, Silverstein JH. The management of type 2 diabetes mellitus in children and adolescents. J Pediatr Endocrinol Metab 2005; 18:111–123.
170. Azziz R, Ehrmann RS, Legro RS, et al. Troglitazone improves ovulation and hirsutism in the polycystic ovary syndrome: a multicenter, double-blind, placebo-controlled trial. J Clin Endocrinol Metab 2001; 86:1626–1632.
171. National Heart, Long, and Blood Institute. Report of the second task force on blood pressure control in children—1987. J Pediatr 1987; 79:1–25.
172. Adler AI. Treating high blood pressure in diabetes: the evidence. Semin Vasc Med 2002; 2:127–137.
173. Haffner SM, Alexander CM, Cook TJ, et al., for the Scandinavian Simvastatin Survival Study Group. Reduced coronary events in Simvastatin treated patients with coronary heart disease and diabetes or impaired fasting glucose levels. Arch Int Med 1999; 59:2661–2667.

10

Maturity-Onset Diabetes of Youth and Other Genetic Conditions Associated with Diabetes

William E. Winter

Department of Pathology, Immunology and Laboratory Medicine, University of Florida, Gainesville, Florida, U.S.A.

INTRODUCTION

This chapter will examine maturity-onset diabetes of youth (MODY) (1) and other genetic forms of diabetes mellitus in the context of normal beta cell function, and the disorder's pathophysiology, presentation, and diagnosis. Initially beta cell disorders will be examined followed by a discussion of insulin-sensitivity disorders. By definition, the topics in this chapter are classified as "other specific types of diabetes" and exclude Type 1 diabetes mellitus (2,3), Type 2 diabetes (4), and gestational diabetes mellitus (GDM). The framework for this discussion will begin with a review of normal beta cell function and peripheral responses to insulin that determine the beta cell response to elevated glucose levels (Table 1).

BETA CELL FUNCTION: A REVIEW OF NORMAL PHYSIOLOGY

Multiple potential defects in beta cell metabolism exist that can cause diabetes (5). Plasma glucose enters and exits the interstitium on the way to and from cells. The transport of glucose across cell membranes is accomplished by energy-dependent or facilitative glucose transporters (Fig. 1).

Glucose in the interstitium enters the beta cell through the facilitative (non-energy-dependent) glucose transporter-2 (GLUT2) (6). The 524 amino acid GLUT2 protein is encoded on chromosome 3q26. GLUT2 is also expressed in intestinal epithelial cells, renal tubular cells, and hepatocytes. In renal tubular cells and intestinal epithelial cells, GLUT2 allows glucose to exit cells into the interstitial space to be taken up by capillaries as opposed to beta cells where glucose enters the cell via GLUT2 (Fig. 2). In hepatocytes, GLUT2 facilitates both uptake and release of glucose across the plasma cell membrane.

Facilitative glucose transporters have an extracellular N-terminal domain, 12 transmembrane domains, and a C-terminal cytoplasmic tail. The transmembrane domains are hypothesized to form a pore through which glucose can travel based upon concentration gradients. The only insulin-responsive glucose transporter is GLUT4 (509 amino acids; chromosome 17p13) expressed on hepatocytes, muscle cells, and adipose cells. With cellular stimulation from insulin, GLUT4 moves from an intracellular pool to fuse with the cell membrane providing more GLUT4 for transport of glucose into cells.

Besides GLUT2 and GLUT4, there are at least 11 other members of the solute carriers 2A family including GLUT1, the red blood cell (RBC) (erythroid)/hepatocyte glucose transporter (492 amino acids, chromosome 1p35–31.3; expressed in: brain, kidney, colon, placenta, and RBC), GLUT3, the brain glucose transporter (496 amino acids, chromosome 12p13; expressed in brain, kidney, and placenta), GLUT5, an intestinal fructose transporter (501 amino acids, chromosome 1p31), and GLUT7, an endoplasmic reticulum(RER)/microsomal glucose transporter moving glucose into the cytoplasm. For example, in the RER of the liver, glucose-6-phosphatase (G-6-P) converts G-6-P to glucose and phosphate. Phosphate leaves the RER via T2beta [a.k.a.: T3, an inorganic phosphate (Pi) transporter] while glucose leaves the RER via GLUT7 (a.k.a.: T2). The "generic" GLUT family can be classified into several subfamilies: class I (GLUT1-4), class II (GLUT5, 7, 9 and 11), and class III (GLUT6, 8, 10, 12, and the Human Myo-Inositol Transporter1) (7,8). GLUT6 is a pseudogene.

In contrast to the facilitative glucose transporters, the sodium-glucose cotransporter of the gut (i.e., SGLT1: sodium-dependent unidirectional transporter) is energy dependent in moving sodium and glucose from the gut lumen into the intestinal epithelial cell against a concentration gradient. The energy driving SGLT1 is provided by the hydrolysis of adenosine triphosphate (ATP) by the sodium-potassium ATPase pump. SGLT1 is also expressed in renal tubular cells to reabsorb glucose from the urine ultrafiltrate in the renal tubules against a concentration gradient.

Interstitial glucose reflects plasma glucose. With wide swings in plasma glucose concentration, there

Table 1 Stages in the Beta-Cell Response to Elevated Glucose

Glucose uptake	GLUT2
Glucose sensing	GCK
Coupling of glucose sensing to insulin release	Mitochondrion
	Potassium channel (Kir6.2 and SUR)
	Calcium channel
Insulin production	Insulin gene and transcription factors

Abbreviations: GLUT2, glucose transporter-2; GCK, glucokinase; SUR, sulfonylurea receptor.

can be a slight delay in the change in interstitial glucose concentration. Upon entry into the beta cell, glucose is phosphorylated to G-6-P by the action of glucokinase [(GCK), a.k.a.: hexokinase D or hexokinase Type IV]. GCK is a special form of hexokinase in that the rate of formation of G-6-P is dependent upon the plasma/ interstitial glucose concentration. Kinetically, GCK has a high K_m and a lower affinity for glucose than other hexokinases. The GCK gene is alternatively transcribed in beta cells and hepatocytes leading to unique isoforms of GCK being expressed in each tissue.

With higher plasma glucose levels, the rate of formation of G-6-P is accelerated. In this manner, GCK has been termed the "glucose sensor" of the beta cell (9). G-6-P proceeds to be metabolized through the glycolytic pathway resulting in the formation of pyruvate molecules and ATP. Pyruvate enters the lumen of the mitochondrion.

The mitochondrion is the power house of the cell (10). Within this unique organelle the Krebs cycle, fatty acid oxidation, and the oxidative respiratory chain take place. In the mitochondrion, pyruvate is converted to acetyl-coenzyme A (acetyl-CoA) through the action of pyruvate dehydrogenase. Acetyl-CoA in turn enters the citric acid cycle to be burned to CO_2 and water (Fig. 3). When glucose is burned completely through the events of the citric acid cycle and oxidative phosphorylation, one glucose molecule yields 38 molecules of ATP. However under anaerobic conditions, each glucose molecule yields only two molecules of ATP plus two molecules of pyruvate, which is converted to lactic acid.

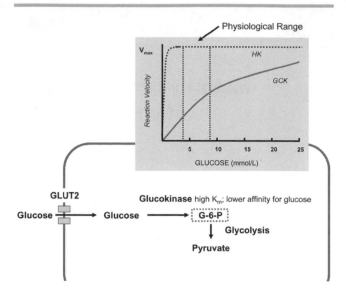

Figure 2 Beta cells take up glucose via their GLUT2 facilitative glucose transporters. Glucose is then phosphorylated by GCK producing G-6-P. This is metabolized via glycolysis to pyruvate, which can then enter into the Krebs cycle (not shown). Compared with other HKs, GCK has a high K_m and a lower affinity for glucose. In this way, over the physiological range of glucose concentrations, the reaction velocity is proportional to the plasma glucose concentration. In this manner, GCK serves as the beta-cell "glucose sensor" producing more G-6-P (and energy) as plasma glucose levels rise. In contrast, for other hexokinases the reaction velocity is maximal at subnormal plasma glucose concentrations (*top right*). *Abbreviations*: GLUT2, glucose transporter-2; GCK, glucokinase; HK, hexokinase; G-6-P, glucose-6-phosphate.

The increased ratio of ATP to adenosine diphosphate plus Pi in the beta cell closes the ATP-sensitive inwardly rectifying potassium channel composed of Kir6.2 (chromosome 11p14.1) and the sulfonylurea receptor (SUR; chromosome 11p15.1). The

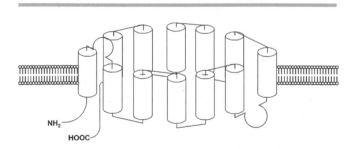

Figure 1 The generic structure of glucose transporters that include 12 transmembrane domains and connecting loops, N-terminal and C-terminal regions.

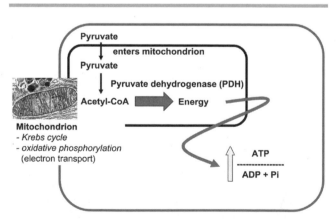

Figure 3 The coupling of glucose detection with insulin release involves the metabolism of pyruvate to CO_2 and H_2O via the Krebs cycle in the mitochondrion. Increased energy production raises the intracellular ratio of ATP to ADP plus Pi. *Abbreviations*: ADP, adenosine diphosphate; ATP, adenosine triphosphate; Pi, inorganic phosphate.

beta cell then depolarizes opening a calcium channel. Increased cytoplasmic calcium stimulates the release of the insulin as insulin-containing secretory vesicles fuse with the plasma membrane. In addition to the release of insulin, C-peptide, small amounts of proinsulin, amylin (islet-associated polypeptide), and carboxypeptidase H exit the beta cell (Fig. 4).

Like other genes, the insulin gene is under the control of numerous transcription factors that operate in hierarchies (11,12). Transcription factors are proteins that regulate DNA transcription by binding to DNA. Transcription factors typically contain domains for (i) binding to ligands (such as metabolites and hormones), (ii) binding to DNA, (iii) transactivation of the DNA, and (iv) binding to other transcription factors (e.g., forming heterodimers) or binding to identical transcription factors (forming homodimers). The DNA regulatory elements that transcription factors can bind to include enhancers, silencers, metabolic response units, and the promoter region. The promoter region encompasses the upstream promoter region (USP) and the TATA box. Examples of the USP include the CAAT box, which binds a CAT-box transcription factor, CCGCCC (a transcriptional response amplifier), the SP1 site that binds SV40 protein 1 and the chicken ovalbumin upstream promoter box. Transcription factors that bind to the USP recruit and stabilize other transcription factors that bind to the TATA box to promote transcription initiation.

Insulin is initially synthesized as preproinsulin by ribosomes associated with RER (i.e., the rough endoplasmic reticulum). With entry into the RER, the pre (leader) -sequence of preproinsulin is cleaved. Proinsulin is then cleaved to insulin and C-peptide prior to release. Insulin is composed of the 21 amino acid A chain and the 30 amino acid B chain that are held together by two disulfide bonds (A7-B7 and A20-B19). There is one A chain intrachain disulfide bond (A6-A11).

Besides elevated plasma glucose concentrations, insulin release is stimulated by amino acids by increasing energy production within the beta cell. Alanine, arginine, and leucine are recognized for their insulin-stimulatory effects. Other energy sources such as free fatty acids and ketone bodies can release insulin although the predominant regulator of insulin release is glucose.

Insulin stimulates the release of somatostatin from islet delta cells. Whereas glucagon stimulates insulin release, both glucagon and insulin release are suppressed by somatostatin. Glucagon is a product of alpha cells. The autonomic nervous system innervates the islets of Langerhans regulating islet hormone release. M3 muscarinic receptor stimulation amplifies insulin secretion. On the other hand with stress and alpha2 adrenergic beta cell stimulation, insulin secretion is inhibited. Gut hormones as incretins significantly influence the sensitivity of the beta cells to stimulation. Specifically, glucagon-like peptide-1 (GLP-1) and gastric inhibitory polypeptide are important regulators of beta cell responsiveness. Other incretins that play a lesser role in fostering insulin release include cholecystokinin, secretin, and gastrin.

Throughout the body, circulating insulin enters the interstitium by diffusion to bind to cell-surface insulin receptors. The insulin receptor is a beta-alpha-alpha-beta tetramer. Both the 135 kDa alpha and 95 kDa beta chains are derived from the insulin receptor precursor protein. The insulin receptor gene is located on the short arm of chromosome 19. The beta chain is transmembrane whereas the alpha chain is completely extracellular. Insulin binds to the extracellular alpha chains. Like other tyrosine kinase receptors, when the insulin receptor binds insulin, its natural ligand, the intracellular domains of the insulin receptor acquire tyrosine kinase activity. The insulin receptor undergoes autophosphorylation and phosphorylates intracellular proteins such as insulin receptor substrate-1 and -2. This initiates a cascade of intracellular second messengers that ultimately signal insulin's actions in target cells.

The insulin-sensitive tissues that express the insulin receptor are hepatocytes, skeletal muscle cells, and adipose cells. In response to insulin, in hepatocytes hepatic GCK expression increases, glycolysis is stimulated, glycogen synthesis is stimulated, triglyceride synthesis is stimulated and gluconeogenesis and lipolysis are suppressed. Overall, there is increased hepatic glucose clearance and suppression of hepatic glucose output although glucose uptake is not directly influenced as in skeletal muscle and adipose tissue via a GLUT. In skeletal muscle and adipose tissue, the insulin-responsive facilitative GLUT4 moves from an intracellular pool to the plasma membrane allowing increased entry of glucose into these tissues. Because normally there is greater skeletal muscle mass than either the mass of the liver or adipose tissue, skeletal

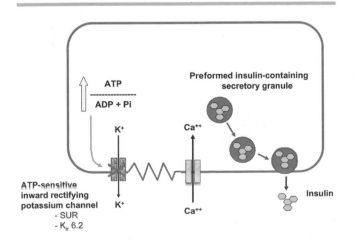

Figure 4 The rise in the ATP to ADP plus Pi ratio closes the potassium channel, depolarizes the beta cell and opens the calcium channel. The rise in the cytoplasmic concentrations of calcium is the signal that stimulates insulin secretion. *Abbreviations*: ADP, adenosine diphosphate; ATP, adenosine triphosphate; Pi, inorganic phosphate.

muscle is the major site of postprandial glucose clearance. Table 1 summarizes these events noting important proteins. Beta cell defects causing diabetes are overviewed in Table 2. With this description of beta cell function and response to insulin as outlined above, discussions of other specific types of diabetes follows.

GENETIC DEFECTS IN BETA CELL FUNCTION
GLUT2—Fanconi-Bickel Syndrome

A loss-of-function mutation in GLUT2 causes a rare, autosomal recessive condition termed the Fanconi-Bickel syndrome (13). Defective uptake of glucose by beta cells leads to relative insulinopenia following meals and consequent postprandial hyperglycemia (14). Because GLUT2 is also expressed in hepatocytes, decreased hepatocyte uptake of glucose following meals also contributes to postprandial hyperglycemia. On the other hand with fasting, because of decreased release of glucose from heptocytes, hypoglycemia can result. Finally because GLUT2 is expressed in renal tubular cells and in intestinal cells, update of glucose by these cells with impaired glucose release leads to defective intestinal epithelial cell function producing diarrhea and/or malabsorption, and defective renal tubular cell function producing a Fanconi-like syndrome.

Although not a beta cell defect, it is instructive to briefly mention glycogen storage disease type 0 (GSD0) which can also manifest fasting hypoglycemia and postprandial hyperglycemia initially between ages 6 and 18 months (15). The name of this disorder is a misnomer because the defect does not concern the excess storage of glycogen in the liver. GSD0 results in defective formation of glycogen due to a deficiency of liver glycogen synthase [(GYS2), chromosome 12p12.2]. On the other hand, GYS1 (chromosome 19q13.3) is expressed in muscle, brain, and kidney. In GYS2 deficiency, while hypoglycemia is the most notable finding accompanied by severe ketosis, postprandial hyperglycemia and hyperlactatemia is noted in 60% of cases presumably due to an inability to clear glucose through its storage as glycogen. Symptoms usually improve spontaneously by age eight years. GYS1 defects can be expressed in a Type 2 diabetes phenotype with polycystic ovary syndrome and hypertension.

Maturity-Onset Diabetes of Youth

MODY is a heterogenous group of autosomal dominant disorders where insulinopenic diabetes typically presents before age 25 (16–18). Therefore, MODY is a form of other specific types of diabetes due to defects in beta cell function (19). Depending upon the specific type of MODY, at least in the first decades of the disease, insulin replacement therapy is usually not required for control of hyperglycemia. As well, ketosis is uncommon and ketoacidosis is not observed. In research studies, MODY is often diagnosed only by oral glucose tolerance testing demonstrating hyperglycemia albeit the patient is asymptomatic. MODY may also present as GDM (20). Distinguishing features of the various MODY syndromes are outlined in Table 3.

Although at one time it was believed that people with MODY were resistant to the development of complications (e.g., Mason-type MODY), complications do occur in MODY patients just as in any other patient with diabetes proportionate to the duration and severity of hyperglycemia (21). In Caucasian children in the United Kingdom lacking autoimmune Type 1 diabetes, MODY is as common as Type 2 diabetes (22). MODY is recognized widely throughout the world. For example, cases of MODY-3 and MODY-6 have been reported in Iceland (23).

There is a unique form of autosomal dominant, insulinopenic diabetes that occurs in African-Americans under age 40 that can be characterized as a form of MODY (24). This disorder has been termed atypical diabetes mellitus (ADM) of African-Americans. These patients lack islet autoantibodies, and lack increased frequencies of high-risk Type-1-diabetes-associated human leukocyte antigen (HLA) alleles such as

Table 2 Beta-Cell Defects Causing Hyperglycemia

Protein/organelle	Disorder	Consequence (mode of inheritance)
GLUT-2	Loss-of-function	Fanconi-Bickel syndrome (AR)
GCK	Loss-of-function	MODY-2 (AD)
Mitochondria	Numerous loss-of-function mutations	Mitochondrial diabetes (mitochondrial inheritance)
Kir6.2	Activating mutations	Neonatal diabetes (variable)
Transcription factors for insulin gene	Various mutations	
HNF-4 alpha		MODY-1 (AD)
HNF-1 alpha		MODY-3 (AD)
IPF-1		MODY-4 (AD)
HNF-1 beta		MODY-5 (AD)
NeuroD1/beta 2		MODY-6 (AD)
Insulin	Point mutations	Insulinopathies (AD), hyperproinsulinemias (AD)

Abbreviations: GLUT2, glucose transporter-2; GCK, glucokinase; AD, autosomal dominant; AR, autosomal recessive; HNF, hepatocyte nuclear factor; MODY, maturity-onset diabetes of youth; PF, insulin promoter factor.

Table 3 Distinguishing Features of MODY-1 Through-5

MODY type	Distinguishing features
1	Progressive beta-cell dysfunction, decreased apo C2, apo C3, lp (a), an uncommon form of MODY
2	Nonprogressive beta-cell dysfunction, mild hyperglycemia from birth; decreased weight at birth, homozygous form: neonatal diabetes; a common form of MODY
3	Progressive beta-cell dysfunction, slightly decreased weight at birth, the most common form of MODY outside France
4	Homozygous form: pancreatic agenesis, heterozygous form: later onset diabetes, a rare form of MODY
5	Renal cysts, vaginal/uterine malformations, abnormal liver function, nondiabetic renal disease, a rare form of MODY
ADM	African-American, initial onset is insulin-requiring with possible ketosis or ketoacidosis, later: a noninsulin-dependent course

Abbreviations: MODY, maturity-onset diabetes of youth; ADM, atypical diabetes mellitus.

HLA-DR3, HLA-DR4, HLA-DQB1∗0201 and HLA-DQB1∗0302 (25,26). There is diminished first-phase insulin response to the intravenous injection of glucose (27). Ketosis is common at onset in ADM and diabetic ketoacidosis is possible. As opposed to MODY described in Caucasians, ADM patients are initially insulin-requiring for control of hyperglycemia and treatment of ketosis. However after one to two years, the requirement for exogenous insulin usually wanes and these patients enter a period of "non-insulin" dependence. Initial insulin dependence may reflect hyperglycemic beta cell toxicity that reverses with a reduction in the degree of hyperglycemia. Because of the initial requirement for exogenous insulin, ADM may be confused with Type 1 diabetes. In one ADM pedigree, a unique GCK mutation has been identified (at codon 108: tyrosine→phenylalanine, Y108F) (28) and in another pedigree a mitochondrial mutation was suggested (29). There is one report of a MODY-3 mutation [hepatocyte nuclear factor-1 alpha (HNF-1 alpha)] in ADM children (30).

Other than ADM in African-Americans, MODY appears to occur rarely in minorities (22). Other than ADM, no documented cases of MODY have been reported in African-Americans. However, in adult diabetic Black Africans from Senegal, 16% carried a Gly574Ser HNF-1alpha gene (MODY-3) mutation (31). Associations between all of the MODY genes and Type 2 diabetes have been sought. However, none of the MODY genes significantly contributes to the development of Type 2 diabetes or GDM (32–42).

Of the six recognized molecular etiologies for MODY, five entities represent mutations in nonubiquitous transcription factors (43) that lead to deficient insulin secretion (44,45). GCK mutations represent the only form of MODY not resulting from transcription factor mutations. An increasing number of genetic conditions are now recognized as resulting from transcription factor mutations including cases of panhypopituitarism (Pit-1 or PROP-1 mutations), X-linked adrenal hypoplasia congenita (DAX-1 mutations), autoimmune polyglandular syndrome Type 1 (autoimmune regulator mutations) (46,47) and some cases of congenital hypothyroidism (thyroid transcription factor mutations).

In 15% to 20% of cases of clinical MODY, the molecular etiology is unknown, e.g., there are no recognized mutations in the genes encoding MODY-1

through MODY-6 (48). Such cases are said to be due to "MODY-X" (49). Recent studies on this topic provided evidence for MODY-X linkage with loci on chromosomes 3, 5, 6, and 10 (48) and chromosome 8 (50).

An earlier study describes MODY-X pedigrees who were negative for MODY-1, MODY-2, and MODY-3 mutations with apparent insulin resistance with insulin doses and insulin levels higher than in MODY-3 subjects, an approximately 50% prevalence of obesity and increased frequencies of hypertriglyceridemia, hypercholesterolemia, hypertension, and nephropathy. Whether such pedigrees fit the MODY phenotype can be questioned (51). In contrast, four other French MODY-X families were not hyperinsulinemic (52). In some populations (e.g., Brazilian MODY families), MODY-X may be more commonly represented than the recognized MODY etiologies.

The following transcription factors have been studied and have not been found to be causes of MODY: Nkx2.2 (chromosome 20p11) (53), HNF-3 alpha (chromosome 14) (54), HNF-3 (chromosome 20p11) (55–57), HNF-4 gamma (chromosome 8q) (58,59), HNF6 (chromosome 15q21.1–21.2) (60), neuroD4 (chromosome 12q13) (61), and neurogenin 3 (chromosome 10q21.2-q21.3) (62).

MODY-2: Glucokinase

In 1992, the first molecular cause of MODY was identified as GCK (e.g., MODY-2) (63). The GCK gene is located on chromosome 7p. In France, MODY-2 is the most common form of MODY (64). Presently more than 130 GCK mutations have been described.

With a loss-of-function mutation in GCK, the beta cell becomes relatively insensitive to glucose (65,66). Elevated glucose levels must be achieved before insulin secretion is triggered leading to modest degrees of hyperglycemia (e.g., fasting plasma glucose approximately 110–145 mg/dL) and mild diabetes.

Studies in nondiabetic carriers of GCK mutations revealed that the beta cell response curve for insulin secretion rate (ISR) versus plasma glucose is "right-shifted" such that rate of insulin secretion is relatively deficient compared with controls, resulting in hyperglycemia. Therefore, the ISR is deficient up to blood-glucose levels of 126 to 144 mg/dL. However above this level, the rate of rise in the ISR is greater than in MODY-1 or MODY-3 but is still less than in normal controls (67). There is potentiation (e.g., improvement) of the ISR with prior glucose priming and insulin responses to nonglucose secretagogues are preserved. Decreased hepatocyte clearance of glucose that is mediated, in part, by a mutated GCK protein may also contribute to hyperglycemia after meals (68).

Insulinopenia is not progressive with advancing age in MODY-2 patients. MODY-2 may only be detected by oral glucose tolerance testing or unmasked during pregnancy as GDM. Less than 50% of GCK mutation gene carriers display clinical diabetes whereas about 50% of women heterozygous for a GCK mutation exhibit gestational diabetes. Because of the milder degree of hyperglycemia observed in MODY-2 compared with other forms of MODY, diabetic complications in MODY-2 are less common than in MODY-1 or MODY-3. Because of presumed in utero insulin deficiency, affected neonates are approximately 500 g lighter than their siblings and exhibit slightly elevated glucose levels from birth.

Molecular diagnosis of MODY-2 is available. Homozygosity for loss-of-function GCK mutations can produce permanent neonatal diabetes (69–71). A gain-of-function mutation in GCK raises the beta cell's sensitivity to glucose and is a cause of autosomal dominant persistent hyperinsulinemic hypoglycemia of infancy (72,73).

Mitochondrial Diabetes

In an increasing number of disorders, a search for mitochondrial dysfunction is being undertaken (74–76). In individuals with various mitochondrial mutations, either as an isolated finding or in association with other clinical defects, diabetes can occur (77). Phenotypically, most cases are "non-insulin-dependent" while a minority of cases have been insulin requiring.

Three percent to 42% of Japanese patients with Type 1 diabetes identified by the presence of islet auto-antibodies have been found to carry mitochondrial mutations (78,79). However, these findings were not duplicated by another Japanese research group (80). The true frequency of mitochondrial diabetes is likely to be very low (81) and will uncommonly be observed in clinical practice even when the treating physician has a high index of suspicion for such disorders (82). Glutamic acid decarboxylase autoantibodies (GADA) and insulin-2-associated autoantibodies (IA-2A) are absent in patients with mitochondrial diabetes and a non-insulin-dependent phenotype (83).

The most common mitochondrial mutation linked to diabetes is the A3243G mutation in the transfer RNA (tRNA)$^{Leu(UUR)}$. Other mutations distinct from A3243G and associated with hyperglycemia or frank diabetes include A3156G, A3252G, C3256T, A3260G, and T3271C in the tRNA$^{Leu(UUR)}$, G3316A in subunit 1 of NADH dehydrogenase (NADH CoQ reductase), A8344G in the tRNA^{Lys} and T14709C in the tRNA^{Glu}. Several mutations can occur together with the A3243G mutation in diabetic individuals such as C946A or A1041G in the 12SrRNA, T3394C in subunit 1 of NADH dehydrogenase, G4491A in the subunit 2 of NADH dehydrogenase, and G11963A in subunit 4 of NADH dehydrogenase. Whereas mitochondrial diabetes can occur in isolation, it can occur together with sensori-neural hearing loss, cardiomyopathy, Leber's hereditary optic neuropathy (LHON), mitochondrial myopathy, encephalopathy, lactic acidosis, stroke-like syndrome (MELAS), and mitochondrial myopathy or the myoclonic epilepsy, ragged-red fiber disorder (MERRF) (84–87).

In cases of mitochondrial diabetes the conceptual basis for diabetes is straightforward: defective energy production within the beta cell will ultimately impair insulin release (77,88,89). Since mitochondria are inherited essentially exclusively from the cytoplasm of the ovum, the inheritance pattern is mitochondrial: mothers pass on the disorder to their offspring yet fathers do not pass on these disorders. A pathologic phenotype is more likely with a higher proportion of mutated mitochondria and this appears to be true for mitochondrial diabetes states (90). Most mitochondria have 6 to 10 copies of the 16,569-base pair (bp) circular mitochondrial genome. Cells can have hundreds of mitochondria. The proportion of mitochondria that carry a mutation is described as the degree of "heteroplasmy" within an individual. Because mitochondria are not equally distributed among all cells or all tissues, in various organs in affected individuals there can be fewer or greater numbers of defective mitochondria. For clinical expression of disease, usually more than 5% of the mitochondria must be mutated.

Mitochondria have a unique genetic code and many unique tRNAs. Despite the presence of the mitochondrial genome that carries genes unique to the mitochondrion, most mitochondrial proteins are encoded by the nuclear genome. Mitochondrial dysfunction has been conceptually implicated in the etiology of Type 2 diabetes (91). Mitochondrial sequence variations have also been implicated as genetic risk factors for autoimmune Type 1 diabetes (92).

Kir6.2 Mutations Causing Neonatal Diabetes

Loss-of-function mutations in Kir6.2 close the potassium channel, depolarizing the beta cell. This is a cause of persistent neonatal hypoglycemia (93,94). On the other hand, gain-of-function mutations in Kir6.2 keep the potassium channel open, preventing depolarization leading to deficient insulin secretion and persistent (e.g., the V59M, Q52R, and I296L mutations) or transient (e.g., the I182V mutation) neonatal diabetes (95). Of clinical interest, despite insulinopenia, some children with neonatal diabetes show a significant reduction in plasma glucose with high-dose sulfonylurea administration, avoiding the necessity of exogenous insulin replacement (96,97). Transient neonatal diabetes mellitus has also been associated with paternal overexpression of an imprinted chromosome 6q24 locus (98). Some Kir6.2 mutations have been associated with childhood diabetes or Type 2 diabetes (99).

MODY-1: Hepatocyte Nuclear Factor-4 Alpha

Mutations in several transcription factors can cause the MODY phenotype (100). Diabetes is believed to result from insufficient insulin production and release although other mechanistic causes of diabetes resulting from such mutations have not been excluded such as pancreatic, islet, or beta cell hypoplasia or aplasia (see the section "MODY-4: Insulin Promoter Factor").

Mutations in HNF-4 alpha (chromosome 20q12-q13.1) cause MODY-1 (101). MODY-1 is an uncommon cause of MODY. The gene for HNF-4 alpha is located on chromosome 20q12-q13.1. HNF-4 alpha is expressed in the liver, kidney, intestine and islets, and serves as a key regulator of hepatic gene expression. GLUT2, aldolase B, glyceraldehyde-3-phosphate dehydrogenase, liver pyruvate kinase, fatty acid binding proteins and cellular retinol binding protein expression are regulated by HNF-1 alpha (the cause of MODY-3) which is controlled, in part, by HNF-4 alpha (the cause of MODY-1).

Fajans and Conn from the University of Michigan in the 1960s first described the MODY phenotype in a pedigree that was found to eventually include over 300 members (102). In 1991 in linkage studies of this RW pedigree, MODY-1 was mapped to chromosome 20 with the gene being in the vicinity of the adenosine deaminase gene. After MODY-3 was identified, a search of chromosome 20 loci near adenosine deaminase revealed mutations in HNF-4 alpha in the RW pedigree but not in unaffected family members or nondiabetic controls. This proved that MODY-1 resulted from HNF-4 alpha mutations.

In MODY-1, modest insulinopenia causes early-onset, autosomal dominant diabetes (103). Many individuals affected with MODY-1 can be controlled for decades through the use of oral sulfonylureas. However, there is progressive insulinopenia with advancing age and 30% to 40% of MODY-1 subjects eventually require insulin replacement therapy.

Evaluation of nondiabetic carriers of MODY-1 mutations revealed that the ISR is normal up to blood-glucose levels of 126 to 144 mg/dL. However above this level the rate of rise in the ISR is deficient to flat (67). There is no potentiation of the ISR with prior glucose priming. Insulin responses to a nonglucose secretagogue such as arginine are deficient (104). Reduced pancreatic polypeptide response to hypoglycemia and amylin response to arginine has also been recognized in MODY-1 subjects (105). Finally demonstrating the broad effects of transcription factor mutations on gene regulation, MODY-1 subjects exhibit reduced levels of apo A2, apo C3, lipoprotein (a) and triglycerides (106,107).

MODY-3: Hepatocyte Nuclear Factor-1 Alpha

MODY-3 results from mutations in HNF-1 alpha (chromosome 12q24.2). Many genes involved in insulin secretion are regulated by HNF-1 alpha (108). Linkage studies initially mapped MODY-3 to chromosome 12 (109). Through detailed analysis of the genes in the vicinity of the chromosome 12 locus linked to MODY-3 in pedigree studies, the cause of MODY-3 was identified as mutations in HNF-1 alpha (110).

Biologically, HNF-1 alpha is expressed in liver, kidney, intestine, and beta cells. Some genes such as amylin are suppressed by HNF-1 alpha expression (111). In a beta cell line, HNF-1 alpha was shown to regulate beta cell growth through altered expression of insulin-like growth factor-1 (112). HNF-1 alpha mutations may function as dominant negatives (113). HNF-4 alpha regulates HNF-1 alpha providing a link between MODY-1 and MODY-3 (114). HNF-α can bind to A3/A4 regulatory region of the insulin gene. Other genetic loci (chromosomes 5p15, 9q22, and 14q24) may influence the age at onset of MODY-3 (115). Greater than 120 HNF-1 alpha mutations have been reported. HNF-1 alpha has an apparent exon 4 mutational hotspot (Pro291fsinsC) (116,117).

MODY-3 is the most common form of MODY worldwide. The higher frequency of MODY-2 reported in France than the United Kingdom (and other parts of the world) may relate to France's case finding approach extensively using oral glucose tolerance testing of asymptomatic first-degree family members of the diabetic proband. Chronic diabetic complications do occur in individuals with MODY-3 (118). There may also be a reduced renal threshold for glycosuria in MODY-3 (119).

Similar to MODY-1, there is progressive insulinopenia with advancing age. Birthweight is reduced by approximately 120 g compared with siblings. Diabetes penetrance in MODY-1 and MODY-3 carriers by age 40 approaches or exceeds 80% (120). Like MODY-1, sulfonylureas can successfully treat MODY-3 (121) although insulin dependence can occur in as many as 30% to 40% of such MODY patients (16).

There are a number of reports of insulin-dependent diabetes patients with MODY-1 mutations (122–126). Therefore, some of the uncommon patients with clinical "Type 1 diabetes" who lack all islet auto-antibodies [such as islet cell autoantibodies, GADA, IA-2A and insulin autoantibodies (IAA)] and lack high-risk HLA Type-1-diabetes alleles may have MODY-3. However, the usual MODY-3 patient is not insulin-requiring early in life.

Studies in nondiabetic carriers of MODY-3 mutations showed that the ISR is normal up to blood glucose levels of 126 to 144 mg/dL, yet above this level the rate of rise in the ISR is deficient (127). There is potentiation of the ISR (e.g., improvement) with prior glucose priming in contrast to MODY-1 where there is no potentiation with glucose priming.

MODY-4: Insulin Promoter Factor-1

Insulin promoter factor-1 (IPF-1) mutations cause MODY-4 (128) by producing insulinopenia (129). IPF-1 is also known as pancreatic duodenal homeobox protein-1 islet duodenum homeobox-1 and STF-1. The gene for IPF-1 is found on chromosome 13q12.1 (130). IPF-1 can bind to the A5, A3/A4, A2, and A1 regulatory regions of the insulin gene. IPF-1 is required for the expression of the fibroblast growth factor receptor-1. IPF-1 activates the transcription of many genes including insulin, somatostatin, islet amyloid polypeptide, GLUT2, and GCK (131).

An infant born with pancreatic aplasia (i.e., small-for-gestational age, neonatal diabetes, and exocrine pancreatic insufficiency) was studied for transcription factor mutations. Insulin deficiency in utero leads to intrauterine growth retardation that is expressed at birth as the infant being "small-for-gestational" age. Exocrine pancreatic insufficiency is manifested as steatorrhea that also contributes to failure to thrive. The infant's father had "Type 2" diabetes and the mother had had "gestational" diabetes. The infant was found to harbor a homozygous mutation in the IPF-1 gene. A single cytosine base pair deletion in code 63 caused a frameshift mutation in IPF-1. It was concluded that the heterozygous parents had MODY (termed "MODY-4") and that homozygosity for the mutation caused pancreatic agenesis. The parents were not related; however, there was a strong family history of diabetes on both sides of the family. Individuals heterozygous for an IPF-1 mutation appear to have a later-onset of diabetes than is usually observed in other types of MODY.

Investigations of carriers of IPF-1 mutations revealed (when compared with controls) hyperglycemia, insulinopenia, a normal early GLP-1 response, elevated nonesterified fatty acids, and elevated glucagon during a five-step hyperglycemic clamp (132). Insulin sensitivity in IPF-1 carriers was enhanced as a possible compensatory response to insulinopenia. Similarly, the expected response of insulin-sensitive tissues to insulinopenia is an increase in insulin receptor number as is observed in cystic fibrosis (CF) (133–135) and anorexia nervosa (136).

The base pair deletion and consequent frameshift mutation in the mutated IPF-1 lead to the production of a dysfunctional protein (mutant isoform-N), which terminated prematurely because of the introduction of a stop codon in the aberrant open reading frame. Instead of the normal-sized IPF-1 protein of 42 to 43 kB, a 13.2-kDa protein resulted which could not translocate to the nucleus. The IPF-1 deletion included the FPWMK motif that is required for interaction of IPF-1 with PBX. Another homeoprotein, PBX1, is "pre-B-cell leukemia transcription factor-1" encoded on chromosome 1q23.

In addition to mutant isoform-N, another mutant protein (mutant isoform-C) was identified that utilized an aberrant translation start site that went "into frame" once the sequence extended past the cytosine deletion, continuing the protein in its normal opening reading frame through to the normal stop codon. This product was 16 kB. Like other transcription factor mutations, IPF-1 mutations may act as dominant negatives (137).

Because pancreatic transcription factors can control pancreatic development in utero in addition to regulating insulin gene expression, transcription factor mutations could lead to diabetes by interfering with normal pancreatic, islet or beta cell development (138). When a knockout mouse is produced lacking IPF-1, pancreatic agenesis results similar to the human "experiment of nature" (139). During embryonic development, IPF-1 transcripts are found in the pancreas, duodenum, and pylorus. Later in development, IPF-1 transcripts are more restricted to the beta cells and a fraction of the delta cells. Similar to the IPF-1 knockout model, PTP-p48 knockout mice also display pancreatic agenesis (140). Of lesser severity, the Isl1 knockout mouse exhibits dorsal pancreatic agenesis. Nkx2.2 is necessary for islet development based upon a knockout of this gene in mice. Based upon other knockout experiments, Pax-4 is crucial for beta and delta cell formation within islets (141), whereas Pax-6 is important for alpha cell development. Knockouts of Nkx6.1 or beta 2/neuro D1 lead to failure of beta cell development (142,143). Various developmental pancreatic islet abnormalities have been described in humans (144–148).

Possibly because of its simplicity (the IPF-1 gene has only two exons), IPF-1 has been examined as a possible contributor to the development of Type 2 diabetes in several studies. While IPF-1 mutations can be found in individuals and families with Type 2 diabetes, IPF-1 is not a major contributor to genetic susceptibility to Type 2 diabetes (149–154). Whereas there is only a single family with MODY-4 with a single IPF-1 mutation, in Type 2 diabetes subjects at least five IPF-1 mutations have been described.

MODY-5: Hepatocyte Nuclear Factor-1 Beta

MODY-5 results from HNF-1 beta mutations. HNF-1 beta (also known as transcription factor-2, hepatic, and as LF-B3; variant hepatic nuclear factor) is found on chromosome 17cen-q21.3. Japanese MODY families screened for mutations in novel transcription factors led to the discovery of mutations in HNF-1 beta in two families (the R177X and A263fsinsGG mutations) (155). MODY-5 is a rare form of MODY (156). MODY-5 does not significantly contribute to the development of Type 2 diabetes (157,158). Mechanistically, HNF-1 beta regulates HNF-4 alpha providing a link between MODY-5 and MODY-1. HNF-1 beta can form homodimers or heterodimers with HNF-1 alpha. At least five mutations affecting HNF-1 beta have now been described.

Clinical hallmarks of MODY-5 include the findings of renal cysts, vaginal aplasia, or rudimentary or bicornuate uterus in affected patients and elevations in liver function tests (159–161). These associated malformations demonstrate the diverse adverse consequences of certain transcription factor mutations.

The renal cysts cause hypoplastic glomerulocystic kidney disease evidenced in proteinuria and nondiabetic renal failure (162,163). Finally, in contrast to MODY-1 and MODY-3 patients that do not exhibit abnormalities in hepatic enzyme release, individuals with the MODY-5 can display elevations in alanine amino transferase, aspartate amino transferase, and gamma glutamyl transpeptidase (164).

MODY-6: Beta 2/NeuroD1

Beta 2/NeuroD1 mutations cause MODY-6. Beta 2/NeuroD1 can bind to the E1 and E2 regulatory regions of the insulin gene. Pancreatic endocrine cells, intestine and brain are the normal sites of expression of NeuroD1. NeuroD1 regulates insulin, cholecystokinin and secretin expression. In nervous tissue, NeuroD1 can induce neuronal differentiation.

MODY-6 is a rare form of MODY (23,165). MODY-6 was not found in any of 57 Japanese MODY families (53). A NeuroD1 mutation has been identified in one Type 2 diabetes family characterized by hyperinsulinism and obesity, suggesting a role for neuroD1 in target sensitivity to insulin (166). However, NeuroD1 was not associated with Type 2 diabetes in France (38). There is controversy concerning the possible role of NeuroD1 polymorphisms in the development of Type 1 diabetes (167–169).

Insulin: Insulinopathies

Diabetes can result from insulinopathies where there are point mutations in the insulin gene causing missense mutations in the insulin molecule (170). Such disorders are exceedingly rare, especially when compared with the high frequency of hemoglobinopathies in various worldwide populations.

The first two mutations described involved serine replacing phenylalanine B24 (amino acid residue number 24 in the B chain; insulin Los Angeles) (171,172) and leucine replacing phenylalanine B25 (insulin Chicago) (173). Normally phenylalanines at B24 and B25 are involved in insulin's interaction with its receptor. The immunoreactivity of theses insulins is normal. Later described was a mutation in the insulin A chain with leucine replacing valine (insulin Wakayama, a.k.a.: Tokyo) (174). Biological activity of insulin Wakayama is reduced (175). All three mutated insulins display in vitro decreased insulin receptor binding, decreased biologic activity, and greatly prolonged half lives (176).

The clinical phenotype of insulinopathies is: (i) glucose intolerance or mild diabetes, (ii) autosomal dominant inheritance, (iii) hyperinsulinemia (a consequence of decreased insulin action and subsequent decreased insulin clearance), and (iv) increased insulin to C-peptide ratios (177). Because the mutated insulin is not cleared normally through receptor-mediated endocytosis, the mutated insulin accumulates in the circulation. Single-strand conformation polymorphism analysis and direct sequencing can detect such mutations (178,179).

Insulin: Familial Hyperproinsulinemias

Mutations in proinsulin at the sites where proinsulin is normally cleaved to insulin plus C-peptide lead to the familial hyperproinsulinemias inherited as autosomal dominant disorders (180,181). Several types of hyperproinsulinemia exist depending upon whether the mutation affects the cleavage site between the B chain and C-peptide or the site between C-peptide and the A chain (182). Failure to normally cleave proinsulin to insulin plus C-peptide leads to high concentrations of partially cleaved proinsulin in the circulation. Proinsulin has approximately 10% the bioactivity of insulin.

The insulin gene mutations result from point mutations where an arginine is replaced by another amino acid at the key cleavage sites between the A and B chains and C-peptide where two arginines or an arginine and a lysine are normally located (183). In at least one family with hyperproinsulinemia, the cause was believed to be due to abnormal cleavage of proinsulin and not a mutation in the proinsulin molecule itself (184). However, later studies suggested that there was a mutation in proinsulin arguing against a pure processing defect (185,186).

Usually hyperproinsulinemia by itself does not cause diabetes (187). However when presumably combined with other risk factors for diabetes such as a genetic predisposition to diabetes, hyperproinsulinemia can be associated with hyperglycemia and a "non-insulin-dependent" diabetes phenotype (188). In at least two families, hyperglycemia became more pronounced with advancing age in adulthood (189,190). It is unlikely that hyperproinsulinemia would be recognized in childhood or adolescence.

A potentially important diagnostic feature of insulinopathies and hyperproinsulinemias in contrast to states of true insulin resistance (e.g., the metabolic syndrome or Type 2 diabetes) is that despite elevated immunoreactive insulin levels in insulinopathies and hyperproinsulinemias, there is a normal decline in glucose when exogenous (normal) insulin is injected in affected patients. Therefore, an insulin tolerance test should be considered in cases of suspected insulinopathy and hyperproinsulinemia. A thorough family history that reveals an autosomal dominant mode of inheritance can also be diagnostically helpful. If immunoassays are used that measure proinsulin and insulin separately, patients with hyperproinsulinemia will have an increased proinsulin to insulin ratio compared with people with insulinopathies.

GENETIC DEFECTS IN INSULIN ACTION: INSULIN RECEPTOR AND POST-RECEPTOR EVENTS

Although insulin resistance is the major predisposing factor causing Type 2 diabetes, insulin resistance in Type 2 diabetes results predominantly from post-receptor defects. Mutations in the insulin receptor in

Type 2 diabetes are extremely rare in the absence of some type of genetic syndrome (191). There is a small group of genetic syndromes where insulin receptor mutations truly occur and many types of individual mutations have been described that can produce an insulin-resistant, diabetic state. The spectrum of clinical expression of these mutations ranges from a nondysmorphic, yet insulin-resistant-diabetic phenotype (Type A insulin resistance) to Rabson-Mendenhall syndrome to the most severe expression: Leprechaunism (Donohue syndrome) (192).

Insulin receptor mutations are found in these disorders that play a significant role in their causation. In the more severe cases there is a marked decline in the cell surface expression of the insulin receptor, while in other less severe cases, the receptor is expressed yet there is an aberrant affinity for insulin leading to decreased receptor stimulation (193). However, a strong correlation between the severity of the insulin receptor mutation and the clinical phenotype has been challenged (194).

Clinical findings associated with Type A insulin resistance include acanthosis nigricans and polycystic-ovary syndrome reminiscent of the metabolic syndrome (195,196) and hyperandrogenism in the absence of obesity or lipodystrophy. Type A insulin resistance has been inherited as either an autosomal recessive trait or an autosomal dominant trait. Nongenetic Type B insulin resistance results from insulin receptor autoantibodies that bind to the receptor but do not activate the receptor. Type B insulin-resistant diabetes is classified as "other specific type of diabetes—uncommon forms of immune mediated diabetes."

Rabson-Mendenhall syndrome and leprachaunism are autosomal recessive conditions that display prenatal and postnatal growth failure and mental retardation. Intrauterine growth retardation is an expected outcome when there is deficient insulin action in utero for any reason. Insulin is a more important and potent growth factor in utero than growth hormone. Growth hormone-deficient neonates are not small at birth.

Rabson-Mendenhall syndrome is characterized by insulin resistance, insulin receptor mutations, short stature, protuberant abdomen, and abnormalities of the nails and teeth (197). Fasting hypoglycemia is a paradoxical feature of this condition. Leptin treatment of such patients has provided some benefit (198). Over time, insulin secretion can decline in Rabson-Mendenhall syndromes producing ketoacidosis (199).

The clinical features of leprachaunism include severe prenatal and postnatal growth failure, developmental delay, adipose tissue deficiency, cutis laxa, hypertrichosis, acanthosis nigricans, distended abdomen, relatively large hands and feet, variable extents of external genitalia hypertrophy, and an elf-like face characterized by hypertelorism, prominent eyes, enlarged ears, and micrognathia (200). Autopsy findings include cystic ovarian changes and pancreatic islet beta cell hyperplasia. Some authors suggest that if a child lives beyond age two, leprachaunism is not an appropriate diagnostic term implying that the diagnosis of Rabson-Mendenhall syndrome should be applied in such cases.

DISEASES OF THE EXOCRINE PANCREAS
Cystic Fibrosis

There are a number of genetic diseases involving the pancreas that can cause diabetes. The best known examples are CF and primary hemochromatosis. CF-related diabetes mellitus (CFRD) is an autosomal recessive disorder caused by mutations in the CF transmembrane conductance regulator, which is a chloride channel. This gene is located on chromosome 7. Seventy percent of mutated CF alleles carry the delta-508 mutation: a 3-bp deletion encoding a phenylalanine (deltaF508). Because the deletion is a multiple of three, a shift does not occur in the reading frame distal to the deletion. The other 30% of CF alleles represent a wide number of possible mutations with the more than 1000 mutations reported. The deltaF508 mutation is the most severe genetic lesion (201–203). In the general population, deltaF508 does not serve as a risk factor for Type 2 diabetes (204).

CFRD is becoming increasingly common as life expectancy in CF has approximately doubled in the last two decades. In 30% to 40% of adult CF patients, some form of dysglycemia is recognized (205). The development of microvascular complications is now a major challenge for long-term CF survivors with CFRD.

CFRD is associated with poor nutrition (206) and an increased risk for pulmonary deterioration (207,208). Deterioration in pulmonary function is much worse in women and men with CF. Screening for diabetes should begin in CF patients at ages 10 (209) to 14 (210). Hemoglobin A_{1c} is not an appropriate screening test for CFRD (211). Presently, the American Diabetes Association does not recommend hemoglobin A_{1c} testing for any type of diabetes screening or diagnosis (212), although some experts recommend revision of the overall diabetes diagnostic guidelines to include elevated hemoglobin A_{1c} (213–215).

The pathogenesis of diabetes in CF appears to be fibrotic damage to the islets of Langerhans consequent to the destruction of the exocrine pancreas from duct obstruction. More than two decades ago, glucagon deficiency, in addition to insulin deficiency, was identified in CFRD (216–219). This can lead to a less severe form of diabetes because hyperglucagonemia is less pronounced than in disorders where only the beta cells are destroyed such as Type 1 diabetes. Similar to Type 2 diabetes, there appears to be a stepwise progression from totally normal glucose tolerance to diabetes leading to the following classification of glucose tolerance in CF: normoglycemic, impaired glucose tolerance, CFRD with post-challenge hyperglycemia, and CFRD with fasting hyperglycemia (205).

Primary Hemochromatosis

Primary hemochromatosis, an inherited autosomal recessive disorder, is characterized by unregulated, hyperabsorption of iron leading to systemic iron load. Hemochromatosis can develop secondarily as a consequence of transfusion therapy for disorders such as chronic anemias. The greatest site of iron deposition is the liver. Excess iron deposition in tissues causes organ damage affecting the heart (heart failure), liver (liver failure), pituitary (hypopituitarism), and pancreas (islet deposition with diabetes). Deposition of iron in the skin causes a darkening of the skin. The combination of skin hyperpigmentation and hyperglycemia has been termed "bronze diabetes." The genetic mutation in primary hemochromatosis involves a class I major histocompatibility complex-like gene named the hemochromatosis gene (HFE).

Primary hemochromatosis affects 1 in every 300 people in the general population. During their reproductive years, women are generally spared the adverse effects of hemochromatosis because of menses. The most sensitive screening test for hemochromatosis is the measurement of transferrin saturation (i.e., serum iron divided by total iron binding capacity). The usual upper limit of the reference interval for saturation is approximately 55%. Whereas symptoms can occur before age 20, between ages 40 and 60 symptoms are most often first apparent when total body iron has reached damaging concentrations.

Pathophysiologically, diabetes in hemochromatosis results from a combination of insulinopenia from beta cell damage and hepatic insulin resistance from liver disease. However, insulin deficiency is more prominent than insulin resistance. In adults, 75% to 90% of affected patients exhibit either impaired glucose tolerance or diabetes. Diabetes resulting from hemochromatosis in children and adolescents must be uncommon, as a recent literature review by the author failed to disclose any such cases reported in PubMed. Cardiac and gonadal problems are more common than liver disease or diabetes in youth with hemochromatosis (219).

Other Forms of Diabetes Including Disorders of the Exocrine Pancreas

Diabetes in the newborn is termed "neonatal diabetes mellitus (NDM)" and can be either transient (TNDM) or permanent (PNDM) (220). Sporadic pancreatic agenesis, pancreatic agenesis secondary to IPF-1 mutations (128) and congenital pancreatic hypoplasia (147) can produce permanent diabetes in infancy. An unbalanced duplication of paternal chromosome 6 and uniparental isodisomy of chromosome 6 have been identified in over 75% of TNDM cases. Autosomal recessive inheritance of PNDM is suggested by the association of PNDM with cerebellar hypoplasia and Wolcott-Rallison syndrome, a rare autosomal recessive

condition characterized by multiple epiphyseal dysplasia and early-infancy-onset diabetes mellitus (221).

A familial form of pancreatic hypoplasia has been described as an autosomal recessive trait (147). Two brothers who exhibited small size at birth suggestive of in utero insulin deficiency, both developed Type 1 diabetes and pancreatic exocrine insufficiency before age one. Neither parent had diabetes thereby negating, MODY-4 as a cause of this disorder. The parents were unrelated.

OTHER GENETIC SYNDROMES ASSOCIATED WITH DM

Diabetes can occur in association with a number of genetic syndromes. Lipodystrophy is the absence of normal subcutaneous fat. This produces a very lean appearance over the parts of the body affected with prominent appearance of the veins and muscles. Lipodystrophy can be generalized or limited to specific areas of the body. The lipodystrophies are remarkable for defective insulin action and subsequent insulin-resistant diabetes. Characteristics shared with the metabolic syndrome [e.g., insulin resistance syndrome; dysmetabolic syndrome X (ICD-9: 277.7)] include hypertriglyceridemia, low high-density lipoprotein cholesterol, hypertension, an accelerated risk for arteriosclerotic cardiovascular disease, and, in women, oligomenorrhea, amenorrhea, and infertility.

One persuasive hypothesis for the metabolic disturbances in the lipodystrophies is that with decreased ability to deposit fat (e.g., triglyceride) in normal adipose tissue, even subnormal amounts of total body fat will lead to fat deposition in ectopic locations such as hepatocytes, skeletal muscle, and beta cells. Fat deposition in liver and skeletal muscle induces insulin resistance. Hepatic glucose output is excessive. As noted above, skeletal muscle is normally responsible for approximately 80% of glucose clearance following meals. Decreased glucose removal by muscle substantially contributes to hyperglycemia. Fat deposition in beta cells contributes to insulinopenia through beta cell dysfunction. The combination of insulin resistance and insulinopenia produces diabetes mellitus.

There are several forms of familial lipodystrophy that display autosomal dominant or autosomal recessive inheritance. For each form, a gene mutation has been identified or is under study. There are several excellent recent reviews that the reader is referred to (222,223). Acquired lipodystrophy is observed in patients receiving treatment for human immunodeficiency virus infection. Reverse-transcriptase inhibitors and protease inhibitors are both associated with lipodystrophy (224).

Diabetes can develop in association with chromosomal aneuploidies of autosomes (e.g., Down syndrome) or sex chromosomes (e.g., Klinefelter and Turner syndromes). Syndromes of disordered aging such as Werner syndrome and Cockayne syndrome are observed where diabetes can be exhibited. Although Prader-Willi syndrome (PWS) patients are massively obese, when diabetes develops it is most commonly due to insulinopenia and not insulin resistance (225,226). Typically children with PWS display hypotonia and failure-to-thrive in the first 18 months of life followed by massive weight gain thereafter due to a voracious appetite and excessive eating. Findings suggestive of PWS include delayed or deficient mental development, a narrow forehead, almond-shaped eyes, small hands and feet, tapered fingers, and hypogonadism.

PWS results from mutations of genes on chromosome 15. Most cases result from a microdeletion event although paternal chromosome 15 imprinting errors without visible microdeletions can cause approximately 5% of cases of PWS. Microdeletions can be sought using fluorescence in situ hybridization studies. Maternal imprinting errors of this same region of the genome produce Angelmann syndrome (also known as the "happy-puppet" syndrome).

Mutations on chromosome 2 can cause Wolfram syndrome which appears to be inherited as an autosomal recessive trait (227). Wolfram syndrome is also knows as the "DIDMOAD" syndrome which summarizes its clinical phenotype of diabetes insipidus (DI), diabetes mellitus (DM), and optic atrophy-deafness (OAD). The gene that causes Wolfram syndrome has been cloned and is WFS1 (228). Ninety percent of affected individuals display compound heterozygous mutations of WFS1.

CLINICAL COMMENTARY

Lean individuals that present with acute-onset, ketotic diabetes usually have autoimmune Type 1 diabetes (229). Typically such patients have short histories of weight loss, polyuria and polydipsia, and are lean (Fig. 5). Because approximately 15% of obese minority adolescents with Type 2 diabetes can present with diabetic ketoacidosis, ketoacidosis by itself is no longer a sine qua non for Type 1 diabetes (230).

In lean individuals who develop early-onset, mild (non-insulin requiring) diabetes who have a family history of diabetes in their parents and grandparents that fits an autosomal dominant pattern of inheritance that is not Type 2 diabetes, MODY should be considered (231). The absence of islet autoantibodies in such circumstances also suggests MODY. In new-onset cases of Type 1 diabetes, 95% or more of individuals will exhibit at least one of the following autoantibodies: ICA, GADA, IA-2A, or IAA (Vol. 1; Chap. 5). African-Americans under age 40 who are diagnosed with ADM and develop acute-onset diabetes that requires insulin initially but later become non-insulin-dependent, often have an autosomal dominant family history of a similar form of diabetes (Fig. 6).

The proposed diagnostic algorithms depicted in Figures 5 and 6 are meant to provide the clinician with an approach to a patient with diabetes. The distinguishing features of the different MODY types are summarized in Table 3. Testing for MODY-3 or MODY-1 through MODY-5 mutations is available from various reference laboratories. New MODY mutations

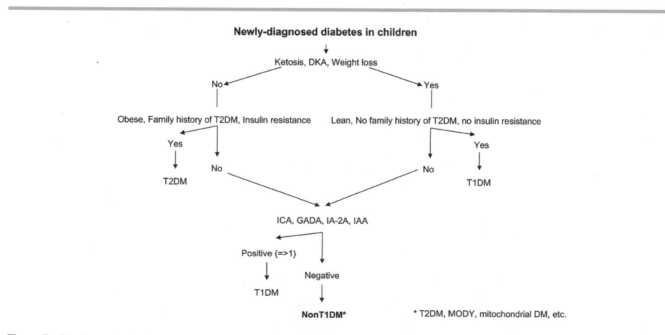

Figure 5 This diagnostic algorithm has been rearranged for emphasis as described: this figure highlights a group of patients who do not clearly have T1DM but may have T2DM or some other form of diabetes such as MODY or mitochondrial diabetes (e.g., nonT1DM). *Abbreviations*: T1DM, Type 1 diabetes mellitus; T2DM, Type 2 diabetes mellitus; MODY, maturity-onset diabetes of youth.

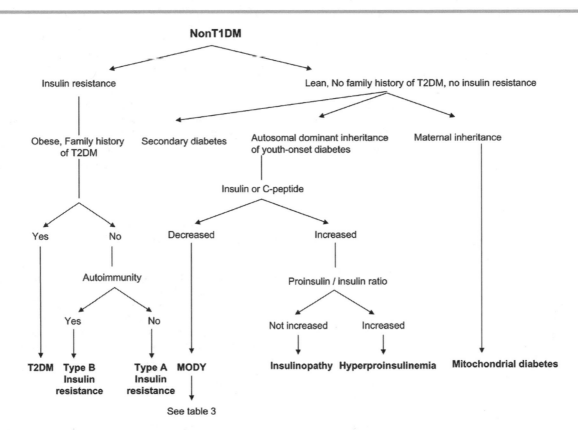

Figure 6 In individuals who do not have Type 1 diabetes but cannot be otherwise classified based upon the investigation utilized in Figure 5 (e.g., individuals with nonT1DM), the algorithm returns to whether the patient is lean or obese, has a family history of T2DM or is insulin-resistant. The presence of diabetes, obesity, a positive family history of T2DM and/or insulin resistance usually supports the diagnosis of T2DM. Patients with nonT1DM and nonT2DM can be affected, in general, with either MODY or mitochondrial diabetes if other causes of secondary diabetes (e.g., "other specific types of diabetes") have been excluded such as steroid-induced diabetes, cystic fibrosis-related diabetes, syndromic diabetes (e.g., Down syndrome, Prader-Willi syndrome, etc.), etc. MODY and mitochondrial diabetes are initially differentiated according to their mode of inheritance. Among the MODY syndromes it is important to recall the following: MODY-3 and MODY-2 are most common. If MODY-3 and MODY-2 have been excluded on a molecular basis, a search for MODY-1 mutations can be pursued. All other forms of MODY are rare. The presence of nondiabetic renal disease and/or vaginal/uterine malformations is highly suggestive of MODY-5. Insulin-resistant patients who are obese and have a family history of Type 2 diabetes likely have Type 2 diabetes themselves. Insulin resistance in the absence of obesity (and lipodystrophy) may be due to type A (inherited) or Type B (autoimmune) insulin resistance (R/o = rule out). *Abbreviations*: T1DM, Type 1 diabetes mellitus; T2DM, type 2 diabetes mellitus; MODY, maturity-onset diabetes of youth.

continue to be described (232–246). Likewise, translocations and gene inversions are now recognized causes of MODY gene mutations (247). This is very important: a normal DNA sequence does not exclude a gene inversion or translocation that can cause, MODY. Genomic evaluations would require the use of restriction fragment length polymorphism analysis for recognition of such mutations (248).

If there is non-insulin-dependent diabetes and a family history of multiple affected siblings with inheritance from the mother, a mitochondrial diabetes syndrome can be considered. Diabetes can occur in a variety of mitochondrial diseases such as LHON, MELAS, and MERRF. Molecular analysis of the mitochondrial genome is available from specialized reference laboratories. In a Scandinavian study of families with diabetes in two or more members with age of onset before 45, 24% had MODY or maternally inherited diabetes and deafness (249).

If insulin resistance is profound, Type A insulin esistance is a clinical consideration. Type B insulin resistance is usually associated with other autoimmune conditions. Insulinopathic and hyperproinsulinemic diabetes does not usually present in childhood. When diabetes is associated with lipodystrophy, CF, hemochromatosis, or other genetic syndromes, the genetic syndrome is almost always clinically recognized before the development of diabetes.

Pediatricians must be able to diagnose and treat Type 1 and Type 2 diabetes. The incidence of Type 2 diabetes in children and adolescents is rising throughout industrialized countries (250–253). If diabetes in a child or adolescent cannot be classified as Type 1 or Type 2, "other specific types of diabetes" must be considered. Among these conditions are several genetic disorders that bear review such as MODY. With the availability of genetic testing for MODY, it is possible that MODY will become more widely recognized.

Although not commonly discussed, clinicians must also consider the possibility that MODY mutations may occur de novo in the absence of a family history of MODY. The degree to which this occurs is yet to be determined. We do know that MODY mutations are uncommon in patients with Type 2 diabetes. Following insulin resistance which is the most common cause of GDM, MODY may be a more common cause of GDM than autoimmune diabetes (254).

The diagnosis of MODY (or ADM) is important because such individuals can generally be managed with oral antidiabetic agents, freeing patients from the requirement for daily insulin injections (255,256). Nevertheless, long-term studies have not been carried out to determine the optimal therapy of MODY. Because of the milder nature of MODY when compared with Type 1 diabetes, self-monitoring for blood-glucose may not be required. This coupled with the use of noninsulin therapies may save money in the care of the diabetic individual, potentially justifying screening for MODY in certain circumstances as discussed above (257).

Regardless of the etiology of the diabetes (e.g., genetic or nongenetic), because the frequency and severity of complications relate to the degree and duration of hyperglycemia, all patients with diabetes should strive to achieve an optimal hemoglobin A_{1c} (e.g., less than 6.5% to 7%) (258,259). For those families diagnosed with a recognized MODY mutation, unaffected family members can undergo genetic screening to determine their risk for MODY (260). Identification of the specific MODY mutation provides important information about the clinical course of the disease, therapy, and prognosis. For example, for individuals with well controlled MODY-3 who are insulin-treated, a trial of sulfonylureas should be considered (261,262).

CONCLUSION

While the general pediatrician will rarely see forms of diabetes other than Type 1 or Type 2 diabetes, these practitioners must be aware that there are a large number of genetic and nongenetic causes of diabetes that are currently classified as "other specific types of diabetes."

REFERENCES

1. Giuffrida FM, Reis AF. Genetic and clinical characteristics of maturity-onset diabetes of the young. Diabetes Obes Metab 2005; 7(4):318–326.
2. Winter WE. Autoimmune disorders that influence carbohydrate metabolism. In: Nakamura RM, Keren DF, Bylund DJ, eds. Clinical and Laboratory Evaluation of Human Autoimmune Diseases. Chapter 24. Chicago, IL: ASCP Press, 2002:345–372.
3. Winter WE. Autoimmune endocrinopathies. In: Lifshitz F, ed. Pediatric Endocrinology. 4th ed. New York, NY: Marcel Dekker Inc., 2003:683–720.
4. Malecki MT. Genetics of type 2 diabetes mellitus. Diabetes Res Clin Pract 2005; 68(Suppl 1):S10–S21.
5. Polonsky KS. The beta-cell in diabetes: from molecular genetics to clinical research. Diabetes 1995; 44:705–715.
6. Bell GI, Kayano T, Buse JB, et al. Molecular biology of mammalian glucose transporters. Diabetes Care 1990; 13(3):198–208.
7. Joost HG, Thorens B. The extended GLUT-family of sugar/polyol transport facilitators: nomenclature, sequence characteristics, and potential function of its novel members (review). Mol Membr Biol 2001; 18(4):247–256.
8. Uldry M, Thorens B. The SLC2 family of facilitated hexose and polyol transporters. Pflugers Arch 2004; 447(5):480–489.
9. Matschinsky FM, Glaser B, Magnuson MA. Pancreatic β-cell glucokinase, closing the gap between theoretical concepts and experimental realities. Diabetes 1998; 47:307–315.
10. Maassen JA, Janssen GM, Lemkes HH. Mitochondrial diabetes mellitus. J Endocrinol Invest 2002; 25(5):477–484.
11. Yamagata K. Regulation of pancreatic beta-cell function by the HNF transcription network: lessons from maturity-onset diabetes of the young (MODY). Endocr J 2003; 50(5):491–499.
12. Rowley CW, Staloch LJ, Divine JK, McCaul SP, Simon TC. Mechanisms of mutual functional interactions between HNF-4 (alpha) and HNF-1(alpha) revealed by mutations that cause maturity onset diabetes of the young. Am J Physiol Gastrointest Liver Physiol 2005; [Epub ahead of print].
13. Santer R, Schneppenheim R, Dombrowski A, Götze H, Steinmann B, Schaub J. Mutations in GLUT2, the gene for the liver-type glucose transporter, in patients with Fanconi-Bickel syndrome. Nat Genet 1997; 17:324–326.
14. Longo N, Elsas LJ. Human glucose transporters. Adv Pediatr 1998; 45:293–311.
15. Orho M, Bosshard NU, Buist NR, et al. Mutations in the liver glycogen synthase gene in children with hypoglycemia due to glycogen storage disease type 0. J Clin Invest 1998; 102(3):507–515.
16. Fajans SS. Scope and heterogeneous nature of MODY. Diabetes Care 1990; 13:49–64.
17. Tattersall RB, Fajans SS. A difference between the inheritance of classical juvenile-onset and maturity-onset type diabetes of young people. Diabetes 1975; 24:44–53.
18. Winter WE, Nakamura M, House DV. Monogenic diabetes mellitus in youth: the MODY syndromes. Endocrinol Metab Clin North Am 1999; 28(4):765–785.
19. American Diabetes Association. Diagnosis and classification of diabetes mellitus. Diabetes Care 2006; 29:S43–S48.
20. Gragnoli C, Stanojevic V, Gorini A, Von Preussenthal GM, Thomas MK, Habener JF. IPF-1/MODY4 gene missense mutation in an Italian family with type 2 and gestational diabetes. Metabolism 2005; 54(8):983–988.
21. Bigler R, Adler S. Diabetic nephropathy in a patient with maturity-onset diabetes of the young. Arch Intern Med 1981; 141:791–792.
22. Ehtisham S, Hattersley AT, Dunger DB, Barrett TG. British Society for Paediatric Endocrinology Diabetes Clinical Trials Group. First UK survey of paediatric type 2 diabetes and MODY. Arch Dis Child 2004; 89(6):526–529.
23. Kristinsson SY, Thorolfsdottir ET, Talseth B, et al. MODY in Iceland is associated with mutations in HNF-1alpha and a novel mutation in NeuroD1. Diabetologia 2001; 44(11):2098–2103.
24. Winter WE, Maclaren NK, Riley WJ, Clarke DW, Kappy MS, Spillar RP. Maturity-onset diabetes of youth in Black Americans. N Engl J Med 1987; 316:285–291.

25. House DV, Nakamura M, Wasserfall C, Maclaren NK, Winter WE. Further evidence that ADM is not an autoimmune disease: studies of GADAb in atypical diabetes (ADM). Clin Chem 1995; 41(S6):S49.

26. Huang W, House DV, Nakamura M, et al. Molecular HLA-DQB1 typing and IA-2 determinations in atypical diabetes mellitus (ADM). Diabetes 1996; 45(Suppl 2):80A.

27. House DV, Nakamura M, Maclaren NK, Winter WE. First phase C-peptide responses to intravenous glucose in atypical diabetes mellitus (ADM) of African Americans: evidence of a severe defect in beta cell function. Clin Chem 1996; 42(6):S235.

28. Nakamura M, House DV, Winter WE. Novel mutation identified in the glucokinase (GCK) gene of a patient with atypical diabetes mellitus (ADM) of African Americans. Diabetes 1996; 45(Suppl 2):76A.

29. Nakamura M, House DV, Winter WE. A novel homoplasmic point mutation at mitochondrial DNA (mtDNA) nucleotide 3308 in a family with atypical diabetes mellitus (ADM) of African Americans (AA). Diabetes 1997; 46(Suppl 1):175A.

30. Boutin P, Gresh L, Cisse A, et al. Missense mutation Gly574Ser in the transcription factor HNF-1alpha is a marker of atypical diabetes mellitus in African-American children. Diabetologia 1999; 42(3):380–381.

31. Collet C, Ducorps M, Mayaudon H, et al. Prevalence of the missense mutation Gly574Ser in the hepatocyte nuclear factor-1alpha in Africans with diabetes. Diabetes Metab 2002; 28(1):39–44.

32. Katagiri H, Asano T, Ishihara H, et al. Nonsense mutation of glucokinase in late-onset non-insulin dependent diabetes mellitus. Lancet 1992; 340:1316–1317.

33. Laakso M, Malkki M, Kekalainen P, Kuusisto J, Mykkanen L, Deeb SS. Glucokinase gene variants in subjects with late-onset NIDDM and impaired glucose tolerance. Diabetes Care 1995; 18(3):398–400.

34. Hani EH, Suaud L, Boutin P, et al. A missense mutation in hepatocyte nuclear factor-4 alpha, resulting in a reduced transactivation activity, in human late-onset non-insulin-dependent diabetes mellitus. J Clin Invest 1998; 101(3):521–526.

35. Sakurai K, Seki N, Fujii R, et al. Mutations in the hepatocyte nuclear factor-4 alpha gene in Japanese with non-insulin-dependent diabetes: a nucleotide substitution in the polypyrimidine tract of intron 1b. Horm Metab Res 2000; 32(8):316–320.

36. Moller AM, Urhammer SA, Dalgaard LT, et al. Studies of the genetic variability of the coding region of the hepatocyte nuclear factor-4 alpha in Caucasians with maturity onset NIDDM. Diabetologia 1997; 40:980–983.

37. Malecki MT, Antonellis A, Casey P, et al. Exclusion of the hepatocyte nuclear factor 4 alpha as a candidate gene for late-onset NIDDM linked with chromosome 20q. Diabetes 1998; 47:970–972.

38. Dupont S, Vionnet N, Chevre JC, et al. No evidence of linkage or diabetes-associated mutations in the transcription factors BETA2/NEUROD1 and PAX4 in Type II diabetes in France. Diabetologia 1999; 42(4):480–484.

39. Lee HJ, Ahn CW, Kim SJ, et al. Mutation in hepatocyte nuclear factor-1 alpha is not a common cause of MODY and early-onset type 2 diabetes in Korea. Acta Diabetol 2001; 38(3):123–127.

40. Zhu Q, Yamagata K, Miura A, et al. T130I mutation in HNF-4alpha gene is a loss-of-function mutation in hepatocytes and is associated with late-onset Type 2 diabetes mellitus in Japanese subjects. Diabetologia 2003; 46(4):567–573.

41. Shiau MY, Huang CN, Liao JH, Chang YH. Missense mutations in the human insulin promoter factor-1 gene are not a common cause of type 2 diabetes mellitus in Taiwan. J Endocrinol Invest 2004; 27(11):1076–1080.

42. Dominguez-Lopez A, Miliar-Garcia A, Segura-Kato YX, et al. Mutations in MODY genes are not common cause of early-onset type 2 diabetes in Mexican families. JOP 2005; 6(3):238–245.

43. Fajans SS, Bell GI, Polonsky KS. Molecular mechanisms and clinical pathophysiology of maturity-onset diabetes of the young. N Engl J Med 2001; 342:971–980.

44. Hansen SK, Parrizas M, Jensen ML, et al. Genetic evidence that HNF-1alpha-dependent transcriptional control of HNF-4alpha is essential for human pancreatic beta cell function. J Clin Invest 2002; 110(6):827–833.

45. Mitchell SM, Vaxillaire M, Thomas H, et al. Rare variants identified in the HNF-4 alpha beta-cell-specific promoter and alternative exon 1 lack biological significance in maturity onset diabetes of the young and young onset Type II diabetes. Diabetologia 2002; 45(9):1344–1348.

46. Su MA, Anderson MS. Aire: an update. Curr Opin Immunol 2004; 16(6):746–752.

47. Villasenor J, Benoist C, Mathis D. AIRE and APECED: molecular insights into an autoimmune disease. Immunol Rev 2005; 204:156–164.

48. Frayling TM, Lindgren CM, Chevre JC, et al. A genome-wide scan in families with maturity-onset diabetes of the young: evidence for further genetic heterogeneity. Diabetes 2003; 52(3):872–881.

49. Johansen A, Ek J, Mortensen HB, Pedersen O, Hansen T. Half of clinically defined maturity-onset diabetes of the young patients in Denmark do not have mutations in HNF4A, GCK, and TCF1. J Clin Endocrinol Metab 2005; 90(8):4607–4614.

50. Kim SH, Ma X, Weremowicz S, et al. Identification of a locus for maturity-onset diabetes of the young on chromosome 8p23. Diabetes 2004; 53(5):1375–1384.

51. Doria A, Yang Y, Malecki M, et al. Phenotypic characteristics of early-onset autosomal-dominant type 2 diabetes unlinked to known maturity-onset diabetes of the young (MODY) genes. Diabetes Care 1999; 22(2):253–261.

52. Dussoix P, Vaxillaire M, Iynedjian PB, et al. Diagnostic heterogeneity of diabetes in lean young adults. Diabetes 1997; 46:622–631.

53. Furuta H, Horikawa Y, Iwasaki N, et al. Beta-cell transcription factors and diabetes: mutations in the coding region of the BETA2/NeuroD1 (NEUROD1) and Nkx2.2 (NKX2B) genes are not associated with maturity-onset diabetes of the young in Japanese. Diabetes 1998; 47(8):1356–1358.

54. Yu L, Wei Q, Jin L, et al. Genetic variation in the hepatocyte nuclear factor (HNF)-3alpha gene does not contribute to maturity-onset diabetes of the young in Japanese. Horm Metab Res 2001; 33(3):163–166.

55. Yamada S, Zhu Q, Aihara Y, et al. Cloning of cDNA and the gene encoding human hepatocyte nuclear factor (HNF) 0 beta and mutation screening in Japanese subjects with maturity-onset diabetes of the young. Diabetologia 2000; 43(1):121–124.

56. Hinokio Y, Horikawa Y, Furuta H, et al. Beta-cell transcription factors and diabetes: no evidence for diabetes-associated mutations in the hepatocyte nuclear factor-3 beta gene (HNF3B) in Japanese patients with maturity-onset diabetes of the young. Diabetes 2000; 49(2):302–305.

57. Abderrahmani A, Chevre JC, Otabe S, et al. Genetic variation in the hepatocyte nuclear factor-3beta gene (HNF3B)

does contribute to maturity-onset diabetes of the young in French Caucasians. Diabetes 2000; 49(2):306–308.

58. Hara M, Wang X, Paz VP, et al. No diabetes-associated mutations in the coding region of the hepatocyte nuclear factor-4gamma gene (HNF4G) in Japanese patients with MODY. Diabetologia 2000; 43(8):1064–1069.

59. Plengvidhya N, Antonellis A, Wogan LT, et al. Hepatocyte nuclear factor-4gamma: cDNA sequence, gene organization, and mutation screening in early-onset autosomal-dominant type 2 diabetes. Diabetes 1999; 48(10):2099–2102.

60. Zhu Q, Yamagata K, Tsukahara Y, et al. Mutation screening of the hepatocyte nuclear factor (HNF)-6 gene in Japanese subjects with diabetes mellitus. Diabetes Res Clin Pract 2001; 52(3):171–174.

61. Horikawa Y, Horikawa Y, Cox NJ, et al. Beta-cell transcription factors and diabetes: no evidence for diabetes-associated mutations in the gene encoding the basic helix-loop-helix transcription factor neurogenic differentiation 4 (NEUROD4) in Japanese patients with MODY. Diabetes 2000; 49(11):1955–1957.

62. del Bosque-Plata L, Lin J, Horikawa Y, et al. Mutations in the coding region of the neurogenin 3 gene (NEUROG3) are not a common cause of maturity-onset diabetes of the young in Japanese subjects. Diabetes 2001; 50(3):694–696.

63. Froguel P, Vaxillaire M, Sun F, et al. Close linkage of glucokinase locus on chromosome 7p to early-onset non-insulin-dependent diabetes mellitus. Nature 1992; 356:162.

64. Froguel P, Zouali H, Vionnet N, et al. Familial hyperglycemia due to mutations in glucokinase. Definition of a subtype of diabetes mellitus. N Engl J Med 1993; 328(10):697–702.

65. Matschinsky F, Liang Y, Kesavan P, et al. Glucokinase as pancreatic beta cell glucose sensor and diabetes gene. J Clin Invest 1993; 92(5):2092–2098.

66. Weir GC. A defective beta-cell glucose sensor as a cause of diabetes. N Engl J Med 1993; 328:729–731.

67. Byrne MM, Sturis J, Fajans SS, et al. Altered insulin secretory responses to glucose in subjects with a mutation in the MODY1 gene on chromosome 20. Diabetes 1995; 44:699–704.

68. Sakura H, Kawamori R, Kubota M, et al. Glucokinase gene mutation and impaired glucose uptake by liver. Lancet 1993; 341(8859):1532–1533.

69. Cerutti F, Rabbone I, Sacchetti C, Matschinsky FM, Barbetti F. Acute and chronic suphonylurea administration in a subject with a homozygous glucokinase mutation. Pediatr Res 2001; 49(abstracts issue):89A.

70. Vagnarelli F, Cianfarani S, Germani D, et al. A case of neonatal diabetes with a novel glucokinase mutation. Pediatr Res 2001; 49(abstracts issue):89A.

71. Porter JR, Shaw NJ, Barrett TG, Hattersley AT, Ellard S, Gloyn AL. Permanent neonatal diabetes in an Asian infant. J Pediatr 2005; 146(1):131–133.

72. Glaser B, Kesavan P, Heyman M, et al. Familial hyperinsulinism caused by an activating glucokinase mutation. N Engl J Med 1998; 338(4):226–230.

73. Gloyn AL. Glucokinase (GCK) mutations in hyper- and hypoglycemia: maturity-onset diabetes of the young, permanent neonatal diabetes, and hyperinsulinemia of infancy. Hum Mutat 2003; 22(5):353–362.

74. Liang P, Hughes V, Fukagawa NK. Increased prevalence of mitochondrial DMA deletions in skeletal muscle of older individuals with impaired glucose tolerance. Diabetes 1997; 46:920–923.

75. (a) Wallace DC. Mitochondrial disease in man and mouse. Science 1999; 283:1482–1488; (b) Maassen JA. Mitochondrial diabetes, diabetes and the thiamine-responsive megaloblastic anaemia syndrome and MODY-2. Diseases with common pathophysiology? Panminerva Med 2002; 44(4):295–300.

76. Enns GM. The contribution of mitochondria to common disorders. Mol Genet Metab 2003; 80(1–2):11–26.

77. Gerbitz KD, Gempel K, Brdiczka D. Mitochondria and diabetes: genetic, biochemical, and clinical implications of the cellular energy circuit. Diabetes 1996; 45: 113–126.

78. Oka Y, Katagiri H, Yazaki Y, Murase T, Kobayashi T. Mitochondrial gene mutation in islet-cell-antibody-positive patients who were initially non-insulin-dependent diabetics. Lancet 1993; 342:527–528.

79. Kobayashi T, Oka Y, Katagiri H, et al. Association between HLA and islet cell antibodies in diabetic patients with a mitochondrial DNA mutation at base pair 3243. Diabetologia 1996; 39:1196–1200.

80. Odawara M, Sasaki K, Nagafuchi S, Tanae A, Yamashita K. Lack of association between mitochondrial gene mutation np 3242 and type 1 diabetes mellitus and autoimmune thyroid disease. Lancet 1994; 344:1086.

81. Matsuura N, Suzuki S, Yokota Y, et al. The prevalence of mitochondrial gene mutations in childhood diabetes in Japan. J Pediatr Endocrinol Metab 1999; 12:27–30.

82. Suzuki S, Oka Y, Kadowaki T, et al. Research Committee or Specific Types of Diabetes Mellitus with Gene Mutations of the Japan Diabetes Society. Clinical features of diabetes mellitus with the mitochondrial DNA 3243 (A–G) mutation in Japanese: maternal inheritance and mitochondria-related complications. Diabetes Res Clin Pract 2003; 59(3):207–217.

83. Taniyama M, Kasuga A, Suzuki Y, et al. Absence of antibodies to ICA512/IA-2 in NIDDM patients with mitochondrial DMA bp 3243 mutation. Diabetes Care 1997; 20:905–906.

84. Reardon W, Ross RJ, Sweeney MG, et al. Diabetes mellitus associated with a pathogenic point mutation in mitochondrial DNA. Lancet 1992; 340(8832):1376–1379.

85. van den Ouweland JM, Lemkes HH, Trembath RC, et al. Maternally inherited diabetes and deafness is a distinct subtype of diabetes and associates with a single point mutation in the mitochondrial tRNA [Leu(UUR))] gene. Diabetes 1994; 43(6):746–751.

86. Kishimoto M, Hashiramoto M, Araki S, et al. Diabetes mellitus carrying a mutation in the mitochondrial tRNA [Leu(UUR)] gene. Diabetologia 1995; 38(2):193–200.

87. Alcolado JC, Thomas AW. Maternally inherited diabetes mellitus: the role of mitochondrial DNA defects. Diabetes Med 1995; 12(2):102–108.

88. Maassen JA, 'T Hart LM, Van Essen E, et al. Mitochondrial diabetes: molecular mechanisms and clinical presentation. Diabetes 2004; 53(Suppl 1):S103–S109.

89. Maassen JA, Janssen GM, 'T Hart LM. Molecular mechanisms of mitochondrial diabetes (MIDD). Ann Med 2005; 37(3):213–221.

90. Ohkubo K, Yamano A, Nagashima M, et al. Mitochondrial gene mutations in the tRNA$^{Leu(UUR)}$ region and diabetes: prevalence and clinical phenotypes in Japan. Clin Chem 2001; 47:1641–1648.

91. Langin. Diabetes, insulin secretion, and the pancreatic beta-cell mitochondrion. N Engl J Med 2001; 354:1772–1774.

92. Uchigata Y, Okada T, Gong J-S, Yamada Y, Iwamoto Y, Tanaka M. A mitochondrial genotype associated with the development of autoimmune-type 1 diabetes. Diabetes Care 2002; 25:2106.

93. Stanley CA. Hyperinsulinism in infants and children. Pediatr Clin North Am 1997; 44(2):363–374.

94. Thomas P, Ye Y, Lightner E. Mutation of the pancreatic islet inward rectifier Kir6.2 also leads to familial persistent hyperinsulinemic hypoglycemia of infancy. Hum Mol Genet 1996; 5(11):1809–1812.

95. Koster JC, Permutt MA, Nichols CG. Diabetes and insulin secretion: the ATP-sensitive K+ channel (KATP) connection. Diabetes 2005; 54(11):3065–3072.

96. Hattersley AT, Ashcroft FM. Activating mutations in Kir6.2 and neonatal diabetes: new clinical syndromes, new scientific insights, and new therapy. Diabetes 2005; 54(9):2503–2513.

97. Klupa T, Edghill EL, Nazim J, et al. Diabetologia 2005; 48(5):1029–1033.

98. Kant SG, van der Weij AM, Oostdijk W, et al. Monozygous triplets discordant for transient neonatal diabetes mellitus and for imprinting of the TNDM differentially methylated region. Hum Genet 2005; 117(4):398–401.

99. Yorifuji T, Nagashima K, Kurokawa K, et al. The C42R mutation in the Kir6.2 (KCNJ11) gene as a cause of transient neonatal diabetes, childhood diabetes, or later-onset, apparently type 2 diabetes mellitus. J Clin Endocrinol Metab 2005; 90(6):3174–3178.

100. Velho G, Froguel P. Genetic, metabolic and clinical characteristics of maturity onset diabetes of the young. Eur J Endocrinol 1998; 138:233–239.

101. Yamagata K, Furuta H, Oda N, et al. Mutations in the hepatocyte nuclear factor-4 alpha gene in maturity-onset diabetes of the young (MODY 1). Nature 1996; 384:458–460.

102. Fajans SS, Conn JW. Tolbutamide-induced improvement in carbohydrate tolerance of young people with mild diabetes mellitus. Diabetes 1960; 9:83–88.

103. Herman WH, Fajans SS, Ortiz FJ, et al. Abnormal insulin secretion, not insulin resistance, is the genetic or primary defect of MODY in the RW pedigree. Diabetes 1994; 43:40–46.

104. Herman WH, Fajans SS, Smith MJ, Polonsky S, Bell GI, Halter JB. Diminished insulin and glucagon secretory responses to arginine in nondiabetic subjects with a mutation in the hepatocyte nuclear factor-4 alpha/MODY1 gene. Diabetes 1997; 46:1749–1754.

105. Ilag LL, Tabaei BP, Herman WH, et al. Reduced pancreatic polypeptide response to hypoglycemia and amyline response to arginine in subjects with a mutation in the HNF-1 alpha/MODY1 gene. Diabetes 2000; 49:961–968.

106. Shih DQ, Dansky HM, Fleisher M, Assmann G, Fajans SS, Stoffel M. Genotype/phenotype relationships in HNF-4 alpha/MODY1. Diabetes 2000; 49:832–837.

107. Pearson ER, Pruhova S, Tack CJ, et al. Molecular genetics and phenotypic characteristics of MODY caused by hepatocyte nuclear factor 4alpha mutations in a large European collection. Diabetologia 2005; 48(5):878–885.

108. Gupta RK, Vatamaniuk MZ, Lee CS, et al. The MODY1 gene HNF-4alpha regulates selected genes involved in insulin secretion. J Clin Invest 2005; 115(4):1006–1015.

109. Menzel S, Yamagata K, Trabb JB, et al. Localization of MODY3 to a 5-cM region of human chromosome 12. Diabetes 1995; 44:1408–1413.

110. Yamagata K, Oda N, Kaisaki PJ, et al. Mutations in the hepatocyte nuclear factor-1 alpha gene in maturity-onset diabetes of the young (MODY3). Nature 1996A; 384: 455–458.

111. Green J, Naot D, Cooper G. Hepatocyte nuclear factor 1 negatively regulates amylin gene expression. Biochem Biophys Res Commun 2003; 310(2):464–469.

112. Yang Q, Yamagata K, Fukui K, et al. Hepatocyte nuclear factor-1 alpha modulates pancreatic beta-cell growth by regulating the expression of insulin-like growth factor-1 in INS-1 cells. Diabetes 2002; 51:1785–1792.

113. Yamagata K, Yang Q, Yamamoto K, et al. Mutation P291fsinsC in the transcription factor hepatocyte nuclear factor-1 alpha is dominant negative. Diabetes 1998; 47:1231–1235.

114. Magenheim J, Hertz R, Berman I, Nousbeck J, Bar-Tana J. Negative autoregulation of HNF-4alpha gene expression by HNF-4alpha1. Biochem J 2005; 388(Pt 1):325–332.

115. Kim SH, Ma X, Klupa T, et al. Genetic modifiers of the age at diagnosis of diabetes (MODY3) in carriers of hepatocyte nuclear factor-1alpha mutations map to chromosomes 5p15, 9q22, and 14q24. Diabetes 2003; 52(8):2182–2186.

116. Kaisaki PJ, Menzel S, Lindner T, et al. Mutations in the hepatocyte nuclear factor-1 alpha gene in MODY and early-onset NIDDM. Diabetes 1997; 46(3):528–535.

117. Glucksmann MA, Lehto M, Tayber O, et al. Novel mutations and a mutational hotspot in the MODY3 gene. Diabetes 1997; 46:1081–1086.

118. Isomaa B, Hemricsson M, Lehto M, et al. Chronic diabetic complications in patients with MODY3 diabetes. Diabetologia 1988; 41:467–473.

119. Menzel R, Kaisaki PJ, Rjasanowski I, Heinke P, Kerner W, Menzel S. A low renal threshold for glucose in diabetic patients with a mutation in the hepatocyte nuclear factor-1alpha (HNF-1alpha) gene. Diabet Med 1998; 15(10):816–820.

120. Miedzybrodzka Z, Hattersley AT, Ellard S, et al. Nonpenetrance in a MODY 3 family with a mutation in the hepatic nuclear factor 1alpha gene: implications for predictive testing. Eur J Hum Genet 1999; 7(6):729–732.

121. Pearson ER, Liddell WG, Shepherd M, Correall RJ, Hattersley AT. Sensitivity to sulphonylureas in patients with hepatocyte nuclear factor-1 alpha gene mutations: evidence for pharmacogenetics in diabetes. Diabet Med 2000; 17:543–545.

122. Yamada S, Nishigori H, Onda H, et al. Identification of mutations in the hepatocyte nuclear factor (HNF)-1 alpha gene in Japanese subjects with IDDM. Diabetes 1997; 46:1643–1647.

123. Miura J, Sanaka M, Ikeda Y, et al. A case of type-1 diabetes mellitus formerly diagnosed as maturity-onset diabetes of the young (MODY) carrying suggestive MODY3 gene. Diab Res Clin Pract 1997; 38:139–141.

124. Moller AM, Dalgaard LT, Pociot F, Nerup J, Hansen T, Pedersen O. Mutations in the hepatocyte nuclear factor-1alpha gene in Caucasian families originally classified as having Type I diabetes. Diabetologia 1998; 41(12):1528–1531.

125. Hathout EH, Cockburn BN, Mace JW, Sharkey J, Chen-Daniel J, Bell GI. A case of hepatocyte nuclear factor-1 alpha diabetes/MODY3 masquerading as type 1 diabetes in a Mexican-American adolescent and responsive to a low dose of sulfonylurea. Diabetes Care 1999; 22(5):867–868.

126. Kawasaki E, Sera Y, Yamakawa K, et al. Identification and functional analysis of mutations in the hepatocyte nuclear factor-1alpha gene in anti-islet autoantibody-negative Japanese patients with type 1 diabetes. J Clin Endocrinol Metab 2000; 85(1):331–335.

127. Byrne MM, Sturis J, Menzel S, et al. Altered insulin secretory responses to glucose in diabetic and nondiabetic subjects with mutations in the diabetes susceptibility gene MODY3 on chromosome 12. Diabetes 1996; 45:1503–1510.

128. Stoffers DA, Zinkin NT, Stanojevic V, Clarke WL, Habener JF. Pancreatic agenesis attributable to a single nucleotide deletion in the human IPF1 gene coding sequence. Nat Genet 1997; 15:106–110.

129. Wang H, Iezzi M, Theander S, et al. Suppression of Pdx-1 perturbs proinsulin processing, insulin secretion and GLP-1 signalling in INS-1 cells. Diabetologia 2005; 48(4):720–731.

130. Inoue H, Riggs AC, Tanizawa Y, et al. Isolation, characterization, and chromosomal mapping of the human insulin promoter factor 1 (IPF-1) gene. Diabetes 1996; 45(6):789–794.

131. Ashizawa S, Brunicardi FC, Wang XP. PDX-1 and the pancreas. Pancreas 2004; 28(2):109–120.

132. Clocquet AR, Egan JM, Stoffers DA, et al. Impaired insulin secretion and increased insulin sensitivity in familial maturity onset diabetes of the young 4 (insulin promoter factor 1 gene). Diabetes 2000; 49:1856–1864.

133. Milunsky A, Bray GA, Londono J, Loridan L. Insulin, glucose growth hormone, and free fatty acids, determinations in patients with cystic fibrosis. Am J Dis Child 1971; 121:15–19.

134. Wilmshurst EG, Soeldner JS, Holsclaw DS, et al. Endogenous and exogenous insulin responses in patients with cystic fibrosis. Pediatrics 1975; 55:75–82.

135. Lippe BM, Kaplan SA, Neufeld ND, Smith A, Scott M. Insulin receptors in cystic fibrosis: increased receptor number and altered affinity. Pediatrics 1980; 65:1018–1022.

136. Wachslicht-Rodbard H, Gross HA, Rodbard D, Ebert MH, Roth J. Increased insulin binding to erythrocytes in anorexia nervosa. N Engl J Med 1979; 300:882–887.

137. Stoffers DA, Stanojevic V, Habener JF. Insulin promoter factor-1 gene mutation linked to early-onset type 2 diabetes mellitus directs expression of a dominant negative isoprotein. J Clin Invest 1998; 102:232–241.

138. Melloul D, Tsur A, Zangen D. Pancreatic Duodenal Homeobox (PDX-1) in health and disease. J Pediatr Endocrinol Metab 2002; 15(9):1461–1472.

139. Jonsson J, Carlsson L, Edlund T, Edlund H. Insulin-promoter-factor 1 is required for pancreas development in mice. Nature 1994; 371:606–609.

140. Krapp A, Knofler M, Ledermann B, et al. The bHLH protein PTF1-p48 is essential for the formation of the exocrine and the correct spatial organization of the endocrine pancreas. Genes Dev 1998; 12(23):3752–3763.

141. Brink C, Chowdhury K, Gruss P. Pax4 regulatory elements mediate beta cell specific expression in the pancreas. Mech Dev 2001; 100(1):37–43.

142. Sander M, Sussel L, Conners J, et al. Homeobox gene Nkx6.1 lies downstream of Nkx2.2 in the major pathway of beta-cell formation in the pancreas. Development 2000; 127(24):5533–5540.

143. Naya FJ, Huang HP, Qiu Y, et al. Diabetes, defective pancreatic morphogenesis, and abnormal enteroendocrine differentiation in BETA2/neuroD-deficient mice. Genes Dev 1997; 11(18):2323–2334.

144. Blum D, Dorchy H, Mouraux T, et al. Congenital absence of insulin cells in a neonate with diabetes mellitus and mutase-deficient methylmalonic acidaemia. Diabetologia 1993; 36:352–357.

145. Dodge JA, Laurence KM. Congenital absence of islets of Langerhans. Arch Dis Child 1977; 52(5):411–413.

146. Voldsgaard P, Kryger-Baggesen N, Lisse I. Agenesis of pancreas. Acta Paediatr 1994; 83(7):791–793.

147. Winter WE, Maclaren NK, Riley WJ, Andres J, Toskes RP, Rosenbloom AL. Congenital pancreatic hypoplasia: a novel diabetes syndrome of exocrine and endocrine pancreatic insufficiency. Pediatrics 1986; 109:465–469.

148. Yorifuji T, Matsumura M, Okuno T, et al. Hereditary pancreatic hypoplasia, diabetes mellitus, and congenital heart disease: a new syndrome? J Med Genet 1994; 31:331–333.

149. Stoffers DA, Ferrer J, Clarke WL, Habener JF. Early-onset type-II diabetes mellitus (MODY4) linked to IPF1. Nat Genet 1997; 17:138–139.

150. Macfarlane WM, Frayling TM, Ellard S, et al. Missense mutations in the insulin promoter factor-1 gene predispose to type 2 diabetes. J Clin Invest 1999; 104(9):R33–R39.

151. Hani EH, Stoffers DA, Chevre JC, et al. Defective mutations in the insulin promoter factor-1 (IPF-1) gene in late-onset type 2 diabetes mellitus. J Clin Invest 1999; 104(9):R41–R48.

152. Weng J, Macfarlane WM, Lehto M, et al. Functional consequences of mutations in the MODY4 gene (IPF1) and coexistence with MODY3 mutations. Diabetologia 2001; 44(2):249–258.

153. Reis AF, Ye WZ, Dubois-Laforgue D, Bellanne-Chantelot C, Timsit J, Velho G. Mutations in the insulin promoter factor-1 gene in late-onset type 2 diabetes mellitus. Eur J Endocrinol 2000; 143(4):511–513.

154. Hansen L, Urioste S, Petersen HV, et al. Missense mutations in the human insulin promoter factor-1 gene and their relation to maturity-onset diabetes of the young and late-onset type 2 diabetes mellitus in Caucasians. J Clin Endocrinol Metab 2000; 85(3): 1323–1326.

155. Horikawa Y, Iwasaki N, Hara M, et al. Mutation in hepatocyte nuclear factor-1 beta gene (TCF2) associated with MODY. Nat Genet 1997; 17(4):384–385.

156. Beards F, Frayling T, Bulman M, et al. Mutations in hepatocyte nuclear factor 1beta are not a common cause of maturity-onset diabetes of the young in the U.K. Diabetes 1998; 47(7):1152–1154.

157. Furuta H, Furuta M, Sanke T, et al. Nonsense and missense mutations in the human hepatocyte nuclear factor-1 beta gene (TCF2) and their relation to type 2 diabetes. J Clin Endocrinol Metab 2002; 87:3859–3863.

158. Selisko T, Vcelak J, Bendlova B, Graessler J, Schwarz PE, Schulze J. Mutations and intronic variants in the HNF-1 beta gene in a group of German and Czech Caucasians with type 2 diabetes mellitus and progressive diabetic nephropathy. Exp Clin Endocrinol Diabetes 2002; 110(3):145–147.

159. Lindner TH, Njolstad PR, Horikawa Y, Bostad L, Bell GI, Sovik O. A novel syndrome of diabetes mellitus, renal dysfunction and genital malformation associated with a partial deletion of the pseudo-POU domain of hepatocyte nuclear factor-1beta. Hum Mol Genet 1999; 8(11):2001–2008.

160. Nishigori H, Yamada S, Kohama T, et al. Frameshift mutation, A263fsinsGG, in the hepatocyte nuclear factor-1 beta gene associated with diabetes and renal dysfunction. Diabetes 1998; 47:1354–1355.

161. Bingham C, Ellard S, Allen L, et al. Abnormal nephron development associated with a frameshift mutation in the transcription factor hepatocyte nuclear factor-1 beta. Kidney Int 2000; 57(3):898–907.

162. Wang C, Fang Q, Zhang R, Lin X, Xiang K. Scanning for MODY5 gene mutations in Chinese early onset or multiple affected diabetes pedigrees. Acta Diabetol 2004; 41(4):137–145.

163. Edghill EL, Bingham C, Ellard S, Hattersley AT. Mutations in hepatocyte nuclear factor-1(beta) and their related phenotypes. J Med Genet 2005; 43:84–90.

164. Iwasaki N, Ogata M, Tomonaga O, et al. Liver and kidney function in Japanese patients with maturity-onset diabetes of the young. Diabetes Care 1998; 21(12):2144–2148.

165. Sagen JV, Baumann ME, Salvesen HB, Molven A, Sovik O, Njolstad PR. Diagnostic screening of NEUROD1 (MODY6) in subjects with MODY or gestational diabetes mellitus. Diabet Med 2005; 22(8):1012–1015.

166. Malecki MT, Jhala US, Antonellis A, et al. Mutations in NEUROD1 are associated with the development of type 2 diabetes mellitus. Nat Genet 1999; 23(3):323–328.

167. Iwata I, Nagafuchi S, Nakashima H, et al. Association of polymorphism in the NeuroD/BETA2 gene with type 1 diabetes in the Japanese. Diabetes 1999; 48(2):416–419.

168. Yamada S, Motohashi Y, Yanagawa T, et al. NeuroD/beta2 gene G→A polymorphism may affect onset pattern of

type 1 diabetes in Japanese. Diabetes Care 2001; 24(8):1438–1441.

169. Marron MP, Hopkins DI, Park YS, She JX. NeuroD/Beta2 polymorphism is not associated with type 1 diabetes in Chinese, Korean, or Caucasian populations. J Endocr Genet 1999; 1:73–77.

170. Gabbay KH. The insulinopathies. N Engl J Med 1980; 302(3):165–167.

171. Haneda M, Chan SJ, Kwok SC, Rubenstein AH, Steiner DF. Studies on mutant human insulin genes: identification and sequence analysis of a gene encoding [SerB24]insulin. Proc Natl Acad Sci USA 1983; 80(20):6366–6370.

172. Haneda M, Polonsky KS, Bergenstal RM, et al. Familial hyperinsulinemia due to a structurally abnormal insulin. Definition of an emerging new clinical syndrome. N Engl J Med 1984; 310(20):1288–1294.

173. Tager HS. Lilly lecture 1983. Abnormal products of the human insulin gene. Diabetes 1984; 33(7):693–699.

174. Steiner DF, Tager HS, Chan SJ, Nanjo K, Sanke T, Rubenstein AH. Lessons learned from molecular biology of insulin-gene mutations. Diabetes Care 1990; 13(6):600–609.

175. Nanjo K, Sanke T, Miyano M, et al. Diabetes due to secretion of a structurally abnormal insulin (insulin Wakayama). Clinical and functional characteristics of [LeuA3] insulin. J Clin Invest 1986; 77(2):514–519.

176. Nanjo K, Kondo M, Sanke T, Nishi M. Abnormal insulinemia. Diabetes Res Clin Pract 1994; 24(Suppl): S135–S141.

177. Sanke T, Nanjo K. Review for clinical molecular genetics of mutant insulin. Nippon Rinsho 1994; 52(10): 2550–2555.

178. Kishimoto M, Sakura H, Hayashi K, et al. Detection of mutations in the human insulin gene by single strand conformation polymorphisms. J Clin Endocrinol Metab 1992; 74(5):1027–1031.

179. Nakashima N, Sakamoto N, Umeda F, et al. Point mutation in a family with hyperproinsulinemia detected by single stranded conformational polymorphism. J Clin Endocrinol Metab 1993; 76(3):633–636.

180. Shibasaki Y, Kawakami T, Kanazawa Y, Akanuma Y, Takaku F. Posttranslational cleavage of proinsulin is blocked by a point mutation in familial hyperproinsulinemia. J Clin Invest 1985; 76(1):378–380.

181. Kanazawa Y, Kuzuya N, Takeuchi Y, Kubo F, Yamamoto W, Noda M. Hyperproinsulinemia in Japan. Diabetes Res Clin Pract 1994; 24(suppl):S143–S144.

182. Gabbay KH, Bergenstal RM, Wolff J, Mako ME, Rubenstein AH. Familial hyperproinsulinemia: partial characterization of circulating proinsulin-like material. Proc Natl Acad Sci USA 1979; 76(6):2881–2885.

183. Robbins DC, Shoelson SE, Rubenstein AH, Tager HS. Familial hyperproinsulinemia. Two cohorts secreting indistinguishable type II intermediates of proinsulin conversion. J Clin Invest 1984; 73(3):714–719.

184. Gruppuso PA, Gorden P, Kahn CR, Cornblath M, Zeller WP, Schwartz R. Familial hyperproinsulinemia due to a proposed defect in conversion of proinsulin to insulin. N Engl J Med 1984; 311(10):629–634.

185. Elbein SC, Gruppuso P, Schwartz R, Skolnick M, Permutt MA. Hyperproinsulinemia in a family with a proposed defect in conversion is linked to the insulin gene. Diabetes 1985; 34(8):821–824.

186. Chan SJ, Seino S, Gruppuso PA, Schwartz R, Steiner DF. A mutation in the B chain coding region is associated with impaired proinsulin conversion in a family with hyperproinsulinemia. Proc Natl Acad Sci USA 1987; 84:2194–2197.

187. Roder ME, Vissing H, Nauck MA. Hyperproinsulinemia in a three-generation Caucasian family due to mutant proinsulin (Arg65-His) not associated with impaired glucose tolerance: the contribution of mutant proinsulin to insulin bioactivity. J Clin Endocrinol Metab 1996; 81(4):1634–1640.

188. Yano H, Kitano N, Morimoto M, Polonsky KS, Imura H, Seino Y. A novel mutation in the human insulin gene giving rise to hyperproinsulinemia (proinsulin Kyoto). J Clin Invest 1992; 89:1902–1907.

189. Oohashi H, Ohgawara H, Nanjo K, et al. Familial hyperproinsulinemia associated with NIDDM. A case study. Diabetes Care 1993; 16(10):1340–1346.

190. Warren-Perry MG, Manley SE, Ostrega D, et al. A novel point mutation in the insulin gene giving rise to hyperproinsulinemia. J Clin Endocrinol Metab 1997; 82:1629–1631.

191. Musso C, Cochran E, Moran SA, et al. Clinical course of genetic diseases of the insulin receptor (type A and Rabson-Mendenhall syndromes): a 30-year prospective. Medicine (Baltimore) 2004; 83(4):209–222.

192. Krook A, O'Rahilly S. Mutant insulin receptors in syndromes of insulin resistance. Baillieres Clin Endocrinol Metab 1996; 10(1):97–122.

193. Taylor SI, Kadowaki T, Kadowaki H, Accili D, Cama A, McKeon C. Mutations in insulin-receptor gene in insulin-resistant patients. Diabetes Care 1990; 13(3): 257–279.

194. Maassen JA, Tobias ES, Kayserilli H, et al. Identification and functional assessment of novel and known insulin receptor mutations in five patients with syndromes of severe insulin resistance. J Clin Endocrinol Metab 2003; 88(9):4251–4257.

195. Flier JS, Kahn CR, Roth J. Receptors, antireceptor antibodies, and mechanisms of insulin resistance. N Engl J Med 1979; 300:413–419.

196. Taylor SI. Insulin action and inaction. Clin Res 1987; 35(5):459–472.

197. Kumar S, Tullu MS, Muranjan MN, Kamat JR. Rabson-Mendenhall syndrome. Indian J Med Sci 2005; 59(2):70–73.

198. Cochran E, Young JR, Sebring N, DePaoli A, Oral EA, Gorden P. Efficacy of recombinant methionyl human leptin therapy for the extreme insulin resistance of the Rabson-Mendenhall syndrome. J Clin Endocrinol Metab 2004; 89(4):1548–1554.

199. Longo N, Wang Y, Pasquali M. Progressive decline in insulin levels in Rabson-Mendenhall syndrome. J Clin Endocrinol Metab 1999; 84(8):2623–2629.

200. Ioan D, Dumitriu L, Belengeanu V, Bistriceanu M, Maximilian C. Leprechaunism: report of two cases and review. Endocrinologie 1988; 26(3):205–209.

201. Gan KH, Veeze HJ, van den Ouweland AM, et al. A cystic fibrosis mutation associated with mild lung disease. N Engl J Med 1995; 333(2):95–99.

202. Cucinotta D, De Luca F, Scoglio R, et al. Factors affecting diabetes mellitus onset in cystic fibrosis: evidence from a 10-year follow-up study. Acta Paediatr 1999; 88(4):389–393.

203. Kulczycki LL, Kostuch M, Bellanti JA. A clinical perspective of cystic fibrosis and new genetic findings: relationship of CFTR mutations to genotype–phenotype manifestations. Am J Med Genet A 2003; 116(3):262–267.

204. Braun J, Arnemann J, Lohrey M, et al. No association between the deltaF508 cystic fibrosis mutation and type 2 diabetes mellitus. Exp Clin Endocrinol Diabetes 1999; 107(8):568–569.

205. Moran A. Diagnosis, screening, and management of cystic fibrosis-related diabetes. Curr Diab Rep 2002; 2(2):111–115.

206. Peraldo M, Fasulo A, Chiappini E, Milio C, Marianelli L. Evaluation of glucose tolerance and insulin secretion in cystic fibrosis patients. Horm Res 1998; 49(2):65–71.

207. Brennan AL, Geddes DM, Gyi KM, Baker EH. Clinical importance of cystic fibrosis-related diabetes. J Cyst Fibros 2004; 3(4):209–222.

208. Tofe S, Moreno JC, Maiz L, Alonso M, Escobar H, Barrio R. Insulin-secretion abnormalities and clinical deterioration related to impaired glucose tolerance in cystic fibrosis. Eur J Endocrinol 2005; 152(2):241–247.

209. Mackie AD, Thornton SJ, Edenborough FP. Cystic fibrosis-related diabetes. Diabet Med 2003; 20(6):425–436.

210. Costa M, Potvin S, Berthiaume Y, et al. Diabetes: a major co-morbidity of cystic fibrosis. Diabetes Metab 2005; 31(3 Pt 1):221–232.

211. Solomon MP, Wilson DC, Corey M, et al. Glucose intolerance in children with cystic fibrosis. J Pediatr 2003; 142(2):128–132.

212. American Diabetes Association. Standards of medical care in diabetes—2006. Diabetes Care 2006; 29:S4–S42.

213. Kilpatrick ES, Maylor PW, Keevil BG. Biological variation of glycated hemoglobin. Implications for diabetes screening and monitoring. Diabetes Care 1998; 21(2):261–264.

214. Takahashi Y, Noda M, Tsugane S, Kuzuya T, Ito C, Kadowaki T. Prevalence of diabetes estimated by plasma glucose criteria combined with standardized measurement of HbA1c among health checkup participants on Miyako Island, Japan. Diabetes Care 2000; 23(8):1092–1096.

215. Perry RC, Shankar RR, Fineberg N, McGill J, Baron AD. Early Diabetes Intervention Program (EDIP). HbA1c measurement improves the detection of type 2 diabetes in high-risk individuals with nondiagnostic levels of fasting plasma glucose: the Early Diabetes Intervention Program (EDIP). Diabetes Care 2001; 24(3):465–471.

216. Redmond AO, Buchanan KD, Trimble ER. Insulin and glucagon response to arginine infusion in cystic fibrosis. Acta Paediatr Scand 1977; 66(2):199–204.

217. Lippe BM, Sperling MA, Dooley RR. Pancreatic alpha and beta cell functions in cystic fibrosis. J Pediatr 1977; 90(5):751–755.

218. Moran A, Diem P, Klein DJ, Levitt MD, Robertson RP. Pancreatic endocrine function in cystic fibrosis. J Pediatr 1991; 118(5):715–723.

219. Haddy TB, Castro OL, Rana SR. Hereditary hemochromatosis in children, adolescents, and young adults. Am J Pediatr Hematol Oncol 1988; 10(1):23–34.

220. Shield JP. Neonatal diabetes: new insights into aetiology and implications. Horm Res 2000; 53(suppl 1):7–11.

221. Iyer S, Korada M, Rainbow L, et al. Wolcott-Rallison syndrome: a clinical and genetic study of three children, novel mutation in EIF2AK3 and a review of the literature. Acta Paediatr 2004; 93(9):1195–1201.

222. Oral EA. Lipoatrophic diabetes and other related syndromes. Rev Endocr Metab Disord 2003; 4(1):61–77.

223. Garg A. Acquired and inherited lipodystrophies. N Engl J Med 2004; 350(12):1220–1234.

224. Grinspoon S, Carr A. Cardiovascular risk and body-fat abnormalities in HIV-infected adults. N Engl J Med 2005; 352(1):48–62.

225. Schuster DP, Osei K, Zipf WB. Characterization of alterations in glucose and insulin metabolism in Prader-Willi subjects. Metabolism. 1996; 45(12):1514–1520.

226. Zipf WB. Glucose homeostasis in Prader-Willi syndrome and potential implications of growth hormone therapy. Acta Paediatr Suppl 1999; 88(433):115–117.

227. Minton JA, Rainbow LA, Ricketts C, Barrett TG. Wolfram syndrome. Rev Endocr Metab Disord 2003; 4(1):53–59.

228. Khanim F, Kirk J, Latif F, Barrett TG. WFS1/wolframin mutations, Wolfram syndrome, and associated diseases. Hum Mutat 2001; 17(5):357–367.

229. Aguilera E, Casamitjana R, Ercilla G, et al. Clinical characteristics, beta-cell function, HLA class II and mutations in MODY genes in nonpaediatric subjects with Type 1 diabetes without pancreatic autoantibodies. Diabet Med 2005; 22(2):137–143.

230. Sapru A, Gitelman SE, Bhatia S, Dubin RF, Newman TB, Flori H. Prevalence and characteristics of type 2 diabetes mellitus in 9 to 18-year-old children with diabetic ketoacidosis. J Pediatr Endocrinol Metab 2005; 18(9):865–872.

231. Hattersley AT. Diagnosis of maturity-onset diabetes of the young in the pediatric diabetes clinic. J Pediatr Endocrinol Metab 2000; 13(Suppl 6):1411–1417.

232. Barrio R, Bellanne-Chantelot C, Moreno JC, et al. Nine novel mutations in maturity-onset diabetes of the young (MODY) candidate genes in 22 Spanish families. J Clin Endocrinol Metab 2002; 87(6):2532–2539.

233. Bulman MP, Harries LW, Hansen T, et al. Abnormal splicing of hepatocyte nuclear factor 1 alpha in maturity-onset diabetes of the young. Diabetologia 2002; 45(10):1463–1467.

234. Shin DQ, Stoffel M. Molecular etiologies of MODY and other early-onset forms of diabetes. Curr Diab Rep 2002; 2:125–134.

235. Hara K, Noda M, Waki H, et al. Maturity-onset diabetes of the young resulting from a novel mutation in the HNF-4alpha gene. Intern Med 2002; 41(10):848–852.

236. Cao H, Shorey S, Robinson J, et al. GCK and HNF1A mutations in Canadian families with maturity onset diabetes of the young (MODY). Hum Mutat 2002; 20(6):478–479.

237. Ikema T, Shimajiri Y, Komiya I, et al. Identification of three new mutations of the HNF-1 alpha gene in Japanese MODY families. Diabetologia 2002; 45(12):1713–1718.

238. Bjorkhaug L, Sagen JV, Thorsby P, Sovik O, Molven A, Njolstad PR. Hepatocyte nuclear factor-1 alpha gene mutations and diabetes in Norway. J Clin Endocrinol Metab 2003; 88(2):920–931.

239. Pruhova S, Ek J, Lebl J, et al. Genetic epidemiology of MODY in the Czech republic: new mutations in the MODY genes HNF-4alpha, GCK and HNF-1alpha. Diabetologia 2003; 46(2):291–295.

240. Kim KA, Kang K, Chi YI, et al. Identification and functional characterization of a novel mutation of hepatocyte nuclear factor-1alpha gene in a Korean family with MODY3. Diabetologia 2003; 46(5):721–727.

241. Mantovani V, Salardi S, Cerreta V, et al. Identification of eight novel glucokinase mutations in Italian children with maturity-onset diabetes of the young. Hum Mutat 2003; 22(4):338.

242. Thomson KL, Gloyn AL, Colclough K, et al. Identification of 21 novel glucokinase (GCK) mutations in UK and European Caucasians with maturity-onset diabetes of the young (MODY). Hum Mutat 2003; 22(5):417.

243. Frechtel GD, Lopez AP, Rodriguez M, Cerrone GE, Targovnik HM. A novel mutation in exon 5 of the glucokinase gene in an Argentinian family with maturity onset diabetes of the young. Mol Diagn 2003; 7(2):129–131.

244. Fehmann HC, Gross U, Epe M. A new mutation in the hepatocyte nuclear factor-1-alpha gene (P224S) in a newly discovered German family with maturity-onset diabetes of the young 3 (MODY 3). Family members carry additionally the homozygous I27L amino acid polymorphism in the HNF1 alpha gene. Exp Clin Endocrinol Diabetes 2004; 112(2):84–87.

245. McKinney JL, Cao H, Robinson JF, et al. Spectrum of HNF1A and GCK mutations in Canadian families with maturity-onset diabetes of the young (MODY). Clin Invest Med 2004; 27(3):135–141.

246. Toaima D, Nake A, Wendenburg J, et al. Identification of novel GCK and HNF1A/TCF1 mutations and poly-

morphisms in German families with maturity-onset diabetes of the young (MODY). Hum Mutat 2005; 25(5): 503–504.

247. Gloyn AL, Ellard S, Shepherd M, et al. Maturity-onset diabetes of the young caused by a balanced translocation where the 20q12 break point results in disruption upstream of the coding region of hepatocyte nuclear factor-4alpha (HNF4A) gene. Diabetes 2002; 51(7):2329–2333.

248. Bellanne-Chantelot C, Clauin S, Chauveau D, et al. Large genomic rearrangements in the hepatocyte nuclear factor-1(beta) (TCF2) gene are the most frequent cause of maturity-onset diabetes of the young type 5. Diabetes 2005; 54(11):3126–3132.

249. Lindgren CM, Widen E, Tuomi T, et al. Contribution of known and unknown susceptibility genes to early-onset diabetes in Scandinavia: evidence for heterogeneity. Diabetes 2002; 51(5):1609–1617.

250. Glaser N, Jones KL. Non-insulin dependent diabetes mellitus in children and adolescents. Adv Pediatr 1996; 43(1):359–396.

251. (a) Pinhas-Hamiel O, Dolan LM, Daniels SR. Increased incidence of non-insulin dependent diabetes mellitus among adolescents. J Pediatr 1996; 128:608–615; (b) Glaser NS. Non-insulin dependent diabetes mellitus in childhood and adolescence. Pediatr Clin North Am 1997; 44(2):307–337.

252. Jones KL. Non-insulin dependent diabetes in children and adolescents: the therapeutic challenge. Clin Pediatr 1998; 2:103–110.

253. Rosenbloom AL, House DV, Winter WE. Non-insulin dependent diabetes mellitus (NIDDM) in minority youth: research priorities and needs. Clin Pediatr 1998; 37(2):143–152.

254. Weng J, Ekelund M, Lehto M, et al. Screening for MODY mutations, GAD antibodies, and type 1 diabetes-associated HLA genotypes in women with gestational diabetes mellitus. Diabetes Care 2002; 25(1):68–71.

255. Timsit J, Bellanne-Chantelot C, Dubois-Laforgue D, Velho G. Diagnosis and management of maturity-onset diabetes of the young. Treat Endocrinol 2005; 4(1):9–18.

256. Shepherd M, Hattersley AT. 'I don't feel like a diabetic any more': the impact of stopping insulin in patients with maturity onset diabetes of the young following genetic testing. Clin Med 2004; 4(2):144–147.

257. Schnyder S, Mullis PE, Ellard S, Hattersley AT, Fluck CE. Related articles, genetic testing for glucokinase mutations in clinically selected patients with MODY: a worthwhile investment. Swiss Med Wkly 2005; 135(23–24):352–356.

258. The Diabetes Control and Complications Trial Research Group. The effect of intensive treatment of diabetes on the development and progression of long-term complications in insulin-dependent diabetes mellitus. N Engl J Med 1993; 329:977–986.

259. UKPDS Group. Intensive blood-glucose control with sulphonylureas or insulin compared with conventional treatment and risk of complications in patients with type 2 diabetes (UKPDS 33). Lancet 1998; 352:837–853.

260. Sheperd M, Sparkes AC, Hattersley AT. Genetic testing in maturity onset diabetes of the young (MODY): a new challenge for the diabetic clinic. Pract Diab Int 2001; 18:16–21.

261. Sheperd M. Genetic testing in maturity onset diabetes of the young (MODY)—practice guidelines for professionals. Pract Diab Int 2003; 20:108–110.

262. Sheperd M. 'I'm amazed I've been able to come off insulin injections': patients' perceptions of genetic testing in diabetes. Pract Diab Int 2003; 20:338–342.

Insulin Resistance Syndrome in Childhood and Beyond

Berrin Ergun-Longmire
*Division of Pediatric Endocrinology, UMDNJ/Robert Wood Johnson Medical School,
New Brunswick, New Jersey, U.S.A.*

Noel K. Maclaren
*Department of Pediatrics, New York-Presbyterian Hospital, Weill Medical College of Cornell
University, and Bioseek Endocrine Clinics, New York, New York, U.S.A.*

INTRODUCTION

Insulin resistance syndrome (IRS), (metabolic syndrome, syndrome X) was first described by Reaven (1) in 1988, as a result of tissue resistance to insulin and the link between insulin resistance (IR) and obesity, Type 2 diabetes (T2DM), coronary artery disease, hypertension, dyslipidemia, and hyperuricemia. IRS has since been expanded from this core phenotype and become known by a variety of names, including metabolic syndrome, dysmetabolic syndrome, and syndrome X. Today, IRS has become increasingly recognized by physicians as a matter of immense public concern because of its frequency and impact upon the health of those affected by it. IRS may affect more than 50% of adults in the United States with even higher prevalences in the highly prone racial groups such as African-Americans, Mexican-Americans, and Native Americans (2). Studies suggest that IRS may originate in utero (3–5). The association of low birth weight and development of IR and, consequently, T2DM has been confirmed in different populations (6,7). Longitudinal studies have shown that children with components of metabolic syndrome in childhood continue with them into adulthood where they acquire more of them (8). Thus, they increase the medical and economic burdens on society with their increased early morbidity and mortality rates (9). Obesity plays a central role in the development of IRS, which increases the risk for development of T2DM and cardiovascular disease (CVD) including hypertension, hypercoagulation, and atherosclerosis (10,11). Diabetes mellitus is rapidly evolving as an epidemic of the 21st century closely following the dramatic rise in obesity rates. The presently estimated worldwide number of 190 million persons afflicted by T2DM is predicted to grow to over 300 million by the year 2025 (12). In the United States, the estimated lifetime risk of diabetes for children born in the year 2000 is more than one in three (13). The increased incidence of T2DM in children parallels the increase in the prevalence and severity of obesity in children (14). According to the third National Health and Nutrition Examination Survey (NHANES), 4% of all adolescents and nearly 30% of overweight adolescents in the United States have IRS (15). IR was found to predict cardiovascular risk factors in young, healthy adolescents, while body weight during childhood was also observed to play an important role in being predictive of risk factors for CVD (16). Thus, current indications suggest that children born today will live less healthy lives and will die earlier than their parents.

EPIDEMIOLOGY

Obesity, which is the most common cause of IRS in children and adolescents, is one of the most serious and urgent public health problems, not only in the United States but worldwide, and its prevalence is increasing dramatically (17) (Vol. 1; Chap. 1). World Health Organization (WHO) declared obesity as a major public health threat not only for industrialized countries but also for developing countries (18,19). Today, WHO finds itself needing to deal with the obesity pandemic and its accompanying noncommunicable diseases while paradoxically, the challenge of childhood malnutrition has far from disappeared (20). Recent data from the 1999–2000 NHANES show that almost 65% of the adult population in the United States is overweight [body mass index (BMI) ranging from 25 to 29.9 kg/m²], compared to 56% seen in NHANES III conducted between 1988 and 1994 (21). The prevalence of obesity (BMI ≥30 kg/m²) has also increased from 23% to 31% over the same time period. NHANES III conducted between 1988 and 1994 also included a group of adolescents aged 12 to 19 years ($n = 2430$) for the estimated prevalence of IRS. According to NHANES III, the prevalence of IR was 6.8% among overweight adolescents and 28.7% among obese adolescents (15).

The telephone survey of 195,005 of those adults aged 18 years or older in 2001 who were overweight or obese showed significant risks for diabetes, hypertension, and high cholesterol levels (22). Since 1991, the prevalence of diabetes has increased by 61%. In the latter study, those with a BMI of 40 or higher when compared to adults with BMIs less than 24.9 kg/m^2, have been found to be 7.4 times more likely to develop diabetes, 6.4 times more likely to have hypertension, and 1.9 times more likely to have hypercholesterolemia (22). In addition, the death rates from all cancers combined were 52% (for men) and 62% (for women) higher in those who had BMIs of 40 or above over the rates in men and women of normal weights (23,24).

The prevalence of childhood obesity continues to increase at a rapid rate as well. Data from the International Obesity Task Force indicate that 22 million of the world's children under five years of age are overweight (BMIs greater than 85th percentile for age and sex) or obese (BMI greater than 95th percentile for age and sex) (25,26). Comparison of cross-sectional data from school-based surveys conducted in 1997 and 1998 describing body size among a total of 29,242 adolescent boys and girls aged 13 and 15 years in 13 European countries plus Israel and the United States, showed that the United States, Ireland, Greece, and Portugal had the highest prevalence of overweight adolescents (27). In China, the prevalence of obesity is also increasing (28). A recent study from China reported that the prevalence of obesity for children was 27.7% in boys and 14.1% in girls (29). In the United States, comparative data obtained in 1965 and 1980 showed a 67% increase in obesity among male children and a 41% increase among female children aged 6 to 11 years (30). The most recent report from NHANES, between 1960 and 2002, indicates that mean weight and BMI have increased dramatically for both sexes, all race/ethnic groups, and all ages (31). The life expectancy in young obese adults is significantly reduced by 5 to 10 years (32). In one study, the risk of adult obesity was at least twice as high for obese children as for nonobese children (33). Other studies also showed that overweight children are more likely to become obese adults (34,35). Thus, most obese children usually do not grow out of it (Vol. 1; Chap. 1)!

Many of the metabolic and cardiovascular complications associated with obesity, namely, hypertension, T2DM, and dyslipidemia, are already present during childhood and are closely linked to concomitant hyperinsulinemia and IR (15,36). In former years, T2DM was predominantly diagnosed in middle-aged or older people. The first alarming effect of increased pediatric obesity was reported in the late 1990s suggesting the increased incidence and prevalence of T2DM in children (37). Impaired glucose intolerance (IGT) is highly prevalent among children and adolescents with severe obesity, irrespective of their ethnic group, and is associated with IR at this time when β-cell function is still relatively well preserved (38). However, severely obese children and adolescents with IGT are at very high risk for developing T2DM

over a short period of time (39). Data from the United States indicated that 8% to 45% of recently diagnosed cases of diabetes in young children were due to T2DM (40). In Japan, the incidence of T2DM increased fourfold in 6 to 15-year-olds, outnumbering those afflicted by T1DM in the United States (41). In March 2004, the Centers for Disease Control and Prevention (CDC) reported that in 2000, deaths due to poor diet and physical inactivity were 16.6% of all deaths, which nearly equaled deaths from cigarette smoking (18.1% of all deaths) as the two leading causes of death (having modifiable behavioral risk factors).

Treatment of overweight and its complications are costly. The increasing prevalence of obesity translates into increasing medical care and disability costs. IR alone is responsible for 46.8%, 6.2%, and 12.5% of the annual coronary heart disease (CHD) events in T2DM, non-T2DM patients, and in the total U.S. population, respectively. The annual total cost of IR-attributable events in the United States was estimated to be $12.5 billion in 1999, of which $6.6 billion were direct medical costs. The annual cost of diabetes in medical expenditures climbed from $98 billion in 1997 to $132 billion in 2002 with additional costs linked to lost productivity. The direct medical costs of diabetes more than doubled in that time, from $44 billion in 1997 to $91.8 billion in 2002 (42). As mentioned, most diabetics have underlying IR. On the other hand, a modest weight reduction of 5% to 10% can significantly decrease the risk of complications from IR (43). Increases in incidences of T2DM may be preventable with simple measures such as age-appropriate exercise and diet programs. When 522 overweight Finns with IGT were randomized to the intervention group (an intensive exercise and diet program), or the control group, there was a 58% reduction in the progression to diabetes in the intervention group over a mean period of 3.2 years (44). Similarly, the Diabetes Prevention Program trial in the United States, which involved 3234 nondiabetic individuals with IGT, showed that the lifestyle intervention reduced the progression of diabetes by 58% and metformin by 31% as compared to placebo-treated control group (45). Thus, a major effort to control childhood obesity and treatment of IRS must be mounted at all levels of health care delivery.

PATHOPHYSIOLOGY OF IR
IR in Relation to Obesity

There is a strong association between obesity and IRS (Fig. 1). Today's diet consists of large amounts of saturated fats and simple carbohydrates that are consumed from early childhood. This diet contributes to the development of hyperinsulinemia and obesity. The epidemic of obesity and diabetes closely follows U.S. commercially driven drink and food sources,

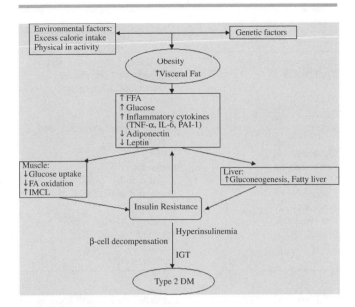

Figure 1 Relationship with obesity and development of IRS and Type 2 DM. *Abbreviations*: FFA, free fatty acids; TNF-α, tumor necrosis factor-α; IL-6, interleukin-6; PAI-1, plasminogen activator inhibitor 1; FA, fatty acid; IMCL, intramyocellular lipids.

leading to the consumption of large amounts of sodas and fruit juices, and foods with a high glycemic index (GI) (Vol. 1; Chap. 2). Dietary carbohydrates (and fats) induce hyperinsulinism, a reduction in fatty acid (FA) oxidation, and hypertryglyceridemia. Diets rich in saturated fats add a strong insulinotropic effect. In many children, obesity and IR can be seen to precede the development of hyperinsulinism; however, others develop IR without first becoming obese. Hyperinsulinemia can thus be seen as a compensatory mechanism for the preexisting, genetically programmed IR, which represents a mechanism for protection against the development of IGT and diabetes.

Increased insulin secretion leads to increased FA synthesis in the liver and adipose tissues. A compensatory increase in glucose oxidation and increased malonyl-coenzyme A (CoA) signaling in the face of abundant FAs direct an FA diversion away from β-oxidation to compensatory increases in long-chain CoA and triglyceride (TG) synthesis in the liver. TG in the blood is a marker of intracellular hepatic long-chain CoA accumulation and increased very-low-density lipoprotein (VLDL) synthesis. Normally, appetite can be suppressed by both leptin and insulin; however, diets high in fat stimulate appetite directly. The liver, in turn, becomes insensitive to compensatory leptin-signaling to increase β-oxidation, which is blocked in IR because of high levels of accumulating malonyl CoA. Elevated levels of malonyl CoA block FA β-oxidation, leading to TG accumulation in muscle and liver, with impaired serine phosphorylation of insulin receptor substrate-1 (IRS-1), decreased glucose transporter (GLUT)-4 translocation to the surface membrane, and thereby decreased glucose entry to

the cell and glucose oxidation. In the islets, these events lead to activation of caspases and increased ceramide levels inducing apoptosis of β-cells. T2DM thus results when there is insufficient insulin secretion to counter preexisting IR. This is consistent with the United Kingdom Prospective Diabetes Study findings of progressive deterioration of β-cell function over time in both obese and nonobese patients with T2DM (46).

In experimental rats and human patients, IR is correlated with total muscle TG, as measured in biopsy samples, especially when intramyocellular fat is the measured variable. Also, tight positive correlations were found between the TG content of skeletal muscle, liver, and whole pancreas, and variables such as the plasma insulin concentration, β-cell function, and IR in a variety of rat models with very different fat contents (47).

Mechanisms Underlying IR

- A central eating disorder versus peripheral metabolic disorder
- Satiety signaling: central vs. peripheral signaling

The regulation of food intake and energy balance is best described as a feedback loop (48). This feedback loop consists of mainly neuroendocrine components.

1. The afferent system, which regulates food intake and satiety via afferent neural (e.g., vagus nerve) and hormonal [leptin, insulin, ghrelin, peptide YY (PYY), etc.] signaling from the gastrointestinal tract to the hindbrain.
2. The central nervous system (CNS) processing unit located in the ventromedial hypothalamus (ventromedial and arcuate nuclei), paraventricular nucleus, and lateral hypothalamus.
3. The efferent system, which coordinates energy expenditure versus energy storage.
4. The nonendocrine component, which is a primary component of energy absorption and metabolism (gut and liver).

The hypothalamus, especially the arcuate nucleus, plays a crucial role in the control of energy balance and the feeding behavior in this loop. The hypothalamus integrates both central and peripheral signals and exerts homeostatic control over food intake and energy expenditure, communicating with the hindbrain structures including the nucleus tractus solitarius for integration of peripheral signals (Fig. 2) (49). The arcuate nucleus of hypothalamus receives signals from anabolic and catabolic pathways. Both anabolic and catabolic pathway neurons in arcuate nucleus of hypothalamus express insulin receptors (IR-1) (50) as well as leptin receptors (51). Insulin and leptin are key factors in circulating signals to the hypothalamus in communicating food intake and energy expenditure to maintain body-fat deposition.

The anabolic pathway neurons coexpress neuropeptide Y/Agouti-related protein (NPY/AgRP) (52).

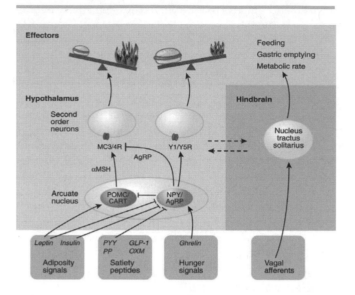

Figure 2 Simplified representation of potential action of gut peptides on the hypothalamus. Access of circulating agents into the arcuate nucleus of the hypothalamus is facilitated by a relaxed blood–brain barrier. Primary neurons in the arcuate nucleus contain multiple peptide neuromodulators. Appetite-inhibiting neurons contain POMC peptides such as α-MSH, which acts on MC3 and MC4 receptors and CART peptide, whose receptor is unknown. Appetite-stimulating neurons in the arcuate nucleus contain NPY, which acts on Y receptors (Y1 and Y5), and AgRP, which is an antagonist of MC3/4 receptor activity. Integration of peripheral signals within the brain involves interplay between the hypothalamus and hindbrain structures including the NTS, which receives vagal afferent inputs. Inputs from the cortex, amygdala, and brainstem nuclei are integrated as well, with resultant effects on meal size and frequency, gut handling of ingested food, and energy expenditure. *Note*: →, direct stimulatory; —|, direct inhibitory; - - ->, indirect pathways. *Abbreviations*: POMC, proopiomelanocortin; α-MSH, α-melanocyte-stimulating hormone; MC, melanocortin; CART, cocaine- and amphetamine-stimulated transcript; NPY, neuropeptide Y; AgRP, agouti-related peptide. *Source*: From Ref. 49.

Table 1 Hypothalamic Orexigenic and Anorexigenic Neuropeptides for the Regulation of Energy Homeostasis

Orexigenic	Anorexigenic
Agouti-related protein	α-Melanocyte-stimulating hormone
Neuropeptide Y	Melanocortin-3 receptor/ melanocortin-4 receptor
GABA	Insulin
Galanin	Amylin
Ghrelin	Cocaine amphetamine-regulated peptide
Glutamate	CRH
Norepinephrine	Bombesin
Melanin concentrating hormone	Angiotensin II
β-endorphin	Glucagon-like peptide-1
Dynorphin	Leptin
Met-enkephalin	Peptide YY
Orexins	Serotonin
	Dopamine
	Neurotensin

Catabolic pathway neurons are called pro-opiomelanocortin (POMC)/cocaine amphetamine-regulated peptide (CART) neurons. Both pathways receive projections from neurons in other brain areas and receive signals from anorexigenic and orexigenic neuropeptides to regulate energy balance (Table 1). Insulin acts as a mediator in the communication between the peripheral endocrine system and the CNS via neuroendocrine axis (53,54). There is growing evidence that there is an intracellular interaction between leptin and insulin signaling, and both insulin and leptin signals circulate in proportion to body adiposity and act in the hypothalamus to stimulate catabolic and inhibit anabolic pathways (55–59). In animal models, injections of insulin into the hypothalamus or ventricles result in inhibition of food intake (anorexigenic effect) with concomitant weight loss (60,61). Like insulin, leptin stimulates POMC/CART receptors and releases α-MSH. The increased α-MSH stimulates melanocortin-3 receptor (MC3R)/melanocortin-4 receptor (MC4R) to reduce food intake and increase energy expenditure by activating the sympathetic nervous

system (62). The central melanocortin system is a key mediator of the catabolic effects of insulin in the brain. Insulin, along with leptin and glucocorticoids, regulates the synthesis and release of NPY in the hypothalamus (63). Insulin and leptin both directly inhibit NPY/AgRP, further limiting feeding and providing for unantagonized MC4R occupancy. Reduced numbers of insulin receptors in experimental animal models result in increased food intake and, consequently, weight gain consistent with elevated NPY levels (60,64). Insulin has both short-term (inhibitory effect on food intake) and long-term (defense energy store) effects, given its responsivity to minimize glucose levels after food intake (65–67).

In addition to this long-term regulation of energy balance with insulin and leptin, short-term regulation on a meal-to-meal basis is secured by several gut hormones such as peptides secreted from the stomach and gut: cholecystokinin, ghrelin, glucagon such as peptide-1 [glucagon-like peptide-1 (GLP-I)], orexins, oxyntomodulin, PYY3–36, pancreatic polypeptide (PP), and gastric inhibitory polypeptide (also known as glucose-dependent insulinotropic polypeptide) (68–71). The gastrointestinal tract uses these peptides and neural pathways (primarily vagus nerve) to communicate with the hypothalamus and the hindbrain to maintain energy balance. For example, PYY3–36 produced by the L-cells of the small intestine reduces food intake by 30% when injected into lean or obese subjects (70). Cholecysokinin is a classical satiety hormone and secreted by duodenum and jejunum in response to the presence of food in the gut lumen (49). In humans, intravenous (IV) infusion of cholecystokinin suppresses food intake and causes earlier meal termination. Ghrelin is produced by the stomach and proximal small intestine during fasting and stimulates NPY/AgRP to antagonize α-MSH. Therefore, lack of anorexigenic pressure on MC4Rs results in increased food intake (69). Several studies demonstrate that glucose and insulin may play a role in the regulation of ghrelin levels (72,73). An inverse relationship between fasting ghrelin and insulin levels, and IR has been reported (74,75). Ghrelin levels are, however, markedly elevated in Prader-Willi syndrome (76) and are dramatically reduced after gastric bypass surgery (77). PP is released from the pancreas in response to ingestion of food. Plasma PP levels have been shown to be reduced in conditions associated with increased food intake and elevated in patients with anorexia nervosa. Peripheral administration of PP has been shown to decrease food intake in rodents (70). The pharmaceutical industry is working to develop analogs at several key points of satiety regulation.

Muscle, Liver, Adipose Tissue, and Adipocytokines and Their Roles in IR

Glucose homeostasis is maintained by three tightly related processes: (i) insulin secretion by pancreatic β-cells, (ii) insulin action on stimulated glucose uptake by liver, gut, and peripheral (primarily muscle) tissues, and (iii) suppression of hepatic glucose output (78). Insulin receptors in the liver, muscle, and adipose tissue are normally exquisitely sensitive to insulin.

The primary site of glucose disposal (approximately 80–85%) after a glucose-containing meal is skeletal muscle, and the primary mechanism of glucose storage is through its conversion to glycogen. Studies using the hyperinsulinemic–euglycemic clamp technique have demonstrated that decreased insulin-stimulated glucose disposal and reduced glycogen synthase activation in subjects with IR could be secondary to a defect in glycogen synthesis (79). The peripheral glucose disposal measured by a hyperinsulinemic–euglycemic clamp technique is lower for the level of hyperinsulinemia in IR subjects with obesity or T2DM (80).

Although skeletal muscle is the principal site of insulin-stimulated glucose uptake in peripheral tissues, adipose tissue, liver, and endothelial cells also develop IR (81). Multiple studies demonstrated that increased fat accumulations in the muscle, liver, and visceral depots are highly correlated with the development and severity of IR (82–84).

Among nondiabetic subjects in the postabsorptive condition, total body endogenous glucose output variability is wide and is largely dependent upon the amount of lean body mass. This in turn explains differences in total endogenous glucose output due to sex, obesity, and age (85). Hyperinsulinemia inhibits hepatic glucose output (86) by acting either directly through the insulin receptor or indirectly as a consequence of a reduced release of gluconeogenic substrates [e.g., lactate, alanine, glycerol, and free FAs (FFAs)], both in the muscle and in the liver (78).

In addition to the muscle and the liver, adipose tissue is the third site of insulin action. Although insulin-stimulated glucose disposal in fat tissue is negligible compared with that in the muscle, the release of glycerol and FFAs following lipolysis has

major implications for glucose homeostasis. Recent studies suggest that an increase in intracellular FFAs alter insulin signaling, resulting in decreased insulin-stimulated IRS-1-associated phosphatidylinositol 3-kinase (PI-3K) activity and decreased glucose transport (87). As visceral fat tissue increases, the rate of lipolysis rises, leading to increased FFAs and glycerol mobilization through its portal drainage, with consequent increase in FFA oxidation in the muscle and the liver. In turn, glucose use by muscle decreases as FFAs are used as an alternate source of energy, hepatic lipogenesis increases, and glucose oxidation decreases (88). Finally, the glycerol released during TG hydrolysis serves as a gluconeogenic substrate (89). Consequently, resistance to the antilipolytic action of insulin in adipose tissue resulting in excessive release of FFAs and glycerol results in hyperglycemia and impaired glucose tolerance.

Adipose tissue is a highly active metabolic and endocrine organ and is critically involved in energy homeostasis by the production of a number of peptide hormones and cytokines (90,91): leptin, adiponectin, resistin, tumor necrosis factor-α (TNF-α), plasminogen activator inhibitor-one (PAI-1), interleukin-6 (IL-6), angiotensinogen, and the peroxisome proliferator-activated receptor-γ (PPAR-γ) (92–97). Of the above, leptin and adiponectin are two of the most important.

Leptin levels are higher in subcutaneous fat and show greater correlations with subcutaneous than with visceral adiposity (98). Animal models clearly demonstrated the relationship between leptin and IR. Leptin-deficient rodents are markedly (five- to sixfold) obese, hyperinsulinemic, and hyperglycemic (99), while administration of leptin reverses hyperglycemia and hyperinsulinemia (100). Recently, it was proposed that leptin might also play a role in the prevention of FFA entry and fat accumulation in peripheral tissues such as skeletal muscle and liver (101). Low leptin levels are found in the absence of adipose tissue in generalized lipodystrophy. As it is well known, low leptin levels correlate with IR, and patients with IR are also leptin-resistant because leptin levels are high in obesity. Studies in animal models of lipodystrophy have shown that exogenous leptin administration (102), or surgical implantation of normal adipose tissue (103), reversed IR and diabetes, and that was independent of caloric restriction. Similar findings were observed in patients with severe lipodystrophy. Chronic leptin treatment in patients with severe IR and lipodystrophy improved insulin-stimulated hepatic and peripheral glucose metabolism, and reduced hepatic and muscle TG content (104).

Adiponectin is highly and specifically expressed in differentiated adipocytes and has insulin sensitizing, anti-inflammatory and antiatherogenic properties (105). There is a strong inverse association between adiponectin and obesity (106,107), and inflammatory states (108). In the liver, adiponectin increases the sensitivity of insulin to inhibit gluconeogenesis (109) and regulates hepatic FFA metabolism in vivo by suppression of lipogenesis and activation of FFA oxidation (110). Circulating adiponectin levels seem to correlate more with hyperinsulinemia and IR than degree of obesity or body fat (107). In case-control studies, low plasma adiponectin was an independent risk factor for future development of T2DM (111) but not for obesity (112). Animal studies have shown decreased adiponectin levels before the onset of obesity and IR (113) and administration of adiponectin ameliorated metabolic parameters in these conditions (114). The mechanisms by which adiponectin may ameliorate IR have not been fully elucidated.

Resistin (a hormone inducing resistance to insulin) is another adipose tissue-derived polypeptide that has effects on insulin action, potentially linked to obesity and IR (115). It is also an effective proinflammatory agent. Resistin levels were found to be elevated in obese mice (93). Administration of resistin in normal mice induces IR in the liver but not in the muscle (110). However, immunoneutralization of resistin reverses IR (110). Some studies showed that exposure to thiazolidinediones (TZDs), PPAR-γ agonists, reduced resistin gene expression (90), but not other studies (116). Similarly, reduced resistin levels were found in obese and IR rodents (116). The role of resistin in obesity-associated IR remains controversial.

TNF-α is an adipocyte-derived proinflammatory cytokine that has a central role in IR. Increased TNF-α production has been observed in adipose tissue derived from animal models of obesity and IR as well as human subjects (117,118) even in the presence of weak correlations between IR and plasma TNF-α. Weight loss decreases TNF-α levels (119). TNF-impairs insulin signaling by inhibiting the function of IRS-1 through serine phosphorylation (120). In vitro and in vivo studies have shown that the inhibitory effects of TNF-α on insulin action are, at least in part, antagonized by TZDs, further supporting the important role of TNF-α in IR (121,122).

IL-6 is one of several proinflammatory cytokines that have been associated with IR. It is secreted by many cell types, including immune cells, fibroblasts, endothelial cells, skeletal muscle, and adipose tissue. The association of IL-6 and IR is supported by epidemiological and genetic studies. Plasma IL-6 levels in humans positively correlate with obesity and IR (112), and the severity of glucose intolerance and inflammation (123,124). Furthermore, plasma IL-6 levels predict future myocardial infarction and T2DM (123–125). IL-6 impairs insulin signaling in hepatocytes (96) and it also decreases adiponectin secretion (126). In addition, IL-6 increases circulating FFAs (from adipose tissue) with their well-described adverse effects on insulin sensitivity (Si) (84).

PPAR-γ is mainly expressed in adipocytes, intestinal endothelium, macrophages, Type II pneumocytes, bladder, breast, and prostate (127–129). PPAR-γ is a potent regulator of adipogenesis (129). The insulin-sensitizing TZDs have been shown to improve insulin action with increased peripheral (primarily muscle) glucose uptake, indicating the presence of skeletal muscle PPAR-γ receptors (130,131). Treatment with TZDs promotes weight gain in humans and, although some have suggested this to be a consequence of improved Si, it is possible that lowering circulating insulin levels per se actually diminishes its anabolic activity. An alternative and more plausible hypothesis is that PPAR-γ agonists improve Si by promoting adipogenesis and postprandial FA/TG storage within adipocytes, both of which are likely to increase adipose tissue mass (132). Several studies have shown that the increase in body weight associated with TZD treatment is mediated principally by accumulation of subcutaneous fat, whereas visceral adipose tissue volume is reduced or unchanged (133).

Pancreatic β-Cell Response to IR

IR and obesity are characterized by increased insulin levels to maintain normal glucose tolerance. Several potential mediators have been suggested to be signals for the β-cells to respond to IR such as glucose, FFAs, autonomic nerves, adipose tissue-derived hormones and the gut hormone GLP-1, and islet cell amylin. Failure of these signals or the pancreatic β-cells to adequately adapt insulin secretion in relation to Si results in inappropriate insulin levels, IGT, and T2DM (134). The response of the β-cells to glucose in the setting of IR is increased insulin levels and insulin secretion rates (135). Further studies have showed that this hyperinsulinemia results from both increased secretion and reduced clearance of insulin. Kahn et al.(136) detected an inverse relationship between Si and insulin secretion, demonstrating β-cell compensation for IR. Furthermore, the relationship between insulin secretion and Si is best described as a hyperbolic function; insulin secretion is increased in reduced Si and decreased in increased Si (136–138) (Fig. 3). The product of Si and insulin secretion is a constant referred to as the glucose disposition index (DI) (136). When IR increases, first-phase insulin release increases proportionately to maintain normal glucose tolerance. This compensatory hypersecretion of insulin reflects expansion of β-cell mass and also expression of key enzymes for glucose metabolism. These mechanisms have been demonstrated in animal models—the Zucker fatty rat is obese and insulin resistant, but has sufficient β-cell compensation to prevent the onset of diabetes. In contrast, the Zucker diabetic fatty rat is obese and insulin resistant and develops overt hyperglycemia associated with a failure of adequate β-cell mass expansion in the face of IR (139).

Similar findings have been observed in humans, that β-cell function initially compensates for IR, but as glucose tolerance deteriorates, early defects in β-cell function appear. By the time diabetes becomes evident, β-cell function is already markedly impaired

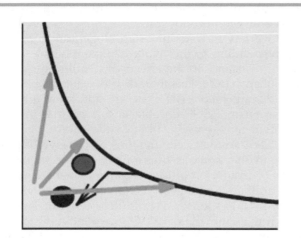

Figure 3 The hyperbolic relation between insulin sensitivity and insulin secretion. Glucose tolerance is impaired if an individual is located below the hyperbolic line and good if an individual is located above the line. This is illustrated as the move from the normal hyperbolic line along the black arrow to the dot (representing impaired glucose tolerance, IGT) or the black dot (representing Type 2 diabetes). Therapeutic approaches should aim at restoring the normal relation between insulin sensitivity and insulin secretion, i.e., to return the subject to the hyperbolic curve, as illustrated by the gray arrows. *Source*: From Ref. 138.

(Vol. 1; Chap. 5). Very early changes in β-cell function can often be demonstrated in subjects with normal glucose tolerance at high risk of diabetes. Normoglycemic women with a history of gestational diabetes are often at high risk of developing T2DM. Studies in those subjects demonstrated reduced first-phase insulin response to normal insulin secretory response to IV glucose infusion, indicating early β-cell dysfunction (140). When IGT develops, first-phase insulin response continues to decrease in relation to degree of insulin resistance, and the coordination of insulin secretory response is lost during oscillatory glucose infusion (141). Although in subjects with IGT, there is a normal ability of a low-dose glucose infusion to prime the insulin secretory response to a subsequent glucose stimulus, in diabetic subjects it is reduced or absent (142).

Evaluation of β-cell dysfunction in individuals at the risk of developing diabetes but with normal glucose levels is difficult. One approach to this problem is administration of glucocorticoids, FFAs, or TZDs, which aggravate or improve IR (143). As described previously, FFAs have an effect on the induction of IR in muscle and liver (84).

Recently, Ahren et al. described a linear relation between fasting PP levels and the Si in Caucasian females with normal glucose tolerance by the hyperinsulinemic, euglycemic clamp technique (134). The gut hormone GLP-1 in humans has been shown to be potent at augmenting glucose-stimulated insulin secretion. In animal models, IV infusions of GLP-1 significantly reduce short-term food intake (144). Similar findings observed in humans suggest an

important role for GLP-1 in the regulation of the early satiety response (145). GLP-1 stimulates differentiation and proliferation of β-cells while inhibiting apoptosis. These actions will increase the β-cell mass and function over a long-term period, which may, in turn, prevent progression to T2DM (146). The neuroendocrine hormone amylin, cosecreted with insulin from pancreatic β-cells in response to nutrient ingestion, is a short-term satiating peptide. However, there is some evidence that basal amylin levels might play a role in the long-term control of food intake and/or body weight. Animal models have shown that amylin decreases food intake, suppresses postprandial glucagon concentrations, and delays gastric emptying (147–149). Amylin seems to be a necessary and complementary factor to insulin, which regulates the rate of glucose disappearance. In this sense, amylin and insulin are adjunctive players in the control of nutrient fluxes, and the control of feeding behavior (150).

Adrenal Glucocorticoids and IRS

Metabolism of the adrenal steroids in adipose tissue may provide an important mechanism for the increase in visceral fat in IR. Excessive glucorticoid exposure as a result of either endogenous overproduction (i.e., Cushing's syndrome) or exogenous administration results in central adiposity, IR, dyslipidemia, hypertension, and glucose intolerance (151). Several steroidogenic enzymes are expressed in adipose tissue including the cytochrome P450-dependent aromatase, 3β-hydroxysteroid dehydrogenase (HSD), 3α-HSD, 11β-HSD1, 17β-HSD, 7α-hydroxylase, 17α-hydroxylase, and 5α-reductase,(152). Importantly, 11β-HSD1 is highly expressed in adipose tissue, particularly in visceral adipose tissue (153). 11β-HSD1 converts inactive 11β-ketoglucocorticoid metabolites (cortisone) to active 11β-hydroxylated metabolites (cortisol) in humans (154). Growth harmone (GH)[and/or insulin-like growth factor (IGF) -1] was suggested recently to inhibit 11β-HSD1, whereas in obesity, GH levels are decreased, leading to higher 11β-HSD1 activity (155). 11β-HSD1 knockout mice have been shown to resist diet-induced IR and hyperglycemia (156). Overexpression of 11β-HSD1 was shown associated with visceral obesity and IR (157). Therefore, dysregulation of glucocorticoid metabolism by 11β-HSD1 has been implicated in obesity, diabetes, hypertension, dyslipidemia, hypertension, polycystic ovarian syndrome (PCOS), etc. (Vol. 2; Chap. 13) (154,158). Clinically, we have repeatedly observed increased abdominal striae and biochemically increased urinary free cortisol levels in obese patients at the time of adrenarche associated with rapid weight gain, suggesting increased cortisol secretion and turnover in obese children approaching their adolescence.

Patients with Cushing's syndrome have high levels of serum cortisol, and the patient with IRS has low-to-normal levels of cortisol, albeit both having increased levels of urinary free cortisol. The explanation lies in the decreased levels of corticosteroid-binding globulin (CBG) found in IRS, where circulating cortisol is disproportionately free and bioactive, with increased conversion of cortisone to the metabolically active cortisol. The clinical distinction between patients with Cushing's syndrome and IRS is that the former patient is invariably growth retarded (Vol. 2; Chap. 8), in contrast to the child with IRS in whom linear growth is excessive as explained below.

The impact of increased adipose 11β-HSD1 in humans remains unclear although we believe that it is of great importance. Pharmacological inhibition of 11β-HSD1 by carbenexolone enhances hepatic Si and it may play a role in the future for the treatment of central obesity/IRS (151).

Puberty and IRS

Puberty is a state of increasing IR. While IR is usually well compensated by hyperinsulinemia in children, we find progressive failure of such compensation through puberty with rising glucose and TG levels, and increasing frequencies of glucose intolerance and T2DM. Weyer et al.(159) followed 48 Pima Indians with normal glucose tolerance for five years, and 17 progressed from normal glucose tolerance through IGT to diabetes. In these progressors, insulin secretion declined by 78%, whereas Si declined by 14%. In the 31 individuals who did not develop diabetes, a similar 11% decrease in Si was associated with a 30% increase in insulin secretion rather than a decrease. The latter 31 individuals had compensated IR. Compensated hyperinsulinism, however, can lead to numerous complications from fatty liver and atherosclerosis to increased cancer risk. It is thus increasingly obvious that this sequence of events will be most easily interrupted at the earliest phases of life, during pre-adolescent childhood.

Ovarian Hormonal Responses to IR

IR can present with premature adrenarche in childhood and later in life as a component of PCOS with signs and symptoms of hyperandrogenism (hirsutism, acne, and/or male pattern balding), menstrual irregularity, and infertility. Both insulin and IGF-1 potentiates ovarian hyperandrogenism by increasing the luteinizing hormone (LH) responsiveness to gonadotropin-releasing hormone (GnRH) to stimulate the production of androgens from ovarian theca cells (160). These effects are mediated through induction of ovarian 17-hydroxylase and 17, 20-lyase activities, suppressing plasma sex hormone–binding globulin (SHBG) and CBG levels, and inhibiting both estradiol- and T4-stimulated SHBG production (161). SHBG levels in the circulation are characteristically low, resulting in increased bioavailability of circulating androgens. Free androgens increase the frequency of GnRH pulses and the ratio of LH to follicle-stimulating hormone, thereby exacerbating thecal androgen production.

Ovarian and adrenal steroidogenesis functions as if responding to the hyperinsulinemic state in IR, despite resistance to the effects of insulin on glucose metabolism (162). This paradox of selective IR has been documented. There is an abnormal glucose disposition in PCOS fibroblasts but normal insulin-mediated mitogenesis (163), while steroidogenesis by PCOS granulosa cells remains responsive to insulin. IR in the ovary is thus related to the metabolic effects of insulin on glucose uptake and metabolism, whereas the steroidogenic action of insulin remains intact (164). Responses of granulosa-lutein cells from women with anovulatory PCOS are relatively resistant to the effects of insulin-stimulated glucose uptake and utilization compared with those from normal and ovulatory PCOS, while maintaining normal steroidogenic output in response to physiological doses of insulin. These studies support the probability of a post-receptor, signalling pathway-specific impairment of insulin action in PCOS (164). Particularly, the P13 kinase, but not mitogen-activated protein (MAP) kinase, pathways have been suggested as a potential mechanism. It is proposed that defective insulin-receptor tyrosine phosphorylation secondary to an increase in competitive serine phosphorylation acts as a mechanism to promote IR while stimulating androgen secretion by the ovaries. All treatments that lower insulin levels reduce levels of androgens. Reducing IR by the administration of metformin, PPAR-γ agonists, D-chiro-inositol, or leptin lowers serum-free testosterone concentrations, reduces cytochrome P450c17 (17-hydroxylase) activity, and improves SHBG levels, resulting in slowed bone maturation and adrenarche (161).

Small for Gestational Age, Prematurity, and IR

The development of adipose tissue in the fetus begins in the mid- to late third trimester. Infants born small for gestational age (SGA) appear to be at an increased risk of metabolic disorders such as T2DM, IRS, visceral obesity, dyslipidemia, and CVD (165,166) (Vol. 1; Chap. 12). In this phenomenon, later amplified as "thrifty-phenotype hypothesis," survival of the undernourished fetus requires endocrinologic and metabolic adaptations that may include shunting of important fuels to the developing brain at the expense of tissues such as muscle and pancreas, resulting in IR and blunting the growth effects of insulin. In our African-American and Hispanic IR patients in particular, moderate SGA has been startlingly common (167). In rat models, intrauterine growth retardation (IUGR) induced an impaired oxidative phosphorylation in skeletal muscle with a diminished uptake of glucose, which contributes to IR and hyperglycemia of T2DM postnatally, particularly if they are fed high calorie diets postnatally (168). Similarly, in humans, the risk of IR is particularly apparent when an SGA newborn undergoes rapid postnatal weight gain to obesity.

The Early Bird Study suggested that IR at five years was related to weight catch-up growth rather than low birth weight, especially in girls (169). Such growth patterns following fetal growth restraints are associated with maternal uterine factors such as primaparity, smoking, calorific restrictions in the maternal diet, maternal IRS, and gestational diabetes. Alternatively, if an inherited IR state was manifested in utero, then diminished fetal growth with SGA might be anticipated because insulin is a powerful prenatal GH. In many of the families we have studied in whom we have documented members with IRS, some 50% of the siblings also develop IRS, and these subjects tend to have been SGA-compared with those siblings with normal birth weights. A recent study indicates that regardless of the birth-weight, prematurity itself may play a role for developing IR (170). However, epidemiologic studies have not yet indicated that there is an increased incidence of T2DM, IR, or other metabolic disorders among long-term survivors of prematurity.

In some populations, the relationships between the prevalence of IR to birth weight appear to be U-shaped (171). A U-shaped relation between birth weight and fasting insulin was also shown in Pima Indian children with both low and high birth weights (172). The same U-shaped relation between birth weight, BMI, and fat mass was demonstrated recently in adolescents (173). In our own experience, large for age (LGA) infants become obese at earlier ages than those who are SGA and have a voracious appetite from early life that suggests an underlying eating disorder.

Gestational diabetes per se significantly increases the subsequent risk of obesity and T2DM (174), with the children of mothers with T1DM being more predisposed to T2DM as adults compared with children born to fathers with T1DM (175).

Serine Protease Inhibitors and IR

It has been shown that high insulin levels suppress hepatic synthesis of multiple-binding proteins including CBG, SHBG, IGF-binding protein-1 (IGFBP-1), thyroid-binding globulin, and vitamin D-binding protein (VitD-BP), which in turn increase biologically active forms of circulating hormones. Several of these hormonal binding proteins belong to the family of serine protease inhibitors or SERPINS. Subsequently, increased active hormone levels become responsible for clinical characteristics: hirsutism and PCOS, Cushing-like features, pseudoacromegaly, thrombosis, inflammation, and even increased cancer risk in cases of IRS.

IGFBP-1 is often strikingly depressed in IRS, producing an excess of free IGF-1, albeit the total level of IGF-1 being usually normal (176,177). IGFBP-1 levels are regulated principally by insulin and, to a lesser extent, by glucose levels. Decreased IGFBP-1 in the face of IR leads to the increased tissue bioavailability of IGF-1 such that it can enhance the glucose-lowering effect of insulin. This can lead to the development of microvascular complications, tall stature, and pseudoacromegaly. We found that low levels of IGFBP-1 are strongly associated with the degree of IR, whereas IGFBP-3 correlates directly with the degree of hyperinsulinism. Furthermore, defective IGFBP-1 expression in childhood is retrospectively associated with SGA births, and an increased subsequent risk for obesity and IR at a later age (178).

SHBG has been found to be negatively correlated with BMI and fasting insulin levels (179). Decreased SHBG increases testosterone bioavailability, leading to the development of hyperandrogenism, even when serum levels of testosterone are normal.

The low levels of CBG found in IRS leads to disproportionately free and active circulating cortisol that can lead to clinical and metabolic overlaps between Cushing's syndrome and IR. Increased conversion of inactive cortisone to active cortisol by 11β-HSD1 in visceral fat compounds the effect. CBG secretion has been shown to be negatively regulated by both insulin and IL-6 (180).

Thyroid-binding globulin levels in IRS are often depressed, leading to diagnostic confusion as to the presence of hypothyroidism. Obese patients are thus often unnecessarily treated for hypothyroidism they do not have. They may, however, develop true hypothyroidism on the basis of associated Hashimoto's disease, which does appear more common in IRS.

The low level of 25-hydroxyvitamin D_3 is associated with IR and obesity (181), and 1,25-dihydroxyvitamin D_3 is essential for normal insulin secretion. VitD-BP is known as a macrophage-activating factor, and polymorphisms of VitD-BP have been linked to diabetes risk in Pima Indians (182). Low levels of IGFBP-1 and 1,25-dihydroxyvitamin D were found in maternal and umbilical cord blood in preeclampsia (183).

CBG, thyroid-binding globulin, and PAI-1 are members of the SERPINS family, and insulin and cytokines levels in IR can regulate their activity. These binding proteins are substrates for elastase that is expressed at the surface of neutrophils. Therefore, the variability in circulating binding protein levels might be linked to their cleavage by activated neutrophils. Increased peripheral white blood cell counts with neutrophilia are often found in both obesity and IR, which might facilitate serine protease availability and binding protein cleavage. This mechanism is likely to contribute to decreased serum-binding globulin levels in obesity and IR. For example, increased PAI-1 has been linked not only to thrombosis and fibrosis, but also to IR itself. Circulating PAI-1 levels correlate strongly with the degree of insulinemia (184). Furthermore, downregulation of PAI-1 in mice ameliorates their diet-induced obesity, hyperglycemia, and hyperinsulinemia. PAI-1 deficiency also enhances basal and insulin-stimulated glucose uptake in adipose cells in vitro. These findings suggest PAI-1 may not merely increase in response to obesity and IR, but may have a direct causal role in inducing them (185).

Fibrinolysis Defect, Thromboses, and Atherosclerosis Acceleration with IR

Maintenance of hemostasis is mediated through such factors as fibrinogen, tissue plasminogen activator (tPA), and PAI-1. Insulin has been shown to increase PAI-1 and tPA levels, diminishing fibrinolytic potential and increasing thrombotic risk secondary to impaired fibrinolysis (186,187). Framingham Offspring Study indicates that elevated fasting insulin levels are associated with increases in serum tPA and PAI-1 levels, thus increasing the risk of thrombosis in both glucose-tolerant and glucose-intolerant patients (186). In the Insulin Resistance Atherosclerosis Study, baseline fibrinogen and PAI-1 levels were significantly associated with risk of diabetes among 1047 nondiabetic individuals (188). Insulin sensitizers such as rosiglitazone and troglitazone have been shown to reduce plasma PAI-1 levels (189). Thus, improving Si with TZDs, as a result improving PAI-1 and fibrinogen levels, may decrease the risk of cardiovascular complications in patients with T2DM.

In recent years, markers of systemic inflammation and certain components of the hemostatic system have been found to predict atherosclerotic risk. The majority of these factors are associated with IR. Endothelial inflammation in obese prepubertal children is mainly associated with IR, lipid levels, and BMI (190). C-reactive protein (CRP) is elevated in IR and was found to be a better predictor of atherosclerosis compared to the total/high-density lipoprotein (HDL) cholesterol ratio (191). In the multiethnic Insulin Resistance Atherosclerosis Study, CRP was found to be independently associated with BMI, IR, and systolic blood pressure (BP) (188). There is growing evidence that adiponectin, the most abundant adipocyte-derived cytokine, also plays a crucial role in atherosclerosis. A study of 145 obese children showed that serum levels of adiponectin were significantly decreased in early stage of atherosclerosis (192).

Endothelial cell dysfunction is among the earliest changes on the arterial wall leading to atherosclerosis that begins in childhood and is associated with IR and hyperinsulinemia (193,194). Under normal conditions, insulin stimulates vasodilatation through induction of nitric oxide synthase and generation of nitric oxide (NO) in vascular endothelial cells. However, in obesity and IR, the production of NO production is disrupted, leading to vasoconstriction and tissue ischemia. The presence of hyperglycemia further contributes to endothelial dysfunction and vascular insufficiency through production of superoxide radicals, which cause direct endothelial damage (195). Together with decrease in NO availability, overexpression of adiposity-related cytokines (IL-1, IL-6, TNF-α), PAI-1, and reduction of adiponectin, stimulate leukocyte adhesion to endothelial surface, promoting platelet aggregation and fibrin deposition on blood vessel walls. Decreased tissue perfusion may limit insulin-mediated glucose disposal and thereby increase circulating glucose levels, creating a vicious cycle (196).

Dyslipidemia and IR

Several population-based studies have demonstrated the evidence of strong association between IR and the development of CVD in individuals without diabetes (197,198) (Vol. 1; Chap. 14). The following factors: Increased thickness of the arterial carotid wall and an atherogenic dyslipidemic profile that includes hypertriglyceridemia, low serum HDL cholesterol concentrations, and atherogenic low-density lipoprotein (LDL) cholesterol particles, compounded by low SHBG levels have been shown to increase the risk of atherosclerosis in adults. In addition, the thickness of the carotid wall, atherosclerosis in teenagers and young adults, is related to their intake of cholesterol, serum levels of cholesterol and TG, BMI, smoking, hypertension, and fasting glucose levels (199).

Moreover, fasting insulin level is an independent cardiovascular risk factor (198,200). The Muscatine Study linked childhood LDL cholesterol and BMI to atherosclerosis in asymptomatic adults. The most predictive childhood risk factor was increased BMI. Coronary artery calcifications were also associated with increased BP and decreased HDL cholesterol levels measured during childhood (201). The Cardiovascular Risk in Young Finns Study also showed that childhood LDL cholesterol and BMI correlated with adult CVD (202). Postmortem studies demonstrated presence of fatty streaks in 50% of children aged 2 to 15 years in their coronary arteries, and 8% of these children had raised fibrous plaques in their coronary arteries (203). The Bogalusa Heart Study confirmed that the same risk factors that are important for adults such as elevated BMI, systolic BP, serum TGs, and LDL, convey greater atherosclerosis risk in the aorta and coronary arteries in children (204). The Pathobiological Determinants of Atherosclerosis in Youth study confirmed the origin of atherosclerosis in childhood, showed that progression toward clinically significant lesions may occur in young adulthood, and demonstrated that the progression of atherosclerosis is strongly influenced by CHD risk factors (205).

A simplified model relating IR to dyslipidemia and CVD was proposed by Ginsberg (187). In physiologic conditions, adipocytes release FFAs to the circulation, which delivers them to the liver and the muscle. In the liver, the majority of FFAs are reesterified to form TGs and only a small amount is oxidized. Thus, FAs and TGs are constantly being transported between the liver and adipose tissue. However, if the transport to adipose tissue is insufficient, then the liver and also muscle may accumulate TG. In the presence of IR, lipolysis in adipocytes is enhanced, which results in increased release of FFAs into the circulation. Increased FFA flux to the liver stimulates TG synthesis and secretion of

VLDL, resulting in hypertriglyceridemia. In addition, VLDL is exchanged for cholesteryl esters in both HDL and LDL for VLDL-TG. TG-enriched LDL and HDL can undergo lipolysis and become smaller. Once HDL is lipolysed, HDL is cleared rapidly from the circulation. The result of these processes is an atherogenic lipid profile with high TGs, low HDL, and high LDL cholesterol.

Fatty Liver, Nonalcoholic Steatohepatitis, and Gallbladder Disease

Recent studies documented a strong relationship between hepatic steatosis and IR (206–208). For a long time, hepatic steatosis was considered to be a benign manifestation. However, recent data indicate that it may progress over years from inflammation and fibrosis [nonalcoholic fatty liver disease, (NAFLD)], to steatohepatitis, fibrosis to cirrhosis, and more rarely to hepatocellular carcinoma (209,210). Tominaga et al. found fatty liver in approximately 22% of obese children aged 4 to 12 years (211). In another study, fatty changes were observed in 10% to 25% of adolescents (212). In adult patients with diabetes and obesity, 100% have some steatosis, 50% have steatohepatitis, and 19% have cirrhosis (213). The disease is usually clinically silent for many years. The underlying mechanism for the association of IR and obesity to hepatic steatosis is the excess of portal or visceral fat, which increases flux of FFAs via portal vein directly to the liver, thereby inducing hepatic steatosis (214). Elevated liver enzymes are observed in overweight and obese individuals with fatty liver (215,216). Kinugasa et al. showed 16% of Japanese obese children with elevated alanine aminotransferase (ALT) had fatty livers with associated fibrosis or cirrhosis on liver biopsy (217). NHANES III study showed elevated levels of ALT in 6% of American overweight and 10% of American obese adolescents (218). Strauss et al. suggested that abnormal liver enzymes in overweight and obese adolescents might result from a combination of hyperinsulinism, hyperlipidemia, and decreased antioxidant levels.

The incidence of cholecystitis and pancreatitis is also higher in obese children. The hypertriglyceridemia may cause increased incidence of pancreatitis particularly in adolescent girls with IRS. TG levels in excess of 500 mg/dL are associated with pancreatitis. Gallstone formation results from increased biliary cholesterol excretion (219).

Uric Acid Metabolism and Gout in IR

The association between hyperuricemia and the IRS as well as obesity is well recognized (220–223). It is being realized that one of the clinical presentations of IRS may be gouty arthritis. Studies in young adults indicated that there is a direct correlation between the risk of developing gout and BMI, weight gain, and waist-to-hip ratio (224,225). Conversely, weight reduction decreases urate levels as well as de novo purine synthesis and the risk of gout (226,227). Insulin enhances renal urate reabsorption and reduces the renal excretion of urate in both healthy and hypertensive individuals (228,229). In the IRS, impaired oxidative phosphorylation may increase systemic adenosine concentrations, which in turn can result in renal retention of sodium, urate, and water (230). Some researchers have speculated that increased extracellular adenosine concentrations over the long term may also contribute to hyperuricemia by increasing urate production (230).

Nephrosis in IR

IR/hyperinsulinemia is associated with increased activity of both renin-angiotensin-aldosterone system and sympathetic nervous system activities, resulting in increased renal sodium reabsorption, fluid retention, and endothelial cell proliferation. The pathogenesis of nephrosis in obese individuals is poorly understood. The main factors such as persistent hyperinsulinemia by promoting angiotensin production, increased plasma levels of free IGF-1 by stimulating glomerular hypertrophy, and hyperlipidemia by promoting glomerulopathy through oxidative cellular injury, may all contribute to the development of glomerulosclerosis and eventually end-stage renal disease (231). This glomerulosclerosis in the hyperinsulinemic/insulin-resistant kidney is peculiar and characterized by lower rate of nephrotic syndrome, fewer lesions of segmental sclerosis, and a greater glomerular size compared with the idiopathic variety (232,233). Microalbuminuria, in addition to being an early marker for nephropathy, is an established marker for increased CVD morbidity and mortality in patients with hyperinsulinemia and hypertension (234). The Insulin Resistance in Atherosclerosis Study revealed that an increasing degree of Si was associated with a decreasing prevalence of microalbuminuria (235). We have found segmental IgA-type glomerulonephritis in several of our own patients with obesity and IR.

Resting Energy Expenditure in IR

Resting Energy Expenditure (REE) accounts for 60% to 75% of total daily energy expenditure, and decreases with age (236,237) and physical inactivity (238). Even small reductions in REE increase the risk of weight gain (239). It is well known that fat-free mass accounts for the majority of interindividual variability in REE (159). In addition to physiologic factors, insulin-related changes are also involved in the regulation of energy balance and contribute to the recovery of body weight stability in a context of long-term positive energy balance.

Carbohydrate "Addiction" in IR

After the industrial revolution, high GI carbohydrates (refined sugars) became available for the large part of populations and resulted in an extraordinary increase in carbohydrate consumption (240). It is well known that high-GI carbohydrates lead to hunger and carbohydrate craving. Ludwig et al. demonstrated in obese adolescents that voluntary food intake after breakfast and lunch was higher after high-glycemic-index meals compared with isocaloric low-glycemic-index meals (241). Studies in adults and adolescents demonstrated increased satiety, delayed return of hunger, and decreased food intake after the ingestion of low-glycemic-index foods compared with high-glycemic-index foods (242,243). Plasma glucose levels are significantly higher following consumption of high-glycemic-index meals, especially when taken with animal fats. Plasma insulin levels and FFA concentrations also elevate after high-glycemic-index meals (242). High-glycemic-index meals increase hepatic secretions of VLDL (244). Taken together, high-glycemic-load carbohydrates promote the development of IR and our dietary advice is always to restrict them in obesity with IR.

Cognition Effects of Insulin

Until recently, the brain was considered to be insensitive to insulin (245). However, this notion has been changed because insulin and its receptors are found widely distributed in the CNS (246–248). Insulin functions through insulin-related peptides synthesized in brain, which serve as neurotransmitters or neuromodulators (248). While the insulin/insulin receptor associated with the hypothalamus plays important roles in regulation of the body energy homeostasis, the hippocampus- and cerebral cortex-distributed insulin/insulin receptors have been shown to be involved in brain cognitive functions (249). In animal models, the expression of insulin receptors or changes in insulin signaling in the hippocampus and temporal cortex is associated with memory and learning (245,250,251). In humans, increased memory capacity has been observed when plasma insulin levels rise acutely (252). Administration of intranasal insulin has been shown to improve verbal memory without the risk of peripheral hypoglycemia (253). However, chronically high insulin levels may potentiate neurodegeneration by increasing oxidative stress and endothelial inflammation, causing microvascular damage or alteration of amyoid β-peptide metabolism with increased amyloid deposition (254–256). Clinical and epidemiologic studies showed the association of IRS and dementia (254,257). Geroldi et al. found significant association between cognitive impairment and IR, and attributed this impairment to microvascular damage and the dyslipidemic effects of IRS (258). A pilot study of 30 subjects with mild Alzheimer's disease or amnestic mild cognitive impairment showed that insulin sensitizer, rosiglitazone, might preserve cognition (259).

PATHOGENESIS AND GENETICS OF IR

Glucose homeostasis is maintained in a narrow range despite wide fluctuations in food intake. Insulin is the master regulator of this homeostasis. In response to the potential hyperglycemic state after food intake, pancreatic β-cells secrete an appropriate amount of insulin resulting in hyperinsulinemia. This compensatory hyperinsulinemia stimulates glucose uptake by skeletal muscle and suppresses endogenous glucose production in the liver (260). In IR, insulin action in these tissues becomes impaired, and results in postprandial hyperglycemia and, consequently, hyperinsulinemia. However, IR is not only a direct consequence of defective insulin action. A number of molecular defects in pathways of insulin action have been associated with the pathogenesis of IR. These include reduced expression of insulin receptors on the surface of insulin-responsive cells (261,262), alterations in the signal-transduction pathways that become activated after insulin binds to its receptor (263,264) and abnormalities in biologic pathways normally stimulated by insulin, including glucose transport (265–267) and glycogen synthesis (268,269). Mutations in the insulin-receptor gene are responsible for severe IR in a limited number of persons (270,271).

Molecular Mechanism of Insulin Action

Insulin signaling is initiated following the interaction of insulin with its specific receptor. The insulin receptor is a glycosylated heterotetrameric complex consisting of two extracellular insulin-binding α-subunits and two β-subunits. Upon binding to its receptor, insulin leads to activation of receptor tyrosine kinase and autophosphorylation of specific tyrosine residues on several substrates, including IRS1–4 (272–274) and stimulation of other signaling molecules such as Shc and Grb, and signal regulatory protein family members, Gab-1, Cbl, CAP, and APS (275) (Fig. 4).

Phosphorylation of IRS family initiates intracellular insulin-signaling chain (260). There are two major, well-described pathways for insulin signaling; the PI-3K-Akt and the MAP kinase pathways (276). Phosphorylation of tyrosine residues of IRS family initiates PI-3K pathway. Following the association of the p85 subunit of PI-3K with the IRS molecules, PI-3K stimulates synthesis of PI-3-,4-,5-phosphate. This results in activation of serine/threonine kinase (Akt), also known as protein kinase B and other downstream effector molecules. Akt in turn phosphorylates a number of proteins that mediate translocation of GLUT-4 transporter to the membrane, and regulates glucose uptake (muscle and adipocyte), glycogen synthesis, protein synthesis, and apoptosis (277).

Several investigators have examined the role of PI-3K and Akt in individuals with IR. However, the results were contradictory with some studies showing a decrease in IRS-associated PI-3K and Akt activity in IR skeletal muscle, while others showed a normal activity of Akt in patients with reduced PI-3K (278,279). Akt deficiency in mice resulted in IR and diabetes (280).

Finally, insulin stimulates translocation of the GLUT-4 from an intracellular pool to the surface of

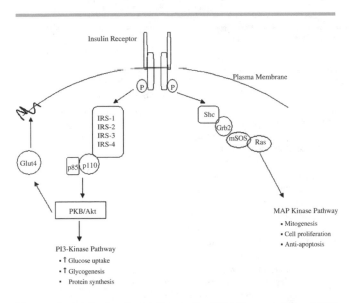

Figure 4 Insulin-signaling pathways: the MAP kinase and the PI-3K. *Abbreviations*: IRS, insulin resistance syndrome; GLUT, glucose transporter; MAP, mitogen-activated protein. *Source*: From Ref. 260.

cells, primarily in skeletal muscle and adipose tissue and heart (281). The mechanism by which the signaling pathways converge on the intracellular GLUT-4–containing vesicles to cause GLUT-4 translocation is not well understood. It appears that the number of GLUTs in skeletal muscle of IR persons is not changed but the ability of insulin to effect this translocation is altered (282,283). Animal models and cellular models of IR showed that insulin-stimulated GLUT-4 translocation to the plasma membrane is reduced (284).

The MAP kinase pathway begins with phosphorylation of collagen-like protein Shc and IRS. IRS and Shc interact with Grb-2 complex and activate the Ras/MAP kinase pathway. Activated MAP kinase mediates the mitogenic and proinflammatory responses of insulin signaling (260). Although the signaling pathways, the MAP kinase and PI-3K, are generally described as acting in a linear fashion, each pathway may activate the other under certain circumstances (276). Therefore, PI-3K/Akt may activate Ras/MAP kinase, and on the other hand, Ras/MAP kinase may stimulate PI-3K pathway.

In insulin-resistant subjects with obesity or T2DM, the pathways leading to activation of PI-3K are blocked, whereas the MAP kinase pathway is normal (285). In normoglycemic subjects with a strong family history of T2DM, despite normal insulin receptor phosphorylation, post-receptor signaling was reduced and was correlated with IR in skeletal muscle (286).

Candidate Genes for IRS

Many studies suggest that genetic factors influence IR; however, despite intensive research there is, so far, no clear understanding of most of the factors involved in

the development of IR. In the insulin-signaling pathway, mutations in insulin receptors, IRS family, PI-3K, and others (GLUT-4, hepatic glucokinase promoter, etc.) have been studied as possible candidate genes.

Many mutations in the insulin receptor gene that affect receptor function are known. Mutations in the insulin receptor are associated with rare forms of IR. These mutations affect insulin receptor number, splicing, trafficking, binding, and phosphorylation. The affected patients demonstrate severe IR, which in most patients results in death during early life (leprechaunism, Rabson-Mendenhall syndrome), or manifest as clinically diverse syndromes including the Type A syndrome and lipoatrophic diabetes (287). Insulin receptor mutations are not commonly found in T2DM, and only small number of individuals (1–5%) may have mutations that could contribute to hyperglycemia and IR (288,289).

Mutations of IRS family of intermediate substrates, especially IRS-1 and IRS-2, were also examined. In animal models, IRS-1 deficiency was associated with IR but not hyperglycemia (290). In contrast, the phenotype of IRS-2 knockout mice is markedly different (291) because they become severely hyperglycemic due to abnormalities of peripheral insulin action and failure of β-cell function (291). This phenotype, with severe hyperglycemia as a consequence of peripheral IR and insufficient insulin secretion, involves a significantly reduced β-cell mass, revealing many similarities to T2DM in man, and outlines the potential role of IRS proteins in the development of cellular IR and β-cell function. However, mutations of IRS-1 and IRS-2 in humans were found with the same frequency in nondiabetics when compared with diabetic individuals (292,293).

PI-3K is another target for gene studies in IRS. However, results in PI-3K mutations in different ethnic groups have been contradictory. Scandinavian IR individuals who were homozygous for p85alpha regulatory subunit of PI-3K had significantly reduced Si (294), whereas this mutation was not found in Japanese patients with T2DM (295). In Pima Indians, this mutation was not associated with Si but rather with an increased acute insulin response (AIR) after a glucose challenge test (296).

Mutations of plasma cell membrane glycoprotein-1, GLUT-4, hepatic glucokinase promoter and PPAR-γ genes have been reported (297). However, in most cases, these mutations are not sufficient to cause IR or T2DM. For example, mutation in PPAR-γ gene causes severe obesity but not IR (297).

Other Molecular Pathways and Their Mutations

In addition to insulin-signaling pathways, several other molecular pathways in energy homeostasis, lipid metabolism, cytokines, hormone-binding proteins including those that are SERPINS, and other protease regulators and their mutations may be responsible for development of IR and obesity (Table 2). In the energy

Table 2 Genetics of Insulin Resistance Syndrome

Insulin receptor pathway defects	Fat cell defects-lipid homeostasis pathway	Hypothalamic level defects-leptin-POMC-MC4R pathway	Miscellaneous
Type A syndrome mutation in the insulin receptor	Congenital generalized lipodystrophy (mutations in 11q13, BSCL2, AGPAT2 gene on 9q34)	POMC mutations; MC4R mutations; MC3R mutations	Proteases–CALP10; impaired processing of prohormones; prohormone convertase deficiency
Leprechaunism	Dunnigan's syndrome (lamin mutation)	Leptin mutations	Estrogen receptor mutations
Rabson–Mendenhall syndrome	Kobberkling's syndrome (mutation in the PPAR-γ gene)	Leptin receptor gene mutation, ghrelin polymorphisms, neuropeptide Y5 receptor polymorphisms, cocaine-and amphetamine-regulated transcript polymorphisms, cholecystokinin A receptor polymorphisms	
Polymorphism in plasma cell membrane glycoprotein-1	Allelic variation in PPAR-γ influence body fat mass by effects on adipocyte; polymorphisms of PPAR-a gene can lead to higher triglyceride and insulin levels; polymorphisms of the lipoprotein lipase gene was both linked and associated with insulin resistance; polymorphisms of UCP1, UCP2, UCP3 genes; polymorphisms of β_2-and β_3-adrenergic receptors	Single gene defects leading to disruption of hypothalamic pathways of energy regulation; Prader-Willi syndrome (15q11.2-q12, uniparental maternal disomy), Alstrom syndrome (ALMS1 gene mutants in the hypothalamus might lead to hyperphagia followed by obesity and insulin resistance), Bardet-Biedl syndrome, Cohen syndrome, Beckwick-Weidermann syndrome, Biemond syndrome II, choroideremia with deafness	

Abbreviations: POMC, proopiomelanocortin; PPAR, peroxisome proliferator-activated receptor; MCR, melanocortin receptor. *Source*: From Ref. 167.

homeostasis pathway, leptin- POMC, ghrelin-NPY, and sympathetic nervous system regulation pathways have proved to be important. In the lipid homeostasis pathway, other than PPAR-γ, PPAR-α, adipocyte-derived hormones, leptin, adiponectin, resistin, etc. are variously involved, as are lipoprotein lipase and genes responsible for adipose tissue formation. Increased availability of FFAs to muscle provokes IR. Proteases contributing to the development of diabetes are represented by CAPN 10 and prohormone convertase deficiencies. The concurrence of several heterozygosities for the mutations described above can have additive adverse effects. In the energy homeostasis, heterozygosity for inactivating mutations of the MC4R results in obesity in both mice and humans (298). Heterozygotes of this most commonly reported form of genetic obesity may also be obese. Heterozygotes for the Bardet-Biedl syndrome have increased frequencies of obesity, renal disease, hypertension, and T2DM (299). Additive adverse effects of heterozygosity are clearly evident in mice carrying heterozygote mutations of the leptin and leptin-receptor genes. Human heterozygotes for a *LEPR* mutation have plasma–leptin concentrations intermediate between wild type and homozygous affected levels (300). Leptin, adipocyte-derived hormone, was identified as an in 1994 by Friedman and coworkers (301). Since then, leptin has gained much attention in the study of the underlying mechanisms of IR in obesity. In rodents, leptin deficiency causes marked obesity, hyperinsulinemia, and hyperglycemia (99). In humans, however, while congenital leptin deficiency or mutations of the leptin receptor have been associated with severe obesity, diabetes was not seen (302,303). However, these few cases reported to date were of young age, and it remains to be seen whether IGT or diabetes may still develop with aging.

In the lipid homeostasis pathway, the PPAR-γ receptor controls the expression of numerous genes. It is assumed that the effect of the TZDs on Si is mediated through altered expression of PPAR-γ-dependent genes (304). Recently, the Pro12Ala and two other polymorphisms were described in the PPAR-γ2 receptor (305). Koch et al. showed that obese individuals carrying heterozygous forms of Pro12Ala polymorphisms appeared to be less insulin resistant compared with individuals without this PPAR-γ2 mutation (306).

Acquired IR

Insulin receptor antibodies, Cushing's syndrome, glucocorticoid steroid therapy, acromegaly, hyperparathyroidism, and exogenous obesity can all produce IR (Table 3) (167). In practice, however, steroid-induced IR in a person who happens to be genetically prone to IR is the most commonly encountered, especially when the obese child also has IR-associated asthma. We find this a frequent occurrence in our clinical practices. GH therapy can provoke transient IR also, but this therapeutic issue needs further study. GH-deficient children tend to have increased fat stores and decreased muscle mass, a situation that reverses after GH therapy. In the SGA disorders without catch-up growth such as the Russell-Silver syndrome, IR may develop even before GH is given.

Defined Syndromes with Severe IR

Numbers of individually rare syndromes characterized by extreme IR have been described over the past 20 years (Table 2) (271). Some of these rare syndromes are linked to mutations of the insulin receptor gene such as Type A syndrome, leprechaunism, and Rabson–Mendenhall syndrome.

Table 3 Acquired Insulin Resistance

Acquired insulin resistance (IR) pathway defects	Acquired fat-cell defects	Miscellaneous
Type B immune-mediated IR	Lipodystrophy associated with HIV protease inhibitors; acquired generalized lipodystrophy-Lawrence syndrome is caused by antibodies against adipocyte-membrane antigens; Barraquer–Simons' syndrome (partial acquired cephalothoracic lipodystrophy) have accelerated complement activation and a serum immunoglobulin-G, called C3 nephritic factor, that is thought to cause lysis of adipose tissue expressing adipsin	Excess counterregulatory hormones; glucocorticoids, catecholamines, PTH, growth hormone, placental lactogen in case of stress, infection, pregnancy, starvation, uremia, cirrhosis, ketoacidosis, aging, inactivity

Source: From Ref. 167.

Type A syndrome is a severe form of inherited IR as a result of mutations in the insulin receptor gene (307). Patients with Type A syndrome present with lean body mass, acanthosis nigricans (ANs), and ovarian hyperandrogenism (acne, hirsutism, oligomenorrhea, elevated testosterone levels, etc.). They may also have short stature, accelerated linear growth, muscle cramps, and retinitis pigmentosa (271).

Rabson–Mendenhall syndrome is another rare syndrome, which presents in childhood with severe IR and T2DM, which is resistant to large doses of insulin (271). In addition to common features of IR, patients with Rabson–Mendenhall syndrome may present in early childhood with accelerated linear growth, precocious pseudopuberty, gingival hyperplasia, and abnormal nails (308). Their prognoses are generally poor. They become constantly hyperglycemic and develop microvascular complications of diabetes (271,308).

Leprechaunism is the most severe form of inherited IR with neonatal onset. It was first described by Donohue and Uchida (309). It is characterized by intrauterine and postnatal growth retardation, hyperinsulinemia, dysmorphic features (prominent eyes, upturned nostrils, low-set posteriorly rotated large ears), and lack of subcutaneous fat (308). These infants have massive hyperinsulinemia, often associated with glucose intolerance or frank diabetes mellitus, in addition to fasting hypoglycemia (308). Most of these infants do not live beyond the first year of life, although a few may survive until adolescence (308).

Both syndromes—Leprechaunism and Rabson–Mendenhall—are inherited as autosomal recessive traits (308).

Type B syndrome patients usually present during middle age. They often demonstrate clinical findings consistent with autoimmunity including vitiligo, chronic thyroiditis, alopecia areata, arthritis, lupus-like feature, etc. in addition to their severe IR (308,310). Postprandial hypoglycemia is a common feature of this syndrome (308,310). The presence of anti-insulin receptor antibodies in the plasma is the diagnostic hallmark of the Type B syndrome (310). In our own experience with obese children with such autoantibodies, about half had other clinical evidence of associated autoimmune disorders while the others did not.

Werner's syndrome, a progeria syndrome, is characterized with bird-like facies, gray hair, cataract formation, slender extremities, and severe IR (311).

The lipodystrophy syndromes consist of a heterogeneous group of disorders and are characterized with severe IR, hypertriglyceridemia leading to pancreatitis, and fatty infiltration of the liver leading to hepatic steatosis, which sometimes can progresses to cirrhosis (307). Leptin levels are low and the clinical features may dramatically reverse with leptin replacement. Lipodystrophies can be genetic or acquired. An increasingly common acquired form of lipodystrophy seen clinically is the one associated with the use of highly active antiretroviral treatment in HIV-infected patients (312). Among the inherited lipodystrophies, the Berardinelli–Seip form of generalized lipodystrophy and the Dunnigan-type familial partial lipodystrophy are the rare forms of syndromic IR (313).

CLINICAL FEATURES

The natural history of IR begins in childhood, from the interplay of genetic and environmental factors (Fig. 5 and 6). Although it is generally unclear in most instances whether a primarily genetically encoded state of IR or a defective satiety disorder appears first, IR results in hyperinsulinism and the precocious

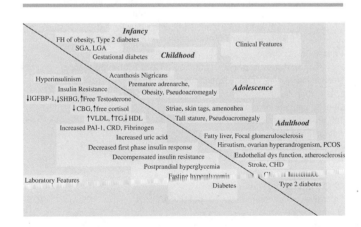

Figure 5 Clinical and laboratory features of IRS with natural history. *Abbreviations*: FGA; LGA, large for age; IGFBP, insulin-like growth factor-binding protein-1; CBG, corticosteroid-binding globulin; VLDL, very low-density lipoprotein; TG, triglyceride; HDL, high-density lipoprotein; PAI, plasminogen activator inhibitor; CRP, C-reactive protein; CHD, coronary heart disease; PCOS, polycycstic ovarian syndrome; FH. *Source*: From Ref. 167.

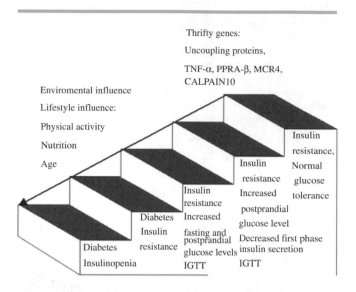

Thrifty genes:

Uncoupling proteins,

TNF-α, PPRA-β, MCR4, CALPAIN10

Figure 6 Natural history of developing diabetes Type 2. *Abbreviations*: TNF, tumor necrosis factor; PPAR, peroxisome proliferator-activated receptor; MCR, melanocortin receptor; IGTT. *Source*: From Ref. 167.

development of atherosclerosis and T2DM (314). The clinical phenotype of IRS includes centrally biased obesity; characteristic skin involvements such as ANs, skin tags, striae, acne, hirsutism, and frontal balding; an allergic diathesis, especially as manifest by asthma; hypertension; an atherogenic dyslipidemia (increased VLDL with raised TGs and reduced levels of the protective HDL cholesterol); early atherosclerosis, tall stature and pseudoacromegaly (with suppressed GH levels); focal segmental glomerulosclerosis; hepatic steatosis; and adrenal and ovarian hyperandrogenism (Table 4). Importantly, IR is not infrequent in the absence of obesity, whereas even considerably obese persons can be insulin sensitive. In the latter instances, we find physical activity to be important in preventing IR.

Obesity

Obese patients represent heterogeneous subgroups of metabolic and phenotypical expressions of IR, whereas individuals with the same BMI can have very different degrees of IR and metabolic (insulin) compensation. However, most individuals with BMIs more than 35 to 40 kg/m² are IR. Adolescents and adults with BMIs of 25 kg/m² or more are at risk for adiposity-related morbidity, whereas those with BMI greater than 30 kg/m² are obese according to the WHO panel. Today, CDC suggests the term of "overweight" instead of "obese" be used for children. According to CDC terminology, overweight children are defined as those with BMI equal to or above the 95th percentile and children at risk of overweight are those with BMI equal to or above the 85th but below the 95th percentile (315) (Vol. 1; Chap. 1).

It is widely believed that obesity itself, especially increased visceral fat accumulation, can lead to IR

Table 4 Comparison of Features of Insulin Resistance Syndrome (IRS) in Children and Adults

Pediatric features of IRS	Adult features of IRS
Family history of diabetes, obesity, hypertension, coronary heart disease, and or stroke	
History of maternal gestational diabetes	
Certain race/ethnicity: African-American and Hispanic, Native Americans	
Small for age (mostly), or large for age (less often)	
Striae: red (new), white (old) from adrenarche onward	Striae: white
Acanthosis nigricans (AN)	AN, skin tags
Premature pubarche	
Hirsutism, polycycstic ovarian syndrome (PCOS) with adolescence	Hirsutism, ovarian hyperandrogenism, PCOS, infertility
Decreasing resting energy expenditure	
Low resting fat to carbohydrate oxidation rates	
Obesity appears or worsens at adrenarche	Central obesity
Tall stature/pseudoacromegaly	Pseudoacromegaly
Adipomastia/gynecomastia	
Asthma/allergic rhinitis	
Acute pancreatitis	Chronic pancreatitis
	Hyperuricemia, gout
Obstructive sleep apnea	Obstructive sleep apnea
Fatty liver, nonalcoholic steatohepatitis (NASH)	Fatty liver, NASH, gallbladder disease
Glomerulonephritis	Focal glomerulosclerosis
Premature atherosclerosis	Premature atherosclerosis
Dyslipidemia	Dyslipidemia
Hypertension	Hypertension
Glucose intolerance	Glucose intolerance
Type 2 diabetes	Type 2 diabetes
	Increased cancer risk
	Increased risk for Alzheimer's disease

Source: From Ref. 167.

(314,316). Genetically induced IR can be the primary mechanism underlying and inducing the progression of obesity. In contrast, nonobese, lean individuals can develop IR also. It has been shown that lean sisters and brothers of patients with obesity complicated by IR and PCOS can have IR, confirming that IR can be a primary mechanism. Generalized lipodystrophy can lead to IRS because of leptin deficiency and is dramatically reversible with leptin therapy.

How IR results in the cluster of the associated symptoms is not clear. One characteristic that associated with IRS is obesity (317). The hyperinsulinemic euglycemic clamp studies clearly demonstrate the relationship between obesity and IRS. Euglycemic insulin clamp studies in children, twin studies, and others indicate that the obese individuals have higher fasting insulin levels and lower Si than the nonobese individuals (16,318,319). Si is inversely correlated with BMI (136,320).

Although obesity is an important factor for IR, the distribution of body fat appears to be of critical importance. For example, Si highly correlates with increased trunk-to-leg fat ratio than BMI (194). Cross-sectional studies in children have confirmed a strong positive relation between body fat distribution and cardiovascular risk factors: greater central adiposity with higher risk factors (321–323). Multiple studies demonstrated that abdominal fat and abdominal sub-cutaneous fat, both of which can exist independent of the degree of general adiposity, can promote IR via the secretion of FFAs and adipocyte-derived cytokines (e.g., PAI-1, TNF-α, leptin, adiponectin) (324,325). Accumulated data suggest that these secreted factors may comprise a mechanistic link among increased abdominal fat, IR, and expression of the IRS (326).

The dramatic rise in obesity-associated IRS reflects environmentally increased availability and consumption of food with high carbohydrate and fat content together with decreased physical activities. Genetic predispositions to obesity favor selection of metabolically advantaged (energy thrifty) traits resulting in an enhanced ability to store excess calories in tissues as fat and to spare protein breakdown for gluconeogenesis, favoring survival in times of hunger. Genotypic factors influence the ability to use food energy efficiently through mechanisms of intra-abdominal fat distribution, resting metabolic rate, changes in energy expenditure, body composition to overfeeding, feeding behavior (including food preferences), adipose tissue lipoprotein lipase activity, and the basal rate of lipolysis. Numerous genes, markers, and chromosome regions have been linked with obesity and its metabolic consequences. In the early phase of obesity, the insulin gene variable number of tandem repeat (VNTR) are associated with different effects of body fatness on insulin secretion. When young, obese patients homozygous for class I VNTR alleles secrete more insulin than those with other genotypes (327). However, overall genetic abnormalities causing obesity account for only 5% of all obese individuals

(328). The incidence of genetic lesions is however greatest in children who present with early onset of obesity.

IGT and T2DM

The majority of persons with IR do not develop T2DM. The genetic backgrounds on which hyperinsulinism and IR develop strongly influence the adequacy of pancreatic β-cell compensation (329). The heritability of β-cell function, assessed in relation to Si [Si × AIR glucose], demonstrated a heritability of 70% in 94 normal glucose-tolerant individuals (330). Pancreatic β-cell failure can represent independent genetic interactions that may be influenced by the human leukocyte antigen genotype.

Reaven et al. found that approximately 25% of nonobese individuals with normal oral glucose tolerance had IR that was of a magnitude similar to that seen in patients with T2DM, but exhibited compensatory hyperinsulinemia to maintain normoglycemia (1). Although IRS individuals who can compensate by hyperinsulinemia may escape hyperglycemia and diabetes, longitudinal studies have clearly shown that they are still prone to other complications of IRS such as early atherosclerosis, progression of obesity (especially central type), hypertension, dyslipidemia, hypercoagulation, stroke, PCOS, fatty liver infiltration, focal segmental glomerulosclerosis, and an increased cancer rate as well (24,331). Thus, IRS is not benign even when diabetes does not develop.

Loss of first phase insulin response to predict development of diabetes: Children affected by IRS are usually hyperinsulinemic individuals in whom carbohydrates can induce a delayed, but excessive, rise in insulin secretion. This may cause an excessive fall in glucose levels later, of sufficient severity to provoke symptoms of hypoglycemia [late reactive (three-five hours) hypoglycemia]. As the ability to secrete insulin declines, postprandial glucose intolerance appears, followed by fasting hyperglycemia and diabetes. On the basis of IV glucose testing, insulin release consists of two phases (332). In individuals with T2DM, the second phase response is diminished, and the first phase response is almost absent. However, the first phase response decreases long before the development of T2DM. In the Insulin Resistance Atherosclerosis Study, 903 subjects were nondiabetic at baseline, 148 had developed diabetes when they were reexamined after five years. Individuals who had a low AIR combined with high proinsulin levels experienced the highest diabetes risk (333). Similar data were supported by the United Kingdom Prospective Diabetes Study (334) and studies in Pima Indians (335), in whom it was shown that a low AIR predicts the development of diabetes at a time when many subjects still have normal glucose tolerance. The DI is an excellent method to detect latent β-cell defects, albeit hyperinsulinism documented by a high AIR is a predictor of the rate of increased fat mass.

Premature Adrenarche

Accumulating data indicate that children with premature adrenarche are at increased risk of developing functional ovarian hyperandrogenism and PCOS (336). The risk is greater in those with a birth history of SGA (336,337). Certain ethnic groups, especially African-American and Hispanic girls with premature adrenarche have a higher risk of developing IRS and PCOS later in life (338,339). In a study, administration of metformin to postmenarchal and IR girls with a history of low birth weight and premature adrenarche improved hyperinsulinemia, dyslipidemia, and body composition within six months. Furthermore, they had significantly decreased serum androgen levels suggesting that early metformin therapy may prevent progression from premature adrenarche to PCOS, in a high-risk group of girls (340). In addition, in a small study, measuring fasting glucose to insulin ratio (<7) appears to be a simple tool for measuring Si for the screening of prepubertal girls with premature adrenarche and/or obesity for IR and its complications (341), despite our increasing reliance on the IR surrogate IGFBP-1 level.

Hyperandrogenism and PCOS

PCOS is probably the most common endocrinopathy of young women and leading endocrine cause of infertility (Vol. 2; Chap. 13) (342). It affects about 6% to 10% of women in childbearing age. Adolescents with PCOS usually present with hirsutism, acne, alopecia, and/or irregular menses. These findings suggest that PCOS usually develops during puberty but may present at a later time as infertility. In addition to elevated testosterone, androstenedione, and DHEA levels, typically there is an increased level of insulin, and decreased SHBG and IGFBP-1 (343). One-third of adults with PCOS have IGT (344) and a similar frequency of IGT has been observed in adolescents with PCOS (345). Girls with PCOS are also at risk of developing CVDs (345). In a clinical study of adolescents with PCOS treated with metformin, menstrual regularity improved (346). Troglitazone is another potent insulin sensitizer that improved hirsutism and ovulation in PCOS in a well-controlled study (347), albeit TZD being subsequently discontinued because of the serious heptic side effects reported. In an in vitro study, troglitazone, but not metformin, directly inhibited the steroidogenic enzymes P450c17 and 3β-HSD (348). We find that PCOS patients usually have IR and respond to metformin, but may relapse when metformin is stopped unless their weight loss has been significant.

Dyslipidemia and Atherosclerosis

The lipid abnormalities in individuals with IRS are highly significant and not limited to an increase in plasma TG (349). The atherogenic dyslipidemia is a triad of hypertriglyceridemia, low HDL cholesterol level, and elevated LDL cholesterol (350). As mentioned previously, hyperinsulinemia is an independent cardiovascular risk factor (351). Children with elevated BMI, systolic BP, serum TG, and LDL lipoproteins, convey greater atherosclerosis risk in the aorta and coronary arteries as adults (Vol. 1; Chap. 14) (204).

Hypertension

Hyperinsulinemia can increase BP by several mechanisms: via its effect to increase renal sodium absorption, via increased activity of the sympathetic nervous system, and via FFA-induced sensitivity to adrenergic stimuli and antagonized nitric oxide vasorelaxation (351). Also, transgenic mice that overexpress leptin develop hypertension. Cruz et al.(352) demonstrated that Si in overweight children was positively related to HDL cholesterol and negatively related to TGs and systolic and diastolic BP. According to National High Blood Pressure Program (353), normal BP is defined as systolic BP and diastolic BP that are below the 90th percentile as per gender, age, and height; hypertension is defined as average systolic BP or diastolic BP that is at the 95th percentile as per gender, age, and height; prehypertension is defined as average systolic BP or diastolic BP levels that are at the 90th percentile but below the 95th percentile on at least three separate occasions. As with adults, adolescents with BP levels equal to or higher than 120/80 mmHg should be considered prehypertensive (Vol. 1; Chap. 13).

Nonalcoholic Steatohepatitis, Nonalcoholic Fatty Liver Disease

Hepatic steatosis is another complication of IR that may progress over years with inflammation and fibrosis into nonalcoholic steatohepatitis. At least 20% of such individuals eventually develop cirrhosis, liver failure, or hepatocellular carcinoma. Fatty liver affects 2.6% of children (211), and 22.5% to 52.8% of obese children and 10% to 25% of adolescents (212). Rashid and Roberts linked it to hyperinsulinemia in pediatric NAFLD after finding that 13 of 36 children with NAFLD had ANs (354). A retrospective analysis of 43 children with biopsy-proven NAFLD showed almost all children had IR (355). The disease is usually silent over many years. Serum levels of ALT, aspartate aminotransferase (AST), alkaline phosphatase, and γ-glutamyltransferase are elevated and have been proposed as surrogate markers of hepatic fat accumulation (86). The ratio of AST to ALT is usually less than 1, but this ratio increases as fibrosis advances. Although there is no accepted pharmacological treatment that can reverse fatty liver disease, insulin sensitizers such as metformin (356,357), and troglitazone (358) have been shown to decrease liver volume and ALT levels. In addition, daily antioxidant therapy in conjunction with weight loss reduces serum aminotransferase levels (359).

Tall Stature and Pseudoacromegaly

Accelerated linear and acral growth that resembles acromegaly is a common feature of patients with IR (Vol. 2; Chap. 7). They have coarse facial features, increased hand and foot size, and tall stature. The levels of GH and IGF-1 are too low to explain this feature in these patients. Thus, it is most likely a result of hyperinsulinism, which promotes linear growth by activating skeletal IGF-1 receptors, whereas low levels of IGFBPs can promote IGF-1 action by allowing it to be freely and metabolically available. Pseudoacromegaly is also well described in patients with severe IR (307,360,361). Previous studies in patients with severe IR and pseudoacromegaly have suggested the presence of unopposed mitogenic and anabolic actions of hyperinsulinemia as the main manifestation of pseudoacromegaly (361,362). Although the primary defect remains unknown, a selective postreceptor defect of insulin signaling may result in the acromegaloid feature of patients with IR (363).

Increased aromatization of androgens to estrogens secondary to obesity may contribute growth acceleration and bone maturation as well as propensity to adipo/gynecomastia in adolescent boys and enhance GH production (364). Estrogens affect longitudinal bone growth through their action on endochondral bone formation (365). Ghrelin is known to stimulate GH secretion, and in obesity, ghrelin levels are decreased (366). However, Korbonits et al. (367) recently identified polymorphism in the ghrelin gene of 14 children who were both tall and obese, suggesting a role of ghrelin in stature and BMI. MC4R gene mutations are present in up to 5.8% of obese children who are tall (>2 SD above the mean for age) (368). Direct action of leptin on bone growth can predispose to pseudoacromegaly (369). Pseudoacromegaly is seen in the face of low plasma GH level secretion typical for obesity. Leptin decreases GHRH-receptor gene transcription, thereby reducing GH levels and responsiveness to GHRH (370).

AN and Skin Tags

AN is a skin lesion that is widely used as a clinical surrogate of laboratory-documented IR/hyperinsulinemia associated with obesity, denoting a subgroup with a high risk of T2DM. AN is characterized by hyperpigmentation and a velvety hyperkeratosis that is mostly seen at axillae, posterior region of the neck, antecubital fossae, and groin. Less commonly, it involves the other flexural areas, umbilicus, submammary region, knuckles, elbows, and, in extreme cases, the entire skin. The severity of AN correlates well with the degree of insulin responses to IR, although AN also persists into the decompensated phase of IR where insulin levels may be normal or low. Another group studied 19 obese children with AN and demonstrated the similar strong association between AN and hyperinsulinemia, IR and T2DM (371), suggesting that AN may be used as a reliable

index of IR. Nearly 40% of Native American teenagers have AN, as do 13% of African-American, 6% of Hispanic, less than 1% of white and non-Hispanic children, aged 10 to 19 years (372). In Caucasian patients, the AN often appears a light yellow/gray color rather than a dark lesion, emphasizing that the lesion represents a thickening of the stratum corneum that becomes pigmented in a racially dependent manner. Both insulin and IGF-1 receptors have been identified in cultured human keratinocytes and dermal fibroblasts (373). High levels of insulin can activate both receptors (308). Likely, hyperinsulinemia induces the mitogenic effects of free IGF-1, which has higher affinity than insulin to IGF-1 receptors on keratinocytes. Additionally, FFAs, TNF-α and interferon-γ (IFN-γ) cytokines that are often elevated in obesity, can induce up-regulation of PPAR-β/δ and thereby keratinocyte proliferation (374,375).

Skin tags (cutaneous papillamos) are hyperproliferative skin lesions that are frequently seen in obese, T2DM, and IR patients (376–378). As with AN, skin tags may result from elevated free IGF-1 and depressed IGFBP-3 levels, acting directly on cutaneous epithelial cells.

Acne

Acne is a common clinical presentation of IRS (379,380). Higher serum androgen levels are associated with increased sebum production, one of the important components of acne development (Vol. 2; Chap. 13) (379). Both insulin and IGF-1 stimulate the synthesis of androgens in ovarian and testicular tissues (381,382), and increase the bioavailability of circulating androgens to tissues by inhibiting the hepatic synthesis of SHBG (240). In addition, decreased IGFBPs in the hyperinsulinemic state may also contribute to unregulated cell proliferation in the follicle, causing large nodular acne (177).

Inflammation, Impaired Immunity, Allergic Diathesis, and Autoimmunity

IRS and T2DM have increased markers of inflammation, such as CRP, erythrocyte sedimentation rates, and TNF-α levels. Data from the NHANES III cohort of 5305 children showed that 24.2% of boys and 31.9% of girls with BMI greater than the 95th percentile had elevated CRP levels (383). The Bogolusa and Pathobiological Determinants of Atherosclerosis in Youth studies confirmed the significance of elevated CRP for future atherosclerosis development in children. BMI (384) and adiposity have been reported to be major determinants of CRP levels in children. In addition, low levels of adipocytokines, especially adiponectin, are described in very young obese children and correlates well with IR (385). Among adults, those with baseline CRP in the top quartile were found to be twice as likely to develop diabetes over three to four years of follow-up as those with lower levels (386). A previous study revealed significantly elevated

TNF receptors Type-2 in obese children compared with lean children, with significantly elevated levels in the group of obese children with IGT (Anhalt et al., personal communication).

Leptin has been shown to up-regulate the production of proinflammatory cytokines, including TNF-α and IL-6, to increase phagocytosis by macrophages, and to increase T-helper cell Type-1 (Th1) levels and suppression of T-helper cell Type-2 (Th2) cytokine production in mice (387).

A connection between leptin and autoimmunity was recently recognized in the light of understanding that leptin could favor proinflammatory cell responses and directly influence the development of autoimmune disease mediated by Th1 responses. Intraperitoneal injections of leptin accelerated autoimmune destruction of insulin-producing β-cells and significantly increased IFN-γ production in peripheral T-cells in nonobese diabetic mice. Similar observations were documented by leptin injections given to C57BL/6J-*ob*/*ob* mice that converted these mice from disease-resistant to susceptible-to-autoimmune encephalomyelitis. This switch was accompanied by a Th2 to Th1 pattern of cytokine release and consequent reversal of Ig subclass production (388). Thus, leptin resistance evident in IR could be biased to Th2-type responses.

The role that leptin plays in the immunosuppression of malnutrition is increasingly recognized. Seven of 11 children in the family with a leptin mutation died of infections in childhood (389). At the same time, it was shown that leptin treatment of human lymphocytes during a mixed lymphocyte reaction in vitro enhanced IFN-γ production and blunted IL-4 production (387).

A significant association between asthma and obesity has been noted, especially during puberty. One of the possible mechanisms is that obesity represents a proinflammatory state, and leptin levels influence Th1/Th2 cytokine responses. Relationships between birth weight and adult BMI, and between obesity and asthma have been well recognized. BMI correlated with the prevalence of asthma in both boys and girls. It was noted that girls who became obese between ages 6 and 11 years were seven times more likely to develop new asthmatic symptoms at ages 11 to 13 years (390). At the same time, intervention trials documented the beneficial effect of weight loss on improvements in forced expiratory volume in one second, forced vital capacity, dyspnea, use of rescue bronchodilators, and the median number of asthma exacerbations in the treatment group compared with the control group (391). We regard IR children to often have an allergic diathesis, with increased rates of allergic rhinitis, eczema, and asthma.

Hypoventilation and Sleep Apnea

Excess body fat leads to a decline in the expiratory reserve volume, vital capacity, total lung capacity, and functional residual volume, probably due to the excess body mass per se, although others implicate excessive leptin levels (392).

Malignancy

The prevalence of endometrial cancer, cervical cancer, and renal cell carcinoma in women increases in proportion to BMI, while liver cancer and some gastrointestinal malignancies are increased markedly in obese men. It is unclear as yet whether childhood obesity predisposes to childhood or adult malignancy, although a retrospective study revealed a 9.1-fold (range 1.1- to 77.5-fold) increase in the incidence of colon cancer among elderly men (not women) who had been obese as adolescents (393). During hyperinsulinemia state, decreased IGFBP-1 and -2 and SHBG levels leading to increasing free IGF-1 and sex steroids may contribute to increased risks of certain malignancies in obese adults (24).

Other Associations

Additional complications of obesity/IR include pseudotumor cerebri, Blount's disease, slipped capital femoral epiphysis, and psychological problems. Manoff et al. compared 106 subjects with radiographically diagnosed SCFE with 46 controls without radiographic evidence of SCFE. In the SCFE group, 81.1% of individuals had a BMI above the 95th percentile; for the control group, the corresponding figure was only 41.3% (394).

DIAGNOSIS
Clinical Diagnosis of IR and IRS

Clinical findings that suggest IRS are the presence of abdominal obesity, ANs in skin fold areas such as the nape of the neck, the axillae, and the groin; acne, hirsutism, and irregular menstrual periods or amenorrhea indicating underlying PCOS. However, a clinical definition of IRS in children currently does not exist. In contrast, clinical definition of IRS in adults was recently proposed by the WHO and the Adult Treatment Panel III of the National Cholesterol Education Program (395). The availability of a clinical definition allows optimal identification of individuals at risk for T2DM and CVD to the investigators. A difficulty on the definition of IRS in children is partly due to growth and developmental changes that occur during childhood and adolescence, which complicate the determination of cut-off points for risk factors that have been used to define adult IR (396). For example, it is difficult to define obesity in children (Vol. 1; Chap. 1). Because children's heights and weights are changing as they grow, it is not possible to give a simple cut-off point to define overweight, or obesity, as is the done for adults (396). As mentioned earlier, today, CDC recommends avoiding using the term "obesity" for children (315). Preferred terms are "overweight" (defined as a BMI $\geq$ 95th percentile for age and sex) and "at risk of overweight" (reserved for children with a BMI ≥85th percentile but < 95th percentile for age and sex) (315). However, BMIs may be misleading in muscular youths.

In a more recent study, to identify children and adolescents with risk factors for obesity and IRS, risk-based, age- and sex-specific thresholds for increased waist circumference were developed (399). Waist circumference is a more specific indicator to assess central obesity in adults than it is for children and adolescents. BMI z-score is another tool that has been used in some studies to assess obesity in children (11).

Laboratory Evaluation

IR is defined as an impaired ability to: promote peripheral glucose disposal at usual blood-glucose concentrations, suppress hepatic glucose, and inhibit VLDL output with the conjunction of clinical evidence and confirmed by measurement of insulin and glucose levels by several tests. Currently available tests for assessing IR include measurement of the fasting insulin to glucose ratios, oral glucose tolerance tests (OGTT) (307), the minimal model frequently sampled IVGTT (FSIVGTT) for Si (398), IV administration of insulin (307), and euglycemic hyperinsulinemic clamp procedure for the measurement of in vivo insulin-mediated glucose disposal (399).

Fasting levels of insulin greater than 15 μU/mL, or insulin peak (post-OGTT) levels of more than 150 μU/mL and/or more than 75 μU/mL at 120 minutes of OGTT are hyperinsulinemic levels, which infer IR (400) in adults.

Numerous indexes have been developed to measure Si from OGTT (Table 5). Such approaches are simple, albeit insensitive, have been validated for epidemiological studies (406,413). They correlate with the indexes of Si obtained from glucose clamp studies and minimal model analysis (414).

The minimal model FSIVGTT is a more accurate method of quantifying Si, AIR, and DI (399). In this test, an IV injection of a fixed amount of glucose is followed by frequent blood sampling over 180 minutes and subsequent modeling of the relevant plasma glucose and insulin data to derive the indexes of Si and glucose effectiveness. The AIR characterizes the first phase of insulin secretion that is a marker of early β-cell compensation (399). In nonobese children, the normal AIR range was recently reported by Gower et al.(415) to be 747 ± 122 μU/mL in Caucasians, 1210 ± 116 μU/mL in African-Americans, and 938 ± 38 μU/mL in Hispanic children at Tanner stages 1 to 3.

IR index (Si), calculated from IVGTT of 2×10^{-4} min^{-1}/(μIU/mL) or less, typically occur in the presence of IR, where values of 5×10^{-4} min^{-1}/(μIU/mL) or more are normal in adults and children (416). Si was reported to be in the range of $6.57\pm0.45\times10^{-4}$ min^{-1}/(μIU/mL) in prepubertal children, $4.63\pm0.86\times10^{-4}$ min^{-1}/(μIU/mL) in postpubertal

adolescents, and $2.92\pm0.45\times10^{-4}$ min^{-1}/(μIU/mL) in pubertal children (417). Gower et al.(415) reported that IR in children at developmental Tanner stages 1 to 3 is different between races: Caucasian children, $6.3\pm0.6\times10^{-4}$ min^{-1}/(μIU/mL); African-American children, $4.1\pm0.6\times10^{-4}$ min^{-1}/(μIU/mL); and Hispanic children, $4.5\pm0.5\times10^{-4}$ min^{-1}/(μIU/mL).

The DI characterizes the relationship of insulin secretion to the degree of IR. The DI calculated by (AIR×Si) describes the hyperbolic relationship between insulin secretion (AIR) and Si from FSIVGTT, which is sensitive to detect even latent β-cell defects (134). Gower et al.(415) reported DI from AIR (minutes^{-1}) to be in the range of 0.29 ± 0.07 in Caucasian, 0.45±0.07 in African-American, and 0.35±0.05 in Hispanic children at Tanner stages 1 to 3.

Hyperglycemic and euglycemic–hyperinsulinemic clamp studies are well established for assessing β-cell function and Si and considered to be the gold standard in the assessment of IR. But these are relatively invasive procedures requiring concurrent IV infusion of insulin at a fixed rate (usually raising plasma insulin levels to either 100 or 1000 μU/mL) and glucose at a variable rate, as necessary to maintain normoglycemi(418). Upon reaching steady state, the glucose disposal rate (*M*) is proportional to the exogenous glucose infusion rate (418). However, all these tests are expensive and invasive, with lack of reference points for children for accurate measurement of IR. Furthermore, current surrogates are not accurate during puberty (419). Thus, additional studies of alternative techniques for evaluating SI are needed. Our own studies suggest that increased hepatic insulin fluxes consequent to IR down-regulate hepatic production of IGFBP-1, which appears to be a useful surrogate marker for IR, which appears to be not depend upon insulin levels in the systemic circulation.

SCREENING

Despite growing evidence that IRS is a risk factor for T2DM and CVD in children and adults, at present there are no guidelines for the screening and management of children or adolescents for IRS. To assess obesity in children, BMI is most commonly used (315). A child or adolescent whose weight is equal to or above the 85th percentile is likely to have the risk factors leading to T2DM or CVD. Therefore, primary care providers must be aware of the following risk factors and screen children during their yearly checkup (420):

1. Birthweight (SGA, LGA).
2. Family history of obesity and T2DM in first- and second-degree relatives.
3. Certain race/ethnic groups (Native Americans, African-Americans, Hispanic-Americans, Asians/South-Pacific Islanders).
4. Signs of IRS or conditions associated with IR (elevated insulin levels, IGT, dyslipidemia, hypertension).
5. Findings from an initial screening may necessitate further investigation and the testing should begin no

Table 5 Methods of Measuring Insulin Resistance from Oral Glucose Tolerance Tests

Indices from oral glucose tolerance tests (OGTT)	Formulae	References
Fasting levels of insulin or insulin peak (post-OGTT)	$\geq$15 and/or peak $\geq$150 mU/mL are hyperinsulinemic levels	401
HOMA	$\dfrac{GluOmin(mmol/L) \times InsOmin(\mu U/mL)}{22.5}$	402
QUICKI	$\dfrac{1}{\log(Ins\,0\,min) + \log(Glu\,0\,min)}$	403
Belfiore	$\dfrac{2}{(AUC\ insulin \times AUC\ Glu) + 1}$	404
Cederholm	$75,000 + (Glu\ 0\ min -2 - hr\ Glu) \times 0.19 \times BW120 \times \log(mean\ Ins) \times mean\ Glu$	405
Gutt	$\dfrac{75,000 + (Glu\ 0\ min -2-hr\ Glu) \times 0.19 \times BW}{120 \times \log(Ins\ 0\ min +2 - hr\ Ins]/2) \times [Glu\ 0\ min +2 - hr\ Glu]/2}$	406
Matsuda	$\dfrac{10,000}{\sqrt{(Ins\ 0\ min \times Glu\ 0\ min) \times (mean\ Glu\ mean\ Ins)}}$	407
Stumvoll	$0.22 - 0.0032 \times BMI - 0.0000645 \times 2\text{-hr Ins} - 0.0037 \times 1.5\text{-hr Glu}$	408
Soonthornpun	$[1.9/6 \times BW\ (kg) \times fasting\ Glu + 520 - 1.9/18 \times BW \times AUC\ Glu$ urinary Glu 1.8] $\div$ [AUC ins $\times$ BW]	409
McAuley	Exp $[2.63 - 0.28 \log_n (ins\ mU/L) - 0.31 \log_n (triglycerides\ mmol/L)]$	410
Oral glucose insulin sensitivity index	Table for calculation is available online (http://www.ladseb.pd.cnr.it/bioing/ogis/home.html)	411, 412

Abbreviations: Glu, Glucose; Ins, insulin; AUC, area under the curve; BMI, body mass index.
Source: From Ref. 167.

later than the age of 10 years, or sooner if puberty already started (396).

Although, American Diabetes Association (ADA) recommends biennial screening of children for diabetes by a fasting plasma glucose level, it is well known that postprandial glycemic levels rise abnormally for long periods before fasting blood-glucose levels become elevated too. American Heart Association (421) and The American Academy of Pediatric Expert Committee on Evaluation and Treatment of Obesity in Children (422) recommend measurement of both fasting glucose and insulin in children at risk for IR. In addition, screening for hypertension and dyslipidemia including low HDL cholesterol and hypertriglyceridemia should be done for children who are overweight and/or at risk for IRS.

TREATMENT

According to the ADA, the first generation of American children is destined to have poorer health and reduced longevity than previous generations. Ten and Maclaren state that: "attention must be urgently given to our nation's children who continue to become more obese and more insulin resistant with the passage of time"

(167). Despite the increased prevalence and incidence of pediatric obesity and IR over the past 15 to 20 years, there remain no practice guidelines for management of these problems in children.

Diet

Lifestyle modifications including diet and physical activity have been shown to improve in Si, dyslipidemia, glucose tolerance, and BP in obese adults with IRS (423). Diabetes Prevention Program and Research Group demonstrated that regardless of ethnic background, a small degree of weight loss (5–7%) with a low-calorie, low-fat diet, plus increased physical activity can prevent progression to T2DM in high-risk individuals (424). Caloric reduction is the essential component of weight loss. In addition to low-calorie, changes in macronutrient composition of diet have been used to promote weight loss and increase Si (Vol. 1; Chap. 2). These diets can range from a proper mix or zone of complex carbohydrates that reduces postprandial serum insulin (Zone diet, the South Beach diet), to very high-fat diets that induce satiety by causing ketogenesis and reducing gastrointestinal motility (the Atkin's diet) (326). Despite a relative lack of scientific data, these diets have become increasingly popular. However, the difficulties their management places in children and adults have not been adequately investigated as yet. The prototypical weight-loss program designed for youths is based on restrictive diets, behavior modification techniques, physical activity, and/or drugs; these approaches, however, generally have not been successful and do not necessarily address insulin resistance and the underlying risks beyond weight loss (425). Some studies have shown that dieting may be ineffective and even counterproductive as it may actually cause weight gain in children and adolescents (426).

Studies in adolescents have demonstrated that a diet that is high in fiber and with a low glycemic index is associated with a lower BMI as well as better insulin sensitivity (427). Such a diet also is associated with reduced risk of developing T2DM and CVD, as well as with improvement of glucose control in diabetic patients (428). Diets containing low glycemic index have been shown to reduce plasma glucose, improve IR in obese children (429,430), and decrease food intake (425,431).

Current recommendations for children and adolescents are made based on the food pyramid, nutritionally balanced meals to support growth (432). Use of the "traffic light diet" helps children and families to differentiate food choices primarily based on fat content that correspond to the three colors on a traffic light (433). Family-based behavioral interventions for obese children are considered safe and useful treatment options. These interventions have been associated with decrease in total cholesterol, increase in HDL cholesterol, decrease in IR and return of ovulatory cycles (434). We are, however impressed by head-to-head studies of low carbohydrate versus low fat diets, which show that the former significantly reduces calorie consumption and induces more weight losses than the latter. Our extensive clinical experience is in line with this also.

Physical Activity

For adults, regular physical activity improves fasting glucose, insulin levels, and dyslipidemia, and decreases the risk of developing T2DM (435–438). Studies in children and adolescents are limited. Some studies did not show any relation to any measure of Si and secretion (439). However, data from 357 nondiabetic children showed that physical activity correlated with lower fasting insulin and greater Si in childhood (440). A cross-sectional study of obese children demonstrated that exercise decreased fasting insulin and improved dyslipidemia in the absence of diet (441). Other studies also showed similar findings with improvement of IRS markers (442) and body composition (443). Regular physical activity may also improve BP, both directly and by increasing Si (444,445). Improvement in endothelial-function has been observed following exercise in overweight children and adolescents (446,447). These results are consistent with the hypothesis that

increasing physical activity may reduce the risk of T2DM in children and adolescents by improving insulin action at the whole body and tissue level. Even with short-term exercise training, Si increases 33% and insulin receptor function improves significantly (448). Improved insulin action by exercise training is associated with increased glucose transport by activation of earlier steps of insulin-signaling pathway and translocation of GLUT-4 to the plasma membrane in muscle (449).

Pharmacological Treatment of IRS
Metformin

Metformin is approved for the treatment of T2DM in children, but is also the drug of choice for IR and IRS. Some have suggested that it is the gastrointestinal side effects of the drug that account for much of its action. However, the drug is effective in T2DM without weight loss, being found to reduce hepatic glucose output in particular. Metformin has various mechanisms of action in IR. It enhances insulin binding to insulin receptor in case of its down-regulation by insulin receptor autoantibodies (450,451), and it otherwise increases binding of insulin to its receptor, with augmented phosphorylation and tyrosine kinase activity of the receptor (452). It is effective even in cases of insulin receptor mutations (453). It increases peripheral utilization of glucose though potentiating the phosphoinositol 3-kinase after engagement of the insulin receptor, increasing translocation of the GLUT-1 and GLUT-4 isoforms to cell membrane in different tissues (452–457); increases the activity of adenosine monophosphate kinase in muscle and liver; and reduces cytochrome P450c17 activity (458). It is considered safe and effective in pregnant women to decrease extreme hyperandrogenemi(459,460). It increases IGFBP-1 (461); decreases endothelin-1, a marker of vasculopathy, and decreases hepatic glucose output. Metformin down-regulates TNF-α expression and uncoupling protein-2 mRNA concentrations in liver, thus decreasing hepatic lipid biosynthesis (358). Metformin is safe for the treatment of IR in pediatric patients (462–465). Our experience in treating obese children and adolescents with IR or PCOS with metformin is, likewise, very positive. We treated 16 females, 15 to 28 years of age, who had IR and hyperandrogenism, with metformin (850 mg, three times daily) for a period of eight months to one year. Si, area under the curve for insulin, SHBG, testosterone and androsterone levels, and levels of TGs improved significantly (466). When gradually increased doses were given to minimize gastrointestinal side effects, this was a safe and effective agent.

Thiazolidinediones

The PPAR-γ agonists are a group of ligand-activated transcription factors that govern energy metabolism, cell proliferation, and inflammation (467). PPAR-γ agonists are effective at insulin sensitization, but are less useful in supporting weight loss. The PPAR-γ isotype is mainly expressed in adipose tissue, where it stimulates adipogenesis and lipogenesis. PPAR-γ agonists have been shown to decrease inflammatory proteins and adhesion molecules, decrease cytokine production, improve lipid oxidation, reduce FFA secretion from adipocytes, decrease 11βHSD1, reduce intramyocellular lipids, and reduce muscle IR (468); decrease PAI-1 expression in endothelial cells (469); decrease testosterone levels in IR females (470); and markedly induce adipocyte glycerol kinase gene expression. By inducing glycerol kinase, TZDs markedly stimulate glycerol incorporation into TGs and reduce FFA secretion from adipocytes (471). Weight gains and fluid retention are troublesome side effects seen with increasing dosages of these agents.

Lipid Lowering Agents

Hypertriglyceridemia raises the risk of fatty liver disease, pancreatitis, and gallstones, while the dyslipidemic profile of IR is also atherogenic. Both are reasons to treat the lipid disorder of IR.

"Fibrates" lower TG levels, as mediated through the PPAR-α transcription factor, mainly in liver, where it has an important role in FA oxidation, gluconeogenesis, and amino acid metabolism. Pretreatment of endothelial cells with a PPAR-α agonist (fenofibrate) reduced markers of inflammation such as vascular cell adhesion molecule-1 expression, CRP, fibrinogen, PAI-1, and IL-6 (472). In cases of combined TG-LDL cholesterol elevations, some combinations of fibrates and statins have been reported to induce serious rhabdomyolysis (473). The use of different combinations or of a cholesterol gastrointestinal uptake inhibitor such as Zetia may be indicated. Fibrates are the drugs of choice in treating the dyslipidemia of IR because they lower TG levels and have a modest effect in raising HDL cholesterol. Some patients happen to have raised LDL cholesterol levels as well as IR-related dyslipidemia. In these patients, combination fibrate and statin therapy may be required. Use of gemfibrozil with a statin raises the risk of muscle necrosis that has not been reported with fenofibrate.

"Statins" inhibit 3-hydroxy-3-methylglutaryl-CoA reductase, the rate-limiting enzyme in the mevalonate pathway through which cells synthesize cholesterol. To compensate for decreased synthesis and to maintain cholesterol homeostasis, cells, particularly hepatocytes, increase the expression of LDL receptors, which increases the uptake of plasma LDL, the main carrier of extracellular cholesterol, resulting in lower plasma LDL concentrations. Decreased plasma LDL levels reduce the progression of atherosclerosis and may even lead to the regression of preexisting atherosclerotic lesions. Statins have important immunomodulatory effects as well and are able to decrease the recruitment of monocytes and T-cells into the arterial wall and inhibit T-cell activation and proliferation in vitro (474).

Treatment for acne, hirsustism, and PCOS when found with IR usually responds to insulin-sensitizing therapy. However, OCPs will raise SHBG and downregulate LH and thus ovarian androgen secretion and may be of adjunctive value. Estrogens, however, raise the possibility of thromboses. The use of antiandrogens sometimes has a place also by blocking androgen binding to receptors on hair follicles. Spironolactone is a general steroid receptor blocker but the one approved for use in the United States by the Food and Drug Administration (FDA). It may cause vaginal bleeding in larger doses as well as hyperkalemia. Flutamide is not approved in the United States but has more specific effects in blocking androgen steroid binding to receptors, but has induced serious hepatic damage in some, and liver enzymes must be closely monitored when using it.

Thrombolytics

Aspirin at low doses inactivates the enzyme cyclooxygenase, which catalyzes the conversion of arachidonic acid to prostaglandins G2 and H2. These prostaglandins are precursors of thromboxane, a potent platelet proaggregant which leads to prothrombotic state in IRS and vasoconstrictor. Aspirin also improves insulin action in vivo by promoting insulin signaling by decreasing inhibitory IRS1 serine phosphorylation (475). Low doses of entericoated aspirin (81 mg/day) are preferred. Aspirin should be used in diabetic individuals over the age of 30 years who are at high risk for cardiovascular events, and may have a place in dyslipidemic children with IRS prone to pancreatitis.

Appetite Suppressants

Orlistat and sibutramine are the only two drugs that are approved for use in obese children. Orlistat is a pancreatic lipase inhibitor and is approved in children older than 12 years in the United States. Studies in obese adolescents with orlistat showed similar results to those in adults with decreased BMI, total and LDL cholesterol levels, and reduced fasting insulin and glucose (476,477). Side effects are usually tolerable and consist mainly of gastrointestinal problems such as flatulence.

The other FDA-approved drug for obesity, sibutramine, is approved for obesity in adolescents older than 16 years. Sibutramine inhibits serotonin reuptake and induces premeal hypophagia. The common side effects are mild elevation of BP (478,479). It may also induce depression, anxiety, and insomnia.

"Rimonabant," a selective canabinoid-1 receptor blocker, is the first new class of appetite suppressant (480). Studies in obese adults showed that rimonabant reduces body weight, waist circumference, and improves lipid and glucose metabolism (481). Rimonabant in Obesity (RIO) trials in Europe and North America demonstrated that rimonabant is well tolerated among patients. The most frequent side effects are nausea, dizziness, and upper respiratory tract infections (482). Rimonabant is about to complete Phase III trial and is under FDA review as Accomplia. There is no study on the effects of Rimonabant in children as yet.

Zhang et al. recently reported "Obestatin" as a new appetite suppressant. Obestatin is derived from the ghrelin gene due to posttranscriptional modification. Contrary to the appetite-stimulating effects of ghrelin, treatment of rats with obestatin had suppressed food intake, inhibited jejunal contraction, and decreased body weight gains (483).

Leptin

Leptin is the first of a group of adipocyte-secreted hormones to be used clinically to treat leptin deficiency. In children with congenital leptin deficiency and extreme obesity, leptin induces satiety and a dramatic loss of weight (484). In hypoleptinemic patients with extreme IR and lipodystrophy, leptin dramatically ameliorates IR, hyperglycemia, hyperinsulinemia, dyslipidemia, and hepatic steatosis (485).

Antiepileptic Drugs (Zonisamide and Topiramate)

Currently, two antiepilepsy drugs, topiramate (Topamax) and zonisamide (Zonegram), are under investigation for their weight-loss effects. During antiseizure trials, it was noted that individuals who took these drugs lost weight compared to the placebo group (486,487). Clinical studies reported that topiramate treatment reduced body weight and decreased fasting blood-glucose levels in obese patients with or without T2DM (488). Studies in ZDF rats and *db/db* mice showed that topiramate ameliorates hyperglycemia by improving glucose-induced insulin release (489). Another study in rats fed with a high-fat diet showed that topiramate treatment markedly lowered glucose and insulin levels during glucose-tolerance tests, and induced increased insulin sensitization in adipose and muscle tissues as assessed by euglycemic clamp studies (490). The most common adverse effects of topiramate are related to the central or peripheral nervous system including paresthesia, difficulty with concentration/attention, depression, memory, language problems, nervousness, and psychomotor slowing. Both loss of weight and side effects are dose-dependent.

Alphaglucosidase Blockers

One of the goals of treating IRS is prevention or delaying of developing diabetes and CVD. Acarbose, an alphaglucosidase inhibitor, reduces postprandial hyperglycemia by delaying carbohydrate absorption from the small intestine. This mechanism of action provides glycemic control without increasing insulin levels and exacerbating coexisting cardiovascular risk factors (491). Studies with acarbose showed significantly increased

reversion of IGT to normal glucose tolerance in a short period (492). The Study to Prevent Noninsulin-Dependent Diabetes Mellitus (STOP-NIDDM), which used acarbose in 1429 individuals with impaired glucose tolerance, showed that acarbose reduced the risk of cardiovascular events by 49% (493).

Bariatric Surgery

Restrictive surgical procedures based on an adjustable silicone band placed around a stomach fundal pouch can create a functional partition of the stomach and diminish the capacity to eat large quantities of food at a sitting. Gastric banding has been shown to be successful for weight loss in adults (494). Whereas restrictive procedures are effective in reducing intake of solid foods, high consumption of more liquid high-calorie foods may prevent weight loss (495). Thus, banding must be seen by the patient to be adjunctive to a low carbohydrate diet and exercise regimen to succeed. Intestinal bypass surgery in children should probably only be used in cases of potentially life-threatening complications such as sleep apnea or seriously impaired venous return from the legs etc. In obese adults, such surgery is increasingly embarked upon and while often successful, is accompanied by a raft of complications such as vitamin deficiencies, liver disease, and stomal ulceration. The degree of T2DM is often mitigated by such surgery.

SUMMARY

The rise in childhood IR-related disorders is closely tracking the obesity epidemic worldwide, creating a serious threat to the current and future health of affected children. Unless ways to prevent obesity and IR in childhood and adolescence at the population level are found, IR and its effect on health, including CVD and T2DM, will continue to increase. More diligence in screening for those at risk, better identification of children and adolescents with IR, and improved support for these children and their families to make healthy lifestyle changes are urgently needed. Practitioner education is also required to alert pediatricians to the problems of childhood IR and to have them initiate therapies before they find that, contrary to expectation, their obese patients failed to "out grow" it during adolescence. The onset of obesity in infancy is associated with a growing number of genetic satiety disorders, while IR occurs in many children who are not obese. Although gaining further knowledge of energy metabolism and satiety is obviously important, strategies involving early lifestyle modifications, aided by targeted pharmaceuticals, are likely to make a more immediate clinical impact.

REFERENCES

1. Reaven GM. Banting lecture. Role of insulin resistance in human disease. Diabetes 1988; 37:1595–1607.

2. Ford ES, Giles WH, Dietz WH. Prevalence of the metabolic syndrome among US adults: findings from the third national health and nutrition examination survey. JAMA 2002; 287:356–359.

3. Ozanne SE, Hales CN. Early programming of glucose-insulin metabolism. Trends Endocrinol Metab 2002; 13:368–373.

4. Levitt NS, Lambert EV. The foetal origins of the metabolic syndrome—a South African perspective. Cardiovasc J S Afr 2002; 13:179–180.

5. Dunger DB, Ong KK. Endocrine and metabolic consequences of intrauterine growth retardation. Endocrinol Metab Clin North Am 2005; 34:597–615.

6. Phipps K, Barker DJ, Hales CN, Fall CH, Osmond C, Clark PM. Fetal growth and impaired glucose tolerance in men and women. Diabetologia 1993; 36:225–228.

7. Eriksson JG, Forsen T, Tuomilehto J, Jaddoe VW, Osmond C, Barker DJ. Effects of size at birth and childhood growth on the insulin resistance syndrome in elderly individuals. Diabetologia 2002; 45:342–348.

8. Frontini MG, Srinivasan SR, Berenson GS. Longitudinal changes in risk variables underlying metabolic Syndrome X from childhood to young adulthood in female subjects with a history of early menarche: the Bogalusa Heart Study. Int J Obes Relat Metab Disord 2003; 27:1398–1404.

9. Gunnel DJ, Frankel SJ, Nanchahal K, Peters TJ, Davey Smith G. Childhood obesity and adult cardiovascular mortality: a 57–y follow-up study based on the Boyd Orr Cohort. Am J Clin Nutr 1998; 67:1111–1118.

10. Kahn CR. Banting Lecture. Insulin action, diabetogenes, and the cause of type II diabetes. Diabetes 1994; 43: 1066–1084.

11. Weiss R, Dziura J, Burgert TS, et al. Obesity and the metabolic syndrome in children and adolescents. N Engl J Med 2004; 350:2362–2374.

12. Zimmet P, Alberti KG, Shaw J. Global and societal implications of the diabetes epidemic. Nature 2001; 414(6865): 782–787.

13. Cheng D. Prevalence, predisposition and prevention of type II diabetes. Nutr Metab (Lond) 2005; 2:29.

14. Aye T, Levitsky LL. Type 2 diabetes:an epidemic disease in childhood. Curr Opin Pediatrics 2003; 15:411–415.

15. Cook S, Weitzman M, Auinger P, Nguyen M, Dietz WH. Prevalence of a metabolic syndrome phenotype in adolescents: findings from the third National Health and Nutrition Examination Survey, 1988–1994. Arch Pediatr Adolesc Med 2003; 157:821–827.

16. Sinaiko AR, Jacobs DR Jr., Steinberger J, et al. Insulin resistance syndrome in childhood: associations of the euglycemic insulin clamp and fasting insulin with fatness and other risk factors. J Pediatr 2001; 139:700–707.

17. Kimm SY, Obarzanek E. Childhood obesity: a new pandemic of the new millennium. Pediatrics 2002; 110: 1003–1007.

18. World Health Organization. Obesity: preventing and managing the global epidemic. Report 894. Geneva, Switzerland: World Health Organization, 1998.

19. World Health Organization.Obesity and Overweight, 2003. http://www.who.int/dietphysicalactivity/publications/facts/obesity/en/index.html.

20. Prentice AM. The emerging epidemic of obesity in developing countries. Int J Epidemiol 2005 Dec 2; [Epub ahead of print].

21. National Center for Health Statistics. Health E-stats. Prevalence of overweight and obesity among adults: United States, 1999. Available online at www.cdc.gov/nchs/products/pubs/pubd/hestats/obese/obse99.htm.

22. Mokdad AH, Ford ES, Bowman BA, et al. Prevalence of obesity, diabetes, and obesity-related health risk factors, 2001. JAMA 2003; 289:76–79.

23. Mokdad AH, Bowman BA, Ford ES, Vinicor F, Marks JS, Koplan JP. The continuing epidemics of obesity and diabetes in the United States. JAMA 2001; 286:1195–1200.

24. Calle EE, Rodriguez C, Walker-Thurmond K, Thun MJ. Overweight, obesity, and mortality from cancer in a prospectively studied cohort of US adults. N Engl J Med 2003; 348:1625–1638.

25. Fox R. Overweight children. Circulation 2003; 108:e9071.

26. Deitel M. The International Obesity Task Force on "globesity." Obes Surg 2002; 12:613–614.

27. Lissau I, Overpeck MD, Ruan WJ, Due P, Holstein BE, Hediger ML. Body mass index and overweight in adolescents in 13 European countries, Israel, and the United States. Arch Pediatr Adolesc Med 2004; 158:27–33.

28. Cheng TO. Childhood obesity in China. Health Place 2004; 10:395–396.

29. Iwata F, Hara M, Okada T, Harada K, Li S. Body fat ratios in urban Chinese children. Pediatr Int 2003; 45:190–192.

30. National Center for Health Statistics. Health E-stats 1999. Prevalence of overweight among children and adolescents: United States. Available online at www. cdc.gov/nchs/products/pubs/pubd/hestats/overwght99.htm.

31. Ogden CL, Fryar CD, Caroll MD, Flegall KM. Mean body weight, height, and body mass index, United States 1960–2002. Adv Data 2004; 347:1–17.

32. St-Onge MP, Heymsfield SB. Overweight and obesity status are linked to lower life expectancy. Nutr Rev 2003; 61:313–316.

33. Serdula MK, Ivery D, Coates RJ, Freedman DS, Williamson DF, Byers T. Do obese children become obese adults? A review of the literature. Prev Med 1993; 22: 167–177.

34. Braddon FE, Rodgers B, Wadsworth ME, Davies JM. Onset of obesity in a 36 year birth cohort study. Br Med J 1986; 293(2):299–303.

35. Guo SS, Roche AF, Chumlea WC, Gardner JD, Siervogel RM. The predictive value of childhood body mass index values for overweight at age 35 y. Am J Clin Nutr 1994; 59:810–819.

36. Kaufman FR. Type 2 diabetes in children and youth. Rev Endocr Metab Disord 2003; 4:33–42.

37. Pinhas-Hamiel O, Dolan LM, Daniels SR, Standiford D, Khoury PR, Zeitler P. Increased incidence of non-insulin-dependent diabetes mellitus among adolescents. J Pediatr 1996; 128:608–615.

38. Sinha R, Fisch G, Teague B, et al. Assessment of skeletal muscle triglyceride content by (1)H nuclear magnetic resonance spectroscopy in lean and obese adolescents: relationships to insulin sensitivity, total body fat, and central adiposity. Diabetes 2002; 51(4):1022–1027.

39. Weiss R, Taksali SE, Tamborlane WV, Burgert TS, Savoye M, Caprio S. Predictors of changes in glucose tolerance status in obese youth. Diabetes Care 2005; 28(4):902–909.

40. American Diabetes Association: type 2 diabetes in children and adolescents. Pediatrics 2000; 105:671–680.

41. Alberti G, Zimmet P, Shaw J, et al. Consensus Workshop Group. Type 2 diabetes in the young: the evolving epidemic: the international diabetes federation consensus workshop. Diabetes Care 2004; 27(7):1798–1811.

42. Benjamin SM, Valdez R, Geiss LS, Rolka DB, Narayan KM. Estimated number of adults with prediabetes in the U.S. in 2000: opportunities for prevention. Diabetes Care 2003; 26:645–649.

43. Long SD, O'Brien K, MacDonald KG, et al. Weight loss in severely obese subjects prevents the progression of

impaired glucose tolerance to type II diabetes. A longitudinal interventional study. Diabetes Care 1994; 17:372–375.

44. Tuomilehto J, Lindstrom J, Eriksson JG, et al. Prevention of type 2 diabetes mellitus by changes in lifestyle among subjects with impaired glucose tolerance. N Engl J Med 2001; 344:1343–1350.

45. DPP Research Group. Reduction in the incidence of type 2 diabetes with lifestyle intervention or metformin. N Engl J Med 2002; 346:393–403.

46. Nathan DM. Some answers, more controversy, from UKPDS. United Kingdom Prospective Diabetes Study. Lancet 1998; 352:832–833.

47. Koyama K, Chen G, Lee Y, Unger RH. Tissue triglycerides, insulin resistance, and insulin production: implications for hyperinsulinemia of obesity. Am J Physiol 1997; 273:E708–E713.

48. Lustig RH. The neuroendocrinology of childhood obesity. Pediatr Clin North Am 2001; 48:909–930.

49. Badman MK, Flier JS. The gut and energy balance: visceral allies in the obesity wars. Science 2005; 307: 1909–1914.

50. Gerozissis K. Brain insulin and feeding: a bi-directional communication. European J Pharmacol 2004; 490:59–70.

51. Kellerer M, Koch M, Metzinger E, Mushack J, Capp E, Haring HU. Leptin activates PI-3 kinase in C2C12 myotubes via janus kinase-2 (JAK-2) and insulin receptor substrate-2 (IRS-2) dependent pathways. Diabetologia 1997; 40:1358–1362.

52. Hahn TM, Breininger JF, Baskin DG, Schwartz MW. Coexpression of Agrp and NPY in fasting-activated hypothalamic neurons. Nat Neurosci 1998; 1:271–272.

53. Woods SC. Insulin and the blood–brain barrier. Curr Pharm Des 2003; 9:795–800.

54. Unger JW, Betz M. Insulin receptors and signal transduction proteins in the hypothalamo-hypophyseal system: a review on morphological findings and functional implications. Histol Histopathol 1998; 13:1215–1224.

55. Schwartz MW, Figlewicz DP, Baskin DG, Woods SC, Porte D Jr., Insulin in the brain: a hormonal regulator of energy balance. Endocrine Rev 1992; 13:387–414.

56. Carvalheira JB, Siloto RM, Ignachitti I, et al. Insulin modulates leptin-induced STAT3 activation in rat hypothalamus. FEBS lett 2001; 500:119–124.

57. Porte D Jr., Baskin DG, Schwartz MW. Leptin and insulin action in the central nervous system. Nutr Rev 2002; 60; S20–29.

58. Niswender KD, Gallis B, Blevins JE, Corson MA, Schwartz MW, Baskin DG. Immunocytochemical detection of phosphotidylinositol 3-kinase activation by insulin and leptin. J Histochem Cytochem 2003; 51:275–283.

59. Schwartz MW, Woods SC, Seeley RJ, Barsh GS, Baskin DG, Leibel RL. Is the energy homeostasis system inherently biased toward weight gain? Diabetes 2003; 52:232–238.

60. McGowan MK, Andrews KM, Kelly J, Grossman SP. Effects of chronic intrahypothalamic infusion of insulin on food intake and diurnal meal patterning in the rat. Behav Neurosci 1990; 104:371–383.

61. Schwartz MW, Sipols AJ, Marks JL, et al. Inhibition of hypothalamic neuropeptide Y gene expression by insulin. Endocrinology 1992; 130:3608–3616.

62. Farooqi IS, Keogh JM, Yeo GS, Lank EJ, Cheetham T, O'Rahilly S. Clinical spectrum of obesity and mutations in the melanocortin 4 receptor gene. N Engl J Med 2003; 348:1085–1095.

63. Kalra SP, Dube MG, Fournier A, Kalra PS. Structure–function analysis of stimulation of food intake by neuropeptideY: effects of receptor agonists. Physiol Behav 1991; 50:5–9.

64. Obici S, Wang JL, Chowdury R, et al. Identification of biochemical link between energy intake and energy expenditure. J Clin Invest 2002; 109:1599–1605.

65. Woods SC. Gastrointestinal satiety signals. An overview of gastrointestinal signals that influence food intake. Am J Physiol Gastrointest Liver Physiol 2004; 286:G7–G13.

66. Air EL, Benoit SC, Blake Smith KA, Clegg DJ, Woods SC. Acute third ventricule administration of insulin decreases food intake in two paradigms. Pharmacol Biochem Behav 2002; 72:423–429.

67. Speakman JR. Obesity: the integrated roles of environment and genetics. J Nutr 2004; 134:S2090–S2105.

68. Moran TH. Cholecystokinin and satiety: current perspectives. Nutritio 2000; 16:858–865.

69. Horvath TL, Diano S, Sotonyi P, Heiman M, Tscop M. Minireview:ghrelin and the regulation of energy balance-a hypothalamic perspective. Endocrinol 2001; 142:4163–4169.

70. Batterham RL, Le Roux CW, Cohen MA, et al. Pancreatic polypeptide reduces appetite and food intake in humans. J Clin Endocrinol Metab 2003; 88: 3989–3992.

71. Konturek SJ, Konturek JW, Pawlik T, Brzozowski T. Brain–gut axis and its role in the control of food intake. J Physiol Parmacol 2004; 55:137–154.

72. Cummings DE, Purnell JQ, Frayo RS, Schmidova K, Wisse BE, Weigle DS. A preprandial rise in plasma ghrelin levels suggests a role in meal initiation in humans. Diabetes 2001; 50:1714–1719.

73. Shiiya T, Nakazato M, Mizuta M, et al. Plasma ghrelin levels in lean and obese humans and the effect of glucose on ghrelin secretion. Clin Endocrinol Metab 2002; 87:240–244.

74. Purnell JQ, Weigle DS, Breen P, Cummings DE. Ghrelin levels correlate with insulin levels, insulin resistance, and high-density lipoprotein cholesterol, but not with gender, menopausal status, or cortisol levels in humans. J Clin Endocrinol Metab 2003; 88:5747–5752.

75. Bacha F, Arslanian SA. Ghrelin suppression in overweight children: a manifestation of insulin resistance?. J Clin Endocrinol Metab 2005; 90:2725–2730.

76. Cummings DE, Clement K, Purnell JQ, et al. Elevated plasma ghrelin levels in Prader Willi syndrome. Nat Med 2002; 8:643–644.

77. Cummings DE, Weigle DS, Frayo RS, et al. Plasma ghrelin levels after diet-induced weight loss or gastric bypass surgery. N Engl J Med 2002; 346:1623–1630.

78. Bugianesi E, McCullough AJ, Marchesini G. Insulin resistance: a metabolic pathway to chronic liver disease. Hepatology 2005; 42:987–1000.

79. Freymond D, Bogardus C, Okubo M, et al. Impaired insulin-stimulated muscle glycogen synthase activation in vivo in man is related to low fasting glycogen synthase phosphatase activity. J Clin Invest 1988; 82:1503–1509.

80. Matthaei S, Stumvoll M, Kellerer M, Haring HU. Pathophysiology and pharmacological treatment of insulin resistance. Endocr Rev 2000; 21:585–618.

81. Beck-Nielsen H. Insulin resistance: organ manifestations and cellular mechanisms. Ugeskr Laeger 2002; 164:2130–2135.

82. Boden G, Lebed B, Schatz M, Homko C, Lemieux S. Effects of acute changes of plasma FFA on intramuscular fat content and insulin resistance in healthy subjects. Diabetes 2001; 50:1612–1617.

83. Kelley DE, McKolanis TM, Hegazi RA, Kuller LH, Kalhan SC. Fatty liver in type 2 diabetes mellitus: relation to regional adiposity, fatty acids, and insulin resistance. Am J Physiol Endocrinol Metab 2003; 285:E906–E916.

84. Boden G, Shulman GI. Free fatty acids in obesity and type 2 diabetes: defining their role in the development of insulin resistance and beta cell dysfunction. Eur J Clin Invest 2002; 32(suppl 3):14–23.

85. Natali A, Toschi E, Camastra S, Gastaldelli A, Groop L, Ferrannini E. Determinants of postabsorptive endogenous glucose output in non-diabetic subjects. European Group for the Study of Insulin Resistance (EGIR). Diabetologia 2000; 43:1266–1272.

86. Marchesini G, Brizi M, Bianchi G, et al. Nonalcoholic fatty liver disease: a feature of the metabolic syndrome. Diabetes 2001; 50:1844–1850.

87. Shulman GI. Cellular mechanism of insulin resistance. J Clin Invest 2000; 106:171–176.

88. Barzilai N, She L, Liu BQ, et al. Surgical removal of visceral fat reverses hepatic insulin resistance. Diabetes 1999; 48:94–98.

89. Nurjhan N, Consoli A, Gerich J. Increased lipolysis and its consequences on gluconeogenesis in non-insulin-dependent diabetes mellitus. J Clin Invest 1992; 89:169–175.

90. Kershaw EE, Flier JS. Adipose tissue as an endocrine organ. J Clin Endocrinol Metab 2004; 89:2548–2556.

91. Hotamisligil GS. Molecular mechanisms of insulin resistance and the role of the adipocyte. Int J Obes Relat Metab Disord 2000; 24:S23–S27.

92. Vozarova B, Stefan N, Lindsay RS, et al. Low plasma adiponectin concentrations do not predict weight gain in humans. Diabetes 2002; 51:2964–2967.

93. Steppan CM, Bailey ST, Bhat S, et al. The hormone resistin links obesity to diabetes. Nature 2001; 409:307–312.

94. Pittas AG, Joseph NA, Greenberg AS. Adipocytokines and insulin resistance. J Clin Endocrinol Metab 2004; 89:447–452.

95. Miyazaki Y, Pipek R, Mandarino LJ, DeFronzo RA. Tumor necrosis factor alpha and insulin resistance in obese type 2 diabetic patients. Int J Obes Relat Metab Disord 2003; 27:88–94.

96. Senn JJ, Klover PJ, Nowak IA, Mooney RA. Interleukin-6 induces cellular insulin resistance in hepatocytes. Diabetes 2002; 51:3391–3399.

97. Ailhaud G, Teboul M, Massiera F. Angiotensinogen, adipocyte differentiation and fat mass enlargement. Curr Opin Clin Nutr Metab Care 2002; 5:385–389.

98. Montague CT, O'Rahilly S. The perils of portliness: causes and consequences of visceral adiposity. Diabetes 2000; 49:883–888.

99. Chen H, Charlat O, Tartaglia LA, et al. Evidence that the diabetes gene encodes the leptin receptor: identification of a mutation in the leptin receptor gene in db/db mice. Cell 1996; 84:491–495.

100. Pelleymounter MA, Cullen MJ, Baker MB, et al. Effects of the obese gene product on body weight regulation in ob/ob mice. Science 1995; 269:540–543.

101. Unger RH, Zhou YT, Orci L. Regulation of fatty acid homeostasis in cells: novel role of leptin. Proc Natl Acad Sci USA 1999; 96:2327–2332.

102. Shimomura I, Hammer RE, Ikemoto S, Brown MS, Goldstein JL. Leptin reverses insulin resistance and diabetes mellitus in mice with congenital lipodystrophy. Nature 1999; 401:73–76.

103. Gavrilova O, Marcus-Samuels B, Graham D, et al. Surgical implantation of adipose tissue reverses diabetes in lipoatrophic mice. J Clin Invest 2000; 105:271–278.

104. Petersen KF, Oral EA, Dufour S, et al. Leptin reverses insulin resistance and hepatic steatosis in patients with severe lipodystrophy. J Clin Invest 2002; 109:1345–1350.

105. Chandran M, Phillips SA, Ciaraldi T, Henry RR. Adiponectin: more than just another fat cell hormone? Diabetes Care 2003; 26:2442–2450.

106. Arita Y, Kihara S, Ouchi N, et al. Paradoxical decrease of an adipose-specific protein, adiponectin, in obesity. Biochem Biophys Res Commun 1999; 257:79–83.

107. Weyer C, Funahashi T, Tanaka S, et al. Hypoadiponectinemia in obesity and type 2 diabetes: close association with insulin resistance and hyperinsulinemia. J Clin Endocrinol Metab 2001; 86:1930–1935.

108. Yamamoto Y, Hirose H, Saito I, et al. Correlation of the adipocyte-derived protein adiponectin with insulin resistance index and serum high-density lipoprotein-cholesterol, independent of body mass index, in the Japanese population. Clin Sci 2002; 103:137–142.

109. Combs TP, Berg AH, Obici S, Scherer PE, Rossetti L. Endogenous glucose production is inhibited by the adipose-derived protein Acrp30. J Clin Invest 2001; 108:1875–1881.

110. Rajala MW, Scherer PE. Minireview: the adipocyte—at the crossroads of energy homeostasis, inflammation, and atherosclerosis. Endocrinology 2003; 144:3765–3773.

111. Spranger J, Kroke A, Mohlig M, et al. Adiponectin and protection against type 2 diabetes mellitus. Lancet 2003; 361:226–228.

112. Vozarova B, Weyer C, Hanson K, Tataranni PA, Bogardus C, Pratley RE. Circulating interleukin-6 in relation to adiposity, insulin action, and insulin secretion. Obes Res 2001; 9:414–417.

113. Hotta K, Funahashi T, Bodkin NL, et al. Circulating concentrations of the adipocyte protein adiponectin are decreased in parallel with reduced insulin sensitivity during the progression to type 2 diabetes in rhesus monkeys. Diabetes 2001; 50:1126–1133.

114. Yamauchi T, Kamon J, Waki H, et al. The fat-derived hormone adiponectin reverses insulin resistance associated with both lipoatrophy and obesity. Nat Med 2001; 7:941–946.

115. Benarjee RR, Lazar MA. Resistin: molecular history and prognosis. J Mol Med 2003; 81:218–226.

116. Way JM, Gorgun CZ, Tong Q, et al. Adipose tissue resistin expression is severely suppressed in obesity and stimulated by peroxisome proliferator-activated receptor agonists. J Biol Chem 2001; 276:25,651–25,653.

117. Hotamisligil GS, Arner P, Caro JF, Atkinson RL, Spiegelman BM. Increased adipose tissue expression of tumor necrosis factor-alpha in human obesity and insulin resistance. J Clin Invest 1995; 95:2409–2415.

118. Fried SK, Bunkin DA, Greenberg AS. Omental and subcutaneous adipose tissues of obese subjects release interleukin-6: depot difference and regulation by glucocorticoid. J Clin Endocrinol Metab 1998; 83:847–850.

119. Kern PA, Saghizadeh M, Ong JM, Bosch RJ, Deem R, Simsolo RB. The expression of tumor necrosis factor in human adipose tissue. Regulation by obesity, weight loss, and relationship to lipoprotein lipase. J Clin Invest 1995; 95:2111–2119.

120. Hotamisligil GS, Peraldi P, Budavari A, Ellis R, White MF, Spiegelman BM. IRS-1–mediated inhibition of insulin receptor tyrosine kinase activity in TNF-alpha- and obesity-induced insulin resistance. Science 1996; 271:665–668.

121. Miles PD, Romeo OM, Higo K, Cohen A, Rafaat K, Olefsky JM. TNF—induced insulin resistance in vivo and its prevention by troglitazone. Diabetes 1997; 46:1678–1683.

122. Peraldi P, Xu M, Spiegelman BM. Thiazolidinediones block tumor necrosis factor—induced inhibition of insulin signaling. J Clin Invest 1997; 100:1863–1869.

123. Pradhan AD, Manson JE, Rifai N, Buring JE, Ridker PM. C-reactive protein, interleukin 6, and risk of developing type 2 diabetes mellitus. JAMA 2001; 286:327–334.

124. Pickup JC, Chusney GD, Thomas SM, Burt D. Plasma interleukin-6, tumour necrosis factor alpha and blood cytokine production in type 2 diabetes. Life Sci 20008; 67:291–300.

125. Ridker PM, Rifai N, Stampfer MJ, Hennekens CH. Plasma concentration of interleukin-6 and the risk of future myocardial infarction among apparently healthy men. Circulation 2000; 101:1767–1772.

126. Fasshauer M, Kralisch S, Klier M, et al. Adiponectin gene expression and secretion is inhibited by interleukin-6 in 3T3–L1 adipocytes. Biochem Biophys Res Commun 2003; 301:1045–1050.

127. Lemberger T, Braissant O, Juge-Aubry C, et al. PPAR tissue distribution and interactions with other hormone-signaling pathways. Ann N Y Acad Sci 1996; 804:231–251.

128. Tafuri SR. Troglitazone enhances differentiation, basal glucose uptake, and Glut 1 protein levels in 3T3–L1 adipocytes. Endocrinology 1996; 137:4706–4712.

129. Rosen ED, Walkey CJ, Puigserver P, Spiegelman BM. Transcriptional regulation of adipogenesis. Genes Dev 2000; 14:1293–1307.

130. Park KS, Abrams-Carter L, Mudalier S, Nikoulina S, Henry RR. Troglitazone effects on gene expression in human skeletal muscle involve regulation of PPAR. Diabetes 1997; 46(suppl):22A.

131. Kruszynska YT, Ranjan M, Lily J, Sharon D, Paterniti JR Jr., Olefsky JM. Skeletal muscle peroxisome proliferator-activated receptor-expression in obesity and non-insulin-dependent diabetes mellitus. J Clin Invest 1998; 101:543–548.

132. Gurnell M, Savage DB, Chatterjee VK, O'Rahilly S. The metabolic syndrome: peroxisome proliferator-activated receptor gamma and its therapeutic modulation. J Clin Endocrinol Metab 2003; 88:2412–2421.

133. Larsen TM, Toubro S, Astrup A. PPAR gamma agonists in the treatment of type II diabetes: is increased fatness commensurate with long-term efficacy? Int J Obes Relat Metab Disord 2003; 27:147–161.

134. Ahren B, Pacini G. Importance of quantifying insulin secretion in relation to insulin sensitivity to accurately assess beta cell function in clinical studies. Eur J Endocrinol 2004; 150:97–104.

135. Jones CN, Pei D, Staris P, Polonsky KS, Chen YD, Reaven GM. Alterations in the glucose-stimulated insulin secretory dose-reponse curve and in insulin clearance in nondiabetic insulin-resistant individuals. J Clin Endocrinol Metab 1997; 82:1834–1838.

136. Kahn SE, Prigeon RL, McCulloch DK, et al. Quantification of the relationship between insulin sensitivity and beta cell function in human subjects. Evidence for a hyperbolic function. Diabetes 1993; 42:1663–1672.

137. Clausen JO, Borch-Johnsen K, Ibsen H, et al. Insulin sensitivity index, acute insulin response, and glucose effectiveness in a population-based sample of 380 young healthy Caucasians. Analysis of the impact of gender, body fat, physical fitness, and life-style factors. J Clin Invest 1996; 98:1195–1209.

138. Ahren B, Pacini G. Islet adaptation to insulin resistance: mechanisms and implications for intervention. Diabetes, Obes Metab 2005; 7:2–8.

139. Pick A, Clark J, Kubstrup C, et al. Role of apoptosis in failure of β-cell mass compensation for insulin resistance and β-cell defects in the male Zucker diabetic fatty rat. Diabetes 1998; 47:358–364.

140. Kousta E, Lawrence NJ, Godsland IF, Penny A, et al. Insulin resistance and β-cell dysfunction in normoglycaemic European women with a history of gestational diabetes. Clin Endocrinol 2003; 59:289–297.

141. O'Meara NM, Sturis J, Van Cauter E, Polonsky KS. Lack of control of ultradian insulin secretory oscillations in impaired glucose tolerance and in non-insulin-dependent diabetes mellitus. J Clin Invest 1993; 92:262–267.

142. Byrne MM, Sturis J, Sobel RJ, Polonsky KS. Elevated plasma glucose 2 h postchallenge predicts defects in β-cell function. Am J Physiol 1996; 270:572–579.

143. Cavaghan MK, Ehrmann DA, Polonsky KS. Interactions between insulin resistance and insulin secretion in the development of glucose intolerance. J Clin Invest 2000; 106:329–333.

144. Donahey JC, van Diijk G, Woods SC, Seeley RJ. Intraventricular GLP-1 reduces short but not long-term food intake or body weight in lean and obese rats. Brain Res 1998; 779:75–83.

145. Gutzwiller JP, Goke B, Drewe J, et al. Glucagon like peptide-1: a potent regulator of food intake in humans. Gut 1999; 44:81–86.

146. Bulotta A, Farilla L, Hui H, Perfetti R. The role of GLP-1 in the regulation of islet cell mass. Cell Biochem Biophys 2004; 40(3 suppl):65–78.

147. Bhavsar S, Watkins J, Young A. Synergy between amylin and cholecystokinin for inhibition of food intake in mice. Physiol Behav 1998; 64:557–561.

148. Gedulin BR, Rink TJ, Young AA. Dose–response for glucagonostatic effect of amylin in rats. Metabolism 1997; 46:67–70.

149. Samsom M, Szarka LA, Camilleri M, Vella A, Zinsmeister AR, Rizza RA. Pramlintide, an amylin analog, selectively delays gastric emptying: potential role of vagal inhibition. Am J Physiol Gastrointest Liver Physiol 2000; 278: 946–951.

150. Lutz TA. Pancreatic amylin as a centrally acting satiating hormone. Curr Drug Targets 2005; 6:181–189.

151. Wake DJ, Walker BR. 11 β-hydroxysteroid dehydrogenase type 1 in obesity and the metabolic syndrome. Mol Cellular Endocrinol 2004; 215:45–45.

152. Meseguer A, Puche C, Cabero A. Sex steroid biosynthesis in white adipose tissue. Horm Metab Res 2002; 34:731–736.

153. Bujalska IJ, Kumar S, Stewart PM. Does central obesity reflect "Cushing's disease of the omentum?" Lancet 1997; 349:1210–1213.

154. Seckle JR, Walker BR. Minireview: 11 β-hydroxysteroid dehydrogenase type-1-α tissue specific amplifier of glucocorticoid action. Endocrinology 2001; 142:1371–1376.

155. Stewart PM, Toogood AA, Tomlinson JW. Growth hormone, insulin-like growth factor-I and the cortisol-cortisone shuttle. Horm Res 2001; 56:1–6.

156. Kotelevtsev Y, Holmes MC, Burchell A, et al. 11β-Hydroxysteroid dehydrogenase type 1 knockout mice show attenuated glucocorticoid-inducible responses and resist hyperglycemia on obesity or stress. Proc Natl Acad Sci USA 1997; 94:14,924–14,929.

157. Masuzaki H, Paterson J, Shinyama H, et al. A transgenic model of visceral obesity and the metabolic syndrome. Science 2001; 294:2166–2170.

158. Walker BR, Best R. Clinical investigation of 11β-hydroxysteroid dehydrogenase. Endocr Res 1995; 21:379–387.

159. Weyer C, Snitker S, Rising R, Bogardus C, Ravussin E. Determinants of age, energy expenditure and fuel utilization in man: effects of body composition, sex, ethnicity and glucose tolerance in 916 subjects. Int J Obes Relat Metab Disord 1999; 23:715–722.

160. Allon MA, Leach RE, Dunbar J, Diamond MP. Effects of chronic hyperandrogenism and/or administered central nervous system insulin on ovarian manifestation and gonadotropin and steroid secretion. Fertil Steril 2005; 83(suppl 1):1319–1326.

161. Dunaif A. Insulin action in the polycystic ovary syndrome. Endocrinol Metab Clin North Am 1999; 28:341–359.

162. Baumann EE, Rosenfield RL. Polycystic ovarian syndrome in adolescence. Endocrinol 2002; 12:333–348.

163. Book CB, Dunaif A. Selective insulin resistance in the polycystic ovary syndrome. J Clin Endocrinol Metab 2001; 86:3115–3119.

164. Rice S, Christoforidis N, Gadd C, et al. Impaired insulin-dependent glucose metabolism in granulosa-lutein cells from an ovulatory women with polycystic ovaries. Hum Reprod 2005; 20:373–381.

165. Barker DJ. In utero programming of cardiovascular disease. Theriogenology 2000; 53:555–574.

166. Kahn IY, Lakasing L, Poston L, Nicolaides KH. Fetal programming for adult disease: where next? J Matern Fetal Neonatal Med 2003; 13:292–299.

167. Ten S, Maclaren N. Insulin resistance syndrome in children. J Clin Endocrinol Metab 2004; 89:2526–2539.

168. Selak MA, Storey BT, Peterside I, Simmons RA. Impaired oxidative phosphorylation in skeletal muscle of intra-uterine growth-retarded rats. Am J Physiol 2003; 285: E130–E137.

169. Wilkin TJ, Metcalf BS, Murphy MJ, Kirkby J, Jeffery AN, Voss LD. The relative contributions of birth weight, weight change, and current weight to insulin resistance in contemporary 5-year-olds: the EarlyBird Study. Diabetes 2002; 51:3468–3472.

170. Hofman PL, Regan F, Jackson WE, et al. Premature birth and later insulin resistance. N Engl J Med 2004; 351: 2179–2186.

171. Mc Cance DR, Pettitt DJ, Hanson RL, Jacobsson LT, Knowler WC, Bennett PH. Birth weight and non-insulin dependent diabetes: thrifty genotype, thrifty phenotype, or surviving small baby genotype? BMJ 1994; 308:942–945.

172. Dabelea D, Pettitt DJ, Hanson RL, Imperatore G, Bennett PH, Knowler WC. Birth weight, type 2 diabetes, and insulin resistance in Pima Indian children and young adults. Diabetes Care 1999; 22:944–950.

173. Murtaugh MA, Jacobs DR, Moran A, Steinberger J, Sinaiko AR. Relation of birth weight to fasting insulin, insulin resistance, and body size in adolescence. Diabetes Care 2003; 26:187–192.

174. Dabelea D, Knowler WC, Pettitt DJ. Effect of diabetes in pregnancy on offspring: follow-up research in the Pima Indians. J Matern Fetal Med 2000; 9:83–88.

175. Sobngwi E, Boudou P, Mauvais-Jarvis F, et al. Effect of a diabetic environment in utero on predisposition to type 2 diabetes. Lancet 2003; 361:1861–1865.

176. Nam SY, Lee EJ, Kim KR, et al. Effect of obesity on total and free insulin-like growth factor (IGF)-1, and their relationship to IGF-binding protein (BP)-1, IGFBP-2, IGFBP-3, insulin, and growth hormone. Int J Obes Relat Metab Disord 1997; 21:355–359.

177. Attia N, Tamborlane WV, Heptulla R, et al. The metabolic syndrome and insulin like growth factor 1 regulation in adolescent obesity. J Clin Endocrinol Metab 1998; 83:1467–1471.

178. Ergun-Longmire B, Sison C, Ten S, Motaghedi R, Maclaren N. Depressed IGFBP-1 levels in obese insulin resistant children are associated with low birth weight [abstr 27662]. Diabetes 2005; 1(suppl 1):A1–A880.

179. Ivandic A, Prpic-Krizevac I, Bozic D, et al. Insulin resistance and androgens in healthy women with different body fat distributions. Wien Klin Wochenschr 2002; 114:321–326.

180. Fernandez-Real JM, Pugeat M, Grasa M, et al. Serum corticosteroid-binding globulin concentration and insulin resistance syndrome: a population study. J Clin Endocrinol Metab 2002; 87:4686–4690.

181. Lind L, Hanni A, Lithell H, Hvarfner A, Sorensen OH, Ljunghall S. 5 Vitamin D is related to blood pressure and other cardiovascular risk factors in middle-aged men. Am J Hypertens 1995; 8:894–901.

182. Pratley RE, Thompson DB, Prochazka M, et al. An autosomal genomic scan for loci linked to prediabetic phenotypes in Pima Indians. J Clin Invest 1998; 101: 1757–1764.

183. Halhali A, Tovar AR, Torres N, Bourges H, Garabedian M, Larrea F. Preeclampsia is associated with low circulating levels of insulin-like growth factor I and 1,25–dihydroxy-vitamin D in maternal and umbilical cord compartments. J Clin Endocrinol Metab 2000; 85:1828–1833.

184. Viitanen L, Pihlajamaki J, Halonen P, et al. Association of angiotensin converting enzyme and plasminogen activator inhibitor-1 promoter gene polymorphisms with features of the insulin resistance syndrome in patients with premature coronary heart disease. Atherosclerosis 2001; 157:57–64.

185. Ma LJ, Mao SL, Taylor KL, et al. Prevention of obesity and insulin resistance in mice lacking plasminogen activator inhibitor 1. Diabetes 2004; 53:336–346.

186. Meigs JB, Mittleman MA, Nathan DM, et al. Hyperinsulinemia, hyperglycemia, and impaired hemostasis: the Framingham Offspring Study. JAMA 2000; 283:221–228.

187. Ginsberg HN. Insulin resistance and cardiovascular disease. J Clin Invest 2000; 106:453–458.

188. Festa A, D'Aotino R Jr., Howard G. Chronic subclinical inflammation as part of the insulin resistance syndrome: the Insulin Resistance Atherosclerosis Study (IRAS). Circulation 2000; 102:42–47.

189. Nesto R. C-reactive protein, its role in inflammation, type 2 diabetes and cardiovascular disease, and the effects of insulin-sensitizing treatment with thiazolidinediones. Diabet Med 2004; 21:810–817.

190. Suheyl Ezgu F, Hasanoglu A, Tumer L, Ozbay F, Aybay C, Gunduz M. Endothelial activation and inflammation in prepubertal obese Turkish children. Metabolism 2005; 54:1384–1389.

191. Ridker PM, Rifai N, Clearfield M. Measurement of C-reactive protein for the targeting of statin therapy in the primary prevention of acute coronary events. N Engl J Med 2001; 344:1959–1965.

192. Pilz S, Horejsi R, Moller R, et al. Early atherosclerosis in obese juveniles is associated with low serum levels of adiponectin. J Clin Endocrinol Metab 2005; 90(8):4792–4796.

193. Tooke JE, Hannemann MM. Adverse endothelial function and the insulin resistance syndrome. J Intern Med 2000; 247:425–431.

194. Paradisi G, Smith L, Burtner C, et al. Dual energy x-ray absorptiometry assessment of fat mass distribution and its association with the insulin resistance syndrome. Diabetes Care 1999; 22:1310–1317.

195. Sowers JR. Insulin resistance and hypertension. Am J Physiol Heart Circ Physiol 2004; 286:H1597–H1602.

196. Artz E, Haqq A, Freemark M. Hormonal and metabolic consequences of childhood obesity. Endocrinol Metab Clin North Am 2005; 34:643–658.

197. Ducimetiere P, Eschwege E, Papoz L, et al. Relationship of plasma insulin levels to the incidence of myocardial infarction and coronary heart disease mortality in a middle-aged population. Diabetologia 1980; 19:205.

198. Despres JP, Lamarche B, Mauriege P, Cantin B, Lupien PJ. Dagenais GR Risk factors for ischaemic heart disease: is it time to measure insulin? Eur Heart J 1996; 17: 1453–1454.

199. Sorof JM, Alexandrov AV, Cardwell G, Portman RJ. Carotid artery intimal-medial thickness and left ventricular hypertrophy in children with elevated blood pressure. Pediatrics 2003; 111:61–66.

200. Fontbonne AM, Eschwege EM. Insulin and cardiovascular disease Paris Prospective Study. Diabetes Care 1991; 14:461–469.

201. Davis PH, Dawson JD, Riley WA, Lauer RM. Carotid intimal-medial thickness is related to cardiovascular risk factors measured from childhood through middle age: The Muscatine Study. Circulation 2001; 104:2815–2819.

202. Raitakari OT, Juonala M, Kahonen M, et al. Cardiovascular risk factors in childhood and carotid artery intima-media thickness in adulthood: the Cardiovascular Risk in Young Finns Study. JAMA 2003; 290: 2277–2283.

203. Tracy RE, Newman WP III, Wattigney WA, Berenson GS. Risk factors and atherosclerosis in youth autopsy findings of the Bogalusa Heart Study. Am J Med Sci 1995; 310(suppl 1): S37–S41.

204. Berenson GS. Childhood risk factors predict adult risk associated with subclinical cardiovascular disease The Bogalusa Heart Study. Am J Cardiol 2002; 90:3L–7L.

205. Strong JP, Malcom GT, McMahan CA, et al. Prevalence and extent of atherosclerosis in adolescents and young adults: implications for prevention from the Pathobiological Determinants of Atherosclerosis in Youth Study. JAMA 1999; 281:727–735.

206. Dixon JB, Bhathal PS, O'Brien PE. Nonalcoholic fatty liver disease: predictors of nonalcoholic steatohepatitis and liver fibrosis in the severely obese. Gastroenterology 2001; 121:91–100.

207. Comert B, Mas MR, Erdem H, et al. Insulin resistance in nonalcoholic steatohepatitis. Dig Liver Dis 2001; 33: 353–358.

208. Pagano G, Pacini G, Musso G, et al. Nonalcoholic steatohepatitis, insulin resistance, and metabolic syndrome: further evidence for an etiologic association. Hepatology 2002; 35:367–372.

209. Matteoni CA, Younossi ZM, Gramlich T, Boparai N, Liu YC, McCullough AJ. Nonalcoholic fatty liver disease: a spectrum of clinical and pathological severity. Gastroenterology 1999; 116:1413–1419.

210. Nair S, Eason JD, Loss GE, Mason AL. Relative risk of hepatocellular carcinoma in cirrhosis due to fatty liver disease: a study based on incidental hepatocellular carcinoma in liver transplant recipients. Hepatology 2001; 34:462A.

211. Tominaga K, Kurata JH, Chen YK, et al. Prevalence of fatty liver in Japanese children and relationship to obesity. An epidemiological ultrasonographic survey. Dig Dis Sci 1995; 40:2002–2009.

212. Oshibuchi M, Nishi F, Sato M, Ohtake H, Okuda K. Frequency of abnormalities detected by abdominal ultrasound among Japanese adults. J Gastroenterol Hepatol 1991; 6:165–168.

213. Silverman JF, Pories WJ, Caro JF. Liver pathology in diabetes mellitus and morbid obesity clinical, pathological, and biochemical considerations. Pathol Annu 1989; 24:275–302.

214. Bjortorp P. "Portal" adipose tissue as a generator of risk factors for cardiovascular disease and diabetes Arteriosclerosis 1990; 10:493–496.

215. Braillon A, Capron JP, Herve MA, Degott, Quenum C. Liver in obesity. Gut 1985; 26:133–139.

216. Tazawa Noguchi H, Nishinomiya F, Takada G. Serum alanine aminotransferase activity in obese children. Acta Paediatr 1997; 86:238–241.

217. Kinugasa A, Tsunamoto K, Furukawa N, Swada T, Kusonoki T, Shimada N. Fatty liver and its fibrous changes found in simple obesity of children. J Pediatr Gastroenterol Nutr 1984; 3:408–414.

218. Strauss RS, Barlow SE, Dietz WH. Prevalence of abnormal serum aminotransferase values in overweight and obese adolescents. J Pediatr 2000; 136:727–733.

219. Ruibal Francisco J, Aleo Lujan E, Alvarez Mingote A, et al. Childhood cholelithiasis. Analysis of 24 patients diagnosed in our department and review of 123 cases. An Esp Pediatr 2001; 54:120–112.

220. Emmerson B. Hyperlipidaemia in hyperuricaemia and gout. Ann Rheum Dis 1998; 57:509–510.

221. Lee J, Sparrow D, Vokonas PS, Landsberg L, Weiss ST. Uric acid and coronary heart disease risk: evidence for a role of uric acid in the obesity-insulin resistance syndrome The Normative Aging Study. Am J Epidemiol 1995; 142:288–294.

222. Cigolini M, Targher G, Tonoli M, Manara F, Muggeo M, De Sandre G. Hyperuricaemia: relationships to body fat distribution and other components of the insulin resistance syndrome in 38-year-old healthy men and women. Int J Obes Relat Metab Disord 1995; 19:92–96.

223. Schmidt MI, Watson RL, Duncan BB, et al. Clustering of dyslipidemia, hyperuricemia, diabetes, and hypertension and its association with fasting insulin and central and overall obesity in a general population. Metabolism 1996; 45:699–706.

224. Roubenoff R, Klag MJ, Mead LA, Liang KY, Seidler AJ, Hochberg MC. Incidence and risk factors for gout in white men. JAMA 1991; 266:3004–3007.

225. Choi HK, Atkinson K, Karlson EW, Curhan G. Obesity, weight change, hypertension, diuretic use, and risk of gout in men: the Health Professionals Follow-up Study. Arch Intern Med 2005; 165:742–748.

226. Emmerson BT. Alteration of urate metabolism by weight reduction. Aust N Z J Med 1973; 3:410–412.

227. Dessein PH, Shipton EA, Stanwix AE, Joffe BI, Ramokgadi J. Beneficial effects of weight loss associated with moderate calorie/carbohydrate restriction, and increased proportional intake of protein and unsaturated fat on serum urate and lipoprotein levels in gout: a pilot study. Ann Rheum Dis 2000; 59:539–543.

228. Ter Maaten JC, Voorburg A, Heine RJ, Ter Wee PM, Donker AJ, Gans RO. Renal handling of urate and sodium during acute physiological hyperinsulinaemia in healthy subjects. Clin Sci (Lond) 1997; 92:51–58.

229. Enomoto A, Kimura H, Chairoungdua A, et al. Molecular identification of a renal urate anion exchanger that regulates blood urate levels. Nature 2002; 417:447–452.

230. Bakker SJ, Gans RO, ter Maaten JC, Teerlink T, Westerhoff HV, Heine RJ. The potential role of adenosine in the pathophysiology of the insulin resistance syndrome. Atherosclerosis 2001; 155:283–290.

231. Sowers JR, Epstein M, Frohlich ED. Diabetes, hypertension, and cardiovascular disease: An update. Hypertension 2001; 37:1053–1059.

232. Hall JE, Crook ED, Jones DW, Wofford MR, Dubbert PM. Mechanisms of obesity-associated cardiovascular and renal disease. Am J Med Sci 2002; 324:127–137.

233. El-Atat FA, Stas SN, McFarlane SI, Sowers JR. The relationship between hyperinsulinemia, hypertension, and progressive renal disease. J Am Soc Nephrology 2004; 15:2816–2827.

234. Yudkin JS. Hyperinsulinemia, insulin resistance, microalbuminuria and the risk of coronary heart disease. Ann Med 1996; 28:433–438.

235. Mykkanen L, Zaccaro DJ, Wagenknecht LE, Robbins DC, Gabriel M, Haffner SM. Microalbuminuria is associated with insulin resistance in nondiabetic subjects: the insulin resistance atherosclerosis study. Diabetes 1998; 7:793–800.

236. Roubenoff R, Hughes VA, Dallal GE, et al. The effect of gender and body composition on the apparent decline

in lean-mass adjusted resting metabolic rate with age. Gerontol A Biol Sci Med Sci 2000; 55:M757–M760.

237. Vaughan L, Zurlo F, Ravussin E. Aging and energy expenditure. Am J Clin Nutr 1991; 53:821–825.

238. Bell C, Day DS, Jones PP, et al. High energy flux mediates the tonically augmented–adrenergic support of resting metabolic rate in habitually exercising older adults. J Clin Endocrinol Metab 2004; 89:3573–3578.

239. Ravussin E, Lillioja S, Knowler WC, et al. Reduced rate of energy expenditure as a risk factor for body-weight gain. N Engl J Med 1988; 318:467–472.

240. Cordain L, Eades MR, Eades MD. Hyperinsulinemic diseases of civilization: more than just Syndrome X. Com Bio Physiol 2003; 136:95–112.

241. Ludwig DS, Majzoub JA, Al-Zahrani A, Dallal GE, Blanco I, Roberts SB. High glycemic index foods, overeating, and obesity. Pediatrics 1999; 103:E26.

242. Ludwig DS. The glycemic index: physiological mechanisms relating obesity, diabetes, and cardiovascular disease. JAMA 2002; 287:2414–2423.

243. Ball SD, Keller KR, Moyer-Mileur LJ, Ding YW, Donaldson D, Jackson WD. Prolongation of satiety after low versus moderately high glycemic index meals in obese adolescents. Pediatrics 2003; 111:488–494.

244. Zammit VA, Waterman IJ, Topping D, McKay G. Insulin stimulation of hepatic triacylglycerol secretion and the etiology of insulin resistance. J Nutr 2001; 131:2074–2077.

245. Craft S, Asthana S, Newcomer JW, et al. Enhancement of memory in Alzheimer disease with insulin and somatostatin, but not glucose. Arch Gen Psychiatry 1999; 56:1135–1140.

246. Havrankova J, Roth J, Brownstein M. Insulin receptors are widely distributed in the central nervous system of the rat. Nature 1978; 272:827–829.

247. Ferrannini E, Galvan AQ, Gastaldelli A, et al. Insulin: new roles for an ancient hormone. Eur J Clin Invest 1999; 29:842–852.

248. Schulingkamp RJ, Pagano TC, Hung D, Raffa RB. Insulin receptors and insulin action in the brain: review and clinical implications. Neurosci Biobehav Rev 2000; 24:855–872.

249. Zhao WQ, Chen H, Quon MJ, Alkon DL. Insulin and the insulin receptor in experimental models of learning and memory. Eur J Pharmacol 2004; 490:71–81.

250. Park CR, Seeley RJ, Craft S, Woods SC. Intracerebroventricular insulin enhances memory in a passive-avoidance task. Physiol Behav 2000; 68:509–514.

251. Zhao W, Chen H, Xu H, Moore E, Meiri N, Quon MJ, Alkon DL. Brain insulin receptors and spatial memory. Correlated changes in gene expression, tyrosine phosphorylation, and signaling molecules in the hippocampus of water maze trained rats. J Biol Chem 1999; 274:34,893–34,902.

252. Singh BS, Rajakumar PA, Eves EM, Rosner MR, Wainer BH, Devaskar SU. Insulin gene expression in immortalized rat hippocampal and pheochromocytoma-12 cell lines. Regul Pept 1997; 69:7–14.

253. Reger MA, Watson GS, Frey WH II, et al. Effects of intranasal insulin on cognition in memory-impaired older adults: modulation by APOE genotype. Neurobiol Aging 2005 [Epub ahead of print].

254. Kuusisto J, Koivisto K, Mykkanen L, et al. Association between features of the insulin resistance syndrome and Alzheimer's disease independently of apolipoprotein E4 phenotype: cross sectional population based study. BMJ 1997; 315:1045–1049.

255. Watson GS, Peskind ER, Asthana S, et al. Insulin increases CSF Abeta42 levels in normal older adults. Insulin increases CSF Abeta42 levels in normal older adults. Neurology 2003; 60:1899–1903.

256. Craft S, Watson GS. Insulin and neurodegenerative disease: shared and specific mechanisms. Lancet Neurol 2004; 3:169–178.

257. Razay G, Wilcock GK. Hyperinsulinemia and Alzheimer's disease. Age Ageing 1994; 23:396–399.

258. Geroldi C, Frisoni GB, Paolisso G, et al. Insulin resistance in cognitive impairment: the In CHIANTI study. Arch Neurol 2005; 62:1067–1072.

259. Watson GS, Cholerton BA, Reger MA, et al. Preserved cognition in patients with early Alzheimer disease and amnestic mild cognitive impairment during treatment with rosiglitazone: a preliminary study. Am J Geriatr Psychiatry 2005; 13:950–958.

260. Miranda PJ, DeFronzo RA, Califf RM, Guyton JR. Metabolic syndrome: definition, pathophysiology, and mechanisms. Am Heart J 2005; 149:33–45.

261. Sun XJ, Rothenberg P, Kahn CR, et al. Structure of the insulin receptor substrate IRS-1 defines a unique signal transduction protein. Nature 1991; 352:73–77.

262. Beck-Nielsen H. The pathogenic role of an insulin-receptor defect in diabetes mellitus of the obese. Diabetes 1978; 27:1175–1181.

263. Maegawa H, Shigeta Y, Egawa K, Kobayashi M. Impaired autophosphorylation of insulin receptors from abdominal skeletal muscles in nonobese subjects with NIDDM. Diabetes 1991; 40:815–819.

264. Freidenberg GR, Henry RR, Klein HH, Reichart DR, Olefsky JM. Decreased kinase activity of insulin receptors from adipocytes of non-insulin-dependent diabetic subjects. J Clin Invest 1987; 79:240–250.

265. Ciaraldi TP, Kolterman OG, Scarlett JA, Kao M, Olefsky JM. Role of glucose transport in the postreceptor defect of non-insulin-dependent diabetes mellitus. Diabetes 1982; 31:1016–1022.

266. Dohm GL, Tapscott EB, Pories WJ, et al. An in vitro human muscle preparation suitable for metabolic studies: decreased insulin stimulation of glucose transport in muscle from morbidly obese and diabetic subjects. J Clin Invest 1988; 82:486–494.

267. Garvey WT, Maianu L, Hancock JA, Golichowski AM, Baron A. Gene expression of GLUT4 in skeletal muscle from insulin-resistant patients with obesity, IGT, GDM, and NIDDM. Diabetes 1992; 41:465–475.

268. Groop LC, Kankuri M, Schalin-Jäntti C, et al. Association between polymorphism of the glycogen synthase gene and non-**insulin**-dependent diabetes mellitus. N Engl J Med 1993; 328:10–14.

269. Vaag A, Henriksen JE, Beck-Nielsen H. Decreased insulin activation of glycogen synthase in skeletal muscles in young nonobese Caucasian first-degree relatives of patients with non-insulin-dependent diabetes mellitus. J Clin Invest 1992; 89:782–788.

270. Taylor SI. Molecular mechanisms of insulin resistance: lessons from patients with mutations in the insulin-receptor gene. Diabetes 1992; 41:1473–1490.

271. Tritos NA, Mantzoros CS. Clinical review 97: syndromes of severe insulin resistance. J Clin Endocrinol Metab 1998; 83:3025–3030.

272. Lavan BE, Lane WS, Lienhard GE. The 60-kDa phosphotyrosine protein in insulin-treated adipocytes is a new member of the insulin receptor substrate family. J Biol Chem 1997; 272:11,439–11,443.

273. White M, Maron R, Kahn C. Insulin rapidly stimulates tyrosine phosphorylation of a Mr 185,000 protein in intact cells. Nature 1985; 318:183–186.

274. Kasuga M, Karlsson FA, Kahn CR. Insulin stimulates the phosphorylation of the 95,000-dalton subunit of its own receptor. Science 1982; 215:185–187.

275. Pessin JE, Saltiel AR. Signaling pathways in insulin action: molecular targets of insulin resistance. J Clin Invest 2000; 106:165–169.

276. Le Roith D, Zick Y. Recent advances in our understanding of insulin action and insulin resistance. Diabetes Care 2001; 24:588–597.

277. Chetham B, Kahn CR. Insulin action and the insulin signaling network. Endocr Rev 1995; 16:117–142.

278. Krook A, Roth RA, Jiang XJ, et al. Insulin-stimulated Akt kinase activity is reduced in skeletal muscle from NIDDM subjects. Diabetes 1998; 47:1281–1286.

279. Kim YB, Nikoulina SE, Ciaraldi TP, et al. Normal insulin-dependent activation of Akt/protein kinase B, with diminished activation of phosphoinositide 3-kinase, in muscle in type 2 diabetes. J Clin Invest 1999; 104:733–741.

280. Cho H, Mu J, Kim JK, et al. Insulin resistance and a diabetes mellitus-like syndrome in mice lacking the protein kinase Akt2 (PKB beta). Science 2001; 292:1728–1731.

281. Zorzano A, Sevilla L, Tomas E, Guma A, Palacin M, Fischer Y. GLUT4 trafficking in cardiac skeletal muscle: isolation characterization of distinct intracellular GLUT4-containing vesicle populations. .

282. Zorzano A, Sevilla L, Tomas E, et al. Trafficking pathway of GLUT4 glucose transporters in muscle. Int J Mol Med 1998; 2:263–271.

283. Garvey WT, Maianu L, Zhu JH, Brechtel-Hook G, Wallace P, Baron AD. Evidence for defects in the trafficking and translocation of GLUT4 glucose transporters in skeletal muscle as a cause of human insulin resistance. J Clin Invest 1998; 101:2377–2386.

284. Patel N, Huang C, Klip A. Cellular location of insulin-triggered signals and implications for glucose uptake. Pflugers Arch 2005 [Epub ahead of print].

285. Cusi K, Maezono K, Osman A. Insulin resistance differentially affects the PI 3-kinase- and MAP kinase-mediated signaling in human muscle. J Clin Invest 2000; 105:311–320.

286. Pratipanawatr W, Pratipanawatr T, Cusi K. Skeletal muscle insulin resistance in normoglycemic subjects with a strong family history of type 2 diabetes is associated with decreased insulin-stimulated insulin receptor substrate-1 tyrosine phosphorylation. Diabetes 2001; 50:2572–2578.

287. Taylor SI. Lilly Lecture: molecular mechanisms of insulin resistance. Lessons from patients with mutations in the insulin-receptor gene. Diabetes 1992; 41:1473–1490.

288. O'Rahilly S, Choi WH, Patel P, Turner RC, Flier JS, Moller DE. Detection of mutations in insulin-receptor gene in NIDDM patients by analysis of single-stranded conformation polymorphisms. Diabetes 1991; 40:777–782.

289. Hart LM, Stolk RP, Heine RJ, Grobbee DE, van-der-Does FE, Maassen JA. Association of the insulin-receptor variant Met-985 with hyperglycemia and non-insulin-dependent diabetes mellitus in the Netherlands: a population-based study. Am J Hum Genet 1996; 59:1119–1125.

290. Tamemoto H, Kadowaki T, Tobe K, et al. Insulin resistance and growth retardation in mice lacking insulin receptor substrate-1. Nature 1994; 372:182–186.

291. Withers DJ, Gutierrez JS, Towery H, et al. Disruption of IRS-2 causes type 2 diabetes in mice. Nature 1998; 391:900–904.

292. Almind K, Bjorbaek C, Vestergaard H, Hansen T, Echwald S, Pedersen O. Aminoacid polymorphisms of insulin receptor substrate-1 in non-insulin-dependentdiabetes mellitus. Lancet 1993; 342:828–832.

293. Bernal D, Almind K, Yenush L, et al. Insulin receptor substrate-2 amino acid polymorphisms are not associated with random type 2 diabetes among Caucasians. Diabetes 1998; 47:976–979.

294. Hansen T, Andersen CB, Echwald SM, et al. Identification of a common amino acid polymorphism in the p85alpha regulatory subunit of phosphatidylinositol 3-kinase: effects on glucose disappearance constant, glucose effectiveness, and the insulin sensitivity index. Diabetes 1997; 46:494–501.

295. Kawanishi M, Tamori Y, Masugi J, et al. Prevalence of a polymorphism of the phosphatidylinositol 3-kinase p85 alpha regulatory subunit (codon 326 Met–>Ile) in Japanese NIDDM patients [letter]. Diabetes Care 1997; 20:1043.

296. Baier LJ, Wiedrich C, Hanson RL, Bogardus C. Variant in the regulatory subunit of phosphatidylinositol 3-kinase (p85alpha): preliminary evidence indicates a potential role of this variant in the acute insulin response and type 2 diabetes in Pima women. Diabetes 1998; 47:973–975.

297. Virkamaki A, Ueki K, Kahn CR. Protein–protein interaction in insulin signaling and the molecular mechanisms of insulin resistance. J Clin Invest 1999; 103:931–943.

298. Dubern B, Clement K, Pelloux V, et al. Mutational analysis of melanocortin-4 receptor, agouti-related protein, and melanocyte-stimulating hormone genes in severely obese children. J Pediatr 2001; 139:204–209.

299. Croft JB, Morrell D, Chase CL, Swift M. Obesity in heterozygous carriers of the gene for the Bardet-Biedl syndrome. Am J Med Genet 1995; 55:12–15.

300. Farooqi IS, Keogh JM, Kamath S, et al. Partial leptin deficiency and human adiposity. Nature 2001; 414:34–35.

301. Zhang Y, Proenca R, Maffei M, Barone M, Leopold L, Friedman JM. Positional cloning of the mouse obese gene and its human homologue. Nature 1994; 372:425–432.

302. Montague CT, Farooqi IS, Whitehead JP, et al. Congenital leptin deficiency is associated with severe early-onset obesity in humans. Nature 1997; 387:903–908.

303. Clement K, Vaisse C, Lahlou N, et al. A mutation in the human leptin receptor gene causes obesity and pituitary dysfunction. Nature 1998; 392:398–401.

304. Spiegelman BM. PPAR-: adipogenic regulator and thiazolidinedione receptor. Diabetes 1998; 47:507–514.

305. Yen CJ, Beamer BA, Negri C, et al. Molecular scanning of the human peroxisome proliferator activated receptor (hPPAR) gene in diabetic Caucasians: identification of a Pro12Ala PPAR 2 missense mutation. Biochem Biophys Res Commun 1997; 241:270–274.

306. Koch M, Rett K, Maerker E, et al. The PPAR2 amino acid polymorphism Pro 12 Ala is prevalent in offspring of Type II diabetic patients and is associated to increased insulin sensitivity in a subgroup of obese subjects. Diabetologia 1999; 42:758–762.

307. Vidal-Puig A, Moller DE. Insulin resistance: classification, prevalence, clinical manifestations, and diagnosis. In: Azziz R, Nestler JE, Dewailly D, eds. Androgen Excess Disorders in Women. Philadelphia: Lippincott Raven, 1997:227–236.

308. Longo N, Wang Y, Smith SA, Langley SD, DiMeglio LA, Giannella Neto D. Genotype-phenotype correlation in inherited severe insulin resistance. Hum Mol Genet 2002; 11:1465–1475.

309. Donohue WL, Uchida I. Leprechaunism: a euphemism for a rare familial disorder. J Pediatr 1954; 45:505–519.

310. Moller DE, Flier JS. Insulin resistance: mechanisms, syndromes, and implications. N Engl J Med 1991; 325:938–948.

311. Uotani S, Yamaguchi Y, Yokota A, et al. Molecular analysis of insulin receptor gene in Werner's syndrome. Diabetes Res Clin Pract 1994; 26:175–176.

312. Barbaro G. HIV-associated lipodystrophy: pathogenesis and clinical features. Adv Cardiol 2003; 40:97–104.

313. Hegele RA. Lamin mutations come of age. Nat Med 2003; 9:644–645.

314. McGarry JD, Dobbins RL. Fatty acids, lipotoxicity and insulin secretion. Diabetologia 1999; 42:128–138.

315. Centers for Disease Control and Prevention. BMI for children and teens. Available at: http://www.cdc.gov/nccdphp/dnpa/bmi/bmi-for-age.htm.

316. St-Pierre J, Lemieux I, Miller-Felix I, et al. Visceral obesity and hyperinsulinemia modulate the impact of the microsomal triglyceride transfer protein-493G/T polymorphism on plasma lipoprotein levels in men. Atherosclerosis 2002; 160:317–324.

317. Bagdade JD, Porte D Jr., Brunzell JD, Bierman EL. Basal and stimulated hyperinsulinism: reversible metabolic sequelae of obesity. J Lab Clin Med 1974; 83:563–569.

318. Ronnemaa T, Koskenvuo M, Marniemi J, et al. Glucose metabolism in identical twins discordant for obesity. The critical role of visceral fat. J Clin Endocrinol Metab 1997; 82:383–387.

319. Bonora E, Del Prato S, Bonadonna RC, et al. Total body fat content and fat topography are associated differently with in vivo glucose metabolism in nonobese and obese nondiabetic women. Diabetes 1992; 41:1151–1159.

320. Bergman RN, Ider YZ, BowdenCR, Cobelli C. Quantitative estimation of insulin sensitivity. Am J Physiol 1979; 236:E667–E677.

321. Daniels SR, Morrison JA, Sprecher DL, Khoury P, Kimball TR. Association of body fat distribution and cardiovascular risk factors in children and adolescents. Circulation 1999; 99:541–545.

322. Morrison JA, Sprecher DL, Barton BA, Waclawiw MA, Daniels SR. Overweight, fat patterning, and cardiovascular disease risk factors in black and white girls: The National Heart, Lung, and Blood Institute Growth and Health Study. J Pediatr 1999; 135:458–464.

323. Morrison JA, Barton BA, Biro FM, Daniels SR, Sprecher DL. Overweight fat patterning, and cardiovascular risk factors in black and white boys. J Pediatr 1999; 135:451–457.

324. Kissebah AH. Insulin resistance in visceral obesity. Int J Obes 1991; 15(suppl 2):109–115.

325. Wajchenberg BL. Subcutaneous and visceral adipose tissue: their relation to the metabolic syndrome. Endocr Rev 2000; 21:697–738.

326. Lara-Castro C, Garvey WT. Diet, insulin resistance, and obesity: zoning in on data for Atkins dieters living in South Beach. J Clin Endocrinol Metab 2004; 89:4197–4205.

327. Le Stunff C, Fallin D, Schork NJ, Bougneres P. The insulin gene VNTR is associated with fasting insulin levels and development of juvenile obesity. Nat Genet 2000; 26:444–446.

328. Clement K, Ferre P. Genetics and the pathophysiology of obesity. Pediatr Res 2003; 53:721–725.

329. Goldfine AB, Bouche C, Parker RA, et al. Insulin resistance is a poor predictor of type 2 diabetes in individuals with no family history of disease. Proc Natl Acad Sci USA 2003; 100:2724–2729.

330. Elbein SC, Hasstedt SJ, Wegner K, Kahn SE. Heritability of pancreatic β-cell function among nondiabetic members of Caucasian familial type 2 diabetic kindreds. J Clin Endocrinol Metab 1999; 84:1398–1403.

331. Facchini FS, Hua N, Abbasi F, Reaven GM. Insulin resistance as a predictor of age-related diseases. J Clin Endocrinol Metab 2001; 86:3574–3578.

332. Daniel S, Noda M, Straub SG, Sharp GW. Identification of the docked granule pool responsible for the first phase of glucose-stimulated insulin secretion. Diabetes 1999; 48:1686–1690.

333. Hanley AJ, D'Agostino R, Wagenknecht LE, et al. Increased proinsulin levels and decreased acute insulin response independently predict the incidence of type 2 diabetes in the insulin resistance atherosclerosis study. Diabetes 2002; 51:1263–1270.

334. Matthews DR, Cull CA, Stratton IM, Holman RR, Turner RC. UKPDS 26: sulphonylurea failure in non-insulin-dependent diabetic patients over six years. UK Prospective Diabetes Study (UKPDS) Group. Diabet Med 1998; 15:297–303.

335. Lillioja S, Mott DM, Spraul M, et al. Insulin resistance and insulin secretory dysfunction as precursors of non-insulin-dependent diabetes mellitus. Prospective studies of Pima Indians. N Engl J Med 1993; 329:1988–1992.

336. Ibanez L, Potau N, de Zegher F. Recognition of a new association: reduced fetal growth, precocious pubarche, hyperinsulinism and ovarian dysfunction. Ann Endocrinol (Paris) 2000; 61:141–142.

337. Ibanez L, Potau N, Francois I, de Zegher F. Precocious pubarche, hyperinsulinism, and ovarian hyperandrogenism in girls: relation to reduced fetal growth. J Clin Endocrinol Metab 1998; 83:3558–3562.

338. Oppenheimer E, Linder B, DiMartino-Nardi J. Decreased insulin sensitivity in prepubertal girls with premature adrenarche and acanthosis nigricans. J Clin Endocrinol Metab 1995; 80:614–618.

339. Ibanez L, Potau N, Zampolli M, et al. Hyperinsulinemia in postpubertal girls with a history of premature pubarche and functional ovarian hyperandrogenism. J Clin Endocrinol Metab 1996; 81:1237–1243.

340. Ibanez L, Ferrer A, Ong K, Amin R, Dunger D, de Zegher F. Insulin sensitization early after menarche prevents progression from precocious pubarche to polycystic ovary syndrome. J Pediatr 2004; 144:23–29.

341. Silfen ME, Manibo AM, McMahon DJ, Levine LS, Murphy AR, Oberfield SE. Comparison of simple measures of insulin sensitivity in young girls with premature adrenarche: the fasting glucose to insulin ratio may be a simple and useful measure. J Clin Endocrinol Metab 2001; 86(6):2863–2868.

342. Bloomgarden ZT. Second World Congress on the Insulin Resistance Syndrome: mediators, pediatric insulin resistance, the polycystic ovary syndrome, and malignancy. Diabetes Care 2005; 28:1821–1830.

343. Lewy VD, Danadian K, Witchel SF, Arslanian S. Early metabolic abnormalities in adolescent girls with polycystic ovarian syndrome. J Pediatr 2001; 138:38–44.

344. Legro RS, Kunselman AR, Dodson WC, Dunaif A. Prevalence and predictors of risk for type 2 diabetes mellitus and impaired glucose tolerance in polycystic ovary syndrome: a prospective, controlled study in 254 affected women. J Clin Endocrinol Metab 1999; 84:165–169.

345. Arslanian SA, Lewy VD, Danadian K. Glucose intolerance in obese adolescents with polycystic ovary syndrome: roles of insulin resistance and beta-cell dysfunction and risk of cardiovascular disease. J Clin Endocrinol Metab 2001; 86:66–71.

346. Ibanez L, Valls C, Ferrer A, Marcos MV, Rodriguez-Hierro F, de Zegher F. Sensitization to insulin induces ovulation in nonobese adolescents with an ovulatory hyperandrogenism. J Clin Endocrinol Metab 2001; 86:3595–3598.

347. Azziz R, Ehrmann D, Legro RS, et al. Troglitazone improves ovulation and hirsutism in the polycystic ovary syndrome: a multicenter, double blind, placebo-controlled trial. J Clin Endocrinol Metab 2001; 86: 1626–1632.

348. Arlt W, Auchus RJ, Miller WL. Thiazolidinediones but not metformin directly inhibit the steroidogenic enzymes P450c17 and 3 beta-hydroxysteroid dehydrogenase. J Biol Chem 2001; 276:16,767–16,771.

349. Reaven GM. Compensatory hyperinsulinemia and the development of an atherogenic lipoprotein profile: the price paid to maintain glucose homeostasis in insulin-resistant individuals. Endocrinol Metab Clin North Am 2005; 34:49–62.

350. Howard BV, Howard WJ. Dyslipidemia in non-insulin-dependent diabetes mellitus. Endocr Rev 1994; 15: 263–274.

351. Despres JP, Lamarche B, Mauriege P, et al. Hyperinsulinemia as an independent risk factor for ischemic heart disease. N Engl J Med 1996; 334:952–957.

352. Cruz ML, Weigensberg MJ, Huang TT, Ball G, Shaibi GQ, Goran MI. The metabolic syndrome in overweight Hispanic youth and the role of insulin sensitivity. J Clin Endocrinol Metab 2004; 89:108–113.

353. National High Blood Pressure Education Working Group. The fourth report on the diagnosis, evaluation, and treatment of high blood pressure in children and adolescents. Pediatrics 2004; 114:555–576.

354. Rashid M, Roberts EA. Nonalcoholic steatohepatitis in children. J Pediatr Gastroenterol Nutr 2000; 30:48–53.

355. Schwimmer JB, Deutsch R, Rauch JB, Behling C, Newbury R, Lavine JE. Obesity, insulin resistance, and other clinicopathological correlates of pediatric nonalcoholic fatty liver disease. J Pediatr 2003; 143(4): 500–505.

356. Schwimmer JB, Middleton M, Deutsch R, Lavine JE. Metformin as a treatment for non-diabetic NASH. J Pediatr Gastroenterol 2003; 37:342.

357. Marchesini G, Brizi M, Bianchi G, Tomassetti S, Zoli M, Melchionda N. Metformin in non-alcoholic steatohepatitis. Lancet 2001; 358:893–894.

358. Lin HZ, Yang SQ, Chuckaree C, Kuhajda F, Ronnet G, Diehl AM. Metformin reverses fatty liver disease in obese, leptin-deficient mice. Nat Med 2000; 6:998–1003.

359. Lavine JE. Vitamin E treatment of nonalcoholic steatohepatitis in children: a pilot study. J Pediatr 2000; 136:734–738.

360. Fukunaga Y, Minamikawa J, Inoue D, Koshiyama H, Fujisawa I. Pseudoacromegaly and hyperinsulinemia: a possibility of premature atherosclerosis? J Clin Endocrinol Metab 1997; 82:3515–3516.

361. Flier JS, Moller DE, Moses AC, et al. Insulin-mediated pseudoacromegaly: clinical and biochemical characterization of a syndrome of selective insulin resistance. J Clin Endocrinol Metab 1993; 76:1533–1541.

362. Kumar S, Durrington PN, O'Rahilly S, et al. Severe insulin resistance, diabetes mellitus, hypertriglyceridemia, and pseudoacromegaly. J Clin Endocrinol Metab 1996; 81: 3465–3468.

363. Dib K, Whitehead JP, Humphreys PJ, et al. Impaired activation of phosphoinositide 3-kinase by insulin in fibroblasts from patients with severe insulin resistance and pseudoacromegaly. A disorder characterized by selective postreceptor insulin resistance. J Clin Invest 1998; 101:1111–1120.

364. Eakman GD, Dallas JS, Ponder SW, Keenan BS. The effects of testosterone and dihydrotestosterone on hypothalamic regulation of growth hormone secretion. J Clin Endocrinol Metab 1996; 81:1217–1223.

365. Nilsson LO, Boman A, Savendahl L, et al. Demonstration of estrogen receptor-β immunoreactivity in human growth plate cartilage. J Clin Endocrinol Metab 1999; 84:370–373.

366. Cowley MA, Smith RG, Diano S, et al. The distribution and mechanism of action of ghrelin in the CNS demonstrates a novel hypothalamic circuit regulating energy homeostasis. Neuron 2003; 37:649–661.

367. Korbonits M, Gueorguiev M, O'Grady E, et al. A variation in the ghrelin gene increases weight and decreases insulin secretion in tall, obese children. J Clin Endocrinol Metab 2002; 87:4005–4008.

368. Farooque SP, Lee TH. Exercise-induced asthma: a review. Practitioner 2003; 247:279–288.

369. Steppan CM, Crawford DT, Chidsey-Frink KL, Ke H, Swick AG. Leptin is a potent stimulator of bone growth in *ob/ob* mice. Regul Pept 2000; 92:73–78.

370. Chen C, Roh SG, Nie GY, et al. The in vitro effect of leptin on growth hormone secretion from primary cultured ovine somatotrophs. Endocrine 2001; 14:73–78.

371. Fu JF, Liang L, Dong GP, Jiang YJ, Zou CC. Obese children with benign acanthosis nigricans and insulin resistance: analysis of 19 cases. Zhonghua Er Ke Za Zhi 2004; 42:917–919.

372. Stuart CA, Driscoll MS, Lundquist KF, Gilkison CR, Shaheb S, Smith MM. Acanthosis nigricans. J Basic Clin Physiol Pharmacol 1998; 9:407–418.

373. Torley D, Munro CS. Genes, growth factors, and acanthosis nigricans. Br J Dermatol 2002; 147:1096–1101.

374. Tan NS, Michalik L, Noy N, et al. Critical roles of PPARβ/ in keratinocyte response to inflammation. Genes Dev 2001; 15:3263–3277.

375. Michalik L, Desvergne B, Tan NS, et al. Impaired skin wound healing in peroxisome proliferator-activated receptor (PPAR) and PPARβ mutant mice. J Cell Biol 2001; 154:799–814.

376. Garcia-Hidalgo L, Orozco-Topete R, Gonzalez-Barranco J, Villa AR, Dalman JJ, Ortiz-Pedroza G. Dermatoses in 156 obese adults. Obese Res 1999; 7:299–302.

377. Hollister DS, Brodell RT. Finger 'pebbles'. A dermatologic sign of diabetes mellitus. Postgrad Med 2000; 107:209–210.

378. Crook MA. Skin tags and atherogenic lipid profile. J Clin Pathol. 2000; 53:873–874.

379. Thiboutot D, Gilliland K, Light J, Lookingbill D. Androgen metabolism in sebaceous glands from subjects with and without acne. Arch Dermatol 1999; 135:1041–1045.

380. Aizawa H, Niimura M. Mild insulin resistance during oral glucose tolerance test (OGTT) in women with acne. J Dermatol 1996; 23:526–529.

381. Nestler JE. Role of hyperinsulinemia in the pathogenesis of the polycystic ovary syndrome, and its clinical implications. Semin Reprod Endocrinol 1997; 15:111–122.

382. Bebakar WM, Honour JW, Foster D, Liu YL, Jacobs HS. Regulation of testicular function by insulin and transforming growth factor-beta. Steroids 1990; 55:266–270.

383. Ford ES, Galuska DA, Gillespie C, Will JC, Giles WH, Dietz WH. C-Reactive protein and body mass index in children: findings from the Third National Health and Nutrition Examination Survey, 1988–1994. J Pediatr 2001; 138:486–492.

384. Visser M, Bouter LM, McQuillan GM, Wener MH, Harris TB. Elevated C-reactive protein levels in overweight and obese adults. JAMA 1999; 282:2131–2135.

385. Valle M, Martas R, Gascan F, et al. Low-grade systemic inflammation, hypoadiponectinemia and high concentration of leptin are present in very young obese children, correlate with metabolic syndrome. Diabetes 2005; 31:55–62.

386. Barzilay JI, Abraham L, Heckbert SR, et al. The relation of markers of inflammation to the development of glucose disorders in the elderly: the Cardiovascular Health Study. Diabetes 2001; 50:2384–2389.

387. Lord GM, Matarese G, Howard JK, Baker RJ, Bloom SR, Lechler RI. Leptin modulates the T-cell immune response and reverses starvation-induced immunosuppression. Nature 1998; 394:897–901.

388. Matarese G, La Cava A, Sanna V, et al. Balancing susceptibility to infection and autoimmunity: a role for leptin? Trends Immunol 2002; 23:182–187.

389. Ozata M, Ozdemir IC, Licinio J. Human leptin deficiency caused by a missense mutation: multiple endocrine defects, decreased sympathetic tone, and immune system dysfunction indicate new targets for leptin action, greater central than peripheral resistance to the effects of leptin, and spontaneous correction of leptin-mediated defects. J Clin Endocrinol Metab 1999; 84:3686–3695.

390. Castro-Rodriguez JA, Holberg CJ, Morgan WJ, Wright AL, Martinez FD. Increased incidence of asthma-like symptoms in girls who become overweight or obese during the school years. Am J Respir Crit Care Med 2001; 163:1344–1349.

391. Stenius-Aarniala B, Poussa T, Kvarnstrom J, Gronlund EL, Ylikahri M, Mustajoki P. Immediate and long term effects of weight reduction in obese people with asthma: randomised controlled study. Br Med J 2000; 320:827–832.

392. Phipps PR, Starritt E, Caterson I, Grunstein RR. Association of serum leptin with hypoventilation in human obesity. Thorax 2002; 57:75–76.

393. Must A, Jacques PF, Dallal GE. Long-term morbidity and mortality of overweight adolescents. A follow-up of the Harvard Growth Study of 1922 to 1935. N Engl J Med 1992; 327:1350–1355.

394. Manoff EM, Banffy MB, Winell JJ. Relationship between body mass index and slipped capital femoral epiphysis. J Pediatr Orthop 2005; 25:744–746.

395. Third Report of the National Cholesterol Education Program Expert Panel on Detection, Evaluation and Treatment of High Blood Cholesterol in Adults (Adult Treatment Panel III) final report. Circulation 2002; 106:3143–3421.

396. Jessup A, Harrel JS. The metabolic syndrome: look for it in children and adolescents, too!. Clinical Diabetes 2005; 23:26–30.

397. Katzmarzyk P, Srinivasan S, Wei C, Malina R, Bouchard C, Berenson G. Body mass index waist circumference clustering of cardiovascular disease risk factors in a biracial sample of children adolescents. Pediatrics 2004; 114:E198–E205.

398. Bergman RN. Toward physiological understanding of glucose tolerance: minimal model approach. Diabetes 1989; 38:1512–1527.

399. Bergman RN, Prager R, Volund A, Olefsky JM. Equivalence of the insulin sensitivity index in man derived by the minimal model method and the euglycemic glucose clamp. J Clin Invest 1987; 79:790–800.

400. Reaven GM, Brand RJ, Chen YD, Mathur AK, Goldfine I. Insulin resistance and insulin secretion are determinants of oral glucose tolerance in normal individuals. Diabetes 1993; 42:1324–1332.

401. Reaven GM, Chen YD, Hollenbeck CB, Sheu WH, Ostrega D, Polonsky KS. Plasma insulin, C-peptide, and proinsulin concentrations in obese and nonobese individuals with varying degrees of glucose tolerance. J Clin Endocrinol Metab 1993; 76:44–48.

402. Matthews DR, Hosker JP, Rudenski AS, Naylor BA, Treacher DF, Turner RC. Homeostasis model assessment: insulin resistance and β-cell function from fasting plasma glucose and insulin concentrations in man. Diabetologia 1985; 28:412–419.

403. Katz A, Nambi SS, Mather K, et al. Quantitative insulin sensitivity check index: a simple, accurate method for assessing insulin sensitivity in humans. J Clin Endocrinol Metab 2000; 85:2402–2410.

404. Belfiore F, Iannello S, Volpicelli G. Insulin sensitivity indices calculated from basal and OGTT-induced insulin, glucose, and FFA levels. Mol Genet Metab 1998; 63: 134–141.

405. Cederholm J, Wibell L. Insulin release and peripheral sensitivity at the oral glucose tolerance test. Diabetes Res Clin Pract 1990; 10:167–175.

406. Young-Hyman D, Schlundt DG, Herman L, De Luca F, Counts D. Evaluation of the insulin resistance syndrome in 5- to 10-year-old overweight/obese African-American children. Diabetes Care 2001; 24:1359–1364.

407. Matsuda M, De Fronzo RA. Insulin sensitivity indices obtained from oral glucose tolerance testing: comparison with the euglycemic insulin clamp. Diabetes Care 1999; 22:1462–1470.

408. Stumvoll M, Mitrakou A, Pimenta W, et al. Use of the oral glucose tolerance test to assess insulin release and insulin sensitivity. Diabetes Care 2000; 23:295–301.

409. Soonthornpun S, Setasuban W, Thamprasit A, Chayanunnukul W, Rattarasarn C, Geater A. Novel insulin sensitivity index derived from oral glucose tolerance test. J Clin Endocrinol Metab 2003; 88:1019–1023.

410. McAuley KA WS, Mann JI, Walker RJ, Ledwis-Barned NJ, Temple LA, Duncan AS. Diagnosing insulin resistance in general population. Diabetes Care 2001; 24:460–464.

411. Mari A, Pacini G, Murphy E, Ludvik B, Nolan JJ. A model-based method for assessing insulin sensitivity from the oral glucose tolerance test. Diabetes Care 2001; 24:539–548.

412. http://www.ladseb.pd.cnr.it/ bioing/ogis/home.html.

413. Hanson RL, Pratley RE, Bogardus C, et al. Evaluation of simple indices of insulin sensitivity and insulin secretion for use in epidemiologic studies. Am J Epidemiol 2000; 15:190–198.

414. Gutt M, Davis CL, Spitzer SB, et al. Validation of the insulin sensitivity index (ISI(0,120)): comparison with other measures. Diabetes Res Clin Pract 2000; 47:177–184.

415. Gower BA, Granger WM, Franklin F, Shewchuk RM, Goran MI. Contribution of insulin secretion and clearance to glucose-induced insulin concentration in African-American and caucasian children. J Clin Endocrinol Metab 2002; 87:2218–2224.

416. Sunehag AL, Treuth MS, Toffolo G, et al. Glucose production, gluconeogenesis, and insulin sensitivity in children and adolescents: an evaluation of their reproducibility. Pediatr Res 2001; 50:115–123.

417. Cutfield WS, Bergman RN, Menon RK, Sperling MA. The modified minimal model: application to measurement of insulin sensitivity in children. J Clin Endocrinol Metab 1990; 70:1644–1650.

418. Elahi D. In praise of the hyperglycemic clamp. A method for assessment of β-cell sensitivity and insulin resistance. Diabetes Care 1996; 19:278–286.

419. Brandou F, Brun JF, Mercier J. Limited accuracy of surrogates of insulin resistance during puberty in obese and lean children at risk for altered glucoregulation. J Clin Endocrinol Metab 2005; 90(2):761–767.

420. American Academy of Pediatric Committee on Nutrition. Prevention of pediatric overweight and obesity. Pediatrics 2003; 112:424–430.

421. Williams CL, Hayman LL, Daniels SR, et al. Cardiovascular health in childhood: a statement for health professionals from the Committee on Atherosclerosis, Hypertension, and Obesity in the Young (AHOY) of the Council on Cardiovascular Disease in the Young, American Heart Association. Circulation 2002; 106:143–160.

422. Barlow SE, Dietz WH. Obesity evaluation and treatment: Expert Committee recommendations. The Maternal and Child Health Bureau, Health Resources and Services Administration and the Department of Health and Human Services. Pediatrics 1998; 102:E29.

423. Grundy SM, Hansen B, Smith SC Jr., Cleeman JI, Kahn RA; American Heart Association; national Heart, Lung, and Blood Institute; American Diabetes Association. Clinical management of metabolic syndrome: report of the American Heart Association/National Heart, Lung, and Blood Institute/American Diabetes Association conference on scientific issues related to management. Circulation 2004; 109:551–556.

424. Diabetes Prevention Program Research Group. Reduction in the incidence of type 2 diabetes with lifestyle intervention or metformin. N Engl J Med 2002; 346: 393–403.

425. Cruz ML, Shaibi GQ, Weigensberg MJ, Spruijt-Metz D, Ball GD, Goran MI. Pediatric obesity and insulin resistance: chronic disease risk and implications for treatment and prevention beyond body weight modification. Annu Rev Nutr 2005; 25:435–468.

426. Field AE, Austin SB, Taylor CB, et al. Relation between dieting and weight change among preadolescents and adolescents. Pediatrics 2003; 112:900–906.

427. Steffen LM, Jacobs DR Jr, Murtaugh MA, et al. Whole grain intake is associated with lower body mass and greater insulin sensitivity among adolescents. Am J Epidemiol 2003; 158:243–250.

428. Murtaugh MA, Jacobs DR Jr., Jacob B, Steffen LM, Marquart L. Epidemiological support for the protection of whole grains against diabetes. Proc Nutr Soc 2003; 62:143–149.

429. Ebbeling CB, Ludwig DS. Treating obesity in youth: Should dietary glycemic load be a consideration? Adv Pediatr 2001; 48:179–212.

430. Ebbeling CB, Leidig MM, Sinclair KB, Hangen JP, Ludwig DS. A reduced-glycemic load diet in the treatment of adolescent obesity. Arch Pediatr Adolesc Med 2003; 157:773–779.

431. Roberts SB. High-glycemic index foods, hunger and obesity: is there a connection? Nutr Rev 2000; 58:163–169.

432. Barlow SE, Dietz WH. Management of child and adolescent obesity: summary and recommendations based on reports from pediatricians, pediatric nurse practitioners, and registered dietitians. Pediatrics 2002; 110:236–238.

433. Epstein LH, Roemmich JN, Raynor HA. Behavioral therapy in the treatment of pediatric obesity. Pediatr Clin North Am 2001; 48:981–993.

434. Pasquali R, Antenucci D, Casimirri F, et al. Clinical and hormonal characteristics of obese amenorrheic hyperandrogenic women before and after weight loss. J Clin Endocrinol Metab 1989; 68:173–179.

435. Irwin ML, Mayer-Davis EJ, Addy CL, et al. Moderate-intensity physical activity and fasting insulin levels in women: the Cross-Cultural Activity Participation Study. Diabetes Care 2000; 23:449–454.

436. Kelley DE, Goodpaster BH. Effects of physical activity on insulin action and glucose tolerance in obesity. Med Sci Sports Exerc 2001; 31:S619–S623.

437. Kriska AM, Pereira MA, Hanson RL, et al. Association of physical activity and serum insulin concentrations in two populations at high risk for type 2 diabetes but differing by BMI. Diabetes Care 2001; 24:1175–1180.

438. Goodpaster BH, Katsiaras A, Kelley DE. Enhanced fat oxidation through physical activity is associated with improvements in insulin sensitivity in obesity. Diabetes 2003; 52:2191–2197.

439. Ball GD, Shaibi GQ, Cruz ML, Watkins MP, Weigensberg MJ, Goran MI. Insulin sensitivity, cardiorespiratory fitness, and physical activity in overweight Hispanic youth. Obes Res 2004; 12:77–85.

440. Schmitz KH, Jacobs DR Jr., Hong CP, Steinberger J, Moran A, Sinaiko AR. Association of physical activity with insulin sensitivity in children. Int J Obes Relat Metab Disord 2002; 26:1310–1316.

441. Ferguson MA, Gutin B, Le NA, Karp W, et al. Effects of exercise training and its cessation on components of the insulin resistance syndrome in obese children. Int J Obes Relat Metab Disord 1999; 23:889–895.

442. Kang HS, Gutin B, Barbeau P, et al. Physical training improves insulin resistance syndrome markers in obese adolescents. Med Sci Sports Exerc 2002; 34:1920–1927.

443. LeMura LM, Maziekas MT. Factors that alter body fat, body mass, and fat-free mass in pediatric obesity. Med SciSports Exerc 2002; 34:487–496.

444. Shoemaker JK, Bonen A. Vascular actions of insulin in health and disease. Can J Appl Physiol 1995; 20:127–154.

445. Akimoto-Gunther L, Hubler M, Santos M, et al. Effects of re-education in eating habits and physical activity on the lipid profile of obese teenagers. Clin Chem Lab Med 2002; 40:460–462.

446. Kelly AS, Wetzsteon RJ, Kaiser DR, Steinberger J, Bank AJ, Dengel DR. Inflammation, insulin, and endothelial function in overweight children and adolescents: the role of exercise. J Pediatr 2004; 145:731–736.

447. Woo KS, Chook P, Yu CW, et al. Effects of diet and exercise on obesity-related vascular dysfunction in children. Circulation 2004; 109:1981–1986.

448. Youngren JF, Keen S, Kulp JL, Tanner CJ, Houmard JA, Goldfine ID. Enhanced muscle insulin receptor autophosphorylation with short-term aerobic exercise training. Am J Physiol Endocrinol Metab 2001; 280:E528–E533.

449. Evans JL, Youngren JF, Goldfine ID. Effective treatments for insulin resistance: trim the fat and douse the fire. Trends Endocrinol Metab 2004; 15:425–431.

450. Cigolini M, Zancanaro C, Benati D, Cavallo E, Bosello O, Smith U. Metformin enhances insulin binding to "in vitro" down regulated human fat cells. Diabetes Metab 1987; 13:20–22.

451. Di Paolo S. Metformin ameliorates extreme insulin resistance in a patient with anti-insulin receptor antibodies: description of insulin receptor and postreceptor effects in vivo and in vitro. Acta Endocrinol (Copenh) 1992; 126:117–123.

452. Matthaei S, Hamann A, Klein HH, et al. Association of metformin's effect to increase insulin-stimulated glucose transport with potentiation of insulin-induced translocation of glucose transporters from intracellular pool to plasma membrane in rat adipocytes. Diabetes 1991; 40:850–857.

453. Rique S, Ibanez L, Marcos MV, Carrascosa A, Potau N. Effects of metformin on androgens and insulin concentrations in type A insulin resistance syndrome. Diabetologia 2000; 43:385–386.

454. Hundal HS, Ramlal T, Reyes R, Leiter LA, Klip A. Cellular mechanism of metformin action involves glucose transporter translocation from an intracellular pool to the plasma membrane in L6 muscle cells. Endocrinology 1992; 131:1165–1173.

455. Hamann A, Benecke H, Greten H, Matthaei S. Metformin increases glucose transporter protein and gene expression in human fibroblasts. Biochem Biophys Res Commun 1993; 196:382–387.

456. Matthaei S, Reibold JP, Hamann A, et al. In vivo metformin treatment ameliorates insulin resistance: evidence

for potentiation of insulin-induced translocation and increased functional activity of glucose transporters in obese (*fa/fa*) Zucker rat adipocytes. Endocrinology 1993; 133:304–311.

457. Matthaei S, Hamann A, Klein HH, et al. Evidence that metformin increases insulin-stimulated glucose transport by potentiating insulin-induced translocation of glucose transporters from an intracellular pool to the cell surface in rat adipocytes. Horm Metab Res 1992; 26(suppl):34–41.

458. Nestler JE, Jakubowicz DJ. Decreases in ovarian cytochrome P450c17 activity and serum free testosterone after reduction of insulin secretion in polycystic ovary syndrome. N Engl J Med 1996; 335:617–623.

459. Sarlis NJ, Weil SJ, Nelson LM. Administration of metformin to a diabetic woman with extreme hyperandrogenemia of nontumoral origin: management of infertility and prevention of inadvertent masculinization of a female fetus. J Clin Endocrinol Metab 1999; 84:1510–1512.

460. Jakubowicz DJ, Iuorno MJ, Jakubowicz S, Roberts KA, Nestler JE. Effects of metformin on early pregnancy loss in the polycystic ovary syndrome. J Clin Endocrinol Metab 2002; 87:524–529.

461. De Leo V, La Marca A, Orvieto R, Morgante. Effect of metformin on insulin-like growth factor (IGF) I and IGF-binding protein I in polycystic ovary syndrome. J Clin Endocrinol Metab 2000; 85:1598–1600.

462. Freemark M, Bursey D. The effects of metformin on body mass index and glucose tolerance in obese adolescents with fasting hyperinsulinemia and a family history of type 2 diabetes. Pediatrics 2001; 107:E55.

463. Morrison JA, Cottingham EM, Barton BA. Metformin for weight loss in pediatric patients taking psychotropic drugs. Am J Psychiatry 2002; 159:655–657.

464. Jones KL, Arslanian S, Peterokova VA, Park JS, Tomlinson MJ. Effect of metformin in pediatric patients with type 2 diabetes: a randomized controlled trial. Diabetes Care 2002; 25:89–94.

465. Kay JP, Alemzadeh R, Langley G, D'Angelo L, Smith P, Holshouser S. Beneficial effects of metformin in normoglycemic morbidly obese adolescents. Metabolism 2001; 50:1457–1461.

466. Ten S, NI, Vogiatzi M, New M, Maclaren N. Adrenal suppressibility by dexamethasone in women with polycystic ovarian syndrome (PCOS) determined by degree of insulin resistance. Program of the 85th Annual Meeting of the Endocrine Society, Philadelphia, PA, 2003:351 [abstr P2–187].

467. Kersten S. Peroxisome proliferator activated receptors and obesity. Eur J Pharmacol 2002; 440:223–234.

468. Aljada A, Ghanim H, Friedman J, Garg R, Mohanty P, Dandona P. Troglitazone reduces the expression of PPAR while stimulating that of PPAR in mononuclear cells in obese subjects. J Clin Endocrinol Metab 2001; 86:3130–3133.

469. Marx N, Bourcier T, Sukhova GK, Libby P, Plutzky J. PPAR activation in human endothelial cells increases plasminogen activator inhibitor type-1 expression: PPAR as a potential mediator in vascular disease. Arterioscler Thromb Vasc Biol 1999; 19:546–551.

470. Dunaif A, Scott D, Finegood D, Quintana B, Whitcomb R. The insulin-sensitizing agent troglitazone improves metabolic and reproductive abnormalities in the polycystic ovary syndrome. J Clin Endocrinol Metab 1996; 81:3299–3306.

471. Guan HP, Li Y, Jensen MV, Newgard CB, Steppan CM, Lazar MA. A futile metabolic cycle activated in adipocytes by antidiabetic agents. Nat Med 2002; 8:1122–1128.

472. Okopien B, Krysiak R, Kowalski J, et al. Monocyte release of tumor necrosis factor-alpha and interleukin-1beta in primary type IIa and IIb dyslipidemic patients treated with statins or fibrates. J Cardiovasc Pharmacol 2005; 46:377–386.

473. Wierzbicki AS, Mikhailidis DP, Wray R, et al. Statin-fibrate combination: therapy for hyperlipidemia: a review. Curr Med Res Opin 2003; 19:155–168.

474. Palinski W, Tsimikas S. Immunomodulatory effects of statins: mechanisms and potential impact on arteriosclerosis. J Am Soc Nephrol 2002; 13:1673–1681.

475. Jiang G, Zhang BB. Modulation of insulin signalling by insulin sensitizers. Biochem Soc Trans 2005; 33:358–361.

476. McDuffie JR, Calis KA, Uwaifo GI, et al. Three-month tolerability of orlistat in adolescents with obesity-related comorbid conditions. Obes Res 2002; 10:642–650.

477. Ozkan B, Bereket A, Turan S, Keskin S. Addition of orlistat to conventional treatment in adolescents with severe obesity. Eur J Pediatr 2004; 163(12):738–741.

478. Berkowitz RI, Wadden TA, Tershakovec AM, Cronquist JL. Behavior therapy and sibutramine for the treatment of adolescent obesity: a randomized controlled trial. JAMA 2003; 289:1805–1812.

479. Derosa G, Cicero AF, Murdolo G, Ciccarelli L, Fogari R. Comparison of metabolic effects of orlistat and sibutramine treatment in Type 2 diabetic obese patients. Diabetes Nutr Metab 2004; 17:222–229.

480. Boyd ST, Fremming BA. Rimonabant-A selective CB1 Antagonist. Ann Pharmacother 2005; 39:684–690.

481. Heshmati HM, Caplain H, Bellisle F, Mosse M, Fauveau C, Le Fur G. SR 141716, a selective cannabinoid CB-1 receptor antagonist, reduces, hunger, caloric intake, and body weight in overweight or obese men [abstr]. Obes Res 2001; 9(suppl 1):S70.

482. Van Gaal L. RIO-Europe: a randomized double-blind study of weight reducing effect and safety of rimonabant in obese patients with or without comorbidities. Program and abstracts from the European Society of Cardiology Congress 2004, August 28–September 1, Munich, Germany.

483. Zhang JV, Ren PG, Avsian-Kretchmer O, et al. Obestatin, a peptide encoded by the ghrelin gene, opposes ghrelin's effects on food intake. Science 2005; 310:996–999.

484. Farooqi IS, Matarese G, Lord GM, et al. Beneficial effects of leptin on obesity, T cell hyporesponsiveness, and neuroendocrine/metabolic dysfunction of human congenital leptin deficiency. J Clin Invest 2002; 110:1093–1103.

485. Gorden P, Gavrilova O. The clinical uses of leptin. Curr Opin Pharmacol 2003; 3:655–659.

486. Faught E, Ayala R, Montouris GG, et al. Randomized controlled trial of zonisamide for the treatment of refractory partial-onset seizures. Neurology 2001; 57(10):1774–1779.

487. Elterman RD, Glauser TA, Wyllie E, et al. A double-blind, randomized trial of topiramate as adjunctive therapy for partial-onset seizures in children. Topiramate YP Study Group. Neurology 1999; 52(7):1338–1344.

488. Wilding J, Van Gaal L, Rissanen A, Vercruysse F, Fitchet M; OBES-002 Study Group. A randomized double-blind placebo-controlled study of the long-term efficacy and safety of topiramate in the treatment of obese subjects. Int J Obes Relat Metab Disord 2004; 28(11):1399–1410.

489. Liang Y, Chen X, Osborne M, DeCarlo SO, Jetton TL, Demarest K. Topiramate ameliorates hyperglycaemia and improves glucose-stimulated insulin release in ZDF rats and db/db mice. Diabetes Obes Metab 2005; 7(4):360–369.

490. Wilkes JJ, Nguyen MT, Bandyopadhyay GK, Nelson E, Olefsky JM. Topiramate treatment causes skeletal muscle insulin sensitization and increased Acrp30 secretion in high-fat-fed male Wistar rats. Am J Physiol Endocrinol Metab 2005; 289(6):E1015-1022.

491. Zeymer U. Cardiovascular benefits of acarbose in impaired glucose tolerance and type 2 diabetes. Int J Cardiol 2006; 107:11–20.

492. Chiasson JL, Josse RG, Gomis R, Hanefeld M, Karasik A, Laakso M; STOP-NIDDM Trail Research Group. Acarbose for prevention of type 2 diabetes mellitus: the STOP-NIDDM randomised trial. Lancet 2002; 359:2072–2077.

493. Chiasson JL, Josse RG, Gomis R, Hanefeld M, Karasik A, Laakso M; STOP-NIDDM Trial Research Group. Acarbose treatment and the risk of cardiovascular disease and hypertension in patients with impaired glucose tolerance: the STOP-NIDDM trial. JAMA 2003; 290:486–494.

494. Pontiroli AE, Pizzocri P, Librenti MC, et al. Laparoscopic adjustable gastric banding for the treatment of morbid (grade 3) obesity and its metabolic complications: a three-year study. J Clin Endocrinol Metab 2002; 87: 3555–3561.

495. Mason EE. Gastric surgery for morbid obesity. Surg Clin North Am 1992; 72:501–513.

12

Low Birth Weight and Endocrine Dysfunction in Postnatal Life

Maria Verónica Mericq G.

*Department of Medicine, Institute of Maternal and Child Research, University of Chile,
Las Condes, Santiago, Chile*

INTRODUCTION

Small size at birth has long been recognized to increase neonatal morbidity and mortality. As early as 1962, Neel, a population geneticist, proposed that changes of in utero environment made to guarantee survival during adverse conditions could become harmful during nutrition abundance (1). This concept is now well established. Reduced growth in early life is strongly linked with a number of endocrine dysfunctions. Included among the most important alterations are insulin insensitivity, gonadal and somatotropic axis abnormalities, and premature adrenarche (2,3). These have been associated with an escalating prevalence of Type 2 diabetes mellitus (T2DM) (4) coronary heart disease (CHD) (5), abnormal gonads and genitalia (6–9), growth hormone (GH) resistance and decreased growth (7,10), and early puberty (8). The usual hypothesis proposed to explain the development of these long-term alterations relates to the thrifty phenotype as an adaptive response to in utero malnutrition (9) and modifications thereof; initially termed "fetal origins" (11) and updated to "developmental origins," which include the additional contributions of the patterns of growth in infancy and childhood (10). Throughout this chapter, we review the current knowledge of the programming of the fetus and infant, which lead to endocrine dysfunction in postnatal life.

GENETIC FACTORS OF FETAL GROWTH

Fetal growth is a delicate controlled process influenced by hormones, growth factors and the intrauterine milieu. Examples of some variables that affect fetal growth are chromosomal abnormalities, genetic diseases, maternal alterations (TORCH, hypertension, nutrition, tobacco, collagen diseases), and placental and demographic factors. The mechanisms that participate in the regulation of size at birth and the later consequences of the intrauterine insult are shown in Figure 1. Insulin trophic actions play a key role in the regulation of fetal growth; this is evidenced by

the severe intrauterine growth impairment occurring in congenital mutations of the insulin structure or of the insulin pathway function (1–3) and by the reduced size of the fetus present at birth in infants with specific gene mutations (10,12,13). The opposite picture develops in diabetic hyperglycemic mothers who give birth to large-for-gestational age infants as a result of chronic in utero fetal hyperinsulinism, which develops to compensate for maternal glycemic fluxes.

Experimental models that retard fetal growth in rats induce modifications of glucose utilization in several fetal tissues (12,14). In addition, insulin-like growth factors (IGFs) and their binding proteins (IGFBPs) are involved in the regulation of fetal growth (13). In fact, the mechanisms of action of IGFs and insulin are shared at several levels in the cell (15). Models that attempt to explain the association of low birth weight (LBW) and postnatal diseases consider as central the action of insulin and related peptides (11,16). Genetically programmed low energy consumers would present resistance to anabolic hormones such as insulin (17). However, no mutation has been identified to explain the strong highly prevalent linkage to insulin resistance genes (18).

The candidate genes associated with reduced size at birth are shown in Table 1. These include homozygous or compound heterozygous insulin receptor (IR) mutations causing Leprechaunism (19), insulin promoter factor-I (IPF1) mutation with pancreatic agenesis (20), and heterozygous glucokinase mutation (14). These mutations may involve alterations in any of the factors that belong to the family of growth receptors with intrinsic tyrosine kinase activity, including the IR, IGF-I, its receptor (IGF-I-R), and the hybrid IR/IGF-I-R (21). These lead to signaling pathway alterations in insulin action and constitute molecular targets of insulin resistance (22). The cellular effectors of insulin participate in intermediary metabolism and in cell proliferation; a disruption in action results in insulin resistance (22,23).

The pattern of insulin secretion per se is able to modify the response of peripheral tissues to this

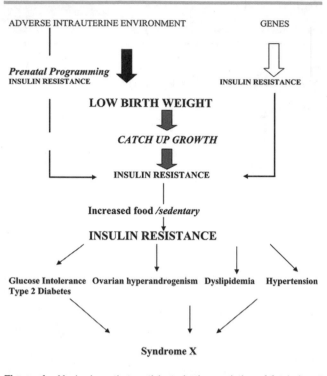

Figure 1 Mechanisms that participate in the regulation of fetal size at birth and later consequences of intrauterine insult.

hormone (24). A relevant factor that determines the pattern of insulin secretion is the short-term insulin gene transcription by glucose in the late phase of Beta cell response (25). In vitro, the gene promoter of variable number of tandem repeat (VNTR) alleles of insulin is able to modify its transcriptional activity through the Pur-1 factor (26). These molecular findings have clear clinical correlations that associate allelic variants of VNTR in the insulin gene with diabetes mellitus (DM), as well as reduced size at birth (27,28). In Caucasian populations, the most frequent allelic VNTR at the insulin gene minisatellite locus (Type I) is associated with an increased risk for Type 1 DM (T1DM), whereas the Type III allelic VNTR is associated with T2DM, obesity and ovarian hyperandrogenism (23,27). The Type III allele is also associated with increased birth weight (28). We

Table 1 Genes Associated with Reduced Growth Utero "Thrifty Genotype"

Homozygote or compound heterozygous insulin receptor mutations	Leprechaunism
IPF1 mutation with pancreatic agenesis	LBW
Heterozygous glucokinase mutation	LBW
IGF-I	LBW
IGF-I receptor	LBW
Insulin gene: polymorphism of tandem repeat in the promoter gene of insulin (VNTR) I/I	LBW
GRB-10 and H19	Russell–Silver syndrome (LBW)

Abbreviations: IGF, insulin-like growth factor; LBW, low birth weight; VNTR, variable number of tandem repeat; IPF-1, insulin promoter factor-1.

recently demonstrated a greater insulin secretion after an intravenous (IV) glucose infusion in a cohort of term one-year-old infants who had the Type III allelic VNTR (29). A second candidate gene, the one encoding calpain (CAPN10), was also identified as being responsible for the T2DM association with the 1 locus in chromosome 2 (30). Other genes that have been proposed to be involved in the association of LBW and later insulin resistance include IGF-1, IRS-1, Glucokinase, H19, preadipocyte factor-1, and growth factor receptor–bound proteins, which constitute a family of structurally related multidomain adapters with diverse cellular functions, which have been implicated in the regulation of IR signaling (14,31).

IN UTERO PROGRAMMING

Several authors have proposed the existence of a prenatal metabolic programming that would promote the development of a "thrifty phenotype" (9). A poor intrauterine nutrition would determine an endocrine adaptation designated to sustain the development of more sensitive organs, such as the central nervous system. This response consists mainly of the inhibition of anabolic factors (insulin and IGFs) in muscle, adipose, and connective tissues during the time of need, which would persist into adult life (11). In animal models there are some examples of prenatal adaptations that persist into postnatal life (32,33). However, in humans, there is no direct evidence to support this theory.

Programming Evidence

Various experimental models have been utilized to study the potential in utero programming mechanisms of a thrifty phenotype. Nutritional restriction of the pregnant animal, in terms of total calories or protein deprivation, is a model that has been utilized to test this hypothesis (32). The human extension of these results has been controversial (34), since LBW due to maternal nutrition deprivation is rare in the occidental world. Another model employed has been the restriction of oxygen delivery to the placental–uterine bed. This model exposes the pregnant animal to low oxygen tension in the environment (35). This model is clearly not applicable to humans.

Wigglesworth developed a model in rats that limits the uteroplacental oxygen delivery (36), and this has also been applied to sheep (37). In this model, partial or total stretching of the uterine artery(s) during the last part of gestation is used. Recent modifications to the technique apply repeated embolization of uterine vessels (38) and systemic use of vasoconstrictor agents such as tromboxan (39). These maneuvers have been used to better reflect what occurs in intrauterine growth restriction (IUGR) due to placental dysfunction, which is the most common cause of small-for-gestational age (SGA) deliveries (50%) (40).

In spite of the differences between the above experimental models, the data have been consistent and provide evidence of the fetal and new born metabolic consequences of the adverse intrauterine environment. Both protein caloric restriction and vascular supply produce a fetus and newborn that develops hypoglycemia, hypoaminoacidemia, and hypoinsulinemia, among the most important metabolic consequences (41,42). Hypoinsulinemia correlated with the alterations in the development of beta cells in the islet of Langerhans (43,44). However there was no glucose intolerance and the glucose uptake in peripheral tissues (muscle and adipose) (45) and insulin/glucose ratios in fetuses and newborns indicated that there was a greater insulin sensitivity compared to control animals (41,42). These findings are in agreement with limited human data provided by chordocentesis (46).

These experimental data have led some authors to cast a note of caution about the Barker's hypothesis, which considers the development of insulin resistance during fetal life (11). Alternatively, it could also be that the resistance is specific to certain tissues. In fact, that is what has been shown when protein-restrictive models are used; namely changes of expression in glucose transporter (GLUT) family proteins in adipose, muscle, and nervous tissues (47). The applicability of these findings to humans was demonstrated (48).

Programming Mechanisms

Insulin sensitivity might be altered during fetal life as a response to endocrine modifications following an adverse intrauterine environment (Fig. 2). One of such

modification could be the increased levels of circulating cortisol, a counter-acting hormone to insulin. In addition, the hyperactivity of the hypothalamic-pituitary-adrenal axis as a consequence of fetal stress (49,50) may be attributable to a decreased activity of the placental enzyme 11β-hydroxysteroid dehydrogenase, which degrades cortisol and thereby alters the maternal impact of the fetal compartment (51). The enhancement of cortisol levels would act in several tissues, including the liver, which is key in determining insulin sensitivity (52). Tumor necrosis factor-α (TNF-α) is also able to induce insulin resistance in several tissues (53). In fact, a certain polymorphism in the promoter region of the TNF-α gene has been linked to the development of insulin resistance in adults (54). Elevated TNF levels are present in fetal blood in several fetal stress situations, such as premature delivery and intrauterine infection (55).

The initial associations of LBW with a decrease in insulin sensitivity were established in studies performed in Hertfordshire, England. In the first studies, 5654 men born between 1911 and 1948 whose birth weights and subsequent growth until one year of age had been registered, were retrospectively analyzed. In this population, those with the lowest birth weight had the highest mortality rates due to cardiovascular disease (5). From the same population, 468 men had a fasting glucose determination and 370 had a complete oral glucose tolerance test (OGTT); 40% of men with birth weights equal to or below 2.5 kg had a glycemia at two and four hours of 140 mg/dL or more compared with only 14% of men born with the highest weights (56). Subsequently, other retrospective studies documented the presence of the other components of the metabolic

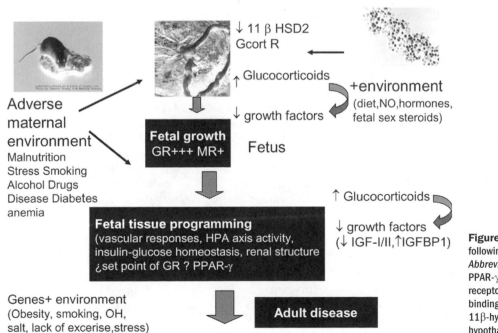

Figure 2 Possible endocrine modifications following an adverse intrauterine environment. *Abbreviations:* IGF, insulin-like growth factor; PPAR-γ, peroxisome proliferator-activated receptors-γ; IGFBP, insulin-like growth factor binding proteins; NO, nitric oxide; 11β-HSD, 11β-hydroxysteroid dehydrogenase; HPA, hypothalamic–pituitary–adrenal.

syndrome, i.e., hypertension and hypercholesterolemia (57,58). These studies confirmed the greater risk of this disease when LBW was present (59,60).

Some of these observations were replicated in different countries and populations of different backgrounds. In India, a study of 517 adults found that the prevalence of CHD was 11% in those with LBW of less than 2500 g whereas in those with a birth weight of 3100 g or more, it was 3%. These associations were independent of other variables associated the CHD such as life style (60,61). The association of T2DM and glucose intolerance with CHD and hypertension suggested that insulin resistance could be present in LBW infants.

POSTNATAL PROGRAMMING OF ENDOCRINE DYSFUNCTION

One of the main limitations of the above-mentioned studies is the retrospective analysis where birth weight is related to the metabolic status or complications detected in later life. These studies did not take into account early growth and metabolic changes that occurred after birth. Since 1998, a number of authors have proposed that postnatal growth of LBW children, as characterized by the body mass index (BMI) at seven to eight years of life, might be an independent factor determining insulin sensitivity (16,62–64). This hypothesis was confirmed in a term cohort of LBW Chilean children (65). Insulin resistance could be programmed in the early postnatal life during the "catch-up growth" (CUG) phase shown by SGA infants. During this phase of CUG, there is an increase in the levels of several anabolic hormones such as insulin and related peptides (IGFs) (66). Insulin resistance could initially develop in SGA to counteract their tendency to hypoglycemia and would then persist during their entire life. CUG could also lead to a disproportionate increase of fat compared to lean mass acquisition (67,68). Some authors propose that suppressed thermogenesis leads to this unequal distribution of fat and lean mass during the CUG period (67). This theory has gained more acceptance because of the current epidemiological data of the explosive worldwide increase in T2DM, which has specially affected those countries where LBW is more prevalent (69).

Ong et al. in the Avon longitudinal study of pregnancy and childhood (ALSPAC) cohort also showed that early CUG predicted increased body fat mass and central fat distribution at five years of age (70). We demonstrated that at one, two, and three years of age, insulin secretion and sensitivity were related to the patterns of CUG. Fasting insulin sensitivity was more closely related to weight CUG and current BMI, whereas insulin secretion appeared to be directly related to length CUG (65). These data were in accordance with previous studies that showed that at later stages of life, those born SGA with early CUG have a greater risk of Syndrome X (71). Recently,

a prospective study of the ALSPAC cohort, which included term newborns with a large variation of normal birth size, confirmed these observations. At eight years of age, those who were lighter and grew faster in early life were the most insulin resistant among the cohort (72). Eriksson et al. analyzed the influence of early CUG and birth weight in CHD deaths (63). Greater mortality rates were present among those subjects who were lighter at birth, but had a normal or increased BMI at seven years of age.

In a pioneering pediatric study by Hofman et al., insulin sensitivity was studied through a long IV glucose tolerance test (IVGTT) in prepubertal short stature children, either born SGA or appropriate for gestational age (AGA) (73). This method allowed the detection of a significant difference in insulin sensitivity; those born SGA had an increased acute phase of insulin release (445 vs.174 µg/mL). Early changes in insulin sensitivity, secretion, and lipid metabolism were associated with being born SGA at term (74). During the first 48 hours of life, SGA infants displayed increased insulin sensitivity with respect to glucose disposal, but showed suppression of lipolysis, ketogenesis, and hepatic production of IGFBP-3, compared with AGA children.

One element of the puzzle not previously clarified was whether the decrease in postnatal insulin sensitivity in SGA children was present only when the adverse condition was present in utero or could also develop when adverse postnatal conditions were present, as in the case of an extremely premature birth. It has been suggested that postnatal morbidity during a critical period of rapid growth might contribute to the metabolic modifications observed in LBW children, independently of the adequacy of their birth weight to gestational age. Another question was the effect of prematurity per se, because in most studies, the birth weight had been evaluated independently of gestational age or preterm infants were excluded. Therefore, the link between LBW and postnatal insulin resistance was assessed regardless of gestational age (63,75,76). The effects of current BMI, birth weight standard deviation score (SDS), postnatal growth rates, and indicators of postnatal morbidity were evaluated in 20 SGA and 40 AGA very-low-birth-weight (VLBW) children (birth weight between 690 and 1500 g; gestational age 25–34 weeks). They were evaluated at five to seven years of age by a short IVGTT. In this cohort of premature, VLBW children, IUGR rather than LBW was associated with reduced sensitivity to insulin. This link was independent of gestational age and other indicators of postnatal stress. In addition, fasting and first-phase insulin secretion were related to postnatal growth rates, which were in accordance with our previous observations (77). However, an opposite finding was reported by Hofman et al., but in their report no comments of the interaction of growth in utero and postnatal growth was described. In addition, the New Zealand cohort was rather small and children had short stature (78).

Several gene polymorphisms involved in the control of intermediary metabolism, such as the insulin gene variable number of tandem repeat (INS VNTR) alleles and Ghrelin $C^{247}A(y)$ leptin $C^{-2549}A$ in peripheral DNA were not related to growth kinetics or to IVGTT response (29). However, at one year, class III/III alleles in the INS VNTR locus were associated with increased fasting as well as poststimulated insulin. These findings were independent of birth weight and postnatal growth kinetics.

One of the important and constant findings regarding the determinants of insulin sensitivity during adulthood is that LBW is not a major determinant of later insulin resistance, except among subjects with the largest current BMI (72). The factors that determine the transition from relatively LBW to childhood overweight are not known, but could be mediated by increased appetite. The regulation of food intake is a complex process involving neural and gut interactions (Vol. 1; Chap. 1). One of the hormones involved in this interplay is Ghrelin (79) and the specific 7 transmembrane G protein–coupled receptor for this hormone present in the hypothalamic arcuate nucleus and pituitary (80). In animal studies, the intracerebrovascular and peripheral administration of Ghrelin induces adiposity and increases appetite, and this orexigenic activity appears to be mediated by increases in NPY (81). In humans, Ghrelin levels are decreased in obesity and increased in anorexia (74).

Because most SGA infants show some degree of postnatal length and weight CUG and because this phenomenon affects postnatal insulin sensitivity independently of birth weight, we postulated that Ghrelin appetite effects could be involved in the CUG. The fasting and post-IVGTT circulating Ghrelin levels in SGA and AGA infants aged one year were not different (82). As seen in older children and adults, circulating Ghrelin concentrations rapidly decreased after IV glucose. Interestingly, postglucose Ghrelin levels, but not fasting values, correlated positively with current length, current weight, and change in weight. In addition, lower reductions in circulating Ghrelin levels following IV glucose were observed in SGA infants who showed greater weight gain during infancy, suggesting that a sustained orexigenic drive could contribute to postnatal growth.

In the literature, only one report addresses the interaction between LBW, postnatal growth, and genetic background. Jaquet et al. (83) investigated the role of several polymorphisms that modulate insulin sensitivity: Proala12 in peroxisome proliferator-activated receptors-γ (PPAR-γ), G+250C in the β3 adrenergic receptor, and G-308A in TNF-α. They genotyped 171 adults who were born SGA and 233 who were born AGA, submitted to an OGTT. The SGA group showed higher serum insulin concentrations at fasting and during stimulation and their fasting glucose–insulin ratios were significantly higher in the TNF/-308, PPAR/ala12, and ADRB3/+250G carriers. Moreover, the effects of these polymorphisms on insulin resistance indexes were significantly potentiated by current BMI in the SGA group (83). In neither the SGA nor AGA group did the polymorphisms affect glucose tolerance.

MECHANISMS OF DEVELOPMENT OF INSULIN RESISTANCE IN SMALL-FOR-GESTATIONAL-AGE SUBJECTS

In young adults with a normal BMI and a similar fat mass, glucose oxidation rate and uptake were diminished in those born SGA as compared with those subjects born AGA (84). In those born SGA, a decreased expression of GLUT-4 in muscle and adipose tissues during an euglycemic hyperinsulinemic clamp was detected (48). Glucose uptake was also reduced during an euglycemic hyperinsulinemic clamp in eight-year-old children (73). These findings reinforce the concept of abnormal glucose transport as an important element in the control of insulin sensitivity. Recently, a study performed in the offspring of young, lean patients with T2DM showed an increase in intramyocellular lipid content, concomitant with impairment of mitochondrial activity in those who were insulin resistant versus insulin-sensitive patients (85).

The adipocyte has been shown to be an active cell that secretes bioactive molecules, termed "adipokines" (86,87). The molecules produced by the adipocyte have autocrine and paracrine actions. These include leptin, TNF-α, plasminogen activator inhibitor Type 1, and adiponectin. Adiponectin is a 244–amino acid protein, product of the most abundant gene transcript-1 expressed in human adipose tissue (88). Recently two adiponectin receptors have been described: adiponectin receptor-1 abundantly expressed in skeletal muscle and adiponectin receptor-2 predominantly expressed in liver (89). Several studies have demonstrated that adiponectin modulates glucose tolerance and insulin sensitivity (90–92). In animal models, this protein decreased circulating free fatty acids by increasing oxidation in muscle and decreasing uptake in liver, with subsequent lower plasma triglyceride levels (93). It also directly activates glucose uptake in adipocytes and muscle through adenosine monophosphate protein kinase. In humans, adiponectin levels predict subsequent changes in insulin resistance, but not lipid profiles or body weight (94,95). Adiponectin mRNA is decreased in the adipose tissue of obese and diabetic patients, but is restored to normal levels after weight loss. Increases in adiponectin levels have been described after weight loss in obese and diabetic subjects. In adult Pima Indians, higher plasma adiponectin levels appeared to protect against the development of T2DM (96). In a small sample of 5- to 10-year-old children, hypoadinectinemia appeared to be the consequence of obesity, but no associations with insulin sensitivity were found (97).

However, it is difficult to assess the effects of weight gain and insulin sensitivity from small cross-sectional studies. We therefore determined whether adiponectin levels were related to patterns of postnatal growth and insulin sensitivity in a prospective cohort of infants followed from birth to two years (98). Serum adiponectin levels at one and two years were higher compared with reported levels in adults and older children and were significantly decreased from one to two years. At two years, adiponectin levels were lower in females as compared with males, but no gender differences were seen in leptin and insulin levels. Also no differences existed in adiponectin levels between SGA and AGA infants at one year or two years. However, in SGA infants, the changes in adiponectin levels from year 1 to year 2 were inversely related to weight gain. Adiponectin levels were not related to insulin levels at one or two years, nor to change in insulin levels. Multiple regression analysis revealed that adiponectin levels were only related to postnatal age. Other determinants of higher adiponectin levels were male gender, lower postnatal body weight, and higher birth weight SDS. In conclusion, changes in serum adiponectin levels during the first two years of life were related to patterns of weight gain in SGA infants, but not to early changes in insulin sensitivity (98).

GONADAL AND ADRENAL AXIS

The child born small is at increased risk for abnormalities of the gonads and genitalia. Francois et al. showed that unexplained, severe hypospadias was related either to restraint of prenatal growth or to complications in early pregnancy (99). This evidence has been supported by the data of Nordic countries where cryptorchidism as well as hypospadias has been found more frequently in SGA babies (100,101).

A conclusive support for the concept of nongenetic pseudohermaphroditism was presented by de Zegher and coworkers (6). This report of monozygotic twins whose gestation was supported by one placenta showed that they were discordant for birth weight and for male differentiation. Detailed studies revealed no evidence for any endocrinopathies. The genitalia of the AGA male were normal, while the SGA male had perineal hypospadias and testes in labia-scrotal folds. It is difficult to conceive an experiment whereby a genetic cause of male pseudohermaphroditism could be more convincingly excluded.

Almost half a century ago, Silver noticed that some men who were born small tended to have high urinary gonadotropin levels and small testes (102). This was the first observation indicating that prenatal growth restraint may be followed by reduced Sertoli-cell function and by subnormal spermatogenesis. More recently, Ibanez et al. assessed the serum concentrations of inhibin B to determine whether there was a relation between reduced prenatal growth and subsequent Sertoli-cell dysfunction in infancy (103). SGA boys appear to need a higher follicle-stimulating

hormone (FSH) drive to generate the normal feedback level of inhibin B.

Premature adrenarche, the prepubertal rise in the secretion of adrenal steroids, occurs in association with decreased insulin sensitivity in the obese and in girls born SGA (104). The presence of premature adrenarche in SGA girls was reported in Spain (2) and in a group of Hispanic and African-American girls living in New York (105). A decrease in insulin sensitivity could be the drive to increased adrenal steroidogenesis. Ibanez et al. also postulated that CRH might be the potent adrenal secretagogue in these girls (106). In addition, exaggerated adrenarche appears as a risk marker of ovarian hyperandrogenism (107). In the northern Spanish girls evaluated by Ibanez et al., the SGA female had smaller ovaries and a smaller uterus in adolescence and also had FSH hypersecretion, first noted during infancy and also present later in adolescence (108,109). However, it is important to note that these studies only evaluated girls from an endocrine clinic, with a similar ethnic background. Treatment with the insulin sensitizer metformin was tried in a Catalunian cohort of nonobese adolescents born SGA with eumenorrheic anovulatory cycles (103). After only six weeks, ovulatory cycles resumed and lipid levels improved. A simultaneous decrease in luteinizing hormone, FSH, insulin, and androgen levels was noted, which suggest that SGA-associated anovulation is a result of hyperinsulinism rather than adrenal and ovarian hyperandrogenism. It remains to be elucidated whether these risks are also present in healthy girls born SGA recruited from the community and from other ethnicities, as studies in France (110) and Holland failed to show such an association (111).

SOMATOTROPIC AXIS

The fetal somatotropic axis is characterized by GH resistance in the SGA fetus. A simple way to understand the somatotropic axis of the SGA fetus is to consider such as being in a fasting condition. SGA fetuses display low serum levels of insulin, IGF-1, IGF-2, and IGFBP-3 and high levels of IGFBP-1, whereas the large-for-gestational age infant shows high insulin and IGF-1 levels and a reverse pattern of IGF binding proteins (7).

After birth, CUG occurs in the vast majority of SGA children (112). Postnatal CUG begins immediately after birth, with a maximum occurring by six months of age. By two years of age, nearly 90% of term or preterm SGA infants achieve a height within the normal range. The age of two years is an important milestone: In SGA children who were born at term, it is quite rare to observe spontaneous CUG after the age of two. Of the SGA infants who fail to show CUG by two years about half remain short even in adulthood. The relative risk for being short at age 18 is 5.2 for children born light and 7.1 for children born short. Failure of CUG could be secondary to altered action of GH, IGF-I, or insulin.

Different series show that there is an increased frequency of growth hormone deficiency (GHD) among SGA with non-CUG (35–53%). Even when GH levels are normal on standard stimulation tests, these children demonstrate abnormalities in the pattern and 24-hour profile of GH and lower IGF-I and IGFBP-3 (113,114). Cutfield, however, in a selected population of short SGA children, found normal or elevated IGF-I levels and postulated that hyperinsulinism could play a role (115). Possible differences among studies could be related to the heterogeneous nature of the SGA condition and some form of IGF-I resistance present in a subset of these children (Vol. 2; Chap. 1).

During the last decade, several investigators studied the effects of therapy with GH for those SGA infants who remained small after two years of age. Over the years, it has become evident that GH administration improved growth velocity, weight gain, height SDS, and final height in SGA children independent of their response to provocative testing. The height gain appears to be related mainly to the total time of GH therapy and the dose employed (116,117). During GH therapy, weight gain is improved, not due to an excess of fat, but to an increase in lean body mass shown by magnetic resonance imaging and levels of serum leptin (118). Importantly, GH stimulation testing is not a requirement prior to therapy and does not predict growth response during therapy. These tests are recommended only if GHD is clinically suspected in an SGA child in view of postnatal growth failure, poor facial development, or poor skeletal growth. Bone age is usually delayed and height prediction is unreliable in children born SGA (119) (Vol. 2; Chap. 5).

In July 2001, a consensus with final Food and Drug Administration (FDA) approval of GH therapy as an indication for non-CUG SGA children emerged (120). Recent reports evaluating the final height of SGA children treated with GH showed that it was significantly improved (121). The standard dose of GH, however, is less effective in assisting short children born SGA to achieve a sufficient CUG. The FDA-approved dose for SGA is 0.48 mg/K/wk. In Europe, a lower starting dose of 0.35 mg/K/wk is recommended. The main determinants of final height are GH dose, duration of treatment, and greater family corrected initial height deficit.

In addition to improvements in height, positive metabolic effects such as lower blood pressure and beneficial effects on craniofacial development, body composition, less atherogenic lipid profile, and psychological well being have been observed (122).

A number of safety issues have been addressed. So far, the evidence continues to be reassuring for GH therapy in these children. In particular, GH does not seem to increase the risk for precocious puberty or glucose intolerance. Benign cranial hypertension, aggravation of scoliosis, jaw prominence, and mild transient hyperglycemia have been reported in recent KIGS data. However, these adverse events were not different from the short stature population given GH therapy (123–125) (Vol. 2; Chap. 5).

CONCLUSIONS

Investigations performed during the last decade have identified the independent association between reduced fetal growth and the later development of endocrine dysfunction primarily manifested by gonadal, adrenal, somatropic, and metabolic abnormalities. Insulin resistance appears to play a critical early role in at least the adrenal and the metabolic alterations associated with frequent diseases, producing increased morbidity and mortality among adults. Data suggest that the link between prenatal growth restriction and postnatal insulin sensitivity is already present at one year of age. On the other hand, IUGR rather than LBW appears to be associated with reduced sensitivity to insulin. Finally, rapid postnatal CUG appears to contribute actively to insulin sensitivity and secretion, at least during the first years of life. We speculate that accelerated CUG during the postnatal period may lead to the development of a metabolically disadvantaged body composition, with an increase, preferentially, in body fat independent of birth weight as has been demonstrated for other conditions where CUG occurs (67,68).

The importance of these data to daily clinical practice is to identify SGA as a risk marker of insulin resistance and T2DM.

On the other hand, there is a clear need to reconcile the contribution of the "thrifty phenotype" and "thrifty genotype" in the generation of adverse health outcomes after a period of nutritional deprivation in early life. The determination of these respective contributions will also clarify the evolutionary adaptations that improve the likelihood of survival of a developing organism that is under duress, but may carry a consequence for poor adult health outcomes after reproductive senescence. It is clear that the use of terms such as programming, plasticity, and predictive adaptative responses may each be hotly debated, particularly as experimental and epidemiological studies investigate the impact of relative nutrition in prenatal life. On the other hand, during postnatal life, the focus of experimental and epidemiological studies will need to investigate the role of environmental factors that modulate rapid CUG. Until these data are available, we will not, in a position to recommend the types of intervention required to improve the efficiency of the growth of these infants to minimize the risk of the morbidity and mortality complications prevalent in adults who were born SGA (Vol. 2; Chap. 5).

REFERENCES

1. Neel JV. Diabetes mellitus: a "thrifty" genotype rendered detrimental by "progress"? Am J Hum Genet 1962; 14: 353–362.
2. Ibanez L, Potau N, de Zegher F. Precocious pubarche, dyslipidemia, and low IGF binding protein-1 in girls: relation to reduced prenatal growth. Pediatr Res 1999; 46(3):320–322.

3. Ibanez L et al. Exaggerated adrenarche and hyperinsulinism in adolescent girls born small for gestational age. J Clin Endocrinol Metab; 1999; 84(12):4739–4741.

4. Hales CN, Barker DJ. Type 2 (non-insulin-dependent) diabetes mellitus: the thrifty phenotype hypothesis. Diabetologia 1992; 35(7):595–601.

5. Barker DJ et al. Growth in utero, blood pressure in childhood and adult life, and mortality from cardiovascular disease. BMJ 1989; 298(6673):564–567.

6. Mendonca BB, Billerbeck AE, de Zegher F. Nongenetic male pseudohermaphroditism and reduced prenatal growth. N Engl J Med 2001; 345(15):1135.

7. Woods KA et al. The somatotropic axis in short children born small for gestational age: relation to insulin resistance. Pediatr Res 2002; 51(1):76–80.

8. Ibanez L et al. Early puberty: rapid progression and reduced final height in girls with low birth weight. Pediatrics 2000; 106(5):E72.

9. Hales CN, Barker DJ. The thrifty phenotype hypothesis. Br Med Bull 2001; 60:5–20.

10. Bateson P et al. Developmental plasticity and human health. Nature 2004; 430(6998):419–421.

11. Barker DJ. Fetal origins of coronary heart disease. BMJ 1995; 311(6998):171–174.

12. Lueder FL et al. Chronic maternal hypoxia retards fetal growth and increases glucose utilization of select fetal tissues in the rat. Metabolism 1995; 44(4):532–537.

13. Accili D et al. Targeted gene mutations define the roles of insulin and IGF-I receptors in mouse embryonic development. J Pediatr Endocrinol Metab 1999; 12(4):475–485.

14. Hattersley AT et al. Mutations in the glucokinase gene of the fetus result in reduced birth weight. Nat Genet 1998; 19(3):268–270.

15. Pessin JE, Saltiel AR. Signaling pathways in insulin action: molecular targets of insulin resistance. J Clin Invest 2000; 106(2):165–169.

16. Cianfarani S, Germani D, Branca F. Low birthweight and adult insulin resistance: the "catch-up growth" hypothesis. Arch Dis Child Fetal Neonatal Ed 1999; 81(1):F71–F73.

17. Hattersley AT, Tooke JE. The fetal insulin hypothesis: an alternative explanation of the association of low birthweight with diabetes and vascular disease. Lancet 1999; 353(9166):1789–1792.

18. Stern MP. Strategies and prospects for finding insulin resistance genes. J Clin Invest 2000; 106(3):323–327.

19. Wertheimer E et al. Homozygous deletion of the human insulin receptor gene results in leprechaunism. Nat Genet 1993; 5(1):71–73.

20. Stoffers DA, et al. Pancreatic agenesis attributable to a single nucleotide deletion in the human IPF1 gene coding sequence. Nat Genet 1997; 15(1):106–110.

21. Longo N et al. Activation of glucose transport by a natural mutation in the human insulin receptor. Proc Natl Acad Sci USA 1993; 90(1):60–64.

22. Virkamaki A, Ueki K, Kahn CR. Protein-protein interaction in insulin signaling and the molecular mechanisms of insulin resistance. J Clin Invest 1999; 103(7):931–943.

23. Waterworth DM et al. Linkage and association of insulin gene VNTR regulatory polymorphism with polycystic ovary syndrome. Lancet 1997; 349(9057):986–990.

24. Nankervis A et al. Hyperinsulinaemia and insulin insensitivity: studies in subjects with insulinoma. Diabetologia 1985; 28(7):427–431.

25. Leibiger B et al. Short-term regulation of insulin gene transcription by glucose. Proc Natl Acad Sci USA 1998; 95(16):9307–9312.

26. Lew A, Rutter WJ, Kennedy GC. Unusual DNA structure of the diabetes susceptibility locus IDDM2 and its effect on transcription by the insulin promoter factor Pur-1/MAZ. Proc Natl Acad Sci USA 2000; 97(23):12508–12512.

27. Bennett ST et al. Susceptibility to human type 1 diabetes at IDDM2 is determined by tandem repeat variation at the insulin gene minisatellite locus. Nat Genet 1995; 9(3):284–292.

28. Dunger DB et al. Association of the INS VNTR with size at birth. ALSPAC Study Team. Avon Longitudinal Study of Pregnancy and Childhood [see comments]. Nat Genet 1998; 19(1):98–100.

29. Bazaes RA et al. Insulin gene VNTR genotype is associated with insulin sensitivity and secretion in infancy. Clin Endocrinol (Oxf) 2003; 59(5):599–603.

30. Horikawa Y et al. Genetic variation in the gene encoding calpain-10 is associated with type 2 diabetes mellitus. Nat Genet 2000; 26(2):163–175.

31. Gicquel C et al. Epimutation of the telomeric imprinting center region on chromosome 11p15 in Silver–Russell syndrome. Nat Genet 2005; 37(9):1003–1007.

32. Holness MJ. Impact of early growth retardation on glucoregulatory control and insulin action in mature rats. Am J Physiol 1996; 270(6 Pt 1):E946–E954.

33. Holness MJ, Sugden MC. Antecedent protein restriction exacerbates development of impaired insulin action after high-fat feeding. Am J Physiol 1999; 276(1 Pt 1):E85–E93.

34. Symonds ME, Budge H, Stephenson T. Limitations of models used to examine the influence of nutrition during pregnancy and adult disease. Arch Dis Child 2000; 83(3):215–219.

35. Tapanainen PJ et al. Maternal hypoxia as a model for intrauterine growth retardation: effects on insulin-like growth factors and their binding proteins. Pediatr Res 1994; 36(2):152–158.

36. Wigglesworth JS. Fetal growth retardation. Animal model: uterine vessel ligation in the pregnant rat. Am J Pathol 1974; 77(2):347–350.

37. Jones CT et al. Studies on the growth of the fetal sheep. Effects of surgical reduction in placental size, or experimental manipulation of uterine blood flow on plasma sulphation promoting activity and on the concentration of insulin-like growth factors I and II. J Dev Physiol 1988; 10(2):179–189.

38. Llanos AJ et al. Increased heart rate response to parasympathetic and beta adrenergic blockade in growth-retarded fetal lambs. Am J Obstet Gynecol 1980; 136(6):808–813.

39. Fukami E et al. Underexpression of neural cell adhesion molecule and neurotrophic factors in rat brain following thromboxane A(2)-induced intrauterine growth retardation. Early Hum Dev 2000; 58(2):101–110.

40. Gaziano E et al. The predictability of the small-for-gestational-age infant by real-time ultrasound-derived measurements combined with pulsed Doppler umbilical artery velocimetry. Am J Obstet Gynecol 1988; 158(6 Pt 1):1431–1439.

41. Ogata S et al. Altered growth, hypoglycemia, hypoalaninemia, and ketonemia in the young rat: postnatal consequences of intrauterine growth retardation. Pediatr Res 1985; 19(1):32–37.

42. Ogata ES, Bussey ME, Finley S. Altered gas exchange, limited glucose and branched chain amino acids, and hypoinsulinism retard fetal growth in the rat. Metabolism 1986; 35(10):970–977.

43. De Prins FA, Van Assche FA. Intrauterine growth retardation and development of endocrine pancreas in the experimental rat. Biol Neonate 1982; 41(1–2):16–21.

44. Garofano A, Czernichow P, Breant B. In utero undernutrition impairs rat beta-cell development. Diabetologia 1997; 40(10):1231–1234.

45. Lueder FL, Ogata ES. Uterine artery ligation in the maternal rat alters fetal tissue glucose utilization. Pediatr Res 1990; 28(5):464–468.

46. Economides DL, Proudler A, Nicolaides KH. Plasma insulin in appropriate- and small-for-gestational-age fetuses. Am J Obstet Gynecol 1989; 160(5 Pt 1):1091–1094.

47. Sadiq HF, deMello DE, Devaskar SU. The effect of intrauterine growth restriction upon fetal and postnatal hepatic glucose transporter and glucokinase proteins. Pediatr Res 1998; 43(1):91–100.

48. Jaquet D et al. Impaired regulation of glucose transporter 4 gene expression in insulin resistance associated with in utero undernutrition. J Clin Endocrinol Metab 2001; 86(7):3266–3271.

49. Goland RS et al. Elevated levels of umbilical cord plasma corticotropin-releasing hormone in growth-retarded fetuses. J Clin Endocrinol Metab 1993; 77(5):1174–1179.

50. Phillips DI et al. Elevated plasma cortisol concentrations: a link between low birth weight and the insulin resistance syndrome? J Clin Endocrinol Metab 1998; 83(3): 757–760.

51. Seckl JR. Glucocorticoids, feto-placental 11 beta-hydroxysteroid dehydrogenase type 2, and the early life origins of adult disease. Steroids 1997; 62(1):89–94.

52. McMillen IC et al. Impact of restriction of placental and fetal growth on expression of 11beta-hydroxysteroid dehydrogenase type 1 and type 2 messenger ribonucleic acid in the liver, kidney, and adrenal of the sheep fetus. Endocrinology 2000; 141(2):539–543.

53. Hotamisligil GS et al. IRS-1-mediated inhibition of insulin receptor tyrosine kinase activity in TNF-alpha- and obesity-induced insulin resistance. Science 1996; 271(5249): 665–668.

54. Day CP et al. Tumour necrosis factor-alpha gene promoter polymorphism and decreased insulin resistance. Diabetologia 1998; 41(4):430–434.

55. Maymon E et al. The tumor necrosis factor alpha and its soluble receptor profile in term and preterm parturition. Am J Obstet Gynecol 1999; 181(5 Pt 1):1142–1148.

56. Hales CN et al. Fetal and infant growth and impaired glucose tolerance at age 64. BMJ 1991; 303(6809):1019–1022.

57. Barker DJ et al. Type 2 (non-insulin-dependent) diabetes mellitus, hypertension and hyperlipidaemia (syndrome X): relation to reduced fetal growth. Diabetologia 1993; 36(1):62–67.

58. Fall CH et al. Relation of infant feeding to adult serum cholesterol concentration and death from ischaemic heart disease. BMJ 1992; 304(6830):801–805.

59. Barker DJ et al. Fetal and placental size and risk of hypertension in adult life. BMJ 1990; 301(6746):259–262.

60. Stein CE et al. Fetal growth and coronary heart disease in south India. Lancet 1996; 348(9037):1269–1273.

61. Law CM et al. Thinness at birth and glucose tolerance in seven-year-old children. Diabet Med 1995; 12(1):24–29.

62. Crowther NJ et al. Association between poor glucose tolerance and rapid post natal weight gain in seven-year-old children. Diabetologia 1998; 41(10):1163–1167.

63. Eriksson JG et al. Catch-up growth in childhood and death from coronary heart disease: longitudinal study. BMJ 1999; 318(7181):427–431.

64. Bavdekar A et al. Insulin resistance syndrome in 8-year-old Indian children: small at birth, big at 8 years, or both? Diabetes 1999; 48(12):2422–2429.

65. Soto N et al. Insulin sensitivity and secretion are related to catch-up growth in small-for-gestational-age infants at age 1 year: results from a prospective cohort. J Clin Endocrinol Metab 2003; 88(8):3645–3650.

66. Colle E et al. Insulin responses during catch-up growth of infants who were small for gestational age. Pediatrics 1976; 57(3):363–371.

67. Crescenzo R et al. A role for suppressed thermogenesis favoring catch-up fat in the pathophysiology of catch-up growth. Diabetes 2003; 52(5):1090–1097.

68. Cettour-Rose P et al. Redistribution of glucose from skeletal muscle to adipose tissue during catch-up fat: a link between catch-up growth and later metabolic syndrome. Diabetes 2005; 54(3):751–756.

69. King H, Aubert RE, Herman WH. Global burden of diabetes, 1995–2025: prevalence, numerical estimates, and projections. Diabetes Care 1998; 21(9):1414–1431.

70. Ong KK et al. Association between postnatal catch-up growth and obesity in childhood: prospective cohort study. BMJ 2000. 320(7240):967–971.

71. Reaven GM. The fourth musketeer—from Alexandre Dumas to Claude Bernard. Diabetologia 1995; 38(1): 3–13.

72. Ong KK et al. Insulin sensitivity and secretion in normal children related to size at birth, postnatal growth, and plasma insulin-like growth factor-I levels. Diabetologia 2004; 47(6):1064–1070.

73. Hofman PL et al. Insulin resistance in short children with intrauterine growth retardation. J Clin Endocrinol Metab 1997; 82(2):402–406.

74. Tschop M et al. Circulating ghrelin levels are decreased in human obesity. Diabetes 2001; 50(4):707–709.

75. Eriksson JG et al. Effects of size at birth and childhood growth on the insulin resistance syndrome in elderly individuals. Diabetologia 2002; 45(3):342–348.

76. Forsen T et al. The fetal and childhood growth of persons who develop type 2 diabetes. Ann Intern Med 2000; 133(3):176–182.

77. Bazaes RA et al. Determinants of insulin sensitivity and secretion in very-low-birth-weight children. J Clin Endocrinol Metab 2004; 89(3):1267–1272.

78. Hofman PL et al. Premature birth and later insulin resistance. N Engl J Med 2004; 351(21):2179–2186.

79. Kojima M, et al. Ghrelin is a growth-hormone-releasing acylated peptide from stomach. Nature 1999; 402(6762):656–660.

80. Howard AD et al. A receptor in pituitary and hypothalamus that functions in growth hormone release. Science 1996; 273(5277):974–977.

81. Nakazato M et al. A role for ghrelin in the central regulation of feeding. Nature 2001; 409(6817):194–198.

82. Iniguez G et al. Fasting and post-glucose ghrelin levels in SGA infants: relationships with size and weight gain at one year of age. J Clin Endocrinol Metab 2002; 87(12):5830–5833.

83. Jaquet D et al. Combined effects of genetic and environmental factors on insulin resistance associated with reduced fetal growth. Diabetes 2002; 51(12):3473–3478.

84. Jaquet D et al. Insulin resistance early in adulthood in subjects born with intrauterine growth retardation. J Clin Endocrinol Metab 2000; 85(4):1401–1406.

85. Petersen KF et al. Impaired mitochondrial activity in the insulin-resistant offspring of patients with type 2 diabetes. N Engl J Med 2004; 350(7):664–671.

86. Trayhurn P, Wood IS. Adipokines: inflammation and the pleiotropic role of white adipose tissue. Br J Nutr 2004; 92(3):347–355.

87. Ahima RS, Osei SY. Molecular regulation of eating behavior: new insights and prospects for therapeutic strategies. Trends Mol Med 2001; 7(5):205–213.

88. Maeda K et al. cDNA cloning and expression of a novel adipose specific collagen-like factor, apM1 (AdiPose Most abundant Gene transcript 1). Biochem Biophys Res Commun 1996; 221(2):286–289.

89. Yamauchi T et al. Cloning of adiponectin receptors that mediate antidiabetic metabolic effects. Nature 2003; 423(6941):762–769.

90. Berg AH et al. The adipocyte-secreted protein Acrp30 enhances hepatic insulin action. Nat Med 2001; 7(8):947–953.

91. Yamauchi T et al. The fat-derived hormone adiponectin reverses insulin resistance associated with both lipoatrophy and obesity. Nat Med 2001; 7(8):941–946.

92. Yamamoto Y et al. Adiponectin, an adipocyte-derived protein, predicts future insulin resistance: two-year follow-up study in Japanese population. J Clin Endocrinol Metab 2004; 89(1):87–90.

93. Chandran M et al. Adiponectin: more than just another fat cell hormone? Diabetes Care 2003; 26(8):2442–2450.

94. Kishida K et al. Disturbed secretion of mutant adiponectin associated with the metabolic syndrome. Biochem Biophys Res Commun 2003; 306(1):286–292.

95. Yu JG et al. The effect of thiazolidinediones on plasma adiponectin levels in normal, obese, and type 2 diabetic subjects. Diabetes 2002; 51(10):2968–2974.

96. Lindsay RS et al. Adiponectin and development of type 2 diabetes in the Pima Indian population. Lancet 2002; 360(9326):57–58.

97. Stefan N et al. Plasma adiponectin concentrations in children: relationships with obesity and insulinemia. J Clin Endocrinol Metab 2002; 87(10):4652–4656.

98. Iniguez G et al. Adiponectin levels in the first two years of life in a prospective cohort: relations with weight gain, leptin levels and insulin sensitivity. J Clin Endocrinol Metab 2004; 89(11):5500–5503.

99. Francois I, van Helvoirt M, de Zegher F. Male pseudohermaphroditism related to complications at conception, in early pregnancy or in prenatal growth. Horm Res 1999; 51(2):91–95.

100. Boisen KA et al. Are male reproductive disorders a common entity? The testicular dysgenesis syndrome. Ann N Y Acad Sci 2001; 948:90–99.

101. Boisen KA et al. Hypospadias in a cohort of 1072 Danish newborn boys: prevalence and relationship to placental weight, anthropometrical measurements at birth, and reproductive hormone levels at three months of age. J Clin Endocrinol Metab 2005; 90(7):4041–4046.

102. Silver HK et al. Syndrome of congenital hemihypertrophy, shortness of stature, and elevated urinary gonadotropins. Pediatrics 1953; 12(4):368–376.

103. Ibanez L et al. Anovulation in eumenorrheic, nonobese adolescent girls born small for gestational age: insulin sensitization induces ovulation, increases lean body mass, and reduces abdominal fat excess, dyslipidemia, and subclinical hyperandrogenism. J Clin Endocrinol Metab 2002; 87(12):5702–5705.

104. Silfen ME et al. Elevated free IGF-I levels in prepubertal Hispanic girls with premature adrenarche: relationship with hyperandrogenism and insulin sensitivity. J Clin Endocrinol Metab 2002; 87(1):398–403.

105. Saenger P, Dimartino-Nardi J. Premature adrenarche. J Endocrinol Invest 2001; 24(9):724–733.

106. Ibanez L et al. Corticotropin-releasing hormone: a potent androgen secretagogue in girls with hyperandrogenism after precocious pubarche. J Clin Endocrinol Metab 1999; 84(12):4602–4606.

107. Ibanez L et al. Polycystic ovary syndrome after precocious pubarche: ontogeny of the low-birthweight effect. Clin Endocrinol (Oxf) 2001; 55(5):667–672.

108. Ibanez L et al. Hypersecretion of FSH in infant boys and girls born small for gestational age. J Clin Endocrinol Metab 2002; 87(5):1986–1988.

109. Ibanez L, Potau N, de Zegher F. Ovarian hyporesponsiveness to follicle stimulating hormone in adolescent girls born small for gestational age. J Clin Endocrinol Metab 2000; 85(7):2624–2626.

110. Jaquet D et al. Intrauterine growth retardation predisposes to insulin resistance but not to hyperandrogenism in young women. J Clin Endocrinol Metab 1999; 84(11):3945–3949.

111. Boonstra VH et al. Serum dehydroepiandrosterone sulfate levels and pubarche in short children born small for gestational age before and during growth hormone treatment. J Clin Endocrinol Metab 2004; 89(2):712–717.

112. Hokken-Koelega AC et al. Children born small for gestational age: do they catch up? Pediatr Res 1995; 38(2):267–271.

113. Boguszewski M et al. Hormonal status of short children born small for gestational age. Acta Paediatr Suppl 1997; 423:189–192.

114. de Waal WJ et al. Endogenous and stimulated GH secretion, urinary GH excretion, and plasma IGF-I and IGF-II levels in prepubertal children with short stature after intrauterine growth retardation. The Dutch Working Group on Growth Hormone. Clin Endocrinol (Oxf) 1994; 41(5):621–630.

115. Cutfield WS et al. IGFs and binding proteins in short children with intrauterine growth retardation. J Clin Endocrinol Metab 2002; 87(1):235–239.

116. Wilton P et al. Growth hormone treatment induces a dose-dependent catch-up growth in short children born small for gestational age: a summary of four clinical trials. Horm Res 1997; 48 Suppl 1:67–71.

117. de Zegher F et al. Growth hormone treatment of short children born small for gestational age: growth responses with continuous and discontinuous regimens over 6 years. J Clin Endocrinol Metab 2000; 85(8):2816–2821.

118. Boguszewski MC, de Zegher F, Albertsson-Wikland K. Serum leptin in short children born small for gestational age: dose-dependent effect of growth hormone treatment. Horm Res 2000; 54(3):120–125.

119. Chaussain L, Colle M, Ducret JP. Adult height in children with prepubertal short stature secondary to intrauterine growth retardation. Acta Paediatr Suppl 1994; 399:72–73.

120. Lee PA et al. International Small for Gestational Age Advisory Board consensus development conference statement: management of short children born small for gestational age, April 24-October 1 2001; Pediatrics 2003; 111(6 Pt 1):1253–1261.

121. Dahlgren J, Wikland KA. Final height in short children born small for gestational age treated with growth hormone. Pediatr Res 2005; 57(2):216–222.

122. Sas T et al. Growth hormone treatment in children with short stature born small for gestational age: 5-year results of a randomized, double-blind, dose-response trial. J Clin Endocrinol Metab 1999; 84(9):3064–3070.

123. Sas T, Mulder P, Hokken-Koelega A. Body composition, blood pressure, and lipid metabolism before and during long-term growth hormone (GH) treatment in children with short stature born small for gestational age either with or without GH deficiency. J Clin Endocrinol Metab 2000; 85(10):3786–3792.

124. Sas T et al. Carbohydrate metabolism during long-term growth hormone treatment in children with short stature born small for gestational age. Clin Endocrinol (Oxf) 2001; 54(2):243–251.

125. van Erum R et al. Craniofacial growth in short children born small for gestational age: effect of growth hormone treatment. J Dent Res 1997; 76(9):1579–1586.

13

Hypertension in Children: Endocrine Considerations

Julie R. Ingelfinger

*Department of Pediatrics, Harvard Medical School and Pediatric Nephrology Unit,
MassGeneral Hospital for Children at Massachusetts General Hospital,
Boston, Massachusetts, U.S.A.*

INTRODUCTION

Considering an endocrine etiology whenever a child presents with hypertension is mandatory, as certain identifiable conditions will otherwise be overlooked. This chapter reviews pediatric hypertension caused either by endocrine abnormalities or by mutations in genes that are modulated by endocrine systems. Endocrine-related hypertension has been thought to account for a minority of those cases of childhood hypertension due to definable causes.

Delineating the pathogenesis and pathophysiology of hypertension is particularly important in managing a child or adolescent with elevated blood pressure; the more specific the diagnosis, the less is the likelihood of placing a child on empirical and often futile regimens. In contrast, the more focused treatment can be, the less is the risk of assigning a child to nonspecific pharmacotherapy, with unknown long-term effects, including those on growth and development.

The alterations in blood pressure regulation that are frequently observed in patients with obesity, insulin resistance/dysmetabolic syndrome, and Type 1 and Type 2 diabetes mellitus are discussed in the respective chapters of this book.

NORMAL BLOOD PRESSURE AND ITS DEFINITION

Hypertension in children was redefined by the most recent update of the National Heart, Lung, and Blood Institute Task Force in Blood Pressure Control in Childhood (1), which not only considered height and weight percentiles but the concept of prehypertension. Tables according to height percentiles are provided, and both 50th and 99th percentiles are added (Table 1) (1–4). While the Task Force data, pooled from measurements in over 12,000 pediatric subjects, are intended as a guideline, the aware clinician must understand that these norms are based on in-office seated blood pressure determinations and do not take into account changes with posture, activity, time of day, or various stresses that occur in daily life (5–7).

A problem in interpreting an in-office blood pressure using available norms when one suspects secondary hypertension is that epidemiologically based normal blood pressure data do not reflect that which may occur in an abnormal state (6). If, for example, blood pressure measurements among children and adolescents with renovascular hypertension are examined, as reported by Hiner and Falkner (7), virtually all subjects have markedly elevated blood pressure. Furthermore, the diurnal pattern of blood pressure elevation in some forms of hypertension may be importantly distinct from a normal blood pressure pattern.

In recent years, much has been learned both about normal blood pressure in disparate ethnic groups and the circadian rhythm of blood pressure response. The reader is referred to reviews on the subject (8–15).

ETIOLOGY OF HYPERTENSION

As noted in the Second Task Force report (3), most pediatric hypertension is not endocrine in nature, yet considering definable causes that are related to adrenal, thyroid, pituitary, and other endocrine organs may identify a cause for hypertension. Additionally, children with specific endocrine disorders and syndromes may have a known increased risk of hypertension and will be able to benefit from specific therapy. Table 2 lists the most common causes of hypertension in each childhood age group, while Table 3 notes those endocrine causes of hypertension most commonly seen in children.

COMPLICATIONS OF HYPERTENSION: PATTERNS AND DIAGNOSIS

By the time a child is referred to a pediatric endocrinologist for hypertension evaluation, it is likely that he or she has already been assessed by a primary care physician, and, possibly, by other specialists such as a pediatric cardiologist or nephrologist. Thus, some referrals will be made for children who have findings in their history, physical examination, or laboratory

Table 1 Blood Pressure Levels for Boys and Girls by Age and Height Percentile

Age (year)	BP percentile	Systolic BP (mmHg)							Diastolic BP ((mmHg)						
		Percentile of height							Percentile of height						
		5th	10th	25th	50th	75th	90th	95th	5th	10th	25th	50th	75th	90th	95th
Boys															
1	50th	80	81	83	85	87	88	89	34	35	36	37	38	39	39
	90th	94	95	97	99	100	102	103	49	50	51	52	53	53	54
	95th	98	99	101	103	104	106	106	54	54	55	56	57	58	58
	99th	105	106	108	110	112	113	114	61	62	63	64	65	66	66
2	50th	84	85	87	88	90	92	92	39	40	41	42	43	44	44
	90th	97	99	100	102	104	105	106	54	55	56	57	58	58	59
	95th	101	102	104	106	108	109	110	59	59	60	61	62	63	63
	99th	109	110	111	113	115	117	117	66	67	68	69	70	71	71
3	50th	86	87	89	91	93	94	95	44	44	45	46	47	48	48
	90th	100	100	103	105	107	108	109	59	59	60	61	62	63	63
	95th	104	105	107	109	110	112	113	63	63	64	65	66	67	67
	99th	111	112	114	116	118	119	120	71	71	72	73	74	75	75
4	50th	88	89	91	93	95	96	97	47	48	49	50	51	51	52
	90th	102	103	105	107	109	110	111	62	63	64	65	66	66	67
	95th	106	107	109	111	112	114	115	66	67	68	69	70	71	71
	99th	113	114	116	118	120	121	122	74	75	76	77	78	78	79
5	50th	90	91	93	95	96	98	98	50	51	52	53	54	55	55
	90th	104	105	106	108	110	111	112	65	66	67	68	69	69	70
	95th	108	109	110	112	114	115	116	69	70	71	72	73	74	74
	99th	115	116	118	120	121	123	123	77	78	79	80	81	81	82
6	50th	91	92	94	96	98	99	100	53	53	54	55	56	57	57
	90th	105	106	108	110	111	113	113	68	68	69	70	71	72	72
	95th	109	110	112	114	115	117	117	72	72	73	74	75	76	76
	99th	116	117	119	121	123	124	125	80	80	81	82	83	84	84
7	50th	92	94	95	97	99	100	101	55	55	56	57	58	59	59
	90th	106	107	109	111	113	114	115	70	70	71	72	73	74	74
	95th	110	111	113	115	117	118	119	74	74	75	76	77	78	78
	99th	117	118	120	122	124	125	126	82	82	83	84	85	86	86
8	50th	94	95	97	99	100	102	102	56	57	58	59	60	60	61
	90th	107	109	110	112	114	115	116	71	72	72	73	74	75	76
	95th	111	112	114	116	118	119	120	75	76	77	78	79	79	80
	99th	119	120	122	123	125	127	127	83	84	85	86	87	87	88
9	50th	95	96	98	100	102	103	104	57	58	59	60	61	61	62
	90th	109	110	112	114	115	117	118	72	73	74	75	76	76	77
	95th	113	114	116	118	119	121	121	76	77	78	79	80	81	81
	99th	120	121	123	125	127	128	129	84	85	86	87	88	88	89
10	50th	97	98	100	102	103	105	106	58	59	60	61	61	62	63
	90th	111	112	114	115	117	119	119	73	73	74	75	76	77	78
	95th	115	116	117	119	121	122	123	77	78	79	80	81	81	82
	99th	122	123	125	127	128	130	130	85	86	86	88	88	89	90
11	50th	99	100	102	104	105	107	107	59	59	60	61	62	63	63
	90th	113	114	115	117	119	120	121	74	74	75	76	77	78	78
	95th	117	118	119	121	123	124	125	78	78	79	80	81	82	82
	99th	124	125	127	129	130	132	132	86	86	87	88	89	90	90
12	50th	101	102	104	106	108	109	110	59	60	61	62	63	63	64
	90th	115	116	118	120	121	123	123	74	75	75	76	77	78	79
	95th	119	120	122	123	125	127	127	78	79	80	81	82	82	83
	99th	126	127	129	131	133	134	135	86	87	88	89	90	90	91
13	50th	104	105	106	108	110	111	112	60	60	61	62	63	64	64
	90th	117	118	120	122	124	125	126	75	75	76	77	78	79	79
	95th	121	122	124	126	128	129	130	79	79	80	81	82	83	83
	99th	128	130	131	133	135	136	137	87	87	88	89	90	91	91
14	50th	106	107	109	111	113	114	115	60	61	62	63	64	65	65
	90th	120	121	123	125	126	128	128	75	76	77	78	79	79	80
	95th	124	125	127	128	130	132	132	80	80	81	82	83	84	84
	99th	131	132	134	136	138	139	140	87	88	89	90	91	92	92
15	50th	109	110	112	113	115	117	117	61	62	63	64	65	66	66
	90th	122	124	125	127	129	130	131	76	77	78	79	80	80	81
	95th	126	127	129	131	133	134	135	81	81	82	83	84	85	85
	99th	134	135	136	138	140	142	142	88	89	90	91	92	93	93

(Continued)

Table 1   Blood Pressure Levels for Boys and Girls by Age and Height Percentile (*Continued*)

Age (year)	BP percentile	Systolic BP (mmHg) Percentile of height							Diastolic BP ((mmHg) Percentile of height						
		5th	10th	25th	50th	75th	90th	95th	5th	10th	25th	50th	75th	90th	95th
16	50th	111	112	114	116	118	119	120	63	63	64	65	66	67	67
	90th	125	126	128	130	131	133	134	78	78	79	80	81	82	82
	95th	129	130	132	134	135	137	137	82	83	83	84	85	86	87
	99th	136	137	139	141	143	144	145	90	90	91	92	93	94	94
17	50th	114	115	116	118	120	121	122	65	66	66	67	68	69	70
	90th	127	128	130	132	134	135	136	80	80	81	82	83	84	84
	95th	131	132	134	136	138	139	140	84	85	86	87	87	88	89
	99th	139	140	141	143	145	146	147	92	93	93	94	95	96	97
Girls															
1	50th	83	84	85	86	88	89	90	38	39	39	40	41	41	42
	90th	97	97	98	100	101	102	103	52	53	53	54	55	55	56
	95th	100	101	102	104	105	106	107	56	57	57	58	59	59	60
	99th	108	108	109	111	112	113	114	64	64	65	65	66	67	67
2	50th	85	85	87	88	89	91	91	43	44	44	45	46	46	47
	90th	98	99	100	101	103	104	105	57	58	58	59	60	61	61
	95th	102	103	104	105	107	108	109	61	62	62	63	64	65	65
	99th	109	110	111	112	114	115	116	69	69	70	70	71	72	72
3	50th	86	87	88	89	91	92	93	47	48	48	49	50	50	51
	90th	100	100	102	103	104	106	106	61	62	62	63	64	64	65
	95th	104	104	105	107	108	109	110	65	66	66	67	68	68	69
	99th	111	111	113	114	115	116	117	73	73	74	74	75	76	76
4	50th	88	88	90	91	92	94	94	50	50	51	52	52	53	54
	90th	101	102	103	104	106	107	108	64	64	65	66	67	67	68
	95th	105	106	107	108	110	111	112	68	68	69	70	71	71	72
	99th	112	113	114	115	117	118	119	76	76	76	77	78	79	79
5	50th	89	90	91	93	94	95	96	52	53	53	54	55	55	56
	90th	103	103	105	106	107	109	109	66	67	67	68	69	69	70
	95th	107	107	108	110	111	112	113	70	71	71	72	73	73	74
	99th	114	114	116	117	118	120	120	78	78	79	79	80	81	81
6	50th	91	92	93	94	96	97	98	54	54	55	56	56	57	58
	90th	104	105	106	108	109	110	111	68	68	69	70	70	71	72
	95th	108	109	110	111	113	114	115	72	72	73	74	74	75	76
	99th	115	116	117	119	120	121	122	80	80	80	81	82	83	83
7	50th	93	93	95	96	97	99	99	55	56	56	57	58	58	59
	90th	106	107	108	109	111	112	113	69	70	70	71	72	72	73
	95th	110	111	112	113	115	116	116	73	74	74	75	76	76	77
	99th	117	118	119	120	122	123	124	81	81	82	82	83	84	84
8	50th	95	95	96	98	99	100	101	57	57	57	58	59	60	60
	90th	108	109	110	111	113	114	114	71	71	71	72	73	74	74
	95th	112	112	114	115	116	118	118	75	75	75	76	77	78	78
	99th	119	120	121	122	123	125	125	82	82	83	83	84	85	86
9	50th	96	97	98	100	101	102	103	58	58	58	59	60	61	61
	90th	110	110	112	113	114	116	116	72	72	72	73	74	75	75
	95th	114	114	115	117	118	119	120	76	76	76	77	78	79	79
	99th	121	121	123	124	125	127	127	83	83	84	84	85	86	87
10	50th	98	99	100	102	103	104	105	59	59	59	60	61	62	62
	90th	112	112	114	115	116	118	118	73	73	73	74	75	76	76
	95th	116	116	117	119	120	121	122	77	77	77	78	79	80	80
	99th	123	123	125	126	127	129	129	84	84	85	86	86	87	88
11	50th	100	101	102	103	105	106	107	60	60	60	61	62	63	63
	90th	114	114	116	117	118	119	120	74	74	74	75	76	77	77
	95th	118	118	119	121	122	123	124	78	78	78	79	80	81	81
	99th	125	125	126	128	129	130	131	85	85	86	87	87	88	89
12	50th	102	103	104	105	107	108	109	61	61	61	62	63	64	64
	90th	116	116	117	119	120	121	122	75	75	75	76	77	78	78
	95th	119	120	121	123	124	125	126	79	79	79	80	81	82	82
	99th	127	127	128	130	131	132	133	86	86	87	88	88	89	90
13	50th	104	105	106	107	109	110	110	62	62	62	63	64	65	65
	90th	117	118	119	121	122	123	124	76	76	76	77	78	79	79
	95th	121	122	123	124	126	127	128	80	80	80	81	82	83	83
	99th	128	129	130	132	133	134	135	87	87	88	89	89	90	91

(*Continued*)

Table 1 Blood Pressure Levels for Boys and Girls by Age and Height Percentile (*Continued*)

Age (year)	BP percentile	Systolic BP (mmHg) Percentile of height							Diastolic BP ((mmHg) Percentile of height						
		5th	10th	25th	50th	75th	90th	95th	5th	10th	25th	50th	75th	90th	95th
14	50th	106	106	107	109	110	111	112	63	63	63	64	65	66	66
	90th	119	120	121	122	124	125	125	77	77	77	78	79	80	80
	95th	123	123	125	126	127	129	129	81	81	81	82	83	84	84
	99th	130	131	132	133	135	136	136	88	88	89	90	90	91	92
15	50th	107	108	109	110	111	113	113	64	64	64	65	66	67	67
	90th	120	121	122	123	125	126	127	78	78	78	79	80	81	81
	95th	124	125	126	127	129	130	131	82	82	82	83	84	85	85
	99th	131	132	133	134	136	137	138	89	89	90	91	91	92	93
16	50th	108	108	110	111	112	114	114	64	64	65	66	66	67	68
	90th	121	122	123	124	126	127	128	78	78	79	80	81	81	82
	95th	125	126	127	128	130	131	132	82	82	83	84	85	85	86
	99th	132	133	134	135	137	138	139	90	90	90	91	92	93	93
17	50th	108	109	110	111	113	114	115	64	65	65	66	67	67	68
	90th	122	122	123	125	126	127	128	78	79	79	80	81	81	82
	95th	125	126	127	129	130	131	132	82	83	83	84	85	85	86
	99th	133	133	134	136	137	138	139	90	90	91	91	92	93	93

Note: The 90th percentile is 1.28 SD, 95th percentile is 1.645 SD, and the 99th percentile is 2.326 SD over the mean.
Abbreviation: BP, blood pressure.
Source: From Ref. 1.

data that specifically suggest an endocrine cause of hypertension. Other referrals, however, will be *de novo* or will be children not referred but who have been found to have hypertension in the course of treatment or evaluation for a known endocrinopathy. Prompt and focused evaluation of elevated blood pressure is critical, given the potential complications of pediatric hypertension.

Certain findings in a hypertensive child imply a role for an endocrinologist. An endocrinologist's first approach should be to seek historical facts that suggest a familial endocrinopathy associated with hypertension, the taking of medications that would be associated with an endocrine-mediated hypertension (e.g., steroids or sympathomimetic agents), or an endocrine diagnosis known to be associated with hypertension (e.g., Turner syndrome). Physical examination will, of course, focus the evaluation further, in that findings may clearly suggest a particular

endocrine diagnosis (clinical hyper- or hypothyroidism, Cushing syndrome). The blood pressure should be determined in both arms and one or both legs,

Table 3 Endocrine Hypertension

Congenital adrenal hyperplasia
    11-β-hydroxylase deficiency
    3-β-hydroxysteroid dehydrogenase
    17-α-hydroxylase deficiency
Hyperaldosteronism and hyperaldosterone-like conditions
    Aldosterone-producing adenoma
    Hyperplasia
    Glucocorticoid responsive aldosteronism
    Apparent mineralocorticoid excess
Salt handling
    Liddle syndrome
    Pseudohypoaldosteronism II (Gordon syndrome)
Catecholamine mediated
    Pheochromocytoma
    Neuroblastoma
Cushing syndrome
Exogenous (due to medication)
    Central
    Adrenal
Thyroid
    Hyperthyroidism
    Hypothyroidism
Parathyroid
    Hyperparathyroidism
    Hypoparathyroidism (related to therapy)
Turner syndrome
Polycystic ovarian syndrome/metabolic syndrome
Diabetes mellitus
Iatrogenic
    Glucocorticoid
    Calcium phosphorus mediated
    Catecholamine mediated
    Thyroid hormone mediated
    Hormone replacement therapy

Table 2 Most Common Causes of Hypertension in Each Age Group

Age group	Etiology
Neonate	Coarctation of the aorta
	Renal artery thromboembolism
	Renal artery stenosis
	Congenital renal abnormalities
Infancy to 6 years	Renal parenchymal disease (including structural, inflammatory disease and tumors)
	Coarctation of the aorta
	Renal artery stenosis
Six to ten years	Renal parenchymal disease (including structural, inflammatory disease and tumors)
	Renal artery stenosis
	Primary hypertension
Adolescence	Primary hypertension
	Renal parenchymal disease

and postural changes should be noted. Additionally, blood pressure after exercise, as well as at several points in the day may be helpful. Ambulatory blood pressure monitoring may be helpful in assessing circadian rhythm and particular patterns that could be associated with endocrine hypertension.

Laboratory data help to hone in on specific forms of hypertension. Thus, the initial endocrine assessment should focus on seeking signs of catecholamine-mediated hypertension, glucocorticoid-related hypertension, or thyroid-mediated hypertension (which are discussed at length in other chapters). Next, a plasma renin level, examined together with a measure of sodium excretion and plasma potassium should provide a basis for a focused endocrine assessment (16–19). A high plasma renin level is unlikely to be associated with endocrine hypertension, though secondary aldosteronism will accompany renovascular hypertension. If plasma renin activity or concentration is low, one should then consider an underlying endocrine basis. As can be seen in Table 4, those forms of low-renin hypertension that have been fully defined are due to mutations on autosomal chromosomes and thus occur equally in males and females (19). Each will be considered in turn. It has been proposed that, in fact, many more cases of "primary hypertension" may be associated with partial defects in steroidogenesis or factors that control steroid effects.

The diagnostic considerations include a variety of inherited disorders that have a very low plasma renin activity as a cardinal feature. These include steroid enzyme abnormalities as well as abnormalities in transporters or in modulating genes. Yiu et al. (16) developed an algorithm for thinking about these entities, which are accompanied by low plasma renin activity, and this is shown in Figure 1 (16). The algorithm is based on the fact that a number of hypertensive syndromes share a low plasma renin as a common feature. Most are inherited either as an autosomal dominant, in which case family history is positive, or as an autosomal recessive, in which case family history is lacking.

STEROIDOGENIC ENZYME DEFECTS

As noted in Volume II, Section II, Chapter 8, steroids are produced in the adrenal cortex, which is divided into zones: the zona glomerulosa (ZG—outer zone), zona fasciculata (ZF—middle zone), and zona reticularis (ZR—inner zone). Normally, the ZG and ZF are functionally separate. Cortisol is synthesized under the control of adrenocorticotropic hormone (ACTH) in the ZF, while aldosterone is synthesized primarily under the influence of angiotensin II and potassium in the ZG. ACTH normally has only a secondary effect on the synthesis of aldosterone. However, when any of the enzymes that control cortisol biosynthesis is defective or acts abnormally, the feedback relationships between the hypophysis and the adrenal are interrupted, with a resultant increase in plasma ACTH. Figure 2 depicts steroidogenesis, indicating enzyme defects that can be associated with hypertension, and Figure 3 outlines the regulation of aldosterone biosynthesis.

Congenital adrenal hyperplasia (CAH) is the general term used to describe those enzyme defects that can occur in steroid biosynthesis, each one causing a characteristic profile of plasma and urinary steroids together with a specific clinical manifestation (18,19). These defects are all autosomal recessive and have varying frequency and a spectrum of clinical manifestations (Volume II, Section II, Chapter 9). Any of the enzymes that are part of the pathways of steroidogenesis may have a mutation, most commonly 21-hydroxylase, which is not generally associated with hypertension. Enzymes with mutations that are associated with hypertension include (in order of frequency) 11-β-hydroxylase $>>$ 3-β-hydroxysteroid dehydrogenase (HSD) $>>>$ 17-α-hydroxylase and cholesterol desmolase. A net salt-retaining propensity and hypertension occur in patients with the 11-β and 3-β-HSD defects. It is also important to remember that individuals with CAH may develop hypertension owing to overzealous replacement therapy.

Steroid 11-β-Hydroxylase Deficiency

Hypertension is one of the cardinal features of 11-β-hydroxylase deficiency (19,21–25), as the abnormal adrenal steroid pattern leads to mineralocorticoid excess, the physiology of which includes decreased renal sodium excretion with consequent volume expansion and hypertension. The virilization seen in 11-β-hydroxylase deficiency and its management are discussed at length in Volume II, Section II, Chapter 9; virilization is universal in this condition. Unless the mother of an affected female fetus is treated during pregnancy, the baby will have ambiguous or masculinized external genitalia, owing to excess of adrenal androgens, while her internal organs will be normal (26). After birth, both affected males and females develop progressive penile or clitoral enlargement, respectively, along with rapid somatic growth. If appropriate treatment is not initiated, early closure of epiphyses will lead to short final stature.

Hypertension is common but not universal in 11-β-hydroxylase deficiency, usually noted in later childhood or adolescence, and this hypertension often has an inconsistent relation to the biochemical profile (18,19). Hypokalemia is only variably present, though it should be remembered that potassium depletion and sodium retention may not be reflected by serum or plasma potassium values, owing to shifts from intracellular potassium to the extracellular space. Thus, total body potassium may be markedly depleted, yet serum or plasma potassium may be in the normal range. The production and release of renin are suppressed by the

Table 4 Low-Renin Hypertension in Childhood

Signs and symptoms	Hormonal findings	Source	Genetics	Comment
Steroidogenic enzyme defects				
Steroid 11-β-hydroxylase deficiency	↓PRA and aldo; high serum androgens/urine 17 ketosteroids; elevated DOC and 11-deoxycortisol	Adrenal: ZF	CYP11B1 mutation (encodes cytochrome P_{450}11b/18 of ZF); impairs synthesis of cortisol and ZF 17-deoxysteroids	Hypertensive virilizing CAH; most patients identified by time they are hypertensive. Increased BP may also occur from medication side effects
Steroid 11-α-hydroxylase/ 17,20-lyase deficiency	↓ PRA and aldo; low serum/ urinary 17-hydroxysteroids; decreased cortisol; ↑ corticosterone (B) and DOC in plasma; serum androgens and estrogens very low; serum gonadotrophins very high	Adrenal: ZF; gonadal: interstitial cells (Leydig in testis; theca in ovary)	CYP17 mutation (encodes cytochrom P_{450}C17) impairs cortisol and sex steroid production	CAH with male pseudohermaphroditism; female external genital phenotype in males; primary amenorrhea in females
Hyperaldosteronism				
Primary aldosteronism	↓ PRA; plasma aldosterone, 18-OH- and 18 oxoF; normal 18-OH/aldo ratio	Adrenal adenoma: clear cell tumor with suppression of ipsilateral ZG	Unknown; very rare in children; female:male ratio is 2.5–3:1	Conn syndrome with aldo producing adenoma; muscle weakness and low K+ in sodium-replete state
Adrenocortical hyperplasia	As above; source of hormone established by radiology or scans	Adrenal: focal or diffuse adrenal cortical hyperplasia	Unknown	As above
Idiopathic primary aldosteronism	High plasma aldo; elevated 18-OHF/aldo ratio	Adrenal: hyperactivity of ZG of adrenal cortex	Unknown	As above
DOC-producing tumor Dexamethasone-suppressible HTN	High plasma DOC	Adrenal: adenoma/carcinoma	Unknown	As above
GRA	Plasma and urinary aldo responsive to ACTH; dexamethasone suppressible within 48 hr; ↑ urine and plasma 18OHS,18-OHF, and 18 oxoF	Adrenal: abnormal presence of enzymatic activity in adrenal ZF, allowing completion of aldo synthesis from 17-deoxy steroids	Chimeric gene that is expressed at high level in ZF [regulated like CYP11B1) and has 18-oxidase activity (CYP11B2 functionality)	Hypokalemia in sodium-replete state
AME	↑ Plasma ACTH and secretory rates of all corticosteroids; nl serum F (delayed plasma clearance)	↑ Plasma F bioactivity in periphery (F→E) of bi-dir. 11-β-HSD or slow clearance by 5 α/β reduction to allo dihydro-F	Type 2 11-β-HSD mutations	Cardiac conduction changes; LVH, vessel remodeling; some calcium abnormalities; nephrocalcinosis; rickets
Nonsteroidal defects				
Liddle's syndrome	Low plasma renin, low or normal K+; negligible urinary aldosterone	Not a disorder of steroidogenesis, but of transport	Autosomal dominant abnormality in epithelial sodium transporter, EnaC, in which channel is constitutively active	Responds to triamterene
Pseudohypoaldosteronism II—Gordon syndrome	Low plasma renin, normal or elevated K+	Not a disorder of steroidogenesis, but of transport	Autosomal dominant abnormality in WNK1 or WNK4	Responds to thiazides

Abbreviations: GRA, glucocorticoid-remediable aldosteronism; AME, apparent mineralocorticoid excess; PRA, plasma renin activity; BP, blood pressure; DOC, deoxycorticosterone; ZF, zona fasciculata; ZG, zona glomerulosa; HTN, hypertension; HSD, hydroxysteroid dehydrogenase; LVH, left ventricular hypertrophy; aldo, aldosterone.
Source: From Ref. 20.

volume expansion. Furthermore, aldosterone production is decreased with relative decrease in circulating potassium. However, in some circumstances, the characteristic findings of low renin and elevated aldosterone have been absent.(24,27–29).

Therapy of 11-β-hydroxylase deficiency should be focused on normalizing steroids. Thus, glucocorticoid administration will not only normalize cortisol function but should reduce ACTH secretion and levels to normal, which should remove the drive for oversecretion of deoxycorticosterone (DOC). Such therapy usually cures the hypertension (21). However, if hypertension is marked, antihypertensive therapy should be used in this disorder to ensure good control of hypertension until control with glucocorticoid therapy.

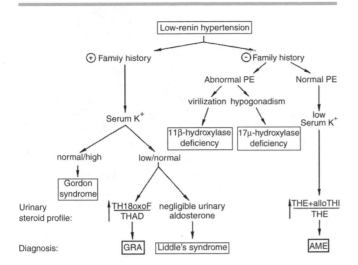

Figure 1 Low-renin hypertension algorithm. *Abbreviations:* GRA, glucocorticoid-responsive aldosteronism; AME, apparent mineralocorticoid excess; THF, tetrahydrocortisol; THE, tetrahydrocortisone. *Source:* From Ref. 16.

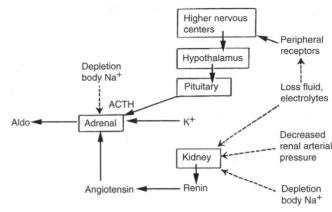

Figure 3 Aldosterone regulation. *Abbreviation:* ACTH, adrenocorticotropic hormone. *Source:* From Ref. 20.

Variants of 11-β-hydroxylase deficiency likely relate to the several mutations that can cause the syndrome. For example, Zachman et al. (25) found a person in whom 11-β-hydroxylation was inhibited for 17-α-hydroxylated steroids but in whom there was intact 17-deoxysteroid hydroxylation. Multiple mutations affecting the expression of the CYP11B1 gene have been described; these include frameshifts,

point mutations, extra triplet repeats, and stop mutations (27–32). A distinct hypotensive disorder, called corticosterone methyloxidase Type II, occurs when a mutation affects CYP11B2 (aldosterone synthase) (33). Clinically, this latter abnormality leads to a problem of terminal aldosterone synthesis and thus is accompanied by salt wasting and hypotension (33).

Steroid 17-α-Hydroxylase Deficiency

Both the adrenals and gonads are affected when the enzyme 17-α-hydroxylase is abnormal and dysfunctional, which results in decreased production of both cortisol and sex steroids (the production of which requires the 17,20 lyase function of the same enzyme) (16,17,29–31). Phenotypically, an affected person, irrespective of genetic sex, appears female, and puberty does not take place. In fact, diagnosis too often occurs late—at the time when puberty should occur but primary amenorrhea and lack of secondary sexual characteristics are noted (19,21,34–36). Another mode of presentation for affected children is the presence of an inguinal hernia. Patients are usually both hypertensive and hypokalemic, owing to huge overproduction of corticosterone (compound B). The biochemical aspects of these defects are described more completely in the chapters on CAH.

This rare type of hypertension was first described in a female patient by Biglieri et al. (34), and then in a feminized male by New and coworkers (25), though since in well over 150 patients (37–40). Treatment is effective if glucocorticoid replacement is initiated before puberty, but this may not always correct the hypertension. If replacement therapy fails to correct the elevated blood pressure, appropriate pharmacotherapy should be used to lower the blood pressure to maintain it within the normal ranges for age and size.

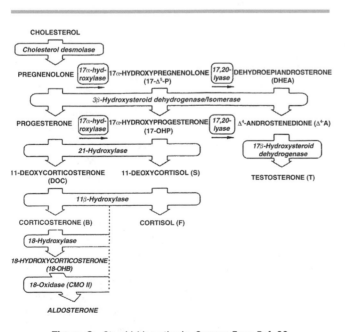

Figure 2 Steroid biosynthesis. *Source:* From Ref. 20.

PRIMARY ALDOSTERONISM: ALDOSTERONE-PRODUCING ADENOMA AND BILATERAL ADRENAL HYPERPLASIA

Aldosterone-producing adenomas (APAs) are rare in children; when these occasionally occur, it is usually as a solitary mass (19,41–49), though bilateral masses may also occur (10% of total). Occasionally, such adenomas produce DOC rather than aldosterone. The hallmarks include hypokalemia and hypertension, and the optimal method for diagnosis can be complex and controversial, even among adults. Rather than primary aldosteronism secondary to adenomas, it is far more likely that a child will have bilateral adrenal hyperplasia (48).

Diagnosis should be possible when the studies for an APA fail to find a definite lesion. The number and type of tests, some invasive, are similar to that for APA and hyperplasia. ACTH sensitivity is assessed by suppression of the adrenal glands. Assessment of aldosterone levels not only peripherally but using bilateral adrenal vein sampling may be helpful. Imaging studies including ultrasonography (47), computed tomography scan (50), scintigraphy using radioiodocholesterol (51), and nuclear magnetic resonance imaging (52) have all been used.

When APA is present, surgery is indicated (19). Surgical therapy with total or subtotal adrenalectomy for bilateral adrenal hyperplasia has been advocated, but hypertension may either continue or return. Instead, management using the nonspecific mineralocorticoid antagonist spironolactone may be more effective (19,43). Eplerenone is the first of the more specific aldosterone receptor antagonists and may prove to have a useful role (53).

GLUCOCORTICOID-RESPONSIVE ALDOSTERONISM–DEXAMETHASONE-SUPPRESSIBLE HYPERALDOSTERONISM (OMIM # 103900)

Glucocorticoid-responsive aldosteronism (GRA) was first reported by Sutherland et al.(54) and New and Peterson (55) in 1966–1967 as a novel form of increased aldosterone secretion accompanied by suppressed renin and treatable by dexamethasone. It is listed in the Online Mendelian Inheritance in Man (OMIM) as #103900. OMIM can be accessed on-line (56). This condition, an autosomal dominant (57), has been reported in numerous pedigrees (58–62) and is due to a chimeric gene duplication (the fusion of 11-β-hydroxylase and aldosterone synthase genes from an unequal crossing-over event) (63,64), leading to the regulation of aldosterone synthesis and secretion solely by corticotropin instead of by angiotensin II and potassium (62,65–67). The chimeric gene product converts cortisol to 18-hydroxy and 18-oxo metabolites that can be measured in urine (68–71).

In GRA patients, both serum and urine aldosterone levels are generally elevated, but not invariably. However, pathognomonic findings are generally that the urinary cortisol metabolites TH18oxoF and 18-hydroxycortisol are very high in GRA, and the ratio of TH18oxoF/THAD is elevated. A commercially available urinary steroid profile can distinguish GRA patients from those with apparent mineralocorticoid excess (AME) or Liddle's syndrome (Nichols Institute, San Juan Capistrano, California, U.S.A.) (71). Specific genetic testing is both sensitive and specific.

Patients have excessive aldosterone secretion, leading to salt and water retention, plasma volume expansion, and then, hypertension. When hypertension occurs, as it often does in GRA, glucocorticoid suppression can control it. GRA appears to be rare, yet it still is not often considered in the course of an evaluation of pediatric hypertension. Affected individuals often have a family history of severe "essential hypertension" that has resisted therapy, or of family members who have had early cardiovascular events including stroke and myocardial infarction.

Dluhy et al. recently reviewed the medical records of 20 children from 10 unrelated pedigrees of GRA to assess their course (72). Of the 20, 16 children developed hypertension, as early as one month of age. Interestingly, four were not hypertensive. Half of those with hypertension were controllable with monotherapy (glucocorticoid suppression or aldosterone receptor/ENaC antagonists). The rest required combination therapy, and three of those were unable to achieve blood pressure control.

Neither hypokalemia nor suppressed plasma renin activity is necessarily present at diagnosis, and thus this diagnosis might be entertained more frequently than it has been. Dexamethasone and other glucocorticoids usually control the hypertension quite easily in young individuals with GRA, though adults with this chimeric gene may not resolve their hypertension when diagnosis has been delayed.

APPARENT MINERALOCORTICOID EXCESS (OMIM # 218030)

AME is marked by low-renin hypertension accompanied by hypokalemia and metabolic alkalosis (27). The syndrome was first delineated in 1977 by New et al. during their evaluation of a young native American girl from the Zuni tribe who presented with this clinical picture (73,74). The hypertension in AME is severe, often accompanied by early end-organ damage (75). The presence of 11-β-HSD is necessary for the prevention of mineralocorticoid activity of cortisol, and when this enzyme is low or absent, cortisol-mediated hypertension can occur. In AME, then, cortisol acts as if it were a potent mineralocorticoid. While initial therapy with spironolactone frequently is effective, patients may well become refractory, and there is an absence of 11-β-HSD.

The microsomal enzyme 11-β-HSD interconverts the active 11-hydroxyglucocorticoids to their inactive ketometabolites. Both aldosterone and cortisol have an affinity for the mineralocorticoid receptor, and under usual circumstances, 11-β-HSD is protective, preventing binding of cortisol to the mineralocorticoid receptor. In AME, the slow metabolism of cortisol to the biologically inactive cortisone, with a prolonged cortisol half-life (76,77) causes cortisol to act as a potent mineralocorticoid. The metabolism of cortisone to cortisol, however, is normal.

There are two forms, kinetically distinct, of the 11-β-HSD enzyme. 11-β-HSD1 is widely distributed and, while its K_m for cortisol is an order of magnitude higher than for 11-β-HSD2, it preferentially requires nicotinamide adenine dinucleotide phosphate, mainly acting as a reductase. In contrast, 11-β-HSD2 is localized mainly to epithelia that transport sodium. It has a high affinity for cortisol and requires nicotinamide adenosine dinucleotide. 11-β-HSD2 is involved in sodium transport, predominantly in the renal distal tubule. Clinical findings have suggested that the 11-β-HSD enzyme was abnormal in AME (78,79). It was postulated that patients with AME had a loss of mineralocorticoid receptor specificity such that cortisol could bind to the mineralocorticoid receptor and act as a mineralocorticoid. Although defective 11-β-HSD seemed a likely explanation, the first form of this enzyme found was normal. However, it is now known that an abnormality in the Type 2 isoform of 11-β-HSD is mutated in AME (80–84). To date, many distinct mutations have been reported. These mutations have been shown to impair the conversion of cortisol to cortisone.

Children with classical AME generally present in early life, often with failure to thrive, severe hypertension and/or persistent polydipsia. These patients are volume expanded and respond to dietary sodium restriction. Plasma renin activity is impressively decreased. The diagnosis can be made biochemically by obtaining the ratio of cortisol to cortisone in the urine. The urinary ratio of tetrahydrocortisol (THF)/tetrahydrocortisone is abnormal, with a predominance of THF. The generation if cortisone from cortisol after 11-tritiated cortisol is injected is only 0% to 6%, compared to normal, which is 90% to 95% (85).

These children often develop cardiovascular complications from their hypertension. In addition, some develop nephrocalcinosis and renal failure (86). Early diagnosis can do much to ameliorate the situation, if the hypertension can be controlled.

A mild form of AME has been reported in a Mennonite kindred, in which there is a P227L mutation in the HSD11B2 gene (87,88). In 2001, New et al. reported two sisters from the Iroquois nation; the proband was referred with mild hypertension as a possible patient with AME, yet she had resistance to glucocorticoids, mineralocorticoids, and androgens (89). Despite significantly elevated glucocorticoids, she had no cushingoid features, and no evidence of masculinization, though her androgen levels were elevated (89). It was proposed that these two young women may have a coactivator defect (89).

Recently, hypertension without the characteristic findings of AME have been described in the heterozygous father and homozygous daughter who have mutations in 11-β-HSD2 (90). Studies in patients with hypertension suggest a deficiency in 11-β-HSD2 activity, along with abnormalities that may be genetically determined (91) The 11-β-HSD2 gene appears to confer specificity for the aldosterone receptor (92).

Licorice-induced hypertension has a pathogenesis similar to that seen in AME (81,82,86). Glycerrhetinic acid, which is the active component of licorice, inhibits 11-β-HSD, leading to increased stimulation of the mineralocorticoid receptor (93).

MUTATIONS IN RENAL TRANSPORTERS CAUSING LOW-RENIN HYPERTENSION

Pseudohypoaldosteronism Type II—Gordon Syndrome (OMIM # 145260)

Pseudohypoaldosteronism Type II is an autosomal dominant condition associated with hyperkalemia, acidemia, and hypertension along with increased salt reabsorption by the kidney (16,94–96). The condition is also known as Gordon's syndrome or familial hyperkalemia and is listed as OMIM # 145260. A hallmark of this disease is low renin hypertension and improvement with the use of thiazide diuretics or with triamterene. Interestingly, aldosterone receptor antagonists do not correct the abnormalities. The pathogenesis long remained elusive, though the physiological studies and response to diuretics strongly indicated a defect in renal ion transport in the presence of normal glomerular filtration rate.

Genes for PHAII were mapped to chromosomes 17, 1, or 12 (97–100). Recently a PHAII kindred in which linkage analysis suggested the involved area was the most telomeric 2-centimorgan segment of chromosome 12p (lod score 5.07) was found to have abnormalities in WNK1. The mutations are large intronic deletions which increase WNK1 expression. Another family has been found with missense mutations in WNK4, which is on chromosome 17. WNK 1 is widely expressed in the body, while WNK4 is mainly expressed in kidney, localized to tight junctions. It is thought that abnormalities in WNKs change the way potassium and hydrogen are handled in the collecting duct, thus increasing salt resorption and intravascular volume. How this occurs is not clear. It is unlikely that these kinases simply increase the activity of ENaC. More likely, they either increase transcellular chloride conductance in the collecting duct or increase paracellular chloride conductance. This may increase salt resorption and intravascular volume and dissipate the electrical gradient and decrease K^+ and H^+ secretion. They might also lead to constitutive increase in activity of the Na-Cl cotransporter in the collecting duct or increase its activity in the distal convoluted tubule.

The lesson inherent in the association of WNK kinases with PHAII is that many people with low renin primary hypertension respond to thiazide diuretics. Might these people have variants in WNK1 or WNK4, which predispose to hypertension? There are some data from linkage studies that suggest such an association might be important (100). Furthermore, the WNK kinases and their signaling pathways may be a fruitful target for future development of antihypertensive drugs.

Liddle Syndrome (OMIM # 177200)

In 1963, Liddle et al. (101) described early onset of hypertension with hypokalemia in a family who had low renin and aldosterone concentrations. Inheritance was as an autosomal dominant. Inhibitors of renal epithelial sodium transport, such as triamterene, worked well in controlling hypertension, but inhibitors of the mineralocorticoid receptor did not. A general abnormality in sodium transport seemed apparent, as the red blood cell transport systems were not normal (102). The concept that a major abnormality was present in renal salt handling was fostered by the fact that a patient with Liddle syndrome who needed a renal transplant had normalization of the blood pressure and serum potassium following the procedure (103).

The abnormality in Liddle syndrome thus looked like aldosterone excess, yet the patients had very low aldosterone as well as renin levels (104–106). Many but not all patients have low potassium. Mineralocorticoid-dependent sodium transport within the renal epithelia requires activation of the epithelial sodium channel, ENaC, which is made up of α, β, and γ subunits, which have been cloned and characterized. The β and γ subunits are in proximity on chromosome 16, and mutations in these subunits have been identified in Liddle syndrome. More information can be found in OMIM, in which Liddle syndrome is listed as OMIM # 177200.

CUSHING SYNDROME AND HYPERTENSION

Glucocorticoid excess leads to a well-described syndrome of weight gain, linear height growth attenuation, myopathy, centripetal obesity, striae, moon facies, and buffalo hump (107–110). Hypertension is part of this constellation, whether due to exogenous glucorticoid therapy or endogenous hypercortisolism from a variety of causes. The hypertension improves upon control of the underlying cause (and therapy is discussed in Volume II, Section II, Chapter 8) It is important that the hypertension be treated and controlled while the cause is being evaluated and treated.

HYPERTENSION IN PHEOCHROMOCYTOMA AND NEURAL CREST TUMORS

Hypertension is nearly universal in pediatric pheochromocytoma, and management is discussed in Volume II, Section II, Chapter 10. Several points concerning the hypertension in children with pheochromocytoma are worth emphasizing in this chapter as well (111–127). The hypertension seen in children and adolescents with pheochromocytoma is often constant rather than episodic; thus the diagnosis should always be ruled out in a child with marked hypertension.

The management of the hypertension in a child with pheochromocytoma should be divided into the preoperative phase, intraoperative phase, and postoperative phase. Preoperatively, it is worthwhile to be certain that the child's blood pressure is controlled and the child stable before surgery is attempted. The doses of medications as used are listed in Table 5. As was pointed out in Volume II, Section II, Chapter 10, while α-blockade is felt to be important, β-adrenoceptor blockade should not be used as sole therapy, as it fails to prevent the effects of catecholamine at α-adrenoceptors and may cause severe hypertension.

Some sources suggest inducing volume expansion along with blood pressure control in the

Table 5 Treatment of Catecholamine Excess Oral Medications to Use Preoperatively

Drug	Indications/pharmacokinetics	Dose	Preparation
α-Adrenergic blockers			
Phenoxybenzamine	Long half-life	Start at 10 mg b.i.d.→20–40 mg b.i.d. or tid	10 mg capsules
Prazosin	Selective α_1-antagonist; short half-life	1 mg q 8 hr, up to 20 mg/day	1,2,and 5 mg capsules
β-Adrenergic blockers	Do not use before full α-blockade		
Propranolol	Nonselective β-antagonist; may induce wheezing; biologic half-life ~4 hr	1 mg/kg/dose b.i.d. to q.i.d.	10,20,40,60,80 mg tabs
Propranolol—long acting	Same as propranolol	1 mg/kg/day	60 and 80 mg capsules
Atenolol	Selective β_1-antagonist; 50% absorbed orally; peaks at 2–4 hr, half-life 6–7 hr; oral duration 24 hr	1–2 mg/kg q.d.	25, 50, and 100 mg tablets
α/β-Adrenergic blockade			
Labetalol	Combined blocker; limited pediatric information	3–4 mg/kg/day in two divided doses; increase to 40 mg/kg/day per oral	100, 200, and 300 mg tablets
Competitive inhibitor of tyrosine hydroxylase			
Metyrosine (Demser)	Competitive inhibitor tyrosine hydroxylase	250 mg b.i.d. to q.i.d.	250 mg capsules

preoperative period—the rationale being that this may help to prevent intraoperative volume instability (128).

Preoperatively, it is wise to premedicate to avoid anxiety, which by itself may precipitate a catecholamine release and crisis (117). Premedication with oral diazepam has been used in children (129). Droperidol should be avoided, as it may increase catecholamine release (130). Glycopyrrolate is an anticholinergic that has little effect on heart rate and works well to reduce secretions (129). Perioperatively, it is important to consider the use of nonexcitatory neuromuscular medications. Accordingly, fentanyl should also be avoided because of the potential of increased catecholamine release. Furthermore, atropine is contraindicated, because this agent may lead to tachycardia in the presence of elevated blood catecholamines.

Monitoring arterial pressure and cardiogram is essential during surgery, and providing muscle relaxants prior to intubation is important. As a muscle relaxant, vecuronium is a good choice, given its minimal influence on the cardiovascular system. One should avoid the use of succinylcholine, which can lead to fasciculations in muscle, leading to catecholamine discharge. Pancuronium is a sympathomimetic that should be avoided, because it can lead to hypertensive crisis in this setting. It may be useful to spray 1% lidocaine into the trachea or give a dose intravenously to decrease sympathetic stimulation just prior to intubation.

Anesthesia with isoflurane or enflurane is usual and well tolerated. If a hypertensive crisis occurs during surgery, prompt therapy with intravenous (IV) phentolamine or nitroprusside is essential, as well as control of any arrhythmias that may develop. In addition to phentolamine and nitroprusside, the calcium channel blocker nicardipine has been used with success, as well as labetalol, esmolol, nitroglycerine, and the dopamine 1 agonist fenoldopam.

Postoperatively, most children with resectable tumors normalize their blood pressure. However, about one-fourth of adults do not, likely because most of these people have concomitant primary hypertension. Those children who require continued antihypertensive therapy after resection are generally those whose tumors are not fully resectable or who have malignant pheochromocytoma. In such situations, a combination of α- and β-blockade can control blood pressure. Additionally, metyrosine (Demser) is useful for inhibiting catecholamine synthesis and the calcium channel blocker nifedipine is successful in decreasing clinical symptoms.

HYPERTENSION IN THYROID DISEASE

Hypertension is widely stated to occur in both hyperthyroidism (131–133) and hypothyroidism (134), not surprisingly via distinctly different mechanisms (Volume II, Section II, Chapters 17 and 18). A considerable body of experimental data demonstrate that models of hyperthyroidism are accompanied by hypertension (135). Activation of the renin–angiotensin system appears important in this form of hypertension, which is ameliorated by the angiotensin II antagonist, e.g., valsartan. Conversely, an older literature showed that spontaneously hypertensive rats had a propensity to have thyroid functional abnormalities.

Clinically, hypertension as part of hyperthyroidism is widely known (131–133). Treatment of the hypertension with antihypertensive agents generally proves to be successful. This form of hypertension has been reported in neonates with hyperthyroidism, as well as in older children.

The circadian rhythm in hyperthyroidism appears to vary compared to normal, with a failure to exhibit nocturnal decrease (dipping) in blood pressure. Systolic hypertension as an isolated finding is more common than elevation of both systolic and diastolic hypertension, particularly in young patients. Increased cardiac output together with decreased total peripheral resistance is observed.

Hypothyroidism has long been reported as associated with hypertension (134). However, few data truly support this claim. Rather, studies note left ventricular hypertrophy post hoc, in autopsy studies, or make this claim without providing control subjects. Therapy of the thyroid deficiency generally decreases the blood pressure for most individuals. The clinical findings include increase in sympathetic nervous system tone, with an augmented α-adrenergic responsiveness. Cardiac output tends to be decreased, while peripheral resistance is increased. If hypertension is present, it is most often diastolic in nature. Once the hypothyroidism is corrected, patients can generally be weaned from hypotensive therapy.

HYPERPARATHYROIDISM AND HYPERTENSION

Hypertension is a frequent occurrence with hyperparathyroidism (136–138). Studies that have considered mechanisms suggest that intracellular ionized calcium is elevated and regulated abnormally in this condition. Additionally, iatrogenic hypertension may occur, as therapy may have side effects leading to hypertension. Similarly, patients with hypoparathyroidism, if treated to excess with vitamin D analogs and calcium, may become hypertensive.

PREVENTION OF HYPERTENSION AND ENDOCRINE SYSTEMS
Expectable Hypertension in the Course of Prescribed Therapy

No discussion of hypertension in children is complete without some mention of iatrogenous forms of hypertension. A number of medications commonly used in endocrine practice may lead to hypertension. These

Table 6   Oral or Topical Antihypertensives

Medication type	Drug	Route	Dose	Adverse effects	Contraindication	Comment
Vasodilator	Minoxidil	PO	0.2 mg/kg to start	Fluid retention, reflex tachycardia	Need to get BP controlled immediately; catecholamine-mediated hypertension	May help in urgencies
	Hydralazine	PO	0.75–3.0 mg/kg/day	Vasodilation symptoms	Tachycardia; sensitivity to hydralazine	Unstable in suspension; consider periodic ANA testing
β-Blockers	Propranolol	PO	0.5–1.90 mg/kg/day divided q 6 hr	Bradycardia, CHF, intensification of AV block; mental depression, visual disturbances, nightmares, hallucinations; bronchospasm; GI symptoms	Asthma, CHF, sinus bradycardia, liver disease, cardiogenic shock, diabetes	May mask signs of hypoglycemia or hyperthyroidism; available in long-acting form
	Atenolol	PO	Once daily; 50 mg q.d. (adult)	Fewer side effects than nonselective β-blockers	Pheochromocytoma	Relatively cardioselective
	Metoprolol	PO	1 mg/kg every 12 hr	Fewer side effects than other β-blockers	Can consider using in patients with reactive airway disease	Relatively cardioselective
	Nadolol	PO	1 mg/kg/24 hr	Same as other β-blockers, but less severe	β-Blocker of choice in asthma	Longer duration of action permits once/day dosing
ACE inhibitors	Captopril	PO	0.05–0.15 mg/kg/dose (low end in infants)	Hyperkalemia, proteinuria, cough, rash, marrow suppression	Use with caution in renal artery disease [bilateral], do not use in pregnancy, or in anyone who has had angioneurotic edema	More rapid onset than other ACE inhibitors
	Enalapril	PO	0.05–0.15 mg/kg/day	Similar to captopril	Similar to captopril-but longer acting. not sulfur containing, so perhaps fewer side effects	Absorption not affected by food
Calcium channel blockers	Nifedipine	PO	0.25 mg/kg/dose, q 4–6 h	Vasoliatation, tachycardia, nausea, vomiting, sweating; cardiac problems	Use with caution in heart failure	Absorption delayed by food
	Verapamil	PO	4–10 mg/kg/day, given t.i.d.	Similar to nifedipine		Can be put into suspension
	Isradipine	PO	0.05–0.83 mg/kg/day	Similar to nifedipine		First dose hypotension may occur
α-Blockers	Prazosin	PO	1 mg to a maximum of 20 mg q 24 hr	Orthostatic hypotension, lethargy, sedation, and fatigue		Specific for catecholamine excess
	Phenoxy-benzamine	PO	0.2 mg/kg/24 hr	Orthostatic hypotension, nasal congestion		
Central adrenergic stimulators	Clonidine	PO or patch	0.05 mg/kg b.i.d. to maximum 2.4 mg/24 hr	Lethargy, sedation, dry mouth, retinal degeneration		

Abbreviations: CHF, congestive heart failure; PO, per oral; BP, blood pressure; ANA, antinuclear antibody; ACE, angiotensin-converting enzyme; GI, gastrointestinal; AV, atrioventricular.

include glucocorticoids and mineralocorticoids, thyroid replacement, and estrogen–progestin combinations (139). Thus, the alert clinician prescribing such medication will monitor any individual for whom such medications are prescribed. Additionally, the self-prescription or inadvertent exposure of patients to such compounds can indeed result in elevated blood pressure.

Glucocorticoid-related hypertension is extremely common among those who are on such preparations for prolonged time periods. It has been estimated that 88% of children receiving glucocorticoids become hypertensive (140). The hypertension related to glucocorticoid use appears irrespective of indication and

has been reported among children with neurological, renal, pulmonary, and gastrointestinal disease. Given a necessary course of steroids, it is imperative that blood pressure be monitored and treated as needed until such time as the glucocorticoid dose can be discontinued.

Expectable Hypertension in the Course of a Known Diagnosis

Certain endocrine diagnoses are associated with hypertension. A child with Turner syndrome has a definitive chance of having renovascular hypertension, owing to renal artery abnormalities or renal malrotation and anatomic problems (141). Children with calcium-regulatory hormone problems may develop hypercalcemia and hypercalciuria and develop nephrocalcinosis with attendant renal calcification and hypertension (142). Children from families affected with a familial endocrinopathy should be followed, given the frequency of neural crest tumors.

Diabetes may be associated with microalbuminuria early, and endocrinologists should, from all that is now known, monitor children with diabetes for microalbuminuria, renal function, and blood pressure. Renoprotective treatment may well be indicated (143–145) (Volume I, Section II, Chapters 4, 6 and 9). The presence of hypertension in obese patients and in those with insulin resistance/dysmetabolic syndrome need also be addressed. Weight loss and behavioral lifestyle changes should be encouraged as the first goal and remain active even when additional medical therapy is instituted.

Those endocrine diagnoses for which monitoring blood pressure levels should be part of routine care are listed in Table 4.

PRIMARY HYPERTENSION: HOW OFTEN ENDOCRINE?

About one-quarter of the adult population has hypertension, and many hypertensive individuals have salt sensitivity—blood pressure increases with a high salt intake and decreases with a lowered salt intake. The delineation of several monogenic forms of low-renin hypertension have raised questions as to whether some individuals with so-called primary hypertension might have abnormalities in those genes that lead to Mendelian forms of low-renin hypertension. Such mutations might not lead inevitably to hypertension but might cause a predisposition to develop hypertension. Interestingly, recent studies of individuals with primary hypertension have detected certain polymorphisms that appear to be associated with differences in function of 11-β-HSD2. Some publications suggest that individuals with either a polymorphism in 11-β-HSD2 or who have an increased cortisol half-life seem to respond differently from others with respect to salt sensitivity. Such findings suggest that some forms of primary

Table 7 Parenteral and Sublingual Drugs for Use in Hypertensive Emergencies and Urgencies in Pediatric Patients

Medication	Route	Dosage	Onset of action	Peak/duration	Adverse effects	Contraindication	Comments
Sodium nitroprusside (Nipride)	IV infusion	0.3–10 µg/kg/min	Immediate	1–2 min/2–3 min	Thiocyanate toxicity	Hepatic insufficiency	Photosensitive preparation; shield from light
Labetalol	IV bolus	0.5 mg/kg over 2 min; if no response, double dose and repeat q 10 min to max dose of 5 mg/kg	1–5 min	5 min/variable (generally 2–6 hr)	Postural hypotension; neurologic symptoms; nausea and vomiting	Bronchial asthma; CHF	
Nifedipine	S.L.	0.25 mg/kg q 4–6 h	10–15 min	60–90 min/ variable, usually 2–4 h	Vasodilatation, headache, cardiac events if preceding heart failure	Cardiomyopathy; concomitant use of β-blockers; cimetidine (relative)	Cardiac concerns less relevant in children than in adults
Esmolol	IV	500 µg/kg over 30 sec, and then infusion of 25 µg/ kg/min increasing dose, e.g. 4 min to max 300 µg/ kg/min	1 min	mins/mins	hypotension, CNS effects, nausea		Good drug for hypertension intra-op
Enalaprilat	IV, over 5 min	0.04–0.8 mg/kg/ dose (child); 0.01 mg/kg starting neonate dosage	15 min	1–4 h/variable	Hypotension, oliguria, hypokalemia	Renal failure; dehydration	Rx hypotension with volume
Diazoxide	IV bolus	1–3 mg/kg repeated every 5–15 min until control of BP	1–5 min	1–5 min/variable (usually < 12 h)	Arrhythmias, hyperglycemia, sodium and water retention	Thiazide sensitivity, diabetes, coarctation	May need diuretics to prevent fluid retention; unpredictable BP drop may occur
Phentolamine	IV bolus	0.05–0.1 mg/kg	within 30 sec	2 min/5–30 min	Tachycardia, arrhythmia, marked hypotension		Specific for pheochromocytoma.

Abbreviation: IV, intravenous.

Table 8 Diuretic Agents for Administration in Pediatric Patients

Medication	Dosage	Onset	Peak/duration	Adverse effects	Relative contraindication
Furosemide (Lasix)	1–2 mg/kg (maximum 6 mg/kg/24 hr)	Oral: 1–2 hr; IV: 5 min (child); 1 hr (neonate)	1–2 h/4–6 hr; 30 min/2 hr (child); 1–2 hr/5–6 hr (neonate)	Hyperuricemia; hyperglycemia; hypokalemia; hyponatremia; fluid depletion, ototoxicity	Sulfonamide sensitivity, anuria, metabolic alkalosis
Ethacrynic acid (Edecrin)	1 mg/kg (maximum, 25 mg total/day)	Oral: ∼30 min; IV: 15–30 min	2 hr/6–8 hr; 45 min/3 hr	Same as for furosemide; ototoxicity more	Anuria, metabolic alkalosis
Bumetanide (Bumex)	Newborn: 0.01–0.05 mg/kg q 24 hr; child: 0.015–0.1 mg/kg/dose q 6–24 hr	Oral:30–60 min; IV: minutes	Oral: 4–6 hr duration; IV: 30–60 min duration	Similar to furosemide; gastrointestinal discomfort	As for furosemide
Hydrochlorothiazide (HydroDiuril)	2 mg/kg b.i.d.	Oral: 2 hr	4 hr/6–12 hr	Electrolyte depletion; hyperuricemia; hypoglycemia	Anuria, sulfonamide sensitivity
Spironolactone (Aldactone); Metolazone (Zaroxolyn, Diulo, Mykrox)	1–3.3 mg/kg; q 6,8,or 12 hr; 1 mg/kg	Oral: gradual; oral: gradual	3 day/2–3 day; gradual	Hyperkalemia, gynecomastia; similar to thiazide; also bloating, chest pain, chills	Anuria, hyperkalemia, decreasing renal fx anuria

Abbreviation: IV, intravenous.

hypertension may be distinguished from others by their 11-β-HSD-2 activity (81,91,146). Because not all studies (147) support such findings, this remains an area of ongoing consideration. Additionally, some studies suggest that metabolic syndrome may have distinct hypertension, differentiable from primary hypertension (148)

TREATMENT

Current evidence supports the concept that blood pressure should be well within normal ranges among adults. For example, the risk of cardiovascular events among adults is higher among individuals with high normal blood pressure when compared to those with mid-range or low normal blood pressure (149). While no such data yet exist for children, it is more likely than not that stringent blood pressure control is important, particularly for children with health problems that can be associated with hypertension. Thus, it is reasonable to control blood pressure into the normal range in any infant, child, or adolescent who has hypertension.

A primary endocrinopathy should be treated; yet, if blood pressure is elevated, either because full therapy is not yet on board, or because therapy includes medications that can raise blood pressure, additional therapy in the form of antihypertensive treatment is indicated. Tables 6–8 lists current oral and IV medications and dosages (1,150–156). One should note that specific pediatric indications are presently evolving, as a result of the Food and Drug Administration Modernization Act of 1997, which has encouraged antihypertensive trials in children (152–154).

REFERENCES

1. Fourth report on the diagnosis, evaluation and treatment of high blood pressure in children and adolescents. Pediatrics 2004; 114:555–576.
2. Report of the Task Force on Blood Pressure Control in Children. Pediatrics 1977; 59(suppl 5):797–820.
3. Task force on blood pressure control in children. Report of the second task force on blood pressure control of children. Pediatrics 1987; 79:1–25.
4. National high blood pressure education program working group on hypertension control in children and adolescents. Update on the 1987 task force report on high blood pressure in children and adolescents: a working group report from the national high blood pressure eduction program. Pediatrics 1996; 98:649–658.
5. Goonasekera CDA, Dillon MJ. Measurement interpretation of blood pressure. Arch Dis Child 2000; 82:261–265.
6. Kay JD, Sinaiko AR, Daniels SR. Pediatric Hypertension. Am Heart J 2001; 142:422–432.
7. Hiner LB, Falkner B. Renovascular hypertension in children. Ped Clin N Am 1993; 40(1):123–140.
8. Wuhl E, Witte K, Soergel M, Mehls O, Schaefer F; German Working Group on Pediatric Hypertension. Distribution of 24-h ambulatory blood pressure in children: normalized reference values and role of body dimensions. J Hypertens 2002; 20(10):1995–2007; erratum. J Hypertens 2003; 21(11):2205–2206.
9. Sorof JM, Portman RJ. Ambulatory blood pressure measurements. Curr Opin Pediatr 2001; 13(2):133–137.
10. Flynn JT. Differentiation between primary and secondary hypertension in children using ambulatory blood pressure monitoring. Pediatrics 2002; 110(1 Pt 1):89–93.
11. Lurbe E, Redon J. Diagnosis of high blood pressure in children by means of ambulatory blood pressure monitoring. Curr Hypertens Rep 2001; 3:89–90.
12. Koch VH, Colli A, Saito MI, et al. Comparison between casual blood pressure and ambulatory blood pressure monitoring parameters in healthy and hypertensive adolescents. Blood Press Monit 2000; 5(5–6):281–289.

13. Khan IA, Gajaria M, Stephens D, Balfe JW. Ambulatory blood pressure monitoring in children: a large center's experience. Pediatr Nephrol 2000; 14:802–805.
14. Simckes AM, Srivastava T, Alon US. Ambulatory blood pressure monitoring in children adolescents. Clin Pediatr (Phila) 2002 Oct; 41(8):549–64.
15. Varda NM, Gregoric A. Twenty-four-hour ambulatory blood pressure monitoring in infants and toddlers. Pediatr Nephrol 2005; 20(6):798–802. Epub 2005 Apr 27.
16. Yiu VW, Dluhy RG, Lifton RP, Guay-Woodford LM. Low peripheral plasma renin activity as a critical marker in pediatric hypertension. Pediatr Nephrol 1997; 11: 343–346.
17. Pratt JH. Low-renin hypertension: more common than we think? Cardiol Rev 2000; 8:202–206.
18. Warnock DG. Genetic forms of human hypertension. Curr Opin Nephrol Hyperten 2001; 138:715–720.
19. New MI. Hypertension in congenital adrenal hyperplasia and apparent mineralocorticoid excess. Ann NY Acad Sci 2002; 970:145–154.
20. New MI, Crawford C, Virdis R. Low renin hypertension in childhood. In: Lifshitz F, ed. Pediatric Endocrinologyed. 3rd. New York: Marcel Dekker, 1996:776.
21. New MI, Seaman MP. Secretion rates of cortisol and aldosterone precursors in various forms of congenital adrenal hyperplasia. J Clin Endocrinol Metab 1970; 30:361.
22. New MI, Levine LS. Hypertension of childhood with suppressed renin. Endocrinol Rev 1980; 1:421–430.
23. New MI, Levine LS. Congenital adrenal hyperplasia. Adv Hum Genet 1973; 4:251–326.
24. Mimouni M, Kaufman H, Roitman A, Morag C, Sadan N. Hypertension in a neonate with 11 beta-hydroxylase deficiency. Eur J Pediatr 1985; 143:231–233.
25. Zachmann M, Vollmin JA, New MI, Curtius C-C, Prader A. Congenital adrenal hyperplasia due to deficiency of 11-hydroxylation of 17a-hydroxylated steroids. J Clin Endocrinol Metab 1971; 33:501.
26. Motaghedi R, Betensky BP, Slowinska B, et al. Update on the prenatal diagnosis and treatment of congenital adrenal hyperplasia due to 11beta-hydroxylase deficiency. J Pediatr Endocrinol Metab 2005; 18(2):133–142.
27. Cerame BI, New MI. Hormonal hypertension in children:11-β-hydroxylase deficiency and apparent mineralocorticoid excess. J Pediatr Endocrinol 2000; 13:1537–1547.
28. White PC, Dupont J, New MI, Lieberman E, Hochberg Z, Rosler A. A mutation in CYP11B1 (Arg448His) associated with steroid 22-β-hydroxylase deficiency in Jews of Moroccan origin. J Clin Invest 1991; 87:1664–1667.
29. Curnow KM, Slutker L, Vitek J, et al. Mutations in the CYP11B1 gene causing congenital adrenal hyperplasia and hypertension cluster in exons 6,7 and 8. Proc Natl Acad Sci USA 1993; 90:4552–4556.
30. Skinner CA, Rumsby G. Steroid 11b-hydroxylase deficiency caused by a 5-base pair duplication in the CYP11B1 gene. Hum Mol Genet 1994; 3:377–378.
31. Helmberg A, Ausserer B, Kofler R. Frameshift by insertion of 2 basepairs in codon 394 of CYP11B1 cuases congenital adrenal hyperplasia due to steroid 11-β-hydroxylase deficiency. J Clin Endocrinol Metab 1992; 75:1278–1281.
32. Zhu YS, Cordero JJ, Can S, et al. Mutations in CYP11B1 gene: phenotype-genotype correlations. Am J Med Genet A 2003; 122(3):193–200.
33. Pascoe L, Curnow KM, Slutsker L, et al. Mutations in the human CYP11B2 (aldosterone synthase) gene causing corticosterone methyloxidase II deficiency. Proc Natl Acad Sci U S A 1992; 89:4996–5000.
34. Biglieri EG, Herron MA, Brust N. 17-hydroxylation deficiency. J Clin Invest 1966; 45:1946.
35. New MI. Male pseudohermaphroditism due to 17-α-hydroxylase deficiency. J Clin Invest 1970; 49:1930.
36. Mantero F, Scaroni C. Enzymatic defects of steroidogenesis:17-α-hydroxylase deficiency. Pediatr Adol Endocrinol 1984; 13:83–94.
37. Wit JM, van Roermund HPC, Oostdik W, et al. Heterozygotes for 17α-hydroxylase deficiency can be detected with a short ACTH test. Clin Endocrinol 1988; 28:657–664.
38. Matteson KJ, Picado-Leonard J, Chung BC, Mohandas TK, Miller WL. Assignment of the gene for adrenal P450c17 to human chromosome 10. J Clin Endocrinol Metab 1986; 63:789.
39. Fan Y-S, Sasi R, Lee C, Winter JSD, Waterman MR, Lin CC. Localization of the human CYP17 gene (cytochrome P45017a) to 10q24.3 by fluorescence in situ hybridization and simultaneous chromosome banding. Genomics 1992; 14:1110–1111.
40. Costa-Santos M, Kater CE, Auchus RJ. Brazilian Congenital Adrenal Hyperplasia Multicenter Study Group. Two prevalent CYP17 mutations and genotype-phenotype correlations in 24 Brazilian patients with 17-hydroxylase deficiency. J Clin Endocrinol Metab 2004; 89(1):49–60.
41. Labhart A. In: Adrenal cortex Labhart A, ed. Clinical Endocrinology: Theory and Practice. New York: Springer-Verlag, 1974:332–339.
42. Stewart PM. Mineralocorticoid hypertension. Lancet 353:1341–1347.
43. Conn JW. Primary aldosteronism, a new clinical entity. J Lab Clin Med 1955; 45:3–17.
44. Young WF. Primary aldosteronism: update on diagnosis and treatment. Endocrinologist 1997; 7:213–221.
45. Kelch RP, Connors MH, Kaplan SL, Biglieri EG, Grumbach MM. A calcified aldosterone-producing tumor in a hypertensive, normokalemic prepubertal girl. J Pediatr 1973; 83:432.
46. Bryer-Ash M, Wilson D, Tune BM, Rosenfeld RG, Shochat SJ, Luetscher JA. Hypertension caused by an aldosterone-secreting adenoma. Am J Dis Child 1984; 138:673–676.
47. Decsi J, Soltesz G, Harangi F, Nemes J, Szabo M, Pinter A. Severe hypertension in a ten-year-old boy secondary to an aldosterone-producing tumor identified by adrenal sonography. Acta Pediatr Hung 1986; 27:233–238.
48. Oberfield SE, Levine LS, Firpo A, et al. Primary hyperaldosteronism in childhood due to unilateral macronodular hyperplasia. Hypertension 1984; 6:75–84.
49. Abdullah N, Khawaja K, Hale J, Barrett AM, Cheetham TD. Primary hyperaldosteronism with normokalaemia secondary to an adrenal adenoma (Conn's syndrome) in a 12 year-old boy. J Pediatr Endocrinol Metab 2005; 18(2):215–219.
50. Prosser PR, Sutherland CM, Scullin DR. Localization of adrenal aldosterone adenoma by computerized tomography. N Engl J Med 1979; 300:1278–1279.
51. Weinberger MH, Grim CE, Hollifield JW, et al. Primary aldosteronism: diagnosis, localization and treatment. Ann Intern Med 1979; 90:386–395.
52. Hietakorpi S, Korhonen T, Aro A, et al. The value of scintigraphy and computed tomography for the differential diagnosis of primary hyperaldosteronism. Acta Endocrinol 1986; 113:118–122.
53. Delyani JA. Rocha R. Cook CS, et al. Eplerenone: a selective aldosterone receptor antagonist (SARA). Cardiovasc Drug Rev 2001; 19(3):185–200.
54. Sutherland DJ, Ruse JL, Laidlaw JC. Hypertension, increased aldosterone secretion and low plasma renin

activity relieved by dexamethasone. Can Med Assoc J 1966; 95:1109–1119.

55. New MI, Peterson RE. A new form of congenital adrenal hyperplasia. J Clin Endocrinol Metab 1967; 27:300–305.

56. http://www.ncbi.nlm.nih.gov/Omim.

57. New MI, Oberfield SE, Levine LS, et al. Demonstration of autosomal dominant transmission and absence of HLA linkage in dexamethasone-suppressible hyperaldosteronism. Lancet 1980; 1:550–551.

58. Miura K, Yoshinaga K, Goto K, et al. A case of glucocorticoid-responsive hyperaldosteronism. J Clin Endocrin Metab 1968; 28(12):1807–1815.

59. New MI, Siegal EJ, Peterson RE. Dexamethasone-suppressible hyperaldosteronism. J Clin Endocrinol Metab 1973; 37:93–100.

60. Giebink GS, Gotlin RW, Biglieri EG, Katz FH. A kindred with familial glucocorticoid-suppressible aldosteronism. J Clin Endocrinol Metab 1973; 36:715–723.

61. Grim CE, Weinberger MH. Familial dexamethasone-suppressible hyperaldosteronism. Pediatrics 1980; 65: 597–604.

62. Oberfield SE, Levine LS, Stoner E, et al. Adrenal glomerulosa function in patients with dexamethasone-suppressible normokalemic hyperaldosteronism. J Clin Endocrinol Metab 1981; 53:158–164.

63. Lifton RP, Dluhy RG, Powers M, et al. Chimeric 11b-hydroxylase/aldosterone synthase gene causes GRA and human hypertension. Nature 1992; 355:262–265.

64. Lifton RP, Dluhy RG, Powers M, et al. Hereditary hypertension caused by chimeric gene duplications and ectopic expression of aldosterone synthetase Nature Genet 1992; 2:66–74.

65. Gill JR Jr., Bartter FC. Overproduction of sodium-retaining steroids by the zona glomerulosa is adrenocorticotropin-dependent and mediates hypertension in dexamethasone-suppressible aldosteronism. J Clin Endocrinol Metab 1981; 53:331–337.

66. Gomez-Sanches CE, Gill JR Jr., Ganguly A, Gordon RD. Glucocorticoid-suppressible aldosteronism: a disorder of the adrenal transitional zone. J Clin Endocrinol Metab 1988; 67:444–448.

67. Ulick S, Chan CK, Gill JR Jr., et al. Defective fasciculate zone function as the mechanims of glucocrticoid-remediable aldosteronism. J Clin Endocrinol Metab 1990; 71:1151–1157.

68. Ulick S, Chu MD. Hypersecretion of a new cortico-steroid, 18-hydroxycortisol in two types of adrenocortical hypertension. Clin Exp Hypertens 1982; Suppl 9/10:1771–1777.

69. Ulick S, Chu MD, Land M. Biosynthesis of 18-oxocortisol by aldosterone-producing adrenal tissue. J Biol Chem 1983; 258:5498–5502.

70. Gomez-Sanchez CE, Montgomery M, Ganguly A, et al. Elevated urinary excretion of 18-oxocortisol in glucocorticoid-suppressible aldosteronism. J Clin Endocrinol Metab 1984; 59:1022–1024.

71. Shackleton CH. Mass Spectrometry in the diagnosis of steroid-related disorders and in hypertension research. J Steroid Biochem Mol Biol 1993; 45:127–140.

72. Dluhy RG, Anderson B, Harlin B, Ingelfinger J, Lifton R. Glucocorticoid-remediable aldosteronism is associated with severe hypertension in early childhood. J Pediatr 2001; 138(5):715–720.

73. New MI, Levine LS, Biglieri EG, Pareira J, Ulick S. Evidence for an unidentified ACTH-induced steroid hormone causing hypertension. J Clin Endocrinol Metab 1977; 44:924–933.

74. New MI, Oberfield SE, Carey RM, Greig F, Ulick S, Levine LS. A genetic defect in cortisol metabolism as the basis for the syndrome of apparent mineralocorticoid excess. In: Mnatero F, Biglieri EG, Edwards CRW, eds. Endocrinology of Hypertension. Serono Symposia No. 50. New York: Academic Press, 1982:85–101.

75. Downey MK, Riddick L, New MI. Apparent mineralocorticoid excess: a genetic form of fatal low-renin hypertension. Program and Abstracts, American Society of Hypertension, Second World Congress on Biologically Active Atrial Peptides, New York, May 1987.

76. Ulick S, Ramirez LC, New MI. An abnormality in steroid reductive metabolism in a hypertensive syndrome. J Clin Endocrinol Metab 1977; 44:799–802.

77. Ulick S, Levine LS, Gunczler P, et al. A syndrome of apparent mineralocorticoid excess associated with defects in the peripheral metabolism of cortisol. J Clin Endocrinol Metab 1979; 44:757–764.

78. Lakshmi V, Monder C. Evidence for independent 11-oxidase and 11-reductase activities of 11b-hydroxysteroid dehydrogenase: enzyme latency, phase transitions, and lipid requirements. Endocrinology 1985; 116: 552–560.

79. Werder EA, Zachmann M, Vollmin JA, Veyrat R, Prader A. Unusual steroid excretion in a child with low renin hypertension. Res Steroids 1974; 6:385–389.

80. White PC, Munte T, Agarwal AK. 11-β-hydroxysteroid dehydrogenase and the syndrome of apparent mineralocorticoid excess. Endocr Rev 1997; 18:135–156.

81. Ferrari P, Lovati E, Frey FJ. The role of the 11-β-hydroxysteroid dehydrogenase type 2 in human hypertension. J Hypertens 2000; 18(3):241–248.

82. Obeyesekere VR, Ferrari P, Andrews RK, et al. The R337C mutation generates a high Km 11 beta-hydroxysteroid dehydrogenase type II enzyme in a family with apparent mineralocorticoid excess. J Clin Endocrinol Metab 1995; 80:3381–3383.

83. Ferrari P, Obeyesekere VR, Li K, et al. Point mutations abolish 11 beta-hydroxysteroid dehydrogenase type II activity in three families with the congenital syndrome of apparent mineralocorticoid excess. Mol Cell Endocrinol 1996; 119:21–24.

84. Mune T, Rogerson FM, Nikkila H, Agarwal AK, White PC. Human hypertension caused by mutations in the kidney isozyme of 11 beta-hydroxysteroid dehydrogenase. Nat Genet 1995; 10:394–399.

85. Dave-Sharma S, Wilson RC, Harbison MD, et al. Examination of genotype and phenotype relationships in 14 patients with apparent mineralocorticoid excess. J Clin Endocrinol Metab 1998; 83(7):2244–2254.

86. Moudgil A, Rodich G, Jordan SC, Kamil ES. Nephrocalcinosis and renal cysts associated with apparent mineralocorticoid excess syndrome. Pediatr Nephrol 2000; 15(1–2):60–62.

87. Mercado AB, Wilson RC, Chung KC, Wei J-Q, New MI. Prenatal treatment and diagnosis of congenital adrenal hyperplasia owing to steroid 21-hydroxylase deficiency. J Clin Endocrinol Metab 1995; 80:2014–2020.

88. Ugrasbul F, Wiens T, Rubinstein P, New MI, Wilson RC. Prevalence of mild apparent mineralocorticoid excess in Mennonites. J Clin Endocrinol Metab 1999; 84:4735–4738.

89. New MI, Nimkarn S, Brandon DD, et al. Resistance to multiple steroids in two sisters. J Ster Biochem Molec Biol 2001; 76:161–166.

90. Li A, Li KXZ, Marui S, et al. Apparent mineralocorticoid excess in a Brazilian kindred: hypertension in the heterozygote state. J Hypertens 1997; 15:1397–1402.

91. Ferrari P, Krozowski Z. Role of the 11-β-hydroxysteroid dehydrogenase in blood pressure regulation. Kidney Int 2000; 57:1374–1381.

92. New MI, Geller DS, Fallo F, Wilson RC. Monoogenic low renin hypertension. Trends Endocrinol Metab 2005; 16(3):92–97.

93. Stewart PM, Wallace AM, Valentino R, Burt D, Shakleton CHL, Edwards CRW. Mineralocorticoid activity of liquorice:11b-hydroxysteroid dehydrogenase deficiency comes of age. Lancet 1987; 2:821–823.

94. Gordon RD, Klemm SA, Tunny TJ, Stowasser M. Genetics of primary aldosteronism. Clin Exp Pharmacol Physiol 1994; 21(11):915–918.

95. Schambelan M, Sebastian A, Rector FC Jr. Mineralocorticoid-resistant renal hyperkalemia without salt wasting (type II pseudohypoaldosteronism): role of increased renal chloride reabsorption.Kidney Int 1981; 19:716.

96. Take C, Ikeda K, Kurasawa T, Kurokawa K. Increased chloride reabsorption as an inherited renal tubular defect in familial type II pseudohypoaldosteronism. N Engl J Med 1991; 324:472–6.

97. Mansfield TA, Simon DB, Farfel Z, et al. Multilocus linkage of familial hyperkalaemia and hypertension, pseudohypoaldosteronism type II, to chromosomes 1q31–42 and 17p11-q21. Nat Genet 1997; 16:202–205.

98. Erdogan G, Corapciolgu D, Erdogan MF, Hallioglu J, Uysal AR. Furosemide and dDAVP for the treatment of pseudohypoaldosteronism type II. J Endocrinol Invest 1997; 20:681–684.

99. Wilson FH, Disse-Nicodeme S, Choate KA, et al. Human hypertension caused by mutations in WNK Kinases. Science 2001; 293:1107–1112.

100. Hadchouel J, Delaloy C, Faure S, Achard JM, Jeunemaitre X. Familial hyperkalemic hypertension. J Am Soc Nephrol 2006; 17(1):208–217. Epub 2005 Oct 12.

101. Liddle GW, Bledsoe T, Coppage WS. A familial renal disorder simulating primary aldosteronism but with negligible aldosterone secretion. Trans Assoc Phys 1963; 76:199–213.

102. Wang C, Chan TK, Yeung RT, Coghlan JP, Scoggins BA, Stockigt JR. The effect of triamterene and sodium intake on renin, aldosterone, and erythrocyte sodium transport in Liddle's syndrome. J Clin Endocrinol Metab 1981; 52:1027–1032.

103. Botero-Velez M, Curtis JJ, Warnock DG. Brief report: Liddle's syndrome revisited—a disorder of sodium reabsorption in the distal tubule. N Engl J Med 1994; 330:178–181.

104. Shimkets RA, Warnock DG, Bositis CM, et al. Liddle's syndrome: heritable human hypertension caused by mutations in the β-subunit of the epithelial sodium channel. Cell 1994; 79:407–414.

105. Hansson JH, Nelson-Williams C, Suzuki H, et al. Hypertension caused by a truncated epithelial sodium channel gamma subunit: genetic heterogeneity of Liddle syndrome. Nat Genet 1995; 11:76–82.

106. Rossier BC. 1996 Homer Smith Award Lecture: cum grano salis: the epithelial sodium channel and the control of blood pressure. J Am Soc Nephrol 1997; 8:980–992.

107. Treadwell BLJ, Sever ED, Savage O, Copeman WSC. Side effects of long term treatment with corticosteroids and corticotrophin. Lancet 1964; 1:1121–1123.

108. Gomez-Sanchez CE. Cushing's syndrome and hypertension. Hypertension 1986; 8:258–264.

109. Ritchie CM, Sheridan B, Fraser R, et al. Studies on the pathogenesis of hypertension in Cushing's disease and acromegaly. Q J Med 1990; 280:855–867.

110. Saruta T, Suzuki H, Handa M, Igarashi Y, Kondo K, Senba S. Multiple factors contribute to the pathogenesis of hypertension in Cushing's syndrome. J Clin Endocrinol Metab 1986; 62:275–279.

111. Mircescu H, Wilkin F, Paquette J, et al. Molecular characterization of a pediatric pheochromocytoma with suspected bilateral disease. J Pediatr 2001; 138(2):269–73.

112. Kinney MA, Warner ME, van Heerden JA, et al. Perianesthetic risks and outcomes of pheochromocytoma and paraganglioma resection. Anesth Analg 2000; 91(5): 1118–1123.

113. Reddy VS, O'Neill JA Jr., Holcomb GW III, et al. Twenty-five-year surgical experience with pheochromocytoma in children. Am Surg 2000; 66(12):1085–1091.

114. Chen TY, Liang CD, Shieh CS, Ko SF, Kao ML. Reversible hypertensive retinopathy in a child with bilateral pheochromocytoma after tumor resection. J Formos Med Assoc 2000; 99(12):945–947.

115. Lertakyamanee N, Lertakyamanee J, et al. Surgery and anesthesia for pheochromocytoma–a series of 40 operations. J Med Assoc Thai 2000; 83(8):921–927.

116. Radmayr C, Neumann H, Bartsch G, Elsner R, Janetschek G. Laparoscopic partial adrenalectomy for bilateral pheochromocytomas in a boy with von Hippel-Lindau disease. Eur Urol 2000; 38(3):344–348.

117. Hack HA. The perioperative management of children with phaeochromocytoma. Paediatr Anaesth 2000; 10(5):463–476.

118. Ross JH. Pheochromocytoma. Special considerations in children. Urol Clin North Am 2000; 27(3):393–402.

119. Laporte R, Godart F, Breviere GM, Vaksmann G, Francart C, Rey C. Severe arterial hypertension and pheochromocytoma in childhood. Case report and review of the literature (French). Arch Mal Coeur Vaiss 2000; 93(5):627–630.

120. Ferragut J, Caimari M, Rituerto B, Gomez-Rivas B, Herrera M, Alonso F. Pheochromocytoma and clear-cell renal carcinoma in a child with von Hippel-Lindau disease: a patient report. J Pediatr Endocrinol 1999; 12(4):579–582.

121. Hack HA, Brown TC. Preoperative management of phaeochromocytoma—a paediatric perspective (letter; comment). Anaesth Intensive Care 1999; 27(1): 112–113.

122. Clements RH, Goldstein RE, Holcomb GW III. Laparoscopic left adrenalectomy for pheochromocytoma in a child. J Pediatr Surg 1999; 34(9):1408–1409.

123. Pretorius M, Rasmussen GE, Holcomb GW. Hemodynamic and catecholamine responses to a laparoscopic adrenalectomy for pheochromocytoma in a pediatric patient. Anesth Analg 1998; 87(6):1268–1270.

124. Eder U, Fischer-Colbrie R, Kogner P, Leitner B, Bjellerup P, Winkler H. Levels and molecular forms of chromogranins in human childhood neuroblastomas and ganglioneuromas. Neurosci Lett 1998; 253(1):17–20.

125. Favia G, Lumachi F, Polistina F, D'Amico DF. Pheochromocytoma, a rare cause of hypertension: long-term follow-up of 55 surgically treated patients. World J Surg 1998; 22(7):689–693; discussion 694.

126. Russell WJ, Metcalfe IR, Tonkin AL, Frewin DB. The preoperative management of phaeochromocytoma. Anaesth Intensive Care 1998; 26(2):196–200.

127. Maher ER, Kaelin WG Jr., Basset A, et al. Renin-angiotensin system contribution to cardiac hypertrophy in experimental hyperthyroidism: an echocardiographic study. J Cardiovasc Pharmacol 2001; 37:163–172.

128. Beck O, Fassbender WJ, Beyer P, et al. Pheochromocytoma in childhood: implication for further diagnostic procedures. Acta Paediatr 2004; 93(12):1630–1634.

129. Matsota P, Avgerinopoulou-Vluahou A, Velegrakis D. Anaesthesia for phaeochromocytoma removal in a 5-year-old boy. Paediatr Anaesth 2002; 12:176–180.

130. Bittar DA. Innovar induced hypertensive crises in patient with pheochromocytoma. Anesthesiology 1979; 50: 366–369.

131. Schonwetter BS, Libber SM, Jones MD Jr., Park KJ, Pictnick LP. Hypertension in neonatal hyperthyroidism Am J Dis Child 1983; 137:954–955.

132. Minami N, Imai Y, Abe K, et al. The circadian variation of blood pressure and heart rate in patients with hyperthyroidism. Tohoku J Exp Med 1989; 159:185–193.

133. Saito I, Saruta T. Hypertension in thyroid disorders. Endocrinol Metab Clin North Am 1994; 23:379–386.

134. Streeten DH, Anderson GH Jr., Howland T, Chiang R, Smulyan H. Effects of thyroid function on blood pressure. Recognition of hypothyroid hypertension. Hypertension 1988; 11:78–83.

135. Vargas F, Moreno JM, Rodriguez-Gomez I, et al. Vascular and renal function in experimental thyroid disorders. Eur J Endocrinol 2006; 154(2):197–212.

136. Lind l, Ridefelt P, Rastad J, Akerstrom G, Ljunghall S. Relationship between abnormal regulation of cytoplasmic calcium and elevated blood pressure in patients with primary hyperparathyroidism. J Hum Hypertens 1994; 8:113–118.

137. Lind L, Ljunghall S. Blood pressure reaction during the intraoperative and early postoperative periods in patients with primary hyperparathyroidism. Exp Clin Endocrinol 1994; 102:409–413.

138. Hedback GM, Oden AS. Cardiovascular disease, hypertension and renal function in primary hyperparathyroidism. J Intern Med 2002; 251:476–483.

139. Scuteri A, Bos AJ, Brant LJ, Talbot L, Lakatta EG, Fleg JL. Hormone replacement therapy and longitudinal changes in blood pressure in postmenopausal women. Ann Int Med 2001; 135(4):229–238.

140. Covar RA, Leung DY, McCormick D, Steelman J, Zeitler JP, Spahn JD. Risk factors assoiated with glucocorticoid-induced adverse effects in children with severe asthma. J Allergy Clin Immunol 2000; 106:651–659.

141. Nathwani NC, Unwin R, Brook CG, Hindmarsh PC. The influence of renal and cardiovascular abnormalities on blood pressure in Turner syndrome. Clin Endocrinol 2000; 52(3):371–377.

142. Jorde R, Sundsfjord J, Haug E, Bonaa KH. Relation between low calcium intake, parathyroid hormone, and blood pressure. Hypertension 2000; 35(5):1154–1159.

143. Balkau B, Tichet J, Caces E, Vol S, Eschwege E, Cahane M. Insulin dose and cardiovascular risk factors in type 1 diabetic children and adolescents. Diabetes Metab 1998; 24(2):143–150.

144. Sochett EB, Poon I, Balfe W, Daneman D. Ambulatory blood pressure monitoring in insulin-dependent diabetes mellitus adolescents with and without microalbuminuria. J Diabetes Complicat 1998; 12(1):18–23.

145. Madacsy L, Yasar A, Tulassay T, et al. Relative nocturnal hypertension in children with insulin-dependent diabetes mellitus. Acta Paediatrica 1994; 83(4):414–417.

146. Brand E, Kato N, Chatelain N, et al. Structural analysis and evaluation of the 11beta-hydroxysteroid dehydrogenase type 2 (11beta-HSD2) gene in human essential hypertension. J Hypertens 1998; 16(11):1627–1633.

147. Donovan SJ. 11 beta-Hydroxysteroid dehydrogenase: a link between the dysregulation of cortisol metabolism and hypertension. Br J Biomed Sci 1999; 56(3):215–25.

148. Bjorntorp P, Holm G, Rosmond R, Folkow B. Hypertension and the metabolic syndrome: closely related central origin? Blood Press 2000; 9(2–3):71–82.

149. Vasan RS, Larson MG, Leip E, et al. Impact of high normal blood pressure on the risk of cardiovascular disease. N Engl J Med 2001; 345:1291–1297.

150. Ingelfinger JR. Hypertensive emergencies in infants and children. In: Grenvik A, Ayres SM, Holbrook PR, Shoemaker WC, eds. Textbook of Critical Care. 4th: WB Saunders, 2000:1087–1098.

151. Wells TG. Trials of antihypertensive therapies in children. Blood Press Monit 1999; 4(3–4):189–192.

152. Chesney RW, Adamson P, Wells T, Wilson JT, Walson PD. The testing of antihypertensive medications in children: report of the Antihypertensive Agent Guidelines Subcommittee of the Pediatric Pharmacology Research Units. Pediatrics 2001; 107(3):558–561.

153. Sinaiko AR, Lauer RM, Sanders SP. End points for cardiovascular drug trials in pediatric patients. Am Heart J 2001; 142(2):229–32.

154. Portman RJ, McNiece KL, Swinford RD, Braun MC, Samuels JA. Pediatric hypertension: diagnosis, evaluation, management, and treatment for the primary care physician. Curr Probl Pediatr Adolesc Health Care 2005; 35(7):262–94.

155. Rowan S, Adrogues H, Mathur A, Kamat D. Pediatric hypertension: a review for the primary care provider. Clin Pediatr (Phila) 2005; 44(4):289–296.

156. Patel HP, Mitsnefes M. Advances in the pathogenesis and management of hypertensive crisis. Curr Opin Pediatr 2005; 17(2):210–214.

14

Lipid Disorders in Children and Adolescents

Hofit Cohen

The Institute of Lipid and Atherosclerosis Research, The Chaim Sheba Medical Center, Tel-Hashomer and Sackler Faculty of Medicine, Tel Aviv University, Tel Aviv, Israel

Raanan Shamir

Division of Gastroenterology and Nutrition, Meyer Children's Hospital of Haifa, and Ruth and Bruce Rappaport Faculty of Medicine, Technion, Haifa, Israel

INTRODUCTION

A body of evidence now shows that elevated levels of plasma cholesterol, especially low-density lipoprotein cholesterol (LDL-C), are associated with an increased probability of premature cardiovascular disease in the adult. This is particularly true for subjects with the common familial hypercholesterolemia (FH) (a dominant disorder of lipoprotein metabolism), who typically manifest atherosclerosis in the fourth to fifth decade. There is also no doubt that the atherosclerotic process begins in childhood and therefore preventive measures should be initiated as early as possible to prevent progression of the disease (1). In 1992, the National Cholesterol Education Program (NCEP) Expert Panel on Blood Cholesterol in Children and Adolescents recommended that selective screening for the diagnosis of hypercholesterolemia should be implemented and that diagnosed children should be treated based on their LDL-C levels and identified risk factors (2). The magnitude of the obesity epidemic, the increasing prevalence of Type II diabetes in children, and recognition of the importance of other risk factors such as sedentary lifestyle, high blood pressure, and smoking are reflected in the recent publications of the American Heart Association (AHA) and the American Academy of Pediatrics, which provides guidelines for primary prevention of atherosclerosis in childhood (3,4).

This chapter provides basic knowledge of lipid metabolism, pediatric lipid disorders, and a review of the currently suggested methods of diagnosis and management of this growing population of children with hyperlipidemia. The management of the prevalent disorders responsible for elevated triglyceride (TG) blood levels in children such as obesity and diabetes are reviewed in Vol. 1; Chaps. 2 and 6.

LIPIDS AND LIPOPROTEINS

Structure of Lipids and Lipoproteins

Lipoproteins serve as carriers of lipids (mostly water insoluble) in body fluids such as blood and lymph. The *outer* surface of the lipoproteins is mainly made up from the water soluble, amphipatic layer of phospholipids and a small amount of free cholesterol molecules. Embedded in the lipid layer of the outer shell are the apoproteins. These proteins serve as structural elements, enzyme cofactors, and ligands for lipoprotein receptors. The *inner* core of the lipoproteins is composed of hydrophobic (water insoluble) lipids, mainly cholesteryl esters and TGs (5).

Lipoproteins can be classified according to their lipid content. Overall, there are four major groups of lipoproteins, two are TG-rich particles [chylomicrons and very low-density lipoprotein (VLDL-C)] and two are cholesterol-rich particles [LDL and high-density lipoprotein (HDL-C)] (5).

The Metabolic Pathways of Lipoproteins

Exogenous Pathway

The exogenous pathway of lipoprotein metabolism begins with the uptake of lipids (predominantly TGs, but also cholesterol and phospholipids) derived mainly from the diet, and also from bile (Fig. 1). The process involves hydrolysis by lipases and formation of micelles, as well as various carrier proteins and ligands. The absorption of dietary and biliary cholesterol plays a role in determining blood cholesterol levels. New insights into this complex process were recently summarized by Lammert and Wang and are beyond the scope of this chapter (6). In the enterocyte, *chylomicrons* are formed and secreted to the systemic circulation through the lymphatic system. From the

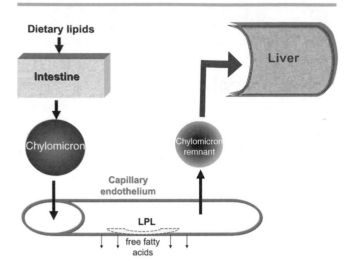

Figure 1 Exogenous pathway of lipoprotein metabolism. *Abbreviation*: LPL, lipoprotein lipase.

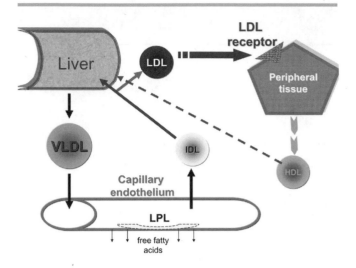

Figure 2 Endogenous pathway lipoprotein metabolism. *Abbreviations*: LDL, low-density lipoprotein; VLDL, very low-density lipoprotein; IDL, intermediate-density lipoprotein; LPL, lipoprotein lipase.

lymphatic vessels, via the thoracic duct, which in turn empties into the vena cava, chylomicrons enter the systemic circulation and peripheral tissues. Chylomicron apolipoproteins are apoC-II, apoB-48, and apoE, and as stated earlier chylomicrons are TG-rich particles (5).

The initial and major step in the metabolism of the chylomicrons is intravascular. The enzyme lipoprotein lipase (LPL) breaks down the TG content of the chylomicrons to monoglycerides and free fatty acids at the capillary endothelium of skeletal muscle, cardiac muscle, and adipose tissue; apoC-II is a *cofactor* of the enzyme LPL. Therefore, deficiency or malfunction of either apoC-II or LPL can lead to abnormalities in chylomicron breakdown. The free fatty acids serve as an energy source for muscle cells, and in the adipocytes, free fatty acids and monoglycerides reassemble as TG to be stored in the adipose tissue. TG-poor chylomicrons are named chylomicron remnants, which after binding to the hepatic remnant receptor are rapidly removed from the plasma. As the clearance of chylomicrons is rapid, in normal circumstances at a *fasting* state, chylomicrons and their remnants are not supposed to be detected in plasma.

Endogenous Pathway

In the endogenous pathway, *VLDL* particles are assembled by the liver (Fig. 2). This particle is a TG-rich particle that also carries free cholesterol on its outer surface and cholesteryl esters in its core. The apolipoproteins of VLDL are apoC-II, apoB-100, and apoE.

Similarly to the initial intravascular metabolism of the chylomicrons, the TG content of the VLDL undergoes hydrolysis by LPL/apoC-II to generate the VLDL remnant or the TG-poor intermediate-

density lipoprotein (IDL) particle. The IDL particle has two optional metabolic pathways—most of it is transformed to LDL, and a smaller amount of the IDL is removed by the hepatic apoE/apoB-100 receptor. *LDL* is the particle that carries cholesterol to peripheral tissues and back to the liver. LDL is almost entirely made of cholesteryl esters and apoB-100. The uptake of cholesterol is dependent on the binding of LDL to its receptor, the apoB-100/LDL receptor, and the cholesterol is used for cell membrane construction, steroid hormone synthesis, and more.

HDL is responsible for transporting cholesterol from the tissues back to the liver (Fig. 3). The liver and the intestine secrete HDL as a nascent particle composed of apoA-IV when secreted by the intestine, and apoA-Ia and apoA-II when secreted by the liver. Acquiring cholesterol requires ATP–binding cassette protein A1ABCA1 (mutations are responsible for

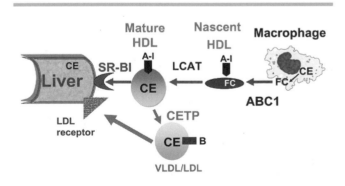

Figure 3 Metabolism of high-density lipoprotein. *Abbreviations*: HDL, high-density lipoprotein; VLDL, very low-density lipoprotein; LDL, low-density lipoprotein; ABC1, ATP binding cassette protein 1; LCAT, lecithin cholesterol acyltransferase; CE, cholesterol ester; CETP, cholesterol ester transfer protein.

Tangier disease where HDL is not detected in the blood). The free cholesterol is esterified by lecithin:cholesterol acyl transferase and the cholesteryl esters are either taken up by the liver or transferred to either VLDL or LDL by cholesteryl ester transfer protein (CETP) (5).

RATIONALE FOR CARDIOVASCULAR DISEASE PREVENTIVE MEASURES DURING CHILDHOOD

Evidence that atherosclerosis begins early in life comes from both clinical evidence and epidemiological data (7,8). The strongest clinical data are provided by children with homozygous FH. These children develop significant coronary heart disease (CHD) in the first decade of life and frequently die from myocardial infarction before the age of 20 (9). Furthermore, blood cholesterol levels measured at 22 years of age predict the risk for CHD over the next 30 to 40 years (10), and data from the Framingham Study show that cholesterol levels measured in young adult males and females predict CHD mortality 30 years later (11). Epidemiological data support the relationship between childhood cholesterol levels and adult levels (12,13), and the relationship between hyperlipidemia in childhood and parental premature CHD (14). Pathological findings provide further evidence about the early development of atherosclerosis: A high frequency of advanced coronary artery lesions was found in young soldiers killed in the Korean War (15). In addition, quantitative postmortem estimation of atherosclerosis in coronary arteries and aortas of children and young adults demonstrated that there is a significant relationship between hyperlipidemia and the extent of atherosclerosis (16).

In agreement with the accumulating evidence, it has been demonstrated that cardiovascular risk factors found in children are related to the severity of atherosclerosis found postmortem in these individuals dying as young adults (17). Thus, identifying risk factors for CHD in children may predict the likelihood of developing CHD as adults, providing the strongest argument for identifying and treating these risk factors.

Screening for Childhood Hypercholesterolemia

Cholesterol screening in childhood is controversial. It has been suggested that childhood screening should not be performed because the outcome of treating children with hyperlipidemia is unknown, cholesterol measurements performed outside of research centers may be inaccurate, and some children found to have elevated plasma cholesterol levels do not continue to have increased levels as adults. However, several studies have demonstrated that childhood rank order of cholesterol is maintained over time (18), and when cholesterol levels in children were greater than the 90th percentile on two occasions, 75% of the children had high cholesterol levels as adults (13). Furthermore, in a study examining adults who initially

were examined as children, it was found that reduced cholesterol levels as adults were partially due to adopting changes of lifestyle in childhood that resulted in modification of risk factors (18).

In the United States, current pediatric recommendations regarding cholesterol screening are to selectively screen children older than two years of age with a positive family history of hypercholesterolemia and/or early heart disease (i.e., a pool of patients enriched in genetic factors predisposing to heart disease) and those children in whom a family history cannot be obtained (i.e., adopted children) (2). Positive family history of premature CHD is defined as a parent, grandparent, or first-degree aunt or uncle who experienced one of the following before the age of 55: myocardial infarction, angina pectoris, peripheral vascular disease, cerebrovascular disease, sudden cardiac death, or documented coronary atherosclerosis. Parental hypercholesterolemia is defined as total blood cholesterol of 240 mg/dL or higher. Presence of other conditions commonly associated with increased risk of CHD, such as smoking, diabetes, obesity, and hypertension are also reasons for checking cholesterol levels.

In this context, it is important to remember that there is low efficacy of the targeted screening. While planned to cover 25% of the population, it is estimated that 35% to 45% of the population would be eligible for these screening recommendations.

Furthermore, the primary focus of the guidelines is on elevated LDL-C levels. They do not address other lipoprotein abnormalities such as decreased HDL levels or hypertriglyceridemia, and they do not address the much more prevalent lipid abnormalities associated with obesity and the metabolic syndrome, such as the presence of small, dense LDL.

Preliminary Assessment of Children with Hyperlipidemia

For children with a positive family history of premature CHD, fasting lipoprotein analysis [total cholesterol (TC), total TGs, HDL-C, and LDL-C] should be performed. Usually, the lipids measured in a routine lipid profile are TC, TG, and HDL-C. LDL-C is calculated utilizing the measurements in the Friedewald equation (can be done only if TG are less than 400 mg/dL). The equation is [LDL-C = TC − (HDL-C + TG/5)], while TG/5 represents the VLDL-C content of serum or plasma. Direct LDL-C measurement is possible but in most circumstances is not necessary, because of the relative accuracy of the calculated LDL-C level. For children, fasting means consuming nothing except water after midnight. Lipoprotein profiles should be performed twice and an average of the two determinations should be used for further evaluation and treatment. This is due to large variability within individuals that may be due to measurement error, regression-to-the-mean, day-to-day variability, seasonal variability and, specifically in children, change with age, growth, and pubertal status.

In the absence of a familial history of premature CHD, but with parental hypercholesterolemia or other risk factors, a nonfasting TC is sufficient as the initial test. Levels of TC and the various lipoproteins are different in children and adolescents compared to those of adults. TC in the umbilical cord blood is approximately 70 mg/dL, and the 50th percentile at two years of age is 162 mg/dL. Acceptable TC levels were set by the NCEP (2) at less than 170 mg/dL (Table 1). If the TC level is elevated, a fasting lipoprotein analysis described above should be performed to confirm the first result, as well as to determine the LDL-C level. Table 1 provides acceptable, borderline, and high LDL-C levels. These NCEP guidelines are based on cholesterol distribution among American children in the Lipid Research Clinics Prevalence study in which the 75th percentile was set as borderline and 95th percentile as high (2). These levels were recently endorsed again by the AHA (4), and serve as the cutoff values for evaluation of children with hypercholesterolemia regardless of age of sex.

For any child with high cholesterol (either TC or LDL-C), screening tests for secondary causes of hypercholesterolemia (in particular, diabetes and diseases of the thyroid, liver, and kidney) should be obtained. Certain medications (such as steroids, anticonvulsants, and oral contraceptives) can also be secondary causes. A list of secondary causes of hypercholesterolemia is given in Table 2.

Elevated TG in children is caused by various conditions detailed in Table 3. These conditions are usually not part of an inherited hyperlipidemia associated with premature CHD (19).

For children and adolescents, the NCEP has not yet defined normal and abnormal TG levels. For adults, NCEP has defined desirable levels of TGs as less than 150 mg/dL, mildly elevated levels are 150 to 199 mg/dL, elevated levels are 200 to 499 mg/dL, and levels at or higher than 500 mg/dL are very high. At the University of Florida (20), hypertriglyceridemia in children is defined as TG levels at or above 125 mg/dL. This value of 125 mg/dL approximates the mean 95th percentile for TGs in boys and girls across childhood and adolescence. Functionally mild hypertriglyceridemia in children is defined as values ranging from 125 to 299 mg/dL, modest

hypertriglyceridemia is from 300 to 499 mg/dL, marked hypertriglyceridemia is from 500 to 999 mg/dL, and values of 1000 mg/dL or more represent massive hypertriglyceridemia. These cut offs can be used when determining treatment approaches to hypertriglyceridemia.

Table 2 Secondary Causes for Hypercholesterolemia

Endocrine
　Hypothyroidism
　Hypopituitarism
　Diabetes mellitus
Metabolic
　Gaucher disease
　Glycogen storage disease
　Tay-Sachs disease
　Niemann-Pick disease
Renal
　Nephrotic syndrome
　Hemolytic uremic syndrome
Liver disease
　Hepatitis
　Cholestasis (benign recurrent intrahepatic cholestasis, congenital biliary atresia, and alagille syndrome)
Medications
　Androgens
　Diuretics (thiazide diuretics and loop diuretics)
　Glucocorticoids
　Immunosuppressive agents and chemotherapy (cyclosporine, tacrolimus, and L-asparaginase)
　Oral contraceptives
　Retinoids
Miscellaneous
　Anorexia nervosa
　SLE
　Klinefelter syndrome
　Idiopathic hypercalcemia

Table 3 Secondary Causes for Hypertriglyceridemia

Endocrine disorders
　Obesity
　Diabetes mellitus
　Insulin resistance
　Cushing syndrome
　Hypothyroidism
　Acromegaly
Renal disease (e.g., chronic renal failure)
Liver disease-hepatocellular
Metabolic disorders
　Lipodystrophy
　Gout
　Glycogen storage disease Type I (Von gierke)
Medications
　Glucocorticoids
　Growth hormone
　Diuretics—thiazides
　Beta-blockers
　Estrogens
　Retinoic acid derivatives
　Antiretroviral HIV therapy
　L-asparaginase
Miscellaneous
　Alcohol abuse
　Pregnancy

Table 1 Cutoff Points of Total and Low-Density Lipoprotein Cholesterol in Children and Adolescents with a Family History of Premature Cardiovascular Disease or Hypercholesterolemia (National Cholesterol Education Program)

Category	Total cholesterol (mg/dL)	LDL-C (mg/dL)
Acceptable	<170	<110
Borderline	170–199	110–129
High	>200	>130

Note: Borderline levels denote the 75th to the 95th percentile. High levels denote those above the 95th percentile (2). The age and sex percentiles for serum lipid levels are shown in Vol. 1; Chap. 30.

MONOGENIC DISORDERS RESULTING IN HIGH LDL-C LEVELS

Familial Hypercholesterolemia

FH is an autosomal dominant disease, characterized by elevated LDL-C levels and premature CHD. FH is caused by mutations in the LDL receptor gene located on chromosome 19. The gene is a housekeeping gene found in almost all tissues, and more than 800 mutations have been described so far. The binding of LDL to its receptor is a complex process in which a defect in any element of that process will present as the phenotype of FH. Figure 4 provides the major possible defects in LDL-R uptake of LDL. In the heterozygote FH, one allele of the LDL-R is defective and this is associated with a 30% increase in LDL production. Homozygous FH is caused when both alleles are mutated causing lack of function of the LDL-R, resulting in ×2- to ×3-fold increase in LDL production. FH is relatively common and, in the heterozygote form, affects approximately 1 in 500 of the general population. Homozygote form is very rare, affecting approximately 1 in 1,000,000 of the general population (21,22).

The diagnostic hallmark of FH is tendon xanthomata. Xanthoma contains infiltrates of lipid-laden foam cells in nonvascular tissues. The most common sites are the Achilles tendon and the tendons overlying the knuckles, but in children, tendon xanthomata are present in a small fraction of heterozygous FH and never before the second decade of life. Corneal arcus and xanthelasma are not specific for FH, but their presence in an adolescent with elevated LDL-C is diagnostic (23).

The diagnosis of heterozygous FH is based on establishing dominantly inherited hyperlipidemia (clear evidence of elevated LDL-C also in one of the parents and either elevated LDL-C or premature CHD in one of the grandparents), and on elevated LDL-C serum levels that are usually twice the normal values. The diagnosis can be confirmed by identifying mutations in the LDL-receptor gene or studying LDL receptor function in cultured cells.

If they remain untreated, subjects with heterozygous FH may experience their first heart attack between the 30th and the 40th year of life. More than 50% of males and about 15% of females with heterozygous FH will die before 60 years of age (24). Homozygous subjects with FH carry two gene mutants from their parents who both must have hypercholesterolemia. They exhibit a 6- to 10-fold elevated LDL-C concentration from birth, develop cutaneous and tendinous xanthoma (Fig. 5) and death from coronary heart disease typically occurs when an individual is aged 20 years or younger (25–27).

Dietary management is usually insufficient for treating children with heterozygous FH and a family history of premature CHD, and the drug treatment options are discussed later.

For homozygous FH, current recommendations and our own experience suggest that LDL-aphaeresis should be performed as early as the first year of life. Heterozygotes of FH that fail to respond adequately to pharmacological treatment are candidates for LDL-apheresis as well (28).

There are few reports of liver transplantation in FH patients. As more than 50% of LDL receptors are located in the liver, liver transplantation has been suggested as a therapeutic option in homozygous FH. Indeed, liver transplantation reverses the metabolic defect but it necessitates chronic immunosuppression. In our opinion, the procedure is indicated if cardiac transplantation is indicated as well due to ischemic

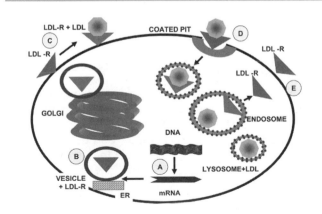

Figure 4 Uptake of LDL by the LDL receptor and potential defects in familial hypercholesterolemia. (**A**) No LDL receptors are synthesized at all. (**B**) LDL receptors are synthesized in the endoplasmic reticulum but fail to migrate to the Golgi apparatus. (**C**) Receptors reach the surface of the cell but fail to bind LDL. (**D**) The mutation is on the cytoplasmic portion of the receptor. The receptor binds LDL but fail to internalize into the coated pit. Receptors cannot recycle after internalization. *Abbreviations*: LDL, low-density lipoprotein; ER, endoplasmic reticulum; LDL-R, LDL-receptor.

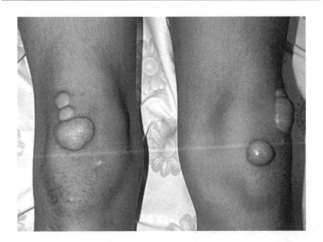

Figure 5 Homozygous familial hypercholesterolemia. Typical xanthomata on the knees of a 10-year-old child with homozygous familial hypercholesterolemia.

cardiomyopathy and would be performed simultaneously (29).

Gene therapy has been attempted in children with homozygous FH, but currently is unavailable worldwide.

Autosomal Recessive Hypercholesterolemia

In this disease, identified in 2001, TC levels approach those of homozygous FH and are differentiated from FH by the normal TC levels of the parents (about 2.5-fold elevated in both parents of homozygous FH). LDL receptor activity is disrupted in liver cells and not in fibroblasts, suggesting a defect only in polarized cells (30).

Familial Defective apoB-100

Phenotypically similar to FH, this syndrome results from a familial defect of apoB-100 at the binding domain, thus diminishing the binding capacity of the LDL particle to its receptor. Therefore, in this syndrome, elevated LDL-C serum levels occur with an intact LDL receptor protein and activity. The single mutation (arg3500gln) in the gene encoding the apoB-100 protein, decreasing the binding of LDL to LDL receptors, was the cause for hyperlipidemia in about 3% of the referrals in pediatric lipid clinics in France (31).

Familial Combined Hyperlipidemia

Familial combined hyperlipidemia (FCHL) is a common lipid disorder that occurs in at least 1% of the population and is found in approximately 10% of patients with premature CHD. Individuals with FCHL have elevated TG levels, LDL-C, or both, and most of the LDL-C is carried in the form of small, dense particles. There are no clinical stigmata for FCHL in childhood, and the diagnosis is based on elevated LDL-C, TG, or both in the child and one of parents (32).

Linkage of FCHL with particular genes or chromosomal regions has been sought, but to date, no consensus implicating a common locus has been obtained. FCHL appears to be a heterogeneous condition associated with several different metabolic alterations. Obesity and insulin resistance coexist with FCHL, but it is unclear whether obesity is responsible for the hypertriglyceridemia observed in FCHL or is a consequence of the basic metabolic defect (33). It has been reported that FCHL is the leading cause for referral to pediatric lipid clinics, but it is unknown whether most cases are expressed in childhood or later in life.

Polygenic Hypercholesterolemia

Polygenic hypercholesterolemia is much more common than FH and is termed polygenic when the clear pattern of autosomal dominant inheritance does not exist. Tendon xanthomata do not appear in polygenic hypercholesterolemia, but corneal arcus and xanthelesma may appear.

INHERITED HYPERTRIGLYCERIDEMIA

Fasting hypertriglyceridemia is encountered more and more among children. Obesity, insulin resistance syndrome, and Type 2 diabetes, with increasing prevalence in the pediatric population, are among the major reasons for fasting hypertriglyceridemia. Despite that observation, no pediatric NCEP recommendations—neither for the pediatric normal levels of TG nor pharmacotherapy of hypertriglyceridemia—have been published up till now.

Elevated TG levels above 1000 mg/dL can be part of the hyperchylomicronemia syndrome (described below), sometimes referred to as Type I hyperlipidemia. It can be caused by increased IDL and LDL levels (Type III hyperlipidemia, or familial dysbetalipoproteinemia, which is rarely seen in children and will not be discussed in this chapter), and in many instances also LDL levels [Type IV hyperlipidemia observed in FCHL that was already discussed, familial hypertriglyceridemia (FHTG), and in diabetes]. Also a combination of increased chylomicrons and VLDL (Type V hyperlipidemia, usually diagnosed by TG levels above 1000 mg/dL), is seen with diabetes, nephritic syndrome, and subjects with mildly elevated TG levels after drug exposure, such as estrogens and alcohol (34).

This chapter describes FHTG and the hyperchylomicronemia syndrome. Since elevated TG in diabetes and obesity are sensitive to controlling glucose homeostasis and weight reduction, respectively, these disorders are not discussed in this chapter despite being one of the most common causes for hyperlipidemia in children.

Familial Hypertriglyceridemia

The disorder is characterized by elevated TG blood levels (above 250 mg/dL and usually below 1000 mg/dL) with a family history of elevated TG blood levels. The prevalence of FHTG in children is about 1 in 500, and it is usually not associated with premature CHD. FHTG may be one of the contributing factors to hypertriglyceridemia in children with additional causes of hypertriglyceridemia (obesity, steroid use, estrogen use, and diabetes). FHTG is an autosomal dominant disease that is usually not expressed until adulthood. In adults, FHTG is the commonest hypertriglyceridemia with an incidence of nearly 1 in 100 persons in the general adult population.

Diagnosis is suggested by TG levels above the 90th percentile with normal cholesterol levels. However, cholesterol levels are mildly elevated in some cases, and FCHL (described in the hypercholesterolemia section of this chapter) should be considered.

Hyperchylomicronemia

The hallmark of this disorder is an extremely high level of TG. Congenital deficiency of LPL, apoC-II, or an LPL inhibitor is responsible for most cases of hyperchylomicronemia (35). Both LPL and apoC-II deficiencies are inherited as autosomal recessive traits. The frequency of either defect is 1 in 1 million in the general population.

The disease is characterized by TG levels greater than 1000 mg/dL, organomegaly (uptake of the chylomicrons by the liver and spleen causes the characteristic hepatosplenomegaly), eruptive xanthomas (yellow orange small papules that appear on the extensor surfaces of the arms and legs, buttocks, and back), and lipemia retinalis (retinal vessels have white/yellowish appearance) (35).

The first clue to the diagnosis is based on the laboratory report of lipemic serum or plasma specimen. Depending on the measurement methods used, the lipemia may interfere with other laboratory tests including electrolytes, hepatic enzymes, and pancreatic amylase levels. The diagnosis of hyperchylomicronemia is easily done even in pediatric wards; fasting plasma is refrigerated overnight, and while normally no lipid layer should be present, plasma from patients with hyperchylomicronemia will have a typical creamy layer on top.

Definite diagnosis can be achieved by measuring postheparin lipase activity or detecting the mutation in the LPL gene. Most patients with LPL deficiency are diagnosed in the first decade of life, while the diagnosis of apoC-II deficiency is typically made later in life (adolescents and adults).

The major risk of the abnormal TG high levels is the occurrence of acute pancreatitis leading to pancreatic insufficiency. The symptoms associated with pancreatitis are severe abdominal pain, nausea, and vomiting. In severe hemorrhagic pancreatitis, death has been reported in adults. However, patients with hyperchylomicronemia syndrome may report episodes of mild abdominal pain, years before the diagnosis. The exact relationship between TG levels and acute pancreatitis is not known. In animal models, blood levels above 1000 mg/dL cause pancreatitis and, in humans, levels are usually above 2000 mg/dL. However, in our experience, children with fasting levels below 1000 mg/dL became pancreatic insufficient with time, while others maintain pancreatic function with much higher levels.

The management of the disease is unique and therefore is described here rather than at the management section of this chapter. The most important treatment is dietary restriction of fat. Restriction of dietary fat to 15% of the total daily energy intake aids in controlling the symptoms, prevents pancreatitis, and reduces TG levels to less than 1000 to 2000 mg/dL. Medium-chain triglycerides (MCTs) are absorbed directly to the intestinal capillaries without creation of chylomicrons and therefore MCT oil can be part of the fat-restricted diet. Care should be taken of total calories to maintain adequate growth, as well as intake of essential fatty acids and fat-soluble vitamins (A, D, E, and K). Premature CHD is usually not a feature of hyperchylomicronemia.

INITIAL EVALUATION OF CHILDREN WITH HYPERLIPIDEMIA
Initial Evaluation of Hypercholesterolemia

This includes a comprehensive family pedigree and assessment for other risk factors. Lipoprotein profile of all immediate family members will help in establishing the mode of inheritance and the etiology (i.e., FH vs. FCHL), as well as identifying undiagnosed family members. Blood chemistry and TSH will identify most cases of secondary hypercholesterolemia and are done routinely in our practice, although the cost effectiveness of such an approach has not been adequately studied (36).

Noninvasive methods such as ultrasound evaluation of carotid-intima medial thickness (CIMT) or flow-mediated dilatation (FMD) of arteries are available mainly as a research tool. Wiegman et al. (37) have recently assessed 201 children heterozygous for FH and 80 unaffected siblings (both age ranges 8–18 years) with B-mode ultrasound to measure CIMT. Mean combined CIMT of heterozygotes was significantly greater than that of unaffected siblings. In that study, a significant deviation in intima-media thickness was noted from age 12 years in children with FH. These and other noninvasive tests have the potential to be used in the future to identify subjects at risk and monitor the response to drug therapy (38).

Before a dietary intervention, an assessment of dietary intake as well as a nutrition evaluation is mandatory.

Initial Evaluation of Hypertriglyceridemia

This includes mainly the identification of secondary causes for the hyperlipidemia, such as obesity and diabetes mellitus, as well as other causes listed in Table 3. Establishing the mode of inheritance as well as the lipid profile in first-degree relatives will help in identifying the etiology of primary hypertriglyceridemia (FHTG vs. FCHL). In cases with TG above 1000 mg/dL, pancreatic function tests are indicated. Again, before a dietary intervention, an assessment of dietary intake as well as a nutrition evaluation is mandatory.

MANAGEMENT OF CHILDREN WITH HYPERCHOLESTEROLEMIA
Dietary Management

The goal of dietary treatment is to reduce LDL-C levels in children and adolescents with elevated LDL-C blood levels (Table 1) (2,4). The recommended initial management to achieve this goal in children is to institute a "heart-healthy diet," i.e., one that is low in cholesterol and saturated fat, high in complex carbohydrates, and adequate in energy for growth and the maintenance of a desirable weight. The AHA Step I diet is well established for this purpose in adults and children older than two years (39). In the Step I diet, no more than 30% of total calories are from fat and less than 10% of total calories are from saturated fat, and cholesterol is restricted to 100 mg/1000 kcal, not to exceed 300 mg/day. Many foods high in cholesterol are also high in saturated fat. A Step I diet substitutes foods rich in monounsaturated and polyunsaturated fats for those rich in saturated fats. The Step I diet does not mention transunsaturated fatty acids, the product of commercial hydrogenation of vegetable oils. These fatty acids increase LDL-C serum levels and decrease serum HDL-C serum levels (saturated fats increase both LDL-C and HDL-C serum levels), and it is reasonable to suggest that their consumption be limited too (40–42). In the most recent guidelines published by the AHA (2005), the recommendations for dietary management of patients older than two years and their families include daily intake of vegetables and fruits, reduced saturated and trans fatty acid intake, increased fiber intake, reduced intake of sugar-sweetened beverages and foods, reduced salt intake, a recommendation to eat more fish (increased intake of Ω-3 polyunsaturated fatty acids), and to use nonfat or low-fat milk and dairy products (4). A complete dietary assessment is required to comprehensively estimate intake of energy and major and minor nutrients. The goal of dietary treatment is to achieve normal LDL-C blood levels. However, in some cases this will not be possible. There are multiple reasons for the failure of dietary intervention; the child may already consume a reasonably heart-healthy diet, the elevation may be high enough so that the percent reduction achieved by dietary modification (typically no more than 20% and frequently less than 10%) still may not lower LDL-C to the target goal, and children with inherited hypercholesterolemia tend to have a smaller response to dietary modification (43). Therefore, a more realistic goal for children and adolescents with a high level of LDL-C is to reduce the level as much as possible, and to consider percentage reduction rather than absolute values. In that context, trials in adults have demonstrated that the risk of death from CHD in adults declines by 2% for every 1 mg% decline in TC levels, and it is reasonable to assume that diet would have a larger impact in children.

To confirm the effectiveness of dietary changes, LDL-C should be checked three to six months after treatment is started and yearly after that. Because lowering LDL-C levels reduces the progression of CHD, the importance of any lowering of LDL-C levels cannot be overemphasized. Nonetheless, if the Step I diet does not achieve even the minimal goal, then the NCEP-recommended dietary approach is for the trial of a more restrictive diet (Step II), which contains less than 7% of total calories from saturated fat and cholesterol less than 75 mg/1000 kcal. Despite the seemingly modest changes relative to the Step I diet, there is the potential to develop nutritional deficiencies (given a more limited food selection), so that these patients should be placed on the Step II diet by someone with considerable nutritional expertise and closely monitored.

When carefully executed, dietary management in children is safe and successful (44,45), and even minor modification may be successful as demonstrated in a study by Dolores Estévez-González et al. (46), where isocaloric substitution of whole milk with low-fat milk containing oleic acid achieved a 7% decrease in TC, 9% decrease in LDL-C, and 13% decrease in TG in children aged three to nine years old.

The effectiveness of dietary treatment is limited by the concomitant reduction observed in HDL-C levels and the observation that long-term adherence is difficult to achieve. Furthermore, at low fat intake, there is higher carbohydrate intake (up to >65% of energy) and there is an increased risk of inadequate vitamin E, alpha linoleic, and linoleic acid intake. The role of carbohydrate intake and health in children, the development of adult onset disease, insulin resistance syndrome, obesity, and the potential value of low glycemic index foods may also play a role, but these have not been adequately studied in children.

Other additives to the diet that have been found to be successful in reducing LDL-C levels are the use of soluble fiber-like psyllium (not demonstrated in all studies), and the use of stanol and sterol esters. The nutritional safety of stanol esters in children is yet to be determined.

Other risk factors for CHD, such as cigarette smoking, physical inactivity, and obesity tend to develop during childhood and adolescence. Recommendations should be made for appropriate lifestyle modifications such as maintaining a desirable weight, increasing exercise, reducing sedentary activities (e.g., television watching), and stop smoking. Treatment programs started in childhood improve the long-term lifestyle adherence and may improve the risk factors in these families. Involving all family members in the dietary changes and lifestyle modifications is important for long-term adherence to these treatment modalities.

Drug Treatment

The NCEP is the only official body that provided guidelines for drug therapy in children. It recommended that drug therapy should be considered for children older than 10 years of age who have had an adequate trial of dietary treatment for 6 to 12 months with LDL-C levels remaining above the 99th percentile (LDL-C above 190 mg/dL). In addition, the

NCEP suggested that drug therapy should be considered when LDL-C levels remain above the 95th percentile (LDL-C above 160 mg/dL) in the presence of a positive family history of premature CHD or if the child has two or more CHD risk factors [these risk factors include cigarette smoking, elevated blood pressure, low HDL-C (lower than 35 mg/dL), severe obesity (above 30% overweight), diabetes mellitus, and physical inactivity]. Other candidates for drug therapy include children with renal disease and hyperlipidemia post organ transplantation.

The only class of drugs that has recommended for children and adolescents at that time was the bile salt sequestrants (cholestyramine). These bile acid–binding resins bind bile salts and increase fecal excretion. The decreased intestinal bile salts available for absorption decrease cholesterol absorption. The reduced cholesterol absorption results also in an increased hepatic LDL receptor activity (resulting in lower LDL-C blood levels), due to the increased hepatic needs for cholesterol to replace the bile salts lost from the enterohepatic circulation. These drugs are not absorbed by the intestine, they lack systemic toxicity, and their usage is considered safe for children and adolescents. A packet of cholestyramine contains 4 g of the resin. It is recommended that cholestyramine be started at 2 g twice a day with the two major meals for maximal effect. The NCEP and others have suggested that the maximal dose of cholestyramine is 16 g/day. However, doses up to 8 g of cholestyramine per day provide the greatest cholesterol reduction, and larger doses increase the prevalence of side effects without a further significant reduction in LDL-C blood levels. In children, cholestyramine reduces LDL-C levels by more than 15% but compliance appears to be a major problem. Despite the lack of systemic effects, nausea, epigastric fullness, bloating, flatulence, and constipation are frequently seen and more than 50% of children discontinue the medication after less than one year (47).

Our experience demonstrated that about 60% of the children stop taking the medication within 24 months, usually because of bad taste, in agreement with the findings of others. Mixing the resin with cold juice, the use of a straw, and taking the resin at the end of the meal may improve compliance. Since fat-soluble vitamins and folic acid absorption may be impaired, their supplementation is recommended. Other medications should be taken one hour before or four hours after the resin, and it should be kept in mind that obese children and children with FCHL may respond with a significant elevation of blood levels of TGs.

The goal of drug therapy is similar to the dietary goals of achieving normal LDL-C levels. However, it is important to emphasize that the percentage of reduction in LDL-C is more important than the absolute blood level achieved, and that normal blood levels cannot be expected in children with LDL-C in the drug therapy–recommended range.

Another inhibitor of cholesterol absorption is *ezetimibe*, but at the time of the writing of this chapter, studies in children are scarce. In adults with heterozygous FH, ezetimibe (10 mg/day) reduces the fractional cholesterol absorption by 54%, with a 15% to 20% reduction in LDL-C serum levels (48). It is of note that the reduction in cholesterol absorption is followed by increased cholesterol synthesis, suggesting the combined need of cholesterol synthesis inhibitors.

Other than cholestyramine, all drugs are absorbed and have systemic effects. *Nicotinic acid* has been used successfully alone or in combination to treat childhood hypercholesterolemia. However, nicotinic acid causes side effects in a significant percentage of children (especially flushing and liver enzyme abnormalities). We do not recommend the use of nicotinic acid and when drug therapy other than cholestyramine is considered, the next step is the usage of *HMG-CoA inhibitors* (*statins*). These drugs inhibit the major step in cholesterol synthesis and cause a significant reduction in LDL-C, a modest decrease in blood levels of TGs, and slightly increased blood levels of HDL-C. In adults, these drugs have proven successful in both secondary and primary prevention of CHD. In children, short-term treatment with various statins reduce LDL-C blood by an average of 40% (49–51) and seems to attenuate the atherosclerotic process as demonstrated by improved FMD in children with heterozygous FH to levels observed in control children (52).

The treatment is safe and elevations of liver enzyme levels and creatine kinase are uncommon, and growth, hormonal, and nutritional status are not impaired during adolescence. The role of statins in adolescent females (after menarche) is currently being investigated, and studies of newer, more-potent statins are in preparation (53–55).

Drug treatment is a commitment for life. Since long-term safety and efficacy of the HMG-CoA reductase inhibitors is limited to a few years, it is our practice to offer statin treatment only to children with LDL-C levels above 200 to 250 mg/dL or to those children who lost a parent due to premature CHD before his/her 40th birthday. Combination of cholestyramine and statins will further decrease LDL-C levels, and as practiced in adults, we believe that the combination of ezetimibe and statins demonstrated to have additive effect in adults will be properly studied in children.

MANAGEMENT OF CHILDREN WITH HYPERTRIGLYCERIDEMIA

In the majority of children with hypertriglyceridemia, obesity or diabetes is the reason for elevated TG blood levels, and the primary cause should be the focus of the treatment efforts. The basis for treatment includes increased exercise, reduced caloric intake, and avoiding alcohol. Fish oil has been shown to have a significant effect on blood TG levels, but the effect is usually modest.

Although some advocate drug therapy in children with serum TG levels of 400 to 500 mg/dL, we believe that the use of drugs should be limited to children at risk for acute pancreatitis (TG serum levels above 1000 mg/dL).

Specific drugs include fibric acid derivatives. Fibrates inhibit lipoprotein production and increase their clearance. No data exist on safety and effectiveness of fibric acid derivatives in pediatric patients and there are no US Food and Drug Administration–approved doses of fibric acid derivatives in children. We have limited experience in children with severe hypertriglyceridemia with the use of bezafibrate in a dose of 5 to 10 mg/kg and up to 20 mg/kg in unresponsive children, without major adverse reactions. Potential side effects of fibrates are hepatic toxicity and muscle injury (myalgia, myopathy, and rhabdomyolysis).

CONCLUSIONS

Atherosclerosis begins in childhood, and therefore efforts to reduce the burden of risk factors should start at the same age range.

In adults, substantial amount of information is now available regarding the target levels for LDL-C (56) and HDL-C levels (57), and recommendations have been made to aggressively reduce these blood levels through lifestyle changes with diet and exercise and, if needed, with drugs such as statins (58–60). Statins reduce the five-year incidence of major coronary events at any given LDL-C level, and their efficacy is correlated with the percent reduction of LDL rather than the initial level (61).

In children, however, there is insufficient data to suggest such an aggressive approach, and until such data become available, we should focus on lifestyle modifications including the dietary modifications suggested above, daily exercise, reduced television, video games, and computer time, and avoidance of smoking. In addition, we should focus on identifying the true impact of preventive measures, such as breast feeding on hyperlipidemia, obesity, and CHD, and define the optimal dietary measures taking into account individual differences as well as the true effect of fat, protein and carbohydrate amount, not only on lipid levels but also on cardiovascular risks such as obesity and diabetes.

Finally, it is reasonable to believe that when data on the long-term efficacy and safety of drugs become available and is not limited to a few years, indications for drug therapy may include lower levels of LDL than currently suggested. Until such data become available, physicians should prescribe statins to children only when a premature CHD seems inevitable without such an intervention, and avoid using lifelong treatment with drugs based on target LDL levels as suggested in adults.

REFERENCES

1. American Academy of Pediatrics. Committee on Nutrition. Cholesterol in childhood. Pediatrics 1998; 101(1 Pt 1): 141–147.
2. National Cholesterol Education Program Coordinating Committee. Report of the Expert Panel on Blood Cholesterol in Children and Adolescents. Bethesda, MD: National Heart, Lung and Blood Institute. NIH Publication No. 91–2732, 1991.
3. Kavey RE, Daniels SR, Lauer RM, et al. American Heart Association guidelines for primary prevention of atherosclerotic cardiovascular disease beginning in childhood. J Pediatr 2003; 142:368–372.
4. Gidding SS, Dennison BA, Birch LL, et al. Dietary recommendations for children and adolescents: a guide for practitioners: consensus statement from the American Heart Association. Endorsed by the American Academy of Pediatrics. Circulation 2005; 112:2061–2075.
5. Havel RJ, Kane JP. Introduction: structure and metabolism of plasma lipoproteins. In: Scriver CR, Beaudet AL, Sly WS, et al., eds. The Metabolic and Molecular Bases of Inherited Disease. 8th ed. McGraw-Hill: New York, NY, 2001: 2705–2716.
6. Lammert F, Wang DQH. New insights into genetic regulation of intestinal cholesterol absorption. Gastroenterology 2005; 129:718–734.
7. Berenson GS. Childhood risk factors predict adult risk associated with subclinical cardiovascular disease. The Bogalusa Heart Study. Am J Cardiol 2002; 90(10C):3L-7L.
8. Raitakari OT, Juonala M, Kahonen M, et al. Cardiovascular risk factors in childhood and carotid artery intima-media thickness in adulthood: The Cardiovascular Risk in Young Finns Study. JAMA 2003; 290:2277–2283.
9. Shamir R, Lerner A, Fisher EA. Hypercholesterolemia in children. Isr Med Assoc J 2000; 2:767–771.
10. Klag MJ, Ford DE, Mead LA, et al. Serum cholesterol in young men and subsequent cardiovascular disease. N Engl J Med 1993; 328:313–318.
11. Anderson KM, Castelli WP, Levy D. Cholesterol and mortality: 30 years of follow-up from the Framingham study. JAMA 1987; 257:2176–2180.
12. Freedman DS, Shear CL, Srinivasan SR, et al. Tracking of serum lipids and lipoproteins in children over an 8-year period: The Bogalusa Heart Study. Prev Med 1985; 14:203–216.
13. Lauer RM, Clarke WR. Use of cholesterol measurements in childhood for prediction of adult hypercholesterolemia: The Muscatine Study. JAMA 1990; 264:3034–3038.
14. Freedman DS, Srinivasan SR, Shear CL, et al. The relation of apolipoprotein A-1 and B in children to parental myocardial infarction. N Engl J Med 1986; 315:721–726.
15. Enos WF, Holmes RH, Beyer J. Coronary disease among United States soldiers killed in action in Korea: preliminary report. JAMA 1953; 152:1090–1093.
16. Pathobiological Determinants of Atherosclerosis in Youth (PDAY) Research Group. Relationship of atherosclerosis in young men to serum lipoprotein cholesterol concentrations and smoking. JAMA 1990; 264:3018–3024.
17. Berenson GS, Srinivasan SR, Bao W, et al. Association between multiple cardiovascular risk factors and atherosclerosis in children and young adults. N Engl J Med 1998; 338:1650–1656.
18. Stuhldreher WL, Orchard TJ, Donahue RP, et al. Cholesterol screening in childhood: sixteen-year Beaver County Lipid Study experience. J Pediatr 1991; 119:551–556.

19. Havel RJ. Approach to the patient with hyperlipidemia. Med Clin North Am 1982; 66(2):319–333.

20. Winter WE, Bertholf RL, Riley WJ, et al. Hypercholesterolemia. A common problem in Florida school-age children and adolescents. Ann N Y Acad Sci 1991; 623:472–475.

21. Kane JP, Havel RJ. Disorders of the biogenesis and secretion of lipoproteins containing the B apolipoproteins. In: Scriver CR, Beaudet AL, Sly WS, et al., eds. The Metabolic and Molecular Bases of Inherited Disease. 8th ed. New York: McGraw-Hill, 2001:2717–2752.

22. Goldstein JL, Hobbs HH, Brown MS. Familial hypercholesterolemia. In: Scriver CR, Beaudet AL, Sly WS, et al., eds. The Metabolic and Molecular Bases of Inherited Disease. 8th ed. New York: McGraw-Hill, 2001:2863–2913.

23. Ose L. Familial hypercholesterolemia from children to adults. Cardiovasc Drugs Ther 2002; 16:289–293.

24. Durrington P. Dyslipidaemia. Lancet 2003; 362:717–731.

25. Marks D, Thorogood M, Neil HA, Humphries SE. A review on the diagnosis, natural history, and treatment of familial hypercholesterolaemia. Atherosclerosis 2003; 168:1–14.

26. Rodenburg J, Vissers MN, Wiegman A, et al. Familial hypercholesterolemia in children. Curr Opin Lipidol 2004; 15:405–411.

27. Marais AD, Firth JC, Blom DJ. Homozygous familial hypercholesterolemia and its management. Semin Vasc Med 2004; 4:43–50.

28. Thompson GR. LDL apheresis. Atherosclerosis 2003; 167:1–13.

29. Castilla Cabezas JA, Lopez-Cillero P, Jimenez J, et al. Role of orthotopic liver transplant in the treatment of homozygous familial hypercholesterolemia. Rev Esp Enferm Dig 2000; 92:601–608.

30. Garcia CK, Wilund K, Arca M, et al. Autosomal recessive hypercholesterolemia caused by mutationsin a putative LDL receptor adaptor protein. Science 2001; 292(5520):1394–1398.

31. Defesche JC, Pricker KL, Hayden MR, et al. Familial defective apolipoprotein B-100 is clinically indistinguishable from familial hypercholesterolemia. Arch Intern Med 1993; 153:2349–2356.

32. Cortner JA, Coates PM, Liacouras CA, et al. Familial combined hyperlipidemia in children: clinical expression, metabolic defects, and management. J Pediatr 1993; 123:177–184.

33. Shamir R, Tershakovec AM, Liacouras CA, et al. The influence of age and relative weight on the expression of familial combined hyperlipidemia in childhood. Atherosclerosis 1996; 121:85–91.

34. Brunzell JD, Deeb SS. Familial LPL deficiency, Apo C-II deficiency and hepatic lipase deficiency. In: Scriver CR, Beaudet AL, Sly WS, et al., eds. The Metabolic and Molecular Bases of Inherited Disease. 8th ed. New York: McGraw-Hill, 2001:2789–2816.

35. Chait A, Brunzell JD. Chylomicronemia syndrome. Adv Intern Med 1992; 37:249–273.

36. Franklin FA, Dashti N, Franklin CC. Evaluation and management of dyslipoproteinemia in children. Endocrinol Metab Clin North Am 1998; 27:641–654.

37. Wiegman A, de Groot E, Hutten BA, et al. Arterial intima-media thickness in children heterozygous for familial hypercholesterolaemia. Lancet 2004; 363(9406):342–343.

38. Schachinger V, Britten MB, Zeiher AM, et al. Prognostic impact of coronary vasodilator dysfunction on adverse long-term outcome of coronary heart disease. Circulation 2000; 101:1899–1906.

39. Fisher EA, Van Horn L, McGill HC Jr. Nutrition and children. Circulation 1997; 95:2322–2333.

40. Expert Panel on Trans Fatty Acids and Coronary Heart Disease. Trans fatty acids and coronary heart disease risk. Am J Clin Nutr 1995; 62:655S–708S.

41. Lichtenstein AH, Ausman LM, Jalbert SM, Schaefer EJ. Effects of different forms of dietary hydrogenated fats on serum lipoprotein cholesterol levels. N Engl J Med 1999; 340:1933–1940.

42. Ascherio A, Katan MB, Zock PL, Stampfer MJ, Willett WC. Trans fatty acids and coronary heart disease. N Engl J Med 1999; 340:1994–1997.

43. Dixon LB, Shannon BM, Tershakovec AM, et al. Effects of family history of heart disease, apolipoprotein E phenotype, and lipoprotein(a) on the response of children's plasma lipids to change in dietary lipids. Am J Clin Nutr 1997; 66:1207–1217.

44. Obarzanek E, Kimm SY, Barton BA, et al. Long-term safety and efficacy of a cholesterol-lowering diet in children with elevated low-density lipoprotein cholesterol: seven-year results of the Dietary Intervention Study in Children (DISC). Pediatrics 2001; 107:256–264.

45. Niinikoski H, Viikari J, Ronnemaa T, et al. Growth until 3 years of age in a prospective, randomized trial of a diet with reduced saturated fat and cholesterol. Pediatrics 1997; 99:687–694.

46. Dolores Estévez-González M, Saavedra-Santana P, Betancor-León P. Reduction of serum cholesterol and low-density lipoprotein cholesterol levels in a juvenile population after isocaloric substitution of whole milk with a milk preparation (skimmed milk enriched with oleic acid). J Pediatr 1998; 132:85–89.

47. Tonstad S, Knudtzon J, Sivertsen M, et al. Efficacy and safety of cholestyramine therapy inperipubertal and prepubertal children with familial hypercholesterolemia. J Pediatr 1996; 129:42–49.

48. Gagne C, et al. Efficacy and safety of ezetimibe co administered with atorvastatin orsimvastatin in patients with homozygous familial hypercholesterolemia. Circulation 2002; 105:2469–2475.

49. Stein EA, Illingworth DR, Kwiterovich PO Jr, et al. Efficacy and safety of lovastatin in adolescent males with heterozygous familial hypercholesterolemia: a randomized controlled trial. JAMA 1999; 281:137–144.

50. Hedman M, Matikainen T, Fohr A, et al. Efficacy and safety of pravastatin in children and adolescentswith heterozygous familial hypercholesterolemia. J Clin Endocrinol Metab 2005; 90:1942–1952.

51. McCrindle BW, Ose L, Marais AD. Efficacy and safety of atorvastatin in children and adolescents with familial hypercholesterolemia or severe hyperlipidemia: a multicenter, randomized, placebo-controlled trial. J Pediatr 2003; 143:74–80.

52. de Jongh S, Lilien MR, op't Roodt J, et al. Early statin therapy restores endothelial function in children with familial hypercholesterolemia. J Am Coll Cardiol 2002; 40:2117–2121.

53. de Jongh S, Ose L, Szamosi T, et al. Efficacy and safety of statin therapy in children with familial hypercholesterolemia: a randomized, double-blind placebo-controlled trial with simvastatin. Simvastatin in Children Study Group. Circulation 2002; 106:2231–2237.

54. Wiegman A, Hutten BA, de Groot E, et al. Efficacy and safety of statin therapy in children with familial hypercholesterolemia: a randomized controlled trial. JAMA 2004; 292:331–337.

55. Rodenburg J, Vissers MN, Trip MD, et al. The spectrum of statin therapy in hyperlipidemic children. Semin Vasc Med 2004; 4:313–320.

56. Mitka M. Guidelines: new lows for LDL target levels. JAMA 2004; 292:911–923.

57. Ashen MD, Blumenthal RS. Clinical practice. Low HDL cholesterol levels. N Engl J Med 2005; 353:1252–1260.

58. Shepherd J, Cobbe SM, Ford I, et al. Prevention of coronary heart disease with pravastatin in men with hypercholesterolemia. West of Scotland Coronary Prevention Study Group. N Engl J Med 1995; 333:1301–1307.

59. The Antihypertensive and Lipid-Lowering Treatment to Prevent Heart Attack Trial (ALLHAT-LLT). Major Outcomes in Moderately Hypercholesterolemic, Hypertensive Patients Randomized to Pravastatin vs Usual Care. JAMA 2002; 288:2998–3007.

60. Athyros VG, Papageorgiou AA, Mercouris BR, et al. Treatment with atorvastatin to the National Cholesterol Educational Program goal versus "usual" care in secondary coronary heart disease prevention. The GREek Atorvastatin and Coronary-heart-disease Evaluation (GREACE) study. Curr Med Res Opin 2002; 18:220–228.

61. Baigent C, Keech A, Kearney PM, et al. Efficacy and safety of cholesterol-lowering treatment: prospective meta-analysis of data from 90,056 participants in 14 randomised trials of statins. Lancet 2005; 366:1267–1278.

15

Hypoglycemia in Children

Joseph I. Wolfsdorf

Department of Medicine, Division of Endocrinology, Children's Hospital Boston, and Department of Pediatrics, Harvard Medical School, Boston, Massachusetts, U.S.A.

David A. Weinstein

Glycogen Storage Disease Program, Department of Pediatrics, University of Florida, College of Medicine, Gainesville, Florida, U.S.A.

INTRODUCTION

Glucose is normally the predominant fuel for mammalian cells. Because the brain cannot synthesize glucose, nor store more than a few minutes supply as glycogen, survival of the brain depends on a continuous supply of glucose (1). Recurrent hypoglycemia during the period of rapid brain growth and differentiation in infancy can result in long-term neurologic sequelae, psychomotor retardation, and seizures (2). Prevention of hypoglycemia and expeditious diagnosis and vigorous treatment is essential to prevent the potentially devastating cerebral consequences of hypoglycemia.

Hypoglycemia is most common in the newborn period. Transient disturbances in neonatal glucose homeostasis are common in the first few days of life, especially where metabolic reserves are low, as in prematurity and intrauterine growth retardation or when energy expenditure is high, as in sepsis, birth asphyxia, and hypothermia (3). Basal energy needs during infancy are high. The ratio of surface area to body mass of a full-term newborn baby is more than twice that of an average adult, necessitating a high rate of energy expenditure to maintain body temperature. Also, the infant brain is large relative to body mass, and its energy requirement is primarily derived from the oxidation of circulating glucose. To meet the high demand for glucose, the rate of glucose production in infants and young children is two to three times that of older children and mature adults (4). Although the demand for glucose is high, the activity of several liver enzymes involved in glucose production is low in the newborn compared to older children and adults (3). In particular, glucose-6-phosphatase activity is diminished in preterm infants (5), and almost one-third of preterm infants at 37 weeks gestation do not have a normal glycemic response to glucagon (6). As a result of these factors, if a feed is delayed, 20% of preterm infants develop hypoglycemia at the time of discharge (7). Until feeding is well established, maintenance of glucose homeostasis in the newborn period is more precarious than later in childhood.

In the postabsorptive state, the rate of glucose turnover in adults is approximately 2 mg/kg/minute (8–10 g/hour); whereas, the average basal (4–6 hours after feeding) rate of glucose turnover is 6 mg/kg/minute in newborns, approximately three times the adult rate (4). During prolonged fasting, infants and children cannot sustain the high rate of glucose production. Normal children, 18 months to 9 years of age, who fasted for 24 hours have a mean blood glucose concentration of 52 ± 14 (SD) mg/dL, and 22% have blood glucose concentrations less than 40 mg/dL; blood glucose values conform to a Gaussian pattern of distribution (8). For these reasons, infants and young children are more prone to develop hypoglycemia than adolescents and adults when normal feeding patterns are disturbed by intercurrent illness.

DEFINITION OF HYPOGLYCEMIA

During acute insulin-induced hypoglycemia in normal adults, symptoms occur at an arterialized venous plasma glucose level of approximately 60 mg/dL (3.3 mmol/L), and impaired brain function occurs at approximately 50 mg/dL (2.8 mmol/L) (9,10). Comparable levels in venous blood are about 3 mg/dL lower (11). In children, functional changes in the central nervous system (brain stem auditory and somatosensory evoked potentials) occur when the venous plasma glucose concentration decreases below 47 mg/dL (2.6 mmol/L) (12). These data suggest that the physiologic threshold is a plasma glucose concentration in the range of 50 to 60 mg/dL (2.8–3.3 mmol/L). Therefore, for clinical care of children, a venous plasma glucose concentration of 60 mg/dL (3.3 mmol/L) or greater may be regarded as normoglycemia, and plasma glucose levels below 50 mg/dL (2.8 mmol/L) as hypoglycemia.

AN OVERVIEW OF FUEL METABOLISM

The physiological mechanisms that normally prevent hypoglycemia ensure that the brain receives a continuous supply of glucose (13). Several tissue-specific glucose transport proteins are responsible for the transport of glucose from the extracellular to the intracellular space (Table 1). GLUT-1 and GLUT-3 transporters are found on most cells and are primarily responsible for basal glucose use by the brain and most other body tissues (14,15). Both GLUT-1 (on glial cells) and GLUT-3 (on neuronal cells) (16) are insulin-independent facilitative glucose transporters. Blood-to-brain glucose transport is a function of the arterial plasma glucose concentration. The supply of glucose to the brain, therefore, is dependent on the precise regulation of systemic glucose balance that maintains the arterial plasma glucose concentration above the critical level that becomes limiting to brain glucose metabolism. None of the glucoregulatory factors, including insulin, modify glucose uptake into the brain. However, chronic exposure to cerebral hypoglycemia results in up-regulation of both these transporters (17–19).

Most body tissues, with the exception of the brain, can use free fatty acids (FFAs) for oxidative metabolism. The heart preferentially uses FFA as an energy source, and skeletal muscle depends upon FFA for energy production during exercise. Under conditions of fasting, the plasma FFA concentration increases and the uptake and oxidation of glucose decreases. The high rate of tissue oxidation of FFA decreases the use of glucose in accordance with Randle's hypothesis (the glucose-fatty acid cycle) (20). Although FFA are not transported across the blood–brain barrier, β-hydroxybutyrate (BOHB) and acetoacetate, the water soluble products of hepatic β-oxidation of FFA, readily cross the blood–brain barrier (21–23).

In the interval between meals and during fasting, maintenance of normal plasma glucose concentrations requires: (i) adequate endogenous substrate (body fat, hepatic and muscle glycogen, and mobilizing amino acids); (ii) intact metabolic and enzymatic pathways; (iii) proper hormonal regulation of the mobilization, interconversion, and use of metabolic fuels. An abnormality in any one of these areas may compromise the homeostatic mechanisms that balance the rate of appearance and disposal of glucose that maintains the plasma glucose concentration in a narrow normal range (24). Glucose is derived from intestinal absorption following digestion of dietary carbohydrate (exogenous glucose delivery) or from endogenous glucose production (glycogenolysis and gluconeogenesis). Gluconeogenesis refers to the formation of glucose from three carbon precursors, including lactate, pyruvate, amino acids (especially alanine and glutamine), and glycerol. The integrated regulatory effects of hormones, neural pathways, and metabolic substrates normally result in the precise matching of glucose utilization and the sum of exogenous glucose delivery and endogenous glucose production. The key glucoregulatory hormones are insulin, glucagon, and epinephrine. Growth hormone (GH) and cortisol modify the effectiveness of these glucoregulatory hormones.

After feeding, glucose absorption from the intestine into the portal circulation occurs via a sodium-dependent transport mechanism. Glucose is then transported into both the liver and pancreas by GLUT-2 transporters (14,15). Unlike the other glucose transporters whose primary function is to deliver glucose into cells for energy production or storage, GLUT-2 is central to the regulation of glucose homeostasis. It is insulin-independent and has a high K_m. Glucose uptake in the liver and pancreas occurs at a rate determined by the plasma glucose concentration, which reflects the carbohydrate content of ingested food and the rate of gastric emptying. Increased plasma insulin levels suppress endogenous glucose production, increase translocation of GLUT-4 transporters in fat and muscle from their intracellular location to the cell membrane, and stimulate glycogen synthesis in muscle and the liver (Table 1). Metabolism of dietary carbohydrate leads to increased cytosolic malonyl coenzyme A (CoA) levels, which

Table 1 Tissue-Specific Glucose Transporters

Glucose transporter	Distribution	Principal function	K_m for glucose (mmol/L)	Gene location	Regulation
GLUT-1	Wide distribution, brain glial cells, erythrocytes, endothelial cells	Constitutive glucose transporter	20	1p35-p31.3	Minimal
GLUT-2	Liver, pancreatic β cells, small intestinal epithelium, kidney	Glucose-sensing in β cells	42	3q26	Zero to minimal
GLUT-3	Wide distribution, CNS neurons, fetal muscle, placenta, kidney	High-affinity glucose transporter	10	12p13	None
GLUT-4	Skeletal muscle, cardiac muscle, adipose cells	Insulin responsive glucose transporter	2–10	17p13	Regulated by insulin
GLUT-5	Liver, small intestine, sperm, adipose cells, brain, muscle	Fructose transporter; very low affinity for glucose	Not defined	1p31	None

inhibit activity of carnitine palmitoyltransferase-I (CPT-I) and diverts fatty acids away from oxidation in peripheral tissues and from β-oxidation and ketogenesis in the liver (25–27). A reduction in β-oxidation also results in decreased production of reduced nucleotides, which are necessary for gluconeogenesis. With decreased circulating plasma concentrations of FFA and ketone bodies, and increased concentrations of glucose and insulin, GLUT-1, GLUT-3, and GLUT-4 transporters efficiently move glucose out of the circulation and into cells.

Despite a substantial increase in glucose influx into the circulation, the increase in plasma glucose concentration is relatively small after a meal, and plasma glucose and insulin concentrations return to basal levels within two to three hours. In healthy children (9–17 years old), venous serum glucose levels fluctuate between approximately 60 and 140 mg/dL (28). When nutrient absorption is complete, flow of glucose from the gut decreases and eventually stops. Plasma glucose concentration frequently decreases to below the premeal value. The relative hypoglycemia, together with the decrease in insulin secretion, triggers release of glucagon, which increases hepatic glucose production (29,30). The transition from endogenous glucose production to exogenous glucose delivery shortly after a meal and the later transition from exogenous glucose delivery back to endogenous glucose production are finely regulated (29,30). Hypoglycemia normally does not occur in the interval between meals, and glucose delivery to the brain continues unabated (Fig. 1A).

Most of the glucose in the body is normally in the extracellular space; the intracellular glucose concentration is low because glucose is rapidly phosphorylated when it enters cells. The extracellular space is approximately 25% of body weight in children and adolescents. The total glucose present in a person with a plasma glucose concentration of 90 mg/dL is 225 mg/kg (1.25 mmol/kg) of body weight. This is equivalent to approximately 5% of a teaspoon of glucose per kilogram of body weight. Thus, the total pool size of a 10-year-old child (30 kg) is approximately 6.75 g of glucose (24), enough to meet the basal needs of the child for approximately 45 minutes. Thus, endogenous glucose production is critical to prevent hypoglycemia. The amount of glycogen stored in the liver is modest—approximately 5% of the wet weight of the liver. In the example of a 10-year-old child, there is about 45 g of glycogen in the liver, which could, theoretically, satisfy the child's basal glucose requirement for only five to six hours. Thus, gluconeogenesis soon plays a major role in maintaining normal blood glucose concentrations (Fig. 1B).

Both the liver and kidney express the critical gluconeogenic enzymes: pyruvate carboxylase, phosphoenolpyruvate carboxykinase (PEPCK), fructose-1,6-bisphosphatase, and glucose-6-phosphatase. Although many tissues are able to convert oxaloacetate to glucose-6-phosphate and glycogen, only the liver and kidney (owing to the presence of the glucose-6-phosphatase system) release glucose into the circulation. In adults, 40% to 50% of glucose is derived from gluconeogenesis in the postabsorptive

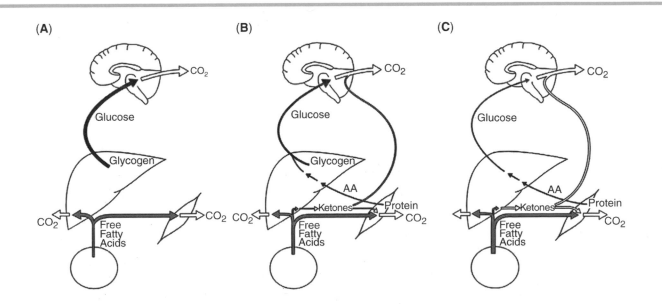

Figure 1 (A) Between meals: glucose is from hepatic glycogenolysis; free fatty acids from adipose tissue are an additional source of fuel for muscle. (B) Overnight fast: liver glycogen is depleted and gluconeogenesis becomes the principal source of glucose. Hepatic ketone production increases and rising plasma ketone body concentrations provide an alternative fuel for brain and muscle. (C) Prolonged starvation: fat-derived fuels are the predominant metabolic substrates. Brain utilization of ketones increases. Glucose is from gluconeogenesis.

state (after an overnight fast), and this increases to approximately 90% after fasting for 48 to 72 hours (31–33). In children and adolescents, the fraction of glucose production from gluconeogenesis after an overnight fast is of the order of 50% to 60% (Fig. 1B) (34); however, the precise fraction of glucose derived from glycogenolysis, as opposed to gluconeogenesis, at any point in time during more prolonged periods of fasting is unknown.

Whereas muscle, which lacks glucose-6-phosphatase, cannot release glucose directly into the circulation, it does indirectly contribute to the maintenance of plasma glucose concentrations during periods of fasting. In muscle, glycogen is metabolized via glycolysis to pyruvate, which can be reduced to lactate, transaminated to form alanine, or undergo oxidation. Lactate and pyruvate released from muscle are transported to the liver and serve as gluconeogenic precursors (the Cori or glucose-lactate-glucose cycle). Alanine, glutamine, and other amino acids also flow from muscle to the liver and serve as gluconeogenic precursors (35). The availability of other fuels (FFA and ketones) for oxidation in muscle affects the activity of pyruvate dehydrogenase and determines whether glucose is completely oxidized to carbon dioxide and water, or is conserved by recycling lactate, pyruvate, and alanine back to glucose in the liver (glucose-lactate-glucose and glucose-alanine-glucose cycles). In addition to releasing precursors for gluconeogenesis during fasting, muscle oxidizes fatty acids and ketones to meet its own energy needs, thereby conserving glucose.

Over periods of more prolonged fasting, fatty acid oxidation becomes the predominant source of fuel accounting for almost 80% of the body's energy source. FFA are released from adipose tissue stores by lipolysis (36,37). FFA provide many tissues (including cardiac and skeletal muscle) with a readily usable energy substrate. A fraction of the FFA undergoes β-oxidation in the liver to form ketone bodies (Fig. 1B,C). High rates of ketone body production are rapidly reached during fasting in children. After fasting for 20 to 22 hours, the ketone body turnover rate in young children is comparable to that achieved by adults fasted for several days (38). During fasting, plasma concentrations of ketone bodies increase dramatically reflecting increased plasma concentrations of FFA and rates of β-oxidation in the liver (36,37,39). Within 30 hours of fasting, normal children achieve plasma total ketone body concentrations of 5 to 6 mmol/L, levels that are seen in adult women after fasting for 2.5 to 3 days, and are not achieved in men even after 84 hours of fasting (39). During prolonged fasting, ketone bodies are the predominant fuel for the brain (which cannot utilize FFA) and may even be more rapidly incorporated into amino acids by the brain than glucose (21,22,40). Normally, the large amounts of ketones generated during fasting results in a decrease in the brain's rate of glucose consumption. In vitro studies in rats have demonstrated that the use of ketones can decrease brain glucose utilization by approximately 50%. Evidence in humans is consistent with these data (41,42).

Prolonged fasting ultimately leads to a decrease to about one-half in the basal rate of glucose turnover, resulting in a gradual decrease in the plasma glucose concentration (43). These metabolic responses to fasting (increased gluconeogenesis, lipolysis, and ketogenesis) are finely regulated by changes in the circulating concentrations of hormones, including decreased insulin secretion and increased plasma concentrations of glucagon, epinephrine, GH, and cortisol, the latter collectively referred to as the counterregulatory hormones.

In summary, the adaptation to fasting involves a major change in the body's fuel economy. As fasting is prolonged, there is decreased dependence on glucose and increased reliance on the products of fat as the primary source of fuel for energy metabolism (Fig. 1C). A failure to oxidize fatty acids or to synthesize or utilize ketones results in greater utilization of glucose, impaired gluconeogenesis, and inability to conserve glucose, which leads to severe hypoglycemia. Examples of these disorders are discussed in detail later.

REGULATION OF INSULIN SECRETION

Insulin secretion is regulated by nutritional, hormonal, metabolic, and autonomic nervous system signals that are transduced by a complex system involving cellular glucose metabolism, depolarization of the cell membrane, regulation of free intracellular cytosolic calcium concentration, and movement of insulin-containing secretory granules to fuse with the plasma membrane to release their contents (Fig. 2) (44). ATP-sensitive potassium channels (K_{ATP} channels) in the plasma membrane, which control the polarity of the β-cell membrane, have a pivotal role in regulating insulin secretion. They are formed from two distinct subunit proteins—the high-affinity sulphonylurea receptor (SUR1) and Kir6.2, a weak inward-rectifier (45–47). The channel's pore is formed by Kir6.2 in a tetrameric arrangement. At rest, K_{ATP} channels are normally kept open maintaining a membrane potential of about –70 mV. A rise in blood glucose concentration increases glucose entry into the cell (via GLUT-2 transport), and the rate of glucose metabolism increases in the β-cell. Intracellular glucose is phosphorylated by glucokinase, the rate-limiting step in glucose metabolism (Fig. 2) (48), and is then metabolized resulting in an increased ratio of ATP:ADP, which leads to closure of the K_{ATP} channels, depolarization of the β-cell membrane, and opening of voltage-dependent L-type calcium channels with influx of extracellular calcium. The increase in cytosolic-free calcium concentration triggers exocytosis of insulin-containing secretory granules (49).

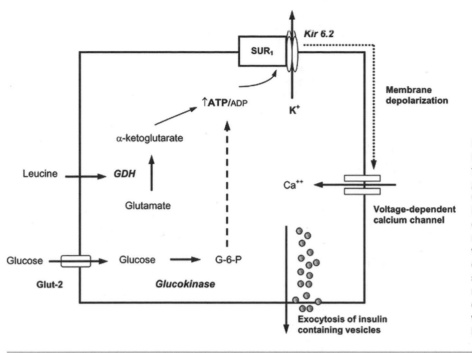

Figure 2 Model of insulin secretion regulation by pancreatic β-cell. Glucose is transported into the β-cell by GLUT-2 and then phosphorylated by glucokinase to glucose-6-phosphate (G-6-P). Glucose metabolism is initiated resulting in an increase in the cytosolic ratio of ATP:ADP, which causes closure of K_{ATP} channels and leads to membrane depolarization and opening of voltage-dependent Ca^{2+} channels. Influx of calcium releases insulin through exocytosis of secretory granules. Leucine stimulates insulin release by allosterically activating glutamate dehydrogenase, increasing glutamate oxidation, which increases the ATP:ADP ratio and closes K_{ATP} channels.

SUR1 encodes for a 39 exon gene with 17 transmembrane domains and produces a 1581 amino acid product; Kir6.2 encodes for a 390 amino acid protein. These genes are located on adjacent regions of chromosome 11p15.1. The SUR protein forms an octameric complex with four SUR1 subunits surrounding four Kir6.2 centrally located channels. ATP acts directly on Kir6.2 resulting in closure of the channel, whereas ADP antagonizes the effect via the SUR receptor. Both SUR1 and Kir6.2 are required for the potassium channel to be membrane-bound and functional. Mutations that alter the function of K_{ATP} channels (see below) lead to continued membrane depolarization and dysregulation of the voltage-dependent calcium channels resulting in uncoupling of insulin secretion from glucose metabolism and congenital hyperinsulinism (50). A constitutive increase in glucokinase activity causes an autosomal dominant form of hyperinsulinism (51–54); whereas decreased glucokinase activity causes an unusual form of maturity onset diabetes in youth characterized by decreased insulin secretion at normal plasma glucose concentrations (55).

CLINICAL MANIFESTATIONS OF HYPOGLYCEMIA

The symptoms of hypoglycemia are not specific. Therefore, when a patient's symptoms are suspected to be caused by hypoglycemia, it is essential to measure the blood glucose concentration, confirm that it is low, and demonstrate that administration of glucose promptly relieves the symptoms.

The symptoms of hypoglycemia (Table 2) are classified into two major categories based on the

mechanism responsible for their generation: autonomic symptoms result from activation of the autonomic nervous system (both sympathetic and parasympathetic divisions); neuroglycopenic symptoms result from the effects of brain glucose deprivation. Symptoms tend to be most severe when hypoglycemia is caused by hyperinsulinism, which prevents formation of alternative fuels (FFA, ketones). Up-regulation of cerebral glucose transporters in response to chronic or recurrent hypoglycemia attenuates clinical symptoms and blunts hypoglycemia awareness in all forms of hypoglycemia (56–58). In newborn babies and infants, hypoglycemia typically manifests as irritability, tremors, feeding difficulty, lethargy, hypotonia, tachypnea, cyanosis, or apnea. Hypoglycemia in this age group is discussed in

Table 2 Signs and Symptoms of Hypoglycemia

Autonomic	Neuroglycopenic
Sweating	Warmth
Hunger	Fatigue
Paresthesias	Weakness
(tingling, numbness)	Dizziness
Tremors	Headache
Pallor	Inability to concentrate
Anxiety	Drowsiness
Nausea	Blurred vision
Palpitations	Difficulty speaking
	Confusion
	Bizarre behavior
	Loss of coordination
	Difficulty walking
	Coma
	Seizures

Vol. 1; Chap. 16. The symptoms of hypoglycemia in children are similar to those in adults.

CAUSES OF HYPOGLYCEMIA IN INFANTS AND CHILDREN

The most common cause of hypoglycemia in children and adolescents is insulin-induced hypoglycemia in individuals with Type 1 diabetes mellitus. This topic is discussed later in the section Hypoglycemia and Diabetes Mellitus. Almost all cases of hypoglycemia fall into one of the five major categories listed in Table 3. Endocrinologic disorders (and particularly hyperinsulinism) are the predominant causes of recurrent or persistent hypoglycemia in the newborn period. In older infants and toddlers, metabolic abnormalities account for most cases of hypoglycemia, and endocrinopathies are relatively uncommon in this age group.

Accelerated Starvation (Idiopathic Ketotic Hypoglycemia; Transient Intolerance of Fasting)

This is the most common noniatrogenic cause of hypoglycemia in children beyond infancy. For more than 40 years, this entity has been referred to as ketotic hypoglycemia (67). Affected children have a characteristic clinical presentation, but it is still unclear whether this is a specific disorder, a common phenotype shared by several disorders, or even a pathologic entity (68). Despite extensive endocrinologic and metabolic investigation, a satisfactory explanation for the hypoglycemia cannot be found in children labeled as having ketotic hypoglycemia.

Hypoglycemia typically first occurs between 18 months and five years of age and remits spontaneously by eight or nine years of age. Many children with accelerated starvation are small and thin for their age and have decreased muscle mass. Many were born small for gestational age and may have had transient neonatal hypoglycemia. Hypoglycemia typically occurs during periods of intercurrent illness when food intake is limited by anorexia or vomiting, and occurs in the morning before breakfast (67,69,70). Manifestations include neurologic symptoms ranging from lethargy to seizures and coma. Sometimes, hypoglycemia occurs in the morning after unusually intense physical exertion on the previous day or after the child has eaten poorly or completely omitted an evening meal.

The precise pathophysiologic cause of accelerated starvation is unclear. Because serum alanine levels are low at the time of hypoglycemia, deficient availability of gluconeogenic substrate, especially alanine from muscle, has been thought to be the cause of hypoglycemia (71). The gluconeogenic pathway is intact, and the serum glucose concentration increases appropriately when alanine is infused at the time of hypoglycemia (72,73). The cause of the hypoalaninemia, however, is controversial (74). It may be the

Table 3   Causes of Hypoglycemia in Children

Accelerated starvation (ketotic hypoglycemia)
Hyperinsulinism
   Congenital hyperinsulinism; persistent hereditary
     hyperinsulinemia of infancy
   Insulinoma
   Beckwith-Wiedemann syndrome (59–61)
   Insulin autoimmunity
   Sulfonylurea ingestion
   Factitious
Hormone deficiency
   ACTH/cortisol
   GH
   Hypopituitarism (ACTH/cortisol and GH)
Metabolic disorders
Disorders of carbohydrate metabolism
   Glycogen synthetase deficiency (type 0 glycogen storage disease)
   Glucose-6-phosphatase deficiency (Type I glycogen storage disease)
   Amylo-1,6-glucosidase deficiency (Type III glycogen storage disease)
   Phosphorylase deficiency (Type VI glycogen storage disease)
   Phosphorylase kinase deficiency (Type IX glycogen storage disease)
   Galactose-1-phosphate uridyltransferase deficiency (galactosemia)
   Fructose-1-phosphate aldolase deficiency (fructose intolerance)
   Defects in gluconeogenesis
     Pyruvate carboxylase deficiency
     Phosphoenolpyruvate carboxykinase deficiency
     Fructose-1,6-bisphosphatase deficiency
Disorders of fatty acid oxidation and ketone synthesis
   Carnitine transport and metabolism
   β-oxidation cycle
   Electron transfer
   Hydroxymethylglutaryl CoA synthase deficiency
   Hydroxymethylglutaryl CoA lyase deficiency
Disorders of protein metabolism
   Maple syrup urine disease (branched-chain ketoacid
     decarboxylase deficiency)
   Methylmalonic acidemia
   Tyrosinemia
Miscellaneous
   Nonpancreatic tumor hypoglycemia (IGF-II) (62,63)
   Salicylate intoxication
   Reye syndrome
   Ethanol intoxication
   Malaria
   Diarrhea
   Malnutrition
   Jamaican vomiting sickness (ingestion of unripe ackee)
   Reactive hypoglycemia (dumping syndrome) (64–66)
   Carbohydrate-deficient glycoprotein syndrome
   Respiratory chain defects

Abbreviations: GH, growth hormone; CoA, coenzyme A.

result of a specific defect in protein catabolism or reflect decreased muscle mass. An alternative explanation is that hypoalaninemia is a consequence of decreased muscle glucose uptake in response to decreasing plasma glucose concentrations and increased levels of FFA and ketone bodies, which inhibit release of alanine from skeletal muscle (75,76). This would affect flux through the glucose-alanine-glucose cycle (74). The plasma epinephrine response to hypoglycemia is reduced in about half the patients with ketotic hypoglycemia (77). It has been suggested that these children may have a deficient catecholamine response to hypoglycemia that results in increased glucose utilization; however, this conclusion is now suspect in light of new knowledge that recent antecedent hypoglycemia elevates the threshold for autonomic, including epinephrine, and symptomatic responses to subsequent hypoglycemia in healthy individuals (78–81).

After 8 to 16 hours, children with accelerated starvation show the same metabolic pattern as normal healthy children fasted for 24 to 36 hours. In many instances, the distinction between accelerated starvation and the normal response to fasting is unclear (82). Because approximately one-fourth of normal children develop hypoglycemia after a fast of 24 to 36 hours duration (8), accelerated starvation may not be a distinct pathological disorder. Rather, it may be one end of the spectrum of the normal child's response to starvation (68,83).

Diagnosis: Because ketosis (and ketonuria) is a normal response to fasting and a falling plasma glucose concentration, ketotic hypoglycemia should not be regarded as a specific diagnosis. The differential diagnosis of the hypoglycemic child with an appropriately suppressed serum insulin concentration and ketosis is shown in Table 4. Accelerated starvation is a diagnosis of exclusion that should only be made when the other causes of "ketotic hypoglycemia" have been considered. In particular, glycogen storage disease (GSD) type 0, GSD IX, and short–chain fatty acid oxidation defects should be considered because they typically present with fasting hyperketonemia and hypoglycemia (86).

Children with accelerated starvation typically become hypoglycemic in 12 to 24 hours and have a normal metabolic and hormonal response to fasting. At the time of hypoglycemia, blood ketone body concentrations are raised, there is ketonuria, plasma alanine concentration is low, and blood lactate and pyruvate levels are normal (73). Plasma insulin levels are appropriately suppressed, and the concentrations of counterregulatory hormones are increased (72,73,83). The glycemic response to glucagon (0.03 mg/kg IM or intravenous (IV); maximum 1 mg) is normal in the fed state, but blunted at the time of hypoglycemia.

Treatment consists of educating parents to ensure that the child avoids prolonged periods of fasting. A bedtime snack consisting of both carbohydrate and protein prevents further episodes of hypoglycemia. During intercurrent illness, carbohydrate-rich drinks at frequent intervals during both the day and night can prevent hypoglycemia. Alternatively, uncooked cornstarch (1 g/kg) in milk given at bedtime can be used to provide a source of slowly absorbed glucose. Parents are instructed to test urine for ketones during intercurrent illnesses. The appearance of ketonuria precedes the onset of hypoglycemia by several hours. When monitoring urine ketones is problematic due to dehydration or the child's age, a blood ketone meter (Precision Xtra®; Abbott Laboratories, Inc.) can be used to accurately measure blood BOHB concentration on a drop of blood (87). This is a useful alternative method of monitoring the development of ketosis during periods of illness or poor food intake in the child with ketotic hypoglycemia. Once ketosis is present, the child must consume adequate amounts of oral carbohydrate and, if this cannot be tolerated, IV glucose is necessary to avert the development of hypoglycemia.

Hyperinsulinism

Hyperinsulinism is the most common cause of persistent hypoglycemia in infants and young children. Islet cell adenomas are rare in children less than one year of age. Hyperinsulinism that presents in an older child is more likely to be caused by an insulinoma or by exogenous insulin administration (factitious hypoglycemia) (88,89) or sulfonylurea ingestion (90,91).

In the past decade, considerable progress has been made toward elucidating the pathophysiology of the heterogeneous disorders that cause hyperinsulinemic hypoglycemia (50,92–94). Several distinct genetic forms of congenital hyperinsulinism have been described (95–97). The most common variety is an autosomal recessive defect caused by either homozygous mutations in the SUR1 gene (ABCC8) (98,99) or in the Kir6.2 gene (KCNJ11) (100,101). Both genes encode components of the K_{ATP} channel involved in glucose-regulated insulin release, and mutations in these genes result in uncoupling of insulin secretion from glucose metabolism. To date, more than 100 mutations have been described in the SUR1 gene and several mutations have been identified in the Kir6.2 gene (50).

The principal clinical and biochemical features of hyperinsulinemic hypoglycemia are shown in Table 5. Patients with autosomal recessive hyperinsulinism due to SUR/Kir6.2 mutations typically present as macrosomic babies with severe intractable hypoglycemia soon after birth.

Table 4 Causes of Ketotic Hypoglycemia

Liver large
  Glycogen storage diseases (Types I, III, VI, and IX)
  Fanconi-Bickel syndrome (GSD XI)
  Disorders of gluconeogenesis (e.g., fructose
    1,6-bisphosphatase deficiency)
Liver normal size
  Accelerated starvation (ketotic hypoglycemia)
  Cortisol/ACTH deficiency
  GH deficiency
  Panhypopituitarism
  Glycogen synthase deficiency (GSD 0)
  Short chain fatty acid oxidation disorders
  Acetoacetyl CoA thiolase deficiency (84)
  Succinyl-CoA:3-oxoacid CoA-transferase deficiency[a]
  Organic acidemias (e.g., maple syrup urine disease
    and methylmalonic acidemia)

[a]A rare cause of hypoglycemia due to inability to utilize ketone bodies.
Abbreviations: CoA, coenzyme A; GSD, glycogen storage disease.
Source: From Ref. 85.

Table 5 Clinical and Biochemical Features of Hyperinsulinemic Hypoglycemia

Usually less than 12 mo of age at time of presentation
Hypoglycemia soon after feeding (0–5.5 hr, average ~2 hr)
Urinary ketones negative, trace, or small
Serum insulin $\geq$2 µU/mL (15 pmol/L) with plasma
  glucose < 45 mg/dL (2.5 mmol/L)
Increased serum C-peptide concentration
Plasma ketone (β-hydroxybutyrate and acetoacetate)
  concentrations inappropriately low
Brisk glycemic response to glucagon > 30 mg/dL (1.7 mmol/L) (102)
Parenteral glucose required to maintain normoglycemia
  is 2–4-fold greater than glucose production rate (~6 mg/kg/min)
Decreased plasma branched chain amino acids
  (valine, leucine, isoleucine)
Decreased IGF-binding protein-1 (103)[a]
Leucine and/or tolbutamide causes an exaggerated
  hyperinsulinemic response
GH, cortisol concentrations usually normal but may be
  inappropriately low if hypoglycemia develops gradually
  or is recurrent (blunted counterregulatory hormone responses)

[a]All other endocrinologic and metabolic abnormalities with fasting hypoglycemia are associated with decreased insulin secretion and increased IGFBP-1 levels.
Abbreviation: GH, growth hormone.

Unlike the autosomal recessive defects of the K_{ATP} channel that result in diffuse β-cell dysfunction, the sporadic form of hyperinsulinemic hypoglycemia can result in either focal or diffuse hyperplasia of β-cells. Focal adenomatous hyperplasia occurs in 40% to 70% of cases requiring pancreatectomy (the remainder are due to diffuse hyperinsulinism) (104–106). It is caused by a specific somatic loss of the maternal allele imprinted at 11p15 in a patient harboring an SUR1 mutation on the paternal allele; i.e., hemizygous germline mutation together with maternal loss of heterozygosity of 11p15 (107–111). Two hypotheses have been proposed to explain focal hyperplasia. The loss of heterozygosity may unmask a recessively inherited SUR1 or Kir6.2 mutation located on the paternal allele. An alternative hypothesis is that this somatic deletion also results in loss of an associated tumor suppressor gene, H19. H19 normally inhibits the actions of IGF-2; unopposed IGF-2 action could lead to β-cell proliferation (112).

Two distinct forms of autosomal dominant hyperinsulinism have been described, both with milder clinical phenotypes than the autosomal recessive form. Patients are not macrosomic at birth and may not present with hypoglycemia until later in childhood or adulthood. Hypoglycemia usually responds well to dietary or pharmacologic therapy (diazoxide) and is generally associated with an excellent prognosis (113,114). One form of autosomal dominant hyperinsulinism is caused by an activating mutation in GCK, the gene encoding β-cell glucokinase, that results in increased affinity of the enzyme for glucose (51–53). The initial report of hyperinsulinism caused by an activating mutation in β-cell glucokinase described a mild clinical phenotype;

however, a case of severe hyperinsulinism unresponsive to medical therapy has recently been described (54). Glucokinase normally has low affinity for glucose and is the rate-limiting step in β-cell glucose metabolism. In the initial description of this disorder, a single base pair change at codon 455 of the gene was found, resulting in substitution of methionine for valine. This alteration increased the activity of the enzyme (a 65% change in enzyme affinity for glucose; K_m 2.9 mM compared to 8.4 mM in wild type). This causes an abnormally low glucose threshold for insulin secretion, 36 to 45 mg/dL (2.0–2.5 mM). A defect in glucokinase can be missed if the critical sample is obtained when the plasma glucose concentration is below the threshold for insulin secretion. If this diagnosis is suspected, a fasting study with serial measurements of plasma insulin levels may be required to document inappropriate insulin secretion.

A distinct form of mild hyperinsulinism is associated with persistent mild asymptomatic hyperammonemia (blood ammonia levels are in the range of 100 to 200 µmol/L or approximately three to five times normal) that is not associated with any abnormality of the amino acids or organic acids characteristic of defects in the urea cycle (115–119). The phenotype is characterized by hypoglycemia following protein meals as well as fasting hypoglycemia (120). Familial cases with an autosomal dominant pattern of inheritance have been documented; however, the majority of cases have been sporadic. The hypoglycemia may go unrecognized until adulthood. It usually responds well to diet and diazoxide. The syndrome is caused by a gain of function mutation in GLUD1, the gene for mitochondrial glutamate dehydrogenase (GDH). GDH catalyzes the oxidative deamination of glutamate to alpha-ketoglutarate and ammonia, using nicotinamide adenine dinucleotide (NAD) or NADP as cofactor. Mutations cause impaired GDH sensitivity to its allosteric inhibitor, GTP, resulting in a gain of enzyme function and increased sensitivity to its allosteric activator, leucine (120). Plasma ammonia levels are increased due to expression of mutant GDH in the liver, probably reflecting increased ammonia release from glutamate as well as impaired synthesis of N-acetylglutamate (an allosteric activator of carbamoyl phosphate synthetase, which catalyzes the first step in ureagenesis) due to reduction of hepatic glutamate pools. Ammonia levels are unaffected by feeding or fasting and appear to cause no symptoms, perhaps due to a protective effect of increased GDH activity in brain (120).

Although glucose is the prime regulator of insulin secretion, fatty acids can increase insulin secretion in vivo and amplify glucose-induced insulin secretion in vitro. Mutations in the gene (HADHSC) encoding short-chain L-3-hydroxyacyl-CoA dehydrogenase (SCHAD) are associated with autosomally recessive inherited hyperinsulinemic hypoglycemia. The clinical presentation is heterogeneous with either mild late onset hypoglycemia or severe neonatal hypoglycemia (121–124). SCHAD is an intramitochondrial enzyme that catalyses the penultimate reaction in the β-oxidation of fatty acids, the NAD$^+$-dependent dehydrogenation of 3-hydroxyacyl-CoA to the corresponding 3-ketoacyl-CoA. The disease is characterized by raised plasma levels of 3-hydroxybutyryl-carnitine and 3-hydroxyglutaric aciduria. The precise mechanism whereby this intramitochondrial metabolic defect causes hyperinsulinism is not yet understood.

An autosomal dominantly inherited form of exercise-induced hyperinsulinism has not been described in the neonatal period. Increased blood pyruvate concentrations induce a brisk insulin secretory response. The phenotype does not include fasting hypoglycemia (125,126). The molecular genetic basis of the disease is still unknown; however, the disorder is not attributable to mutations in the monocarboxylate transporter genes MCT1–MCT8 (126).

Despite extraordinary advances in our understanding of the pathophysiology of hyperinsulinism, only 30% to 50% of patients have a definable genetic abnormality (96,97,127). It is likely that other abnormalities will be revealed as the search continues for new defects in the secretory apparatus, including defects in the intracellular control of calcium signaling of exocytosis (127).

Diagnosis: Hyperinsulinism should be considered in any infant or child with hypoketotic hypoglycemia and is the probable diagnosis when the concomitant serum insulin level is greater than 2 μU/mL (Table 5). Malicious insulin administration should be suspected if severe hypoglycemia is associated with a very high serum insulin concentration (greater than 100 μU/mL), and is confirmed by finding concomitantly low or suppressed serum C-peptide levels.

The patient with focal adenomatous hyperplasia cannot be differentiated clinically from the patient with diffuse disease. Patients who fail to respond to pharmacological therapy, and especially those without a family history of hyperinsulinism, should be referred to a specialized center for evaluation before undergoing a 95% to 99% (near-total) pancreatectomy. It is crucial to distinguish between focal and diffuse forms of hyperinsulinism because, in the former, local resection of the lesion is usually associated with minimal morbidity and cures most patients, whereas near-total pancreatectomy frequently results, eventually, in insulin-dependent diabetes and pancreatic exocrine insufficiency (128–131). Sonography and computerized axial tomography are both insensitive imaging modalities. Pancreatic venous sampling and intraoperative histopathologic examination of the pancreas (evaluation of β-cell nuclear radius and cell density) have been successfully used to distinguish between the two (104,132). Recently, positron emission tomography with 18F-fluoro-l-DOPA has been successfully used to distinguish between focal and diffuse forms of hyperinsulinism (133) and promises to be a reliable noninvasive method to distinguish between focal adenomatous hyperplasia and diffuse β-cell dysfunction.

A possible genotype–phenotype correlation has recently been described (134), and mutation analysis [Athena Diagnostics, Worcester, Massachusetts, U.S.A.; (135)] should be performed as a part of the evaluation of these patients.

Treatment: The goal of therapy is to prevent hypoglycemia in order to protect the developing brain. Successful treatment should maintain the plasma glucose concentration greater than 60 mg/dL (3.3 mmol/L) on a feeding schedule appropriate for the age of the child. Prompt effective treatment is necessary to minimize the risk of long-term adverse neurological sequelae (2,127,136,137).

The patient should be given a trial of oral diazoxide, which opens normal K$_{ATP}$ channels and thereby suppresses insulin secretion, at a starting dose of 10 mg/kg/day in three doses at eight-hour intervals (127). If no effect is observed at a dose of 15 mg/kg/day, increasing the dose is not recommended because this will aggravate side-effects (edema, hypertrichosis) without improving efficacy. The effect of diazoxide may be potentiated by the addition of a thiazide diuretic (chlorothiazide 7–10 mg/kg/day divided b.i.d.), which acts synergistically with diazoxide (activates potassium channels by a different mechanism) and decreases edema (127). Diazoxide is ineffective in infants whose hyperinsulinism is caused by mutations resulting in complete functional inactivation of the K$_{ATP}$ channel.

A long-acting injectable somatostatin analog (Octreotide) may be successful in maintaining normoglycemia in up to 50% of cases of congenital hyperinsulinism. Octreotide inhibits insulin secretion by decreasing intracellular translocation of calcium ions into β-cells and through a direct effect on secretory granules. It may also mediate G-protein activity in the potassium channel (138). The starting dose is 5 μg/kg every six to eight hours. If glucose is not maintained greater than or equal to 60 mg/dL, the dose of Octreotide is increased up to a maximum of 40 to 60 μg/kg daily, divided into three to six doses. Gastrointestinal side-effects usually limit the tolerable dose of Octreotide. Because of the marked variability of response to Octreotide, the therapeutic regimen has to be adapted for each individual patient and its effects closely monitored (139).

More recently, nifedipine (a calcium channel blocker) has been used to treat hyperinsulinemic hypoglycemia that is unresponsive to conventional therapy (140–143). Experience is still very limited; however, after failure of diazoxide and/or somatostatin analogue to restore euglycemia, nifedipine (0.7–2.5 mg/kg/day) has been used successfully to maintain normoglycemia in at least three patients (141,143). The clinical response to this drug is highly variable, and it is currently not possible to predict which child will respond without a trial.

Continuous subcutaneous infusions of Octreotide (5–20 µg/kg/day) or glucagon (1–10 µg/kg/hour) IV or subcutaneous (SC) infusion can be used to stabilize plasma glucose levels within the normal range in patients prior to surgery. They should be used when the orally administered drugs have been shown not to be effective, particularly if the child remains dependent on a glucose infusion to maintain normoglycemia. When used in high doses, both drugs cause tachyphylaxis. Many infants fail medical therapy and require near-total pancreatectomy to prevent hypoglycemia (104,128,129,144).

Hormone Deficiency
ACTH/Cortisol Deficiency

Cortisol limits glucose utilization in several tissues, including skeletal muscle, by directly opposing the action of insulin and, secondarily, by promoting lipolysis. It stimulates protein breakdown and release of gluconeogenic precursors from muscle and fat. Cortisol stimulates hepatic gluconeogenesis and glycogen synthesis and has a permissive effect on the gluconeogenic and glycogenolytic actions of glucagon and epinephrine. As a result of all these effects, cortisol tends to raise the plasma glucose concentration.

Hypoglycemia is an uncommon presentation of primary adrenal failure. Nevertheless, adrenocortical insufficiency should be considered in the differential diagnosis of patients who present with hypoglycemia and ketosis. In infancy and early childhood, adrenocortical insufficiency may be secondary to congenital adrenal hypoplasia or, rarely, congenital adrenal hyperplasia. The hypoglycemia may be severe (145) because both cortisol and epinephrine secretion are impaired (146). In older children, adrenocortical insufficiency is more likely to be caused by Addison's disease, exogenous glucocorticoids, or X-linked adrenoleukodystrophy (147). ACTH deficiency or panhypopituitarism usually presents with neonatal hypoglycemia, but hypoglycemia may first be observed in infancy or in later childhood. Hypoglycemia caused by isolated deficiency of ACTH is rare (148,149); it is more common in children with multiple pituitary hormone (including GH and ACTH) deficiencies (150,151). Oral glucocorticoids (152) or high doses of inhaled corticosteroids for treatment of asthma are the most common causes of adrenal insufficiency in childhood (153–156).

Diagnosis: A serum cortisol concentration less than 10 µg/dL at the time of hypoglycemia should suggest the diagnosis. The diagnosis is confirmed by a low or high dose cosyntropin (Cortrosyn) stimulation test that evaluates the hypothalamo-pituitary-adrenal axis. Hyperkalemia and hyponatremia occurs in primary adrenal insufficiency, but serum potassium concentration is usually normal when adrenal insufficiency is secondary to primary or secondary ACTH deficiency.

Treatment consists of physiological replacement of cortisol and mineralocorticoids (when necessary).

Hypopituitarism (Isolated Growth Hormone Deficiency, Multiple Pituitary Hormone Deficiencies)

GH decreases sensitivity to insulin, stimulates lipolysis, and decreases glucose utilization. Congenital hypopituitarism often presents in the newborn period with hypoglycemia, persistent hyperbilirubinemia, and a microphallus (157–159). About 20% of children with isolated GH deficiency or multiple anterior pituitary hormone deficiencies present with fasting hypoglycemia and ketosis (150). The occurrence of hypoglycemia in children with GH deficiency is inversely related to age and GH deficiency seldom causes hypoglycemia in older children and adolescents (150,160). The combination of low serum GH and cortisol concentrations at the time of hypoglycemia suggests hypopituitarism; however, serum GH levels during spontaneous hypoglycemia do not correlate well with GH levels obtained by stimulation tests of pituitary GH secretory reserve. Therefore, a single low serum GH concentration cannot be relied on to make the diagnosis of GH deficiency (161–163). Patients with IGF-1 deficiency (Laron syndrome) have high GH levels, but are otherwise indistinguishable from patients with isolated GH deficiency and are prone to symptomatic hypoglycemia in infancy (164). The tendency to develop hypoglycemia ameliorates with advancing age. Pituitary GH secretory reserve should be formally tested if there is any suspicion of GH insufficiency.

Treatment of panhypopituitarism consists of replacing thyroxine, cortisol, and GH.

Disorders of Glycogen Synthesis and Glycogen Degradation
Glycogen Synthase Deficiency (Type 0 Glycogen Storage Disease)

Type 0 glycogen storage disease (GSD 0) is a rare autosomal recessive disorder caused by mutations in the hepatic glycogen synthase (GYS2) gene (165) located on chromosome 12p12.2. To date, 15 different mutations have been documented (86). Mutations in GYS2 result in impaired hepatic glycogen synthesis and shunting of glucose into the glycolytic pathway. The disorder causes a unique metabolic disturbance characterized by fasting hypoglycemia and hyperketonemia alternating with daytime hyperglycemia and hyperlacticacidemia after meals.

Fasting ketotic hypoglycemia is the cardinal feature of GSD 0. The disorder is usually asymptomatic during infancy, but weaning from overnight feeds often proves difficult. Patients may be relatively asymptomatic despite severe hypoglycemia because hyperketonemia provides the brain with an alternative energy source. Consequently, many patients are investigated for short stature, failure to thrive, or other disorders, and are more than two years old before hypoglycemia is found and the diagnosis is made (86). The postprandial hyperglycemia and keto-nuria characteristic of this disorder may be confused with early diabetes mellitus. GSD 0 should be considered in any child with asymptomatic hyperglycemia or glucosuria (166).

Diagnosis: Home blood glucose and urine ketone monitoring may be used to screen for this disorder because fasting hypoglycemia and ketonemia are universal in children less than five years of age. If fasting ketotic hypoglycemia is demonstrated, frequent measurements of blood glucose, lactate, and ketones during fasting and after an oral glucose load or a carbohydrate containing breakfast should be performed to look for the characteristic biochemical disturbances. Mutation analysis of GYS2 is now the preferred method for confirming the diagnosis [Prevention Genetics, Marshfield, Wisconsin, U.S.A. (167)].

Treatment: The goal of treatment is to prevent hypoglycemia and ketosis during the night and hyperglycemia and hyperlacticacidemia during the day. Fasting hypoglycemia is prevented by administration of uncooked cornstarch (1 g/kg) at bedtime. During the day, patients are fed frequently (e.g., every four hours), and cornstarch may be useful when children are physically active. The diet should contain increased amounts of protein to provide substrate for gluconeogenesis (168) and a correspondingly reduced amount of carbohydrate to minimize postprandial hyperglycemia and hyperlacticacidemia (169).

Glucose-6-Phosphatase Deficiency (Type I Glycogen Storage Disease)

Type I glycogen storage disease (GSD I) is an autosomal recessive disorder that results from lack of glucose-6-phosphatase activity, the enzyme that catalyzes the final step in the production of glucose from glucose-6-phosphate (Fig. 3) (170). Glucose production from both glycogenolysis and gluconeogenesis is severely impaired resulting in fasting hypoglycemia and increased production of lactic acid, uric acid, and triglycerides (Fig. 3). Glycogen and fat accumulate in the liver resulting in hepatomegaly and a protuberant abdomen. Symptomatic hypoglycemia may be detected soon after birth; however, most infants are asymptomatic as long as they receive frequent feeds containing sufficient glucose to prevent hypoglycemia. Symptoms of hypoglycemia usually appear when the interval between feeds increases and the infant begins to sleep through the night.

Characteristic manifestations in untreated patients are a progressive decrease in linear growth, muscle wasting, delayed motor development, and the development of a cushingoid appearance (171). The kidneys are enlarged; renal tubular dysfunction and

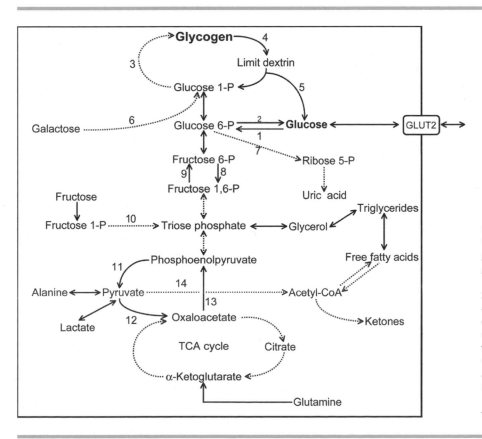

Figure 3 Schematic outline of glucose metabolism shows pathways of glycogen synthesis, glycogen degradation, glycolysis, and gluconeogenesis. Key enzymes are designated by number as follows: 1—hexokinase/glucokinase; 2—glucose-6-phosphatase; 3—glycogen synthase; 4—phosphorylase; 5—amylo-1,6-glucosidase (glycogen debrancher); 6—galactose-1-phosphate uridyl transferase; 7—pentose phosphate pathway; 8—phosphofructokinase; 9—fructose-1, 6-bisphosphatase; 10—fructose-1-phosphate aldolase; 11—pyruvate kinase; 12—pyruvate carboxylase; 13—phosphoenolpyruvate carboxykinase; 14—pyruvate dehydrogenase. *Abbreviation*: TCA, tricarboxylic acid cycle.

glomerular hyperfiltration are common in childhood. Increased urinary albumin excretion may be observed in adolescents (172,173). More severe renal injury (proteinuria, hypertension, and decreased creatinine clearance) due to focal segmental glomerulosclerosis and interstitial fibrosis is associated with suboptimal control, and nephrocalcinosis is common in young adults secondary to hypercalciuria and hypocitraturia (174–176). Inadequate therapy causes severe retardation of physical growth and delayed puberty. Hepatic adenomas usually develop in the second and third decades of life, and may be associated with an iron-resistant anemia, malignant degeneration, or hemorrhage (177–179).

Patients with Type Ib GSD (deficiency of the glucose-6-phosphate transporter required to move glucose-6-phosphate across the microsomal membrane into the lumen of the endoplasmic reticulum where it is exposed to the hydrolytic function of the glucose-6-phosphatase enzyme system) have similar clinical manifestations (180). In addition, they have either constant or cyclic neutropenia associated with recurrent bacterial infections. Neutropenia of varying severity is a consequence of disturbed myeloid maturation, and it is accompanied by functional defects of circulating neutrophils and monocytes (181). Most patients develop an inflammatory bowel disease resembling Crohn's disease that is responsive to treatment with granulocyte colony stimulating factor (182,183).

Diagnosis: In infancy, severe hypoglycemia accompanied by marked hyperlacticacidemia develops three to four hours after a feed. The serum is often cloudy or milky with very high triglyceride and moderately increased levels of cholesterol. Serum uric acid is increased, and serum aspartate aminotransferase (AST) and alanine aminotransferase (ALT) levels are moderately elevated. Glucagon causes either no increase or only a small increase in blood glucose, whereas the already elevated blood lactate level increases further. GSD Ia and Ib are usually suspected on the basis of their characteristic clinical and biochemical abnormalities. The diagnosis usually can be confirmed by mutation analysis (184) and commercially available tests identify more than 95% of mutations for GSD Ia and 80% of mutations for GSD Ib [Duke University School of Medicine Glycogen Storage Disease Laboratory, Durham, North Carolina, U.S.A. (185)]. A liver biopsy and assay of glucose-6-phosphatase activity should seldom be necessary to confirm the diagnosis.

Treatment consists of providing a continuous dietary source of glucose at a rate that prevents the blood glucose level from falling below the threshold for glucose counterregulation, approximately 70 mg/dL. When hypoglycemia is prevented by providing an appropriate amount of glucose throughout the day and night, the biochemical abnormalities are ameliorated, the liver size decreases, the bleeding tendency reverses, and the growth improves (186). The amount of glucose required varies among patients, but can be approximated, initially, by using the formula for calculating basal glucose production rate as a guide: $y = 0.0014x^3 - 0.214x^2 + 10.411x - 9.084$, where $y = $ mg glucose per minute, and $x = $ body weight in kilograms (4). Glucose itself or glucose-containing polymers can be given intermittently during the day and continuously (via a nasogastric tube or gastrostomy) at night. Alternatively, after six to eight months of age, intermittent feedings of uncooked cornstarch can be used as the source of continuous glucose administration (187,188). Orally administered uncooked cornstarch appears to act as an intestinal reservoir of glucose that is slowly absorbed into the circulation. It is given in a slurry of water or artificially flavored drink, or a lactose and sucrose-free formula at three- to five-hour intervals during the day, and four- or five-hour intervals overnight (187,189–191).

Amylo-1,6-Glucosidase Deficiency (Type III Glycogen Storage Disease; Glycogen Debranching Enzyme Deficiency)

Release of glucose from glycogen stores requires the combined actions of glycogen phosphorylase and glycogen debranching enzyme, which consists of two independent catalytic activities on a single polypeptide chain, an oligo-1,4→1,4 glucan transferase and amylo-1,6-glucosidase. After phosphorylase has acted exhaustively on the outer branches of glycogen, four glucosyl residues remain distal to the branch point (limit dextrin). Transferase activity transfers three glucose residues from one short outer branch to the end of another thus exposing the branch-point (an α-1,6-linkage). Glucosidase then hydrolyzes the branch-point permitting phosphorylase access to the α-1,4-linkages. The transferred dextrin may be further depolymerized by phosphorylase. Full debranching enzyme activity requires both the transferase and glucosidase activities. In the absence of debrancher activity, breakdown of glycogen is arrested when the outermost branch points are reached. Only 1,4 segments distal to the outermost branch points are accessible to phosphorylase and can yield glucose. This results in accumulation of an abnormal form of glycogen, phosphorylase limit dextrin, in affected tissues.

Deficiency of debranching enzyme activity due to mutations in the AGL gene, located on chromosome 1p21, impairs glycogenolysis, but gluconeogenesis is unaffected. There are several subtypes of Type III glycogen storage disease (GSD III), and all are transmitted in an autosomal recessive fashion. About 80% to 85% of patients with GSD III lack glycogen debranching enzyme (GDE) activity in both liver and muscle (GDE IIIa); about 15% of patients have GDE deficiency only in the liver (GSD IIIb) (170). In rare cases, there is selective loss of only one of the two GDE activities, glucosidase (type IIIc) or transferase (type IIId) (192,193).

GSD Types IIIa and IIIb have different prognoses and outcomes. Myopathy and cardiomyopathy is common in GSD IIIa and can lead to early death or debilitation in adult life. Muscle involvement can be inferred from high plasma creatine kinase concentrations, but normal values do not rule out muscle involvement.

Because glucose can be produced from 1,4-segments beyond the outermost branch points and from gluconeogenesis, patients with GSD III often develop less severe hypoglycemia than patients with glucose-6-phosphatase deficiency. Fasting causes hypoglycemia with ketosis and hyperlipidemia without elevation of blood lactate and serum uric acid concentrations. Liver enzymes (AST, ALT, alkaline phosphatase, and LDH) are consistently elevated in children (194). The kidneys are not enlarged, nor does renal dysfunction occur. In 85% of patients with skeletal muscle involvement, muscle disease is usually not clinically significant in childhood. Myopathy usually becomes prominent in the third or fourth decades of life, manifesting as slowly progressive muscle weakness involving the large proximal muscles of the shoulders and hips (195). Abnormal glycogen (limit dextrin) may also accumulate in the heart. Subclinical evidence of cardiac involvement is common and manifests as ventricular hypertrophy on EKG and an abnormal echocardiograph (196). Some patients develop a cardiomyopathy similar to hypertrophic obstructive cardiomyopathy (197). Hepatic adenomata occur less frequently in GSD III than in GSD I, but hepatic fibrosis, cirrhosis, and malignant transformation can occur (177,198).

Diagnosis: After an overnight fast, the low blood glucose and normal blood lactate concentrations do not increase after administration of glucagon (0.03 mg/kg, maximum dose 1 mg IM or IV). When the test is repeated two hours after a high-carbohydrate meal, which lengthens the outer branches of glycogen, a glycemic response does occur. Definitive diagnosis and sub-typing formerly required a biopsy of both liver and muscle for assay of enzyme activity, but GSD Type IIIb can now be diagnosed noninvasively by mutation analysis of exon 3 [Duke University School of Medicine Glycogen Storage Disease Laboratory, Durham, North Carolina, U.S.A. (185)]. Mutation analysis is not yet available for the diagnosis of GSD Type IIIa.

Treatment: As in GSD I, continuous provision of an adequate amount of glucose, using uncooked cornstarch, combined with a normal intake of total calories, protein, and other nutrients corrects the clinical and biochemical disorder and restores normal growth. Uncooked cornstarch, 1.75 g/kg at six-hour intervals maintains normoglycemia, increases growth velocity, and decreases serum aminotransferase concentrations (199,200). The lowest dose of cornstarch that maintains normoglycemia should be used. For patients who have significant growth retardation and myopathy, continuous nocturnal feeding of a nutrient mixture composed of glucose, glucose oligosaccharides, and amino acids combined with meals

that have a high protein content has been shown to improve muscle strength (201). The diet should contain at least 2 to 3 g/kg of protein and there is no need to restrict dairy products or fruit.

Hepatic Phosphorylase Complex Deficiency (Glycogen Storage Diseases VI and IX)

The GSDs caused by a reduction in liver phosphorylase activity are a heterogeneous group of disorders that includes autosomal recessive liver glycogen phosphorylase deficiency (Type VI or Hers disease) and phosphorylase kinase deficiency (Type IX), which can be either autosomal recessive or X-linked (171). They are all mild forms of hepatomegalic glycogenosis, and patients seldom have symptomatic hypoglycemia during infancy unless they fast for a prolonged period. Prebreakfast ketosis, as in GSD 0, is almost universal. These disorders present in infancy or early childhood with ketotic hypoglycemia, growth retardation, and prominent hepatomegaly. Delayed motor development is common in patients with reduced enzyme activity in both muscle and liver. Blood lactate and uric acid levels are normal, but mild hyperlipidemia and elevated hepatic transaminases are common biochemical abnormalities (202). Clinical and biochemical abnormalities gradually disappear with increasing age. Hepatomegaly decreases at puberty, and most adult patients are asymptomatic (202).

Diagnosis: Functional tests are not especially useful in evaluating these patients and cannot distinguish between GSD VI and IX. Glucagon administered after an overnight fast usually elicits a brisk glycemic response without a rise in the blood lactate level. Assessment of phosphorylase kinase activity can be performed on whole blood, but confirmation of GSD VI, and often GSD IX, requires assaying enzyme activity on a liver biopsy specimen.

Treatment: Prolonged fasting should be avoided. A bedtime snack may be sufficient to prevent morning hypoglycemia, but ketosis is prevented and patients feel better with uncooked cornstarch supplementation at bedtime (1.5–2 g/kg). Improved growth has been reported in children receiving cornstarch supplementation (203).

Fanconi-Bickel Syndrome (Glycogen Storage Disease Type XI)

Fanconi-Bickel syndrome (FBS) is a rare autosomal recessive disorder due to mutations in the GLUT-2 gene located at 3q16.1-q26.3. GLUT-2 is a facilitative monosaccharide transporter that mediates transport of d-glucose and, to a lesser extent, d-galactose across the cell membrane of hepatocytes, pancreatic β-cells, enterocytes, and the basolateral membrane of renal proximal tubular cells (15). Deficiency of GLUT-2 is characterized by glucose and galactose intolerance and accumulation of glycogen in the liver and kidney. Impaired insulin secretion results in postprandial hyperglycemia leading to a pattern of fasting ketotic hypoglycemia alternating with postprandial hyperglycemia, which can be confused with GSD 0. The absence of hepatomegaly in GSD 0 and the presence of chronic glucosuria in FBS are features that help to distinguish between the disorders.

As with the other forms of GSD, patients with FBS present in infancy when overnight feeds are spaced, and they have fasting ketotic hypoglycemia. Patients may present with chronic diarrhea (from carbohydrate malabsorption), failure to thrive, hypophosphatemic rickets, and developmental delay. Presence of a "moon facies" and a protuberant abdomen may lead to confusion with GSD I. Short stature persisting into adulthood is almost universal in FBS (204,205).

Diagnosis: The diagnosis of FBS should be considered when postprandial hyperglycemia alternates with fasting ketotic hypoglycemia. Mutation analysis can be used to confirm the diagnosis (206), but testing is not yet commercially available.

Treatment: The goal of treatment is to prevent hypoglycemia and ketosis. Frequent small meals supplemented with uncooked cornstarch (1.5–2 g/kg given b.i.d.) improves growth and stamina (207). Because fructose transport into cells is facilitated by GLUT-5, fructose can be used as an alternative source of carbohydrate. High concentrations of glucose, sucrose, and galactose should be avoided because they exacerbate hyperglycemia and aggravate malabsorption.

Disorders of Gluconeogenesis

Disorders of gluconeogenesis may be caused by deficiency of one of the key gluconeogenic enzymes (pyruvate carboxylase, PEPCK, fructose-1,6-bisphosphatase, and glucose-6-phosphatase) (Fig. 3) (208). In addition to these inborn errors of metabolism, gluconeogenesis is impaired in hereditary fructose intolerance, by ingestion of ethanol, in children with Jamaican vomiting sickness, falciparum malaria, severe diarrhea, and in salicylate intoxication. Hypoglycemia caused by disorders of gluconeogenesis is characteristically accompanied by hyperlacticacidemia and hyperalaninemia.

Phosphoenolpyruvate Carboxykinase Deficiency

PEPCK is a unidirectional rate-limiting enzyme of gluconeogenesis that converts oxaloacetate to phosphoenolpyruvate (Fig. 3). Hypoglycemia is seen in infancy and may be severe. Fatty infiltration of the liver, kidney, and other organs occurs because there is increased formation of acetyl CoA. Laboratory evaluation reveals high concentrations of lactate and pyruvate, a normal lactate:pyruvate ratio, and ketosis. The definitive diagnosis of PEPCK deficiency depends on the demonstration of impaired enzyme activity on a liver biopsy. Treatment consists of frequent feedings and avoiding fasting.

Fructose-1,6-Bisphosphatase Deficiency

The block in gluconeogenesis resulting from failure to convert fructose-1,6-bisphosphate to fructose-6-phosphate causes fasting hypoglycemia and lactic acidosis (Fig. 3) (208,209). Hypoglycemia occurs during fasting and intercurrent illness, and is associated with ketosis, hypertriglyceridemia, and hyperuricemia. In the immediate postprandial period, glucagon elicits a glycemic response (210). The biochemical abnormalities caused by fructose-1,6-bisphosphatase deficiency are similar to those of glucose-6-phosphatase deficiency. Affected children typically fail to thrive. Hepatomegaly is caused by fatty infiltration of the liver. Diagnosis is based on demonstrating decreased enzyme activity in the liver. Treatment consists of eliminating dietary fructose and sucrose and avoiding prolonged fasts. During intercurrent illness, IV glucose must be given to arrest catabolism.

Hereditary Fructose Intolerance

This rare disorder is caused by deficiency of fructose-1-phosphate aldolase (Fig. 3). Nursing infants are asymptomatic until fruits and juices are added to their diet. It usually presents following the introduction of a commercial formula containing sucrose, or at the time of weaning when fructose or sucrose are ingested for the first time. Fructose causes vomiting, diarrhea, and hypoglycemia. Chronic exposure to fructose causes hepatomegaly, jaundice, failure to thrive, and renal tubular dysfunction with aminoaciduria. Older children have an aversion to sweets. Fructose-1-phosphate accumulates in the liver and acutely inhibits glycogenolysis via the phosphorylase system and gluconeogenesis at the level of fructose-1,6-bisphosphatase (209). Chronic fructose intoxication can occur after infancy without causing symptoms of acute fructose intoxication and can be expressed as an apparently isolated, reversible retardation of somatic growth. The diagnosis is suggested by fructosuria after meals; a fructose tolerance test results in hypoglycemia. In the past, the diagnosis was based on the response to an IV fructose challenge or was made by liver biopsy, which are both difficult and risky invasive tests. Mutation analysis has become the preferred method for diagnosing hereditary fructose intolerance (HFI), and more than 20 different mutations have been described (211,212). The two most common mutations in HFI in North America and Western Europe are both in exon 5; sequencing of this exon will detect mutations in more than 70% of cases (213).

Alcohol Intoxication

Ingestion of alcohol by children and adolescents can cause hypoglycemia several hours after its consumption as a result of inhibition of gluconeogenesis (214). Ethanol inhibits gluconeogenesis because its metabolism by alcohol dehydrogenase depletes hepatic NAD, a cofactor critical to the entry of most precursors into the gluconeogenic pathway. It does not inhibit glycogenolysis (215). Ethanol also inhibits cortisol and GH responses to hypoglycemia (214). When hepatic glycogen stores are adequate, ethanol does not cause hypoglycemia. However, severe hypoglycemia occurs when glycogen is depleted as a result of ethanol consumption without food, or after accidental alcohol ingestion after an overnight fast in a young child. Glucagon cannot raise the blood glucose level; treatment of ethanol-induced hypoglycemia should always be with administration of IV glucose.

Salicylate Poisoning

Large doses of salicylates can lower the plasma glucose concentration (216). Both hyperinsulinemia and reduced gluconeogenesis have been observed following acute ingestion of aspirin (216). However, the precise mechanism causing hypoglycemia is unclear. Experimentally, salicylates may decrease gluconeogenesis via their ability to uncouple oxidative phosphorylation.

Malaria

Hypoglycemia is common in children with severe falciparum malaria in the absence of treatment with quinine (217–220). Impaired gluconeogenesis is suggested by the presence of high blood levels of ketones, lactate, and alanine at the time of hypoglycemia. Gluconeogenesis appears to be limited by an insufficient supply of precursors and is unable to compensate for the decreased availability of glucose from glycogen (221). Hypoglycemia has also been described during treatment with quinine and has been attributed to quinine's hyperinsulinemic effect (216). It has been suggested that the frequency of hypoglycemia in malaria may be no higher than in other serious illnesses associated with severe calorie deprivation (220). Treatment of hypoglycemia associated with malaria is with IV glucose.

Reye Syndrome

This syndrome typically follows viral infections with varicella and influenza A and B. Aspirin has been implicated in its pathogenesis. It is characterized by recurrent vomiting, an altered level of consciousness, hyperpnea, and hypoglycemia that is mainly the result of altered gluconeogenesis (222). Hypoglycemia occurs most often in children less than five years of age. Increased plasma levels of ammonia and FFAs suggest impaired ureagenesis and fatty acid oxidation (223,224). Recurrent episodes that mimic Reye syndrome should raise suspicion for a fatty acid oxidation defect. Treatment is supportive (225,226).

Diarrhea and Malnutrition

In developing countries, hypoglycemia is a common complication of infectious diarrhea in both well-nourished and poorly nourished children (227–230), and is a major cause of death (230,231). Children with kwashiorkor frequently suffer from severe hypoglycemia (232–234). Infants with acquired monosaccharide intolerance after an episode of gastroenteritis are also at increased risk of developing severe and even fatal hypoglycemia when fed a carbohydrate-free diet (235,236).

Depletion of hepatic glycogen together with hepatic steatosis is observed in children with fatal hypoglycemia and diarrhea (237). Serum insulin levels are appropriately suppressed and glucose counterregulatory hormone concentrations are appropriately elevated in children with diarrhea and hypoglycemia, whereas gluconeogenic substrates are low suggesting that the hypoglycemia may be due to failure of gluconeogenesis (231). Reduced availability of fat-derived fuels (FFA and ketones) may play an important role in the development of hypoglycemia. In children who developed hypoglycemia during acute diarrheal illness, BOHB concentrations were not significantly higher than in normoglycemic children with diarrhea, suggesting deficient generation of ketones, either because fat stores were diminished as a result of malnutrition or because the oxidation of fat was impaired (231). If fatty acids are less available (as may occur in malnutrition) or when oxidation of fatty acids is defective (e.g., as a result of acquired carnitine deficiency), hypoglycemia is more likely to occur because body tissues and brain (secondary to hypoketonemia) are more dependent on glucose. The failure of gluconeogenesis in diarrheal illness, therefore, may be a consequence of depleted fat stores, defective fatty acid oxidation and ketogenesis, or a defect in the hepatic enzymatic pathways required for gluconeogenesis (238).

Frequent feeding of children during diarrhea may help to prevent hypoglycemia. When patients with diarrhea require parenteral therapy, dextrose-containing electrolyte solutions should be used and the child's blood glucose level must be carefully monitored.

Disorders of Amino Acid Metabolism

Several disorders of amino acid metabolism result in hypoglycemia with organic aciduria. These patients typically have a delay in growth and development, recurrent vomiting, and may have hepatomegaly. Laboratory features include hyperammonemia and hyperchloremic metabolic acidosis. Diagnosis depends on identification of specific organic acids in the urine and analysis of liver biopsy specimens or cultured fibroblasts (239,240).

Methylmalonic Acidemia

Methylmalonic acidemia results from a deficiency of methylmalonyl-CoA mutase, a cobalamin-dependent enzyme involved in the carboxylation of propionyl-CoA. Patients typically present in the newborn period with ketoacidosis, hyperammonemia, hypoglycemia, and acute encephalopathy. Hypoglycemia is due to impaired gluconeogenesis (241). Asymptomatic and benign variants are also detected by the analysis of urine organic acids. Plasma amino acid profile shows an increased concentration of glycine.

3-Hydroxy-3-Methyl Glutaric Acidemia

3-Hydroxy-3-methylglutaryl CoA lyase catalyzes the last step of leucine degradation and ketogenesis. Deficiency of this enzyme results in a clinical presentation that includes episodes of hypoketotic hypoglycemia, fatty liver, coma, and mental delay (242).

Maple Syrup Urine Disease

Maple Syrup Urine Disease (MSUD) is caused by a deficiency of branched-chain ketoacid dehydrogenase, the enzyme that decarboxylates the α-ketoacids of leucine, isoleucine, and valine (243). The classic clinical presentation consists of failure to thrive, acidosis, hypoglycemia, and neurologic symptoms with rapid deterioration when left untreated. The pathogenesis of hypoglycemia is not entirely clear, although it appears to result from defective gluconeogenesis (244). The levels of the branched-chain amino acids (leucine, isoleucine, and valine), particularly leucine, are elevated in plasma and urine. Increased plasma and urine concentrations of leucine, isoleucine, and valine with accumulation of branched-chain ketoacids and 2-hydroxy acids are essential for making the diagnosis. Additional metabolites of the branched-chain amino acids may be detected. The enzymatic defect can be detected in leukocytes. Treatment of MSUD aims to inhibit endogenous protein catabolism, sustain protein synthesis, prevent deficiencies of essential amino acids, and maintain normal serum osmolarity. Acute illnesses precipitate a catabolic state that must be promptly arrested (245).

Hereditary Tyrosinemia (Tyrosinemia Type I)

This disorder is caused by deficiency of fumarylacetoacetate hydrolase. Infants present with vomiting, diarrhea, and failure to thrive. Liver disease and hypoglycemia are consistent findings. A large amount of succinylacetone is excreted in the urine. Diagnosis is confirmed by measurement of fumarylacetoacetate hydrolase in the liver. Treatment consists of a diet low in tyrosine and phenylalanine in addition to the administration of 2-(2-nitro-4(trifluoromethyl) benzoyl) -1,3-cyclohexandione. Liver transplant is an effective therapy.

Miscellaneous Causes of Hypoglycemia
Galactosemia

Galactosemia is caused by deficiency of galactose-1-phosphate uridyl transferase (Fig. 3) resulting in inability to convert galactose-1-phosphate to glucose-1-phosphate (246). A defect in UDP-galactose-4-epimerase may cause a similar presentation (246). Hypoglycemia occurs following milk feedings. Although the precise mechanism causing hypoglycemia is unclear, there is evidence suggesting that the accumulation of galactose-1-phosphate inhibits phosphoglucomutase activity, thereby inhibiting glycogenolysis. Patients may present with neonatal *Escherichia coli* sepsis, diarrhea, vomiting, failure to thrive, hepatomegaly, jaundice, ascites, cataracts, and mental retardation. The urine contains a reducing substance that is not glucose (urine gives a positive Clinitest reaction but is negative with Clinistix) while the patient is receiving galactose. The increased concentration of galactose-1-phosphate leads to intellectual impairment, cataracts, hepatic dysfunction, renal tubular disease (Fanconi syndrome), and ovarian failure (247). Diagnosis is confirmed by identifying a marked increase in blood levels of galactose and galactose-1-phosphate and near absent galactose-1-phosphate uridyl transferase activity in red blood cells (246). Treatment consists of eliminating galactose from the diet.

Liver Disease

Fasting hypoglycemia may occur in patients with a variety of diseases and ingestions that cause extensive severe damage to the liver parenchyma, resulting in fulminant hepatic necrosis and liver failure (248). Hypoglycemia results from impaired glycogenolysis and gluconeogenesis. Treatment is supportive.

Jamaican Vomiting Sickness

The unripe ackee fruit of the Blighia surpida tree contains a water-soluble toxin, hypoglycin, which produces vomiting, central nervous system depression, acute fatty liver, and severe hypoglycemia. Hypoglycemia is caused by hypoglycin A, which inhibits gluconeogenesis secondary to its interference with oxidation of long chain fatty acids (249). The disease is endemic in Jamaica where ackee is part of the diet of the poor. It has been reported in the United States resulting from the consumption of canned ackee (250).

Glucose Transporter Defects

Hypoglycorrhachia, despite normal plasma glucose concentrations, has been described in infants with a seizure disorder, developmental delay and acquired microcephaly, caused by a defect in the blood–brain glucose transporter (GLUT-1). Glucose and lactate concentrations in the cerebrospinal fluid are low. Two distinct classes of mutations cause the functional defect of glucose transport: hemizygosity of GLUT-1 and nonsense mutations resulting in truncation of the GLUT-1 protein (251). Treatment is with a ketogenic diet to provide the brain with an alternative fuel source (252).

Congenital Disorders of Glycosylation (Carbohydrate-Deficient Glycoprotein Syndrome)

Congenital disorders of glycosylation (CDG) are due to several distinct genetic defects in the synthesis of the glycan moiety of glycoproteins or other glycoconjugates (253). CDGs affect many organs and have diverse clinical manifestations. In addition to failure to thrive and developmental delay, some patients exhibit characteristic dysmorphic features: large ears, a prominent forehead, inverted nipples, and abnormal fat distribution, but these features are not invariably present. Both CDG-Ia (phosphomannomutase 2 deficiency) (254) and CDG-Ib (phosphomannose isomerase deficiency) are associated with hypoglycemia; however, in CDG-Ib, hyperinsulinemic hypoglycemia is responsive to treatment with oral mannose (255). Serum transferrin isoelectrofocusing is used to screen for *N*-glycosylation defects associated with sialic acid deficiency; however, a normal pattern does not exclude these defects (253).

Respiratory Chain Defects

Hypoglycemia occasionally occurs in children with defects of oxidative phosphorylation associated with liver failure (256–258). Hypoglycemia may, however, be the presenting symptom in some cases of respiratory chain defect without any obvious hepatic dysfunction. The mechanism underlying the hypoglycemia is incompletely understood. It has been suggested that hypoglycemia in the absence of hepatic failure may be due to impairment of either gluconeogenesis or fatty acid oxidation or glycogenolysis as a result of reduced cofactors, ATP, NAD, or FAD, which may interfere with the different pathways involved in glucose homeostasis (259).

Insulin Autoimmune Hypoglycemia (Hirata Syndrome)

Initially reported from Japan in 1970, this rare disorder, which is exceedingly uncommon in whites and in children, is characterized by hyperinsulinemic hypoglycemia and high titers of antibodies to human insulin in the absence of pathologic abnormalities of the pancreatic islets and prior exposure to exogenous insulin (260,261). More than 90% of cases have been reported in the Japanese literature. Patients are typically middle aged, although children as young as three years and elderly patients have been reported.

Insulin autoimmune hypoglycemia (IAH) is caused by interaction of endogenous autoantibodies with insulin and causes severe postprandial and/or fasting neuroglycopenia that may be confused with an insulinoma or other cause of hyperinsulinemic hypoglycemia (260,261). Its frequency is increased in patients with autoimmune diseases (e.g., Graves disease, systemic lupus erythematosus, ulcerative colitis, and with use of sulfhydryl-containing drugs such as methimazole) (262). Postprandial hypoglycemia has been attributed to a buffering effect of insulin antibodies causing prolonged elevations of postprandial total and free insulin concentrations with release of free insulin out of synchrony with the ambient glucose concentration (261,263).

Diagnosis: During spontaneous episodes of hypoglycemia, serum insulin, C-peptide and proinsulin concentrations are elevated. As a result of interference by the autoantibodies in the immunoassay, serum insulin may be dramatically increased to concentrations of the order of 100 to 1000 μU/mL or higher (264). IAH can be readily detected by high titers of insulin antibodies (measured by ^{125}I-labeled insulin binding in polyethylene glycol precipitated samples or by ELISA), which may also bind to C-peptide and proinsulin and interfere with their immunoassays resulting in spuriously elevated concentrations.

Treatment: Most cases occur in the setting of autoimmune disease with or without precipitating medications. The hypoglycemia is usually transient and resolves spontaneously within three to six months of diagnosis (260). Possible offending medications should be stopped. The most consistent benefit has been obtained from high doses of prednisone and plasmapheresis (263) in conjunction with a diet consisting of frequent small meals low in either total or readily absorbable carbohydrate, together with acarbose to reduce postprandial hyperglycemia and the stimulus to insulin secretion (261).

Disorders of Carnitine Metabolism, Fatty Acid β-Oxidation, and Ketone Synthesis

Disorders of carnitine metabolism and fatty acid β-oxidation (FAO) are characterized by impaired ability to metabolize FFAs to acetyl CoA in various tissues and to synthesize ketones in the liver. During periods of fasting, mitochondrial oxidation of fatty acids becomes the major source of energy. Fatty acids with a chain length of less than or equal to 18 carbons undergo a series of reactions that produce acetyl CoA, a Krebs cycle intermediate and a precursor of hepatic ketone body synthesis. Normally, ketones are an alternative fuel for a variety of tissues, thereby conserving glucose for oxidation by the brain and heart (23). The paucity of ketones in FAO disorders results in continued utilization of glucose resulting in inability to maintain fasting plasma glucose concentrations and accumulation of intermediates of β-oxidation, which cause encephalopathy, arrhythmias, cardiac arrest, and sudden death (265,266).

The oxidation of fatty acids begins with the formation of acyl-coenzyme A (acyl-CoA), which is transported across the mitochondrial membrane by a carnitine-mediated transport mechanism. Within the mitochondrion, carnitine is removed and four reactions, catalyzed by membrane-bound enzymes,

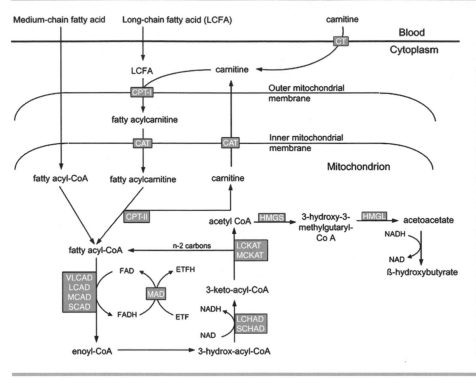

Figure 4 Schema of carnitine metabolism, fatty acid ß-oxidation, and ketone synthesis. Reactions associated with known metabolic defects are shown in shaded boxes. *Abbreviations*: CAT, carnitine-acylcarnitine translocase; CT, carnitine transporter; CPT-I, carnitine palmitoyltransferase-I; CPT-II, carnitine palmitoyltransferase-II; ETF(H), electron transfer flavoprotein (reduced); FAD(H), flavin adenine dinucleotide (reduced); HMGL, 3-hydroxy-3-methylglutaryl-CoA lyase; HMGS, 3-hydroxy-3-methylglutaryl-CoA synthetase; LCAD, long-chain acyl-CoA dehydrogenase; LCFA, long-chain fatty acid; LCHAD, long-chain hydroxyacyl-CoA dehydrogenase; LCKAT, long-chain 3-ketoacyl-CoA thiolase; MAD, multiple acyl-CoA dehydrogenase; MCAD, medium-chain acyl-CoA dehydrogenase; MCKAT, medium-chain 3-ketoacyl-CoA thiolase; NAD(H), nicotinamide adenine dinucleotide (reduced); SCAD, short-chain acyl-CoA dehydrogenase; SCHAD, short-chain hydroxyacyl-CoA dehydrogenase; VLCAD, very-long chain acyl-CoA dehydrogenase.

result in sequential removal of two carbon moieties (Fig. 4). Although defects in the formation of CoA esters, transport, or β-oxidation all result in impaired energy metabolism, there is a wide spectrum of clinical phenotypes. To date, at least 22 distinct disorders of fatty acid oxidation or transport have been described. Clinical manifestations may appear at any age between birth and adulthood; approximately 70% of patients manifest symptoms before one year of age (267). Clinical manifestations usually develop during periods of catabolic stress or reduced caloric consumption (268). Symptoms of an acute metabolic crisis vary in severity and include nausea, vomiting, lethargy, confusion, coma, seizures, or sudden death. Patients may have hypoglycemia (usually, but not always hypoketotic), liver disease ranging in severity from increased serum transaminase levels to fulminant hepatic failure, skeletal myopathy, or cardiac dysfunction caused by cardiomyopathy (Tables 6 and 7).

Approximately one-third of patients with FAO disorders present in the newborn period with lethargy, hypotonia, and neurologic depression (267). Developmental abnormalities (including facial dysmorphism, renal dysplasia or cysts, and developmental brain malformations caused by defects in neuronal migration) have been observed in multiple acyl-CoA dehydrogenase deficiency (MAD, glutaric acidemia Type II) (272,276), in CPT-II deficiency (277), and long-chain hydroxyacyl-CoA dehydrogenase (LCHAD) deficiency (278). Other disorders that may present in the neonatal period, but are not typically associated with developmental abnormalities

include translocase deficiency, trifunctional protein deficiency, CPT-I deficiency, and very long-chain acyl-CoA dehydrogenase (VLCAD) deficiency. Cardiac manifestations, including conduction disturbances and arrhythmias, are common in all of the disorders that present in the newborn period, but are particularly characteristic of the long-chain fatty acid oxidation disorders. Although hypoglycemia is a feature of these disorders, severely ill infants usually die within a few days of birth despite treatment of hypoglycemia (272,279). About 5% of cases of sudden infant death syndrome (SIDS) are thought to be caused by defects in carnitine transport and/or FAO, including deficiencies of medium-chain acyl-CoA dehydrogenase (MCAD), VLCAD, LCHAD, MAD, and carnitine transport defects (280).

In infancy and childhood, hypoglycemia is the most common presenting abnormality; more than 80% of patients have hypoglycemia at diagnosis (267). Hypoglycemia typically is associated with hypoketosis. In patients with short chain fatty acid disorders, however, ketogenesis may be sufficient to cause moderate or large (appropriate) ketonuria at the time of presentation with hypoglycemia. Moderate hepatomegaly at presentation is caused by fatty infiltration (micro- and macrovesicular steatosis), which may lead to the erroneous impression that the patient has a GSD or Reye syndrome (281,282). Hepatomegaly rapidly resolves with treatment. Most patients have hepatic dysfunction during episodes of acute metabolic decompensation (266,268). A moderate increase in serum transaminase concentrations (100–800 U/L) is common, and patients with MAD

Table 6 Disorders of Carnitine Metabolism

Enzyme deficiency	CT	CAT	CPT-I	CPT-II
Clinical				
Fasting intolerance	+	+	+	+
Acute episodes	+	+	+	+
Coma/seizures	+	+	+	+
Muscle weakness/myopathy	+	+	+	+
Muscle pain/myoglobinuria				+
Cardiomyopathy/arrhythmia	+	+		±
Hepatopathy	+	+	+	±
Nephropathy			+	
Congenital anomalies				+
Biochemical				
Hypoglycemia	+	+	+	+
Ketones	Low	Low	Low	Low
Ammonia	+/−High	+/−High	+/−High	+/−High
AST, ALT	Abnormal	Abnormal	Abnormal	Abnormal
Plasma carnitine	Very low	Low/normal	High/normal	Low/normal
Plasma acylcarnitines	Normal	Abnormal	Normal	Abnormal
Dicarboxylic aciduria	No	Yes	Yes	No
Other abnormal organic acids	No	No	No	No
Urine acylglycines	Normal	Normal	Normal	Normal

Abbreviations: CT, carnitine transporter; CAT, carnitine acylcarnitine translocase; CPT-I, carnitine palmitoyltransferase-I; CPT-II, carnitine palmitoyltransferase-II; ±, not common but occasionally reported; +/−high, plasma ammonia level is not invariably high.
Source: From Refs. 265,266,268-271.

and translocase deficiency may present with hepatic failure. Hepatocyte mitochondria may be abnormal in shape and size in both disorders. Electron microscopy may reveal differences: dense condensation of mitochondria with inclusion bodies in FAO defects in contrast to mitochondrial swelling in Reye syndrome (283).

Patients with defects in carnitine transport (primary carnitine deficiency) and metabolism (other than CPT-I deficiency) or in the oxidation of longer

Table 7 Disorders of Fatty Acid Oxidation and Ketone Synthesis

Enzyme deficiency	MAD	VLCAD	MCAD	SCAD	LCHAD	SCHAD	KAT	HMGS	HMGL
Clinical									
Fasting intolerance	+	+	+	+	+	+	+	+	+
Acute episodes	+	+	+	+	+	+	+	+	+
Coma/seizures	+	+	+	+	+	+	+	+	+
Myopathy/weakness	+	+		+	+	+	+		+
Myoglobinuria/pain		+			+	+			
Neuropathy		+			+				
Retinopathy					+				
Cardiomyopathy	+	+			+	±	+		
Hepatopathy	+	+	+	+	+	±	+	+	+
Nephropathy		+							
Congenital anomalies	+								
Biochemical									
Hypoglycemia	+	+	+	+	+	+	+	+	+
Ketones	Low	Low	Low	High	Low	High	Low	Low	Low
Ammonia	+/−High	+/−High	+/−High	+/−High	+/−High			N	+/−High
AST, ALT	Abnl	Abnl	Abnl	Abnl	Abnl		Abnl	Abnl	Abnl
Plasma carnitine	Low	Low	Low	Low	Low	Low	Low[a]	N	N
Plasma acylcarnitines	Abnl	Abnl	Abnl	Abnl	Abnl	N	Abnl	N	N
Dicarboxylic aciduria	Yes	Yes	Yes	Yes	Yes	Yes	Yes	Yes/no	No
Other abnormal OA	Yes	Yes	Yes	Yes	Yes	Yes	Yes	Yes[b]	Yes
Urine acylglycines	Abnl	N	Abnl	Abnl	N	N	N	N	N

[a]May be normal.
[b]During acute episodes or after MCT loading.
Abbreviations: Abnl, abnormal; N, normal; OA, organic acids; ±, not common but occasionally reported; KAT, 3-ketoacyl-CoA thiolase; HMGS, 3-hydroxy-3-methylglutaryl-CoA synthase; HMGL, 3-hydroxy-3-methylglutaryl-CoA lyase; SCHAD, short-chain hydroxyacyl-CoA dehydrogenase; MAD, multiple acyl-Co-A dehydrogenase; VLCAD, very long-chain acyl-CoA dehydrogenase; MCAD, medium-chain acyl-CoA dehydrogenase; SCAD, short-chain acyl-CoA dehydrogenase; LCHAD, long-chain hydroxyacyl-CoA dehydrogenase.
Source: From Refs. 265,266,268,272-275.

chain fatty acids (long-chain acyl-CoA dehydrogenase (LCAD), VLCAD, LCHAD, and MAD deficiency) characteristically have hypertrophic or dilated cardiomyopathy (266,268,284) and often present with congestive heart failure or cardiac arrest. Arrhythmias have been reported without cardiomyopathy. Conduction disturbances are thought to be due to accumulation of toxic intermediates and can occur before the development of severe hypoglycemia.

Muscle symptoms are the hallmark of FAO defects that present in adulthood. Progressive muscle weakness, episodic muscle pain, rhabdomyolysis, and myoglobinuria after strenuous physical activity occur in adults with CPT-II, translocase, LCHAD, and VLCAD deficiency (Tables 6 and 7). Symptoms may occur after prolonged exercise or exposure to cold, during fasting or an intercurrent infection. Hypoglycemia and alterations in mental status are unusual in the late onset disorders.

The characteristic biochemical features of disorders of carnitine metabolism and FAO are summarized in Tables 6 and 7. Acute metabolic crises are frequently, but not invariably, associated with hypoglycemia and metabolic acidosis. Hypoglycemia results from a combination of failure to decrease utilization of glucose (because of the lack of an alternative energy source) and impaired gluconeogenesis. Metabolic acidosis is accompanied by an increased anion gap. Mild to marked hyperammonemia may occur as a result of secondary inhibition of N-acetylglutamate synthesis in the urea cycle. Hepatic dysfunction generally manifests with increases in serum AST and ALT concentrations. When muscle is affected, serum creatine kinase increases during symptomatic episodes. The cause of the increased serum uric acid level is unclear.

Urinalysis shows an inappropriately low level of ketonuria relative to the duration of fasting and/or degree of hypoglycemia. Ketones are seldom completely absent from the urine. Ketonuria may be abundant in patients with defects limited to the oxidation of short chain fatty acids (particularly short-chain acyl-CoA dehydrogenase (SCAD) and SCHAD deficiency) because most of the long chain fatty acid is oxidized to ketones; only the metabolism of the short chain remnants is impaired.

Quantitative assays of plasma carnitine concentrations measure total carnitine as well as free and bound (or esterified) carnitine. Normally, the free fraction comprises about 80% of total carnitine. Carnitine transport defects (primary carnitine deficiency) are rare, and are characterized by extremely low total and free carnitine levels in blood and urine (generally less than 10 µmol/L) (269). Carnitine loading (for example with 100 mg/kg) raises the blood level of carnitine, but causes inappropriate carnitinuria. Secondary carnitine deficiency is much more common. A low level of total plasma carnitine is usually the result of an inadequate supply of dietary carnitine and the ratio of the free and esterified fractions to total

carnitine generally remains intact. A low free/total carnitine ratio can occur for a number of reasons including physiologic ketosis (when acetyl CoA binds free carnitine to form acetylcarnitine), and with certain medications (e.g., valproate binds carnitine forming valproylcarnitine). In disorders of FAO, carnitine binds with intermediate compounds in the pathway (e.g., octanoylcarnitine) resulting in decreased total and free carnitine and increased esterified fractions.

Diagnosis: All children with hypoglycemia should be screened for FAO disorders. Failure to make the correct diagnosis in a timely fashion increases the risk of hepatic failure or sudden death. During an episode of hypoglycemia, screening for a FAO defect should routinely include urinalysis for measurement of ketones and an analysis of urinary organic acids. Urinary ketones are usually inappropriately low for the degree of hypoglycemia; complete absence of ketones is unusual. Hypoketosis (unless clearly explained by hyperinsulinism) always warrants an investigation for FAO defects. Moderate or large ketonuria does not exclude the diagnosis of a FAO disorder.

Analysis of a urine sample (obtained as soon as possible after presentation) for organic acids by gas chromatography/mass spectrometry is a useful method to screen for FAO disorders. The urinary excretion of ketones is reduced (except in the short chain variants). In all defects characterized by impaired β-oxidation of fatty acids, intermediate compounds accumulate and undergo ω-oxidation resulting in the production of dicarboxylic acids (adipic, suberic, and sebacic acids, corresponding to the saturated fatty acids hexanoate, octanoate, and decanoate, respectively). The excretion of dicarboxylic acids is not necessarily pathological because this may occur to a limited degree during physiologic ketosis. Also, patients receiving medium chain triglycerides (MCT), e.g., in a formula, have dicarboxylic aciduria. Defects in carnitine transport and metabolism do not directly disrupt β-oxidation and are not generally associated with dicarboxylic aciduria. In 3-hydroxy-3-methylglutaryl-CoA lyase deficiency, only adipic acid is found in urine during a metabolic crisis. Other metabolites in the organic acid analysis may help to identify the specific site of the metabolic block.

Glycine and carnitine are normal cellular constituents that displace CoA from organic acyl and fatty acyl intermediates, producing acylglycines and acylcarnitines, respectively. The former is analyzed in urine (285), the latter in plasma or in blood filter paper specimens (286,287). Certain compounds have a higher affinity for glycine, others for carnitine. The specific pattern of unusual compounds identified by these techniques, in concert with urine organic acid findings, increases the likelihood of making a specific diagnosis. Quantitative FFA profiles allow direct analysis of all fatty acid intermediates and appears to be the most sensitive test for diagnosing disorders of FAO (265). Because deficiency of carnitine and disorders of carnitine transport do not cause abnormal patterns of fatty acyl-CoA intermediates, measurement of total, free, and esterified carnitine concentrations should be included in the investigation of a suspected FAO disorder.

The importance of obtaining diagnostic specimens during the acute catabolic phase of illness (or as soon as possible after the patient has been treated) cannot be overstated. Once treatment is begun with oral and/or IV glucose, fatty acid flux through the defective pathway decreases, and the characteristic biochemical abnormalities necessary to establish a diagnosis may no longer be evident. Consequently, specimens obtained after treatment is well underway may be normal, necessitating a more invasive and potentially dangerous approach to investigating these patients (37,288).

Several American states and European regions are using tandem mass spectrometry to screen for FAO disorders and CPT-II deficiency on filter paper blood specimens obtained during the newborn period (287,289–291).

There are several options for investigating the asymptomatic patient who has a history suggestive of a defect in carnitine metabolism or FAO. Plasma acylcarnitine and urinary acylgycine should be obtained before breakfast after a routine overnight fast of 8 to 10 hours duration when the child is well. Arrangements can be made for diagnostic blood and urine specimens to be obtained when the patient is under catabolic stress (e.g., during a febrile or other intercurrent illness). The patient can be admitted to the hospital to monitor the response to fasting (37,288). Because of the potential hazard of inducing an arrhythmia, hepatic failure, or sudden death, a monitored fast should be performed as a last resort in the child with hypoglycemia in whom all noninvasive methods have failed to yield a diagnosis. A supervised oral fat load has been used to identify defects affecting longer chain fatty acid metabolism (292). In all cases of potential carnitine transport defects and FAO defects, especially in very young patients or when it is inappropriate for a patient to fast or undergo a provocative study, skin fibroblasts may be obtained for FAO studies and for analysis of enzyme activity. In addition, mutational analysis can be performed for diseases with common mutations, e.g., MCAD and LCHAD deficiency.

Treatment: The specific treatment of disorders of carnitine metabolism and defects of FAO depends upon the individual defect. The primary recommendation for all disorders of FAO is to avoid prolonged fasting and ensure a frequent feeding regimen when patients are at risk for acute metabolic decompensation. Provision of a continuous exogenous source of carbohydrate obviates dependence on fatty acids and ketones for energy. During intercurrent illnesses or when calorie intake decreases for any

reason, patients should be fed every four hours around-the-clock until a normal diet is resumed and symptoms of the illness abate. When vomiting prevents dependable consumption of food or fluids, 10% dextrose solution must be given intravenously at a rate approximately 1.5 times the hepatic glucose production rate to prevent glucose counterregulation.

Dietary therapy for defects of FAO is controversial. For the young child (more than one year of age) who is otherwise well, raw cornstarch at night decreases dependence on fatty acids as a source of energy. Restriction of fat has been used; however, overzealous fat restriction may lead to deficiencies of essential fatty acids. In defects of long chain fatty acid oxidation, supplemental dietary MCT allows ketone synthesis to occur. The availability of fat as a substrate for energy may be of therapeutic benefit even during an acute metabolic crisis.

Carnitine supplementation (usually 100 mg/kg/day) is indicated for carnitine transport defects. Whether carnitine supplementation is beneficial for other defects of FAO is controversial. Carnitine may displace toxic intermediates bound to CoA, thereby liberating CoA to participate in other metabolic reactions and enhancing excretion of acylcarnitines.

Patients with later onset MAD deficiency (glutaric acidemia Type II) may respond to high dose (100–200 mg/kg/day) riboflavin supplementation.

Because defects in carnitine metabolism and FAO may be asymptomatic, the siblings of probands should be screened and parents should be counseled regarding the autosomal recessive pattern of inheritance of these diseases. Prenatal diagnosis may be available depending on the specific disorder of concern.

DETERMINING THE CAUSE OF HYPOGLYCEMIA

The cause of hypoglycemia is often readily apparent; for example, in the child with Type 1 diabetes mellitus treated with insulin or when hypoglycemia occurs in a child with fulminant hepatitis or Reye syndrome. When the cause of hypoglycemia is not obvious, following the diagnostic approach outlined below will usually lead to the specific cause. Determining the cause begins with a detailed history and physical examination. Important features of the history and physical examination are shown in Tables 8 and 9, and a diagnostic algorithm based on key clinical and biochemical features is shown in Figure 5. Infants with hyperinsulinism who do not present in the newborn period usually present within the first 6 to 12 months of life. Mild forms of congenital hyperinsulinism may present for the first time in childhood or adolescence. When hyperinsulinemic hypoglycemia presents after infancy an islet cell adenoma (often part of multiple endocrine neoplasia Type 1 syndrome) should be suspected (293). GH and/or cortisol deficiency usually presents in the newborn period or in early childhood. Accelerated starvation usually

Table 8 History

Birth weight, gestational age, maternal health and medications
Symptoms of hypoglycemia at birth or during neonatal period
Prolonged neonatal jaundice
Age at onset of symptoms
Family history of hypoglycemia
History of consanguinity
Frequency of hypoglycemia
Temporal relationship to feedings
    Less than 4 hours suggests a defect in glycogenolysis
    or hyperinsulinism
    10–12 hours suggests a defect in gluconeogenesis
    or fatty acid β-oxidation
Specific content of feedings and relationship to onset of symptoms
Food intolerance or aversion
Unexplained infant deaths or sudden infant death syndrome in
    family; Reye syndrome, cardiomyopathy, myopathy
Potential drug exposure (sulfonylurea, insulin)
Hypoglycemia after an adult party: alcohol ingestion
Recurrent "pneumonia": episodes of hyperventilation
    from metabolic acidosis
Unusual odors, especially when sick

presents at 18 months to five years old. Hepatomegaly, ketosis, and metabolic acidosis suggests an inborn error of metabolism, which may present either in the neonatal period or later in infancy, usually

Table 9 Findings on Physical Examination

Examination	Possible causes
Short stature; growth failure	GH deficiency, hypopituitarism
Microphallus	GH deficiency, hypopituitarism
Midline facial defects	GH deficiency, hypopituitarism
Cleft lip and palate	
Single central incisor	
Optic nerve hypoplasia	
Abnormal skin pigmentation	Addison's disease
Large liver	Glycogen storage disease
	Disorder of gluconeogenesis
	Galactosemia
	Disorder of fatty acid β-oxidation
	Disorder of carnitine metabolism
	Tyrosinemia Type I
Macrosomia	Beckwith-Wiedemann syndrome
Large tongue	
Omphalocele/umbilical hernia	
Visceromegaly	
Horizontal grooves	
on ear lobes	
Hyperventilation	Metabolic acidosis, hyperammonemia
Odor	Maple syrup urine disease, isovaleric acidemia, 3-methylcrotonyl-CoA carboxylase deficiency, multiple acyl-CoA dehydrogenase deficiency (glutaric acidemia Type II)
Heart	Disorder of fatty acid β-oxidation
Gallop or murmur	Disorder of carnitine transport or metabolism
Cardiomyopathy	

Abbreviation: GH, growth hormone.

precipitated by cessation of overnight feeding or an infection that interrupts the child's normal feeding pattern and causes catabolic stress.

Glucose meters are widely used in newborn nurseries, emergency departments, and intensive care units to screen for hypoglycemia. These instruments are not consistently reliable at low blood glucose concentrations; therefore, any value below 60 mg/dL (3.3 mmol/L) should be confirmed by a laboratory measurement of the plasma glucose concentration (294,295). In addition, a simultaneous "critical" blood sample should be obtained for the measurement of hormones, metabolic substrates, and serum chemistries (Table 10).

The first urine sample obtained after the episode of hypoglycemia should be tested for the presence of ketones (ketotic vs. nonketotic hypoglycemia), reducing sugars (suggest galactosemia or fructose intolerance), and glucose using a glucose-specific method. An aliquot should be saved and frozen for possible later analysis of amino acids, organic acids, and acylglycines after the initial laboratory investigations have been completed.

The initial laboratory evaluation should include measurement of serum insulin to determine whether the hypoglycemia is associated with a normal (suppressed) or inappropriate hyperinsulinemia and measurement of urinary ketones to determine if the hypoglycemia is associated with ketosis. Absence of urinary ketones or their presence in only trace or small amounts, i.e., nonketotic or hypoketotic hypoglycemia, is characteristic of hyperinsulinism and disorders of carnitine metabolism, disorders of FAO and ketogenesis. The serum C-peptide concentration is low or undetectable when hyperinsulinism is caused by exogenous insulin administration (e.g., Munchausen by proxy); but is increased when hyperinsulinemia is caused by malicious administration or accidental ingestion of sulfonylureas (88,90). If the serum insulin concentration is appropriately suppressed (less than 2 μU/mL with a highly sensitive insulin assay), the diagnosis is likely to be a disorder of FAO. Encephalopathy is common at the time of acute metabolic decompensation; the liver may be moderately enlarged from acute fatty infiltration (microvesicular steatosis), and liver enzymes (AST and ALT) and plasma ammonia levels are increased during acute episodes of catabolic stress (267,268). If a disorder of FAO is suspected, plasma total and esterified carnitine, plasma (or filter paper) acylcarnitines (286), and plasma FFAs should be measured, and urine analyzed for organic acids and acylglycines (285).

Ketosis with hypoglycemia is a normal physiological response to a falling blood glucose concentration. The differential diagnosis of the hypoglycemic child with an appropriately suppressed serum insulin concentration and ketosis can be further delineated depending on whether or not the liver is large (Fig. 5). Elevated levels of GH and

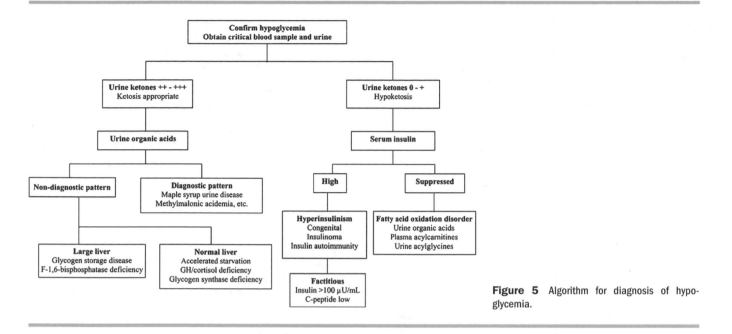

Figure 5 Algorithm for diagnosis of hypoglycemia.

cortisol exclude deficiency of these counterregulatory hormones and obviate the need for further testing. This is in contrast to random values that appear to be inappropriately low during a spontaneous episode of hypoglycemia, which do not constitute definitive evidence of deficient secretion (161,162). Specific testing must be performed.

A large liver suggests a GSD or disorder of gluconeogenesis (e.g., fructose 1,6-bisphosphatase deficiency). The liver size is normal in patients with accelerated starvation, cortisol deficiency, GH deficiency, glycogen synthase deficiency, maple syrup urine disease, and the other conditions listed in Table 3. Transient enlargement of the liver during an acute metabolic crisis can occur in organic acidemias, FAO disorders, and in disorders of carnitine metabolism, as a result of acute fat deposition in the cytosol associated with impaired mitochondrial function.

A specific diagnosis of the cause of the hypoglycemia is usually evident from the analysis of the results of the so-called critical blood sample obtained at the time of hypoglycemia (Table 10) and application of the diagnostic algorithm is shown in Figure 5. If the laboratory data required to make a diagnosis are not available, it may be necessary to perform a comprehensive evaluation of intermediary metabolism by reproducing the conditions that caused the hypoglycemia. This involves measurement of hormones and metabolic substrates that reflect carbohydrate, fat and amino acid metabolism during a monitored fast of specified duration depending on the age of the child (37,288). Fasting may be hazardous and can even be lethal in patients with a disorder of FAO. Before a child is subjected to a monitored fast, first attempt to rule out a disorder of FAO by measuring nonfasting plasma acylcarnitines (by tandem mass spectrometry) (286) and urinary acylglycines (285).

TREATMENT

Immediately after the critical blood sample has been obtained, 0.3 g/kg glucose is injected intravenously over 10 minutes to restore the plasma glucose concentration to normal. A continuous infusion of 10% dextrose solution at a rate of approximately 6 to

Table 10 Laboratory Investigation of Unexplained Hypoglycemia

Blood				
Metabolites	Insulin secretion	Counterregulation	Fatty acid oxidation	Urine
Glucose	Insulin	Cortisol	Free fatty acids	Ketones
Lactate/pyruvate	C-peptide	Growth hormone	Fatty acid profile	Reducing sugars
Amino acids (alanine)	Proinsulin	Glucagon	β-hydroxybutyrate	Organic acids
Ammonia	Insulin antibodies[a]	Epinephrine	Acetoacetate	Acylglycines
Uric acid			Total and free carnitine	
Serum electrolytes (anion gap)			Acylcarnitines	
pH, bicarbonate				
AST, ALT, CPK				

[a]Measure insulin antibodies when serum insulin concentration is markedly increased.
Abbreviations: AST, aspartate aminotransferase; ALT, alanine aminotransferase; CPK, cretine phosphokinase.

8 mg/kg/minute is given to maintain normoglycemia. This rate of glucose infusion is usually sufficient to reverse catabolism. The plasma glucose concentration is monitored, and the infusion rate is adjusted to maintain a level of approximately 80 mg/dL (4.5 mmol/L). Valuable diagnostic information can be obtained from the response to treatment. Infants and children with hyperinsulinism characteristically require considerably higher rates (14.5 ± 1.7 mg/kg/minute) of glucose infusion to prevent hypoglycemia (127,296). In disorders of FAO, administration of glucose at approximately 1.5 times basal glucose production (10 mg/kg/minute) stimulates insulin secretion, inhibits lipolysis, reverses the acute metabolic disorder, and leads to a decrease in liver size to normal over several days.

HYPOGLYCEMIA AND DIABETES MELLITUS

Hypoglycemia is the most frequent acute complication of the treatment of diabetes mellitus in children and adolescents, and is the principal factor that limits the ability to achieve normoglycemia (297–299). Recent population-based data indicate that hypoglycemia continues to be a major problem for children and adolescents with Type 1 diabetes; however, insulin pump treatment may be associated with a decreased risk of severe hypoglycemia while allowing improved metabolic control to be achieved (Vol. 1; Chaps. 6 and 7) (300).

Hypoglycemia results from the interplay of relative or absolute insulin excess and compromised physiological defenses against falling plasma glucose concentrations (299,301). Patients with Type 1 diabetes mellitus are susceptible to hypoglycemia for many reasons, including the nonphysiological nature of insulin replacement therapy, the pharmacokinetic imperfections of all insulin preparations, variability in food intake and exercise, defective counterregulatory hormone responses to hypoglycemia (301), and other reasons as shown in Table 11. Because the glucagon response to hypoglycemia is lost early in the course of the disease (302,303), patients with diabetes mellitus are dependent on sympathoadrenal responses to prevent or correct hypoglycemia (299,301). Recent mild hypoglycemia blunts the sympathoadrenal response to and symptomatic awareness of subsequent episodes of hypoglycemia (78,81,304,305) (Vol. 1; Chapters 6 and 7).

Causes of Hypoglycemia in Diabetes Mellitus

In addition to these pathophysiologic disturbances, patient errors relating to insulin dosage, decreased food intake, or unplanned exercise contribute to or account for 50% to 85% of episodes of hypoglycemia in children and adolescents (306–311). After several years of living with diabetes, some patients and/or their parents conduct their routine diabetes self-care practices without carefully considering the

Table 11   Causes of Hypoglycemia in Diabetes Mellitus

Insulin errors (inadvertent or deliberate)
   Reversal of morning and evening dose
   Reversal of short- or rapid-acting insulin and
   intermediate- or long-acting insulin
   Improper timing of insulin in relation to food
   Excessive insulin dosage
   Surreptitious insulin administration, suicide gesture or attempt
Erratic or altered absorption
   Inadvertent intramuscular injection
   More rapid absorption from exercising limbs
   Unpredictable absorption from lipohypertrophy at injection sites
   More rapid absorption after sauna, hot bath, sunbathing
Diet
   Omission or reduced size of meals or snacks
   Delayed snacks or meals
   Eating disorders
   Gastroparesis
   Malabsorption (e.g., gluten enteropathy)
Exercise
   Unplanned moderate or intensive physical activity
   Prolonged duration and/or increased intensity of physical activity
   Failure to reduce the dose of basal insulin to
   combat the lag effect of exercise
Alcohol and/or drugs
   Impaired gluconeogenesis from excessive consumption of ethanol
   Impaired cognition from use of ethanol, marijuana,
   cocaine, other recreational drugs
Hypoglycemia-associated autonomic failure
   Defective glucose counterregulation
   Hypoglycemia unawareness
Miscellaneous uncommon causes of hypoglycemia
   Adrenocortical insufficiency
   Hypothyroidism
   Growth hormone deficiency
   Renal failure
   Decreased insulin requirement in first trimester of pregnancy
Insulin antibodies

intricate interplay among insulin, food, and exercise (312) (Table 11).

Symptoms and Signs

Symptoms of hypoglycemia are caused by neuronal deprivation of glucose and are autonomic (sweating, palpitations, tremor, and hunger) or neuroglycopenic (difficulty thinking, confusion, drowsiness, behavioral changes, speech difficulty, incoordination, seizures, and coma) (313). Common signs and symptoms of hypoglycemia in diabetic children are pallor, weakness, tremor, hunger, fatigue, drowsiness, sweating, and headache (306,314). In contrast to adolescents and insulin-treated adults, autonomic symptoms are less common in children less than six years old (314). Autonomic and neuroglycopenic symptoms reported by children and their parents tend to cluster, which contrasts with adult patients, who are usually able to distinguish between these two types of symptoms. The coalescence of autonomic and neuroglycopenic symptoms in children may indicate that both types of symptoms are generated at similar glycemic thresholds. Because behavioral changes are a primary feature of hypoglycemia in children, this difference from adults has important implications for educating parents about the recognition of hypoglycemia (315).

Hypoglycemia in diabetes is classified in terms of its severity as either symptomatic or asymptomatic (also referred to as biochemical hypoglycemia), defined as plasma glucose less than or equal to 70 mg/dL, which is common. Symptomatic hypoglycemia is further classified as mild, moderate, or severe (defined as requiring the assistance of another person to administer carbohydrate or glucagon, seizure or coma) (316). Most symptomatic episodes in children and adolescents are mild (314). Parents are usually alerted to the presence of hypoglycemia in a young child by noting pallor, drowsiness, or unexplained irritability. By definition, cognitive deficits do not accompany mild reactions, and older children with mild hypoglycemia are able to treat themselves. Mild symptoms abate within 10 to 15 minutes after consuming an appropriate amount of rapidly absorbed carbohydrate. Moderate hypoglycemia has neuroglycopenic (e.g., headache, mood changes, irritability, decreased attentiveness, and drowsiness) as well as autonomic symptoms. Young children require assistance with treatment because they are often confused; weakness and poor coordination makes self-treatment difficult. Moderate hypoglycemia produces longer-lasting symptoms and may require a second dose of rapidly absorbed carbohydrate. Severe hypoglycemia is characterized by unresponsiveness, unconsciousness, or convulsions and requires emergency treatment with glucagon or IV glucose given by an emergency medical technician in the field or in a hospital emergency department.

Patients with longer duration of diabetes describe a change in their symptoms over time, characterized by reduced occurrence of autonomic symptoms and increased frequency of neuroglycopenic symptoms (drowsiness, difficulty concentrating, and lack of coordination). Patients must learn to recognize the change in symptoms to prevent severe episodes (317). The blood glucose concentration at which symptoms occur varies among patients. This threshold may also vary in the same individual as a consequence of antecedent glycemic control. As plasma glucose concentrations decrease toward normal, children and adults with chronically poor glycemic control may experience symptoms of hypoglycemia at plasma glucose concentrations well above 70 mg/dL (318,319).

Impact of Hypoglycemia

Occasional, mild symptomatic hypoglycemia may be the price one has to pay for near-normal glycemic control (320–324); however, it must be recognized that cognitive function deteriorates and motor processing speed slows at low blood glucose levels even in the absence of typical symptoms (325,326). The psychological reaction to hypoglycemia can be frightening and extend beyond the patient to include family, friends, teachers, and coaches (327). Moderate and severe hypoglycemia is disabling, affects school performance, and makes driving a car or operating dangerous machinery hazardous (325,328–330). Repeated or prolonged severe hyperinsulinemic hypoglycemia can cause permanent central nervous system damage (331), especially in very young children (2,332). Fortunately, hypoglycemia is an unusual cause of death in children with Type 1 diabetes (333). Although diabetes is not typically associated with reduced intelligence in children, subtle neurocognitive impairments may develop if onset occurs before five years (334), or the child has seizures from hypoglycemia (335,336). The hippocampus is particularly vulnerable to prolonged severe hypoglycemia (337–340). Repeated severe hypoglycemia (more than three episodes and particularly when this begins before the age of five years) negatively affects spatial long-term memory performance (341). The neurocognitive sequelae of intensive diabetes management in children whose brains are still developing are still largely unknown. Preliminary findings suggest poorer memory skills, presumably the consequence of recurrent and severe hypoglycemia (342). A recent study of children with onset of Type 1 diabetes before six years with a prospectively documented history of seizure or coma were compared with their peers with no history of severe hypoglycemia. There was no clear evidence that episodes of seizures or coma in early childhood resulted in cognitive dysfunction or memory difficulties at the time of testing (343).

The confidence of the patient and members of the patient's family is often shaken after an episode of severe hypoglycemia. The rational fear of hypoglycemia may cause the patient or physician to change the diabetes management strategy to avoid subsequent episodes of hypoglycemia (344). Fear of hypoglycemia, therefore, can become a barrier to attaining and maintaining optimal glycemic control. Examples of altered patient/family or physician behaviors that result in worsening metabolic control include chronic overeating or selection of inadequate doses of insulin to maintain higher blood glucose levels that are perceived as being safe (327,344–346). Concern about nocturnal hypoglycemia causes more anxiety for some parents than any other aspect of diabetes, including the fear of long-term complications. Parents may fear that an episode of severe hypoglycemia during the nighttime may not be treated in a timely fashion or that an episode could go entirely undetected and lead to permanent brain damage or death (347).

Frequency of Hypoglycemia

The true frequency of mild (self-treated) symptomatic hypoglycemia is almost impossible to ascertain because mild episodes are quickly forgotten or are not recorded. In a random sample of 47 children attending a diabetes clinic, the average incidence of symptomatic hypoglycemia was once every 33 days (range 0–5.2 times per month), and occurred more frequently in children with the lowest glycated hemoglobin levels (321). In a 12-month population-based study, Aman et al. found that mild episodes (managed by the child without assistance) occurred in 97% of children and occurred at least once a week in 53% (306). More recently, Tupola et al. prospectively examined the frequency of hypoglycemia [blood glucose less than 3 mmol/L (54 mg/dL)] in 161 children and adolescents predominantly treated with multiple doses of insulin, who were asked to document hypoglycemia episodes in a three-month diary (314). Fifty-two percent of the clinic population experienced episodes of hypoglycemia (0.6 hypoglycemia events per patient per month), of which 77% were mild.

The literature is replete with reports of the frequency of severe hypoglycemia in children and adolescents with diabetes (300,307–311,320,322,323, 348–358). Various methods of collecting data and different definitions of hypoglycemia and methods of insulin replacement make comparisons among the reports difficult (359). For example, in some studies, severe hypoglycemia is defined as loss of consciousness, whereas others include children who required assistance with treatment. In young children, all episodes of hypoglycemia require the assistance of a third party for treatment regardless of the severity of the symptoms. It is not surprising, therefore, that the reported incidence of moderate or severe hypoglycemia in the pediatric diabetes population varies widely. The incidence of severe hypoglycemia varies from 3.1 (356) to 134 per 100 patient-years (324); most studies document a range of 10 to 40 episodes per 100 patient-years (358–360). The adolescent cohort of the diabetes control and complications trial (DCCT) had a frequency of severe hypoglycemia of 27.8 and 85.7 episodes per 100 patient-years for the conventional and intensive treatment groups, respectively (323). It is also likely that severe hypoglycemia in pediatric studies has been underreported. This is suggested by the fact that the rate of severe hypoglycemia in conventionally treated adolescents in the year before the DCCT started was 15.7 per 100 patients, but increased to 27.8 per 100 patients during the course of the study, whereas hemoglobin A1c did not decrease (9.20% ± 1.8% before and 9.76% ± 0.12% during the study) (298,323).

Many, but not all, studies have found an increased frequency of severe hypoglycemia in younger children (311,322,351,352,354,357,358) and in association with lower hemoglobin A1c concentrations (308,309,320,322,323,351,352,354,356). Other factors associated with a higher risk of moderate and severe hypoglycemia are a prior history of severe hypoglycemia (298,309,350,354), relatively higher doses of insulin and low C-peptide secretion (298,350,354,356), longer duration of diabetes (310,352,355,358), and male gender (298,349,358).

Nocturnal Hypoglycemia

Hypoglycemia, often asymptomatic, frequently occurs during sleep. Moderate and severe (with coma and seizures) hypoglycemia is more common during the night and early morning (before breakfast) than during the daytime (352,361). In the DCCT, 55% of severe hypoglycemia events occurred during sleep and 43% occurred between midnight and 8 a.m.(298,361).

Studies of diabetic children and adolescents, in the hospital or at home, in which blood glucose concentrations were measured frequently during the night, show a high incidence (14–47%) of asymptomatic hypoglycemia. Such episodes during sleep often exceed four hours in duration (362–368). Up to half of these episodes may be undetected because the subject does not wake from sleep. The incidence of hypoglycemia on any given night may be affected by numerous factors, including the insulin regimen, the timing and content of meals and snacks, and antecedent physical activity (369). The highest frequency of asymptomatic nocturnal hypoglycemia occurs in children less than 10 years old (364,366–368). Low blood glucose concentrations in the early morning (before breakfast) are associated with a higher frequency of preceding nocturnal hypoglycemia. This knowledge is useful in counseling patients to modify the evening insulin regimen and bedtime snack to prevent more severe nocturnal hypoglycemia.

Sleep impairs counterregulatory hormone responses to hypoglycemia in normal subjects and in patients with diabetes mellitus (370,371). Because a rise in plasma epinephrine concentration is normally the main hormonal defense against hypoglycemia, impaired counterregulatory hormone responses to hypoglycemia explains the increased susceptibility to hypoglycemia during sleep and high frequency of nocturnal hypoglycemia in Type 1 diabetes. Asymptomatic nocturnal hypoglycemia may itself result in further deficits in counterregulatory hormone responses (372). Thus, impaired defenses against hypoglycemia during sleep may contribute to the cycle of hypoglycemia, impaired counterregulatory responses, and unawareness of hypoglycemia either awake or asleep. Recurrent asymptomatic nocturnal hypoglycemia is an important cause of hypoglycemia unawareness, which, in turn, leads to more frequent and severe hypoglycemia because of failure to experience autonomic warning symptoms before the onset of neuroglycopenia (297,301).

Treatment

Most episodes of symptomatic hypoglycemia are self-treated (except in preschool age children) with rapidly absorbed carbohydrate such as glucose tablets, fruit juices, soft drinks, candy, crackers, and milk. Glucose tablets raise blood glucose levels more rapidly than does orange juice or milk, and the dosage is easily calibrated (373). Glucose tablets are the treatment of choice for children old enough to safely chew and swallow large tablets. The recommended dose is 0.3 g glucose per kg body weight. The glycemic response to oral glucose usually lasts less than two hours (374). Therefore, unless a scheduled meal or snack is due within an hour of the episode of hypoglycemia, immediately after treatment with oral glucose the patient should be given either a snack containing both carbohydrate and protein or a meal.

Severe reactions (unresponsiveness, unconsciousness, or convulsions) require emergency treatment with parenteral (IM or SC) glucagon. Buccal and rectal administration of glucose is ineffective (375). Parenteral glucagon is as effective in treating severe hypoglycemia in children (376) as it is in adults (374,377). Glucagon raises blood glucose levels within 5 to 15 minutes and usually relieves the symptoms of hypoglycemia (374,377). In healthy adults (377) there appears to be no important difference between the effects of glucagon injected either SC or IM. Likewise, symptoms of experimentally induced hypoglycemia in diabetic children are relieved within 10 minutes of giving glucagon either by SC or IM injection; and mean blood glucose and plasma glucagon levels are slightly but not significantly higher after IM than SC injection (376). In diabetic children, both 10 and 20 $\mu g/kg$ of glucagon relieve clinical signs and symptoms caused by insulin-induced hypoglycemia, but the increment in blood glucose concentration after 10 minutes is less after the 10 $\mu g/kg$ dose (1.1 ± 0.3 vs. 1.7 ± 0.7 mmol/L). However, after 20 and 30 minutes, the differences in blood glucose concentrations are not significant. Nausea and/or vomiting can be expected to occur after the injection in a minority of children who receive a dose of 20 $\mu g/kg$, but usually do not occur after 10 $\mu g/kg$. Excessively high plasma glucagon levels are more likely to cause nausea and/or vomiting (376). The recommended dose, therefore, is 15 $\mu g/kg$ to a maximum of 1.0 mg.

The increase in blood glucose concentration after glucagon administration is sustained for at least 30 minutes; therefore, it is unnecessary to repeat the dose or force the child to eat or drink for at least 30 minutes. Intranasal glucagon has a similar effect, but is not available in the United States (378). In an emergency department or hospital, the preferred treatment is IV glucose (0.3 g/kg). Because the glycemic response is transient after bolus administration of glucose, the patient should continue to receive IV glucose infusion until the patient is able to swallow safely.

If severe hypoglycemia was prolonged, and the patient had a seizure, complete recovery of normal mental and neurologic function may take many hours despite restoration of a normal blood glucose level (379). Permanent hemiparesis, or other neurologic sequelae, is rare (380,381). The post-ictal period may be complicated by headache, lethargy, nausea, vomiting, and aching muscles.

REFERENCES

1. Sokoloff L. Circulation and energy metabolism of the brain. In: Siegel G, Agranoff B, Albers R, Molinoff P, eds. Basic Neurochemistry. New York: Raven Press, 1989:565–590.
2. Menni F, de Lonlay P, Sevin C, et al. Neurologic outcomes of 90 neonates and infants with persistent hyperinsulinemic hypoglycemia. Pediatrics 2001; 107:476–479.
3. Hume R, Burchell A, Williams FL, Koh DK. Glucose homeostasis in the newborn. Early Hum Dev 2005; 81(1):95–101.
4. Bier DM, Leake RD, Haymond MW, et al. Measurement of "true" glucose production rates in infancy and childhood with 6,6-dideuteroglucose. Diabetes 1977; 26:1016–1023.
5. Hume R, Burchell A. Abnormal expression of glucose-6-phosphatase in preterm infants. Arch Dis Child 1993; 68(2):202–204.
6. Jackson L, Burchell A, McGeechan A, Hume R. An inadequate glycemic response to glucagon is linked to insulin resistance in preterm infants? Arch Dis Child Fetal Neonatal Ed 2003; 88(1):F62–F66.
7. Hume R, McGeechan A, Burchell A. Failure to detect preterm infants at risk of hypoglycemia before discharge. J Pediatr 1999; 134(4):499–502.
8. Chaussain J. Glycemic response to 24 hour fast in normal children and children with ketotic hypoglycemia. J Pediatr 1973; 82:438–443.
9. Schwartz NS, Clutter WE, Shah SD, Cryer PE. Glycemic thresholds for activation of glucose counterregulatory systems are higher than the threshold for symptoms. J Clin Invest 1987; 79(3):777–781.
10. Mitrakou A, Ryan C, Veneman T, et al. Hierarchy of glycemic thresholds for counterregulatory hormone secretion, symptoms, and cerebral dysfunction. Am J Physiol 1991; 260(1 Pt 1):E67–E74.
11. Liu D, Moberg E, Kollind M, Lins PE, Adamson U, Macdonald IA. Arterial, arterialized venous, venous and capillary blood glucose measurements in normal man during hyperinsulinaemic euglycemia and hypoglycaemia. Diabetologia 1992; 35(3):287–290.
12. Koh T, Aynsley-Green A, Tarbit M, Eyre J. Neural dysfunction during hypoglycaemia. Arch Dis Child 1988; 63:1353–1358.
13. Cryer PE. Hypoglycemia: pathophysiology, diagnosis, and treatment. New York: Oxford University Press, 1997.
14. Shepherd PR, Kahn BB. Glucose transporters and insulin action–implications for insulin resistance and diabetes mellitus. N Engl J Med 1999; 341(4):248–257.
15. Brown GK. Glucose transporters: structure, function and consequences of deficiency. J Inherit Metab Dis 2000; 23(3):237–246.
16. Vannucci SJ, Maher F, Simpson IA. Glucose transporter proteins in brain: delivery of glucose to neurons and glia. Glia 1997; 21(1):2–21.
17. Simpson IA, Appel NM, Hokari M, et al. Blood–brain barrier glucose transporter: effects of hypo- and hyperglycemia revisited. J Neurochem 1999; 72(1):238–247.
18. Kumagai AK, Kang YS, Boado RJ, Pardridge WM. Upregulation of blood–brain barrier GLUT1 glucose transporter protein and mRNA in experimental chronic hypoglycemia. Diabetes 1995; 44(12):1399–1404.
19. Uehara Y, Nipper V, McCall AL. Chronic insulin hypoglycemia induces GLUT-3 protein in rat brain neurons. Am J Physiol 1997; 272(4 Pt 1):E716–E719.
20. Randle PJ. Regulatory interactions between lipids and carbohydrates: the glucose fatty acid cycle after 35 years. Diabetes Metab Rev 1998; 14(4):263–283.

21. Settergren G, Lindblad B, Persson B. Cerebral blood flow and exchange of oxygen, glucose, ketone bodies, lactate, pyruvate, and amino acids in infants. Acta Paediatr Scand 1976; 65:343–353.

22. Hasselbalch SG, Knudsen GM, Jakobsen J, Hageman LP, Holm S, Paulson OB. Blood–brain barrier permeability of glucose and ketone bodies during short-term starvation in humans. Am J Physiol 1995; 268(6 Pt 1):E1161–E1166.

23. VanItallie TB, Nufert TH. Ketones: metabolism's ugly duckling. Nutr Rev 2003; 61(10):327–341.

24. Haymond MW, Sunehag A. Controlling the sugar bowl: regulation of glucose homeostasis in children. Endocrinol Metab Clin North Am 1999; 28(4):663–694.

25. McGarry JD, Leatherman GF, Foster DW. Carnitine palmitoyltransferase I The site of inhibition of hepatic fatty acid oxidation by malonyl-CoA. J Biol Chem 1978; 253(12):4128–4136.

26. McGarry JD, Foster DW. Regulation of hepatic fatty acid oxidation and ketone body production. Annu Rev Biochem 1980; 49:395–420.

27. Ruderman NB, Saha AK, Kraegen EW. Minireview: malonyl CoA, AMP-activated protein kinase, and adiposity. Endocrinology 2003; 144(12):5166–5171.

28. Mauras N, Beck RW, Ruedy KJ, et al. Lack of accuracy of continuous glucose sensors in healthy, nondiabetic children: results of the Diabetes Research in Children Network (DirecNet) accuracy study. J Pediatr 2004; 144(6):770–775.

29. Tse TF, Clutter WE, Shah SD, Cryer PE. Mechanisms of postprandial glucose counter regulation in man. Physiologic roles of glucagon and epinephrine vis-a-vis insulin in the prevention of hypoglycemia late after glucose ingestion. J Clin Invest 1983; 72(1):278–286.

30. Tse TF, Clutter WE, Shah SD, Miller JP, Cryer PE. Neuroendocrine responses to glucose ingestion in man. Specificity, temporal relationships, and quantitative aspects. J Clin Invest 1983; 72(1):270–277.

31. Landau BR, Wahren J, Chandramouli V, Schumann WC, Ekberg K, Kalhan SC. Contributions of gluconeogenesis to glucose production in the fasted state. J Clin Invest 1996; 98(2):378–385.

32. Hellerstein MK, Neese RA, Linfoot P, Christiansen M, Turner S, Letscher A. Hepatic gluconeogenic fluxes and glycogen turnover during fasting in humans. A stable isotope study. J Clin Invest 1997; 100(5):1305–1319.

33. Katz J, Tayek JA. Gluconeogenesis and the Cori cycle in 12-, 20-, and 40-h-fasted humans. Am J Physiol 1998; 275(3 Pt 1):E537–E542.

34. Sunehag AL, Treuth MS, Toffolo G, et al. Glucose production, gluconeogenesis, and insulin sensitivity in children and adolescents: an evaluation of their reproducibility. Pediatr Res 2001; 50(1):115–123.

35. Felig P, Pozefsky T, Marliss E, Cahill GF Jr. Alanine: key role in gluconeogenesis. Science 1970; 167(920):1003–1004.

36. Wolfsdorf J, Sadeghi-Nejad A, Senior B. Fat derived fuels during a 24 hour fast in children. Eur J Pediatr 1982; 138:141–144.

37. Bonnefont J, Specola N, Vassault A, et al. The fasting test in paediatrics: application to the diagnosis of pathological hypo- and hyperketotic states. Eur J Paediatr 1990; 150:80–85.

38. Bougneres PF, Ferre P. Study of ketone body kinetics in children by a combined perfusion of 13C and 2H3 tracers. Am J Physiol 1987; 253(5 Pt 1):E496–E502.

39. Haymond M, Karl I, Clarke W, Pagliara A, Santiago J. Differences in circulating gluconeogenic substrates during short-term fasting in men, women, and children. Metabolism 1982; 31:33–41.

40. Persson B, Settergren G, Dahlquist G. Cerebral arteriovenous difference of acetoacetate and d-hydroxybutyrate in children. Acta Paediatr Scand 1972; 61(3):273–278.

41. Owen O, Morgan A, Kemp H, Sullivan J, Herrera M, Cahill G Jr. Brain metabolism during fasting. J Clin Invest 1967; 46:1589–1595.

42. Amiel S, Archibald H, Chusney G, Williams A, Gale E. Ketone infusion lowers hormonal responses to hypoglycaemia: evidence for acute cerebral utilisation of a non-glucose fuel. Clin Sci 1991; 81:189–194.

43. Haymond M, Howard C, Ben-Galim E, DeVivo D. Effects of ketosis on glucose flux in children and adults. Am J Physiol 1983; 245:E373–E378.

44. Matschinksy F. Banting lecture 1995 A lesson in metabolic regulation inspired by the glucokinase glucose sensor paradigm. Diabetes 1996; 45:223–241.

45. Aguilar-Bryan L, Bryan J. Molecular biology of adenosine triphosphate-sensitive potassium channels. Endocr Rev 1999; 20(2):101–135.

46. Dunne MJ, Cosgrove KE, Shepherd RM, Ammala C. Potassium channels, sulphonylurea receptors and control of insulin release. Trends Endocrinol Metab 1999; 10(4):146–152.

47. Ashcroft FM. ATP-sensitive potassium channelopathies: focus on insulin secretion. J Clin Invest 2005; 115(8):2047–2058.

48. Matschinsky FM, Glaser B, Magnuson MA. Pancreatic beta-cell glucokinase: closing the gap between theoretical concepts and experimental realities. Diabetes 1998; 47(3):307–315.

49. Shepherd RM, Cosgrove KE, O'Brien RE, Barnes PD, Ammala C, Dunne MJ. Hyperinsulinism of infancy: towards an understanding of unregulated insulin release. European Network for Research into Hyperinsulinism in Infancy. Arch Dis Child Fetal Neonatal Ed 2000; 82(2):F87–F97.

50. Dunne MJ, Cosgrove KE, Shepherd RM, Aynsley-Green A, Lindley KJ. Hyperinsulinism in infancy: from basic science to clinical disease. Physiol Rev 2004; 84(1):239–275.

51. Glaser B, Kesavan P, Heyman M, Davis E, Cuesta A, Buchs A, et al. Familial hyperinsulinism caused by an activating glucokinase mutation. N Engl J Med 1998; 338:226–230.

52. Christesen HB, Jacobsen BB, Odili S, et al. The second activating glucokinase mutation (A456V): implications for glucose homeostasis and diabetes therapy. Diabetes 2002; 51(4):1240–1246.

53. Gloyn AL, Noordam K, Willemsen MA, et al. Insights into the biochemical and genetic basis of glucokinase activation from naturally occurring hypoglycemia mutations. Diabetes 2003; 52(9):2433–2440.

54. Cuesta-Munoz AL, Huopio H, Otonkoski T, et al. Severe persistent hyperinsulinemic hypoglycemia due to a de novo glucokinase mutation. Diabetes 2004; 53(8):2164–2168.

55. Froguel P, Zouali H, Vionnet N, et al. Familial hyperglycemia due to mutations in glucokinase. Definition of a subtype of diabetes mellitus. N Engl J Med 1993; 328(10):697–702.

56. McCall AL. Effects of glucose deprivation on glucose metabolism in the central nervous system. In: Frier BM, Fisher BM, eds. Hypoglycaemia and Diabetes: Clinical and Physiological Aspects. London: Edward Arnold, 1993:56–71.

57. Boyle PJ, Kempers SF, O'Connor AM, Nagy RJ. Brain glucose uptake and unawareness of hypoglycemia in patients with insulin-dependent diabetes mellitus (see comments). N Engl J Med 1995; 333(26):1726–1731.

58. Boyle PJ, Nagy RJ, O'Connor AM, Kempers SF, Yeo RA, Qualls C. Adaptation in brain glucose uptake following

recurrent hypoglycemia. Proc Natl Acad Sci USA 1994; 91(20):9352–9356.

59. DeBaun MR, King AA, White N. Hypoglycemia in Beckwith-Wiedemann syndrome. Semin Perinatol 2000; 24(2):164–171.

60. Munns CF, Batch JA. Hyperinsulinism and Beckwith-Wiedemann syndrome. Arch Dis Child Fetal Neonatal Ed 2001; 84(1):F67–F69.

61. Hussain K, Cosgrove KE, Shepherd RM, et al. Hyperinsulinemic hypoglycemia in Beckwith-Wiedemann syndrome due to defects in the function of pancreatic beta-cell adenosine triphosphate-sensitive potassium channels. J Clin Endocrinol Metab 2005; 90(7):4376–4382.

62. Agus MS, Katz LE, Satin-Smith M, Meadows AT, Hintz RL, Cohen P. Non-islet-cell tumor associated with hypoglycemia in a child: successful long-term therapy with growth hormone. J Pediatr 1995; 127(3):403–407.

63. Teale JD. Non-islet cell tumour hypoglycaemia. Clin Endocrinol (Oxf) 1999; 51(2):147.

64. Gitzelmann R, Hirsig J. Infant dumping syndrome: reversal of symptoms by feeding uncooked cornstarch. Eur J Pediatr 1986; 145:504–506.

65. Rivkees SA, Crawford JD. Hypoglycemia pathogenesis in children with dumping syndrome. Pediatrics 1987; 80(6):937–942.

66. Ng DD, Ferry RJ Jr., Kelly A, Weinzimer SA, Stanley CA, Katz LE. Acarbose treatment of postprandial hypoglycemia in children after Nissen fundoplication. J Pediatr 2001; 139(6):877–879.

67. Colle E, Ulstrom R. Ketotic hypoglycemia. J Pediatr 1964; 64:632–651.

68. Senior B. Ketotic hypoglycemia. J Pediatr 1973; 82:555–556.

69. Grunt JA, Howard RO. Findings in children with ketotic hypoglycemia. Can J Ophthalmol 1972; 7(2):151–156.

70. Daly LP, Osterhoudt KC, Weinzimer SA. Presenting features of idiopathic ketotic hypoglycemia. J Emerg Med 2003; 25(1):39–43.

71. Haymond M, Karl I, Pagliara A. Ketotic hypoglycemia: an amino acid substrate limited disorder. J Clin Endocrinol Metab 1974; 38:521–530.

72. Senior B, Loridan L. Gluconeogenesis and insulin in the ketotic variety of childhood hypoglycemia and in control children. J Pediatr 1969; 74:529–539.

73. Pagliara AS, Karl IE, De Vivo DC, Feigin RD, Kipnis DM. Hypoalaninemia: a concomitant of ketotic hypoglycemia. J Clin Invest 1972; 51(6):1440–1449.

74. Wolfsdorf J, Sadeghi-Nejad A, Senior B. Hypoalaninemia and ketotic hypoglycemia: Cause or consequence? Eur J Paediatr 1982; 138:28–31.

75. Sherwin RS, Hendler RG, Felig P. Effect of ketone infusions on amino acid and nitrogen metabolism in man. J Clin Invest 1975; 55(6):1382–1390.

76. Fery F, Balasse EO. Ketone body turnover during and after exercise in overnight-fasted and starved humans. Am J Physiol 1983; 245(4):E318–E325.

77. Hansen I, Levy M, Kerr D. Differential diagnosis of hypoglycemia in children by responses to fasting and 2-deoxyglucose. Metabolism 1983; 32:960–970.

78. Heller SR, Cryer PE. Reduced neuroendocrine and symptomatic responses to subsequent hypoglycemia after 1 episode of hypoglycemia in nondiabetic humans. Diabetes 1991; 40(2):223–226.

79. Widom B, Simonson DC. Intermittent hypoglycemia impairs glucose counter regulation. Diabetes 1992; 41(12):1597–1602.

80. Davis MR, Shamoon H. Counterregulatory adaptation to recurrent hypoglycemia in normal humans. J Clin Endocrinol Metab 1991; 73(5):995–1001.

81. Davis SN, Shavers C, Mosqueda-Garcia R, Costa F. Effects of differing antecedent hypoglycemia on subsequent counter regulation in normal humans. Diabetes 1997; 46(8):1328 1335.

82. Chaussain J, Georges P, Olive G, Job J. Glycemic response to a 24-hour fast in normal children and children with ketotic hypoglycemia II. Hormonal and metabolic changes. J Pediatr 1974; 85:776–781.

83. Dahlquist G, Gentz J, Hagenfeldt L, et al. Ketotic hypoglycemia of childhood–a clinical trial of several unifying etiological hypotheses. Acta Paediatr Scand 1979; 68(5):649–656.

84. Leonard J, Middleton B, et al. Acetoacetyl CoA thiolase deficiency presenting as ketotic hypoglycemia. Pediatr Res 1987; 21:211.

85. Berry GT, Fukao T, Mitchell GA, et al. Neonatal hypoglycaemia in severe succinyl-CoA: 3-oxoacid CoA-transferase deficiency. J Inherit Metab Dis 2001; 24(5): 587–595.

86. Weinstein DA, Correia CE, Saunders AC, Wolfsdorf JI. Hepatic glycogen synthase deficiency: an infrequently recognized cause of ketotic hypoglycemia. Molecular Genetics Metabolism 2006; 87(4): 284–288.

87. Byrne H, Tieszen K, Hollis S, Dornan T, New J. Evaluation of an electrochemical sensor for measuring blood ketones. Diabetes Care 2000; 23:500–503.

88. Marks V, Teale JD. Hypoglycemia: factitious and felonious. Endocrinol Metab Clin North Am 1999; 28(3):579–601.

89. Dershewitz R, Vestal B, Maclaren NK, Cornblath M. Transient hepatomegaly and hypoglycemia. A consequence of malicious insulin administration. Am J Dis Child 1976; 130(9):998–999.

90. Hussain K, Mundy H, Aynsley-Green A, Champion M. A child presenting with disordered consciousness, hallucinations, screaming episodes and abdominal pain. Eur J Pediatr 2002; 161(2):127–129.

91. Giurgea I, Ulinski T, Touati G, et al. Factitious hyperinsulinism leading to pancreatectomy: severe forms of Munchausen syndrome by proxy. Pediatrics 2005; 116(1):e145–e148.

92. Stanley CA. Hyperinsulinism in infants and children. Pediatr Clin North Am 1997; 44(2):363–374.

93. de Lonlay P, Fournet JC, Touati G, et al. Heterogeneity of persistent hyperinsulinaemic hypoglycaemia. A series of 175 cases. Eur J Pediatr 2002; 161(1):37–48.

94. Meissner T, Mayatepek E. Clinical and genetic heterogeneity in congenital hyperinsulinism. Eur J Pediatr 2002; 161(1):6–20.

95. Thomas PM. Genetic mutations as a cause of hyperinsulinemic hypoglycemia in children. Endocrinol Metab Clin North Am 1999; 28(3):647–656.

96. Glaser B, Thornton P, Otonkoski T, Junien C. Genetics of neonatal hyperinsulinism. Arch Dis Child Fetal Neonatal Ed 2000; 82(2):F79–F86.

97. Fournet JC, Junien C. The genetics of neonatal hyperinsulinism. Horm Res 2003; 59(suppl 1):30–34.

98. Thomas P, Cote G, Wohlik N, et al. Mutations in the sulfonylurea receptor gene in familial persistent hyperinsulinemic hypoglycemia of infancy. Science 1995; 268:426–429.

99. Dunne M, Kane C, Shepherd R, et al. Familial persistent hyperinsulinemic hypoglycemia of infancy and mutations in the sulfonylurea receptor. N Engl J Med 1997; 336:703–706.

100. Thomas P, Ye Y, Lightner E. Mutations of the pancreatic islet inward rectifier Kir6.2 also leads to familial persistent hyperinsulinemic hypoglycemia of infancy. Hum Mol Genet 1996; 5:1809–1812.

101. Nestorowicz A, Inagaki N, Gonoi T, et al. A nonsense mutation in the inward rectifier potassium channel gene, Kir6.2, is associated with familial hyperinsulinism. Diabetes 1997; 46(11):1743–1748.

102. Finegold D, Stanley C, Baker L. Glycemic response to glucagon during fasting hypoglycemia: an aid in the diagnosis of hyperinsulinism. J Pediatr 1980; 96:257–259.

103. Levitt Katz L, Satin-Smith M, Collett-Solberg P, et al. Insulin-like growth factor binding protein-1 levels in the diagnosis of hypoglycemia due to hyperinsulinism. J Pediatr 1997; 131:193–199.

104. de Lonlay-Debeney P, Poggi-Travert F, Fournet JC, et al. Clinical features of 52 neonates with hyperinsulinism. N Engl J Med 1999; 340(15):1169–1175.

105. Stanley CA. Advances in diagnosis and treatment of hyperinsulinism in infants and children. J Clin Endocrinol Metab 2002; 87(11):4857–4859.

106. Stanley CA, Thornton PS, Ganguly A, et al. Preoperative evaluation of infants with focal or diffuse congenital hyperinsulinism by intravenous acute insulin response tests and selective pancreatic arterial calcium stimulation. J Clin Endocrinol Metab 2004; 89(1):288–296.

107. de Lonlay P, Fournet JC, Rahier J, et al. Somatic deletion of the imprinted 11p15 region in sporadic persistent hyperinsulinemic hypoglycemia of infancy is specific of focal adenomatous hyperplasia and endorses partial pancreatectomy. J Clin Invest 1997; 100(4):802–807.

108. Verkarre V, Fournet JC, de Lonlay P, et al. Paternal mutation of the sulfonylurea receptor (SUR1) gene and maternal loss of 11p15 imprinted genes lead to persistent hyperinsulinism in focal adenomatous hyperplasia. J Clin Invest 1998; 102(7):1286–1291.

109. Ryan F, Devaney D, Joyce C, et al. Hyperinsulinism: molecular aetiology of focal disease. Arch Dis Child 1998; 79(5):445–447.

110. Glaser B, Ryan F, Donath M, et al. Hyperinsulinism caused by paternal-specific inheritance of a recessive mutation in the sulfonylurea-receptor gene. Diabetes 1999; 48(8):1652–1657.

111. Fournet JC, Mayaud C, de Lonlay P, et al. Unbalanced expression of 11p15 imprinted genes in focal forms of congenital hyperinsulinism: association with a reduction to homozygosity of a mutation in ABCC8 or KCNJ11. Am J Pathol 2001; 158(6):2177–2184.

112. Rahier J, Guiot Y, Sempoux C. Persistent hyperinsulinaemic hypoglycaemia of infancy: a heterogeneous syndrome unrelated to nesidioblastosis. Arch Dis Child Fetal Neonatal Ed 2000; 82(2):F108–F112.

113. Thornton PS, Satin-Smith MS, Herold K, et al. Familial hyperinsulinism with apparent autosomal dominant inheritance: clinical and genetic differences from the autosomal recessive variant. J Pediatr 1998; 132(1):9–14.

114. Hufnagel M, Eichmann D, Stieh J, Santer R. Further evidence for a dominant form of familial persistent hyperinsulinemic hypoglycemia of infancy: a family with documented hyperinsulinemia in two generations (letter). J Clin Endocrinol Metab 1998; 83:2215–2216.

115. Stanley CA, Lieu YK, Hsu BY, et al. Hyperinsulinism and hyperammonemia in infants with regulatory mutations of the glutamate dehydrogenase gene. N Engl J Med 1998; 338(19):1352–1357.

116. Zammarchi E, Filippi L, Novembre E, Donati M. Biochemical evaluation of a patient with a familial form of leucine-sensitive hypoglycemia and concomitant hyperammonemia. Metabolism 1996; 45:957–960.

117. Weinzimer S, Stanley C, Berry G, Yudkoff M, Tuchman M, Thornton P. A syndrome of congenital hyperinsulinism and hyperammonemia. J Pediatr 1997; 130:661–664.

118. Kitaura J, Miki Y, Kato H, Sakakihara Y, Yanagisawa M. Hyperinsulinaemic hypoglycaemia associated with persistent hyperammonaemia. Eur J Pediatr 1999; 158(5):410–413.

119. Miki Y, Taki T, Ohura T, Kato H, Yanagisawa M, Hayashi Y. Novel missense mutations in the glutamate dehydrogenase gene in the congenital hyperinsulinism-hyperammonemia syndrome. J Pediatr 2000; 136(1):69–72.

120. Stanley CA. Hyperinsulinism/hyperammonemia syndrome: insights into the regulatory role of glutamate dehydrogenase in ammonia metabolism. Mol Genet Metab 2004; 81(suppl 1):S45–S51.

121. Clayton PT, Eaton S, Aynsley-Green A, et al. Hyper insulinism in short-chain L-3-hydroxyacyl-CoA dehydrogenase deficiency reveals the importance of beta-oxidation in insulin secretion. J Clin Invest 2001; 108(3):457–465.

122. Eaton S, Chatziandreou I, Krywawych S, Pen S, Clayton PT, Hussain K. Short-chain 3-hydroxyacyl-CoA dehydrogenase deficiency associated with hyperinsulinism: a novel glucose-fatty acid cycle? Biochem Soc Trans 2003; 31(Pt 6):1137–1139.

123. Molven A, Matre GE, Duran M, et al. Familial hyperinsulinemic hypoglycemia caused by a defect in the SCHAD enzyme of mitochondrial fatty acid oxidation. Diabetes 2004; 53(1):221–227.

124. Hussain K, Clayton PT, Krywawych S, et al. Hyperinsulinism of infancy associated with a novel splice site mutation in the SCHAD gene. J Pediatr 2005; 146(5):706–708.

125. Meissner T, Otonkoski T, Feneberg R, et al. Exercise induced hypoglycaemic hyperinsulinism. Arch Dis Child 2001; 84(3):254–257.

126. Otonkoski T, Kaminen N, Ustinov J, et al. Physical exercise-induced hyperinsulinemic hypoglycemia is an autosomal-dominant trait characterized by abnormal pyruvate-induced insulin release. Diabetes 2003; 52(1):199–204.

127. Aynsley-Green A, Hussain K, Hall J, et al. Practical management of hyperinsulinism in infancy. Arch Dis Child Fetal Neonatal Ed 2000; 82(2):F98–F107.

128. Lovvorn HN III, Nance ML, Ferry RJ Jr., et al. Congenital hyperinsulinism and the surgeon: lessons learned over 35 years. J Pediatr Surg 1999; 34(5):786–792; discussion 792–793.

129. Fekete CN, de Lonlay P, Jaubert F, Rahier J, Brunelle F, Saudubray JM. The surgical management of congenital hyperinsulinemic hypoglycemia in infancy. J Pediatr Surg 2004; 39(3):267–269.

130. Adzick NS, Thornton PS, Stanley CA, Kaye RD, Ruchelli E. A multidisciplinary approach to the focal form of congenital hyperinsulinism leads to successful treatment by partial pancreatectomy. J Pediatr Surg 2004; 39(3):270–275.

131. Cretolle C, de Lonlay P, Sauvat F, et al. Congenital hyperinsulinism of infancy: surgical treatment in 60 cases of focal form. Arch Pediatr 2005; 12(3):258–263.

132. Sempoux C, Guiot Y, Lefevre A, et al. Neonatal hyperinsulinemic hypoglycemia: heterogeneity of the syndrome and keys for differential diagnosis. J Clin Endocrinol Metab 1998; 83(5):1455–1461.

133. Ribeiro MJ, De Lonlay P, Delzescaux T, et al. Characterization of hyperinsulinism in infancy assessed with PET and 18F-fluoro-l-DOPA. J Nucl Med 2005; 46(4):560–566.

134. Henwood MJ, Kelly A, Macmullen C, et al. Genotype-phenotype correlations in children with congenital hyperinsulinism due to recessive mutations of the adenosine triphosphate-sensitive potassium channel genes. J Clin Endocrinol Metab 2005; 90(2):789–794.

135. www.athenadiagnostics.com.

136. Meissner T, Brune W, Mayatepek E. Persistent hyperinsulinaemic hypoglycaemia of infancy: therapy, clinical outcome and mutational analysis. Eur J Pediatr 1997; 156(10):754–757.

137. Meissner T, Wendel U, Burgard P, Schaetzle S, Mayatepek E. Long-term follow-up of 114 patients with congenital hyperinsulinism. Eur J Endocrinol 2003; 149(1):43–51.

138. Kane C, Lindley KJ, Johnson PR, et al. Therapy for persistent hyperinsulinemic hypoglycemia of infancy. Understanding the responsiveness of beta cells to diazoxide and somatostatin. J Clin Invest 1997; 100(7):1888–1893.

139. Thornton P, Alter C, Levitt Katz L, Baler L, Stanley C. Short- and long-term use of octreotide in the treatment of congenital hyperinsulinisim. J Pediatr 1993; 123:637–643.

140. Lindley K, Dunne M, Kane C, et al. Ionic control of β-cell function in nesidioblastosis. A possible therapeutic role for calcium channel blockade. Arch Dis Child 1996; 74:373–378.

141. Bas F, Darendeliler F, Demirkol D, Bundak R, Saka N, Gunoz H. Successful therapy with calcium channel blocker (nifedipine) in persistent neonatal hyperinsulinemic hypoglycemia of infancy. J Pediatr Endocrinol Metab 1999; 12(6):873–878.

142. Suprasongsin C, Suthutvoravut U, Mahachoklertwattana P, Preeyasombat C. Combined raw cornstarch and nifedipine as an additional treatment in persistent hyperinsulinemic hypoglycemia of infancy. J Med Assoc Thai 1999; 82(suppl 1):S39–S42.

143. Eichmann D, Hufnagel M, Quick P, Santer R. Treatment of hyperinsulinaemic hypoglycaemia with nifedipine. Eur J Pediatr 1999; 158(3):204–206.

144. Spitz L, Bhargava RK, Grant DB, Leonard JV. Surgical treatment of hyperinsulinaemic hypoglycaemia in infancy and childhood. Arch Dis Child 1992; 67(2):201–205.

145. Mackinnon J, Grant DB. Hypoglycaemia in congenital adrenal hyperplasia. Arch Dis Child 1977; 52(7):591–593.

146. Weise M, Mehlinger SL, Drinkard B, et al. Patients with classic congenital adrenal hyperplasia have decreased epinephrine reserve and defective glucose elevation in response to high-intensity exercise. J Clin Endocrinol Metab 2004; 89(2):591–597.

147. Sadeghi-Nejad A, Senior B. Adrenomyeloneuropathy presenting as Addison's disease in childhood. N Engl J Med 1990; 322(1):13–16.

148. Aynsley-Green A, Moncrieff MW, Ratter S, Benedict CR, Storrs CN. Isolated ACTH deficiency. Metabolic and endocrine studies in a 7-year-old boy. Arch Dis Child 1978; 53(6):499–502.

149. al Jurayyan NA. Isolated adrenocorticotropin deficiency as a rare cause of hypoglycaemia in children. Further studies and report of an additional case. Horm Res 1995; 44(5):238–240.

150. Hopwood NJ, Forsman PJ, Kenny FM, Drash AL. Hypoglycemia in hypopituitary children. Am J Dis Child 1975; 129(8):918–926.

151. Haymond MW, Karl I, Weldon VV, Pagliara AS. The role of growth hormone and cortisone on glucose and gluconeogenic substrate regulation in fasted hypopituitary children. J Clin Endocrinol Metab 1976; 42(5):846–856.

152. Carrel AL, Somers S, Lemanske RF Jr., Allen DB. Hypoglycemia and cortisol deficiency associated with low-dose corticosteroid therapy for asthma. Pediatrics 1996; 97(6 Pt 1):921–924.

153. Hollman GA, Allen DB. Overt glucocorticoid excess due to inhaled corticosteroid therapy. Pediatrics 1988; 81(3):452–455.

154. Todd GR, Acerini CL, Ross-Russell R, Zahra S, Warner JT, McCance D. Survey of adrenal crisis associated with inhaled corticosteroids in the United Kingdom. Arch Dis Child 2002; 87(6):457–461.

155. Todd GR, Acerini CL, Buck JJ, et al. Acute adrenal crisis in asthmatics treated with high-dose fluticasone propionate. Eur Respir J 2002; 19(6):1207–1209.

156. Mahachoklertwattana P, Sudkronrayudh K, Direkwattanachai C, Choubtum L, Okascharoen C. Decreased cortisol response to insulin induced hypoglycaemia in asthmatics treated with inhaled fluticasone propionate. Arch Dis Child 2004; 89(11):1055–1058.

157. Lovinger R, Kaplan S, Grumbach M. Congenital hypopituitarism associated with neonatal hypoglycemia and microphallus. J Pediatr 1975; 87:1171–1181.

158. Copeland KC, Franks RC, Ramamurthy R. Neonatal hyperbilirubinemia and hypoglycemia in congenital hypopituitarism. Clin Pediatr (Phila) 1981; 20(8):523–526.

159. Kaufman FR, Costin G, Thomas DW, Sinatra FR, Roe TF, Neustein HB. Neonatal cholestasis and hypopituitarism. Arch Dis Child 1984; 59(8):787–789.

160. Wolfsdorf J, Sadeghi-Nejad A, Senior B. Hypoketonemia and age-related fasting hypoglycemia in growth hormone deficiency. Metabolism 1983; 32:457–462.

161. Aynsley-Green A, McGann A, Deshpande S. Control of intermediary metabolism in childhood with special reference to hypoglycaemia and growth hormone. Acta Paediatr Scand Suppl 1991; 377:43–52.

162. Hussain K, Hindmarsh P, Aynsley-Green A. Spontaneous hypoglycaemia in childhood is accompanied by paradoxically low serum growth hormone and appropriate cortisol counterregulatory hormonal responses. J Clin Endocrinol Metab 2003; 88(8):3715–3723.

163. Crofton PM, Midgley PC. Cortisol and growth hormone responses to spontaneous hypoglycaemia in infants and children. Arch Dis Child 2004; 89(5):472–478.

164. Laron Z. Prismatic cases: Laron syndrome (primary growth hormone resistance) from patient to laboratory to patient. J Clin Endocrinol Metab 1995; 80(5):1526–1531.

165. Orho M, Bosshard N, Buist N, et al. Mutations in the liver glycogen synthase gene in children with hypoglycemia due to glycogen storage disease type 0. J Clin Invest 1998; 102:507–515.

166. Bachrach BE, Weinstein DA, Orho-Melander M, Burgess A, Wolfsdorf JI. Glycogen synthase deficiency (glycogen storage disease type 0) presenting with hyperglycemia and glucosuria: report of three new mutations. J Pediatr 2002; 140(6):781–783.

167. www.preventiongenetics.com.

168. Aynsley-Green A, Williamson DH, Gitzelmann R. The dietary treatment of hepatic glycogen synthetase deficiency. Helv Paediat Acta 1977; 32:71–75.

169. Gitzelmann R, Spycher M, Feil G, et al. Liver glycogen synthase deficiency: a rarely diagnosed entity. Eur J Pediatr 1996; 155:561–567.

170. Chen Y-T. Glycogen storage diseases. In: Scriver C, Beaudet A, Sly W, et al., eds. The Metabolic and Molecular Bases of Inherited Disease. 8th ed. New York: McGraw-Hill, 2001:1521–1555.

171. Wolfsdorf JI, Holm IA, Weinstein DA. Glycogen storage diseases. Phenotypic, genetic, and biochemical characteristics, and therapy. Endocrinol Metab Clin North Am 1999; 28(4):801–823.

172. Chen Y-T. Type 1 glycogen storage disease: kidney involvement, pathogenesis and its treatment. Pediatr Nephrol 1991; 5:71–76.

173. Wolfsdorf JI, Laffel LMB, Crigler JF Jr. Metabolic control and renal dysfunction in type I glycogen storage disease. J Inherit Metab Dis 1997; 20(4):559–568.

174. Chen Y-T, Coleman RA, Scheinman JI, Kolbeck PC, Sidbury JB. Renal disease in type glycogen storage disease. N Engl J Med 1988; 318:7–11.

175. Lee PJ, Dalton RN, Shah V, Hindmarsh PC, Leonard JV. Glomerular and tubular function in glycogen storage disease. Pediatr Nephrol 1995; 9(6):705–710.

176. Weinstein DA, Somers MJ, Wolfsdorf JI. Decreased urinary citrate excretion in type 1a glycogen storage disease. J Pediatr 2001; 138(3):378–382.

177. Labrune P, Trioche P, Duvaltier I, Chevalier P, Odievre M. Hepatocellular adenomas in glycogen storage disease type I and III: a series of 43 patients and review of the literature. J Pediatr Gastroenterol Nutr 1997; 24(3):276–279.

178. Franco LM, Krishnamurthy V, Bali D, et al. Hepatocellular carcinoma in glycogen storage disease type Ia: a case series. J Inherit Metab Dis 2005; 28(2):153–162.

179. Weinstein DA, Roy CN, Fleming MD, Loda MF, Wolfsdorf JI, Andrews NC. Inappropriate expression of hepcidin is associated with iron refractory anemia: implications for the anemia of chronic disease. Blood 2002; 100(10):3776–3781.

180. Hiraiwa H, Pan CJ, Lin B, Moses SW, Chou JY. Inactivation of the glucose 6-phosphate transporter causes glycogen storage disease type 1b. J Biol Chem 1999; 274(9):5532–5536.

181. Gitzelmann R, Bosshard NU. Defective neutrophil and monocyte functions in glycogen storage disease type Ib: a literature review. Eur J Pediatr 1993; 152(suppl 1):S33–S38.

182. Roe TF, Coates TD, Thomas DW, Miller JH, Gilsanz V. Treatment of chronic inflammatory bowel disease in glycogen storage disease type 1b with colony-stimulating factors. N Engl J Med 1992; 326(18):1666–1669.

183. Visser G, Rake JP, Labrune P, et al. Granulocyte colony-stimulating factor in glycogen storage disease type 1b. Results of the European Study on Glycogen Storage Disease Type 1. Eur J Pediatr 2002; 161(suppl 1):S83–S87.

184. Rake JP, ten Berge AM, Visser G, et al. Glycogen storage disease type Ia: recent experience with mutation analysis, a summary of mutations reported in the literature and a newly developed diagnostic flow chart. Eur J Pediatr 2000; 159(5):322–330.

185. http://medgenetics.pediatrics.duke.edu/.

186. Wolfsdorf JI, Crigler JF Jr. Effect of continuous glucose therapy begun in infancy on the long-term clinical course of patients with type I glycogen storage disease. J Pediatr Gastroenterol Nutr 1999; 29(2):136–143.

187. Chen Y-T, Cornblath M, Sidbury JB. Cornstarch therapy in type 1 glycogen storage disease. N Engl J Med 1984; 310:171–175.

188. Wolfsdorf JI, Keller RJ, Landy H, Crigler JF Jr. Glucose therapy for glycogenosis type 1 in infants: comparison of intermittent uncooked cornstarch and continuous overnight glucose feedings. J Pediatr 1990; 117(3):384–391.

189. Wolfsdorf JI, Plotkin RA, Laffel LMB, Crigler JF Jr. Continuous glucose for treatment of patients with type 1 glycogen-storage disease: comparison of the effects of dextrose and uncooked cornstarch on biochemical variables. Am J Clin Nutr 1990; 52:1043–1050.

190. Wolfsdorf JI, Ehrlich S, Landy HS, Crigler JF Jr. Optimal daytime feeding regimen to prevent postprandial hypoglycemia in type 1 glycogen storage disease. Am J Clin Nutr 1992; 56:587–592.

191. Weinstein DA, Wolfsdorf JI. Effect of continuous glucose therapy with uncooked cornstarch on the long-term clinical course of type 1a glycogen storage disease. Eur J Pediatr 2002; 161(suppl 1):S35–S39.

192. Ding JH, de Barsy T, Brown BI, Coleman RA, Chen YT. Immunoblot analyses of glycogen debranching enzyme in different subtypes of glycogen storage disease type III. J Pediatr 1990; 116(1):95–100.

193. Van Hoof F, Hers H. The subgroups of type III glycogenosis. Eur J Biochem 1967; 2:265–270.

194. Coleman RA, Winter HS, Wolf B, Chen YT. Glycogen debranching enzyme deficiency: long-term study of serum enzyme activities and clinical features. J Inherit Metab Dis 1992; 15(6):869–881.

195. Moses S, Gadoth N, Bashan E, Ben-David E, Slonim A, Wanderman K. Neuromuscular involvement in glycogen storage disease type III. Acta Paediatr Scand 1986; 75:289–296.

196. Moses S, Wanderman K, Myroz A, Frydman M. Cardiac involvement in glycogen storage disease type III. Eur J Pediatr 1989; 148:764–766.

197. Lee PJ, Deanfield JE, Burch M, Baig K, McKenna WJ, Leonard JV. Comparison of the functional significance of left ventricular hypertrophy in hypertrophic cardiomyopathy and glycogenosis type III. Am J Cardiol 1997; 79(6):834–838.

198. Markowitz AJ, Chen YT, Muenzer J, Delbuono EA, Lucey MR. A man with type III glycogenosis associated with cirrhosis and portal hypertension. Gastroenterology 1993; 105(6):1882–1885.

199. Borowitz SM, Greene HL. Cornstarch therapy in a patient with type III glycogen storage disease. J Pediatr Gastroenterol Nutr 1987; 6(4):631–634.

200. Gremse DA, Bucuvalas JC, Balistreri WF. Efficacy of cornstarch therapy in type III glycogen storage disease. Am J Clin Nutr 1990; 52(4):671–674.

201. Slonim A, Weisberg C, Benke P, Evans O, Burr I. Reversal of debrancher deficiency myopathy by the use of high-protein nutrition. Ann Neurol 1982; 11:420–422.

202. Willems PJ, Gerver WJ, Berger R, Fernandes J. The natural history of liver glycogenosis due to phosphorylase kinase deficiency: a longitudinal study of 41 patients. Eur J Pediatr 1990; 149(4):268–271.

203. Nakai A, Shigematsu Y, Takano T, Kikawa Y, Sudo M. Uncooked cornstarch treatment for hepatic phosphorylase kinase deficiency. Eur J Pediatr 1994; 153:581–583.

204. Santer R, Steinmann B, Schaub J. Fanconi-Bickel syndrome–a congenital defect of facilitative glucose transport. Curr Mol Med 2002; 2(2):213–227.

205. Manz F, Bickel H, Brodehl J, et al. Fanconi-Bickel syndrome. Pediatr Nephrol 1987; 1(3):509–518.

206. Sakamoto O, Ogawa E, Ohura T, et al. Mutation analysis of the GLUT2 gene in patients with Fanconi-Bickel syndrome. Pediatr Res 2000; 48(5):586–589.

207. Lee PJ, Van't Hoff WG, Leonard JV. Catch-up growth in Fanconi-Bickel syndrome with uncooked cornstarch. J Inherit Metab Dis 1995; 18(2):153–156.

208. van den Berghe G. Disorders of gluconeogenesis. J Inherit Metab Dis 1996; 19(4):470–477.

209. Steinmann B, Gitzelman R, Van den Berghe G. Disorders of fructose metabolism. In: Scriver C, Beaudet A, Sly W, et al., eds. The Metabolic and Molecular Bases of Inherited Disease. 8th ed. New York: McGraw-Hill, 2001:1489–1520.

210. Pagliara AS, Karl IE, Keating JP, Brown BI, Kipnis DM. Hepatic fructose-1,6-diphosphatase deficiency. A cause of lactic acidosis and hypoglycemia in infancy. J Clin Invest 1972; 51(8):2115–2123.

211. Kaiser UB, Hegele RA. Case report: heterogeneity of aldolase B in hereditary fructose intolerance. Am J Med Sci 1991; 302(6):364–368.

212. Kullberg-Lindh C, Hannoun C, Lindh M. Simple method for detection of mutations causing hereditary fructose intolerance. J Inherit Metab Dis 2002; 25(7):571–575.

213. Tolan DR, Brooks CC. Molecular analysis of common aldolase B alleles for hereditary fructose intolerance in North Americans. Biochem Med Metab Biol 1992; 48(1):19–25.

214. Lecavalier L, Bolli G, Cryer P, Gerich J. Contributions of gluconeogenesis and glycogenolysis during glucose counterregulation in normal humans. Am J Physiol 1989; 256(6 Pt 1):E844–E851.

215. Marks V, Teale JD. Drug-induced hypoglycemia. Endocrinol Metab Clin North Am 1999; 28(3):555–577.

216. Chan JC, Cockram CS, Critchley JA. Drug-induced disorders of glucose metabolism. Mechanisms and management. Drug Saf 1996; 15(2):135–157.

217. White NJ, Warrell DA, Chanthavanich P, et al. Severe hypoglycemia and hyperinsulinemia in falciparum malaria. N Engl J Med 1983; 309(2):61–66.

218. White NJ, Miller KD, Marsh K, et al. Hypoglycaemia in African children with severe malaria. Lancet 1987; 1(8535):708–711.

219. Taylor TE, Molyneux ME, Wirima JJ, Fletcher KA, Morris K. Blood glucose levels in Malawian children before and during the administration of intravenous quinine for severe falciparum malaria (published erratum appears in N Engl J Med 1989; 320(10):676). N Engl J Med 1988; 319(16):1040–1047.

220. Kawo NG, Msengi AE, Swai AB, Chuwa LM, Alberti KG, McLarty DG. Specificity of hypoglycaemia for cerebral malaria in children. Lancet 1990; 336(8713):454–457.

221. Dekker E, Hellerstein MK, Romijn JA, et al. Glucose homeostasis in children with falciparum malaria: precursor supply limits gluconeogenesis and glucose production. J Clin Endocrinol Metab 1997; 82(8):2514–2521.

222. Davis LE, Woodfin BM, Tran TQ, et al. The influenza B virus mouse model of Reyes syndrome: pathogenesis of the hypoglycaemia. Int J Exp Pathol 1993; 74(3): 251–258.

223. Corkey BE, Hale DE, Glennon MC, et al. Relationship between unusual hepatic acyl coenzyme A profiles and the pathogenesis of Reye syndrome. J Clin Invest 1988; 82(3):782–788.

224. Yoshida Y, Singh I, Singh AK, Tecklenberg FW, Brown FR III, Darby CP. Reye syndrome: rate of oxidation of fatty acids in leukocytes and serum levels of lipid peroxides. J Exp Pathol 1989; 4(3):133–139.

225. Haymond MW, Karl IE, Keating JP, DeVivo DC. Metabolic response to hypertonic glucose administration in Reye syndrome. Ann Neurol 1978; 3(3):207–215.

226. DeVivo DC, Keating JP, Haymond MW. Reye syndrome: results of intensive supportive care. J Pediatr 1975; 87(6 Pt 1):875–880.

227. Hirschhorn N, Lindenbaum J, Greenough WB III, Alam SM. Hypoglycemia in children with acute diarrhoea. Lancet 1966; 2(7455):128–132.

228. Jones R. Hypoglycaemia in children with acute diarrhea. Lancet 1966; 2:643.

229. Molla AM, Hossain M, Islam R, Bardhan PK, Sarker SA. Hypoglycemia: a complication of diarrhea in childhood. Indian Pediatr 1981; 18(3):181–185.

230. Osier FH, Berkley JA, Ross A, Sanderson F, Mohammed S, Newton CR. Abnormal blood glucose concentrations on admission to a rural Kenyan district hospital: prevalence and outcome. Arch Dis Child 2003; 88(7):621–625.

231. Bennish ML, Azad AK, Rahman O, Phillips RE. Hypoglycemia during diarrhea in childhood. Prevalence, pathophysiology, and outcome. N Engl J Med 1990; 322(19):1357–1363.

232. Slone D, Taitz L, Gilchrist G. Aspects of carbohydrate metabolism in kwashiokor: with special reference to spontaneous hypoglycaemia. Br Med J 1961; 1:32–34.

233. Hadden D. Glucose, free fatty acid, and insulin interrelations in kwashiokor and marasmus. Lancet 1967; 1:589–593.

234. Wharton B. Hypoglycaemia in children with kwashiorkor. Lancet 1970; 1:171–173.

235. Lifshitz F, Coello-Ramirez P, Gutierrez-Topete G. Monosaccharide intolerance and hypoglycemia in infants with diarrhea. I. Clinical course of 23 infants. J Pediatr 1970; 77(4):595–603.

236. Lifshitz F, Coello-Ramirez P, Gutierrez-Topete G. Monosaccharide intolerance and hypoglycemia in infants with diarrhea. II. Metabolic studies in 23 infants. J Pediatr 1970; 77(4):604–612.

237. Butler T, Arnold M, Islam M. Depletion of hepatic glycogen in the hypoglycaemia of fatal childhood diarrhoeal illnesses. Trans R Soc Trop Med Hyg 1989; 83(6):839–843.

238. Haymond MW. Diarrhea, malnutrition, euglycemia, and fuel for thought (editorial). N Engl J Med 1990; 322(19):1390–1391.

239. Shih VE. Detection of hereditary metabolic disorders involving amino acids and organic acids. Clin Biochem 1991; 24(4):301–309.

240. Saudubray JM, Nassogne MC, de Lonlay P, Touati G. Clinical approach to inherited metabolic disorders in neonates: an overview. Semin Neonatol 2002; 7(1):3–15.

241. Cheema-Dhadli S, Leznoff CC, Halperin ML. Effect of 2-methylcitrate on citrate metabolism: implications for the management of patients with propionic acidemia and methylmalonic aciduria. Pediatr Res 1975; 9(12):905–908.

242. Gibson KM, Breuer J, Nyhan WL. 3-Hydroxy-3-methylglutaryl-coenzyme A lyase deficiency: review of 18 reported patients. Eur J Pediatr 1988; 148(3):180–186.

243. Chuang D, Shih V. Disorders of branch chain amino acid and ketoacid metabolism. In: Scriver C, Beaudet A, Sly W, Valle D, eds. The Metabolic and Molecular Bases of Inherited Disease. 7th ed. New York: McGraw-Hill, 1995:1239–1277.

244. Haymond MW, Ben-Galim E, Strobel KE. Glucose and alanine metabolism in children with maple syrup urine disease. J Clin Invest 1978; 62(2):398–405.

245. Morton DH, Strauss KA, Robinson DL, Puffenberger EG, Kelley RI. Diagnosis and treatment of maple syrup disease: a study of 36 patients. Pediatrics 2002; 109(6):999–1008.

246. Holton J, Walter J, Tyfield L. Galactosemia. In: Scriver C, Beaudet A, Sly W, et al., eds. The Metabolic and Molecular Bases of Inherited Disease. 8th ed. New York: McGraw-Hill, 2001:1553–1587.

247. Holton JB, Leonard JV. Clouds still gathering over galactosaemia. Lancet 1994; 344(8932):1242–1243.

248. Zimmerman HJ, Lewis JH. Chemical- and toxin-induced hepatotoxicity. Gastroenterol Clin North Am 1995; 24(4):1027–1045.

249. Tanaka K, Ikeda Y. Hypoglycin and Jamaican vomiting sickness. Prog Clin Biol Res 1990; 321:167–184.

250. McTague JA, Forney R Jr. Jamaican vomiting sickness in Toledo, Ohio. Ann Emerg Med 1994; 23(5):1116–1118.

251. Seidner G, Alvarez MG, Yeh JI, et al. GLUT-1 deficiency syndrome caused by haploinsufficiency of the blood–brain barrier hexose carrier. Nat Genet 1998; 18(2):188–191.

252. De Vivo DC, Trifiletti RR, Jacobson RI, Ronen GM, Behmand RA, Harik SI. Defective glucose transport across the blood–brain barrier as a cause of persistent hypoglycorrhachia, seizures, and developmental delay. N Engl J Med 1991; 325(10):703–709.

253. Jaeken J. Congenital disorders of glycosylation (CDG): update and new developments. J Inherit Metab Dis 2004; 27(3):423–426.

254. Babovic-Vuksanovic D, Patterson MC, Schwenk WF, et al. Severe hypoglycemia as a presenting symptom of carbohydrate-deficient glycoprotein syndrome. J Pediatr 1999; 135(6):775–781.

255. de Lonlay P, Cuer M, Vuillaumier-Barrot S, et al. Hyperinsulinemic hypoglycemia as a presenting sign in phosphomannose isomerase deficiency: a new manifestation of carbohydrate-deficient glycoprotein syndrome treatable with mannose. J Pediatr 1999; 135(3):379–383.

256. Yoon KL, Ernst SG, Rasmussen C, Dooling EC, Aprille JR. Mitochondrial disorder associated with newborn cardiopulmonary arrest. Pediatr Res 1993; 33(5):433–440.

257. Maaswinkel-Mooij PD, Van den Bogert C, Scholte HR, Onkenhout W, Brederoo P, Poorthuis BJ. Depletion of mitochondrial DNA in the liver of a patient with lactic acidemia and hypoketotic hypoglycemia. J Pediatr 1996; 128(5 Pt 1):679–683.

258. Freckman M-L, Thorburn D, Kirby D, et al. Mitochondrial electron transport chain defect presenting as hypoglycemia. J Pediatr 1997; 130:431–436.

259. Mochel F, Slama A, Touati G, et al. Respiratory chain defects may present only with hypoglycemia. J Clin Endocrinol Metab 2005; 90(6):3780–3785.

260. Uchigata Y, Eguchi Y, Takayama-Hasumi S, Omori Y. Insulin autoimmune syndrome (Hirata disease): clinical features and epidemiology in Japan. Diabetes Res Clin Pract 1994; 22(2–3):89–94.

261. Redmon JB, Nuttall FQ. Autoimmune hypoglycemia. Endocrinol Metab Clin North Am 1999; 28(3):603–618.

262. Uchigata Y, Kuwata S, Tsushima T, et al. Patients with Graves' disease who developed insulin autoimmune syndrome (Hirata disease) possess HLA-Bw62/Cw4/DR4 carrying DRB1*0406. J Clin Endocrinol Metab 1993; 77(1):249–254.

263. Dozio N, Scavini M, Beretta A, et al. Imaging of the buffering effect of insulin antibodies in the autoimmune hypoglycemic syndrome. J Clin Endocrinol Metab 1998; 83(2):643–648.

264. Basu A, Service FJ, Yu L, Heser D, Ferries LM, Eisenbarth G. Insulin autoimmunity and hypoglycemia in seven white patients. Endocr Pract 2005; 11(2):97–103.

265. Rinaldo P, Raymond K, al-Odaib A, Bennett MJ. Clinical and biochemical features of fatty acid oxidation disorders. Curr Opin Pediatr 1998; 10(6):615–621.

266. Roe C, Ding J. Mitochondrial fatty acid oxidation disorders. In: Scriver C, Beaudet A, Sly W, et al., eds. The Metabolic and Molecular Bases of Inherited Disease. 8th ed. New York: McGraw-Hill, 2001:2297–2326.

267. Saudubray JM, Martin D, de Lonlay P, et al. Recognition and management of fatty acid oxidation defects: a series of 107 patients. J Inherit Metab Dis 1999; 22(4):488–502.

268. Hale D, Bennett M. Fatty acid oxidation disorders: a new class of metabolic diseases. J Pediatr 1992; 121:1–11.

269. Stanley CA. Carnitine deficiency disorders in children. Ann NY Acad Sci 2004; 1033:42–51.

270. Olpin SE, Allen J, Bonham JR, et al. Features of carnitine palmitoyltransferase type I deficiency. J Inherit Metab Dis 2001; 24(1):35–42.

271. Bonnefont JP, Demaugre F, Prip-Buus C, et al. Carnitine palmitoyltransferase deficiencies. Mol Genet Metab 1999; 68(4):424–440.

272. Frerman F, Goodman S. Defects of electron transfer flavoproteins and electron transfer flavoprotein-ubiquinone oxidoreductase: glutaric acidemia type II. In: Scriver C, Beaudet A, Sly W, et al., eds. The Metabolic and Molecular Bases of Inherited Disease. 7th ed. New York: McGraw-Hill, 2001:2357–2366.

273. Bennett MJ, Sherwood WG. 3-Hydroxydicarboxylic and 3-ketodicarboxylic aciduria in three patients: evidence for a new defect in fatty acid oxidation at the level of 3-ketoacyl-CoA thiolase. Clin Chem 1993; 39(5):897–901.

274. Kamijo T, Indo Y, Souri M, et al. Medium chain 3-ketoacyl-coenzyme A thiolase deficiency: a new disorder of mitochondrial fatty acid beta-oxidation. Pediatr Res 1997; 42(5):569–576.

275. Mitchell G, Fukao T. Inborn errors of ketone body metabolism. In: Scriver C, Beaudet A, Sly W, et al., eds. The metabolic and molecular bases of inherited disease. 8th ed. New York: McGraw-Hill, 2001:2327–2356.

276. Bohm N, Uy J, Kiessling M, Lehnert W. Multiple acyl-CoA dehydrogenation deficiency (glutaric aciduria type II), congenital polycystic kidneys, and symmetric warty dysplasia of the cerebral cortex in two newborn brothers. II. Morphology and pathogenesis. Eur J Pediatr 1982; 139(1):60–65.

277. Hug G, Bove KE, Soukup S. Lethal neonatal multiorgan deficiency of carnitine palmitoyltransferase II. N Engl J Med 1991; 325(26):1862–1864.

278. Oey NA, den Boer ME, Wijburg FA, et al. Long-chain fatty acid oxidation during early human development. Pediatr Res 2005; 57(6):755–759.

279. North KN, Hoppel CL, De Girolami U, Kozakewich HP, Korson MS. Lethal neonatal deficiency of carnitine palmitoyltransferase II associated with dysgenesis of the brain and kidneys. J Pediatr 1995; 127(3):414–420.

280. Boles RG, Buck EA, Blitzer MG, et al. Retrospective biochemical screening of fatty acid oxidation disorders in postmortem livers of 418 cases of sudden death in the first year of life. J Pediatr 1998; 132(6):924–933.

281. Orlowski JP. Whatever happened to Reye's syndrome? Did it ever really exist? Crit Care Med 1999; 27(8):1582–1587.

282. Alonso EM. Acute liver failure in children: the role of defects in fatty acid oxidation. Hepatology 2005; 41(4):696–699.

283. Treem WR, Witzleben CA, Piccoli DA, et al. Medium-chain and long-chain acyl CoA dehydrogenase deficiency: clinical, pathologic and ultrastructural differentiation from Reye's syndrome. Hepatology 1986; 6(6):1270–1278.

284. Stanley C, DeLeeuw S, Coates P, et al. Chronic cardiomyopathy and weakness or acute coma in children with a defect in carnitine uptake. Ann Neurol 1991; 30:709–716.

285. Rinaldo P, O'Shea J, Coates P, Hale D, Stanley C, Tanaka K. Medium-chain acyl-CoA dehydrogenase deficiency. Diagnosis by stable isotope dilution measurement of urinary n-hexanoylglycine and 3-phenylpropionylglycine. N Engl J Med 1988; 319:1308–1313.

286. Van Hove J, Zhang W, Kahler S, et al. Medium-chain acyl-CoA dehydrogenase (MCAD) deficiency: Diagnosis by acylcarnitine analysis in blood. Am J Hum Genet 1993:958–966.

287. Millington D. Newborn screening for metabolic diseases. American Scientist 2002; 90:40–47.

288. Morris A, Thekekara A, Wilks Z, Clayton P, Leonard J, Aynsley-Green A. Evaluation of fasts for investigating

hypoglycaemia or suspected metabolic disease. Arch Dis Child 1996; 75:115–119.

289. Ziadeh R, Hoffman EP, Finegold DN, et al. Medium chain acyl-CoA dehydrogenase deficiency in Pennsylvania: neonatal screening shows high incidence and unexpected mutation frequencies. Pediatr Res 1995; 37(5):675–678.

290. Seymour CA, Thomason MJ, Chalmers RA, et al. Newborn screening for inborn errors of metabolism: a systematic review. Health Technol Assess 1997; 1(11):1–95.

291. Shekhawat PS, Matern D, Strauss AW. Fetal fatty acid oxidation disorders, their effect on maternal health and neonatal outcome: impact of expanded newborn screening on their diagnosis and management. Pediatr Res 2005; 57(5 Pt 2):78R–86R.

292. Parini R, Garavaglia B, Saudubray JM, et al. Clinical diagnosis of long-chain acyl-coenzyme A-dehydrogenase deficiency: use of stress and fat-loading tests. J Pediatr 1991; 119(1 Pt 1):77–80.

293. Thakker RV. Multiple endocrine neoplasia type 1. Endocrinol Metab Clin North Am 2000; 29(3):541–567.

294. Trajanoski Z, Brunner GA, Gfrerer RJ, Wach P, Pieber TR. Accuracy of home blood glucose meters during hypoglycemia. Diabetes Care 1996; 19(12): 1412–1415.

295. Ho HT, Yeung WK, Young BW. Evaluation of "point of care" devices in the measurement of low blood glucose in neonatal practice. Arch Dis Child Fetal Neonatal Ed 2004; 89(4):F356–F359.

296. Antunes JD, Geffner ME, Lippe BM, Landaw EM. Childhood hypoglycemia: differentiating hyperinsulinemic from nonhyperinsulinemic causes. J Pediatr 1990; 116(1):105–108.

297. Cryer PE. Banting Lecture. Hypoglycemia: the limiting factor in the management of IDDM. Diabetes 1994; 43(11):1378–1389.

298. Diabetes Control and Complications Trial Research Group. Hypoglycemia in the Diabetes Control and Complications Trial. Diabetes 1997; 46(2):271–286.

299. Cryer PE, Davis SN, Shamoon H. Hypoglycemia in diabetes. Diabetes Care 2003; 26(6):1902–1912.

300. Bulsara MK, Holman CD, Davis EA, Jones TW. The impact of a decade of changing treatment on rates of severe hypoglycemia in a population-based cohort of children with type 1 diabetes. Diabetes Care 2004; 27(10):2293–2298.

301. Cryer PE. Diverse causes of hypoglycemia-associated autonomic failure in diabetes. N Engl J Med 2004; 350(22):2272–2279.

302. Gerich JE, Langlois M, Noacco C, Karam JH, Forsham PH. Lack of glucagon response to hypoglycemia in diabetes: evidence for an intrinsic pancreatic alpha cell defect. Science 1973; 182(108):171–173.

303. Bolli G, Calabrese G, De Feo P, et al. Lack of glucagon response in glucose counter-regulation in type 1 (insulin-dependent) diabetics: absence of recovery after prolonged optimal insulin therapy. Diabetologia 1982; 22(2):100–105.

304. Cryer PE. Iatrogenic hypoglycemia as a cause of hypoglycemia-associated autonomic failure in IDDM. A vicious cycle. Diabetes 1992; 41(3):255–260.

305. Dagogo-Jack SE, Craft S, Cryer PE. Hypoglycemia-associated autonomic failure in insulin-dependent diabetes mellitus. Recent antecedent hypoglycemia reduces autonomic responses to, symptoms of, and defense against subsequent hypoglycemia. J Clin Invest 1993; 91(3):819–828.

306. Aman J, Karlsson I, Wranne L. Symptomatic hypoglycaemia in childhood diabetes: a population-based questionnaire study. Diabet Med 1989; 6(3):257–261.

307. Bergada I, Suissa S, Dufresne J, Schiffrin A. Severe hypoglycemia in IDDM children. Diabetes Care 1989; 12(4):239–244.

308. Egger M, Gschwend S, Smith GD, Zuppinger K. Increasing incidence of hypoglycemic coma in children with IDDM. Diabetes Care 1991; 14(11):1001–1005.

309. Bhatia V, Wolfsdorf JI. Severe hypoglycemia in youth with insulin-dependent diabetes mellitus: frequency and causative factors. Pediatrics 1991; 88(6):1187–1193.

310. Limbert C, Schwingshandl J, Haas J, Roth R, Borkenstein M. Severe hypoglycemia in children and adolescents with IDDM: frequency and associated factors. J Diabetes Complications 1993; 7(4):216–220.

311. Bognetti F, Brunelli A, Meschi F, Viscardi M, Bonfanti R, Chiumello G. Frequency and correlates of severe hypoglycaemia in children and adolescents with diabetes mellitus. Eur J Pediatr 1997; 156(8):589–591.

312. Jacobson AM, Hauser ST, Wolfsdorf JI, et al. Psychologic predictors of compliance in children with recent onset of diabetes mellitus. J Pediatr 1987; 110(5):805–811.

313. Hepburn DA, Deary IJ, Frier BM, Patrick AW, Quinn JD, Fisher BM. Symptoms of acute insulin-induced hypoglycemia in humans with and without IDDM. Factor-analysis approach. Diabetes Care 1991; 14(11):949–957.

314. Tupola S, Rajantie J. Documented symptomatic hypoglycaemia in children and adolescents using multiple daily insulin injection therapy. Diabet Med 1998; 15(6):492–496.

315. McCrimmon RJ, Gold AE, Deary IJ, Kelnar CJ, Frier BM. Symptoms of hypoglycemia in children with IDDM. Diabetes Care 1995; 18(6):858–861.

316. Defining and reporting hypoglycemia in diabetes: a report from the American Diabetes Association Workgroup on Hypoglycemia. Diabetes Care 2005; 28(5):1245–1249.

317. Dammacco F, Torelli C, Frezza E, Piccinno E, Tansella F. Problems of hypoglycemia arising in children and adolescents with insulin-dependent diabetes mellitus. The Diabetes Study Group of The Italian Society of Pediatric Endocrinology & Diabetes. J Pediatr Endocrinol Metab 1998; 11(suppl 1):167–176.

318. Boyle PJ, Schwartz NS, Shah SD, Clutter WE, Cryer PE. Plasma glucose concentrations at the onset of hypoglycemic symptoms in patients with poorly controlled diabetes and in nondiabetics. N Engl J Med 1988; 318(23):1487–1492.

319. Amiel SA, Sherwin RS, Simonson DC, Tamborlane WV. Effect of intensive insulin therapy on glycemic thresholds for counterregulatory hormone release. Diabetes 1988; 37:901–907.

320. Goldstein DE, England JD, Hess R, Rawlings SS, Walker B. A prospective study of symptomatic hypoglycemia in young diabetic patients. Diabetes Care 1981; 4(6): 601–605.

321. Macfarlane PI, Walters M, Stutchfield P, Smith CS. A prospective study of symptomatic hypoglycaemia in childhood diabetes. Diabet Med 1989; 6(7):627–630.

322. Daneman D, Frank M, Perlman K, Tamm J, Ehrlich R. Severe hypoglycemia in children with insulin-dependent diabetes mellitus: frequency and predisposing factors. J Pediatr 1989; 115(5 Pt 1):681–685.

323. Diabetes Control and Complications Trial Research Group. Effect of intensive diabetes treatment on the development and progression of long-term complications in adolescents with insulin- dependent diabetes mellitus: Diabetes Control and Complications Trial. J Pediatr 1994; 125(2):177–188.

324. Boland EA, Grey M, Oesterle A, Fredrickson L, Tamborlane WV. Continuous subcutaneous insulin infusion. A

new way to lower risk of severe hypoglycemia, improve metabolic control, and enhance coping in adolescents with type 1 diabetes. Diabetes Care 1999; 22(11):1779–1784.

325. Ryan C, Becker D. Hypoglycemia in children with type 1 diabetes mellitus: risk factors, cognitive function, and management. Endocrinol Metab Clin North Am 1999; 28:883–900.

326. Pramming S, Thorsteinsson B, Theilgaard A, Pinner EM, Binder C. Cognitive function during hypoglycaemia in type I diabetes mellitus. Br Med J (Clin Res Ed) 1986; 292(6521):647–650.

327. Clarke WL, Gonder-Frederick A, Snyder AL, Cox DJ. Maternal fear of hypoglycemia in their children with insulin dependent diabetes mellitus. J Pediatr Endocrinol Metab 1998; 11(suppl 1):189–194.

328. Frier BM, Matthews DM, Steel JM, Duncan LJ. Driving and insulin-dependent diabetes. Lancet 1980; 1(8180): 1232–1234.

329. Songer TJ, LaPorte RE, Dorman JS, et al. Motor vehicle accidents and IDDM. Diabetes Care 1988; 11(9):701–707.

330. Ratner RE, Whitehouse FW. Motor vehicles, hypoglycemia, and diabetic drivers. Diabetes Care 1989; 12(3):217–222.

331. Brierley J. Brain damage due to hypoglycaemia. In: Marks V, Rose C, eds. Hypoglycaemia 2nd ed. Oxford: Blackwell Scientific Publications, 1981:488–494.

332. Aynsley-Green A, Soltesz G. Hypoglycaemia in infancy and childhood. 1st ed. Edinburgh: Chuchill Livingstone, 1985.

333. Edge JA, Ford-Adams ME, Dunger DB. Causes of death in children with insulin dependent diabetes 1990–1996. Arch Dis Child 1999; 81(4):318–323.

334. Ryan C, Vega A, Drash A. Cognitive deficits in adolescents who developed diabetes early in life. Pediatrics 1985; 75(5):921–927.

335. Rovet JF, Ehrlich RM, Hoppe M. Intellectual deficits associated with early onset of insulin-dependent diabetes mellitus in children. Diabetes Care 1987; 10(4):510–515.

336. Rovet JF, Ehrlich RM. The effect of hypoglycemic seizures on cognitive function in children with diabetes: a 7-year prospective study. J Pediatr 1999; 134(4):503–506.

337. Auer RN. Progress review: hypoglycemic brain damage. Stroke 1986; 17(4):699–708.

338. Fujioka M, Okuchi K, Hiramatsu KI, Sakaki T, Sakaguchi S, Ishii Y. Specific changes in human brain after hypoglycemic injury. Stroke 1997; 28(3):584–587.

339. Holemans X, Dupuis M, Misson N, Vanderijst JF. Reversible amnesia in a Type 1 diabetic patient and bilateral hippocampal lesions on magnetic resonance imaging (MRI). Diabet Med 2001; 18(9):761–763.

340. Chalmers J, Risk MT, Kean DM, Grant R, Ashworth B, Campbell IW. Severe amnesia after hypoglycemia. Clinical, psychometric, and magnetic resonance imaging correlations. Diabetes Care 1991; 14(10):922–925.

341. Hershey T, Perantie DC, Warren SL, Zimmerman EC, Sadler M, White NH. Frequency and timing of severe hypoglycemia affects spatial memory in children with type 1 diabetes. Diabetes Care 2005; 28(10):2372–2377.

342. Hershey T, Bhargava N, Sadler M, White NH, Craft S. Conventional versus intensive diabetes therapy in children with type 1 diabetes: effects on memory and motor speed. Diabetes Care 1999; 22(8):1318–1324.

343. Strudwick SK, Carne C, Gardiner J, Foster JK, Davis EA, Jones TW. Cognitive functioning in children with early onset type 1 diabetes and severe hypoglycemia. J Pediatr 2005; 147(5):680–685.

344. Tupola S, Rajantie J, Akerblom HK. Experience of severe hypoglycaemia may influence both patient's and physician's subsequent treatment policy of insulin-dependent diabetes mellitus. Eur J Pediatr 1998; 157(8):625–627.

345. Cox DJ, Irvine A, Gonder-Frederick L, Nowacek G, Butterfield J. Fear of hypoglycemia: quantification, validation, and utilization. Diabetes Care 1987; 10(5):617–621.

346. Gonder-Frederick LA, Clarke WL, Cox DJ. The emotional, social, and behavioral implications of insulin-induced hypoglycemia. Semin Clin Neuropsychiatry 1997; 2(1):57–65.

347. Santiago JV. Nocturnal hypoglycemia in children with diabetes: an important problem revisited. J Pediatr 1997; 131(1 Pt 1):2–4.

348. Soltesz G, Acsadi G. Association between diabetes, severe hypoglycaemia, and electroencephalographic abnormalities. Arch Dis Child 1989; 64(7):992–996.

349. Dumont RH, Jacobson AM, Cole C, et al. Psychosocial predictors of acute complications of diabetes in youth. Diabet Med 1995; 12(7):612–618.

350. Verrotti A, Chiarelli F, Blasetti A, Bruni E, Morgese G. Severe hypoglycemia in insulin-dependent diabetic children treated by multiple injection insulin regimen. Acta Diabetol 1996; 33(1):53–57.

351. Mortensen HB, Hougaard P. Comparison of metabolic control in a cross-sectional study of 2873 children and adolescents with IDDM from 18 countries. The Hvidore Study Group on Childhood Diabetes (published erratum appears in Diabetes Care 1997; 20(7):1216). Diabetes Care 1997; 20(5):714–720.

352. Davis EA, Keating B, Byrne GC, Russell M, Jones TW. Hypoglycemia: incidence and clinical predictors in a large population-based sample of children and adolescents with IDDM. Diabetes Care 1997; 20(1):22–25.

353. Nordfeldt S, Ludvigsson J. Severe hypoglycemia in children with IDDM. A prospective population study, 1992–1994. Diabetes Care 1997; 20(4):497–503.

354. Davis EA, Keating B, Byrne GC, Russell M, Jones TW. Impact of improved glycaemic control on rates of hypoglycaemia in insulin dependent diabetes mellitus. Arch Dis Child 1998; 78(2):111–115.

355. Rosilio M, Cotton JB, Wieliczko MC, et al. Factors associated with glycemic control. A cross-sectional nationwide study in 2579 French children with type 1 diabetes. The French Pediatric Diabetes Group. Diabetes Care 1998; 21(7):1146–1153.

356. Tupola S, Rajantie J, Maenpaa J. Severe hypoglycaemia in children and adolescents during multiple-dose insulin therapy. Diabet Med 1998; 15(8):695–699.

357. Lteif AN, Schwenk WF II. Type 1 diabetes mellitus in early childhood: glycemic control and associated risk of hypoglycemic reactions. Mayo Clin Proc 1999; 74(3):211–216.

358. Rewers A, Chase HP, Mackenzie T, et al. Predictors of acute complications in children with type 1 diabetes. Jama 2002; 287(19):2511–2518.

359. Clarke WL, Gonder-Frederick L, Cox DJ. The frequency of severe hypoglycaemia in children with insulin-dependent diabetes mellitus. Horm Res 1996; 45(suppl 1):48–52.

360. Aynsley-Green A, Eyre J, Soltesz G. Hypoglycaemia in diabetic children. In: Frier BM, Fisher BM, eds. Hypoglycaemia Diabetes: Clinical Physiological Aspects. 1st ed. London: Edward Arnold, 1993:228–240.

361. Diabetes Control and Complications Trial Research Group. Epidemiology of severe hypoglycemia in the diabetes control and complications trial. Am J Med 1991; 90(4):450–459.

362. Gale EA, Tattersall RB. Unrecognised nocturnal hypoglycaemia in insulin-treated diabetics. Lancet 1979; 1(8125):1049–1052.

363. Winter RJ. Profiles of metabolic control in diabetic children-frequency of asymptomatic nocturnal hypoglycemia. Metabolism 1981; 30(7):666–672.

364. Shalwitz RA, Farkas-Hirsch R, White NH, Santiago JV. Prevalence and consequences of nocturnal hypoglycemia among conventionally treated children with diabetes mellitus. J Pediatr 1990; 116(5):685–689.

365. Porter PA, Byrne G, Stick S, Jones TW. Nocturnal hypoglycaemia and sleep disturbances in young teenagers with insulin dependent diabetes mellitus. Arch Dis Child 1996; 75(2):120–123.

366. Porter PA, Keating B, Byrne G, Jones TW. Incidence and predictive criteria of nocturnal hypoglycemia in young children with insulin-dependent diabetes mellitus. J Pediatr 1997; 130(3):366–372.

367. Beregszaszi M, Tubiana-Rufi N, Benali K, Noel M, Bloch J, Czernichow P. Nocturnal hypoglycemia in children and adolescents with insulin-dependent diabetes mellitus: prevalence and risk factors. J Pediatr 1997; 131(1 Pt 1):27–33.

368. Lopez MJ, Oyarzabal M, Barrio R, et al. Nocturnal hypoglycaemia in IDDM patients younger than 18 years. Diabet Med 1997; 14(9):772–777.

369. Tsalikian E, Mauras N, Beck RW, et al. Impact of exercise on overnight glycemic control in children with type 1 diabetes mellitus. J Pediatr 2005; 147(4):528–534.

370. Jones TW, Porter P, Sherwin RS, et al. Decreased epinephrine responses to hypoglycemia during sleep. N Engl J Med 1998; 338(23):1657–1662.

371. Banarer S, Cryer PE. Sleep-related hypoglycemia-associated autonomic failure in type 1 diabetes: reduced awakening from sleep during hypoglycemia. Diabetes 2003; 52(5):1195–1203.

372. Veneman T, Mitrakou A, Mokan M, Cryer P, Gerich J. Induction of hypoglycemia unawareness by asymptomatic nocturnal hypoglycemia. Diabetes 1993; 42(9):1233–1237.

373. Brodows RG, Williams C, Amatruda JM. Treatment of insulin reactions in diabetics. JAMA 1984; 252(24):3378–3381.

374. Wiethop BV, Cryer PE. Alanine and terbutaline in treatment of hypoglycemia in IDDM. Diabetes Care 1993; 16(8):1131–1136.

375. Aman J, Wranne L. Treatment of hypoglycemia in diabetes: failure of absorption of glucose through rectal mucosa. Acta Paediatr Scand 1984; 73(4):560–561.

376. Aman J, Wranne L. Hypoglycaemia in childhood diabetes II. Effect of subcutaneous or intramuscular injection of different doses of glucagon. Acta Paediatr Scand 1988; 77(4):548–553.

377. Muhlhauser I, Koch J, Berger M. Pharmacokinetics and bioavailability of injected glucagon: differences between intramuscular, subcutaneous, and intravenous administration. Diabetes Care 1985; 8(1):39–42.

378. Slama G, Alamowitch C, Desplanque N, Letanoux M, Zirinis P. A new non-invasive method for treating insulin-reaction: intranasal lyophylized glucagon. Diabetologia 1990; 33(11):671–674.

379. Lala VR, Vedanarayana VV, Ganesh S, Fray C, Iosub S, Noto R. Hypoglycemic hemiplegia in an adolescent with insulin-dependent diabetes mellitus: a case report and a review of the literature. J Emerg Med 1989; 7(3):233–236.

380. Wayne EA, Dean HJ, Booth F, Tenenbein M. Focal neurologic deficits associated with hypoglycemia in children with diabetes. J Pediatr 1990; 117(4):575–577.

381. Shehadeh N, Kassem J, Tchaban I, et al. High incidence of hypoglycemic episodes with neurologic manifestations in children with insulin dependent diabetes mellitus. J Pediatr Endocrinol Metab 1998; 11(suppl 1):183–187.

16

Hypoglycemia in the Newborn

Hussien M. Farrag
Baystate Medical Center, Tufts University School of Medicine,
Springfield, Massachusetts, U.S.A.

Richard M. Cowett
CIGNA Insurance, Pittsburgh, Pennsylvania, U.S.A.

INTRODUCTION

Relative to glucose homeostasis, the neonate is considered to be in a transition between the complete dependence of the fetus and the complete independence of the adult. The neonate must become independent after birth, balancing between glucose deficiency and excess to maintain euglycemia. The dependence of the conceptus on the mother for continuous substrate delivery in utero contrasts with the variable and intermittent exogenous intake orally, which is the hallmark of the neonatal period and beyond. The maintenance of euglycemia especially in the sick/or low-birth-weight (LBW) neonate is difficult. This is especially true in the so-called micropremies [birth weight (BW) < 1000 g], who represent a majority of the patient days in the neonatal intensive care nursery (1). Maturation of neonatal homeostasis is influenced by the integrity of the specific pathways of intermediary metabolism important in glucose metabolism. The heterogeneity, which is the hallmark of neonatal glucose metabolism, is illustrated by the multiplicity of conditions producing or associated with neonatal hypo-and hyperglycemia. This reinforces the concept that the neonate is vulnerable to carbohydrate disequilibrium. This topic has been the subject of a number of recent evaluations (2–7). Management of both hypo- and hyperglycemia during the neonatal period should be a primary goal of those caring for these neonates to insure the absence of long-term sequelae (8).

NEONATAL EUGLYCEMIA AND HYPOGLYCEMIA

A prime example of the heterogeneity that exists in neonatal glucose metabolism is that there are no uniform standards accepted for specific limits for euglycemia. It is well accepted that glucose is the major substrate for carbohydrate metabolism. At birth, the maternal supply of glucose to the neonate ceases abruptly. Although the neonatal plasma glucose concentration is usually in the normoglycemic range at delivery, its actual concentration depends on factors such as the last maternal meal, the duration of labor, the route of delivery, and the type of intravenous (IV) fluid administered to the mother.

As an example, Figure 1 depicts the mean plasma glucose and insulin concentrations of mothers and their neonates who received either no glucose (Ringer's lactate) ($n = 14$) or glucose (Ringer's lactate +5% dextrose) ($n = 15$) as a bolus infusion during anesthesia for elective cesarean section (9). Blood samples for plasma glucose and insulin concentrations were taken prior to IV fluid administration and at the time of delivery. Corresponding samples were taken from the neonate's umbilical vein and artery at 30 minutes and hourly after birth for four hours. As noted in Figure 1, all mothers and infants receiving glucose had hyperglycemia and hyperinsulinemia at delivery. The neonatal plasma glucose concentration declined rapidly during the first four hours of life. With one exception, all neonates evidenced normal plasma glucose concentrations repeatedly and all were clinically asymptomatic. The changes in the neonate following glucose infusion to the mother reflect the differences that can occur in the neonate, depending on the type of IV infusion administered at delivery. After normal delivery, the plasma glucose concentration declines to approximately 50 mg/dL by two hours of age, but equilibrates at approximately 70 mg/dL at 72 hours after birth.

Their data suggested that concentrations below 40 mg/dL or greater than 125 mg/dL are abnormal after three days after birth. Critical adjustments are required by the neonate in the first 72 hours after birth to maintain glucose homeostasis.

Srinivasan et al. evaluated plasma glucose concentrations in normal full-term neonates who weighed between 2500 and 4000 g and were appropriate for age between 37 and 42 completed weeks of gestation (10). The predicted glucose concentrations

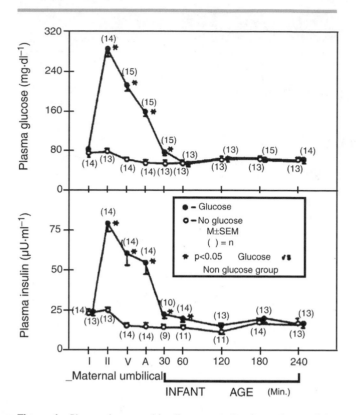

Figure 1 Plasma glucose and insulin concentration for mothers and the neonates. Maternal I and II, samples obtained prior to fluid infusion and at delivery of infants, respectively. *Abbreviations*: V, umbilical venous; A, umbilical arterial samples; *n*, number of determinations. *Source*: From Ref. 9.

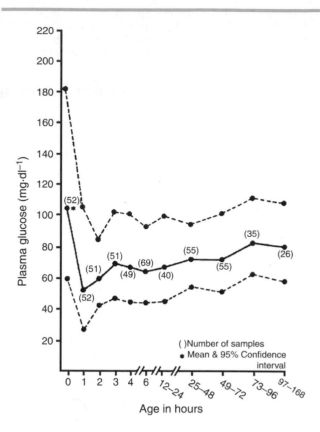

Figure 2 Plasma glucose concentrations in term neonates weighing 2.5 to 4.0 kg. *Source*: From Ref. 10.

during the first week of life are noted in Figure 2. All neonates were fed after three hours. The data indicated that the nadir in plasma glucose concentration is between one and two hours and that a significant rise occurs during the third hour. The mean glucose concentration in this study ranged from 50 to 80 mg/dL during the first week of life.

No similar evaluation of the limits of euglycemia has been reported for the preterm neonate. This difficult study is clearly necessary because of the general lack of consensus that exists relative to definition of euglycemia. What should be apparent from this discussion is the variation not only in the definition of euglycemia but also in the so-called normal concentration of glucose at any particular time. An obvious example of this latter situation is noted in Figure 3. In the four types of neonates commonly cared for in a neonatal unit, the term appropriate for gestational age (AGA), term small for gestational age (SGA), preterm AGA, and preterm SGA, plasma glucose concentration changed constantly and in an apparent random fashion (11). This chapter will catalog the various causes of hypoglycemia as well as the mechanisms controlling neonatal glucose homeostasis.

Definition of Hypoglycemia in the Human Neonate

Transiently low blood-glucose concentrations are common in the neonatal period and may be considered a normal feature of adaptation to extra uterine life (12). However, there is controversy involving the definition, method/site of sampling, symptoms, significance of asymptomatic status, management, and its effect on neurodevelopmental outcome (7,13). Koh et al., who surveyed the definition of hypoglycemia in pediatrics textbooks as well as the opinion of over 200 consultant pediatricians in the United Kingdom, considered the controversy relative to the definition (14). They documented substantial variation in the definition of hypoglycemia not only among the pediatricians surveyed but also among caregivers within the same nursery.

One can postulate four possible approaches to the definition of hypoglycemia in the neonate: statistical, clinical, neurophysiological, and neurodevelopmental. First, from a statistical standpoint, if a normally distributed curve of glucose concentration exists for the healthy term and preterm neonate, a glucose concentration less than 2 standard deviations of the mean would represent hypoglycemia. Most term neonates had blood-glucose concentration greater than 30 mg/dL, whereas 98% of the preterm infants

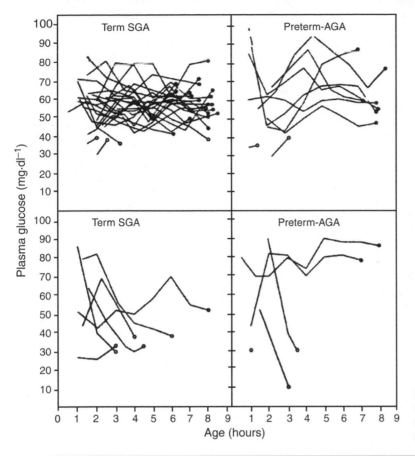

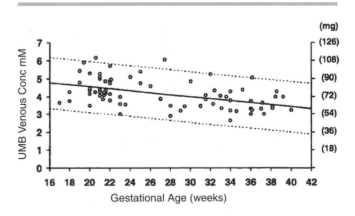

Figure 3 Plasma glucose concentration for the four groups of neonates studied during the first nine hours of life. *Abbreviations*: SGA, small for gestational age; AGA, appropriate for gestational age. *Source*: From Ref. 11.

had values greater than 20 mg/dL. Hypoglycemia in the preterm neonate (BW < 2.5 kg) was defined as blood-glucose concentration of less than 20 mg/dL. It has been suggested that an average lower limit of 95% CI for neonatal blood-glucose concentration is probably 45 mg/dL or greater (10,15). However, generalization of this knowledge is an inaccurate approach to the problem for multiple reasons. The population studied in these reports varied relative to the following: the source of the blood samples; the methods of assay; whether blood or plasma glucose concentration was measured (i.e., plasma glucose concentration is up to 18% higher than that of the blood) (13); feeding schedules (i.e., early vs. late feeding); whether the neonate was fed formula or breast milk (i.e., formula induced a higher insulin response than breast milk and may cause lower glucose concentration in formula-fed neonates) (16); cross-sectional versus longitudinal design; and other metabolic fuels provided at the time of the study, among other issues.

Marconi et al. reported fetal glucose concentration obtained during chordocentesis using venous blood samples (17). We can extrapolate from the data obtained at different gestational ages (GAs) that venous blood-glucose concentrations ranged from 54 to 108 mg/dL (Fig. 4). That study is probably of greater importance and relevance to the healthy term and

preterm neonate. It is clear that blood-glucose concentration was rarely less than 54 mg/dL. This is in agreement with venous cord blood concentrations reported from the neonate by Hawdon et al. that were greater than 47 mg/dL (18).

Figure 4 Umbilical venous glucose concentrations and gestational age for AGA pregnancies (*n*=77). Dashed lines, mean =/-2 SDs of fetal glucose concentration during pregnancy. Glucose concentrations are noted in mmol/L. Each mmol/L of glucose=18 mg/dL. *Abbreviations*: UMB VENOUS CONC, umbilical venous glucose concentrations; AGA, appropriate for gestational age. *Source*: From Ref. 17.

Second, a clinical approach considers a glycemic concentration to be safe, if clinical symptoms associated with hypoglycemia (Table 1) are not observed, or if these symptoms have disappeared at that concentration. A classic report, published in 1959 and based on this definition, continues to be influential in clinical practice currently. In that report, clinical manifestations of hypoglycemia (i.e., including tremors, irritability, limpness, apnea, seizures, and coma) were observed at a glucose concentration of less than 25 mg/dL; these resolved by increasing the blood glucose concentration to greater than 40 mg/dL (19).

There are many concerns with this approach, including the observation of extremely low-blood concentrations in asymptomatic neonates, especially after glucose screening became a routine clinical practice. If we accept the argument presented in that analysis, we should then consider these extremely low blood-glucose concentrations, as observed in the asymptomatic neonates, to be acceptable. The nonspecificity of the symptoms associated with hypoglycemia is another concern, especially when these symptoms are also associated with many other neonatal illnesses. Most of these studies did not evaluate the availability of other energy substrates to the neonate that may compensate for the lower glucose concentration. The availability of other substrates may have a protective effect on the brain.

Third, a neurophysiological definition of hypoglycemia was introduced, based on alteration of neurophysiological functions relative to different glycemic concentrations. Koh et al. evaluated the latency of the auditory-evoked response waveform, based on the fact that the inferior colliculus has one of the highest obligatory rates of glucose utilization in the brain (20). They reported that as blood-glucose concentration declines (i.e., below 47 mg/dL), the latency between waves 1 and 5 gradually increased until wave 5 disappeared. Restoration of wave 5 was documented when hypoglycemia was corrected; however, it took a few hours, in some instances, before this restoration was achieved. Among the 17 children they studied, there were only 5 neonates. Other studies have failed to demonstrate similar effect of hypoglycemia not only on auditory-evoked

response but also on electroencephalographic signals as well as visual-evoked potential (21,22).

Fourth, an approach can be based on neurodevelopmental outcome of the neonate relative to symptomatic or asymptomatic hypoglycemia. The study reported by Lucas et al. provides the most helpful information in this area (23). In their study, 661 neonates, all preterm, were evaluated at 18 months of age for neurodevelopmental outcome. Bayley motor and mental developmental scores were blindly assigned to the infants and then these scores were correlated with their neonatal glycemic concentrations. Data were adjusted for gender, GA, BW, days of mechanical ventilation, and other social risks. The observed low-glucose concentration ranged from 9 to 72 mg/dL. These investigators demonstrated that two-thirds of the neonates had a blood-glucose concentration of less than 47 mg/dL for a period of time ranging from 3 to 30 days. They found the highest regression coefficient at plasma glucose concentration less than 47 mg/dL. A more important finding was that if hypoglycemia (level < 47 mg/dL) existed for five or more consecutive or separate days, the risk of neurodevelopmental deficit (scores < 70) significantly increased, regardless of the severity of hypoglycemia during that time. They also suggested that even at lower blood-glucose concentration, transient hypoglycemia was tolerated.

These data reflect the relative inability of the clinician to diagnose hypoglycemia in the neonatal period. However, there are enough data to support a definition based on the above approaches to the understanding of hypoglycemia in the neonate. A blood-glucose concentration of 54 to 108 mg/dL may represent a more desirable euglycemic range for the term and preterm neonate including the micropremie.

Measurement of Neonatal Glucose Concentration

Problems in the definition of euglycemia are accentuated by the lack of attention given to details of measurement of neonatal glucose concentration. Failure to measure the glucose concentration rapidly enough would allow red blood cell oxidation of glucose, resulting in falsely low values. In the past, Dextrostix® was used, despite the caution that the reagent strips were not intended for use with neonatal blood. This point is moot because Dextrostix is no longer on the market. However, we suggest that abnormal values, obtained by any strip or meter method either in the hypoglycemic or hyperglycemic range, need to be corroborated with laboratory determination of glucose concentration prior to correction of the suspected disequilibrium, unless the patient is symptomatic (3).

Furthermore, more recent investigations allow one to question if glucose strips should be used at all. Several studies have evaluated various means of assessing blood-glucose concentration. Lin et al. evaluated four glucose reflectance meters in use at the

Table 1 Signs and Symptoms Associated with Hypoglycemia in the Neonate

Apnea
Bradycardia
Cyanosis
Tachypnea
Abnormal cry
Hypothermia
Hypotonia
Lethargy
Apathy
Jitteriness
Seizures

time of their study (24). The manufacturers claimed that these meters could reliably measure whole blood-glucose concentrations as low as 20 mg/dL. To determine whether the accuracy of the determination would be affected by the technique of obtaining capillary blood by heel stick, the investigators used cord arterial blood from a separate group of neonates for comparison. All blood was sequentially analyzed five different times on each meter and the YSI analyzer. Evaluation of the data showed that accuracy was limited in heel stick blood whether one evaluated the percentage of difference between the means or the least-squares regression for all the meters tested. The use of cord blood appeared to be associated with greater accuracy than the use of capillary blood obtained by heel stick in the analyses. The reason for the poor correlations with capillary samples and the high variability in the values of blood-glucose concentrations remains unclear. There was no relationship between accuracy and reliability of the various glucose reflectance meters. The Diascan S meter, which seemed to have accuracy closest to that of the YSI analyzer, was clearly not the most reliable in comparison with the YSI analyzer. However, the One Touch meter, which had the best reliability among the four glucose reflectance meters tested, was the least accurate. The investigators concluded that contrary to the manufacturers' claims, glucose reflectance meters should probably not be used for evaluation of capillary blood-glucose concentrations in the high-risk neonate.

Holtrop et al. evaluated the sensitivity and specificity of glucose oxidase peroxidase chromogen test strips by comparing values of 272 samples of serum glucose concentration with values obtained by Chemstrip bG (25). The diagnostic sensitivity of a test strip of 40 mg/dL or less, to predict a serum glucose concentration of 34 mg/dL or less, was 86% with 78% specificity. The positive predictive value with a 21% prevalence of serum glucose less than or equal to 34 mg/dL was 52% with a negative predictive value of 95%. Fifty-eight of the serum glucose concentrations were/= 34 mg/dL, and the strips reported values greater than 40 mg/dL in eight. The investigators concluded that more sensitive and specific methods are required for the neonate.

More recent methods comparing bedside blood-glucose testing with laboratory measurements for the assessment of neonatal hypoglycemia continue to demonstrate that low-sugar concentrations might be missed (26). The Accutrend sensor glucose analyzer measurements varied by more than 20% as compared with quantitative laboratory measurements. The Glucometer Elite XL device for point of care testing was found to have a better sensitivity and specificity for hypoglycemia detection at a threshold of 3.2 mmol/L. Importantly, confirmation by valid clinical laboratory measurements was recommended (27). The feasibility of continuous glucose monitoring sensors in the neonatal intensive care unit is now being investigated (28).

GLUCOSE METABOLISM
Methods of Evaluation

Metabolic research in the human neonate is generally limited by several basic ethical constraints, as discussed in a recent review (29). First, the studies must be noninvasive or minimally so. Second, blood samples should be invariably small, particularly those obtained from the very-LBW neonate. Third, given the limited direct access to most organ systems, the approaches used must allow extrapolation from the sampled data to events occurring in otherwise inaccessible areas. Fourth, the maximal information possible must be obtained from any given study owing to the difficulty of recruiting and the need to study the smallest number of subjects necessary to evaluate the proposed hypotheses adequately.

Many of the above constraints on perinatal metabolic research have been reduced or eliminated by methodological advances in the field. Kinetic studies utilizing stable isotopic tracers in conjunction with mass spectrometric quantification have been the most popular technique in investigating glucose metabolism in the human neonate. This technique is advantageous because both the substrate and the tracer are measured simultaneously with high precision and that minimizes measurement errors. The sample size required for the measurement is small, compared to other analytical methods, which is a major advantage in studies performed in the neonate.

Kinetic studies have been long used to evaluate glucose production and utilization (30–32), gluconeogenesis (33), oxidative and nonoxidative disposal of glucose (34–36), insulin sensitivity via the euglycemic hyperinsulinemic clamp (37), and other aspects of glucose energy metabolism especially during total parenteral nutrition in the human neonate (38).

Evaluation of Hepatic Glucose Production

During kinetic studies utilizing stable isotopic methodology, glucose infusion, glucose absorbed from the gastrointestinal tract, glycogenolysis, and gluconeogenesis may collectively contribute to the rate of glucose appearance in the metabolic pool (i.e., plasma). Only the latter two variables reflect the endogenous rate of glucose production, primarily from the liver.

Measurement of the true rate of glucose production usually gives a good estimate of the glucose requirement of the body and the rate of its utilization under basal conditions (39). To measure the true rate of endogenous glucose production, the neonate has to be fasted for at least three hours prior to the study, resulting in minimal glucose being absorbed from the gastrointestinal tract during the study. No exogenous glucose should be infused during the basal period of the study, except for the tracer isotope that is usually infused at a very slow rate. In investigations involving the micropremie (BW = 1000 g), the endogenous glucose production rate under basal conditions cannot be measured for obvious ethical considerations. The rate of glucose infusion, glycemic concentration achieved, and the pancreatic β-cell response to the infused glucose during any given study would individually or collectively affect the measured rate of glucose production. The dichotomy that exists in the neonatal literature relative to the endogenous glucose production rate response to plasma insulin concentration, glycemic concentration and, correspondingly, to the rate of glucose infused, is probably secondary to many of these issues (40).

Our laboratory as well as others has previously demonstrated, in the preterm neonate, that persistent glucose production (glucose production 1 mg/kg/min) exists during glucose infusion at rates similar to or slightly greater than the basal glucose production rate of the human neonate (i.e., 4–7 mg/kg/min) (30,31,41). Developmentally this is in marked contrast with the adult, in whom glucose production can be suppressed when glucose is infused at a rate equal to or slightly greater than the basal endogenous glucose production rate (i.e., 2–3 mg/kg/min) (Fig. 5) (42). Other investigators have suggested that plasma glucose concentration of the human neonate, rather than the rate of glucose infusion to the neonate, has an important regulatory effect on the rate of endogenous glucose production (43). When the results of glucose kinetics studies in three groups of neonates (i.e., the

AGA term, the SGA term, and the LBW preterm neonate) were combined, Kalhan et al. reported a linear and negative correlation between plasma glucose concentration and endogenous glucose production (31). Complete suppression of glucose production was not achieved in their study.

We have previously studied, in a comparable group of neonates, the glucose production response to three different glycemic concentrations (150, 200, and 250 mg/dL), utilizing the hyperglycemic clamp technique (44). A significant reduction in the rate of endogenous glucose production was observed in all groups. Complete suppression of glucose production was not consistent within or among the groups, except in the 250 mg/dL group. To achieve this glycemic level, glucose was infused at an average rate of 16 mg/kg/min.

The dichotomy in results also exists in studies that involve the micropremie. Hertz et al. showed a correlation between glucose production and glycemic concentration in the very LBW (VLBW) neonate (43). They reported a reduction in endogenous glucose production at moderate glucose infusion rate. Complete suppression of glucose production was achieved at a relatively high glucose infusion rate and plasma glucose concentration.

Other investigations that evaluated relatively similar groups of VLBW neonates have reported a higher glucose production rate and persistent glucose production during glucose infusion. Sunehag et al. studied 10 neonates born at less than or equal to 30 weeks gestation (41). They reported a persistent glucose production during glucose infusion at two consecutive rates of 1.7 and then 6.5 mg/kg/min. Although there was incomplete suppression of glucose production, it is evident that the neonate can partly reduce endogenous glucose production in response to higher rates of glucose infusion. A significant correlation was found between glucose production and plasma insulin concentration but not with glucose concentration. The investigators suggested that insulin plays a more important role in the control of endogenous glucose production.

In two groups of smaller AGA neonates (GA, 25–27 weeks), Farrag et al. demonstrated persistent glucose production when glucose was infused at 4 and 8 mg/kg/min. There was no significant correlation between endogenous glucose production and either glycemic concentration or plasma insulin concentration. At the higher glucose infusion rate (8 mg/kg/min), the rate of endogenous glucose production was almost double that reported by Sunehag et al. The data were in agreement with those reported by Keshen et al. and demonstrated a negative correlation between glucose production rate and body weight in the VLBW neonate (33). Table 2 summarizes the results of these three studies.

Although there were differences among the data sets (in weight, GA, glycemic concentration, and rate of glucose infused), there is a general agreement that the

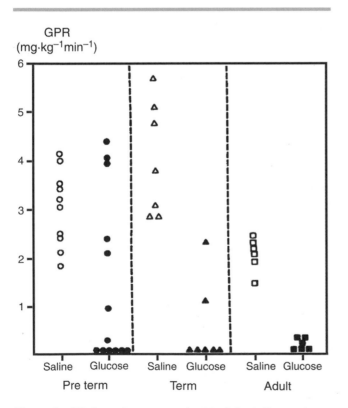

Figure 5 GPR for each neonate and adult during saline or glucose infusion. *Abbreviation*: GPR, glucose production rate. *Source*: From Ref. 30.

Table 2 Comparison of Three Studies Evaluating Glucose Production Rate in the Micropremie During Two Different Glucose Infusion Rates for Each Study

Reference	Study weight (g)	Glucose infusion rates (GIR$_1$ and GIR$_2$) (mg/kg/min)	Plasma glucose concentration (mg/dl)	Glucose production rate after infusion (mg/kg/min)
43	854 ± 51	GIR$_1$ = 6.2 ± 0.4	113 ± 12	1.67 ± 0.45
		GIR$_2$ = 9.5 ± 0.5	136 ± 15	0.32 ± 0.07
41	976 ± 262	GIR$_1$ = 1.7 ± 0.2	65 ± 20	4.3 ± 1.3
		GIR$_2$ = 6.5 ± 0.3	110 ± 23	1.4 ± 1.1
Farrag et al., in progress	708 ± 39	GIR$_1$ = 4.0 ± 0	58 ± 9	3.0 ± 0.8
	677 ± 39	GIR$_2$ = 8.0 ± 0	83 ± 13	2.5 ± 1.0

neonate is able, at least partly, to decrease the rate of endogenous glucose production when receiving glucose infusion. However, there is no agreement as to whether glycemic concentration plays a more important role in the control of hepatic glucose production than plasma insulin concentration or vice versa.

Relative to the effect of insulin on glucose production, Farrag et al. also reported in the preterm neonate that endogenous glucose production persisted during a wide range of insulin infusion rates (Fig. 6) (37).

In that study, the investigators applied the euglycemic hyperinsulinemic clamp technique to evaluate insulin sensitivity in the human neonate. When insulin was infused at rates that ranged from 0.5 to 4.0 mU/kg/min, which resulted in physiological and pharmacological plasma insulin concentrations (i.e., ranged from 10–89 mU/ml), only a reduction of 41% to 58% of preinsulin glucose production rate was achieved. In a subsequent study, this concept was noted to be true for the term as well

as the smaller preterm neonate (28–31 weeks gestation) immediately after birth and in the same preterm neonate restudied after the conclusion of the neonatal period (≥28 days of age) (45). In that study, endogenous glucose production was comparably reduced by 36% to 60% during insulin infusion at a rate of 2 mU/kg/min. This is again in marked contrast with what is known to be the adult glucose production response to insulin infusion. Our laboratory as well as others has demonstrated complete suppression of glucose production in the adult at low plasma insulin concentration and/or minimal insulin infusion rate (30).

Many factors are known to play an important role in glucose homeostasis: glucose infusion rate, glycemic concentration, insulin, and contrainsulin-regulatory hormones. There is no evidence that any of these factors plays a dominant role in the control of hepatic glucose production in the human neonate. Most of the differences between the neonate and the adult in glucose homeostasis are believed to be related to the stress of labor (46). This concept is clearly important in the transition, in the regulation of glucose homeostasis, from the complete dependence of the fetus to the complete independence of the neonate in the immediate neonatal period (40). However, there is evidence that these distinctive physiological and metabolic differences between the neonate and the adult continue through the neonatal period and for months afterwards (13). There is also evidence that this pattern of neonatal glucose homeostasis is consistent with the ontogeny of the glucose transporters (GLUTS), i.e., GLUT-2, which occurs both at the hepatocyte and at the pancreatic β-cell (47).

Thus the control of glucose production in the neonate is a complex process that is only partially controlled by insulin and glycemic concentrations. This unique response of the liver to insulin and glucose may be of physiological relevance in the human neonate. It is clearly important to ensure adequate glucose delivery to the brain under different metabolic circumstances. This may be of particular importance for the neonate who lacks the autonomy to do so during this critical stage of development. The ontogeny of this process requires further evaluation at both the physiological and molecular levels. The developmental switch to an

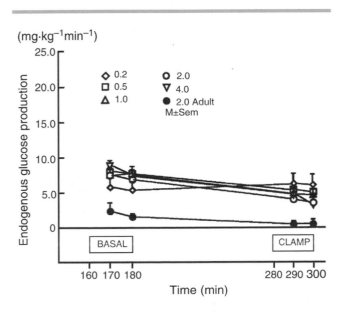

Figure 6 Endogenous glucose production over time subdivided by the various insulin infusion rates (i.e., 0.2, 0.5, 1.0, 2.0, and 4.0 mU/kg/min) administered to the neonate, as well as the 2 mU/kg/min rate administered to the adult. *Abbreviation*: SEM, standard error of the mean. *Source*: From Ref. 37.

Table 3 Distribution of Glucose Transporters

Glucose transporter isoform	Primary site of expression	Affinity to glucose
GLUT-1	All fetal tissues, erythrocytes and blood-tissue barriers	High affinity (+++)
GLUT-2	Hepatocyte, pancreatic beta cell and small intestine	Low affinity (+)
GLUT-3	Neurones and testis	Highest affinity (++++)
GLUT-4	Adipose tissue, skeletal muscle and cardiac muscle	Moderate affinity (++)
GLUT-5	Small intestine and sperm	Fructose uptake (+)
GLUT-6	Pseudogene	None
GLUT-7	Liver (endoplasmic reticulum)	Unknown

Abbreviation: GLUT, glucose transporter.

adult-like response, as has been demonstrated in some of its aspects, most probably requires maturation past the neonatal period (45,48).

Evaluation of Glucose Utilization

It is important to recognize that glucose is utilized by a variety of tissues with different metabolic characteristics (42). First, there are tissues that utilize glucose, independent of insulin (e.g., brain). Second, there are tissues that increase their glucose utilization with increments in plasma glucose concentration independent of increments in insulin concentration (e.g., liver, gut, and the red blood cell). Third are tissues dependent on insulin for glucose utilization (e.g., adipose tissues and skeletal and cardiac muscles). It is also important to recognize that these tissues host different GLUTS that are expressed in a tissue-specific pattern (Table 3).

The factors that control the gene expression and function of these transporters probably dictate the metabolic characteristics of the corresponding host tissue (49). The ontogeny of these transporters within any given tissue can explain some of the developmental differences between the neonate and the adult. GLUT-1 is the predominant isoform of the fetus; it is found in virtually all tissues (49,50). It has a very high affinity for glucose and can effectively transport glucose to organs across the blood–tissue barrier. This may be crucial to meet the energy requirement of the fetal tissues during this stage of rapid growth and differentiation. After birth, GLUT-1 decreases and other isoforms such as GLUT-2 in the liver, GLUT-3 in the brain, and GLUT-4 in the muscle increase (51,52).

There are two facilitative GLUTS involved in the brain uptake of glucose. GLUT-1 is primarily responsible for transport of glucose across the blood–brain barrier, and GLUT-3 is responsible for the uptake of glucose into the neuron. Evidence from animal studies suggests that GLUT-1 is downregulated by high glucose concentrations, whereas GLUT-3 is not (50). There is otherwise little information available relative to the regulation of GLUT-3. Insulin regulates the expression of GLUT-4 in insulin-sensitive tissues such as adipose tissue and skeletal and cardiac muscle (49).

The effect of insulin is rapid and reversible, because it primarily translocates intracellular vesicles of GLUTS to the plasma membrane (53). This step can be rate-limiting for insulin-induced glucose uptake under most conditions (54,55). Except for GLUT-1, which is abundant in fetal life and decreases after birth, some of the other transporters appear to be developmentally regulated. They are found in fetal tissues in smaller amounts that increase after birth and reach adult levels later in life (51,56).

On the physiological level, there is an agreement that neonatal glucose utilization positively correlates to the increase in glucose infusion, glycemic concentration, and plasma insulin concentration (37–39). However, it is not clear when this positive correlation would reach plateau in response to each of these factors. In the larger preterm neonate, we have demonstrated that endogenous glucose production is sensitive to low insulin concentration, reaches plateau quickly, and then becomes nonresponsive to higher insulin concentrations (Fig. 7) (37).

Relative to glucose utilization, although we established a strong positive correlation between insulin concentration and glucose utilization, a plateau was not reached with insulin infusion up to 4.0 mU/kg/min, which resulted in a plasma insulin concentration of 89 mU/ml (Fig. 8) (37).

In a comparable group of neonates, we have recently demonstrated that glucose utilization was not significantly different among three groups of neonates evaluated at three glycemic concentrations: 150, 200, and 250 mg/dL (37). We utilized the hyperglycemic clamp technique in that study. To achieve these glycemic concentrations, glucose was infused at an average rate of 12.8, 14.4, and 16.0 mg/kg/min, respectively. At least in this group of preterm neonates, there was no added benefit, in terms of glucose utilization (i.e., glucose utilization reached plateau), in increasing glucose infusion from 12.8 to 16.0 mg/kg/min or glycemic concentration from 150 to 250 mg/dL. Similar studies will be important to duplicate in the micropremie to determine the optimal rates of glucose infusion and the appropriate glycemic concentration for these neonates.

Oxidative and Nonoxidative Disposal of Glucose

It is important not only to evaluate the overall ability of the neonate to utilize glucose but also to understand how the utilized glucose contributes to energy metabolism. Glucose is generally utilized by either a nonoxidative or an oxidative disposal (40,57). Nonoxidative disposal represents glucose utilized for structural or energy-storage purposes. Only glucose utilized by oxidative disposal will contribute to the energy expenditure of the neonate (57,58). In the preterm neonate, van Goudoever et al. evaluated the contribution of glucose oxidation to total energy expenditure at glucose infusion rate of 4 mg/kg/min (59). They found that glucose was oxidized at a rate

(A)

(B)

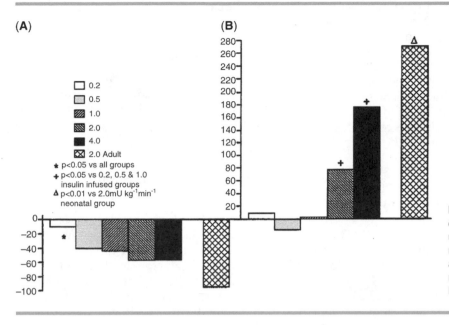

Figure 7 **(A)** Percentage decrease in endogenous glucose production and **(B)** percentage increase in glucose utilization subdivided by the various insulin infusion rates (i.e., 0.2, 0.5, 1.0, 2.0, and 4.0 mU/kg/min) administered to the neonate, as well as the 2 mU/kg/min insulin rate administered to the adult. *Source*: From Ref. 37.

of 2.9 mg/kg/min, which represents 50% of the total glucose utilized by the neonate. They concluded, based on arithmetic calculations, that the contribution of glucose oxidation to total energy expenditure was limited. Other studies evaluating glucose oxidation in the preterm neonate while receiving total parenteral nutrition reported oxidation of up to 65% of total glucose utilized (36,60). Because glucose represents the main source of energy for the preterm neonate during most of the neonatal period, it is important to determine the extent of glucose oxidation and its contribution to total glucose utilization. It is also important to understand if the preterm neonate can adapt to progressive increases in the amount of glucose infused with corresponding increases in the rate

of glucose oxidation (61). This knowledge will assist clinically in the determination of the optimal rate of glucose infusion, which is the rate appropriate to the neonate's capacity to oxidize glucose.

To answer some of the above questions, we evaluated glucose utilization, both oxidative and nonoxidative, in the preterm neonate (48). We also wanted to determine if hyperglycemia is partly related to diminished glucose oxidation capacity in the preterm neonate. We used stable isotopic infusion of $NaH^{13}CO_3$, followed by [U-^{13}C]-glucose, and then analyzed breath and plasma samples to determine glucose oxidation and total glucose utilization, respectively. This was done over the range of glucose infusion commonly provided clinically in neonatal intensive care units (i.e., 4–8 mg/kg/min). We compared the data obtained within the first four days after birth to those obtained from the same neonate at a postnatal age of at least one month at the same glucose infusion rates. Thus, we could evaluate the developmental contribution of glucose utilization, both oxidative and nonoxidative, to glucose metabolism in the micropremie.

In that study, we established a significant linear and negative correlation between glycemic concentration and the percentage of glucose utilized by oxidation. We also found that the percentage of glucose oxidized was significantly higher in the immediate neonatal period (68%) than that oxidized at about five weeks of life (47%) by the same neonate. This was true at both glucose infusion rates with each micropremie serving as both subject and control at the same glucose infusion (4.0 or 8.0 mg/kg/min). We also found that, soon after birth, the micropremie was able to oxidize significantly higher rates of glucose when glucose was infused at a rate of 8.0 versus 4.0 mg/kg/min. We found that the preterm neonates were

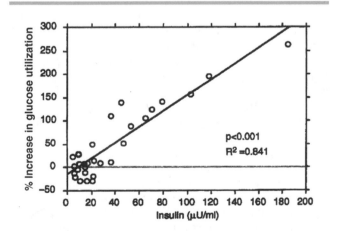

Figure 8 Regression plot correlating the percentage increase in glucose utilization relative to plasma insulin concentration in the neonate. *Source*: From Ref. 37.

able, soon after birth, to oxidize glucose at rates up to 7.5 mg/kg/min (95%, CI: 5.5–9.4 mg/kg/min) when they received glucose infusion at a rate of 8 mg/kg/min. The glucose oxidation rate may exceed the rate of glucose infusion, reflecting the contribution of endogenous glucose production to the total pool of glucose available for oxidation. None of these neonates developed hyperglycemia during glucose infusion at 8.0 mg/kg/min, and at that rate, blood-glucose concentration averaged 83 ± 14 mg/dL [mean (M)± standard error of the mean] (48).

These results should encourage the use of glucose infusion at a rate of 8 mg/kg/min in the preterm neonate after the first day of life: the study age ranged from 27 to 96 hours. The clinical practice of using as low a glucose infusion rate as possible in the preterm neonate to avoid hyperglycemia limits energy intake, not only from glucose but also from fat and protein, because the composition of parenteral alimentation is usually administered proportionally. Hyperglycemia did not result from the rates of glucose infusion employed in these studies. However, the addition of fat and/or amino acids (AAs) can increase the risk of this complication (29,62). The risk of hyperglycemia should be weighed against the benefit of providing adequate energy, especially when insulin infusion has been shown to improve peripheral glucose utilization and enhance glucose tolerance significantly in the preterm neonate (37,63).

We found nonoxidative disposal to be significantly higher in the older neonates when they were studied after the conclusion of the neonatal period (the late study) compared to themselves when they were studied in the immediate neonatal period (the early study). It is important to recognize that the metabolic state of the neonate is different during these two periods. Early after birth, the caloric intake of the micropremie is insufficient to satisfy his or her energy expenditure, because he/she is in a catabolic state. If the neonate is medically stable after the conclusion of the neonatal period (i.e., similar to our study population) and receiving adequate caloric intake, he/she will be in an anabolic state.

The nonoxidative disposal of glucose represents its utilization by different metabolic pathways (40,57). In an anabolic state, lipogenesis is a major route for nonoxidative disposal (36). Other nonoxidative pathways for glucose may include glycogenesis, cycling in the pentose phosphate pathway, and/or formation of a carbon skeleton for AAs (57,58,60). The extrauterine developmental switch from a catabolic state (the early study) to an anabolic one (the late study) during the course of the current investigation can, at least in part, explain the significant increase in the contribution of the nonoxidative disposal of glucose to total energy metabolism in the late studies. Other factors, such as the change in the substrate available for energy metabolism from primarily glucose to a mixture of fat and carbohydrates, may play an equally important role in that phenomenon.

CLINICAL ASSESSMENT
Incidence

It is not surprising that variations in the estimated incidence of hypoglycemia exist in the neonatal literature. Different reports vary relative to populations, definitions, screening methods, clinical status, and strategies for nutrition and fluid management. The incidence ranges from 7% to 57% based on these variations (13).

General Pathophysiological and Metabolic Considerations

The close relationship between maternal and fetal glucose, the repetitive occurrence of wide swings of neonatal glucose concentration, and the retarded disappearance of an acute glucose load in both term and preterm neonates indicate that the regulation of neonatal carbohydrate metabolism is poorly developed 72 hours after birth, as shown several years ago (64). The birth process brings the necessity of a period of readjustment to allow subsequent control. In the LBW neonate, especially, this adjustment is delicate and may result in abnormal consequences. We have already discussed the difficulties in the definition of hypoglycemia. One of the main clinical difficulties with the definition is the nonspecific symptoms, which include the signs and symptoms listed in Table 1. These difficulties are compounded by the occurrence of symptoms at different concentrations of blood-glucose in different neonates and the lack of a universal threshold below or above which symptoms may occur (2,7).

During steady-state glucose metabolism, glucose production equals glucose utilization, and glycemic concentration is maintained within a narrow range. A simplistic approach will attribute hypoglycemia to decreased glucose production and/or increased glucose utilization. As discussed earlier, the neonate, on a per kilogram body weight basis, is able to produce glucose at adequate rates. There is evidence that the enzymatic pathways for glucose production via glycogenolysis as well as gluconeogenesis are intact in the term and preterm neonate (40). It is also recognized that the glycogen stores are limited in the preterm neonate as glycogen accumulation primarily takes place in the third trimester (13,40). Based on that, gluconeogenesis is the major route of glucose production in these neonates.

The change in metabolic milieu that occurs at birth, including the reduction of plasma insulin concentration as well as the elevation of cortisol, catecholamine, and glucagon levels, favors the induction of gluconeogenesis. Of course, the clamping of the cord and the termination of maternal glucose supplementation initiate and enhance these changes. The time necessary to induce and transcript the involved enzyme's protein of gluconeogenesis, in metabolically functioning amounts (about two hours), coincides with the clinical observation that the lowest blood-glucose concentrations in the neonate occur between one and two hours after birth. The absence of stored glycogen in the LBW neonate makes hypoglycemia almost inevitable in the first few hours after birth if exogenous glucose is not provided.

The brain is the major site of glucose utilization in the neonate and the major site of concern as well. The neonate has the greatest brain to body weight ratio during human development. Some investigations have concluded that up to 90% of the glucose produced is utilized by the brain, via oxidation (65). Other investigations conclude that the entire amount of glucose oxidized, in the term neonate, is insufficient to satisfy brain glucose requirements (66). There is evidence that the neonatal brain utilizes other metabolic substrates soon after birth, including lactate and ketones (57,67,68). There is evidence from animal and human studies that during hypoglycemia, the brain reduces its glucose consumption by more than 50% and increases its utilization of other substrates (e.g., ketones and lactate) by 15-fold or greater (57,68,69). There is also evidence that the term neonate can efficiently mobilize similar substrates during fasting (70). Furthermore, free fatty acids (FFAs), glycerol, and ketone concentrations were negatively correlated with blood-glucose concentration in these term neonates (18). This ability to mobilize other energy substrates to adapt to hypoglycemia has a protective effect on the brain.

There is evidence that the preterm neonate lacks this protective ability (71). The lack of energy stores in the form of glycogen, as discussed earlier, and adipose tissue is prominent in these neonates. Although fat cannot substitute glucose for brain energy metabolism, its mobilization and oxidation reduce glucose uptake by other tissues and make more glucose available for the brain (13). Levistky et al. demonstrated that nonesterified fatty acids and ketone body concentrations of the preterm infant are significantly lower than those of the term infant (68). Moreover, preterm infants with low blood-glucose concentrations did not show increased ketone body concentrations, as did their term counterparts. This discussion emphasizes that, in the micropremie, cerebral defenses against hypoglycemia are limited, and prolonged episodes, even of milder nature, of hypoglycemia may have a more significant effect on the brain of the preterm than that of the term neonate.

There is evidence, as reviewed by Simmons, that the immaturity of GLUT-2 function in the hepatocyte as well as in the pancreatic β-cell may play a role in the pathophysiology of neonatal hypoglycemia (49). GLUT-2 is a low-affinity GLUT that occurs only in the hepatocyte and pancreatic β-cell. In the mature hepatocyte, the low affinity of this transporter allows glucose release into the plasma in response to small reductions, in plasma glucose concentration. This process is sensitive even within the normal glucose concentration range, resulting in maintenance of euglycemia.

In the newborn period, studies in multiple species demonstrate that the hepatocyte expresses a relatively high amount of GLUT-1 but relatively low levels of GLUT-2 (47). Decreased GLUT-2 expression may limit the hepatocyte sensitivity and responsiveness to changes in glucose and insulin concentration during hypoglycemia (37). This is in agreement with data from our laboratory demonstrating that the preterm neonatal liver was nonresponsive to progressive increments in insulin rates of infusion and plasma concentrations. We attributed this nonresponsiveness to insulin to intracellular mechanism(s) that probably involve a defect in GLUT rather than insulin receptors (37).

In the pancreatic β-cell GLUT-2, in concert with glucokinase, functions as a glucose sensor that allows the β-cell to recognize modest changes in plasma glucose concentration and appropriately secrete insulin (49,50). Although the β-cell of the neonate responds to changes in the glycemic level, this process is diminished, in part due to decreased expression and/or function of the immature glucose sensor, and in part due to decreased activity of other metabolic linkages in the β-cell. Thus, the immature glucose sensor in the pancreatic β-cell may contribute to its inability to downregulate insulin secretion during hypoglycemia. There is evidence that this phenomenon is developmentally regulated (50). This is in agreement with reports suggesting that the basal insulin/glucose ratio is significantly higher in the preterm than in the term neonate.

Pryds et al. reported some evidence of increased cerebral blood flow in preterm infants to support cerebral metabolism during hypoglycemia (<30 mg/dL) (72). They also reported decreased cerebral blood volume during restoration of hypoglycemia in the preterm neonate (73). They concluded from these observations and the rapidity of adjustment of cerebral blood vessels to alteration in glucose concentration that a cerebral glucose sensor exists in the preterm neonate (74). They suggested that this sensor functions by recruiting brain capillaries to maintain adequate glucose transport to the brain during hypoglycemia.

Causes of Hypoglycemia

A number of different classifications have been used to categorize the various causes of hypoglycemia seen in the neonatal period. Table 4 lists the mechanisms known to be associated with hypoglycemia in the human neonate. One or a combination of the following three mechanisms generally causes neonatal hypoglycemia: diminished hepatic glucose production; depletion of glycogen stores; and increased rate of glucose utilization. Extreme prematurity is a prime example of hypoglycemia due to primary failure to produce and/or store glycogen. Hypoglycemia secondary to depletion of glycogen stores is evident in the prematurely born AGA and/or SGA

Table 4 Conditions Associated with Hypoglycemia in the Neonate

Mechanism and/or origin	Condition, disease, and/or syndrome
Primary failure to produce and/or store glycogen	Extreme prematurity
Depletion of glycogen stores	Prematurity, intrauterine growth restriction/ small for gestational age, postmaturity, and congenital heart disease/congestive heart failure
Increased rate of glucose utilization	Perinatal stress/hypoxia, cold stress, and sepsis
Hyperinsulinemia	Infant of diabetic mother, large for gestational age, Rh incompatibility, following exchange transfusion, malposition of umbilical artery catheter, nesidioblastosis, exposure to β-adrenergic agonists and others
Inherited diseases	Malformation syndromes (e.g., Beckwith–Wiedemann syndrome), autosomal-recessive hyperinsulinism, inborn errors of carbohydrate, protein, and lipid metabolism
Endocrine deficiency	Hypopituitarism, growth hormone deficiency, glucagon deficiency, cortisol deficiency/adrenocorticotropic hormone unresponsiveness
Newly described syndromes	Specific glucose transporter deficiency (neuroglucopenia during euglycemia), neonatal hyperinsulinemia-hypoglycemia and isoimmune thrombocytopenia association

neonate as well as the one with congenital heart disease. Increased rate of glucose utilization, without hyperinsulinism, may explain the hypoglycemia seen in the perinatally stressed and asphyxiated neonate, cold-stressed neonate, and the neonate with congestive heart failure (e.g., hemodynamically significant patent ductus anteriosus and/or sepsis). The common thread in all these conditions is poor peripheral circulation and tissue perfusion associated with hypoxemia and lactic acidosis. This will lead to diminished mobilization of substrates as well as energy-inefficient anaerobic glycolysis. Neonatal hyperinsulinemic syndromes, including the infant of a diabetic mother, can be associated with significant and/or persistent neonatal hypoglycemia. Neonates may also be hypoglycemic because of deficits in intermediary metabolic pathways such as glycogen storage disease Type I, fructose 1,6 diphosphatase deficiency, or primary glucagon deficiency, reflecting a series of hereditary metabolic and endocrinological disorders in which hypoglycemia may be the initial or most obvious presenting feature (Vol. 1; Chap. 15).

PRETERM AGA NEONATES

The AGA neonates born before term may develop hypoglycemia. While the first report of this entity concerned small for GA neonates (19), it has long been documented that hypoglycemia also occurs in the LBW AGA neonate. In 1968, Raivio and Hallman

reported a frequency of 1.4% of hypoglycemia in these neonates (75). Fluge reported that as many as 14% of AGA neonates evidenced neonatal hypoglycemia (76). Transient neonatal hypoglycemia occurring in infants with no clear risk factors may have long-term effects on neurodevelopmental outcome (77).

The diminished oral and parenteral intake in the LBW neonate in combination with the decreased concentration of substrates may explain the lower plasma glucose seen in these neonates and their propensity to hypoglycemia. Indeed preterm infants remain at risk for the development of hypoglycemia once they are discharged home if a feeding is omitted or delayed (78). Functionally immature gluconeogenic and glycogenolytic enzyme systems present in the neonate potentiate these difficulties. The relatively increased size of the brain (13% of the body mass in the newborn vs. 2% in the adult) may be responsible for the greater proportion of glucose consumption during periods of fasting. This effect is magnified in the LBW neonate. However, there are a number of perinatal factors that influence hepatic glucose-6-phosphatase enzyme activity, including the mode of delivery and the presence of pathogenic bacteria in high vaginal bacterial swabs, among others (79). Hepatic glucose production is essential to maintain glucose homeostasis in newborns, though cortisol, corticotrophin, and epinephrine levels are higher in the infant with hypoglycemia, but insulin, glucagons, and growth hormone do not differ from normoglycemic infants (80). Infants born vaginally were found to have higher plasma resistin levels compared with those born by cesarean section (81). The association among resistin, leptin, and anthropometric indexes suggests that these hormones are gestationally related and that high resistin levels at term gestation are advantageous to the infant by promoting glucose production and preventing hypoglycemia (81). Resistin levels are also increased by the vaginal birth process.

SMALL FOR GESTATIONAL AGE INFANTS

Many centers have reported a relatively high frequency of hypoglycemia in SGA neonates ever since Cornblath et al. in 1959 described its occurrence in eight infants born to mothers with toxemia (19). Lubchenco and Bard (82), deLeeuw and deVries (83), and others have all substantiated the occurrence of hypoglycemia in these neonates. The neonatal management of the growth-restricted infant requires special consideration to a number of other significant morbidities in addition to hypoglycemia that are usually present in such neonates. The contribution of each of these may play a role in the alterations of glucose homeostasis that lead to hypoglycemia (84). The frequent comorbidities include asphyxia, meconium aspiration, respiratory distress syndrome, hypothermia, and polycythemia–hyperviscosity, among others. It has long been known that toxemia has been associated with hypoglycemia, and its incidence has been shown to be highest (61%) in neonates born to mothers with relatively low urinary estriol, compared to a frequency of 19% in neonates born to mothers with normal estriol levels (85). Reduction in energy reserves in the form of decreased glycogen deposition, combined with increased utilization of substrate, may account for the appearance of hypoglycemia.

Kliegman studied the effect of maternal nutritional deprivation on fetal/neonatal metabolism in dogs (86). Besides reduced fetal weight at term (251 ± 7 vs. 277 ± 7 g), the growth-retarded pups evidenced lower glucose concentrations after three, six, and nine hours of fasting, reduced plasma concentrations of FFAs at 9 and 24 hours, and lower ketone bodies at 24 hours compared to controls. Although the systemic rates of palmitate and alanine turnover were not affected, systemic glucose production was reduced for three to nine hours after birth, which resulted in the observed hypoglycemia. The investigator speculated that reduced rates of gluconeogenesis from alanine and reduced oxidation of fuels such as FFAs contributed to the hypoglycemia. FFA recycling to triglyceride rather than oxidation contributed to the observed hypoglycemia.

Plasma insulin and blood-glucose concentrations were measured in umbilical venous samples from 42 SGA and 68 AGA fetuses by cordocentesis at 17 to 38 weeks of gestation (87). In the AGA fetus, plasma insulin and the insulin/glucose ratio increased exponentially with gestation, suggesting maturation of the pancreas. The major determinant of fetal blood-glucose concentration was maternal blood-glucose concentration. The insulin/glucose ratio in the SGA fetuses was lower than in the AGA fetuses, suggesting that hypoinsulinemia in the former was the result of hypoglycemia and pancreatic dysfunction. The degree of SGA status did not correlate with plasma insulin or the insulin/glucose ratio, which suggested to the authors that insulin is not the primary determinant of fetal size.

However, the endocrine regulation of human fetal growth depends on the role of the mother, placenta, and fetus (88). The placenta is the site where growth-regulating hormones are processed, and placental transport responds as nutrient sensors (89). Elevated circulating insulin-like growth factor–binding protein-1 is sufficient to cause fetal growth restriction (90). The endocrine profile of children with intrauterine growth retardation is altered; there are low cortisol levels (91), and the serum adiponectin levels are decreased in subjects born small for GA, which determines insulin sensitivity (92). Although this effect in adiponectin production and its insulin sensitizing action remains to be elucidated at the molecular level, it strengthens the critical contribution of the adipose tissue in the metabolic complications associated with reduced fetal growth. In contrast, ghrelin in preterm and term newborns remains

relatively constant at birth, between 23 and 42 weeks of gestation, a phenomenon that may be beneficial to stimulate appetite and thereby to maintain blood sugar concentration during the most critical period when nutrients from the mother are abruptly terminated after birth (93).

Following bilateral maternal uterine artery ligation, Bussey et al. studied the sequential changes in plasma glucose, insulin, and glucagon concentrations, hepatic glycogen, and phosphoenolpyruvate carboxykinase (PEPCK) during the first four hours in growth-retarded rat pups (94). Hypoglycemia was noted in SGA pups compared to control (AGA pups), as well as reduced hepatic glycogen stores at birth. Plasma glucagon rose, but plasma insulin fell. PEPCK levels did not rise in either. The investigators concluded that SGA pups developed hypoglycemia because of limited glycogen stores and retarded gluconeogenesis. They speculated that delayed PEPCK induction in these animals may result from inadequate glycogen release at birth or decrease sensitivity to glucagon.

A number of studies have evaluated the intermediary metabolism of substrate available postnatally. A functional delay in the development of PEPCK, thought to be the rate-limiting enzyme of gluconeogenesis, in SGA neonates was suggested by Haymond et al. (95). This was substantiated by Williams et al., who studied the effect of oral alanine feeding on glucose homeostasis in the SGA neonate compared to AGA neonates (96). Oral alanine feeding enhanced plasma glucagon in both groups, but stimulated hepatic glucose output only in the AGA infants.

The effect of intravenously administered glucagon on plasma AAs has been evaluated in various types of neonates including the SGA neonate. SGA neonates in the first hours of life had significantly lower total AAs compared to a comparable group of AGA neonates, although the response to glucagon in the SGA neonates mimicked the control (AGA) group. It was speculated that the inability of the SGA neonate to extract specific gluconeogenic AAs could account for the susceptibility to hypoglycemia in these stressed neonates (97).

Twenty-five SGA neonates received 0.5 mg/day glucagon to treat hypoglycemia (98). Of the 25, 20 responded within three hours with a rise in blood-glucose to greater than 72 mg/dL. Five subsequently required hydrocortisone to maintain euglycemia. Rebound hypoglycemia occurred in nine, following discontinuation of the glucagon. The response was poor after maternal b-blockade. More recently, IV glucagon infusions were successful in the treatment of resistant neonatal hypoglycemia (99).

Mestyan et al. also evaluated the role of glucagon by measuring 17 AAs before and during glucagon infusion in normoglycemic and hypoglycemia SGA neonates (100). In the normoglycemic group, most AA concentrations declined significantly, but this did not occur in the SGA neonates who were hypoglycemic.

Although the effect was transient, these results reflect the ability of glucagon to produce acute changes in hepatic glucose homeostasis. This was demonstrated in neonatal lambs between one and three days of age with infusions of somatostatin alone, or which received insulin and glucagon during a two-hour interval. Plasma glucose concentration fell when both insulin and glucagon were suppressed acutely, suggesting that the latter is of importance in maintaining glucose concentration during short-term fasting. It was suggested that the ratio between the two hormones acutely affected glucose homeostasis (101).

The secretion of glucagon and insulin has been evaluated in SGA neonates. Both SGA and AGA neonates, after being fed oral glucose and protein (1 g/kg each after a four-hour fast), had similar secretion of both pancreatic hormones. The investigators speculated that the instability of glucose metabolism in the SGA neonate resulted from the rapid fall of glucose and probably because of a transient deficiency of hepatic gluconeogenic enzymes, but not from altered secretory patterns of the hormones (102).

The adequacy of the hormonal response was reinforced in a study of glucose-infused SGA neonates who were evaluated by stable isotope kinetic analysis. Under stimulation of glucose infusion, the SGA neonate and his AGA counterpart had similar regulatory responses as well as functional integrity in handling glucose during the second day after birth (103).

Using the newborn piglet model, Flecknell et al. studied the effects of an IV glucose infusion on glucose homeostasis in normal and growth-restricted newborn piglets using non–steady-state tracer technique (104). Suppression of hepatic glucose output was noted, but hyperglycemia (plasma glucose >180 mg/dL) developed in the majority of study subjects. The mechanism of the hyperglycemia was thought to be failure to increase glucose utilization in response to the glucose infusion.

The possibility of hormonal excess, producing growth retardation, has been emphasized by Ogata et al. (105). The investigators adapted methodology to produce maternal hyperinsulinemia in a rat model. This resulted in decreased concentrations of glucose and AAs in both the mother and the fetus, which produced retarded fetal growth, limited hepatic glycogen deposition, and delayed neonatal PEPCK induction.

Sann et al. evaluated the effect of hydrocortisone on IV glucose tolerance (1 gm/kg) in eight term SGA neonates compared to seven AGA neonates at mean of 41 hours of age (106). The rate of glucose disappearance was decreased in the SGA neonates compared to control neonates. Plasma glucose concentrations were similar in both groups, while plasma insulin concentration did not change in the control group. After hydrocortisone administration, plasma insulin concentration increased. The investigators concluded that hydrocortisone induced a reduced peripheral uptake of glucose independent of insulin secretion. Congenital isolated adrenocorticotropic hormone

deficiency has also been recognized as a cause of hypoglycemia and death in neonates (107). These patients carried TPIT genes mutations, which may be recognized in utero by measurements of maternal serum estriol levels during the third trimester of pregnancy. This is important in families with a history of infants who succumbed with hypoglycemia. Additionally the infant born to a mother who was on steroids during pregnancy may become hypoglycemic (Vol. 2; Chap. 8).

CONGENITAL HEART DISEASE/CONGESTIVE HEART FAILURE

Hypoglycemia is a frequent complication of critically ill patients requiring resuscitation care (108). Many years ago, Benzing et al. reported on a series of 27 patients in whom the simultaneous occurrence of hypoglycemia and acute congestive heart failure was noted in association with congenital heart disease (109,110). An inverse relationship has been noted between the concentration of cardiac glycogen and the level of maturity of the neonate, exemplified by the low levels in the offspring of mammalian species more mature at birth (i.e., human, monkey, sheep, etc.). These reserves are rapidly depleted during anoxia (111). Reduced dietary intake in association with diminished hepatic glycogen resulted in hypoglycemia. This has been further substantiated by Amatayakul et al., who noted the association of hypoglycemia with congestive heart failure in neonates without significant heart defects (110). The pathophysiology of hypoglycemia in cyanotic congenital heart disease was studied by Haymond et al. (112). Six subjects were evaluated between 13 and 67 months of age. Glucose and alanine turnover studies utilizing stable isotope labeling in these neonates were compared to controls. A subtle defect in hepatic extraction of gluconeogenic substrates was suspected, possibly secondary to decreased hepatic blood flow. It is apparent that the presence of either hypoglycemia or congestive heart failure should be considered when one or the other appears.

The interrelationship of hypoglycemia and pulmonary edema has been emphasized. Unfortunately, it was unclear whether the pulmonary edema was secondary to the hypoglycemia or due to treatment of the hypoglycemia, since D20W was administered through an umbilical venous catheter into a branch of the left pulmonary vein (113).

Nineteen neonates with symptomatic ventricular septal defect (VSD) were examined by means of an IV glucose tolerance test and compared to 14 neonates who were healthy (114). The VSD neonates were growth retarded with lower weight for age and length for age. Glucose tolerance was similar in both groups. Plasma insulin concentration was low in the VSD neonates, but insulin secretion, as measured by C-peptide concentration, was elevated. The authors speculated that increased insulin extraction occurs in the liver, but the mechanism was unknown. Hypoglycemia may also result as a complication of indomethacin therapy for patent ductus arteriosus in the very LBW (115).

PERINATAL STRESS/HYPOXIA

Neonates who utilize glucose at an increased rate may be prone to hypoglycemia. Because the LBW neonate is subject to hypoxia, the combination of decreased substrate availability and increased rate of utilization may result in hypoglycemia. An increased rate of anaerobic glycolysis in combination with an increased rate of glycogenolysis is probably the underlying biochemical mechanism. Two moles of adenosine triphosphate (ATP) are generated by the Embden–Meyerhof anaerobic pathway, whereas aerobic oxidation results in 36 moles of ATP; thus, 18 times more glucose is required to generate the same amount of ATP. In addition, increased lactate production may result in an associated acidosis. Beard has emphasized the association between hypoxia and hypoglycemia in the LBW neonate and noted increased metabolic needs out of proportion to substrate availability (116,117). The difficulties are all accentuated in neonates who are unable to replace substrate from the usual exogenous (oral) sources because of hypoxia or other clinical problems. Metabolic acidosis and lactic acidemia were noted during the first 24 hours of life in 4 term and 11 preterm neonates whose Apgar score had been 5 at one minute after birth and who were fed oral glucose loads (118). Thus, not only may endogenous stores be depleted but also these neonates may be unable to tolerate an exogenous load.

Another complication of perinatal stress is the presence of hyperinsulinism. In a report by Collins and Leonard, hyperinsulinism was noted unequivocally in three SGA neonates and in three who were asphyxiated (119). The cause of the hyperinsulinism was unclear. However, it is known that acute pulmonary edema may ensue with insulin overdose (120).

Jansen et al. undertook a further evaluation of the metabolic effects of neonatal asphyxia (121). Using a rat preparation, they showed that hypoxia drastically altered both metabolic fuel and glucoregulatory hormone availability. They suggested that persistence of the catecholamine surge and tissue hypoxia and acidosis are responsible for the transient surge in glucose and subsequent delay in decrease of insulin and increase of glucagon in the asphyxiated neonatal rat. That is consistent with the clinical observation that the asphyxiated neonate's initial glucose concentration may be elevated and falsely reassuring. However, it is not unusual for the neonate to drop glucose concentrations to significantly hypoglycemic levels soon after this initial surge. This emphasizes the importance of careful monitoring of the asphyxiated neonate's blood-glucose concentration in the first few hours of life, even if the initial values were reassuring.

COLD INJURY AND SEPSIS

Hypoglycemia has been identified in neonates who experience cold injury. Mann and Elliott described 14 neonates who suffered neonatal cold injury following prolonged exposure to environmental temperatures below 90°F (122). Marked hypoglycemia was documented in three of six neonates in whom it was measured. The hypoglycemia was presumed to be the result of FFA elevation secondary to a cold-induced norepinephrine response (123). Recognition of the potential association of hypoglycemia following cold stress should result in parenteral treatment, if necessary, in conjunction with warming of the neonate. In addition, this relationship needs to be considered in the evaluation of blood-glucose levels in neonates with either temperature instability or who are in a suboptimal thermal environment.

Close et al. evaluated the influence of environmental temperature on glucose tolerance and insulin response in the neonatal piglet (124). Temperatures were maintained at 17°C, 24°C, and 33°C during which an IV infusion of 1 g glucose/kg body weight was administered. Rectal temperatures were maintained in all of the piglets subjected to the two higher temperatures but not the lowest one in which 6 of 18 became hypothermic. A higher glucose disappearance rate was noted—KG: 2.00%/min and 2.32%/min was recorded for animals maintaining homeothermic temperatures during 17°C and 24°C temperature conditions compared to those kept at thermal neutrality (1.66%/min). The insulin response was comparable. During hypothermia, both KG: $0.76 \pm 0.12\%$/min and the insulin response were decreased. Glucose uptake by skeletal muscle was increased in environmentally cold-exposed homeothermic animals, resulting in an increased metabolic rate.

Neonatal sepsis has been identified with increased frequency in association with hypoglycemia. Yeung noted the association in 20 of 56 neonates with signs of sepsis (125). He suggested that inadequate caloric intake in these infected neonates may predispose to hypoglycemia. The possibility of an increased metabolic rate was considered, because these neonates were infused with 100 kcal/kg/day intravenously. A decreased rate of gluconeogenesis has been documented in laboratory animals following gram-negative bacterial infection (126). The possibility of increased peripheral utilization because of enhanced insulin sensitivity in sepsis has been considered (127). It is likely that one or more of these factors will operate to produce the resultant hypoglycemia. In an experimental model in rats given salmonella intraperitoneally leading to septic shock and hypoglycemia, polyclonal antitumor necrosis factor-a antibody ameliorated the hypoglycemia and lactic acidemia and reduced the mortality rates (128).

HYPERINSULINISM: THE INFANT OF THE DIABETIC MOTHER

Hypoglycemia following increased plasma insulin concentration has now been associated with several discrete disorders of the islets. It may be found in the infants of diabetic mothers, neonates with hemolytic diseases of the newborn, neonates with pancreatic nesidioblastosis, discrete or multiple islet cell adenomatosis, and neonates undergoing exchange transfusion. The Beckwith–Wiedemann syndrome should be considered along with other causes of hyperinsulinemic hypoglycemia, β-sympathomimetic treatment to the mother, following high umbilical artery catheter placement, and following maternal ethanol consumption.

The infant of the diabetic mother (IDM) is the premier metabolic example of the morbidity that may exist in the neonate secondary to maternal disease (i.e., diabetes). Although the IDM may have greater morbidity than the neonate of the nondiabetic woman, many infants of insulin-dependent diabetic women experience an uneventful clinical course, and even more infants of women with gestational diabetes do well (129,130).

The obstetric and diabetic care for pregnancy in diabetic women has improved over the years and this has resulted in better outcomes for both the mother and the infant. In theory, the more closely metabolically controlled the diabetic pregnant patient is, the greater the potential for producing a normal neonate. Since the early 1980s, it was shown that with improved control of the disease, the perinatal mortality, except for congenital anomalies, approached that for the neonate born to a nondiabetic mother (131,132). However, the improved maternal and fetal outcome of diabetic pregnancy is usually achieved in specialized centers caring for the diabetic mother, but problems arise when transfers occur midpregnancy (133). Recent reports continue to show that even in Western countries, spontaneous abortions may be as high as 17%, stillbirth's rates are five times higher, neonatal mortality 15 times greater, and that infant mortality might be trebled as a result of diabetic pregnancies (134). Additionally the pregnancy can complicate diabetes. Retinopathy and nephropathy may worsen (135,136), and preeclampsia and hypertension may worsen (137). Fetal monitoring and tight metabolic control of the diabetes are considered mandatory, but there are limitations to the predictive power of many fetal monitoring methods and a lack of randomized trials to assess the validity of the interventions and protocols for use in the context of the diabetic pregnancy (138). The best outcomes are usually achieved in diabetic women who undergo preconception planning and maximize their glycemic control before pregnancy (139–141). Preconception intervention is most beneficial as it positively impacts the critical periods of embryogenesis and organogenesis. Malformation rates dropped from 14% to 2.2%, and mortality rates dropped from 7% to 2%. Glycohemoglobin levels are lower in women who attend such programs and correlate with better glycemic control during conception.

Of special consideration is the pregnancy in adolescents with Type 1 diabetes mellitus. In these patients, medical intervention usually begins after the critical period of embryogenesis and organogenesis, as planned pregnancies are not relevant for most teenagers, and pregnancy is usually unintended (142,143). Additionally the burgeoning public health problem of overweight and obesity in children will likely result in an increased incidence of metabolic syndrome characterized by insulin resistance, gestational diabetes (144), and Type 2 diabetes (Vol. 1; Chaps. 9 and 11) with the undesirable consequences when pregnancy occurs (145). Knowledge of the character of the maternal diabetes, prior pregnancy history, and complications occurring during pregnancy allows the physician caring for the neonate to anticipate many of the potential fetal and neonatal complications that are reported in the IDM (Table 5). Macrosomia poses a major problem, ranging from 20% in gestational diabetes to 35% or more in pre-existing diabetes.

It is generally considered that good glycemic control of the diabetic women was not achieved or that good was not necessarily optimal when alterations occur in the offspring of a diabetic pregnancy.

Table 5 Neonatal Morbidities Associated with the Infant of the Diabetic Mother

Asphyxia
Birth injury
Caudal regression
Congenital anomalies
Double-outlet right ventricle
Heart failure
Hyperbilirubinemia
Hypocalcemia
Hypoglycemia
Hypomagnesemia
Increased blood volume
Macrosomia
Neurological instability
Organomegaly
Polycythemia and hyperviscosity
Renal vein thrombosis
Respiratory distress
Respiratory distress syndrome
Septal hypertrophy
Small left colon syndrome
Transient hematuria
Transposition of the great vessels
Truncus arteriosus

Note: In addition oculoauriculovertebral sequence abnormalities occur
Source: From Ref. 146.

Alternatively, it can be argued that there are other metabolic fuels, besides glucose operating at different developmental stages of pregnancy that account for the etiopathogenesis of the whole syndrome of the IDM. There has been increasing evidence to support the theory that, in addition to sugar, other metabolic fuels, from ketones to deranged lipid peroxidation, may be responsible for the pathogenic mechanisms of the congenital malformations, each playing a role at crucial periods during development (134). Multifactorial influences at critical gestational stages may also play a role in the development of macrosomia, respiratory complications, hypoglycemia, and the metabolic disturbances of the diabetic pregnant woman. Nonetheless a strict diabetes control begun as early as possible should always be implemented (147).

Factors known to influence the degree of hypoglycemia in the IDM include prior maternal glucose homeostasis and maternal glycemia during delivery. An inadequately controlled pregnant diabetic will have stimulated the fetal pancreas to synthesize excessive insulin, which may be readily released. Administration of IV dextrose during the intrapartum period, which results in maternal hyperglycemia (> 125 mg/dL), will be reflected in the fetus and will exaggerate the normal postdelivery fall in plasma glucose concentration. In addition, hypoglycemia may persist for 48 hours or may develop after 24 hours. Fetal hyperinsulinemia is associated with a suppressed concentration of plasma FFAs and/or variably diminished hepatic glucose production in the neonate (Fig. 9). Thus, not only is peripheral glucose utilization increased due to hyperinsulinemia, but hepatic glucose production is also diminished, and other energy substrates are lacking as well (129).

Other factors that may contribute to the development of hypoglycemia include defective counter-regulation by catecholamines and glucagon. The neonate exhibits transitional control of glucose metabolism, which suggests that a multiplicity of factors affects homeostasis. Many of the factors are similar to those that influence homeostasis in the adult. What is different in the neonate are the various stages of maturation that exist. Prior work in conjunction with glucose infusion studies can be summarized to suggest that there is blunted splanchnic (hepatic) responsiveness to insulin in the neonate both in the IDM and in the preterm and term neonate of the nondiabetic mother, compared to the adult (30).

Of particular interest are the many contrainsulin hormones that influence glucose metabolism. If insulin is the primary glucoregulatory hormone, then contrainsulin hormones assist in balancing the effect of insulin and other factors. In the IDM, the sympathoadrenal neural axis plays an important role. Many studies have evaluated epinephrine and norepinephrine concentrations in the IDM, and hypoglycemia may be secondary to an adrenal medullary exhaustion phenomenon (148). Elevated concentrations of epinephrine and norepinephrine were

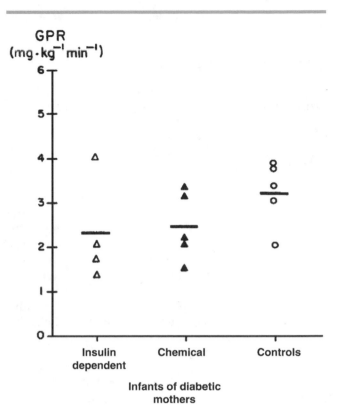

Figure 9 GPR for the infant of the diabetic mother (chemical- and insulin-dependent diabetic mothers) versus healthy control. The solid bar indicates the mean rate of production within each group. *Abbreviation*: GPR, glucose production rate. *Source*: From Ref. 30.

reported, although variation was markedly increased in the IDM. The investigators speculated that hypoglycemia after birth may be secondary to adrenal exhaustion, producing temporary depletion later in the neonatal period.

Other factors related to sympathoadrenal activity in the neonate may be of importance. In a continuing evaluation of the transitional nature of neonatal glucose metabolism, both of insulin and of contrainsulin factors, epinephrine was infused in two dosages (50 mg or 500 mg/kg/min) in a newborn lamb model, and glucose kinetics (turnover) were measured with [6-^{3}H]glucose. The newborn lamb showed a blunted response to the lower dosage of epinephrine infused. The investigators speculated that the newborn lamb evidenced blunted responsiveness to this important contrainsulin stimulus (149,150). It is possible that if this occurs in the diabetic state, it would partially account for the presence of hypoglycemia noted clinically.

Thus, the IDM is a prime example of the potential of glucose disequilibrium in the neonate. Because of the transitional nature of glucose homeostasis in the neonatal period in general, accentuation of the disequilibrium may be enhanced in the IDM secondary to metabolic alterations present in the diabetic mother.

A great deal of work is necessary to appreciate fully the operative mechanisms.

RH INCOMPATIBILITY AND HYPOGLYCEMIA

Hyperinsulinism has long been implicated as the cause of the hypoglycemia seen in neonates with severe Rh isoimmunization (151,152). These children are invariably severely affected by their disease, with profound anemia and hepatosplenomegaly at birth. The shock and collapse seen on occasion may be caused primarily by the profound hypoglycemia and, under such circumstances, glucose administration in addition to measures taken to correct the anemia may be critical. The IDM and severely Rh-affected neonate share several pathological hallmarks. In addition to the hyperinsulinism and islet cell hyperplasia, both show almost identical edematous placental changes. Both have excessive islands of extramedullary hematopoiesis in both liver and spleen. Although this latter finding may be the result of insulin stimulation, the precise cause of the hyperinsulinism itself in the Rh-affected neonate is uncertain. It has been suggested that an increase in reduced glutathione resulting from massive hemolysis of red blood cells may act as a stimulus to insulin release.

EXCHANGE TRANSFUSION AND UMBILICAL CATHETER

Hypoglycemia, although not often considered, may be a significant problem following exchange transfusion. In this connection, the exchange blood and its preservatives are more critically important in the neonate, in whom a double-volume washout is being undertaken, than in an adult who is receiving 450 mL the blood/preservative mixture to be diluted in a total 5 L or more solvent.

Heparinized blood contains no added glucose. Moreover, the heparin, by raising the FFA levels, contributes to the hypoglycemic potential of the transfusion blood, so that under some circumstances (e.g., severe Rh incompatibility with hyperinsulinism), its use would be contraindicated unless a concomitant IV glucose infusion is administered to prevent and/or treat hypoglycemia (153). With citrated blood, acid citrate dextrose or citrate phosphate dextrose, the added dextrose will yield a blood preservative mixture containing as much as 300 mg % glucose. In this situation, although immediate hypoglycemia is not a problem, the high glucose load may result in a reactive insulin response. This response lags behind the glucose infusion so that when the glucose bolus is suddenly terminated at the end of the exchange procedure, a state of hyperinsulinism ensues. Studies performed 40 years ago documented a precipitous two-hour postexchange fall in blood-glucose to levels below that prior to the exchange procedure (154). Once again, the severely Rh-affected neonate is at greatest risk, but even mildly affected and nonerythroblastotic neonates who undergo an exchange transfusion may respond in such a manner. Recognition of this possibility should lead to its detection and treatment.

Another cause of relative hyperinsulinism was reported secondary to malposition of an umbilical artery catheter. In a neonate requiring supplemental oxygen because of increasing respiratory distress, hypoglycemia was relieved only when a high catheter was repositioned from T11–T12 to L4. Following repositioning of the catheter, the child became euglycemic (155). Malik and Wilson reported on two neonates who developed hyperinsulinism secondary to malposition of the umbilical arterial catheter. Repositioning resulted in creation of the hyperinsulinemia (156). Puri et al. reported on the association of neonatal hypoglycemia associated with position of an umbilical catheter between the eighth and ninth thoracic vertebrae that is the normal position. In this report, the catheter was moved, and neonatal hypoglycemia resolved (157). Three neonates were reported, whose catheter were placed between the eighth and ninth thoracic vertebrae. They were noted to have hypoglycemia, which responded to catheter withdrawal to the third to fourth lumbar region. The investigators speculated that the cause was a high streaming of glucose to the celiac axis. The mechanism of the hypoglycemia was postulated to be excessive insulin secretion following infusion into the celiac axis (158). This was studied using a neonatal lamb model, and the clinical suspicion was confirmed. The mechanism was thought to be decreased production of hepatic glucose secondary to the presumed increased portal insulin, following high catheter placement (159).

Jacob and Davis studied differences in serum glucose concentrations from different extremities in neonates with umbilical arterial catheter through which dextrose was being infused. Neonates without catheter had no differences in simultaneous capillary glucose concentrations, obtained from both lower extremities, while neonates with catheters did. Neonates with a high catheter did not. As expected, the highest values were in those extremities into which the catheter was placed. This is another study pointing out the heterogeneity possible in glucose determinations depending on the location from which the blood is taken (160).

PERSISTENT HYPERINSULINEMIC HYPOGLYCEMIA

Persistent hyperinsulinemic hypoglycemia of infancy (PHHI) consists of persistent neonatal hyperinsulinemia for more than several weeks (Vol. 1; Chap. 15). Although the IDM is the premier example of hyperinsulinemia in the newborn, the hyperinsulinemia is usually transient and resolves after few or several days. PHHI is a heterogeneous group of disorders and has been given a number of different names in the medical literature (154,155): leucine-sensitive hypoglycemia, nesidioblastosis (161–163), β-cell hyperplasia, congenital hyperinsulinism, and discrete islet cell adenoma (164,165), or adenomatosis (166,167). The term "leucine-sensitive hypoglycemia" disappeared when leucine was found to function as an insulin secretagogue in patients with PHHI as well as in the healthy infant. Nesidioblastosis (meaning neoformation of islets) refers to the histological finding of newly formed islets budding from pancreatic ductal cells in histopathological specimens from patients who have PHHI. These findings explain the other names used in the literature to describe the syndrome of PHHI as discussed earlier. However, controlled studies have since shown that these histological findings are not unique to PHHI patients. Similar findings do exist in normal controls at different stages of maturation and are quite prominent in the term neonate (168).

PHHI is a heterogeneous disorder; it is characterized by hyperinsulinemic hypoglycemia and presents a varied clinical presentation, molecular biology, genetic etiology, and response to medical therapy (168). The biochemical profile includes hypoketotic, hypofattyacidemic hypoglycemia. Until recently, its pathophysiology was an enigma, although it was thought to be due to an anatomical abnormality of the islet of Langerhans, the so-called nesidioblastosis (169). Several distinct genetic forms of congenital hyperinsulinism have been described (170–172). Most cases are caused by mutations in genes coding for either of two subunits of the β-cell KATP channel (ABCC* and KCNJ11) (168). Two histological subtypes of the disease—diffuse and focal—have been described (Vol. 1; Chap. 15). Most patients share a common target protein, the ATP-sensitive K^+ channel, from gene defects in ion-channel subunits to defects in β-cell metabolism and anaplerosis (170). Until recently, congenital hyperinsulinism in infancy was considered an orphan disease, but now is known to share parallel defects in ion channels, enzymes, and metabolic pathways that give rise to diabetes and impaired insulin release. The treatment of these patients must be prompt and aggressive (171).

Both autosomal recessive and autosomal dominant forms of PHHI have been described (172,173). The autosomal recessive form is common in Saudi Arabia, with an incidence of 1:2675, most probably due to high rates of consanguinity in that country. Genetic mapping linked the disorder to chromosome 11p14 to 15.1 (172). This finding excluded the involvement of glucokinase gene in chromosome 7 and/or GLUT-2 gene on chromosome 3. Of particular interest was that both the insulin gene and the Beckwith–Wiedemann's gene are located on chromosome 11. In 1995, the sulfonylurea receptor (SUR) was cloned and mapped to chromosome 11p15 (174). Subsequently, some cases of PHHI were attributed to mutations in the SUR gene (175). Absence of KATP activity in the pancreatic β-cell has been documented in patients PHHI (176,177). The absence of this function was attributed in some cases to SUR mutations, but in other cases mutations other than that of the SUR (e.g., inward rectifier K^+ channel defect) were identified as well (177–179). Of clinical relevance is that patients with PHHI who have these two later mutations usually do not respond well to diazoxide therapy (180).

An autosomal dominant form of hyperinsulinism in infancy has been reported in several families (173). These patients usually have a milder variant of the disease than those with the autosomal recessive form. They often present after the neonatal period and respond well to diazoxide therapy. Treatment has been successfully discontinued after 2 to 14 years of therapy in many patients. A mutation of the glucokinase gene was reported in one family with an autosomal dominant variant of hyperinsulinism (181). Increased rate of insulin secretion was attributed to greater affinity of glucokinase for glucose, leading to higher rates of glycolysis.

Although rare in the neonatal period, insulin-secreting adenomas have been reported in cases of PHHI. They are usually resistant to diazoxide therapy. Focal adenomatous hyperplasia (FoPHHI) as well as diffuse β-cell hyperplasia (DiPHHI) has been described (182). Differentiating between these two variants of PHHI has important implications for therapy. Of interest in the cases of FoPHHI is that a paternal uniparental disomy was confirmed (183). In these cases, both alleles in the chromosome 11p15 region were found to be from a paternal origin with loss of maternal alleles. A similar defect was not found in cases of DiPHHI. It is also fascinating to know that uniparental paternal disomy was reported in some cases of Beckwith–Wiedemann syndrome (184).

Reports described several years ago showed the potential for hypoglycemia after b-sympathomimetic tocolytic therapy, which has been used increasingly to inhibit the premature onset of labor. A possible explanation of the relationship involves increased pancreatic secretion of insulin in response to a specific glucose concentration (185,186). A prospective double-bind study of 35 patients in preterm labor with and without ruptured membranes was conducted. Leake et al. evaluated the neonatal metabolic and cardiovascular effects of Ritodine administration to the mother (187). Patients received IV and/or oral ritodrine or a placebo. The shortest time from drug administration to delivery was six hours. No differences were noted in the Ritodrine versus the control groups relative to glucose and cardiovascular determinations. The investigators concluded that chronic oral administration did not significantly affect the neonate. In an investigation of the causes of the clinical situation, a neonatal lamb model was used to evaluate the drug (188). Administration of Ritodrine produced both increased insulin secretion from the β-cell and glucose production from the liver. It would follow that the presence of clinical hypoglycemia would depend on the time of administration prior to delivery. However, severe hyperinsulinemic hypoglycemia in infants born to mothers taking oral ritodrine therapy for preterm labor continues to be reported (189).

HYPOGLYCEMIA FOLLOWING MATERNAL ETHANOL CONSUMPTION AND MISCELLANEOUS CAUSES

The association between neonatal hypoglycemia and maternal ethanol ingestion has been known. Singh et al. evaluated glucose metabolism in neonatal rats exposed to maternal ethanol ingestion (190). Blood glucose concentration, liver glycogen, and plasma insulin concentrations were decreased in ethanol-treated mothers, as was litter size and average fetal body weight. The pups from ethanol-fed mothers evidenced hypoglycemia and hypoinsulinemia. Within one hour after birth, an elevation in blood-glucose concentration was followed by a decline to hypoglycemic concentrations. Liver glycogen stores were reduced and they were quickly mobilized. The hypoglycemic tendency in pups of ethanol-treated mothers disappeared after four days.

Witer-Janusek examined the effect of maternal ethanol ingestion on the maternal and neonatal glucose balance in a rat model (191). Controls included an isocaloric liquid pair–fed diet or ad libitum rat chow. Blood for glucose concentration and liver was sampled on days 21 to 22, and pups were studied up to 24 hours after birth. Ethanol depressed not only maternal liver glycogen stores, but also liver glycogen in the neonatal liver. Ethanol had no effect on plasma insulin concentrations. Postnatal hypoglycemia could be observed, following maternal ethanol ingestion. Singh et al. evaluated the combined effect of chronic ethanol ingestion in pregnant rats and three offspring (192). Fetal body weight and liver weight were reduced in fetuses of alcohol-fed mothers. Blood glucose concentrations were also lower, as was liver glycogen.

Isolated instances have been reported, which mimic insulin excess and resultant hypoglycemia. Zucker et al. have reported symptomatic neonatal hypoglycemia in association with maternal administration of chlorpropamide (193). This resulted in stimulation of both maternal and fetal β-cells. Because teratogenicity of the drug is a concern, its use is limited, especially since it provides poor control of glucose for the management of diabetes in pregnancy. Benzothiadiazide (thiazide) diuretics have been implicated in producing insulin secretion (194). It has been suggested that these drugs produce elevated maternal blood-glucose concentrations and result in stimulation of the fetal islets with subsequent neonatal hypoglycemia.

Neonatal hypoglycemia has followed administration of salicylates, the suggested mechanism being an uncoupling of mitochondrial oxidative phosphorylation (195). Actavia-Loria et al. reported a survey of the frequency of hypoglycemia in 165 children with primary adrenal insufficiency (196). Of these children, 118 had congenital adrenal hyperplasia, 47% had Addison's disease, and 18% had hypoglycemia. One-half of the episodes occurred in the neonatal period. The episodes of hypoglycemia were isolated in 13 children, 4 neonates with congenital adrenal hyperplasia, and in 1 male with 11B-OH deficiency. A significant mechanistic correlation was noted between plasma glucose concentration and cortisol concentration during the episodes of hypoglycemia (Vol. 2; Chaps. 8 and 9).

BECKWITH–WIEDEMANN SYNDROME

In 1964, Beckwith et al. described a syndrome characterized by omphalocele, muscular macroglossia, and visceromegaly (197). Wiedemann almost simultaneously described a similar clinical picture in three siblings (198). The cause of the syndrome remains unclear, though it has been described to be more prevalent in children conceived by invitro fertilization (IVF) (199). De novo DNA methylation on the maternal allele and the allele-specific acquisition of histone methylation lead to aberrant Igf2/H19 imprinting in IVF-derived ES cells. This has been suggested as the cause of imprinting errors that lead to the development of this syndrome and in patients with Angelman and Prader Willi syndrome. Abnormal DNA methylation accompanies imprinting of certain human genes on chromosome 11p15.5 in Beckwith–Wiedemann syndrome and Wilms' tumors and on chromosome 15q11 to 15q13 in the Prader Willi and Angelman syndromes (200). On pathologic examination, islet cell hyperplasia of the pancreas has been demonstrated in these neonates. It was subsequently shown that hypoglycemia may be an associated metabolic component of this syndrome, occurring in approximately 50% of cases reported, with hyperinsulinism responsible for both the hypoglycemia and the somatic and visceral growth abnormalities. The hypoglycemia is ultimately self-limiting, but may be protracted and difficult to control. In a patient with resistant hypoglycemia and hyperinsulinism, Schiff et al. (201) were ultimately able to achieve adequate control of glucose levels with a combination of Susphrine and diazoxide therapy, which suppressed the release of basal and postprandial insulin. The neonate presented at birth with an umbilical hernia, macroglossia, hepatosplenomegaly, and hyperinsulinism and severe, persistent hypoglycemia. Normal glucose control was achieved by one month of age. At six months, somatic growth was normal, hepatosplenomegaly had receded, but the macroglossia was still present. At two years of age, growth was normal, and the tongue, although still large, could be kept within the mouth without any evidence of malocclusion. Genetic mapping linked the disorder to a defect in chromosome 11p15, as noted earlier (184).

DEFECTIVE GLUCONEOGENESIS/GLYCOGENOLYSIS

Hypoglycemia has been noted in neonates unable to sustain normal gluconeogenesis. Glucagon is influential in hepatic glucose production because it enhances glycogenolysis and gluconeogenesis. An old report documented a neonate with isolated glucagon deficiency and neonatal hypoglycemia (202). The diagnosis was based on a low basal glucagon concentration as well as a diminished response to hypoglycemia and alanine infusion, both of which are potent stimulators of glucagon secretion, in a neonate in whom normal insulin secretion was present. Vidnes has reported three neonates with persistent neonatal hypoglycemia, one of whom evidenced an abnormal subcellular distribution of PEPCK in the extramitochondrial fraction (203,204). More recent reports documented glucagon deficiency (205) and were treated with glucagon given via subcutaneous infusion system (206).

Galactosemia may present in neonates who are septic and/or have hepatocellular jaundice. Later (one month), galactosemic infants may present with cataract formation. In some neonates, hypoglycemic symptoms have been reported, and a positive reducing test in the urine (to copper or iron) noted. The usual biochemical defect is in galactose-1-phosphate uridyl transferase. The diagnosis involves the demonstration of a low true glucose concentration (glucose oxidase) in the presence of normal total hexoses, together with the determination of the enzymatic defect, which can be analyzed in both red and white blood cells. Exclusion of milk and milk products (lactose) is the treatment of choice. Because early intervention is preventive, routine neonatal screening has been recommended, because it is inherited as an autosomal-recessive condition (207).

Hereditary fructose intolerance may be diagnosed in neonates who are old enough to ingest fruits or juices. The major intolerance is due to fructose-1-phosphate accumulation secondary to fructose-1-phosphate aldolase deficiency. The hypoglycemia is secondary to an inhibition of hepatic glucose release and absence of a hyperglycemic response to glucagons, following ingestion or parenteral administration of fructose (208).

In neonates, inborn errors of metabolism can produce all the major signs of liver dysfunction—jaundice, coagulopathy, splenomegaly, ascites, and encephalopathy. The significance of encephalopathy in the neonate is different from that of older children and adults; it is usually due to a specific abnormality such as hypoglycemia, rather than being a nonspecific indicator of liver failure (209). The neonate with an inborn error often presents with unconjugated hyperbilirubinemia, cholestatic jaundice with otherwise normal liver function, hepatomegaly with hypotonia, and cardiopathy (Vol. 1; Chap. 17). The prompt diagnosis may lead to specific treatment often with dramatic results, e.g., withdrawal of galactose in galactosemia. Inborn errors of AA metabolism, which may present as hypoglycemia in the neonatal period, include maple syrup urine disease, propionic acidemia,

methyl-malonic acidemia, tyrosinemia, and/or 3-hydroxy-3-methylglutaryl CoA lyase deficiency. Disorders of fatty acid metabolism, which may present as hypoglycemia in the neonatal period, include medium-chain and long-chain acyl CoA dehydrogenase deficiency (Vol. 1; Chap. 17).

Glycogen storage diseases that may affect gluconeogenesis in the neonate include Type I glycogen storage disease (glucose-6-phosphatase deficiency). The deficiency is an autosomal-recessive genetic defect, which may occasionally present in the neonatal period with severe hypoglycemia and hepatomegaly. A second enzymatic defect, fructose-1,6-diphosphatase deficiency, has also been associated with hypoglycemia. The details of these alterations are reviewed in other publications.

EVALUATION

Current perinatal clinical practice has significantly reduced hypoglycemia associated with conditions such as the use of glucose infusion during labor, erythroblastosis fetalis, double-volume exchange transfusion, cold stress, and delay of starting enteral feed in the larger neonate or glucose infusion in the LBW neonate. As noted with other diagnostic dilemmas in neonatology, a detailed maternal history and thorough physical examination are required to determine the probable cause of neonatal hypoglycemia. Maternal history including family history of diabetes or other glucose intolerance, drug ingestion (chloropropamide, benzothiadiazide diuretics, salicylates, and/or ethanol), blood group incompatibility, preeclampsia or pregnancy-induced hypertension, and the rate of dextrose administered to the mother during labor should alert the physician to the potential mechanism of the observed hypoglycemia.

A thorough physical examination of the neonate will indicate if the neonate is AGA, SGA, or LGA, as well as the GA. The appearance of the infant of the well-controlled diabetic mother of classes A, B, and C can usually be differentiated from that of the infant of classes D, E, and F (who may be SGA). The neonate with Beckwith–Wiedemann is usually obvious, with evidence of a protuberant tongue, umbilical hernia, and macrosomia. Prolonged jaundice and cataracts are suggestive of galactosemia, as are reducing substances in the urine, while unexplained hepatomegaly may indicate glycogen storage disease. Abnormalities, which may indicate central defects, include abnormal genitalia indicative of pituitary abnormalities and cleft lip and palate. Often the presence of an underlying defect is brought to the attention of the clinician by an abnormal metabolite detected through the neonatal screening program (Vol. 1; Chap. 17).

Treating the underlying condition, providing the optimal thermal environment, and supporting the cardiocirculatory system, if indicated, are basic concepts in the management of hypoglycemia. Appropriate laboratory evaluation should include the evaluation of the following: glucose, insulin, growth hormone, cortisol, and thyroid function. Evaluation of pH, lactate, pyruvate, and ketones is indicated for glycogen storage disease. Studies are usually performed when hypoglycemia is present or at a time following a fast of at least three to four hours. Tolerance tests are reserved for confirmation of suspected diagnosis such as a glucagon tolerance test if glycogen storage disease is suspected. Further details of the clinical evaluation of the child with hypoglycemia are in Vol. 1; Chap. 15.

TREATMENT

Treatment of neonatal hypoglycemia begins with the identification of its potential in the neonate at risk, documentation of its existence by appropriate laboratory measurement, and determination of appropriate corrective measures (210). Oral administration of nutrients generally is advocated, as either 5% dextrose or formula, in the neonate with mild hypoglycemia (glucose concentration 35–45 mg/dL). It should be used only in the neonate who is quickly able to achieve and maintain a glucose concentration in the euglycemic range during oral feedings. It is unreasonable to expect that oral feedings alone will provide for adequate glucose intake in the neonate whose hypoglycemia does not respond quickly to this approach.

In the case of moderate or severe hypoglycemia, we advocate parenteral (IV) treatment with a constant infusion pump to avoid fluctuations in the rate of infusion that would result in irregular rates of endogenous insulin release. Oral feedings should be allowed as tolerated, whenever clinically appropriate. Repeated documentation of blood or plasma glucose concentration should be an integral part of the treatment of any neonate. The glucose infusions should be gradually reduced rather than abruptly terminated, so that sudden reactive hypoglycemia is avoided. Once oral feedings are initiated, evaluation of the glucose concentration just before a subsequent feeding provides an analysis of the neonate's status.

Parenteral therapy should begin with 6 mg/kg/min followed by graded increases to achieve euglycemia with the minimal concentration of glucose required. A peripheral vein rather than an umbilical vessel is the preferred route of infusion (159). However, other than in an emergency, rates greater than 15 mg/kg/min should be given only when a central venous line is being used. Rates greater than 25 mg/kg/min are usually contraindicated by either route.

There is disagreement about the beneficial effect of a glucose bolus prior to the administration of continuous glucose infusion (211). Most authorities appropriately agree that there is no place for a large bolus (i.e., ≥500 mg/kg or 5 mL/kg D10W) in the treatment of hypoglycemia in the neonate, because of the high likelihood of pancreatic β-cell stimulation and rebound hypoglycemia (40). Some investigators (Lilien and Hawdon) recommend a so-called minibolus of 2 to 3 mL/kg D10W (i.e., 200–300 mg/kg) given at a rate of 1 mL/kg/min and followed by continuous glucose infusion at a rate of 5 to 8 mg/kg/min (Fig. 10) (210,211). The currently popular approach involves the infusion of 2 mL/kg 10% dextrose in H_2O (200 mg/kg) given over one minute, followed by a continuous dextrose infusion of 8 mg/kg/min. However, the concept of the minibolus was challenged based on the potential for hyperosmolar cerebral edema at that extremely rapid administration rate, as reported in older children (212). Additionally, at this high-administration rate, glucose entry far exceeds glucose uptake; the potential for provoking excessive insulin secretion and inhibition of glucagon secretion may, in fact, aggravate the existing hypoglycemia.

Based on this discussion, we recommend the use of a minibolus (200 mg/kg or 2 mL/kg D10W, over 5–10 minutes) only in cases of severe hypoglycemia (i.e., glucose concentration £ 24 mg/dL), followed by continuous glucose infusion at a rate of 6 to 8 mg/kg/min. For milder cases or for improving (i.e., partial correction after an initial bolus) hypoglycemia (i.e., glucose concentration of 25–45 mg/dL), a continuous glucose infusion alone at a rate of 5 to 8 mg/kg/min is an appropriate approach. In all cases, blood-glucose concentration should be closely monitored every 30 to 60 minutes, and glucose infusion rate should be gradually adjusted until hypoglycemia resolves. Calculation of parenteral glucose therapy must include the actual concentration of glucose present in the administered fluids. A hydrated form of dextrose ($C_6H_{12}O_6H_2O$) (molecular weight of 198) is used by most manufacturers to prepare the parenteral fluid, so that the actual amount of glucose available is approximately 10% less (213,214). This is

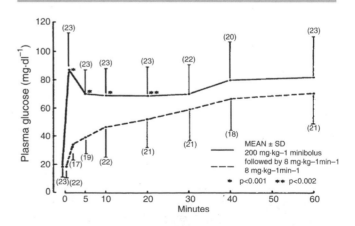

Figure 10 Plasma glucose concentrations in neonate treated with 200 mg/kg minibolus followed by 5 to 8 mg/kg/min constant infusion compared with plasma glucose concentrations treated with constant infusion alone. *Source*: From Ref. 211.

of particular concern when very LBW or severely hypoglycemic neonates are being treated. Lipid infusion is also used to assist in the prevention of hypoglycemia. Sann et al. evaluated the effect of oral lipid supplementation on the prevention of neonatal hypoglycemia in 28 LBW neonates whose mean GA was 36 ± 1 week and whose BW was 1778 ± 230 g compared to a control group of 23 neonates with comparable demographic data (215). Hypoglycemia < 31 mg/dL occurred in 8 of 23 neonates in the control group compared with 2 of 28 in the supplemented group receiving 2.9 g/day of a solution containing 67% medium-chain triglycerides. Prospectively, this study showed that lipid supplementation can prevent the occurrence of hypoglycemia in the LBW neonate.

A number of specific medications are usually recommended when continuous glucose infusion at a rate of greater than 15 mg/kg/min is not effective in maintaining euglycemia (40). Corticosteroids have been shown to be effective in the therapy of hypoglycemia. Although steroids enhance several glucose-producing reactions, the major effect is probably that of gluconeogenesis from noncarbohydrate (protein) sources and decreased peripheral glucose utilization. Hydrocortisone is given at a dosage of 5 mg/kg/day either intravenously or orally every 12 hours, or prednisone is used at a dosage of 2 mg/kg/day orally. As with all forms of steroid therapy, a gradual diminution of the dosage administered should be followed (Vol. 2; Chap. 8), in concert with decreasing parenteral concentrations of glucose and increasing oral intake of nutrients, should successfully allow for weaning.

The use of glucagon provides a highly effective method of releasing glycogen from the liver and can be a therapeutic means of assessing whether or not the liver contains adequate stores. Its failure in some growth-retarded neonates is considered to be evidence for a lack of hepatic glycogen stores (84). In the IDM, there is often a failure to respond to the usual dosages (30 mg/kg), despite the presence of more than adequate hepatic glycogen stores. These neonates will frequently respond to higher dosages (300 mg/kg) with a prolonged and sustained hyperglycemia, so that the higher dosage might well be used as initial therapy. Because glucagon may stimulate insulin release, its administration in all probability should be accompanied by an IV glucose infusion. The rate and risk of hypoglycemia in the large-for-age newborn infant of nondiabetic mothers is also high, and similar considerations to those infants of diabetic mothers should be followed for the treatment (216).

Like glucagon, epinephrine is capable of promoting glycogen to glucose conversion, but in far smaller quantities. For this effect, glucagon is the drug of choice. The hyperglycemic potential of epinephrine in blocking glucose uptake by peripheral muscle presupposes an adequate blood level initially and is of little practical benefit in the hypoglycemia state. Epinephrine is a powerful anti-insulin hormone, a fact that explains its success as an effective antihypoglycemic agent in the IDM as well as in other hyperinsulinemic neonates. The agent most commonly used is a 1:200 epinephrine in aqueous suspension (Sus-Phrine), which can be readily administered subcutaneously (201).

In cases of transient or persistent hyperinsulinism, diazoxide, Octreotide (217), calcium channel blockers, and/or partial pancreatectomy have been used as therapeutic modalities (Table 6).

It is important to summarize the metabolic signals that lead to insulin gene transcription and then insulin secretion by the pancreatic β-cell, so that the mechanism of action of these therapeutic agents may be understood. Glucose enters the β-cell via the GLUT-2 isoform of GLUTS. Glycolysis begins with glucokinase, which metabolizes glucose to glucose-6-phosphate. Further glycolysis, including interactions in the tricarboxylic acid (TCA) cycle, results in ATP production. AAs and FFA also contribute to ATP production through metabolism in the TCA cycle. Different intermediate signals from glycolysis lead to insulin gene transcription. Increase of the intracellular ATP/ADP ratio activates the SUR. The KATP channel then closes, the cell membrane depolarizes, and Ca^{2+} influx through the voltage-gated calcium channel (VGCC) triggers insulin secretion. Figure 11 depicts the metabolic signals involved in insulin production and the sites of action for various drugs used in the treatment of PHHI.

Diazoxide, in a dosage of 10 to 15 mg/kg/day divided every eight hours, is the first drug of choice in the hyperinsulinemic neonate who cannot be weaned from IV glucose. Diazoxide causes hyperglycemia by stabilizing the β-cell KATP channel in the open state, thereby inhibiting membrane depolarization and insulin secretion. An intact SUR and inward rectifier K^+ channel are necessary for full action of the drug. Insulin synthesis is uncompromised by this therapy. A secondary hyperglycemic mechanism is via stimulation of catecholamine; this may reduce insulin secretion and counter its actions peripherally as well. A response to diazoxide is usually evident within the first 48 hours of therapy. Diazoxide has several important side effects that should be carefully monitored; in some cases, the severity of these side effects may necessitate termination of diazoxide therapy. Fluid retention, hypertricosis, and coarse facial changes have been reported. Diazoxide therapy can result in hyperglycemia and even diabetic ketoacidosis, if the infant is unable to secrete insulin appropriately during time of stress. Uricemia, leukopenia, and thrombocytopenia are rare side effects of this therapy.

Diazoxide is effective in only 22% to 50% of the patients with PHHI, and it is less likely to work in patients presenting in the immediate neonatal period (218–221).

Table 6 Therapeutic Modalities for the Treatment of Infants and Children with PHHI

Therapy	Mechanism of action	Dosage	Efficacy and side effect
Diazoxide	Opens K_{ATP} channels	5–20 mg/kg/day orally every 8 h	*Effective in 22–50% of cases* Hypotension, fluid retention, hyperuricemia, hypertrichosis, coarse facial features, leukopenia, thrombocytopenia
Octreotide	Activates a G-protein-coupled inward rectifier K^+ channel	5–40 mg/kg/day subcutaneously every 4–6 h	*Effective in 25–80% of cases* Abdominal distention, steatorrhea, cholelithiasis, possible suppression of other hormones: growth hormone, thyroid-stimulating hormone, adrenocorticotropic hormone
Calcium channel blockers	Inhibits Ca^{2+} influx via voltage-gated calcium channels	Nifedipine 0.25–0.7 mg/kg/day orally every 8 h	*Case reports suggest efficacy* Potential hypotension, lack of long-term experience
Surgery	Reduction of β-cell mass	Surgical removal of 95% of the pancreas	*Indicated in cases of failure of medical therapy, effective in 75–95% of cases* *Immediate*: injury to the common bile duct and other surgical complications *Long term*: failure to achieve euglycemia; diabetes mellitus and exocrine pancreatic insufficiency

Somatostatin has a very short half-life (one to three minutes), which prohibits its clinical use. Somatostatin acts via a G-protein–coupled inward rectifier K^+ channel. The activation of this channel results in

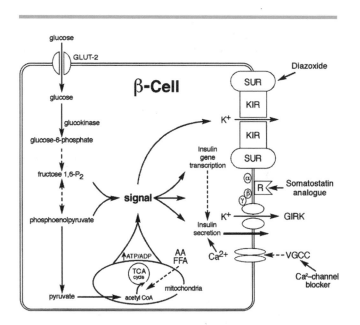

Figure 11 Metabolic signals involved in insulin gene transcription and insulin secretion in the β-cell. Dashed lines represent pathways with intermediate steps, GLUT-2, TCA cycle. The right side of the cell membrane represents the sites of action for various drugs used in the treatment of PHHI. Diazoxide binds to the SUR and opens the KIR. Somatostatin analogs bind to the somatostatin receptor (R) and activate a with its α, β, and γ sub units. These two drugs serve to hyperpolarize the β-cell membrane, which inhibits Ca^{2+} influx and therefore insulin secretion. Ca^{2+} channel blockers inhibit Ca^{2+} influx through VGCC. *Abbreviations*: GLUT-2, glucose transporter isoform 2; TCA, tricarboxylic acid; PHHI, persistent hyperinsulinemic hypoglycemia of infancy; SUR, sulfonylurea receptor; KIR, inward rectifier K^+ channel; GIRK, G-protein–coupled inward rectifier K^+ channel; VGCC, voltage-gated calcium channel; R, receptor; ATP, adenosine triphosphate; ADP, adenosine diphosphate; AA, amino acid; FFA, free fatty acid.

hyperpolarization of the β-cell, which inhibits Ca^{2+} influx, thereby inhibiting insulin release (Fig. 4). The synthetic analog octreotide, however, has a half-life of 1.5 hours, and it has been successfully used at intervals of up to six to eight hours in cases of hyperinsulinemia. A starting dosage of 5 to 10 mcg/kg/day produces favorable initial responses, but because of the development of tolerance, the dosage sometimes has to be increased to as much as 40 mcg/kg/day. Although Thornton et al. advocate octreotide use as an adjunct therapy during the pre- and postoperative period of partial pancreatectomy, Glaser et al. demonstrated that aggressive octreotide therapy alone was successful in almost 50% of the cases of PHHI that were resistant to other medical therapy (217,222). The side effects reported during the course of therapy include vomiting, steatorrhea, and abdominal distention; these were self-limiting within the initial few weeks of therapy (223). Asymptomatic cholelithiasis was reported, and concerns relative to the effect of octreotide on other hormonal axies require more careful evaluation.

Because Ca^{2+} influx is required for insulin secretion, calcium channel blockers have been used in the treatment of selective cases of hyperinsulinism. Although there are few encouraging case reports in the literature in which nifedipine was successfully used as adjunct therapy for PHHI, further experience is needed to assess the efficacy of this approach (224).

Surgical intervention is indicated when euglycemia cannot be maintained by medical therapy alone (Vol. 1; Chap. 15). A 95% pancreatectomy is the surgical procedure of choice. Medical therapy may need to be continued postoperatively, if hypoglycemia persists. If hypoglycemia persists despite added medical therapy, as is the case in 5% to 25% of the patients, a second surgery would be indicated to remove 99% of the pancreas. Risks associated with surgery other than failure to achieve euglycemia include injury to the common bile duct, exocrine pancreatic insufficiency, and diabetes mellitus. The latter may be transient or persist (225).

This review has evaluated the current knowledge of the kinetics of glucose homeostasis in the neonate. Glucose production, glucose utilization, and glucose oxidation have been reviewed in detail. The relationship of the developmental regulation of glucose homeostasis and some of the fundamental differences known to exist in the neonate were compared to the adult. The pathophysiological basis and the clinical aspects of neonatal hypoglycemia were discussed. Conditions associated with neonatal hyperinsulinemia, including the IDM, were also comprehensively reviewed (226,227).

REFERENCES

1. Cowett RM. Introduction. In: Cowett RM, Hay WW Jr., eds. The Micropremie: The Next Frontier. Report of the ninety-ninth Ross Conference on Pediatric Research. Columbus, OH: Ross Laboratories, 1990:1–3.
2. Farrag HM, Cowett RM. Glucose homeostasis in the micropremie. Clin Perinatol 2000; 27(1):1–22.
3. Cowett RM. Hypo and hyperglycemia in the newborn. In: Polin RA, Fox WW, eds. Neonatal and Fetal Medicine; Physiology and Pathophysiology. Philadelphia: WB Saunders, 1998:594–608.
4. Battagliia FC, Thureen PJ. Nutrition of the fetus and premature infant. Nutrition 1997; 13:903–906.
5. Ogata ES. Problems of glucose metabolism in the extremely-low birth weight infant. In: Cowett RM, Hay WW Jr., eds. The Micropremie: The Next Frontier. Report of the Ninety-Ninth Ross Conference on Pediatric Research. Columbus, OH: Ross Laboratories, 1990:55–63.
6. Cowett RM. Carbohydrate metabolism in the premature and compromised infant. In: Lebenthal E, ed. Textbook of Gastroenterology and Nutrition in Early Childhood. 2nd ed. New York: Raven Press, 1989:311–326.
7. Aynsley-Green A, Hawdon JM. Hypoglycemia in the neonate: current controversies. Acta Paediatr Jpn 1997; 39:S12–S16.
8. Flykanaka-Gauntenbein C. Hypoglycemia in childhood: long-term effects. Pediatr Endocrinol Rev 2004; suppl 3:530–536.
9. Cowett RM, Barcohana Y, Oh W. Human fetal and neonatal insulin response to maternal hyperglycemia at cesarean section (C/S). Pediatr Res 1981; 15:506A.
10. Srinivasan G, Pildes RS, Cattamanchi G. Plasma glucose values in normal neonates: a new look. J Pediatr 1986; 109:114–117.
11. Stanley CA, Anday EX, Baker L. Metabolic fuel and hormone response to fasting in newborn infants. Pediatrics 1979; 64:613–619.
12. William AF. Neonatal hypoglycemia: clinical and legal aspects. Semin Fetal Neonatal Med 2005; 10:363–368.
13. Williams AF. Hypoglycaemia of the newborn: a review. Bull WHO 1997; 75(3):261–290.
14. Koh T, Eyre JA, Aynsley-Green A. Neonatal hypoglycemia: the controversy regarding definition. Arch Dis Child 1988; 63:1386–1388.
15. Heck LJ, Erenburg A. Serum glucose levels in term neonates during the first 48 hours of life. J Pediatr 1987; 110:119–122.
16. Lucas A. Metabolic and endocrine responses to a milk feed in six-day-old term infants: differences between breast and cow's milk formula feeding. Acta Paediatr Scand 1981; 70:195–200.
17. Marconi AM, Paolini C, Buscaglia M, Zerbe G, Battaglia F, Pardi G. The impact of gestational age and fetal growth on the maternal-fetal glucose concentration difference. Obstet Gynecol 1996; 87:937–942.
18. Hawdon JM, Ward Platt MP, Aynsley-Green A. Patterns of metabolic adaptation for preterm and term infants in the first neonatal week. Arch Dis Child 1992; 67:357–365.
19. Cornblath M, Odell GB, Levin EY. Symptomatic neonatal hypoglycemia associated with toxemia of pregnancy. J Pediatr 1959; 55:545–562.
20. Koh T, Eyre JA, Aynsley-Green A. Neural dysfunction during hypoglycemia. Arch Dis Child 1988; 63:1353–1358.
21. Greisen G, Pryds O. Neonatal hypoglycaemia. Lancet 1989; 1:332–333.
22. Phillips DI, Barker DJ, Fall CH. Elevated plasma cortisol concentrations: a link between low birth weight and the insulin resistance syndrome? J Clin Endocrinol Metabol 1998; 83(3):757–760.
23. Lucas A, Morley R, Cole TJ. Adverse neurodevelopmental outcome of moderate neonatal hypoglycemia. Br Med J 1988; 297:1304–1308.
24. Lin HC, Maguire C, Oh W. Accuracy and reliability of glucose reflectance meters in the high risk neonate. J Pediatr 1989; 115:998–1000.
25. Holtrop PC, Madison KA, Kiechle FL. A comparison of chromagen test strip (Chemstrip bG) and serum glucose values in newborns. Am J Dis Childhood 1990; 144:183–185.
26. Rosenthal M, Ugele B, Lipowsky G Kuster H. The Accu-trend sensor glucose analyzer may not be adequate in bedside testing for neonatal hypoglycemia. Eur J Pediatr 2006; 165:99–103.
27. Michel A, Kuster H, Krebs A, Kadow I, Nauck, Fush C. Evaluation of the glucometer Elite XL device for screening for neonatal hypoglycemia. Eur J Pediatr 2005; 164:660–664.
28. Beardsall K, Oglyvy-Stuart AL, Ahluwalia J, Thompson M, Dunger DB. The continuous glucose monitoring sensor in neonatal intensive care. Arch Dis Child Fetal Neonatal Ed 2005; 90:F307–F310.
29. Bier DM. Methodology for the study of metabolism: kinetic techniques. In: Cowett RM, ed. Principles of Perinatal-Neonatal Metabolism. 2nd ed. New York: Springer-Verlag, 1998:3–15.
30. Cowett RM, Oh W, Schwartz R. Persistent glucose production during glucose infusion in the neonates. J Clin Invest 1983; 71:467–475.
31. Kalhan SC, Oliven A, King KC. Role of glucose in the regulation of endogenous glucose production in the human newborn. Pediatr Res 1986; 20:49–52.
32. Tyrala EE, Chen X, Boden G. Glucose metabolism in the infant weighing less than 1100 grams. J Pediatr 1994; 125:283–287.
33. Keshen T, Miller R, Jahoor F. Glucose production and gluconeogenesis are negatively related to body weight in mechanically ventilated, very low birth weight neonates. Pediatr Res 1997; 41:132–138.
34. Glamour TS, McCullough AJ, Sauer PJJ. Quantification of carbohydrate oxidation by respiratory gas exchange and isotopic tracers. Am J Physiol 1995; 258:E789–E796.
35. Jacot E, Defronzo A, Jequier E. The effect of hyperglycemia, hyperinsulinemia and route of glucose administration on glucose oxidation and glucose storage. Metabolism 1982; 31:922–930.
36. Sauer PJ, Van Aerde JEE, Pencharz PB. Glucose oxidation rates in newborn infants measured with indirect calorimetry and [U-13C] glucose. Clin Sci 1986; 70:587–593.

37. Farrag HM, Nawrath LM, Healey JE, Oh W, Cowett RM. Persistent glucose production and greater peripheral sensitivity to insulin in the neonate vs the adult. Am J Physiol 1997; 272:E86–E93.

38. Savich RD, Finley SL, Ogata ES. Intravenous lipid and amino acids briskly increase plasma glucose concentrations in small premature infants. Am J Perinat 1988; 5:201–205.

39. Bier DM, Leake RD, Haymond MW. Measurement of true glucose production rules in infancy and childhood with 6,6 dideutero glucose. Diabetes 1977; 26:1016–1023.

40. Cowett RM, Farrag HM. Neonatal glucose metabolism. In Cowet RM, ed., Principles of Perinatal Medicine. 2nd ed. New York, NY: Springer-Verlag, 1998:683–722.

41. Sunehag A, Gustafsson J, Ewald U. Very immature infants (≤30 wk) respond to glucose infusion with incomplete suppression of glucose production. Pediatr Res 1994; 36:550–555.

42. Vranic M. Banting lecture: glucose turnover: A key to. Am J Physiol 1992; 263:E102–E106.

43. Hertz DE, Karn CA, Liu YM, Denne S. Intravenous glucose suppresses glucose production but not proteolysis in extremely premature newborns. J Clin Invest 1993; 92:1752–1758.

44. Farrag HM, Hamill SA, Gelardi NL, Cowett RM. Hyperglycemic clamp studies of pancreatic Beta Cell sensitivity in the human preterm neonate. Pediatr Res 1999; 45:281A.

45. Farrag HM, Dorcus EJ, Cowett RM. Maturation of the glucose utilization response to insulin occurs before that of glucose production in the preterm neonate. Pediatr Res 1996; 39:308A.

46. Hay WW. Assessing the effect of disease on nutrition of the preterm infant. Clin Biochem 1996; 29:399–417.

47. Lane RH, Simmons RA. Hyperglycemia and other consequences of aggressive intravenous glucose administration. Semin Neonatal Nutr Metab 1997; 4:3–7.

48. Farrag HM, Nawrath LM, Dorcus EJ, Oh W, Cowett RM. 593. Ontogeny of glucose production and glucose oxidation in.

49. Simmons R. Glucose transporters: molecular, biochemical, and physiologic aspects. In: Cowett RM, ed. Principles of Perinatal-Neonatal Metabolism. 2nd ed. New York: Springer-Verlag, 1998:121–133.

50. Simmons RA, Flozak AS, Ogata ES. Glucose regulated Glut 1 function and expression in fetal rat lung and muscle in vitro. Endocrinology 1993; 132:2312–2318.

51. Simmons RA, Flozak AS, Ogata ES. Glut 1 gene expression in growth-retarded juvenile rats. Pediatr Res 1994; 35:382A.

52. Studelska DR, Campbell C, Pary S. Developmental expression of insulin-regulatable glucose transporter Glut 4. Am J Physiol 1992; 263:E102–E106.

53. Slot JW, Gevze HJ, Gigengack S. Immuno-localization of the insulin regulatable glucose transporter in brown adipose tissue of the rat. J Cell Biol 1991; 113:123–135.

54. Eriksson J, Koranyi L, Bourey R. Insulin resistance in type 2 (non-insulin-dependent) diabetic patients and their relatives is not associated with a defect in the expression of the insulin-responsive glucose transporter (Glut-4) gene in human skeletal muscle. Diabetologia 1992; 35:143–147.

55. Koranyi LI, Bouney RE, Vuorinen MH. Levels of skeletal muscle glucose transporter protein correlates with insulin-stimulated whole body glucose disposal in man. Diabetologia 1991; 34:763–765.

56. Hughes SJ. The role of reduced glucose transporter content and glucose metabolism in the immature secretory responses of fetal rat pancreatic islets. Diabetologia 1994; 37:134–140.

57. Vannucci RC. Perinatal brain metabolism. In: Polin RA, Fox WW, eds. Fetal and Neonatal Physiology. Philadelphia: WB Saunders, 1992:1510–1519.

58. Altman DI, Perlman JM, Volpe JJ. Cerebral oxygen metabolism in newborns. Pediatrics 1993; 92:99–104.

59. van Goudoever JB, Sulkers EJ, Chapman TE, Sauer P. Glucose kinetics and glucoregulatory hormone levels in ventilated preterm infants on the first day of life. Pediatr Res 1993; 33:583–589.

60. LaFeber HN, Sulkers EJ, Chapman TE, Sauer PJJ. Glucose production and oxidation in preterm infants during total parenteral nutrition. Pediatr Res 1990; 28:153–157.

61. Wolfe RR, O'Donell TF, Stone MD. Investigation of factors determining the optimal glucose infusion rate in total parenteral nutrition. Metabolism 1980; 29:892–900.

62. Yunis KA, Oh W, Kalhan S, Cowett RM. Glucose kinetics following administration of an intravenous fat emulsion to low birth weight neonates. Am J Physiol 1992; 283:E844–E849.

63. Pollak A, Cowett RM, Schwartz R, Oh W. Glucose disposal in low birth weight infants during steady state hyperglycemia: effects of exogenous insulin administration. Pediatrics 1978; 61:546–549.

64. Shelley HJ, Bassett JM. Control of carbohydrate metabolism in the fetus and newborn. Br Med Bull 1975; 31:37–43.

65. McGowan J. The role of glucose in cerebral function. Semin Neonatal Nutr Metab 1997; 4:2–3.

66. Denne SC, Kalhan SC. Glucose carbon recycling and oxidation in human newborns. Am J Physiol 1986; 251: E71–E77.

67. Fernandes J, Berger R, Smit GPA. Lactate as a cerebral metabolic fuel for glucose-6-phosphatase deficient children. Pediatr Res 1984; 18:335–339.

68. Levistky LL. Fasting plasma levels of glucose acetoacetate, D-hydroxybutyrate, glycerol and lactate in the baboon infant: correlation and cerebral uptake of substrates and oxygen. Pediatr Res 1977; 11:298–302.

69. Hernandez MJ, Vannucci RC, Salcedo A, Brennan RW. Cerebral blood flow and metabolism during hypoglycaemia in newborn dogs. J Neurochem 1980; 35:622–628.

70. Bougneres PF. Ketone body transport in the human neonate and infant. J Clin Invest 1986; 77:42–48.

71. Cornblath M. Neonatal hypoglycemia 30 years later: does it injure the brain? Historical summary and present challenges. Acta Paediatr Jpn 1997; 39(1):S7–S11.

72. Pryds O, Greisen G, Friis-Hansen B. Compensatory increase of CBF in preterm infants during hypoglycaemia. Acta Paediatr Scand 1988; 77:632–637.

73. Pryds O, Christensen NJ, Friis-Hansen B. Increased cerebral blood flow and plasma epinephrine in hypoglycemic preterm neonates. Pediatrics 1990; 85:172–176.

74. Skov L, Pryds O. Capillary recruitment for preservation of cerebral glucose influx in hypoglycemic preterm newborns: evidence for a glucose sensor? Pediatrics 1992; 90:193–195.

75. Raivio KO, Hallman N. Neonatal hypoglycemia: Occurrence of hypoglycemia in patients with various neonatal disorders. Acta Paediatr Scand 1968; 57:517–521.

76. Fluge G. Clinical aspects of neonatal hypoglycemia. Acta Paediatr Scand 1974; 63:826–832.

77. Dalgic N, Ergenekon E, Soysal S, Koc E, Atalay Y, Gucuyener K. Transient neonatal hypoglycemia—long-term effects on neurodevelopmental outcome. J Pediatr Endocrinol Metab 2002; 15:319–324.

78. Hume R, McGeechan A, Burchell A. Failure to detect preterm infants at risk of hypoglycemia before discharge. J Pediatr 1999; 134:499–502.

79. Hume R, McGeechan A, Burchell A. Perinatal factors influencing hepatic glucose-6-phosphatase enzyme activity. J Perinatol 2000; 20:301–306.

80. Hume R, Burchell A, Williams FI., Koh DK. Glucose homeostasis in the newborn. Early Hum Dev 2005; 81: 95–101. (Epub 2004 Nov 19).

81. Ng PC, Lee CH, Lam CW, Chan IH, Wong E, Fok TF. Resistin in preterm and term newborns: relation to anthropometry, leptin, and insulin. Pediatr Res 2005; 58: 725–730.

82. Lubchenco LO, Bard H. Incidence of hypoglycemia in newborn infants classified by birth weight and gestational age. Pediatrics 1971; 47:831–838.

83. deLeeuw R, deVries IL. Hypoglycemia in small for dates newborn infants. Pediatrics 1976; 58:18–22.

84. Yu VY, Upadhyay A. Neonatal management of the growth-restricted infant. Semin Fetal Neonatal Med 2004; 9:403–409.

85. Koivisto M, Jouppila P. Neonatal hypoglycemia and maternal toxaemia. Acta Paediatr Scand 1974; 63:743–749.

86. Kliegman R. Alterations of fasting glucose and fat metabolism in intrauterine growth retarded newborn dogs. Am J Physiol 1989; 256:E380–E385.

87. Economides DL, Proudler A, Nicolardes KH. Plasma insulin in appropriate and small for gestational age fetuses. Am J Obstet Gynecol 1989; 160:1091–1094.

88. Murphy VE, Smith R, Giles WB, Clifton VL. Endocrine regulation of human fetal growth: the role of the mother, placenta and fetus. Endocr Rev 2006 Jan 24; [Epub ahead of print].

89. Jansson T, Powell TL. Human placental transport in altered fetal growth: does the placenta function as a nutrient sensor? A review. Placenta 2006 Jan 24; [Epub ahead of print].

90. Watson CS, Bialek P, Anzo M, Khosravi J, Yee SP, Han VK. Elevated circulating insulin-like growth factor binding protein-1 is sufficient to cause fetal growth restriction. Endocrinology. 2006; 147:1175–1186. (Epub 2005 Nov 17).

91. Fattal-Valevski A, Toledano-Alhadef H, Golander A, Leitner Y, Harel S. Endocrine profile of children with intrauterine growth retardation. J Pediatr Endocrinol Metab 2005; 18:671–676.

92. Jaquet D, Deghmoun S, Chevenne D, Czernichow P, Levy-Marchal C. Low serum adiponectin levels in subjects born small for gestational age: impact on insulin sensitivity. Int J Obes (Lond) 2006; 30:83–87.

93. Ng PC, Lee CH, Lam CW, Chan IH, Wong E, Fok TF. Ghrelin in preterm and term newborns: relation to anthropometry, leptin and insulin. Clin Endocrinol (Oxf) 2005; 63:217–222.

94. Bussey ME, Finley S, LaBarbera A. Hypoglycemia in the newborn growth retarded rat delayed phosphoenol pyruvate carboxy kinase induction despite increased glucagon availability. Pediatr Res 1985; 19:363–367.

95. Haymond MW, Karl IE, Pagliara AS. Increased gluconeogenic substrate in the small gestation age infant. N Engl J Med 1974; 291:322–328.

96. Williams PR, Fiser RH Jr., Sperling MA. Effects of oral alanine feeding of blood glucose, plasma glucagon, and insulin concentrations in small for gestational age infants. N Engl J Med 1975; 292:612–614.

97. Reisner SH, Aranda JV, Colle E. The effect of intravenous glucagon on plasma amino acids in the newborn. Pediatr Res 1973; 7:184–191.

98. Carter PE, Lloyd DJ, Duffty P. Glucagon for hypoglycemia in infants small for gestational age. Arch Dis Child 1988; 63:1264–1266.

99. Miralles RE, Lodha A, Perlman M, Moore AM. Experience with intravenous glucagon infusions as a treatment for resistant neonatal hypoglycemia. Arch Pediatr Adolesc Med 2002; 156:999–1004.

100. Mestyan MJ, Schultz K, Soltesz G. The metabolic effects of glucagon infusion in normoglycemic and hypoglycemic small for gestational age infants. Changes in plasma amino acids. Acta Paediatr Acad Sci Hung 1976; 17:245–253.

101. Sperling MA, Grajwer L, Leake RD. Effects of somatostatin (SRIF) infusion on glucose homeostasis in newborn lambs: evidence for a significant role of glucagon. Pediatr Res 1977; 11:962–967.

102. Salle BL, Ruiton-Ugliengo A. Effects of oral glucose and protein load on plasma glucagon and insulin concentrations in small for gestational age infants. Pediatr Res 1977; 11:108–112.

103. Cowett RM, Susa JB, Oh W. Glucose kinetics in glucose infused small for gestational age infants. Pediatr Res 1984; 18:74–79.

104. Flecknell PA, Wootton R, Royston JP. Glucose homeostasis in the newborn: effects of an intravenous glucose infusion in normal and intrauterine growth retarded neonatal piglets. Biol Neonate 1987; 52:205–215.

105. Ogata ES, Paul RI, Finley SL. Limited maternal field availability due to hyperinsulinemia retards fetal growth and development in the rat. Pediatr Res 1987; 22:432–437.

106. Sann L, Morel Y, Lasne Y. Effect of hydrocortisone on intravenous glucose tolerance in small for gestational age infants. Helv Paediatr Acta 1983; 38:475–482.

107. Vallete-Kasic S, Brue T, Pulichino AM, et al. Congenital isolated adrenocorticotrophin deficiency: an underestimated cause of neonatal death, explained by TPIT gene mutations. J Clin Endocrinol Metab 2005; 90:1323–1331.

108. Losek JD. Hypoglycemia and the ABC'S (sugar) of pediatric resuscitation. Ann Emerg Med 2000; 35:43–46. Comment in: Ann Emerg Med 2000; 36:278–279.

109. Benzing G, Schubert W, Hug G. Simultaneous hypoglycemia and acute congestive heart failure. Circulation 1969; 40:209–216.

110. Amatayakul O, Cumming GR, Haworth JC. Association of hypoglycemia with cardiac enlargement and heart failure in newborn infants. Arch Dis Child 1970; 45:717–720.

111. Shelley HJ. Glycogen reserves and their changes at birth and in anoxia. Br Med Bull 1972; 17:137–143.

112. Haymond MW, Strauss AW, Arnold KJ. Glucose homeostasis in children with severe cyanotic heart disease. J Pediatr 1979; 95:220–227.

113. Kerkering KW, Robertson LW, Kodroff MB. Grand round. N Engl J Med 1967; 277:394–398.

114. Lindell KH, Sabel KG, Eriksson BD. Glucose metabolism and insulin secretion in infants with symptomatic ventricular septal defect. Acta Paediatr Scand 1989; 78: 620–626.

115. Hosono S, Ohono T, Kimoto H, Nagoshi R, Shimizu M, Nozawa M. Preventive management of hypoglycemia in very low-birthweight infants following indomethacin therapy for patent ductus arteriosus. Pediatr Int. 2001; 43:465–468.

116. Beard AG, Panos TC, Marasigan BV. Perinatal stress and the premature neonate. Effect of fluid and caloric deprivation on blood glucose. J Pediatr 1966; 68: 329–343.

117. Beard AG. Neonatal hypoglycemia. J Perinat Med 1975; 3:219–225.

118. Tejani N, Lifshitz F, Harper RG. The responses to an oral glucose load during convalescence from hypoxia in newborn infants. J Pediatr 1979; 94:792–796.

119. Collins JE, Leonard JV. Hyperinsulinism in the asphyxiated lamb. Metabolism 1988; 37:831–836.

120. Uchida D, Ohigashi S, Hikita S, Kitamura N, Motoyoshi M, Tatsuno I. Acute pulmonary edema caused by hypoglycemia due to insulin overdose. Intern Med 2004; 43: 1056–1059.

121. Jansen RD, Hayden MK, Ogata ES. Effects of asphyxia at birth on postnatal glucose regulation in the rat. J Dev Physiol 1984; 6:473–484.

122. Mann TP, Elliott RIK. Neonatal cold injury due to accidental exposure to cold. Lancet 1957; 1:229–234.

123. Schiff D, Stern L, Leduc J. Chemical thermogenesis in newborn infants: catecholamine excretion and the plasma nonesterified fatty acid response to cold exposure. Pediatrics 1966; 37:577–582.

124. Close WH, LeDividish J, Dulee PH. Influence of environmental temperature on glucose tolerance and insulin response in the newborn piglet. Biol Neonate 1985; 47: 84–91.

125. Yeung CY. Hypoglycemia in neonatal sepsis. J Pediatr 1970; 77:812–817.

126. LaNaoue KF, Mason AD Jr., Daniels JP. The impairment of glucogenesis by gram negative infection. Metabolism 1968; 17:606–611.

127. Yeung CY, Lee VMY, Yeung CM. Glucose disappearance rate in neonatal infection. J Pediatr 1973; 83:486–489.

128. Bhola M, Goto M, Chen HY, Myers TF. Effect of polyclonal anti-TNFalpha antibody on endotoxic shock in suckling rats. Biol Neonate 2000;78:207–211.

129. Cowett RM. The infant of the diabetic mother. In: Cowett RM, ed. Principles of Perinatal-Neonatal Metabolism, 2nd ed. New York: Springer-Verlag, 1998:1105–1129.

130. Kitzmiller JL, Cloberty IP, Younger MD. Diabetic pregnancy and perinatal morbidity. Am J Obstet Gynecol 1978; 131:560–568.

131. Jovanovic L, Druzin M, Peterson CM. Effects of euglycemia on the outcome of pregnancy in insulin-dependent diabetic women as compared with normal control subjects. Am J Med 1980; 68:105–112.

132. Pedersen J, Molsted-Pedersen L, Andersen B. Assessors of fetal perinatal mortality in diabetic pregnancy. Analyses of 1332 pregnancies in the Copenhagen series 1946–1972. Diabetes 1974; 23:302–305.

133. Hadden DR, Alexander A, McCance DR, Traub AI. Northern Ireland Diabetes Group; Ulster Obstetrical Society. Obstetric and diabetic care for pregnancy in diabetic women: 10 years outcome analysis, 1985–1995. Diabet Med 2001; 18:546–553.

134. Carrapato MR, Marcelino F. The infant of the diabetic mother: the critical developmental windows. Early Pregnancy 2001; 5:57–58.

135. The DCCT Research Group. Diabetes Care 1999; 23: 1084–1091.

136. Purdy LP, Hantsch CE, Molitch ME, et al. Effect of pregnancy on renal function in patients with moderate-to-severe diabetic renal insufficiency. Diabetes Care 1996; 19:1067–1074.

137. Yucesoy G, Ozkan S, Bodur H, et al. Maternal and perinatal outcome in pregnancies complicated with hypertensive disorder of pregnancy: a seven year experience of a tertiary care center. Arch Gynecol Obstet 2005; 273(1):43–49. Epub 2005 Apr 15.

138. Siddiqui F, James D. Fetal monitoring in type 1 diabetic pregnancies. Early Hum Dev 2003; 72:1–13.

139. Roland JM, Murphy HR, Ball V, Northcote-Wright J, Temple RC. The pregnancies of women with Type 2 diabetes: poor outcomes but opportunities for improvement. Diabet Med 2005; 22(12):1774–1777.

140. Rosenberg TJ, Garbers S, Lipkind H, Chiasson MA. Maternal obesity and diabetes as risk factors for adverse pregnancy outcomes: differences among 4 racial/ethnic groups. Am J Public Health 2005; 95(9):1545–1551.

141. Dunne F. Type 2 diabetes and pregnancy. Semin Fetal Neonatal Med 2005; 10(4):333–339.

142. McGrew MC, Shore WB. The problem of teenage pregnancy. 32:17–21 J Fam Pract 1991; 32(1):17–21, 25.

143. St James PJ, Younger MD, Hamilton BD, Waisbern SE. Unplanned pregnancies in young women with diabetes. An analysis of psychosocial factors. Diabetes Care 1993; 16:1572–1578.

144. Garcia-Carrapato MR. The Offspring of gestational diabetes. J Perinat Med 2003; 31:5–11.

145. Nold JL, Georgieff MK. Infants of diabetic mothers. Pediatr Clin North Am 2004; 51:619–37, viii.

146. Wang R, Martinez-Frias ML, Graham JM Jr. Infants of diabetic mothers are at increased risk for the oculo-auriculo-vertebral sequence: A case-based and case-control approach. J Pediatr 2002; 141:611–617.

147. The Diabetes Control and Complication Trial Research Group. Am J Obstet Gynecol 1996; 174:1343–1353.

148. Artel R, Platt LD, Kurnmula RK. Sympatho-adrenal activity in infants of diabetic mothers. Am J Obstet Gynecol 1982; 142:436–439.

149. Cowett RM. Decreased response to catecholamines in the newborn: effect on glucose kinetics in the lamb. Metabolism 1988; 37:736–740.

150. Cowett RM. Alpha adrenergic agonists stimulate neonatal glucose production less than beta adrenergic agonists in the lamb. 1988; 37:831–836.

151. Barrett CT, Oliver TK Jr. Hypoglycemia and hyperinsulinism in infants with erythroblastosis fetalis. N Engl J Med 1968; 278:1260–1263.

152. Molsted-Pedersen L, Trautner H, Jorgensen KR. Plasma insulin and K values during intravenous glucose tolerance test in newborn infants with erythroblatosis fetalis. Paediatr Scand 1973; 62:11–16.

153. Schiff D, Aranda JV, Chan G. Metabolic effects of exchange transfusions. Effect of citrated and of heparinized blood on glucose, non-esterified fatty acids, 2-(4 hydroxybenzeneazo) benzoic acid binding and insulin. J Pediatr 1971; 78:603–609.

154. Schiff D, Aranda JC, Colle E. Metabolic effects of exchange transfusion. Delayed hypoglycemia following exchange transfusion with citrated blood. J Pediatr 1971; 79:589–593.

155. Nagel JW, Sims JS, Aplin CE. Refractory hypoglycemia associated with a malpositioned umbilical artery catheter. Pediatrics 1979; 64:315–317.

156. Malik M, Wilson DP. Umbilical artery catheterization. A potential cause of refractory hypoglycemia. Clin Pediatr 1987; 26:181–182.

157. Puri AR, Alkalay AL, Pomerance JJ. Neonatal hypoglycemia associated with umbilical artery catheter positioned at eighth to ninth thoracic vertebrae. Am J Perinatol 1987; 4:195–197.

158. Carey BE, Zeilinger TC. Hypoglycemia due to high positioning of umbilical artery catheters. J Perinatol 1989; 9:407–410.

159. Cowett RM, Tenenbaum D, Fatoba O. The effects of glucose infusion above the celiac axis in the newborn lamb. Biol Neonate 1985; 47:179–185.

160. Jacob J, Davis RF. Differences in serum glucose determinations in infants with umbilical artery catheters. J Perinatol 1988; 8:40–42.

161. Heitz PU, Kloppel G, Hacki WH. Nesidioblastosis: the pathologic basis of persistent hyperinsulinemic hypoglycemia in infants. Diabetes 1977; 26:637–642.

162. Schwartz SS, Rich BH, Lucky AW. Familial nesidioblastosis: severe neonatal hypoglycemia in two families. Pediatrics 1979; 95:44–53.

163. Woo D, Scopes JW, Polak JM. Idiopathic hypoglycemia in situ with morphological evidence of nesidioblastosis of the pancreas. Arch Dis Child 1976; 51:528–531.

164. Baerentsen H. Case report: neonatal hypoglycemia due to an islet cell adenoma. Acta Paediatr Scand 1973; 62:207–210.

165. Burst NRM, Campbell JR, Castro A. Congenital islet cell adenoma causing hypoglycemia in a newborn. Pediatrics 1971; 47:605–610.

166. Habbick BJ, Cram RW, Miller KR. Neonatal hypoglycemia resulting from islet cell adenomatosis. Am J Dis Child 1977; 131:210–212.

167. Gruppuso PA, DeLuca F, O'Shea PA. Near total pancreatectomy for hyperinsulinism. Spontaneous remission or resultant diabetes. Acta Paediatr Scand 1985; 74:311–315.

168. Hussain K. Congenital hyperinsulinism. Semin Fetal Neonatal Med 2005; 10:369–370.

169. Hussain K, Aynsley-Green. A hyperinsulinaemic hypoglycemia in infancy and childhood-resolving enigma. J Pediatr Endocrinol Metab 2004; 17:1375–1384.

170. Dunne MJ, Cosgrove KE, Shepherd RM, Aynsley-Green A, Lindley KJ. Hyperinsulinism in infancy: from basic science to clinical disease. Physiol Rev 2004; 84:239–275.

171. Hussain K, Aynsley-Green A, Stanley CA. Medications used in the treatment of hypoglycemia due to congenital hyperinsulinism in infancy. Pediatr Endocrinol Rev 2004; 1(suppl 2):163–167.

172. Fournet JC, Junien C. The genetics of neonatal hyperinsulinism. Horm Res 2003; 59(suppl 1):30–34.

173. Thornton PS, Satin-Smith MS, Herold K. Familial hyperinsulinism with apparent autosomal dominant inheritance: clinical and genetic differences from the autosomal recessive variant. J Pediatr 1998; 132:9–14.

174. Aguilar-Bryan L, Nichols CG, Wechsler SW. Cloning of the β-cell high-affinity sulfonylurea receptor: a regulator of insulin secretion. Science 1995; 268:423–429.

175. Thomas PM, Cote GJ, Wohllk N. Mutations in the sulfonylurea receptor gene in familial persistent hyperinsulinemic hypoglycemia of infancy. Science 1995; 268:426–431.

176. Kane C, Shepherd RM, Squires PE. Loss of functional ATP channels in pancreatic β-cells causes persistent hyperinsulinemic hypoglycemia of infancy. Nat Med 1996; 2:1344–1348.

177. Nestorowicz A, Wilson BA, Schoor KP. Mutations in the sulfonylurea receptor gene are associated with familial hyperinsulinism in Ashkenazi Jews. Hum Mol Genet 1996; 5:1813–1818.

178. Dunne MJ, Kane C, Shepherd RM. Familial persistent hyperinsulinemic hypoglycemia of infancy and mutations in the sulfonylurea receptor. N Engl J Med 1997; 336:703–708.

179. Suzuki M, Fujikura K, Inagaki N. Localization of the ATP-sensitive K+ channel subunit Kir6.2 in mouse pancreas. Diabetes 1997; 46:1440–1445.

180. Nichols CG, Shyng SL, Nestorowicz A. Adenosine diphosphate as an intracellular regulator of insulin secretion. Science 1996; 272:1785–1790.

181. Glaser B, Kesavan P, Heyman M. Familial hyperinsulinism caused by an activating glucokinase mutation. N Engl J Med 1998; 338:226–231.

182. Dubois J, Brunelle F, Touati G. Hyperinsulinism in children: diagnostic value of pancreatic venous sampling correlated with clinical, pathological and surgical outcome in 25 cases. Pediatr Radiol 1995; 25:512–517.

183. de Lonlay P, Foumet JC, Rahier J. Somatic deletion of the imprinted 11p15 region in sporadic persistent hyperinsulinemic hypoglycemia of infancy is specific of focal adenomatous hyperplasia and endorses partial pancreatectomy. J Clin Invest 1997; 100:802–806.

184. Weksberg R, Shen OR, Fei YL. Disruption of insulin-like growth factor 2 imprinting in Beckwith-Wiedemann syndrome. Nat Genet 1993; 5:143–147.

185. Epstein MF, Nicholls E, Stubblefield PG. Neonatal hypoglycemia after beta-sympathomimetic tocolytic therapy. J Pediatr 1979; 94:449–453.

186. Procianoy RS, Pinheiro CEA. Neonatal hyperinsulinism after short term maternal beta sympathomimetic therapy. J Pediatr 1982; 101:612–614.

187. Leake RD, Hobel CJ, Okada DM. Neonatal metabolic effects of oral retodrine hypochloride administration. Pediatr Pharm 1983; 3:101–106.

188. Tenenbaum D, Cowett RM. The mechanisms of beta sympathomimetic action on neonatal glucose homeostasis in the lamb. J Pediatr 1985; 107:588–592.

189. Kurtoglu S, Akcakus M, Keskin M, Ozcan A, Hussain K. Severe hyperinsulinaemic hypoglycemia in a baby born to a mother taking oral ritodrine therapy for preterm labor. Horm Res 2005; 64:61–63.

190. Singh SP, Sayder AK, Singh SF. Effects of ethanol ingestion on maternal and fetal glucose homeostasis. J Lab Clin Med 1984; 104:176–184.

191. Witer-Janusek L. Maternal ethanol ingestion: effect on maternal and neonatal glucose balance. Am J Physiol 1986; 251:E178–E184.

192. Singh SP, Snyder AK, Pullen GL. Fetal alcohol syndrome: glucose and liver metabolism in term rat fetus and neonate. Alcoholism 1986; 10:54–58.

193. Zucker P, Simon G. Prolonged symptomatic neonatal hypoglycemia associated with maternal chloropropamide therapy. Pediatrics 1968; 42:824–825.

194. Senior B, Slone D, Shapiro S. Benzothiadiazides and neonatal hypoglycemia. Lancet 1976; 2:377–381.

195. Pickering D. Neonatal hypoglycemia due to salicylate poisoning. Proc R Soc Med 1968; 61:1256.

196. Actavia-Loria E, Chaussain JL, Bougneres PF. Frequency of hypoglycemia in children with adrenal insufficiency. Acta Endocrinol Suppl (Copenh) 1986; 279:275–278.

197. Beckwith JB, Wang CI, Donel GN. Hyperplastic fetal visceromegaly with macroglossia, omphalocele, cytomegaly of adrenal fetal cortex, postnatal somatic gigantism, and other abnormalities. Newly recognized syndrome. Proceedings, American Pediatrics Society, Seattle, 1964, June 16–18 (abstr 41).

198. Wiedemann HR. Complexe malformatif familiale avec hernie ombilicale et macroglossie un syndrome nouveau? J Genet Hum 1964; 13:223–225.

199. Li T, Vu TH, Ulaner GA, Littman E, Ling JQ, Chen HL, Hu JF, Behr B, Giudice L, Hoffman ARIVF results in de novo DNA methylation and histone methylation at an Igf2-H19 imprinting epigenetic switch. Mol Hum Reprod. 2005; 11:631–40. Epub 2005 Oct.

200. Tycko B. DNA methylation in genomic imprinting. Mutat Res 1997; 386:131–140. Comment in Mutat Res 1997; 386):103–105.

201. Schiff D, Colle EC, Wells D. Metabolic aspects of the Beckwith-Wiedemann syndrome. J Pediatr 1973; 82:258–267.

202. Vidnes J, Oyasaeter S. Glucagon deficiency causing severe neonatal hypoglycemia in a patient with normal insulin secretion. Pediatr Res 1977; 11:943–949.

203. Vidnes J, Sovik O. Gluconeogenesis in infancy and childhood. Studies on the glucose production from alanine in three cases of persistent neonatal hypoglycaemia. Acta Paediatr Scand 1976; 65:297–305.

204. Vidnes J, Sovik O. Gluconeogenesis in infancy and childhood. Deficiency of the extramitochondrial form of hepatic phosphoenolpyruvate carboxykinase in a case of persistent neonatal hypoglycemia. Acta Paediatr 1976; 65:307–312.

205. Davidson MB. Glucagon deficiency associated with hypoglycaemia. Diabetologia 1984; 26:473.

206. Abs R, Verbist L, Moeremans M, Blockx P, DeLeeuw I, Bekaert J. Hypoglycemia owing to inappropriate glucagon secretion treated with a continuous subcutaneous glucagon infusion system. Acta Endocrinol 1990; 122:319–322.

207. Levy HL, Hammersen G. Newborn screening for galactosemia and other galactose metabolic defects. J Pediatr 1978; 92:871–878.

208. Baerlocher K, Gitzelmann R, Steinmann B, Gitzelmann-Cumarasamy N. Hereditary fructose intolerance in early childhood: a major diagnostic challenge. Survey of 20 symptomatic cases. Helv Paediatr Acta 1978; 33:465–487.

209. Clayton PT. Inborn errors presenting with liver dysfunction. Semin Neonatol 2002; 7:49–63.

210. Hawdon JM, Ward Platt M, Aynsley Green A. Prevention and management of neonatal hypoglycaemia. Arch Dis Childh 1994; 70:F60–F65.

211. Lilien LD. Treatment of neonatal hypoglycemia with minibolus and intravenous glucose infusion. J Pediatr 1980; 97:295–298.

212. Settergren G, Lindblad BS, Persson B. Cerebral blood flow and exchange of oxygen, glucose, ketone bodies, lactate, pyruvate and amino acids in infants. Acta Paediatr Scand 1976; 65:343–353.

213. Mehta A. Prevention and management of neonatal hypoglycaemia. Arch Dis Childhood 1994; 70:F54–F59.

214. Cowett RM, Susa JB, Schwartz R. Concentration of parenteral glucose solution. Pediatrics 1977; 59:791–794.

215. Sann L, Mousson B, Rousson M. Prevention of neonatal hypoglycemia by oral lipid supplementation in low birth weight infants. Eur J Pediatr 1988; 147:158–161.

216. Schaefer-Graf UM, Rossi R, Buhrer C, et al. Rate and risk factors if hypoglycemia in large-or-gestational-age newborn infants and nondiabetic mothers. Am J Obst Gynecol 2002; 187:913–917.

217. Glaser B, Hirsch HJ, Landau H. Persistent hyperinsulinemic hypoglycemia of infancy: long-term Octreotide treatment without pancreatectomy. J Pediatr 1993; 123:644–651.

218. Grant DB, Dunger DB, Burns EC. Long-term treatment with diazoxide in childhood hyperinsulinism. Acta Endocrinol Suppl (Copenh) 1986; 279:340–344.

219. Labrune P, Bonnefont JP, Nihoul-Fekete C. Evaluation of diagnostic and therapeutic methods in hyperinsulinism in newborn infants and infants. Apropos of a retrospective study of 26 cases. Arch Fr Pediatr 1989; 46:167–173.

220. Thornton PS, Sumner AE, Ruchelli ED. Familial and sporadic hyperinsulinism: histopathologic findings and segregation analysis support a single autosomal recessive disorder. J Pediatr 1991; 119:721–728.

221. Woolf OA, Leonard IV, Trembath RC. Nesidioblastosis: evidence for autosomal recessive inheritance. Arch Dis Child 1991; 66:529–534.

222. Thornton PS, Alter CA, Katz LE. Short-and long-term use of octreotide in the treatment of congenital hyperinsulinism. J Pediatr 1993; 123:637–642.

223. Stanley CA. Hyperinsulinism in infants and children. Pediatr Clin North Am 1997; 44:363–377.

224. Lindley K, Dunne MJ, Kane C. Ionic control of β-cell function in nesidioblastosis: a possible therapeutic role for calcium channel blockade. Arch Dis Child 1996; 74:373–377.

225. Leibowitz G, Glaser B, Higazi AA. Hyperinsulinemic hypoglycemia of infancy (nesidioblastosis) in clinical remission: high incidence of diabetes mellitus and persistent β-cell dysfunction at long-term follow-up. J Clin Endocrinol Metab 1995; 80:386–393.

226. Permutt MA, Nestorowicz A, Glaser B. Familial hyperinsulinism: An inherited disorder of spontaneous hypoglycemia in neonates and infants. Diabetes Rev 1996; 4:347–353.

227. Milner RD. Nesidioblastosis unraveled [comment]. Arch Dis Child 1996; 74:369.

17

Emergencies of Inborn Metabolic Disease

Jose E. Abdenur

Division of Metabolism, PSF-Children's Hospital of Orange County, Orange, California, U.S.A.

INTRODUCTION

Baby JO was born full term, after an uneventful pregnancy and delivery. He had a normal physical examination and was discharged home at 36 hours of age. Twelve hours later, the mother noted poor sucking and a weak cry. He was brought to the hospital and found to be lethargic. A sepsis work-up was performed and, as a blood gas revealed respiratory alkalosis, an ammonium level was obtained. The value was 1600 mM (normal up to 80). Blood for plasma amino-acids (AAs) was sent out and he was treated with sodium benzoate, sodium phenylacetate, arginine, and a high glucose infusion. Citrulline levels were 2300 mM and arginine dose was adjusted for the treatment of argininosuccinic acid synthetase (AS) deficiency. The patient improved and was discharged after two weeks on a special diet. The family history of JO revealed that a brother had died at five days of age. He had also presented with poor suck and lethargy early in life, was admitted into a hospital, had seizures, and lapsed into coma. The diagnosis was sepsis.

This story shows two dramatically different outcomes for two siblings who had the same disease. Inborn metabolic diseases (IMDs) are a group of genetic disorders in which there is a block in a metabolic pathway. They are usually the product of a single gene defect that affects the activity of an enzyme either directly or through abnormalities in its cofactors or activating proteins. IMD comprise a variety of disorders affecting the metabolism of small (i.e., AAs) or large molecules (i.e., sphingolipids). Many patients present with a catastrophic collapse in the neonatal period. However, the age and clinical presentation of IMD are highly variable. Therefore a disease-free period of months or years, or a subacute presentation does not rule out the possibility of an IMD (1). A variable phenotype can be seen in patients with the same enzyme deficiency, and clinical heterogeneity has even been observed between siblings carrying the same mutations. Nevertheless, when possible, the molecular defect of a patient should be identified. This information is useful for prenatal diagnosis and, in some cases, may allow predicting the clinical course of the disease (genotype–phenotype correlation), helping to find the best therapeutic option for each individual.

The increasing availability of newborn screening (NBS) programs using tandem mass spectrometry (TMS) allows presymptomatic diagnosis and early treatment of affected children, changing what we know today as the natural course of the disease (2).

A complete description of the different IMD can be found in excellent textbooks (3,4). In this chapter, we will describe the most common IMD that can present with acute, life-threatening illness, focusing on the diagnosis and treatment of these emergencies.

UREA CYCLE DEFECTS

Pathophysiology: The Urea Cycle

High ammonium levels can be found in a variety of diseases, but the most severe causes of hyperammonemia are the urea cycle defects (UCDs) (Table 1).

The urea cycle prevents the toxic accumulation of ammonium and other nitrogen compounds by incorporating nitrogen not used for protein synthesis into urea. Each molecule of urea contains two atoms of waste nitrogen, one derived from ammonia and the other from aspartate (Fig. 1) (5,6). The urea cycle is also responsible for the biosynthesis of arginine. Abnormalities in the urea cycle produce hyperammonemia and elevation of glutamine. The former may have a deleterious effect on the central nervous system (CNS) through different mechanisms, including alteration in trafficking of AAs and monoamines between neurons and astrocytes, and deficit in cerebral energy metabolism due to inhibition of 2-ketoglutarate-dehydrogenase (5–8). Additionally, high levels of glutamine produce an intracellular osmotic effect with secondary swelling of astrocytes and increased intracranial pressure, leading to cerebral edema encephalopathy (5,7–10).

There are five enzymes involved in the urea cycle: carbamylphosphate synthetase (CPS), ornithine transcarbamylase (OTC), arginosuccinic acid synthetase (AS), argininosuccinic acid lyase (AL), and arginase (Fig. 1). As *N*-acetylglutamate (NAG) is required for the activity of CPS, the enzyme

Table 1 Causes of Hyperammonemia

Inborn errors of metabolism
  Urea cycle defects
    N-acetylglutamate synthetase deficiency
    Carbamylphosphate synthetase deficiency
    Ornithine transcarbamylase deficiency
    Argininosuccinic acid synthetase deficiency
    Argininosuccinic acid lyase deficiency
    Arginase deficiency
  Organic acidemias
    Propionic acidemia, methylmalonic acidemia,
      isovaleric acidemia and others.
  Fatty acid oxidation defects
    Medium-chain acyl-CoA-dehydrogenase deficiency,
      long-chain 3-hydroxyacyl-CoA-dehydrogenase and others.
  Transport defects of urea cycle intermediates
    Citrin deficiency
    Lysinuric protein intolerance
    Hyperammoniemia–hyperornithinemia–homocitrullinuria syndrome
  Mitochondrial diseases
    Mitochondrial DNA depletion, and others
  Pyruvate carboxylase deficiency(neonatal form)
  Hepatic glutamine synthetase deficiency
  Glutamate dehydrogenase hyperactivity
    (hyperamonemia and hyperinsulinism)
Acquired
  Transient hyperammonemia of the newborn
  Muscular hyperactivity (seizures, respiratory distress syndrome)
  Infections with urease positive bacteria (skin, intestine, urinary tract)
  Asparaginase treatment
  Deficient arginine supply in diet
  Valproate and other anticonvulsants treatment
  Hepatocellular carcinoma
  Liver insufficiency
    Reye's syndrome, infections, intoxication, etc.
  Portocavashunt (liver bypass)
    Vascular malformations, cirrhosis

responsible for NAG biosynthesis (NAG synthetase) is also considered to be a part of the pathway (5,6). Defects for each of these enzymes have been described. Except for OTC deficiency, which is X linked, inheritance in all UCD is autosomal recessive.

Clinical Presentation

Neonatal Form

Patients with UCD can present with symptoms from birth to adulthood. The neonatal presentation is the most common and is due to a complete deficiency of NAGS, CPS, OTC, AS, or AL, which have almost identical clinical expression (5,6,11). These patients are usually full term and have a normal physical exam at birth. Between the first 24 and 72 hours, depending on protein intake, the neonate presents with poor suck, vomiting and hypotonia followed by lethargy, seizures, vasomotor instability, hypothermia, and coma. Slight liver enlargement and hyperventilation are also constant findings. AS-deficient patients may present with hypertonicity and trismus, and pulmonary hemorrhage has been described as a complication of OTC deficiency (6). If hyperammonemia is not detected, the patient might die with a suspected diagnosis of sepsis, respiratory distress, and/or intracranial bleeding (5,6).

Late-Onset Form

Clinical presentation beyond the neonatal period is seen in approximately 40% of the UCD patients (12). Clinical expression in this group is highly variable, depending on the degree of the enzyme defect, nitrogen intake, and endogenous

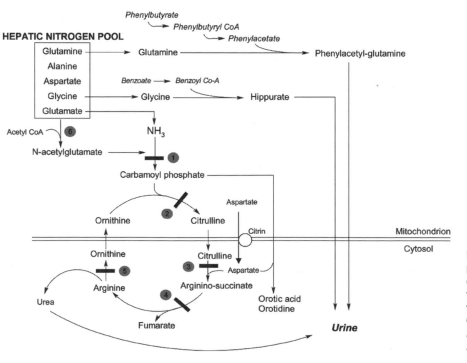

Figure 1 The urea cycle and alternative pathways of nitrogen excretion. Enzymes: **1**, carbamyl phosphate synthetase; **2**, ornithine transcarbamylase; **3**, argininosuccinate synthetase; **4**, argininosuccinate lyase; **5**, arginase; **6**, N-acetylglutamate synthetase. Enzyme defects are shown by solid bars across the arrows. *Source:* Modified from Ref. 6.

catabolism. Common presentations are intermittent episodes of vomiting associated with headaches, irritability, agitation, ataxia, and/or lethargy, sometimes progressing to coma (5,6,12). Recovery of these episodes may be complete, or with different degrees of neurological sequelae. These crises can be triggered by an exogenous protein load or increased endogenous catabolism (i.e., fever, fasting, steroid treatment, surgery, etc.). A history of anorexia, poor weight gain, and a self-imposed protein restriction is frequently overlooked. Stroke-like episodes and central pontine myelinolysis have been reported in patients with OTC and CPS deficiencies (13–15). Hepatomegaly is common in AS deficiency, and severe liver involvement, mimicking a Reye's syndrome, has been described in several UCDs (5,6,12). Brittle hair (trichorrhexis nodosa) is characteristic of AS- and AL-deficient patients.

Female carriers for OTC deficiency can have a similar variability in clinical presentation, ranging from being completely asymptomatic to presenting with severe neonatal hyperammonemia, due to the different degree of Lyonization in the hepatocytes (5,16). Some of these women have presented with severe hyperammonemia in the postpartum period (17).

Common misdiagnoses of the late presentation of UCD include migraine, cyclic vomiting, esophageal reflux, food allergies, behavioral problems, and hepatitis (5,6).

Clinical presentation of arginase deficiency differs from the other UCDs. The disease is characterized by chronic encephalopathy progressing to spastic tetraplegia, seizures, and microcephaly. Episodic vomiting and hyperammonemia are less common (5,18) and neonatal onset has exceptionally been described (10).

Diagnosis

The most important biochemical finding in patients with NAGS, CPS, OTC, AS, or AL deficiency is severe hyperammonemia (usually greater than 300 mM), with low blood urea nitrogen (BUN) and mildly elevated transaminases. These abnormalities are present in the severe neonatal forms, or during the acute decompensation in the late-onset forms. It is important to note that in common diseases of the neonatal period such as sepsis, seizures, or asphyxia, ammonia levels rarely exceed 200 uM. Also, ammonia can be falsely elevated (two to three times normal) if specimens are not collected properly (on ice) and processed immediately. Respiratory alkalosis, due to the toxic effect of the ammonia to the respiratory center, is another key to the diagnosis (5), but this sign is frequently overlooked. More rarely, patients with UCD can present with metabolic acidosis, probably secondary to dehydration. When severe hyperammonemia in a sick neonate is found, samples for quantitative plasma and urine AAs, acylcarnitines (ACs), urine organic acids (UOA) analysis, and orotic acid should be obtained as soon as possible. Diagnosis of the specific blockade in the urea cycle is determined by the AA and orotic acid results. Low or undetected citrulline levels are present in NAGS, CPS, and OTC deficiencies (Fig. 1) (5,6). Differential diagnosis among these three conditions depends on the levels of orotic acid. The latter derives from carbamyl phosphate, which is diverted to the pyrimidine synthetic pathway when accumulated. Therefore, orotic acid will be absent in NAGS or CPS deficiencies (5,6) and will be increased in OTC and, to a lesser degree, in AS, AL, and arginase deficiencies. Additionally uracil, another pyrimidine, may be found in the UOA of these enzyme deficiencies. An oral N-carbamyl glutamate (analog of N-acetyl glutamate) test is useful to differentiate between patients with NAGS (who normalize ammonia after the test) and patients with CPS deficiency, who may need assessment of CPS activity in hepatocytes for confirmation (6,11,19,20).

Patients with AS deficiency have markedly increased citrulline levels (usually more than 1000 mM) and patients with AL deficiency have milder elevations of citrulline (100–300 mM) and increased argininosuccinic acid (5). The latter is detected more easily in urine than in serum AAs. Other abnormalities in the AA profile, common to all of the above-mentioned enzyme deficiencies, are increased glutamine, lysine, and alanine, due to nonspecific nitrogen accumulation, and decreased arginine and ornithine, due to the impaired arginine biosynthesis (5,6).

In arginase deficiency, in contrast, hyperammonemia is uncommon and the AA profile shows a marked elevation of arginine (18).

The most common differential diagnoses of UCD are transient hyperammonemia of the newborn (THAN), organic acidemias (OA), and fatty acid oxidation (FAO) defects. Patients with THAN are usually preterm babies who present in the first 24 hours of life with respiratory distress and severe hyperammonemia (even higher than the UCD) (21). Neonates with OA (mainly propionic and methylmalonic) classically present with metabolic acidosis with high anion gap, ketonuria, and hyperammonemia. The latter can be as severe as in the UCD. Exceptionally, metabolic acidosis and ketonuria may be absent but UOA and/or ACs are diagnostic (see section Organic Acidemias). Children with FAO defects can have mild hyperammonemia and neonatal presentation. However, other distinctive features in these patients, such as hypoketotic hypoglycemia and severe liver or cardiac involvement, are useful to differentiate them from the UCD patients. ACs are the main tool for the diagnosis of FAO defects (see below).

Other causes of hyperammonemia are outlined in Table 1 (5,6,22–24).

Diagnosis of UCD in patients out of crisis is more difficult, especially for the female heterozygous for OTC deficiency. AA levels in these female patients are slightly different from normal controls (17,25), but might still fall within the normal range, even during a mild crisis. Additionally, enzyme activity measured in liver biopsy samples is unreliable in these patients (5). The allopurinol test is useful for diagnosis and carrier detection, but it might not be completely specific (5,25,26). When possible, mutation analysis of the OTC gene should be done. Even though the majority of mutations are private, recent information allows establishing some degree of genotype to phenotype correlations (27,28). This information is also essential for prenatal diagnosis.

Treatment: The Acute Episode

For teaching purposes, we divide treatment of this emergency into three areas: supportive therapy, anabolism, and detoxification.

Supportive Therapy

A hyperammonemic episode is a life-threatening condition with risk for severe brain damage. Protein intake should be discontinued. A central line should be placed for intravenous (IV) infusion and an arterial line is useful for blood drawing and blood pressure monitoring. The hemodialysis team should be alerted. Blood samples for ammonium, blood gas, electrolytes, BUN, glucose, and calcium should be obtained prior to the beginning of the treatment and every four to six hours thereafter. If intracranial pressure is elevated, therapy with mannitol can be started. Corticosteroids should be avoided, because they will produce protein catabolism (5). Many patients are dehydrated due to the previous history of vomiting and poor feedings. However IV fluids should be cautiously given, as cerebral edema is frequently present in severely ill patients. Infections should be searched for and treated accordingly and inotropics may be used as needed.

Anabolism

To decrease endogenous protein catabolism, calories to cover at least the basal energy expenditure should be provided (60 cal/kg/day in newborns) (29) but, when possible, a higher caloric intake (100–120 cal/kg/day) is desirable. This requires the use of a high glucose infusion rate (GIR). The different GIR and calories delivered using different concentrations of dextrose can be seen in Tables 2 and 3. In less severely ill patients, who can tolerate per oral (PO)/nasogastric (NG) feedings, IV calories can be supplemented by using one of the protein-free formulas available: Duocal® (SHS North America, Gaithersburrg, Maryland, U.S.A.), Pro-Phree® (Ross Laboratories, Columbus, Ohio, U.S.A.), Mead-Johnson 80056® (Mead Johnson Laboratories, Evansville, Indiana, U.S.A.). If the gastrointestinal (GI) tract cannot be used, IV lipids (Intralipid® Baxter, Ontario, California, U.S.A.) should be given at 0.5 to 2 g/kg/day, as long as triglycerides are not severely elevated.

Table 2 Glucose Infusion Rates (GIR) Calculated from Different Dextrose Concentrations (D%) and IU Infusion Rates (cc/kg)

cc/kg	D5%	D7.5%	D10%	D12.5%	D15%	D20%
40	1.4	2.1	2.8	3.5	4.2	5.6
50	1.7	2.6	3.5	4.3	5.2	6.9
60	2.1	3.1	4.2	5.2	6.2	8.3
67	2.3	3.5	4.6	5.8	7.0	9.3
75	2.6	3.9	5.2	6.5	7.8	10.4
100	3.5	5.2	6.9	8.7	10.4	13.9
120	4.2	6.2	8.3	10.4	12.5	16.7
150	5.2	7.8	10.4	13.0	15.6	20.8
180	6.2	9.4	12.5	15.6	18.8	25.0

Detoxification

Hemodialysis is the treatment of choice for severe hyperammonemia and can usually normalize ammonium levels in less than 24 hours (5, 30, and 31). If the former is not possible, continuous hemodiafiltration, hemofiltration, peritoneal dialysis, or exchange transfusion, in that order, are the alternatives (30,31). Pharmacologic treatment with sodium benzoate and sodium phenylacetate should be carried on until dialysis procedures are available. These drugs provide alternative pathways for nitrogen excretion. After esterified to their CoA esters, sodium benzoate and phenylacetate will produce hippurate and phenylacetylglutamine, respectively. The latter two compounds are excreted through the urine, diverting nitrogen from the urea cycle (Fig. 1) (5,32–34). IV preparations, of sodium benzoate and sodium phaylacetate, recommended for the acutely ill patient, can be obtained for emergency treatment through a pharmaceutical company (35). For CPS, OTC, and AS deficiencies, both drugs are given with a priming infusion of 250 mg/kg in 25 to 35 mL/kg over 90 to 120 minutes, followed by a sustaining infusion of 250 mg/kg given over 24 hours (5,34). Lower doses (5.5 g/m^2 in 400–600 mL/m^2) are used in older patients. It has been recommended that the priming infusion be prepared in 10% dextrose (D10%); however, the resulting GIR infusion is very high (28–39 mg/kg/min), and we have observed hypoglycemia with hyperinsulinism

Table 3 Calories/kg/Day Provided at Different GIRs

mg/kg/min	cal/kg/day
4.0	19.6
5.0	24.5
6.0	29.4
7.0	34.3
8.0	39.2
9.0	44.0
10.0	49.0
11.0	53.9
12.0	58.8
13.0	63.6
14.0	68.5
15.0	73.4
16.0	78.3
17.0	83.2
18.0	88.1

as a result of the sudden change in IV glucose infusion when the priming dose finishes. To avoid this problem, we dilute the drugs in D5%. Repeat priming doses are not recommended due to the potential toxic effect of these drugs. It is also important that doses of the IV medications be carefully calculated as cases of overdose with toxic effects have been reported (36). The levels of these drugs in blood should be measured when possible. Alternatively, we have followed levels of benzoylcarnitine by TMS as a rapid and simple estimation of the benzoate levels.

Sodium benzoate and sodium phenylacetate provide 6.9 and 6.4 mEq of sodium per gram, respectively. Therefore, the amount of sodium given to the patient with both drugs in 24 hours will be approximately 6.7 mEq/kg. The use of these salts can produce potassium loss (5), which, in association with the increased cellular potassium uptake secondary to the high GIR, may result in hypokalemia. Therefore, serum electrolytes must be followed closely and IV fluids adjusted accordingly. Nausea and vomiting are frequent side effects of the treatment and could be avoided by using antiemetics (5). As an alternative to the IV medications, sodium benzoate can be given via a NG tube. Recommended doses are up to 500 mg/kg/day (5,6,32).

Arginine, which becomes an essential AA in UCD, should also be provided. The recommended dose is 210 mg/kg/day for CPS, OTC, and AS deficiencies and of 660 mg/kg day for AL deficiency (4 and 12 g/m² respectively, for older patients). It is also recommended to give a priming infusion over 90 minutes followed by a sustaining infusion of a similar dose, given over a 24-hour period (5). An IV preparation of arginine–HCl (10% solution) is available. Alternatively, oral arginine can be given diluted in water via a NG tube. A side effect of the treatment with arginine–HCl is the development of hyperchloremic metabolic acidosis, which may require treatment with sodium bicarbonate (5). The use of potassium acetate, rather than KCl, is useful to decrease the hyperchloremia resulting from the arginine administration.

Long-Term Management

When ammonium levels are close to normal, protein can be added to the parenteral nutrition at an initial dose of 0.5 gm/kg/day. NG or PO feeds can be started as soon as the clinical condition is stable. Whole protein can be then provided by an infant formula, increasing the intake gradually according to ammonium levels. Protein tolerance varies from patient to patient; in general 1 to 1.5 g/kg/day can be given to newborns and young infants, but protein tolerance decreases after six months of age. The use of special formulas with essential AAs mixtures to provide about 50% of the total protein intake is recommended for OTC and CPS and could also be used in AS and AL deficiencies. This approach is used to meet the requirements for essential AAs and to reutilize

waste nitrogen for the synthesis of the nonessential ones (6). To achieve the desired caloric intake (120–140 cal/kg for a newborn), the formula should be supplemented with one of the protein-free formulas available (see above). If the latter are not available, glucose polymers and oil can be added to the formula as an alternative source of calories. Requirements of minerals, vitamins, and trace elements should be covered and enough water has to be added to meet the patient's needs and to maintain the caloric density at 20 to 24 cal/oz. Hyperosmolar preparations may cause diarrhea. The diet should be frequently adjusted to ensure weight gain and growth. Protein and calorie requirements per kilogram of body weight will decrease with age and vary from patient to patient according to the disease, growth rate, and residual enzyme activity. Fasting plasma ammonium, branched-chain AA (BCAA), arginine, and serum protein should be maintained within normal limits and plasma glutamine should be below 1000 mM (5).

As carnitine deficiency may develop in patients with UCD (32), carnitine should be given to these patients (50–100 mg/kg/day, divided in three doses). The dose should be adjusted according to free carnitine levels.

When PO intake is satisfactory, the appropriate medicines for long-term treatment (sodium phenylbutyrate, arginine, and/or citrulline) can be given orally, mixed with the formula. Sodium phenylbutyrate is converted into phenylacetate in the organism and is twice as effective as sodium benzoate on a molar basis; recommended doses are 0.45 to 0.60 g/kg/day for newborns and young children and 9.9 to 13.0 g/kg/day for older patients (5,6,32). Sodium benzoate 0.25 to 0.5 g/kg/day can be alternatively prescribed. These detoxifying agents might not be needed in AL deficiency (5,6).

Arginine (free base) is given at a dose of 0.40 to 0.70 g/kg/day for young children and 0.8 to 15.4 g/kg/day for older patients. The dose can be adjusted to maintain normal arginine levels for age. Patients with AS and AL deficiencies require the higher doses. In patients with severe CPS or OTC deficiencies, arginine can be substituted by citrulline, 0.17 g/kg/day or 3.8 g/m²/day, according to age. Citrate has also been used to provide a substrate for Krebs-cycle intermediates and might be useful in the treatment of AL deficiency (6).

NAGS deficiency might only require treatment with oral N-carbamyl glutamate (100–300 mg/kg/day) (6).

If anticonvulsant agents are needed, valproic acid should be avoided (37).

The outcome of patients with UCD remains very guarded. It depends on the disease, age at diagnosis, residual enzyme activity, and compliance with treatment (5,6,8,12,38). Neurological damage may be directly related to the duration and degree of the hyperammonemic episodes; therefore neurological impairment is common in almost all patients with neonatal presentation. Patients with AS deficiency seem to have better prognosis than OTC- or CPS-deficient patients (5). Surprisingly AL patients appear to have poor outcome in spite of infrequent decompensations (39). Prospective treatment of children with confirmed prenatal diagnosis or at risk of having UCD has been more effective in patients with AS and AL than in those with OTC and CPS deficiencies (40). Alternative therapies such as liver transplantation or hepatocyte infusion should be considered for patients with severe CPS or OTC deficiency, for patients with AL who develop cirrhosis, and for any patient who has recurrent hyperammonemia despite optimal medical treatment (41). Liver transplantation has been performed in several patients (39,42,43). Correction of the hyperammonemia can be obtained but neurological outcome is mainly related to the condition of the patient prior to transplant (39,42). Experience with hepatocytes infusion is still limited (43,44) Further studies are still needed to confirm long-term benefits for these therapeutic approaches. Efforts to develop gene therapy for UCD are under way, but the outcome is still uncertain (41,45).

ORGANIC ACIDEMIAS
Pathophysiology

OAs are a group of IMDs characterized by an abnormal accumulation of one or more organic acids in body fluids. The majority of OA are due to defects in the catabolic pathways of AA. However, as the site of the enzymatic blockade is far from the step where the amino group is lost, AA do not accumulate. The FAO defects and the primary lactic acidemias (PLAs), which can also produce abnormal organic acid profiles, are described in different sections of this chapter.

For teaching purposes, we can divide the OA into three groups (Table 4). The first one includes OA due to defects in the metabolism of BCAAs. They usually present with acute "intoxication-like" symptoms dominated by metabolic acidosis with increased anion gap and have dietary treatment (1,53,77).

The second group is called "cerebral OAs." In this group, the clinical picture is characterized by a progressive neurological deterioration (65,68–70,72). These patients appear to be normal in infancy or early childhood. Thereafter, mental retardation, movement disorders, ataxia, and/or seizures become apparent. Some of these OA have characteristic neuroradiological findings (65,66,71,73). The most common of these conditions, and one of the most common OAs, is glutaric aciduria Type 1 (glutaryl-CoA dehydrogenase deficiency) (45,66,67). Clinical presentation of these OA highlights the importance of requesting organic acid analysis in every patient with mental retardation, movement disorder, dystonia, and/or macrocephaly of unknown origin, even if metabolic acidosis or episodes of acute decompensation are absent (78).

In the third group, we listed miscellaneous disorders that are usually diagnosed through the UOA

analysis but have a clinical presentation that differs from the other two groups or have a still unknown enzymatic defect.

For the purpose of this chapter, we will focus on the OAs due to defects in BCAA metabolism. The metabolic pathway alterations are shown in Figure 2 .

These inborn defects are inherited as autosomal recessive conditions and have a variable phenotype. The most common disorders of this group are isovaleric acidemia (IVA), propionic acidemia (PA), and methylmalonic acidemia (MMA); therefore, we will mainly address these conditions (Table 4).

IVA, a defect of leucine (Leu) metabolism, results from the deficiency of isovaleryl-CoA dehydrogenase. Patients with IVA accumulate isovaleric acid and isovaleryl-CoA. The former is a volatile compound and is responsible for the characteristic sweaty feet odor found in the urine and skin of affected patients.

PA results from a defect in propionyl-CoA carboxylase, a biotin-dependent enzyme and MMA from a deficiency of methylmalonyl-CoA mutase (53,77). Activity of the latter could be impaired due to complete or partial defects in the mutase itself (mut^0 or mut^- respectively) or due to defects in the synthesis of its cofactor, adenosylcobalamin (53,54,62). Both PA and MMA accumulate propionyl-CoA, which derives from the catabolism of valine (Val), isoleucine (Ileu), threonine and methionine, odd-chain fatty acids (FAs), and cholesterol side-chain, and it is also produced by the anaerobic gut flora (79,80). Patients with OA accumulate acyl-CoA esters and organic acids in the mitochondria. These abnormal metabolites inhibit several mitochondrial enzymes, leading to a series of secondary biochemical abnormalities (54). Inhibition of N-acetyl-glutamate-synthetase and carbamyl phosphate synthetase is responsible for the hyperammonemia, which usually correlates with the level of organic acid accumulation (81,82). Impairment of pyruvate carboxylase (PC) and the shunt of malate explain the hypoglycemia and ketosis found in these patients, and inhibition of the glycine cleavage system may be responsible for the hyperglycinemia (54). Additionally, decreased adenosine triphosphate (ATP) synthesis and hyperlactacidemia may result from inhibition of citrate synthase and pyruvic dehydrogenase (53).

Clinical Manifestations

The clinical presentation of patients with OA can be divided schematically into a severe neonatal form with metabolic distress, a chronic intermittent late-onset form, and a chronic progressive form (53). Additionally, asymptomatic patients have been found as a result of NBS programs and studies performed in relatives of affected individuals (46–48).

Neonatal Form

Neonatal form is the most common and severe. The usual presentation is a neonate with a history of normal pregnancy, delivery, and a short disease-free

Table 4 Organic Acidemias

Organic acidemias due to defects in branched-chain amino acids

Common name	Enzyme deficiency	Pathway involved	Comments
Isovaleric aciduria	Isovaleryl-CoA dehydrogenase	Leu	"Sweaty feet" odor. Asymptomatic forms detected by newborn screening in patients and relatives (46)
3-Methyl crotonylglycinuria	3-Methyl crotonyl-CoA carboxylase	Leu	"Cat urine" odor. Severe forms with hypoglycemia and metabolic acidosis. Asymptomatic and "maternal" forms of 3-MCC detected through newborn screeening (47)
3-Methyl glutaconic aciduria Type I[a]	3-Methyl glutaconyl CoA hydratase	Leu	Speech delay
3-OH 3-methyl glutaric aciduria	3-OH 3-methyl glutaryl-CoA lyase	Leu, ketone bodies synthesis	Metabolic decompensation with severe acidosis and hypoketotic hypoglycemia due to impaired leucine catabolism and ketone bodies synthesis
2-Methyl butyrylglycinuria	2-Methylbutyryl-CoA-dehydrogenase/short-branched-chain acyl-CoA dehydrogenase	Ileu	Few cases reported with cerebral palsy and movement dissorders. Mild/asymptomatic forms detected by NBS, common in the Hmong population (48)
2-Methyl-3-hydroxybutyric aciduria	2-Methyl-3-hydroxybutyryl-CoA dehydrogenase	Ileu, 2-methyl fatty acids	Few patients reported. Progressive neurodegeneration. X-linked (49)
2-Methyl acetoacetic aciduria	2-Methyl acetoacetyl-CoA thiolase (B-keto-thiolase)	Ileu, ketolysis	Recurrent episodes of ketoacidosis. Can present with hyperglycemia mimicking DKA (50)
	Succynyl-CoA: 3-ketoacid CoA transferase	Ileu, ketolysis	Recurrent crises of emesis with dehydration and ketoacidosis. Differential diagnosis of cyclic vomiting (50)
3-OH-isobutyric aciduria	Isobutyryl-CoA dehydrogenase	Val	Few patients reported. Mild forms detected through NBS (51)
	3-OH isobutyryl-CoA deacilase? 3-OH isobutyric-acid dehydrogenase? Methylmalonate semialdehyde dehydrogenase	Val	Rare. It could be due to 3 different enzyme defects, but only methylmalonate semialdehyde dehydrogenase deficiency has been well documented. Patients described with cetoacidosis, facial dysmorphisms, severe neurological damage and brain dysgenesis (52)
Propionic aciduria	Propionyl-CoA carboxylase	Val, Ileu, Met, Treo, OCFA, Ch.	One of the most common OA. Some patients present with severe hyperammonemia, without metabolic acidosis. Cardiomyopathy (53–56)
Methylmalonic aciduria	Methylmalonyl-CoA mutase (mut⁰/mut⁻)	Val, Ileu, Met, Treo, OCFA, Ch.	Frequent. Methylmalonic aciduria without homocystinuria. Differential diagnosis with cobalamin defects A and B. Frequent renal involvement (tubular defects, chronic renal failure) requiring dialysis/transplant (53,54,57–61). May respond to hydroxocobalmin in high doses
Methylmalonic aciduria	Cbl-B: adenosyltransferase deficiency; bl-A: reductase deficiency	AdoCbl. synthesis defect. Val, Ileu, Met, Treo, OCFA, Ch.	Methylmalonic aciduria without homocystinuria. May respond to high doses of hydroxocobalamin (62)
Methylmalonic aciduria	Cobalamin defects C, D and F	AdoCbl and MetCbl synthesis. Val, Ileu, Met, Treo, OCFA, Ch.	Homocystinuria and methylmalonic aciduria. Treatment with hydroxocobalamin and betaine (62). Cbl-C is the most frequent, associated with retinopathy
Malonic aciduria	Malonyl-CoA decarboxylase	Leu, Ileu	Rare. Metabolic acidosis, hypoglycemia, dev. delay, seizures, cardiomyoopathy. Secondary inhibition fatty acid oxidation and methylmalonyl CoA mutase (combined malonic/methylmalonic aciduria) (53,63)
Biotinidase deficiency	Affects activity of 3-methyl crotonyl-CoA carboxylase, propionyl-CoA carboxylase and pyruvate carboxylase	Leu, Val, Ileu, Met, Threo, AGCl, Ch, Pyr.	Frequent (1:40,000). Presents in infants (3–6 mo) with alopecia and rash, developmental delay and seizures. Good response to biotin. Newborn screening requires enzymatic measurement (not detectable by tandem mass spectrometry) (64)
Holocarboxylase synthetase deficiency	Affects activity of 3-methyl crotonyl-CoA carboxylase, propionyl-CoA carboxylase and pyruvate carboxylase	Leu, Val, Ileu, Met, Threo, AGCl, Ch, Pyr.	Rare. Earlier and more severe presentation than biotinidase deficiency. Some patients respond to biotin (64)

(Continued)

Table 4   Organic Acidemias (*Continued*)

Common name	Enzyme deficiency	Pathway involved	Comments
Cerebral organic acidemias			
Glutaric aciduria Type I	Glutaryl-CoA dehydrogenase	Lys, Try	Frequent. Macrocephaly (may be present from birth). Acute onset dystonia and movement disorder in infancy due to basal ganglia involvement (putamen and caudate). Fronto-temporal atrophy. Non-secretory forms (normal urine OA) described (65–67). False negatives reported in NBS.
4-OH butyric aciduria	Succinic semialdehyde dehydrogenase	Glu, GABA	Affects GABA metabolism (neurotransmitter defect). Marked speech delay. Hypotonia, dev. delay, hyperactivity, ataxia, ocular apraxia, movement disorder. Limited response to treatment with Vigabatrim® [68]
N-acetylaspartic aciduria (Canavan disease)	Aspartoacylase deficiency	N-acetyl-aspartic acid	Prevalent in Ashkenazi Jewish population. Neonatal or infantile presentation. Irritability, progressive encephalopathy, loss of vision, nystagmus, optic atrophy, retinal degeneration. Magnetic resonance imaging (MRI): subcortical demyelination and basal ganglia involvement. Magnetic resonance Spectroscopy: increased N-acetyl aspartic in brain (69)
L-2-hydroxyglutaric aciduria	L-2-hydroxyglutarate dehydrogenase	Lys, Try	Rare. Onset in infancy. Dev. delay, extrapyramindal signs, seizures. Macrocephaly in some patients. MRI: subcortical demyelination (70,71)
D-2-hydroxyglutaric aciduria	D-2-hydroxyglutaric dehydrogenase?	Unknown	Variable clinical presentation from severe infantile with seizures and dysmorphic features to late onset, slowly progressive neurological disease. Cardiomyopathy.(72,73)
Encephalopathy, petechiae and ethylmalonic aciduria syndrome	ETHE-1 gene defect. Unknown protein targeted to mitochondrial matrix	Unknown	Severe. Early infantile onset with dev. Delay, hypotonia, pyramidal signs, chronic diarrhea. Ortostatic acrocyanosis. Equimoses after minimal trauma. Biochemically can be confused with SCAD and mild MAD (74,75). Might respond to methionine restriction (76)
Miscellaneous organic acidemias			
Hyperoxaluria Type I	Alanine:glyoxylate aminotransferase	Oxalate	Peroxisomal defect
Hyperoxaluria Type II	D-Glyceric dehydrogenase	Oxalate	Peroxisomal defect
Glyceroluria	Glycerol kinase (isolated or as a contiguous gene defect)	Glycerol	X-linked. As a contiguous gene defect can be associated to Duchenne's muscular dystropy, adrenal hypoplasia and OTC deficiency
Alkaptonuria	Homogentisic acid oxidase	Tyrosine, homogentisic acid	Rare. Abnormal (gray) pigmentation of sclerae, cartilagues (oocronosis) and skin. Arthritis.
Pyroglutamic aciduria	Glutathione synthetase	Gamma glutamyl cycle	Rare. Neonatal onset. Hemolitic anemia, acidosis, dev. delay, seizures.
Mevalonic aciduria/hyper-IgD and periodic fever syndrome	Mevalonate kinase	Cholesterol and nonsterol isoprenes	Developmental delay. Periodic fever of unknown etiology with rash and abdominal pain. Hepatosplenomegaly, FTT. Increased IgD (100%) and IgA (80%). Intermittent mevalonic aciduria

aOther metabolic diseases can present with mild/intermittent increase in 3-methylglutaconic acid. They include Barth Syndrome (X-linked cardiomyopathy and neutropenia, also known as 3-methylglutaconic aciduria Type II), Pearson syndrome, Costeff syndrome, ATPase synthase deficiency and other mitochondrial defects. In all of the above the activity of 3-methylglutaconyl-CoA hydratase is normal.

Abbreviations: Val, valine; Ileu, isoleucine; Met, methionine; Treo, treonine; Lys, lysine; Try, tryptophan; Glu, glutamic acid; GABA, 4-aminobutyric acid; FA, fatty acids; OCFA, odd-chain fatty acids; Ch, Cholesterol (side-chain); Cbl, cobalamin; AdoCbl, adenosylcobalamin; MetCbl, methylcobalamin; FAO, fatty acid oxidation; SCAD, short-chain acyl-CoA dehydrogenase deficiency; MAD, multiple acyl-CoA dehydrogenase deficiency.

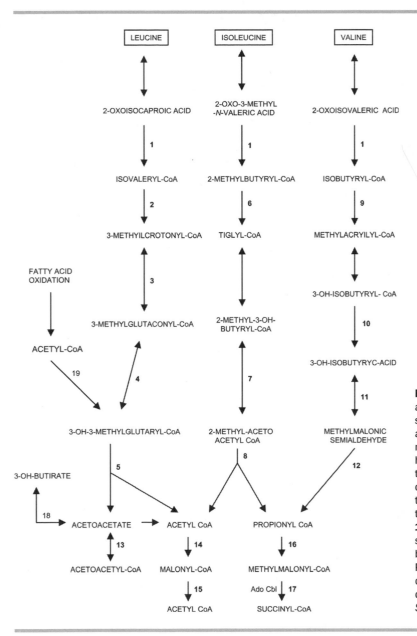

Figure 2 Metabolic pathway of the branched-chain amino-acid catabolism and related compounds. Numbers denote sites of the known enzymatic blocks. **1**, branched-chain-oxo-acid dehydrogenase; **2**, isovaleryl-CoA dehydrogenase; **3**, 3-methylcrotonyl-CoA-carboxylase; **4**, 3-methylglutaconyl-CoA-hydratase; **5**, 3-OH 3-methyl glutaryl-CoA lyase; **6**, 2-methylbutyryl-CoA-dehydrogenase; **7**, 2-methyl-3-hydroxybutyryl-CoA dehydrogenase; **8**, 2-methyl acetoacetyl-CoA thiolase (B-keto-thiolase); **9**, Isobutyryl-CoA-dehydrogenase; **10**, 3-OH isobutyryl-CoA deacylase; **11**, 3-OH isobutyric-acid dehydrogenase; **12**, methylmalonate semialdehyde dehydrogenase; **13**, succinyl-CoA: 3-ketoacid CoA transferase; **14**, acetyl CoA carboxylase (cytosolic); **15**, malonyl-CoA decarboxylase; **16**, Propionyl-CoA carboxylase; **17**, methylmalonyl-CoA mutase, cobalamin defects A, B, C, D, and F; **18**, 3-OH-butyric-acid dehydrogenase; **19**, 3-OH 3-methyl glutaryl-CoA synthase. *Source:* Adapted from Ref. 36.

period, who presents with poor sucking, vomiting, respiratory distress, hypotonia or dystonia, lethargy, and coma. These symptoms are usually attributed to sepsis or, in less severe cases, to gastroesophageal reflux or pyloric stenosis. Mild dehydration is frequent, due to vomiting and osmotic diuresis. A strong "sweaty feet" odor in urine and skin is present in IVA. Seizures and a Reye-like syndrome can be present in severely ill patients (1,53).

Late-Onset Form

In the intermittent, late-onset form, the patients present with recurrent attacks of coma, or lethargy with ataxia or dystonia. Acute hemiplegia, hemianopsia, and cerebellar hemorrhage have also been described (53,77). Increased protein intake or endogenous catabolism due to an intercurrent illness may trigger these crises.

The first attack may present at several months or years of age, even in adolescence or adulthood, and has frequently been preceded by episodes of dehydration, anorexia, vomiting, failure to thrive, hypotonia, developmental delay, and/or other symptoms (53,83,84). In between attacks, clinical and laboratory evaluations may appear normal. However, the laboratory profile obtained during the attacks is similar to the one found in the severe neonatal form, with the exception of hyperammonemia, which is less frequent (53).

Chronic Form

The chronic progressive form is characterized by persistent anorexia, failure to thrive, and vomiting. These symptoms are frequently attributed to GI problems. Renal Fanconi syndrome or osteoporosis may develop. Hypotonia and muscle weakness can be present, mimicking congenital or metabolic myopathies. Developmental delay, progressive mental retardation, self-mutilation, and seizures sometimes accompany the above-mentioned symptoms (1,53,77,85).

Common Laboratory Abnormalities

The most characteristic biochemical abnormalities are metabolic acidosis, with elevated anion gap and ketosis. Mild hyperammonemia (200–500 mM) is usually present, but levels could be as high as those seen in patients with UCD (>1000 mM) (81,82). Exceptionally, patients with PA can present with severe hyperammonemia without metabolic acidosis, mimicking a UCD (55). Lactic acid is only mildly elevated, unless there is thiamine deficiency (86). Severe lactic acidosis can also be been found due to glutathion deficiency, which responds to vitamin-C supplementation (87). Hypocalcemia, associated with PTH resistance has been reported (88). We have also documented low calcium associated with a defect in renal hydroxylation of vitamin-D. Amylase and lipase are increased if pancreatitis is present (89–91). Blood-glucose is usually low, but in some patients may be high, even before IV fluids are started (92,93). This is particularly frequent in patients with ketolysis defects (i.e., β-keto-thiolase or succinyl-acetoacetate (AcAc)-CoA-transferase deficiencies), who can present with hyperglycemia and ketosis resembling an episode of diabetic ketoacidosis (50). In contrast, patients with 3-OH 3-methyl glutaryl-CoA lyase deficiency, a defect affecting Leu catabolism and ketone bodies synthesis, present with metabolic acidosis (characteristic of OA) and hypoketotic hypoglycemia (characteristic of FA oxidation defects) (50).

Diagnosis

The most important test is the analysis of UOAs performed by gas chromatography and mass spectrometry (GC/MS). Diagnostic possibilities of this test increase if the urine is collected during the acute episode, when the characteristic profile for each OA is most likely to be recognized (78). In an acutely ill patient, the laboratory performing the test must be alerted, so that the result can be available as soon as possible. UOA show increased levels of 3-OH-isovaleric acid and isovalerylglycine in IVA; 3-OH-propionic acid, 3-hydroxyvaleric acid, methylcitrate, tiglylglycine, and propionylglycine in PA; and a large increase of methylmalonic acid, with or without mild elevation of some of the propionate metabolites in MMA (78). Ketone bodies (3-OH-butirate and AcAc) may also be increased in decompensated patients. Another reliable and fast methodology for the diagnosis of several OA is the analysis of ACs by TMS. This methodology is highly sensitive and can be performed in blood spots on filter paper (Guthrie card), plasma, urine, or cerebrospinal fluid (94,95). AC analysis allows the diagnosis of more than 20 different diseases (OA, FAO defects, and aminoacidopathies) and is being used for the diagnosis of symptomatic patients as well as for mass NBS (97). Abnormal profiles can even be obtained from cord blood in asymptomatic newborns (see section Newborn Screening) (98,99). In IVA, a typical AC profile shows a large increase of isovalerylcarnitine (IVC). However, other AC species, like pivaloylcarnitine and 2-methylbutyrylcarnitine, have the same molecular weight and should be considered when the profile is being interpreted (100,101). In PA and MMA, there is a large increase of propionylcarnitine. Additionally, a slight increase of methylmalonylcarnitine may be present in the latter. It is important to consider that the elevations in diagnostic AC species may be less pronounced in patients with severe carnitine deficiencies. Acylglycines by GC/MS stable isotope dilution or TMS may also be used for diagnosis (102). Quantitative AA usually shows a nonspecific elevation of glycine. Glutamine is also elevated, usually correlating with the degree of hyperammonemia, although exceptions have been reported in PAs (55,103). Total and free carnitine are low, with elevation of the AC/free carnitine ratio (53).

Treatment: The Acute Episode

Rapid recognition and treatment of the acute metabolic decompensation in patients with OA can be lifesaving. Treatment should provide supportive therapy, promote anabolism, and remove the offending toxins and should be carried out in specialized centers (53).

Supportive Therapy

The treatment will depend on the patient's clinical condition. A central line to assure IV access is needed and an arterial line for blood pressure monitoring and frequent blood drawing should be considered. Assisted ventilation, inotropics, albumin, and/or blood products are frequently needed. Gastric protection with H2 blockers should be provided.

Acutely ill patients with OA are usually dehydrated due to poor intake, vomiting, hyperventilation, and increased urinary losses. After fluid resuscitation is provided, IV hydration should be aimed at correcting dehydration over a period of 24 to 48 hours. Rapid rehydration should be avoided due to the risk of cerebral edema. If pH is less than 7.25, metabolic acidosis should be partially corrected with sodium bicarbonate at a dose of 1 to 3 mEq/kg, which can be repeated as needed. Overcorrection of the metabolic acidosis should be avoided, as it can increase cerebral edema. In severely acidotic patients, there is the risk of sodium overload due to frequent corrections with bicarbonate. This complication can be prevented by giving the sodium requirements in the IV fluids as sodium bicarbonate, instead of sodium chloride, at 40 to 60 mEq/L. Blood gases, electrolytes, BUN, glucose, calcium, ammonium, and urine ketones should be monitored every two to four hours. Initial potassium levels are usually normal or high in the acutely ill patients, but these levels might be artificially increased due to the acidosis. In fact, potassium requirements are elevated due to the usual history of vomiting that precedes the admission and also due to the treatment with a high GIR and insulin (see below). Patients with MMA may have tubular dysfunction and renal insufficiency leading to hyperkalemia (57–59). Liver function tests, creatinine, amylase, and lipase should be checked initially and repeated as needed. Acute pancreatitis should be treated when present (89–91). Cultures should be obtained and antibiotics should be started. Staphylococcal and candida infections should be considered in the differential diagnosis, and CBC and platelet count should be followed daily.

Anabolism

It has been shown that endogenous production is an important source of abnormal metabolites in nonacutely ill patients with OA. This production is probably due to protein turnover (104,105) and it is also increased by FA breakdown and intestinal production of propionate in patients with PA and MMA (79,80). These endogenous sources of toxic metabolites become even more important in severely ill patients and treatment should be aggressive to decrease their production (53). Oral intake is usually not possible and IV nutrition should be used to promote anabolism. Initially, this goal can be partially achieved by giving high GIR to provide at least 8 to 10 mg/kg/min (Table 2). It is important to note that even with such a GIR, caloric intake is not sufficient to cover the patient's needs (Table 3), which are increased during the decompensation (106). When patients are acidotic, it is common to observe hyperglycemia and glycosuria in response to the GIR. We have documented an inadequate insulin response to hyperglycemia during the acute decompensation. If hyperglycemia develops, the GIR should not be lowered, instead, the patient should be started on insulin (53,107). The requirements vary depending on the severity of the patient's condition and the GIR. In our experience, in a severely ill patient receiving a GIR of 8 to 10 mg/kg/min, a dose of 0.10 to 0.25 U/kg/hr is required to control hyperglycemia, but it is advisable to start with a lower dose (0.05 U/Kg/hr) and to adjust the insulin drip according to blood sugar levels. Insulin requirements decrease rapidly when acidosis improves.

Plasma ammonium levels decrease in parallel with those of the organic acids (82). Once acidosis has been corrected, fat can be added to the treatment. If amylase and lipase are high, or oral intake is not possible, IV lipids (Intralipid® Baxter, Ontario, California, U.S.A.) should be used, starting at 1 g/kg/day and increasing to 2 to 3 g/kg/day. When the oral route cannot be used for more than 48 hours, total parenteral nutrition (TPN) should be considered. TPN has been successfully used in chronic and acutely ill

patients with OA and allows an effective anabolism, which cannot be achieved with glucose and lipids alone (107,108). Ideally, the IV AA mixture should contain a lower concentration of those AAs that are precursors of the increased organic acid (i.e., Leu in IVA). Such preparations are not available in the majority of the medical centers. Alternatively, any available AA solution can be used cautiously. We start with an amount that provides ∼50% of the recommended intake of the AA involved in the metabolic block (109). This amount can be increased gradually depending on the results of blood gases, ammonium, and plasma AA. Essential AA deficiency (especially of Val and Ileu in PA and MMA) should be rapidly corrected because they can be associated with severe skin lesions that can lead to sepsis. Levels of the abnormal metabolites in urine (UOA) or blood (ACs) should also be followed up to monitor the response to treatment. With a high calorie supply from carbohydrates and fat, an IV AA dose of 1 to 1.5 g/kg/day can be achieved, but special mixtures, deprived of the offending AAs might be required to supply more protein. As the patient improves, the oral/NG tube route can be restarted (See section Long-Term Treatment).

Detoxification

In IVA and MMA, the organic acids are effectively excreted through the urine. Therefore, detoxification procedures should be indicated only in those severely ill patients who do not respond rapidly to treatment in spite of maintaining a good urinary output (53). In contrast, urinary excretion of propionic acid is poor; therefore, detoxifying procedures should be considered early in the treatment in patients with PA (53,110). In our experience, with aggressive nutritional management and insulin, detoxifying procedures are seldom required. When needed, the most effective detoxification method is hemodialysis, which allows a high clearance of organic acids, AAs, and ammonium. Continuous venovenous hemofiltration is an alternative that is well tolerated by newborns or infants and allows rapid toxin removal (111). Peritoneal dialysis is available in most centers and is more effective in newborns than children. The dialysate should be warmed and buffered with bicarbonate. Hypertonic solutions can be used when overhydration is present. In those circumstances, hyperglycemia can develop, which will require insulin treatment.

In order to treat the hyperammonemia, sodium benzoate (250 mg/kg/day) can be used alone or with sodium phenylacetate, in conjunction with any of the above-mentioned detoxification procedures (53,112). The amount of sodium provided by this source should be accounted for when the daily sodium requirements are calculated (see section on Treatment of Urea Cycle Defects). More recently, the use of carbamyl glutamic acid (100–270 mg/kd) has been tried for the treatment of hyperammonemia in PA and MMA (113,114). Initial results are encouraging but further studies are needed to validate its use.

IV carnitine is another important tool for toxin removal. This therapy will correct the free carnitine deficiency, provide enough substrate for the synthesis of nontoxic AC compounds (i.e., IVC and propionylcarnitine), which are excreted through the urine, and restore the intramitochondrial levels of CoA (53,77). After obtaining a baseline sample, a dose of 100 to 200 mg/kg/day (divided every four to six hours) should be given intravenously. The highest dose should be used in newly diagnosed patients who may have severe carnitine depletion. When the IV preparation is not available, higher doses should be used via NG tube.

In patients with IVA, treatment with l-glycine increases the conversion of isovaleryl-CoA to the nontoxic compound isovalerylglycine, which is excreted through the urine (77,115). Oral or NG-tube supplementation of l-glycine (250 to 600 mg/kg/day, divided in four to eight doses) prepared in a 100 mg/mL water solution should be given during the acute episode (53,77). Another potential resource for toxin removal is the administration of cofactors: biotin (10–20 mg/day) in PA and hydroxocobalamin (1 mg/day-IM) in MMA (53). However, patients with severe neonatal presentation rarely respond to vitamin treatment.

Clinical improvement correlates with correction of the metabolic acidosis, hyperammonemia, and ketonuria.

Complications During the Acute Episode

Acute complications include bone marrow suppression (neutropenia, thrombocytopenia, or pancytopenia) (53), pancreatitis (89–91), and infections such as generalized staphylococcal epidermolysis and alopecia (53,116,117). Acute basal ganglia dysfunction can develop after a severe crisis and should be suspected in any patient with sudden onset of dystonia and/or movement disorder. Interestingly, the globus pallidum is more frequently affected in MMA and PA (118–120) while abnormalities in the caudate and putamen are the most frequent basal ganglion involved in patients with glutaric aciduria Type I (65–67).

Clotting abnormalities, such as thrombosis with secondary DIC and bleeding (Abdenur J. Unpublished.), pulmonary hypertension secondary to microemboli (121), and microangiopathy/hemolytic uremic syndrome (HUS) (122), have been described in cobalamin defects with associated MMA and homocystinuria. Hydrocephalus has also been associated with cobalamin defects and methylenetetrahydrofolate reductase deficiency (123,124), and cardiomyopathy has been described in PA (56).

Long-Term Management

When the patient's condition permits, PO or NG feedings can be started. Natural protein is restricted to meet the recommended amounts of the AAs involved in the metabolic blockade, and can be initially provided with an infant formula. Total protein requirements for age and sex are achieved by adding special formulas

devoid of the offending AAs (53,77,109). Recent studies suggest that energy requirements might be normal or even low in OA patients out of crisis (125). However, energy intake should be adequate to meet the patient's needs for normal growth, to maintain anabolism when poor appetite is present, and should also cover the increased requirements during intercurrent illnesses (53). Caloric requirements can be met with the use of protein-free powders such as Duocal, Pro-Phree, or Mead-Johnson 80056. Alternatively, carbohydrate supplements or oil (except for olive oil in PA and MMA patients) can be added to the formula when the above-mentioned protein-free products are not available. Osmolarity of the final preparation should be considered to prevent diarrhea.

Long fasting periods (104) and constipation (126) should be avoided and dietary treatment should meet all the requirements for micronutrients and minerals. Iron, calcium, and multivitamin supplements are frequently needed. Treatment with carnitine should continue with oral preparation at 100 to 200 mg/kg/day, divided into three doses in patients with PA and MMA. Carnitine or glycine supplementation can be used in IVA (see above). Specific coenzyme therapy should only continue if a positive response has been documented. Metronidazole has been shown to be effective in decreasing the production of propionate by the gut flora (53,80,127). Due to the possible side effects of metronidazole, (leucopenia, peripheral neuropathy, and pseudomembranous colitis), it has been recommended to restrict its use to 10 mg/kg/day × 10 on 10 consecutive days every month (53). We have not seen adverse effects using the drug 10 mg/kg/day, daily for prolonged periods of time.

The long-term prognosis varies depending upon the particular OA, age at diagnosis, response to vitamin therapy, and residual enzyme activity. Several mutations have been described in IVA, MMA, and both genes involved in PA, allowing genotype/phenotype correlations for milder cases (46,128–132).

Family compliance, psychological adjustment, and education are important for successful treatment. NG or gastrostomy feedings are usually needed and frequent hospitalizations are common in the most severe cases. Guidelines should be given to parents and primary physicians for special situations like intercurrent illnesses, immunizations, anesthesia, or surgery (53,133,134).

Reported long-term outcome has varied from a normal development to different degrees of neurological involvement, including mental retardation and movement disorders (135–141). Other long-term complications such as poor growth, malnutrition, cutaneous lesions (142), trace metal deficiency (143), and osteoporosis can be prevented if good metabolic control and proper nutritional treatment can be achieved. Cardiomyopathy has been reported in some OA (53,56,144,145). Tubular dysfunction and progressive renal insufficiency are common in MMA patients (53,57–61), and it is not clear if these long-term manifestations can be prevented with optimum metabolic control. Kidney transplant or combined kidney and liver transplant has been performed in several patients with MMA. In general, better metabolic control and higher protein tolerance were obtained, but decompensations, CNS involvement, or acute basal ganglia lesions could not be prevented with these treatments (146–148). Similar experience has been reported for PA patients undergoing liver transplant (141,149).

Early diagnosis and intensive treatment are key factors to improve long-term prognosis, therefore the availability of NBS with TMS opens a new chapter for the future outcome of these diseases (see section Newborn Screening).

MAPLE SYRUP URINE DISEASE
Pathophysiology

MSUD is an autosomal recessive disease affecting the metabolism of the BCAAs, Leu, Ileu, and Val. BCAAs play an important role in intermediate metabolism. They are substrates for gluconeogenesis and ketogenesis, and their end-catabolic product, acetyl-CoA, is precursor for FA and cholesterol synthesis. The defect in MSUD is located in the branched-chain 2-ketoacid dehydrogenase (BCKD) complex, which is made of three catalytic components, encoded by four different genes (E_1-α, E_1-β, E_2, and E_3), and two regulatory proteins.

BCKD deficiency results in the elevation of Leu, Ileu, and Val and their corresponding branched-chain 2-ketoacids (BCKAs): 2-ketoisocaproic, 2-keto-3-methylvaleric, and 2-ketoisovaleric (Fig. 2) (150). Accumulation of BCKAs may lead to reduced glutamate, glutamine, and gamma-aminobutyrate in the brain cortex, which is believed to be the cause of the MSUD encephalopathies (151).

Clinical and Laboratory Manifestations

Five phenotypes have been described, based on the clinical presentation and response to thiamine therapy: classic, intermediate, intermittent, thiamine-responsive, and E_3 (dihydrolipoamide dehydrogenase) deficiency (150,151). The classical form is the most common. Children appear normal at birth, but between the first and the second week of life present with poor feedings, lethargy, dystonic posturing, seizures, and apneas. The characteristic "maple syrup" odor can easily be identified in urine. This "intoxication-like" encephalopathy resembles that of the OAs. Biochemical abnormalities include ketoacidosis and hypoglycemia. Hyperammonemia may be mild or absent (53,150). Diagnosis can be made by either plasma AAs or UOA. Typical findings in the former are elevated levels of the BCAAs, mainly Leu (500–5000 mM/L), and the presence of l-alloisoleucine, which is a transamination product of the 2-keto-3-methylvaleric acid. Routine UOA analysis shows an elevation of branched-chain 2-OH-acids and BCKAs. The latter is better detected when the sample is previously oximated. Ketone bodies are also usually present (150).

The intermediate form of MSUD presents in infancy to young adulthood with neurological impairment, seizures, failure to thrive, and ataxia. Ketoacidosis is less severe and acute crisis may be absent. In these patients, BCAA are always abnormal, with Leu levels ranging between 400 and 2000 mM/L (151,152).

The intermittent form presents in children or adults with episodes of acute decompensation (ataxia, dystonia, seizures, coma, and ketoacidosis) triggered by infections or high protein ingestion (150,153). Plasma Leu values are mildly elevated during the crisis, but they can be normal while compensated.

The "thiamine-responsive" patients are heterogeneous and have mutations in the E2 component of the enzyme (151). Their clinical presentation resembles that of the intermediate form of the disease. Treatment with thiamine (50–1000 mg/day) tends to normalize the BCAAs levels a few days or weeks after starting the treatment, and some patients can be completely off diet (53,150,152).

The E_3 component of the BCKD is common to the other three enzymatic complexes: pyruvate dehydrogenase complex (PDHC), α-ketoglutarate dehydrogenase (α-KGD), and the glycine cleavage system (involved in glycine catabolism). Clinical presentation of patients with E_3 deficiency is variable, combining features of BCKDs and PLAs (see below).

MSUD can be detected by TMS-based NBS, which allows presymptomatic treatment (154) (see section Newborn Screening).

The disease is transmitted as an autosomal recessive trait and it has been diagnosed in all ethnic groups. Incidence has been estimated in 1:185,000 in the general population, but the incidence is much higher for some communities such as the Mennonites (155). More than 100 different mutations have been identified in the genes encoding for the four different subunits of the BCKD (151,156,157).

Treatment: The Acute Episode

Acute management follows the same principles outlined for the treatment of OAs (see section Organic Acidemias). Prevention of cerebral edema with slow correction of dehydration and metabolic acidosis is important. Patients with MSUD usually require less bicarbonate than OA to correct the metabolic acidosis. High glucose infusion and insulin drip are required to correct acidosis and to decrease Leu levels. Dialysis should be considered for patients with severe encephalopathy, or in cases when acidosis does not improve in few hours. These patients usually have Leu levels above 1,500 mMol (53). Hemodialysis and hemofiltration are the preferred methods for toxin removal (96,111,158–160). Pancreatitis and brain edema have been reported in acutely ill MSUD patients (53,161–163). Abnormalities consistent with edema and dysmyelination of several areas of the brain have been reported in computed tomography (CT), magnetic resonance imaging (MRI), magnetic resonance (MR) diffusion imaging, and MR spectroscopy studies in patients with acute encephalopathy or poor metabolic control (164–168). Secondary carnitine deficiency can be present but is not as common as it is in OA patients.

Long-Term Management

Long-term treatment of MSUD patients is based on the same principles as the OAs (see above). As Leu is considered the most toxic of the BCAA, Leu-recommended intakes for MSUD patients are followed to prescribe the diet (109). The Leu-restricted diet is supplemented with special formulas devoid of BCAA's (53,109,169). In order to maintain near-normal levels of Leu, it is frequent to observe low levels of Val and Ileu. To avoid the deficiency of those essential AAs, they can be added to the formula in small amounts (5–20 mg/kg/day each). Thiamine should be tried in all patients for at least three weeks at doses of 50 to 1,000 mg/day. Administration should continue over time in thiamine-responsive patients. Prognosis of MSUD patients has dramatically improved due to the early diagnosis through NBS programs, intensive treatment, and availability of special formulas (154). For children treated in specialized centers, survival is 100% (53,150). However, even with early diagnosis and treatment, some degree of psychomotor impairment can be found (170,171), which may correlate with long-term metabolic control (172). Orthotopic liver transplantation has been performed in few patients, allowing improved metabolic control, and protein tolerance, without completely normalizing BCAA's levels (173,174). Successful pregnancies have

been reported in intermediate MSUD female patients who were followed with close monitoring (150).

FATTY ACID OXIDATION DEFECTS
Pathophysiology: Mitochondrial Fatty Acid Oxidation

Mitochondrial FAO disorders are a relatively new group of IMD of increasing relevance. FAO is the major source of energy for skeletal muscle and the heart, while liver oxidizes FA primarily during fasting (175,176). Understanding the FAO process is essential to interpret the pathophysiology of these diseases and to develop adequate strategies for treatment.

The FAO process begins when triglycerides, stored in adipose tissue, are broken down to glycerol and FAs, mainly long chain. The latter are transported in blood bound to albumin and enter liver cells through a specific transport system (177–179). Once inside the cell, FFA of carbon length 18 or shorter are oxidized in the mitochondria, while longer-chain fats are metabolized in the peroxisomes (180). To undergo mitochondrial oxidation, FAs are activated to their corresponding acyl-CoA by specific acyl-CoA synthetases. The resulting acyl-CoAs enter into the mitochondria in different ways, depending on their chain length. Short- (4–6 carbons), and medium-chain (6–10 carbons) acyl-CoAs directly enter the mitochondrial matrix. In contrast, long-chain acyl-CoAs (12–18 carbons) enter the mitochondria through a complex active transport system (Fig. 3).

Initially, long-chain acyl-CoAs are conjugated to carnitine by carnitine palmitoyl transferase I (CPT-I), in the outer mitochondrial membrane. There are three tissue-specific isoforms of CPT-I, hepatic, muscular,

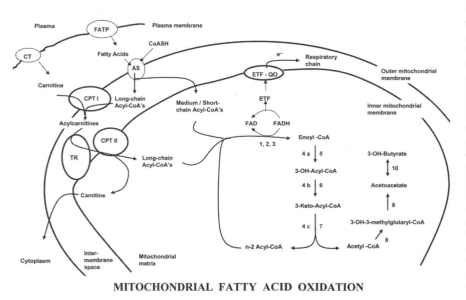

MITOCHONDRIAL FATTY ACID OXIDATION

Figure 3 Enzymes and transporter proteins involved in mitochondrial oxidation of saturated straight-chain fatty acids. **1,** very long-chain acyl-CoA-dehydrogenase; **2,** medium-chain acyl-CoA-dehydrogenase; **3,** short-chain acyl-CoA-dehydrogenase; **4,** mitochondrial trifunctional protein; **4a,** long–chain-enoyl-CoA-hydratase; **4b,** long-chain 3-hydroxy-acyl-CoA-dehydrogenase; **4c,** long–chain-ketoacyl-CoA thiolase; **5,** short-chain-enoyl-CoA-hydratase (crotonase); **6,** short-chain 3-hydroxy-acyl-CoA-dehydrogenase; **7,** medium-chain 3-ketoacyl-CoA thiolase; **8,** hydroxymethylglutaril-CoA-synthetase; **9,** hydroxymethylglutaril-CoA-lyase (enzyme involved in ketogenesis and leucine metabolism); **10,** 3-OH-butyric-acid dehydrogenase. *Abbreviations*: CoA, coenzyme A; CoASH, free CoA; FAD, flavin adenine dinucleotide; FADH, reduced form of FAD; CT, carnitine transporter; FATP, Fatty acid transport proteins; AS, acyl-CoA synthetase(s); CPT I, carnitine palmitoyltransferase I; TR, carnitine-acylcarnitine translocase; CPT II, carnitine palmitoyltransferase II; ETF, electron transfer flavoprotein; ETF-QO, ETF-ubiquinone-oxidoreductase.

and cerebral, but only patients with the hepatic form have been described so far (181–183). Long-chain ACs are passed by a carnitine-AC translocase (translocase) to carnitine palmitoyl-transferase II (CPT II), bound to the inner mitochondrial membrane, which releases carnitine and long-chain acyl-CoAs into the mitochondrial matrix (175,181). Carnitine itself is transported into the tissues by a plasma membrane CT specific for kidney, muscle, and heart (176).

In the mitochondrial matrix, Acyl-CoAs of all chain lengths undergo a series of cyclic enzymatic reactions (β-oxidation) (Fig. 3). The first step is a dehydrogenation of the acyl-CoA to enoyl-CoA. This reaction is catalyzed by four FAD-dependent enzymes: very long-, long-, medium-, and short-chain acyl-CoA dehydrogenases (VLCAD, LCAD, MCAD, and SCAD, respectively), which differ in their chain-length specificity (175,180). Nevertheless, there is some degree of overlap in their activity. The main enzyme involved with long-, straight-chain FAs metabolism is VLCAD, while LCAD may play a role in the metabolism of branched-chain FAs (184). Electrons released during these reactions are channeled by the electron transfer flavoprotein (ETF), and the ETF-ubiquinone oxidoreductase (ETF-QO), to produce ATP (180,185). ETF and ETF-QO defects impair not only the dehydrogenases involved in FA oxidation, but also those involved in the metabolism of BCAAs (Val, Ileu, and Leu), lysine, hydroxylysine, tryptophan, and sarcosine (185).

The enoyl-CoAs produced by the Acyl-CoA dehydrogenases are further metabolized in three enzymatic reactions to release acetyl-CoA and a new acyl-CoA molecule that is two carbons shorter (Fig. 3) (175,180). The exact mechanism of the last three steps varies for substrates of different chain length. For long-chain acyl-CoA substrates, the reactions are carried by a mitochondrial trifunctional protein (MTP) with enoyl-CoA-hydratase, hydroxyacyl-CoA dehydrogenase, and ketoacyl-CoA thiolase activities (186,187). This protein is composed of four α- and four β-subunits. The α-subunits contain the long-chain 3-enoyl-CoAA hydratase activity and the long-chain 3-hydroxy-acyl-CoA dehydrogenase (LCHAD) activities and the β subunit has the long-chain 3-ketoacyl-CoA thiolase activity (180,186–188). Biochemical studies have identified two groups of LCHAD-deficient patients. The first one, most common, has an isolated LCHAD deficiency due to mutations in the LCHAD coding region of the α-subunit gene. In the second group, all three enzyme activities are deficient (186–190).

For shorter-chain FAs, individual enzymes, each one with a single activity, have been identified: short-chain-enoyl-CoA-hydratase (crotonase), short-chain 3-hydroxyacyl-CoA dehydrogenase (SCHAD), and medium-chain 3-ketoacyl-CoA thiolase (175,180).

The acetyl-CoA moieties produced during the FAO are used as a source of energy through the tricarboxylic acid cycle (TCA). Under fasting conditions, acetyl-CoA also becomes the substrate for ketone bodies synthesis, which are used as fuel by several tissues, including the brain. Two enzymes are involved in ketone bodies synthesis: hydroxymethylglutaryl CoA-synthase and hydroxymethylglutaryl-CoA lyase (Fig. 3) (191–194). The latter is also the final enzyme of Leu catabolic pathway.

Clinical Presentation

Several enzymatic defects in FAO and ketogenesis have been found in humans, all inherited as autosomal recessive diseases. These defects have become one of the most important group of IMD, due to the number of patients and the severe outcome (175). In a series of 107 patients, Saudubray et al. found that 50 patients and 47 siblings died, 60% before one year of life (195).

Main Clinical Features

The most common diseases are MCAD, LCHAD, and MAD deficiencies, but it is possible that many patients with other long-chain FAO defects still die without recognition. Table 5 summarizes the known defects in saturated straight-chain FA metabolism found in humans and their most distinctive features. Clinical presentation ranges from completely asymptomatic to severe malformations or unexplained sudden death in infancy or adulthood. As expected by the important role of FAO in liver, heart, and muscle, the main clinical presentation of FAO defects is dominated by symptoms related to these organs. Neurological symptoms are also found during the acute crisis, and they might be in part related to hypoglycemia and impaired ketogenesis.

Neonatal presentations were thought to be limited to CPT-II, translocase and MAD deficiencies (185,195,196), but neonatal cases of MCAD, LCHAD, and VLCAD deficiencies have also been reported (195,197,198). Overall mortality in the neonatal period has been estimated in 30% (195). Clinical manifestations in newborns include lethargy, hypotonia, liver involvement (with or without cholestasis), or sudden death. Heart beat abnormalities (supraventricular and ventricular tachycardia, ventricular fibrillation, AV blocks, or nodal dysfunctions) are particularly frequent in CPT-II, translocase, and LCHAD deficiencies (196). Most common dysmorphic features are a high forehead, wide spaced eyes, and low set ears, resembling a Zellweger syndrome. Renal dysplasia (polycystic kidneys) and brain malformations have also been reported (175,185,195).

Biochemical manifestations in these neonates can be extremely severe including hypoglycemia, acidosis, and abnormalities related to liver failure.

Infantile presentation usually follows a symptom-free period of few months followed by a "metabolic crisis," which is usually triggered by an intercurrent infection or a fasting period longer than usual. The metabolic crisis is characterized by vomiting,

Table 5 Fatty Acid Oxidation Defects

Known enzyme deficiencies in humans	Main organ involved			Distinctive features
	Liver	Muscle	Heart	
Defects in plasmatic membrane transport				
Carnitine transporter	Yes	Yes	Yes	Impaired metabolism of long-chain fatty acid, hypoglycemia, hyperammonemia; cardiomyopathy, muscle weakness; severe carnitine deficiency
Fatty acid transport protein	Yes	No	No	Severe episodic liver failure; two patients reported.
Defects in mitochondrial transport				
Carnitine palmitoyltransferase I	Yes	No	No	Severe hypoglycemia with hypoketosis; plasma carnitine elevated or normal; renal tubular acidosis reported
Carnitine-acylcrnitine translocase (translocase)	Yes	Yes	Yes	Neonatal presentation: arrhythmias, cardiomyopathy, muscle weakness. hypoketotic hypoglycemia, hyperammonemia, increased creatine kinase (CK)
Carnitine palmitoyltransferase II				
Perinatal	Yes	Yes	Yes	Severe, fatal renal and brain abnormalities are common. Severe hypoglycemia, acidosis, hyperammonemia; cardiomyopathy and arrhythmias. oligohydramnios reported
Infantile	Yes	No	Yes	Less frequent; hepatomegaly, liver failure, arrhythmias, cardiomyopathy, sudden death; hypoglycemia, acidosis hyperammonemia increased transaminases and CK
Late onset (most frequent)	No	Yes	No	Most common cause of rhabdomyolysis and myoglobinuria; cardiac arrest after exercise reported
Mitochondrial beta oxidation				
Very long-chain acyl-CoA-dehydrogenase	Yes	Yes	Yes	Neonatal form with cardiomyopathy, arrhythmias, pericardial effusion. Infantile form with liver failure, late-onset form with skeletal muscle involvement. Sudden death; hypoketotic hypoglycemia, acidosis, hyperammonemia
Medium-chain acyl-CoA-dehydrogenase	Yes	No	No	Most frequent fatty acid oxidation defect; Reyes-like episodes; sudden death.
Short-chain acyl-CoA-dehydrogenase	Yes	Yes	No	Variable phenotype. FTT, dev, delay, hypotonia, ophthalmoplegia, muscle weakness, metabolic acidosis
Long-chain 3-hydroxy-acyl-CoA-dehydrogenase (LCHAD)	Yes	Yes	Yes	Liver failure, Reye-like syndrome, cholestasis. Hypotonia, muscle weakness; cardiomyopathy, pericardial effusion; retinitis pigmentosa and peripheral neuropathy described; sudden death; hypoketotic hypoglycemia, lactic acidosis, elevated CK and transaminases.
Mitochondrial trifunctional protein	Yes	Yes	Yes	Few cases reported; more severe than LCHAD deficiency; cardiomyopathy
Short-chain 3-hydroxy-acyl-CoA-dehydrogenase	Yes	Yes	Yes	Few cases reported; variable phenotype, hypoglycemia; liver and muscle isoforms (cardiomyopathy in the latter).
Medium-chain 3-ketoacyl-CoA-thiolase deficiency	Yes	Yes	Yes	Few patients known
Electron transfer				
Multiple acyl-CoA-dehydrogenase deficiency				
Electron transfer flavoprotein (ETF)	Yes	Yes	Yes	Affects catabolism of fatty acids (all carbon lengths) and some aminoacids (leucine, isoleucine, valine, lysine, hydroxylysine, tryptophan, and sarcosine). Great phenotypic variation from severe neonatal form with malformations to progressive muscle weakness with lipidic myopathy; cardiomyopathy, pericardial effusion
ETF-ubiquinone-oxidoreductase (ETF-QO)	Yes	Yes	Yes	
Ketone body synthesis				
Hydromymethylglutaryl-CoA synthetase	Yes	No	No	Few patients reported
Hydromymethylglutaryl-CoA lyase	Yes	No	No	Hypoketotic hypoglycemia and metabolic acidosis; enzyme involved in ketogenesis and leucine catabolism

followed by lethargy, hypotonia, and slight liver enlargement. Respiratory distress due to cardiac insufficiency and/or metabolic acidosis can be present. Symptoms are usually erroneously attributed to an intercurrent illness or cyclic vomiting syndrome (175,195). Patients can recover from the initial crisis, and repeat another episode, remaining asymptomatic in between. Liver insufficiency can be severe, leading to a Reyes-like syndrome, complicated by hypothermia and GI bleeding (199). Cholestasis has been reported in patients with LCHAD deficiency (186,195,200,201).

Cardiac involvement is characterized by hypertrophic, less common, dilated cardiomyopathy, or arrhythmias (see above) leading to cardiac insufficiency. Arrhythmias are particularly common in patients with CPT-II, translocase, and LCHAD deficiencies (176,181,195,196), diseases where there is an accumulation of long-chain-acyl-CoAs and long-chain-ACs. In contrast, heart beat abnormalities have not been observed in CT, CPT-I, or MCAD deficiencies. Pericardial effusion and endocardial fibroelastosis have been described (202). Symptoms of skeletal muscle involvement have been described for the majority of the FAO defects at this age and are manifested by hypotonia, decreased DTRs, and muscle (leg) pain.

In adolescents and adults, FAO defects present mainly with skeletal muscle involvement, which is particularly common in CPT II-adult type, LCHAD, and mild MAD deficiencies (175). Usual manifestations are hipotonia and/or progressive proximal weakness. Acute episodes of muscle pain or cramps, fatigue, and/or exercise intolerance with rhabdomyolysis can appear in response to stress, prolonged exercise, or cold, and can produce acute renal failure (176,181,195).

Retinitis pigmentosa and peripheral neuropathy have been found in patients with LCHAD deficiency (187,188,203). Mental retardation and/or other neurological sequelae are observed mostly in patients who had severe encephalopathy associated with Reye-like syndrome (195,199). Other manifestations, specific for a given defect, are outlined in Table 5.

Maternal Complications During Pregnancy of Affected Fetuses

The association between LCHAD deficiency in the fetus, and maternal preeclampsia, the syndrome of hemolysis, elevated liver enzymes and low platelets (HELLP) or acute fatty liver of pregnancy (AFLP) has been well documented (204). These complications have been reported in up to 79% of the pregnancies with fetuses affected with LCHAD, while there were no complications if the carrying fetus was heterozygous or normal. Additionally, Ibdah et al. reported that the complications were related to the presence of the prevalent E474Q mutation on one or both alleles (homozygous or compound heterozygous) of the LCHAD-affected fetus (204). However another report describes three families with trifunctional enzyme deficiency and maternal hepatic dysfunction in pregnancy not associated with the common E474Q mutation (205).

Affected LCHAD patients show a higher incidence of prematurity, asphyxia, intrauterine growth retardation, and intrauterine death than their unaffected siblings (204,206). These findings highlight the importance of obtaining molecular diagnoses for patients and parents, and to provide adequate genetic counseling and molecular prenatal diagnosis when indicated (207). AFLP has also been reported in pregnancies with fetal CPT-1, MCAD, and SCAD deficiencies using the possibility of a common mechanism producing liver disease in mothers carrying fetuses affected with FAO defects (208–210).

Sudden Infant Death

Many FAO defects have been associated with episodes of sudden, unexpected, infant death. Different studies analyzing postmortem specimens of liver, bile, cultured fibroblasts, or blood spots in filter paper have estimated that 2% to 5% of SIDS can be attributed to FAO defects (211,212). They include deficiencies of the CT, translocase, VLCAD, LCHAD, MCAD, SCHAD, and MAD (211–218). The mechanism of sudden death in these patients is not clear, but acute arrhythmia may account for the unexpected deaths in children with abnormalities in long-chain FA metabolism (196). AC analysis by TMS in postmortem bile or in the NBS samples (Guthrie card) stored by the State programs have significantly expanded the retrospective diagnosis of FAO disorders (217–220). With the availability of NBS by TMS and early treatment, it is reasonable to expect that the number of patients with sudden death due to FAO defects will decrease significantly.

Other metabolic diseases, not involving the FA metabolism, have also been found in children with sudden or unexpected death in infancy. Among others they include glutaric aciduria Type I, myophosphorilase deficiency, lysinuric protein intolerance, and defects of the respiratory chain (218,221–224).

Laboratory Abnormalities

The most common laboratory abnormality found during an acute episode is hypoglycemia. Ketone bodies can be detected in urine, but in smaller amounts than expected for the degree of hypoglycemia (hypoketotic hypoglycemia). Total nonesterified FAs (NEFA) are increased, and the NEFA to ketone body ratio is abnormally high (>3) when the sample is obtained before the IV glucose is started. Some patients with suspected SCHAD deficiency have been described as presenting with large amounts of ketones in urine (225,226). Interestingly, patients with proven molecular defects in the SCHAD gene have been described with hyperinsulinemic hypoglycemia (227–229).

Elevated liver enzymes, mild hyperammonemia, and slight metabolic acidosis are common. Abnormal clotting factors are rarely observed. Very high levels of creatine kinase (CK)(several thousands) reveal muscle involvement. The latter is characteristically found in long-chain defects and may also be found in MCAD deficiency during mild decompensations.

Hyperuricemia appears to be a common finding in MCAD deficiency and mild elevation of lactic acid is present in LCHAD deficiency (198,200). Myoglobinuria can be present in any FAO defect affecting skeletal muscle, and is a common presentation in the adult form of CPT II deficiency (175,176,195).

Muscle or liver biopsies are rarely indicated for diagnosis. During the acute episode, a liver biopsy under light microscopy shows micro- and macrovesicular steatosis. These abnormalities usually lead to the diagnosis of Reye syndrome. However, the electron microscopy will lack the characteristic mitochondrial changes of Reye syndrome (230). Fibrosis and cirrhosis have been described in liver biopsies of VLCAD and LCHAD deficiencies. Pathology of skeletal and cardiac muscle shows fatty infiltration (lipidic myopathy) (175,185).

Diagnosis

Once the diagnosis of a FAO defect is suspected, samples should be immediately obtained for specialized metabolic studies. Analysis of ACs by TMS in plasma or blood spots in filter paper have become the most important tool for diagnosis of FAO defects. This methodology is highly sensitive and abnormal profiles can be obtained even when samples are collected out of crisis. Rarely, an AC profile can be misinformed as normal when free carnitine levels are very low, when the patient has been on IV with high GIR, or when the sample is obtained out of crisis in nonfasting conditions. Typical AC profiles can be identified for CPT-II/translocase, LCAD/VLCAD, MCAD, SCAD, LCHAD, and MAD as well as for 3-hydroxy-3-methylglutaryl-CoA-lyase (HMG-CoA-lyase) deficiencies (94,231–233). More difficult is the diagnosis of the carnitine uptake deficiency, where the marker is a low free carnitine level (234) and in CPT-I deficiency, where low levels of all AC species (including acetylcarnitine), combined with high levels of free carnitine, are suggestive of the defect (235,236). In the transport defects of long-chain FAs, ACs are uninformative and ACs have been reported as normal in children with SCHAD (213) and HMG-CoA-synthase deficiencies (237). AC analysis performed in the NBS card have allowed retrospective diagnosis in patients who died of MCAD, CPT II, VLCAD, translocase, and MAD deficiencies (199,214,217,238–240). TMS is also being employed by many screening programs around the world for the neonatal detection of FAO defects as well as other IMD (see section Newborn Screening). It is likely that early diagnosis and treatment will change the natural history of the disease for many patients (241,242).

Urine OA profile may be informative for the diagnosis of FAO defects, but it is important that analysis and interpretation be performed in an experienced center. Several defects can be diagnosed if samples are obtained during the acute episode; they include HMG-CoA-lyase, MCAD, LCHAD, SCAD, MCKAT, SCHAD and MAD and CPT 1 (175,183,233). However, frequently the results may be suggestive, but nonspecific for a FAO defect, or give a false-negative result when samples are collected after the patient has been started on supportive therapy. Therefore, patients with FAO defects can be misdiagnosed if only OA analysis is performed.

Quantitative analysis of acylglycines by GC/MS (by stable isotope dilution or TMS) is an alternative method for diagnosis and it is useful for the evaluation of MAD and differential diagnoses of SCAD (233,243). Carnitine levels are informative. Total and free carnitine are normal or high in CPT-I deficiency and extremely low in the CT defect. In all other FAO diseases, total and free carnitine are usually decreased, and the percentage of ACs is increased (195,233). Another method for the diagnosis of FAO defects is to measure the levels of individual free FAs in plasma by GC/MS (244). This method is sensitive but time consuming and it is not routinely used, except when the diagnosis of SCHAD is suspected (short-chain-3-hydroxy FAs are not esterified with carnitine) (245).

In vitro flux studies with labeled FAs in lymphocytes of fibroblasts are another useful tool for diagnosis of the more difficult patients (246–249). Fasting or loading tests are rarely needed and should only be performed in experienced centers if the above-mentioned specialized tests are not informative (195,249). It is usually not necessary to measure enzyme activity to confirm diagnosis. Eventually, enzymatic studies can be performed for the majority of these conditions in cultured fibroblasts, except for SCAD activity, which is only reliable in muscle. Tissue specificity is known for CT, and CPT-I, and has also been postulated for SCHAD, while HMG-CoA-synthase is only expressed in liver.

Molecular studies are available for most of the FAO defects and should be performed to establish genotype phenotype correlations and also as a tool for genetic counseling. Common mutations have been described in MCAD and LCHAD deficiencies (250). Several studies have shown that a missense mutation 985 A > G accounts for the majority of the mutant alleles in MCAD deficiency, being more prevalent in Northern Europeans (250,251). In LCHAD deficiency, a common 1528G > C mutation has been identified (186,250,252). Molecular studies for some disorders, like SCAD deficiency, are complicated by the presence of common variant alleles. Homozygosity and compound heterozygosity for SCAD gene sequence variants 625G–>A and 511C–>T are associated with ethylmalonic aciduria and mild increase in butyril carnitine, which are potential biochemical indicators of SCAD deficiency. Additionally, mild increase in butyrylcarnitine can be detected by some NBS programs. The clinical and biochemical implications of these variants are not fully understood (247,253).

Treatment: The Acute Episode

Acutely ill patients with suspected FAO defect should be treated in an experienced pediatric intensive care unit. Delay in proper treatment may result in death or permanent brain damage (195).

Supportive Therapy

IV hydration should be cautiously given as patients with hyperammonemia may have cerebral edema and patients with heart involvement may develop cardiac insufficiency. Clotting factors and vitamin K may be required in patients with severe liver dysfunction, and H2 blockers should be given to prevent GI bleeding.

Salicylates and valproic acid are contraindicated due to their potential mitochondrial toxicity and should be investigated as a potential cause of the metabolic crisis (254). Epinephrine and glucagon have a lipolytic effect and therefore should be avoided.

Pivalic acid–containing drugs should also be avoided as they can cause secondary carnitine deficiency (255).

Anabolism

To suppress lipolysis, IV fluids should provide a GIR of 6 to 10 mg/kg/min or more, which may require placement of a central line. High GIR should be used regardless of the blood sugar levels found on admission (195). If patients develop hyperglycemia, IV insulin should be started, titrating the dose according to hourly glucose levels. Alternatively glucose can be provided via a NG tube (10% glucose polymers solution). In known patients with long-chain FA defects, medium-chain triglycerides (1–3 g/kg/day) can be added via a NG tube as soon as the GI tract allows it.

Detoxification

Treatment with IV carnitine (200–300 mg/kg/day PO, 70–100 mg/kg/day IV) is life saving for the carnitine transport defect. Regarding other FAO defects, there is general agreement in the use of carnitine (50–100 mg/kg/day PO, 15–30 mg/kg/day IV) in patients with short- and medium-chain defects (175,180,195). The use of carnitine for defects involving long-chain FAs is more controversial, due to the possible role of long-chain ACs in the development of heart beat abnormalities and/or their inhibitory effect of FAO in vitro (195,256). However, despite theoretical considerations, experienced centers routinely use carnitine in long-chain FA defects and have not reported adverse effects (257). Our approach is to start treatment with 50% of the usual dose and adjust treatment to maintain free carnitine levels within normal limits.

Riboflavin (100–200 mg/day) should be tried in patients with MAD and SCAD deficiencies, even though only a few patients with mild variants have been reported to respond to it (175).

Long-Term Management
Carnitine

Carnitine is the only treatment needed for the CT defect (200–400 mg/kg/day PO). Long-term carnitine supplementation for the other disorders should be provided (see above) and dose should be adjusted according to free carnitine levels.

Diet

Dietary guidelines for the treatment of other FAO defects are outlined in Table 6. Different degrees and types of fat restriction are indicated depending on the enzymatic defect. There is a rationale for the use of medium chain triglycerides (MCTs) in patients with impaired metabolism of long chain FAs (FATP, CPT-I, translocase, CPT-II, VLCAD, LCHAD, MTP). In contrast, the use of MCT is contraindicated for all other metabolic blocks. Enough essential FAs (linoleic and a-linolenic acids) should be provided to avoid

Table 6 Dietry Treatment of FAO Defects

Diet	Long-chain FAO defects (%)	Medium- and short-chain FAO defects (%)	Electron transfer (MAD) (%)
Calories	> 10 RDA	> 10 RDA	> 10 RDA
Protein	RDA	RDA	7
Fat	25–30	20–30	15–20
MCT	15–20 (1–3 g/kg/day)	Contraindicated	Contraindicated
LCFA	±10	–	–
EFA	4	4	4
CHO	60–65	60–70	73–78

Abbreviations: FAO, fatty acid oxidation; MAD: multiple acyl CoA dehydrogenase deficiency; MCT, medium-chain triglycerides, LCFA, long-chain fatty acids; EFA, essential fatty acids; CHO, carbohydrates.

deficiencies. Usefulness of supplementation with docosohexaenoic acid to prevent retinal damage has been proposed for LCHAD-deficient patients (258,259). In addition to the low-fat diet, patients with MAD may benefit from mild protein restriction and patients HMG-CoA-lyase may also benefit from Leu restriction.

Fasting

Besides the composition of the diet, another key for the treatment of FAO defects is to avoid prolonged fasting by providing frequent feedings around the clock. Infant formulas can be supplemented with carbohydrates to meet caloric needs and to decrease postabsorptive fasting. Glucose polymers are well tolerated (i.e., Moducal® or Polycose®) and can provide a safe fasting period of three to four hours. Treatment of infants and young children with severe enzyme deficiencies needs to be aggressive and may require frequent feedings during the day and overnight NG or G-tube feedings (195).

After two years of age, the diet can be supplemented with uncooked cornstarch (CS). This provides a sustained release of glucose, preventing hypoglycemia. Additionally, CHO stimulate insulin secretion, which prevents lipolysis. In most patients, CS (1–2 g/kg) is used during the night-time feedings. CS, plain or flavored, can be given mixed with water, formula, or juices and it is generally well tolerated. We usually start with lower doses (i.e., 0.5 g/kg) and increase the amount gradually while monitoring for possible diarrhea. In children with severe enzyme deficiencies or poor appetite, CS can be given at regular intervals throughout the 24 hours, as used in the treatment of glycogen storage diseases. The beneficial effect of uncooked CS has been documented in MCAD, MAD, and LCHAD and severe CPT I deficiencies (182,242,260,261). In children between one and two years, who may not have enough amylase activity, CS can be tried at smaller doses, which can be increased slowly according to efficacy and tolerance or can also be given with exogenous amylase (242).

Monitoring Treatment

Individual response to dietary treatment and fasting can be evaluated by measuring ACs, which are very sensitive markers. It is important to remember that AC levels tend to rapidly increase during short fasting periods, reflecting the accumulation of toxic metabolites (242,260,261). Therefore AC should be obtained always with the same time interval after a meal in order to compare results. Blood-glucose, liver enzymes, uric acid, ammonia or CK are *late* markers of metabolic decompensation and cannot be used to monitor long-term response. Optimal interval between meals may vary for the different diseases, for different patients and age groups in dietary treatment.

Education and family compliance are essential to avoid life-threatening decompensation, which can occur very rapidly in young patients.

Other Treatments

Treatment of long-chain FA defects with triheptanoate has been proposed as a source of medium chain FAs (odd-numbered), which can also provide anaplerotic substrates to the Krebb's cycle (262). Further controlled studies are needed to validate its use.

Other experimental treatments include dl-3-hydroxybutryrate, which has been used in patients with severe MAD deficiency (263) and fibrates, which are being considered for clinical trials (264).

Prognosis

Long-term prognosis varies according to the disease, age at diagnosis, residual enzyme activity, and long-term management. Mortality rate has been estimated at 25% for MCAD deficiency, and the majority of these patients die in the initial episode (199). Long-term complications in MCAD deficiency include developmental delay, muscle weakness, failure to thrive, and cerebral palsy (199). Early diagnosis by NBS can prevent the mortality and severe morbidity of MCAD (241,265).

Limited information is still available for the long-term prognosis of patients with other FAO defects, but it is likely that, as shown for MCAD deficiency, NBS may change the natural history of these diseases (186,242).

NEWBORN SCREENING WITH TANDEM MASS SPECTROMETRY

NBS has been applied worldwide for the early diagnosis of metabolic and endocrine diseases for many years. It was initially developed for the detection of phenylketonuria (PKU), a disorder of AA metabolism that, unrecognized, could lead to severe mental retardation. It is now clear that with early diagnosis and treatment, neurological damage can be prevented in PKU patients.

Over time other endocrine and metabolic disorders were added to the NBS panels, including congenital hypothyroidism, galactosemia, MSUD, hemoglobinopathies, biotinidase deficiency, etc. In general, the disorders selected for NBS programs fulfill the following traditional criteria related to the disease and methodology.

Related to the disease:
■ Relatively frequent (i.e., 1:10:000 newborns)
■ Known clinical course with initial symptom-free period
■ Significant morbidity/mortality if untreated
■ Early treatment (newborn period) required to change the outcome
■ Health benefits for patients and families, which outweigh the burden of NBS
■ Availability of resources for confirmatory testing, treatment, and follow-up
■ Total costs of diagnosis, treatment and follow up must be reasonable and outweigh the cost of potential disabilities

Relative to the methodology:
■ Massive screening should be possible using a reliable methodology
■ Sample must be small, easy to collect, transport, and store
■ Test must be reasonably simple, allowing for high throughput
■ Test should be sensitive (no false negatives) and specific enough (few false positives)

Traditionally, for each disorder, a different blood sample and test methodology are needed; therefore the addition of new diseases to a NBS program is limited by the amount of sample and testing costs. In the 1990s, the method to measure AA and AC by TMS in a small blood sample collected in filter paper was developed by D. Millington at Duke University. The AA levels allow the NBS of many aminoacidopathies (Table 7), while AC allow the neonatal detection of several OAs and the vast majority of the FAO defects (Table 7) (266).

More than 30 different diseases can be detected with a combined frequency of approximately 1:4000 (271). However, not all those conditions fulfill the criteria (for disease or methodology) traditionally accepted for NBS (see above). More recently, TMS and other technologies have been applied for the neonatal detection of lysosomal storage disorders. This approach is particularly exciting as enzyme replacement therapy is available for some of these disorders (i.e., mucopolysaccharidosis I, II, and VI, Gaucher, Fabry, and Pompe diseases) and others may benefit from early bone marrow transplant (i.e., Krabbe disease). Pilot studies are under way, but no state has started offering NBS for those disorders yet (266). For the purpose of this chapter, we will focus on the diseases that can potentially be detected by measuring AA and AC.

As of January 2006, in the United States, 36 out of the 51 state programs as well as a few private- and University-based laboratories offer TMS-based NBS (National Newborn Screening Status Report (272)). Several review papers have been published, highlighting the success of this technology (241,271,273–276). Some concerns have been raised regarding parental stress

(Text continues on p. 385)

Table 7   Newborn Screening with Tandem Mass Spectrometry

Amino acid (AA) disorders (enzyme deficiency)	Markers	Effectiveness of TMS	Suggested confirmatory evaluation	Symptoms if untreated	Treatment	Effectiveness of early treatment	Risk for acute crisis
Argininemia (arginase)	Arg	(+)	Plasma AA's, ammonia	Hyperammonemia, protein intolerance, episodic vomiting, FTT. Neurologic damage, spastic quadriplegia if undiagnosed	Low protein diet, restricted in arginine (Special medical diet). Sodium phenylbutyrate	+++	(+/−)
Argininosuccinic aciduria (argininosuccinic acid lyase)	Cit	+	Plasma AA's, ammonia, urine AA's (RBC enzyme activity)	Hyperammonemia, lethargy, vomiting, hypothermia, hyperventilation, hepatomegaly, trichorexis nodosa (brittle hair; pili torti), coma and death	Low protein diet (Special medical diet). Arginine supplementation	++	+
Citrullinemia Type I (argininosuccinic acid synthetase)	Cit	+	Plasma AA's, ammonia	Clinical picture varies: hyperammonemia, vomiting, diarrhea. Mental retardation, hypotonia, lethargy, coma, seizures and death can occur	Sodium benzoate and/or sodium phenylacetate. Supplementation with arginine. Protein restriction (Special medical diet)	++	+
Citrullinemia Type II (citrin)	Cit?, Met, Phe, Tyr?	(+)	Plasma AA's, chemistry panel, liver function tests. Galactose in blood/urine (confrimation requires DNA analysis)	Infancy: ketotic hypoglycemia, cholestatic liver disease, mild hyperammonemia, anemia. Adults: hyperammonemia, lethargy, coma, and death can occur	Treatment of cholestasis (vit A,D,E, and K, MCT containing formulas), frequent feedings, uncooked corn starch?, Arginine supplementation	?	(+/−)
Gyrate atrophy of the choroid and retina (ornithine aminotransferase)	Orn	(+)	Plasma AA's	Progressive loss of vision (early myopia and decreased night vision). Mild muscle weakness	Arginine restricted diet (special medical diet). Creatine. Some patients may respond to pyridoxine	?	−
Hyperammonemia, hyperornithinemia, homocitrullinuria syndrome (ornithine transporter)	Orn	(+)	Plasma AA's, ammonia, urine AA's	Hyperammonemia, protein intolerance, episodic vomiting, FTT. Neurologic damage if undiagnosed. Ataxia, choreoathetosis, seizures	Low protein diet. Arginine supplementation?	?	+
Phenylketonuria (PKU) and hyperphenylalaninemias (phenylalanine hydroxylase)	Phe, Phe/Tyr	+	Plasma AA's, urine pterin studies, bloodspot DHPR studies	Classic PKU: Microcephaly, mental retardation, seizures, autistic-like behavior, and fair-light hair and eye color; "mousy/musty" odor	Phenylalanine restriction, tyrosine supplementation (Special medical diet). Tetrahydrobiopterin supplementation in some	+++	−
Biopterin defects (GTPCH, PTPS, DHPR, PH)	Phe, Phe/Tyr	+	Plasma AA's, urine pterin studies, bloodspot DHPR studies	Hypotonia, dystonia, myoclonic seizures, temperature instability, developmental delay	Depending on the defect: phenylalanine restriction, tetrahydrobiopterin, L-Dopa/carbidopa	+	−

(Continued)

Table 7 Newborn Screening with Tandem Mass Spectrometry (Continued)

Amino acid (AA) disorders (enzyme deficiency)	Markers	Effectiveness of TMS	Suggested confirmatory evaluation	Symptoms if untreated	Treatment	Effectiveness of early treatment	Risk for acute crisis
Tyrosinemia Type I (fumarylacetoacetate hydrolase)	Tyr, Met	(+/−)[a]	Plasma AA's, succinylacetone (blood or urine), urine organic acids, urine AA's, renal function tests, liver function tests. (enzyme activity in RBC)	Liver failure with ascites, jaundice, coagulopathy; renal enlargement, renal Fanconi syndrome, rickets, neurologic porphyria-like crises; "boiled cabbage" odor. Chronic patients develop cirrhosis and hepatomas,	Phenylalanine and tyrosine restriction (Special medical diet). NTBC (inhibitor of 4-hydroxyphenylpyruvate dioxygenase) to decrease formation of fumarylacetoacetate. Liver transplant if NTBC is ineffective	+++	(+/−)
Tyrosinemia Type II (tyrosine aminotransferase)	Tyr	(+)	Plasma AA's, urine organic acids. (confirmatory diagnosis by enzyme activity in liver)	Corneal ulcers, hyperkeratosis in palms and soles. Mental retardation may be present in some patients	Low phenylalanine and tyrosine diet	+++	−
Tyrosinemia Type III (4-hydroxyphenyl-pyruvate dioxygenase)	Tyr	(+)	Plasma AA's. Urine organic acids (confirmation by enzyme assay in liver)	Mental retardation. Ataxia	Low phenylalanine and tyrosine diet?	?	−
Homocystinuria (cystathionine beta synthase)	Met	(+)	Plasma AA's, total homocysteine, urine organic acids	Marfanoid appearance and lens dislocation. Mild to moderate mental retardation in some patients; thromboembolism and osteoporosis may occur	Methionine restriction with cystine supplementation (Special medical diet). Betaine supplementation. Vitamin B6 may benefit milder forms	+++	−
Maple syrup urine disease (branched chain keto acid decarboxylase)	Leu, Leu/Ala, Val	+	Plasma AA's, urine organic acids, serum chemistry panel	Poor feedings, vomiting, lethargy, hypertonia, seizures, coma and death; "maple syrup" odor. May have a later age of onset	Evaluate for possible thiamin responsiveness (rare). Leucine, isoleucine, and valine restriction (Special medical diet)	+++	+
Methionine adenosyltransferase deficiency	Met	(+)	Plasma AA's, total HCY, organic acids	Neurological involvment, demyelination. Cabbage-like odor	Dietary methionine restriction and/or supplementation with adenosylmethionine	?	−
Nonketotic hyperglycinemia (glycine cleavage system)	Gly	(+/−)	Simultaneous plasma and CSF AA's	Neonatal onset lethargy, hypotonia, hiccups, seizures (unresponsive to treatment), apnea. EEG: burst -suppresion pattern. Severe mental retardation, spastic quadriplegia. Transient and late-onset forms known	Low glycine diet, sodium benzoate, dextromethorphan	−	−
Prolinemia Type I (proline oxidase) and Type II (pyrroline-5-carboxylate dehydrogenase)	Pro	?	Plasma and urine AA's	Prolinemia Type I may be no have distinctive clinical manifestations. Prolinemia Type II has been asssociated to seizures and MR, but clinical presentation is unclear	Not established	?	−

Organic acid (OA) disorders (enzyme deficiency)	Marker	Effectiveness of TMS	Suggested initial evaluation	Symptoms if untreated	Treatment	Effectiveness of early treatment	Risk for acute crisis
2-Methyl butyrylglycinuria (2-methylbutyryl-CoA dehydrogenase)	2-Me-C4^c	+	Blood acylcarnitines, plasma carnitine, urine organic acids (urine acylglycines)	Few cases reported with cerebral palsy and movement disorders. Mild/asymptomatic forms detected by NBS, common in the Hmong population (48)	Carnitine supplementation. Dietary isoleucine restriction	?	?
2-Methyl-3-hydroxybutyric aciduria (2-methyl-3-hydroxybutyryl CoA dehydrogenase)	2-Me-3H-C4	?	Blood acylcarnitines, urine organic acids, plasma carnitine	Few patients reported. Progressive neurodegeneration. X-linked (49)	Carnitine supplementation. Dietary isoleucine restriction	?	?
3-Hydroxy-3-methylglutaric aciduria (3-hydroxy-3-methylglutaryl CoA lyase)	C5OH^c 3Me-C5DC	+	Blood acylcarnitines, urine organic acids, plasma carnitine, serum chemistry panel	Severe metabolic acidosis without ketosis; hypoglycemia with fasting; "cat's urine" odor	Avoidance of fasting; aggressive intervention during intercurrent illness. Low leucine, high carbohydrate diet (Special medical diet). Carnitine supplementation	+	+
2-Methyl acetoacetic aciduria (3-ketothiolase or beta-ketothiolase)	C5:1^c, C5OH	(+)	Blood acylcarnitines, urine organic acids, serum chemistry panel	Recurrent severe ketoacidosis, vomiting, Reyes-like episodes	Carnitine supplementation, low protein diet. Avoidance of fasting	?	+
3-Methyl crotonylglycinuria (3-methylcrotonyl-CoA carboxylase)(3MCC)	C5OH^c	+	Blood acylcarnitines, urine organic acids, plasma carnitine, serum chemistry panel	Metabolic acidosis and hypoglycemia. Some asymptomatic and "maternal" forms of 3-MCC can be detected through NBS (47)	Low protei/leucine restricted diet. Carnitine supplementation. Avoid long fasting periods	+++	+
3-Methylglutaconic aciduria (Type I)(3-Methylglutaconyl-CoA hydratase)(AUH gene)	C5OH^c	(+/−)	Blood acylcarnitines, urine organic acids, plasma carnitine, serum chemistry panel	Variable clinical presentation from asymptomatic to severe neurological impairment or acidosis. Speech delay	Leucine restricted diet for severe forms. Carnitine supplementation	?	(+/−)
Ethylmalonic encephalopathy (ETHE 1-gene defect)	C4^c	(+)	Blood acylcarnitines, urine organic acids or urine acylglycines. Lactic acid	Severe. Developmental delay, hypotonia, pyramidal signs, orthostatic acrocyanosis, petechiae, diarrhea. Abnormal magnetic resonance imaging (demyelination) (74–76)	Methionine restriction? Carnitine supplementation? Avoid long fasting periods	−	(+/−)
Glutaric acidemia Type I (glutaryl-CoA dehydrogenase deficiency)	C5DC	(+/−)	Blood and urine acylcarnitines, plasma carnitine, urine organic acids. Some patients may have normal	Macrocephaly at birth; sudden onset dystonia or progressive neurological deterioration. Movement disorders. Episodes of decompensation with vomiting,	Diet restricted in lysine and tryptophan (Special medical diet). Carnitine supplementation. Intensive treatment during intercurrent illnesses	++	+

(Continued)

Table 7 Newborn Screening with Tandem Mass Spectrometry (*Continued*)

Organic acid (OA) disorders (enzyme deficiency)	Marker	Effectiveness of TMS	Suggested initial evaluation	Symptoms if untreated	Treatment	Effectiveness of early treatment	Risk for acute crisis
			organic acid analysis (low excreters) and can be missed by NBS (281,282). Confirmatory diagnosis by enzyme activity in fibroblasts	lethargy and Reye's-like syndrome. Subdural and retinal hemorrhages, mimicking shaken baby syndrome			
Isobutyryl CoA dehydrogenase deficiency	Iso C4[c]	+	Blood acylcarnitines, urine organic acids or urine acylglycines	Few patients reported. FTT, cardiomyopathy? Mild forms may be detected through NBS (51)	Low protein/valine restriction? Carnitine supplementation	?	?
Isovaleric acidemia (isovaleryl-CoA dehydrogenase deficiency)	C5[c]	+	Blood acylcarnitines, urine organic acids, plasma carnitine, serum chemistry panel, CBC	Poor feedings, vomiting, acidosis, lethargy, seizures, coma and death. "Sweaty feet" odor. Asymptomatic forms detected by newborn screening in patients and relatives (46)	Low leucine diet (Special medical diet). Carnitine supplementation. Glycine supplementation	+++	+
Malonic aciduria	C3DC	+	Blood acylcarnitines, urine organic acids, plasma carnitine, serum chemistry panel	Rare. Metabolic acidosis, hypoglycemia, dev. delay, seizures, cardiomyopathy (53,63)	High CHO, low fat diet. Carnitine supplementation	?	+
Methylmalonic acidemia (methylmalonyl-CoA mutase deficiency or cobalamin synthesis defects -Cbl A,B,C,D or F)	C3, C4DC	+	Blood acylcarnitines, plasma homocysteine, AA's, ammonia, carnitine, CBC, blood gases and chemistry panel. Urine organic acids	Life threatening/fatal ketoacidosis and hyper-ammonemia may appear during first week of life; later symptoms include failure to thrive, developmental delay and episodes of acidosis and coma with risk of death. Increased risk of thrombosis and hydrocephalus in cobalamin defects (53,62)	Low protein diet, restricted in isoleucine, valine, methionine, threonine (Special medical diet). Carnitine supplementation. Cobalamin (vitamin B12) useful in some cases. Betaine for cobalamin C, D and F defects	+++	+
Multiple carboxylase deficiency (holocarboxylase synthetase or biotinidase)	C5OH[c]	(+/−)	Blood acylcarnitines, biotinidase, carnitine, blood gases and serum chemistry panel. Urine organic acids	Alopecia, rash, developmental delay and seizures. Metabolic acidosis. Good response to biotin (64). Many NBS programs have separate screening for biotinidase deficiency	Biotin (10–50 mg/day)	+++	(+/−)
Propionic acidemia (Propionyl-CoA carboxylase deficiency)	C3	+	Blood acylcarnitines, plasma AA's, ammonia, carnitine, CBC, blood gases and serum chemistry panel. Urine organic acids	Feeding difficulties, vomiting, lethargy, coma with or without acidosis. Seizures and developmental delay are common (53,55)	Low protein diet, restriction of isoleucine, valine, methionine, threonine (Special medical diet). Carnitine supplementation	+++	+

Fatty acid oxidation disorders	Marker	Effectiveness of TMS	Suggested initial evaluation	Symptoms if untreated	Treatment	Effectiveness of early treatment	Risk for acute crisis
Carnitine uptake/transport deficiency	Low C0	(+/−)	Plasma carnitine, urine carnitine, serum chemistry panel, creatine kinase (CK)(confirmatory studies in fibroblasts)	Hypoketotic hypoglycemia, cardiomyopathy, skeletal myopathy. Potential liver failure and hyperammonemia (234)	Carnitine supplementation. Avoidance of fasting	+++	+
Carnitine palmitoyltransferase i deficiency	High C0, C0//(C16 + C18:1)	(+)	Blood acylcarnitines, urine organic acids, plasma carnitine, serum chemistry panel	Hypoketotic hypoglycemia, hepatomegaly, coma, seizures (181,182)	Avoidance of fasting, aggressive treatment during intercurrent illness. Low fat, high CHO diet with medium chain triglycerides supplementation	+/+++	+
Carnitine/acylcarnitine translocase deficiency	C16, C18:1, C18	+	Blood acylcarnitines, plasma carnitine, serum chemistry panel, CK	Hypoketotic hypoglycemia, hepatomegaly, cardiomyopathy, arrhythmias, muscle weakness, cardiorespiratory collapse, death. May present with severe hypoglycemia and hyperammonemia in the newborn period. Risk for SIDS (214)	Avoidance of fasting. Low -fat, high-carbohydrate diet, supplemented with MCT oil. Carnitine supplementation. Effectiveness of treatment is variable and not well known	+/?	+
Carnitine palmitoyltransferase II deficiency neonatal onset/infantile	C16, C18:1, C18	+	Blood acylcarnitines, plasma carnitine, serum chemistry panel, CK	Severe hypoglycemia with hypoketosis, cardiomyopathy, hepatomegaly, hyperammonemia, hypotonia, seizures. Polycystic/dysplastic kidneys in neonatal cases	Avoidance of fasting. Low -fat, high-carbohydrate diet, supplemented with MCT oil. Carnitine supplementation	−/?	+[b]
Carnitine palmitoyltransferase II deficiency late onset	C16, C18:1, C18	+	Blood acylcarnitines, plasma carnitine, serum chemistry panel, CK	Excercise intolerance, rhabdomyolysis, myoglobinuria (risk of renal failure)	High carbohydrate, limited fat diet. Avoidance of fasting. May include supplementation with MCT and carnitine. (Triheptanoate?)	+	+
Multiple acyl-CoA dehydrogenase deficiency, glutaric acidemia Type II	C4[c], C5[c], C8, C12, C14, C16	+	Blood acylcarnitines, plasma carnitine, AA's, ammonia, chemistry panel and CK. Urinary organic acids/urine acylglycines	Severe neonatal form: hypoglycemia, hyperammonemia, hepatomegaly, cardiomyopathy, "sweaty feet" odor, often with polycycstic kidneys. Later onset form generally milder, may have hypoglycemia, Reye-like symptoms	Avoidance of fasting; aggressive intervention when hypoglycemia and/or acidosis. Low fat, high CHO, low protein diet, Carnitine supplementation. Riboflavin	+	+
Medium-chain acyl-CoA dehydrogenase deficiency	C8, C6, C10:1. C8/C10	+	Blood acylcarnitines, plasma carnitine, serum chemistry panel (mutation analysis)	Fasting intolerance, hypoglycemia, hyperammonemia, acute encephalopathy, liver failure, Reye's like syndrome SIDS	Avoidance of fasting; aggressive intervention during intercurrent illneses. Carnitine supplementation. Moderate fat restriction with high CHO diet	+++	+

(Continued)

Table 7 Newborn Screening with Tandem Mass Spectrometry (*Continued*)

Fatty acid oxidation disorders	Marker	Effectiveness of TMS	Suggested initial evaluation	Symptoms if untreated	Treatment	Effectiveness of early treatment	Risk for acute crisis
Short-chain acyl-CoA dehydrogenase deficiency	C4[c]	+	Blood acylcarnitines and carnitine. Chemistry panel. Urine acylglycines or organic acids. Confirmation may require fibroblast assays and/or mutation analysis	Variable phenotype. Lethargy, vomiting, delayed development, muscle weakness, hypotonia. May be asymptomatic	Avoidance of fasting; aggressive intervention during intercurrent illness. Carnitine supplementation. Low fat diet?	+	+
Long chain acyl-CoA dehydrogenase deficiency (trifunctional protein deficiency)	C16OH, C18:1OH, C18OH	(+)	Blood acylcarnitines, urine organic acids, serum chemistry panel, CK	Clinical variability: hypoglycemia, vomiting, lethargy, coma, seizures, hepatic disease, cardiomyopathy, rhabdomyolysis, progressive neuropathy; in some older patients, pigmentary retinopathy	Avoidance of fasting; aggressive intervention during intercurrent illnesses. Low fat, high CHO diet supplemented with MCT. Carnitine supplementation. DHA (docosahexanoic acid) may prevent retinal disease	+	+
Very long-chain acyl-CoA dehydrogenase deficiency	C14:1, C14, C16 (C14:2)	(+)	Blood acylcarnitines, serum chemistry panel, urine organic acids	Hypoketotic hypoglycemia with cardiomyopathy and/or liver failure; rhabdomyolysis	Avoidance of fasting; aggressive intervention during intercurrent illness. Low fat, high carbohydrate diet, supplemented with MCT. Carnitine supplementation (controversial)	+	+

[a] Tyrosine levels are mildly elevated in tyrosinemia Type I and can be missed if cut-off is set above 100 uMol. Effective screening of tyrosinemia Type I may require assay of fumarylacetoacetate hydrolase in filter paper, or a two-tier approach, with tyrosine as first marker and succinylacetone as second test.

[b] Risk for rhabdomyolysis

[c] This marker has at least another analyte with the same M/Z ratio (isomer).

generated by false-positive results and also regarding the lack of information among pediatricians (277,278).

Following are some important considerations for the understanding of NBS detection of AA, organic acid, and FAO disorders:

Initial Evaluation

In the majority of the state NBS programs, a positive result is communicated simultaneously to the primary physician as well as the closest designated metabolic center. Both should work together to ensure that the patient's initial evaluation, confirmatory testing, and treatment are carried out appropriately, following the guidelines of each state NBS program.

Emergency

While the confirmatory testing for a positive NBS should be obtained as soon as possible, not all the diseases detected by TMS present with acute metabolic crisis or require immediate treatment. Table 7 summarizes information about the majority of the diseases that could potentially be detected measuring AA and AC, their suggested initial evaluation, symptoms, treatment, effectiveness of early treatment, and risk for an acute crisis. The table should be used as a guide and it is always advised that the patient be referred to an experienced metabolic center.

It is important to understand that there is a great phenotypic variation within the same disorder, ranging from neonatal crisis to asymptomatic forms (i.e., MCAD). For management of patients presenting with metabolic crisis, see corresponding sections above.

Impact of Early Discharge

In the majority of the NBS programs, the samples are collected between 24 and 48 hours of life. Early discharge affects the NBS by TMS in different ways. In general, AC levels increase very rapidly and it is therefore likely that diagnosis of OAs or FAO defects can be established before 24 hours. For some disorders, TMS screening in cord blood may be possible (279). For PKU, diagnosis in samples obtained before 24 hours has been established, but early diagnosis for other AA disorders (i.e., mild forms of MSUD) may require a longer period or a higher protein intake (268,279).

Frequent False Positives
Premature Babies
Premature babies have different normal values than full-term babies (269). However not all NBS programs have adjusted cut-offs for newborns of different gestational ages. Additionally, in extreme premise or sick neonates, samples are frequently obtained too early (less than 12 hours of age), or very soon (less than four hours) after a blood transfusion. Additionally, there is a tendency to use TPN with lipids and high dose AAs (2–3 g/kg/day) early in life, which often results in false-positive results for several diseases. Data from the California NBS program shows that, while 7.4% of all NBS samples come from the neonatal intensive care unit, these samples account for 43.4% of the initial positive results (280). Confirmatory studies in a patient with a positive result obtained while on TPN are complicated if the patient continues to be on TPN. One possibility is to wait until the patient is off parenteral nutrition and receiving full feeds before obtaining the confirmatory samples. However, that could take several weeks for some patients. Our approach depends on the confirmatory sample needed. For organic acids, the urine sample can be obtained while the patient continues on TPN. In contrast, for quantitative plasma AA or AC, we advise to discontinue the infusion of AAs and lipids for four to six hours before obtaining a confirmatory sample. During that period of time the patient should be maintained on IV fluids with a similar GIR to avoid hypoglycemia. This approach avoids repeat false-positive results for aminoacidopathies or FAO disorders.

Liver Disease

Cholestatic liver disease is a relatively common finding in sick neonates. In those patients, there is frequently a nonspecific elevation of methionine, tyrosine, and phenylalanine, which can be detected by NBS. While the same profile can be found in patients with liver disease of any etiology (infectious, metabolic, etc), it is important to remember that galactosemia, tyrosinemia Type 1, citrin deficiency (citrullinemia Type 2), and some FAO defects can present in the neonatal period, with significant liver involvement and cholestasis. Therefore, appropriate work-up should be obtained to rule out those disorders. Additionally, it is important to highlight that the cut-off used for tyrosine by the majority of the NBS programs is too high to detect tyrosinemia Type I, which should be screened for by measuring succinylacetone in blood or urine in every patient with liver disease of unknown etiology.

Possible False Negatives

Not all the diseases that are listed as screened for by an NBS program are going to be detected. For some, the markers are very elevated in the newborn period and are easy to detect: i.e., IVC in patients with IVA or octanoylcarnitine (C8) in patients with MCAD deficiency. In contrast, other analytes are only marginally elevated in affected newborns and can be missed (270). As an example, glutarylcarnitine can be only marginally elevated in affected patients with glutaric aciduria Type I, and false-negative results have been reported (267,281,282). Additionally, some diseases have only been diagnosed by TMS when patients were symptomatic (sick) and had abnormal ACs profiles at the time. Therefore, while it is expected that the analytes would also be found in an asymptomatic newborn, the true efficacy of NBS for those diseases has not been proved yet. The "effectiveness" of NBS for each disease is listed in Table 7.

One Result, More Than One Disease?

Some analytes can be markers of more than one disease. For example, citrulline is elevated in argininosuccinic acidemia and also in citrullinemia. Similarly, 3-hydroxyIVC can be elevated in 3-methylcrotonyl-CoA carboxylase, HMG, and 3-methylglutaconic aciduria and can also be elevated as secondary marker in multiple carboxylase deficiencies and B-ketothyolase deficiency (97,283). The NBS program may list all these disorders in the differential diagnosis. It is therefore important to emphasize the need for rapid and appropriate confirmatory testing.

Confirmatory Samples

Table 7 provides a guide to the suggested confirmatory evaluation. The list includes specific confirmatory tests (i.e., organic acids, AAs) as well as common tests that are useful to assess the patient's clinical condition (i.e., chemistry panel). Some states provide strict guidelines regarding laboratories in charge of confirmatory testing. It is always advisable to choose a laboratory with experience in the diagnosis and follow-up of metabolic diseases. Age-appropriate normal values, fast turn around, and experienced interpretation are mandatory. It is also important to consider that for some FAO defects, ACs can normalize at the time of the confirmatory sample, which could be misinterpreted as an initial false-positive result (284).

Need for Enzymatic/Molecular Studies?

For the majority of the diseases screened by TMS, biochemical diagnosis can be confirmed in blood and urine samples. Enzyme activity is rarely needed. Molecular studies are available for most disorders, and common mutations have been described for some conditions (i.e., MCAD, LCHAD). It is always advisable to obtain confirmatory molecular diagnosis to establish genotype/phenotype information that could help in the management and prognosis of the disease, as well as for genetic counseling. Prenatal diagnosis is available for the majority of the diseases.

Asymptomatic "Patients"

The availability of NBS with TMS has allowed the identification of affected family members (siblings and parents) of the positive newborn. These findings have uncovered many "asymptomatic" or mild forms for MCAD, 3-methylcrotonylCoAcarboxylase deficiency, IVA, and 2-methylbutyryl-CoA dehydrogenase deficiency (48,285–287). In general, those mild/asymptomatic forms are associated with specific mutations. However, it is important to remember that a disease may remain "silent" until a significant stress (illness/surgery) occurs. Therefore, caution is advised in the counseling and follow-up of these patients.

For conditions where asymptomatic forms are known, it is advisable to screen siblings and parents.

Effectiveness of Treatment

For the vast majority of diseases detected by TMS, early treatment is effective in preventing morbidity and mortality (i.e., MCAD deficiency). However, it is known that treatment is not effective in preventing neurological impairment for some disorders (i.e., biopterin defects, nonketotic hyperglycinemia) and effectiveness of early treatment has not yet been established for others (i.e., 3-methylglutaconic aciduria or 2-methylbutyryl-CoA dehydrogenase deficiency). Nevertheless, it is important to remember that diagnosis of an affected individual allows genetic counseling.

Long-Term Management

Metabolic diseases require follow-up by a multidisciplinary team, involving the metabolic specialist, dietitian, nurse, and social worker. Education of parents/patients and health-care providers on treatment is essential. Preventive health measures and early identification of warning signs that require immediate medical attention should be addressed by a short and clear emergency letter. Treatment during intercurrent illness may require short hospital admissions during the period of decreased PO intake or vomiting to assure hydration and glucose infusion. Detailed emergency treatment is provided above for each group of diseases mentioned.

Technical and Methodological Considerations
Different Programs
There is a great diversity of NBS systems and programs in different countries and even within the same country. As an example, in the United States, all 51 NBS programs follow different protocols and only 36 of them routinely use TMS (National Newborn Screening Status Report, January 2006).

Different Methods

Different NBS programs using TMS may detect or report different analytes. The analytes that are measured depend on the methodology used to acquire the data, and it may be determined by the state legislature. For example, some states measure only octanoylcarnitine (C8) for the diagnosis of MCAD deficiency. In contrast other states measure more than 30 different analytes (including AAs and ACs).

Different Diseases

The number of diseases listed as screened for by a NBS program varies, even among programs measuring the same analytes. This variation is somewhat artificial as NBS programs list the conditions in different ways; for example, in one NBS, "tyrosinemia" is listed as one condition, while another program may disclose tyrosinemia Type 1, Type 2, and Type 3 (and count them three different diseases). Other examples are biopterin defects, which could be listed as one disorder under "biopterin defects" or subdivided into four different diseases (all screened using the same marker).

Different Acylcarnitines with Same Molecular Weight

Another consideration is that different ACs have the same mass/charge ratio. As an example, a peak detected at the mass/charge ratio of 302 could be due to increased IVC (indicative of IVA), pivaloylcarnitine (indicative of treatment with pivalic acid–containing drugs), or 2-methyl-butyrilcarnitine (indicative of 2 methylbutyryl-CoA dehydrogenase deficiency) (48,255,288).

	Corresponding analytes observed by mass spectrometry	Abbreviation
288	Butyryl canitine or iso-butyryl carnitine	C4
300	Tiglyl carnitine or 3-methyl-crotonyl carnitine	C5:1
302	Isovaleryl carnitine, pivaloyl carnitine, or 2-methyl-butyryl canitine	C5 or 2Me–C4
318	3-Hydroxy-isovaleryl carnitine, or 3-hydroxy-2-methyl-butyryl carnitine	3–OH–C5 or 2–Me–3–OH–C4
402	Adipyl carnitine or HMG-carnitine	C6DC or 3–Me–C5DC

Useful websites for further information about NBS programs, diseases and initial treatment are:

1. http://www.genes-r-us.uthscsa.edu (289)
2. http://www.childrenshospital.org/newenglandconsortium/ (290)
3. www.dhs.ca.gov/gdb (291)
4. http://www.baylorhealth.com/medicalspecialties/metabolic/newbornscreening.htm (292)
5. http://www.mayoclinic.org/laboratorygenetics-rst/newbornscreening.html (293)

PRIMARY LACTIC ACIDEMIAS

The PLAs are a group of IMD with variable clinical presentation, including life-threatening episodes of metabolic acidosis, and complex biochemical, enzymatic, and molecular diagnosis. They represent abnormalities in pyruvate metabolism that is recognized biochemically by hyperlactacidemia and, clinically, by symptoms reflecting "energy deficiency" (1,294). Pyruvic acid produced by the glycolytic pathway can follow different metabolic fates. To produce energy, pyruvate enters the mitochondria and undergoes aerobic catabolism via acetyl-CoA, the TCA, cycle and the respiratory chain (Fig. 4).

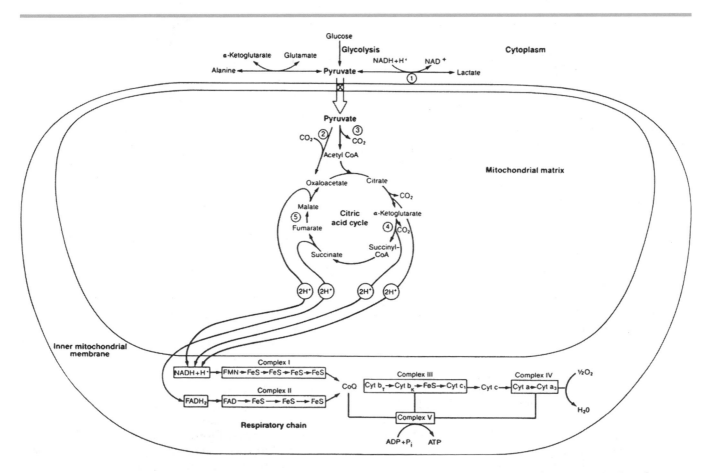

Figure 4 Pyruvate metabolism, the tricarboxylic acid cycle and the respiratory chain. Enzymes: **1**, lactate dehydrogenase; **2**, pyruvate carboxylase; **3**, pyruvate dehydrogenase complex; **4**, α-ketoglutarate dehydrogenase; **5**, fumarase. *Source*: From Ref. 295.

During fasting periods, pyruvic acid can also be an intermediary substrate for gluconeogenesis, via oxaloacetic acid. A block in any of the many enzymatic steps involved in those pathways can increase pyruvic acid levels, with simultaneous elevation of lactic acid and alanine, and limit the production of energy or glucose synthesis.

PLA can be divided into four groups:

- Defects in PDHC
- Defects in the TCA cycle
- Defects in gluconeogenesis
- Defects in oxidative phosphorylation (OXPHOS) (respiratory chain)

Pathophysiology and Clinical Presentations

Correlation between symptoms and enzymatic block is difficult as one enzymatic defect can present with different phenotypes and different enzyme deficiencies can give a similar clinical presentation. A detailed description of each enzymatic defect is beyond the scope of this chapter; so we will mainly address those conditions that can present with severe hyperlactacidemia, requiring emergency treatment.

Pyruvate Dehydrogenase Complex

Deficiency of PDHC is one of the most frequent causes of PLA. This thiamine-dependent enzymatic complex is responsible for the decarboxylation of pyruvate to acetyl-CoA (Fig. 4) and is made of four different catalytic components: E_1-α, E_1-β, E_2, and E_3. Additionally two regulatory proteins at the E_1level (pyruvate dehydrogenase kinase and pyruvate dehydrogenase phosphatase) and an E_3-binding protein (X-lipoate protein) are also part of the complex (294–296).

Three different clinical presentations are known: The most severe is the neonatal, characterized by overwhelming lactic acidosis. These children present soon after birth with poor feeding, hypotonia, lethargy, and respiratory distress. Mild dysmorphism (frontal bossing, low nasal bridge, upturned nose, and tented lips) has been described, and death occurs within few weeks (294,296,297). A less severe picture appears in infants and young children with hypotonia, developmental delay, and seizures. The third form presents with acute, intermittent episodes of ataxia, which can be triggered by a high carbohydrate intake (294,296,299). Deficiencies in different components of the PDHC have been reported, but the most common is the deficiency of the E_1-α subunit, which is encoded by an X-linked gene (294,296,297). However, due to the important role of the PDHC in energy metabolism, males as well as females can be affected. Most defects of E_1-α gene are de novo, with point mutations being more common in males and deletions or insertions in females (296,297). This information is extremely important for genetic counseling.

Defects in the E_2 component, the E_3-binding protein and the pyruvate dehydrogenase phosphatase, while rare, have been reported (294,298–301). Their phenotypes have ranged from severe mental retardation to Leigh syndrome and refractory lactic acidosis. The E_3 component (dihydrolipoamide dehydrogenase) is common to other 3 enzymatic complexes: the α-KGD (involved in TCA cycle), the BCKD, which is the enzyme deficient in MSUD, and the glycine cleavage system (involved in glycine catabolism). Few patients with deficiency of the E_3 component (lipoamide dehydrogenase) are known. Their clinical and biochemical presentation is variable, with a combination of the different manifestations of the PDHC, α-KGD, and BCKD deficiencies. Recurrent episodes of liver failure, cardiomyopathy, and myoglobinuria have also been reported (294,302–304).

Progressive involvement of the basal ganglia and brain stem are frequent in PDHC-deficient patients and can lead to nystagmus, dystonia, apnea, or sudden, unexpected death. MRI findings in these patients are suggestive of subacute necrotizing encephalopathy (Leigh syndrome). However, it is important to note that Leigh syndrome has also been described in patients with PC, the TCA cycle, and respiratory chain deficiencies (see below), as well as in other IEM (1,305,306). Other frequent abnormalities of the CNS in PDHC deficiency are congenital malformations of the brain, including agenesis or hypoplasia of the corpus callosum (294,296).

Defects in the Tricarboxylic Acid Cycle

The TCA cycle is responsible for the oxidative decarboxylation of citrate to oxaloacetate (Fig. 4). Several enzymes are involved, and defects in α-KGD, fumarase, and succinate dehydrogenase (SDH) have been characterized.

Structure of α-KGD is similar to that of the PDHC and the BCKD, sharing with them the E_3 component. Therefore, the three enzymes can be affected in E_3 deficiency (see PDHC deficiency above) (307). Additionally, a few patients with isolated α-KGD have been reported. They present in infancy or early childhood with severe neurological involvement, including developmental delay, hypo- or hypertonia, and ataxia. Structural brain abnormalities can be present (308,309).

Fumarase deficiency appears to be more common. Clinical presentation ranges from severe neurological involvement, seizures and death in childhood, to mild mental retardation and survival into adulthood (310–312). Dysmorphic facial features and neonatal polycythemia have been recently reported. Structural brain malformations like diffuse polymicrogyria, hypomyelination, agenesis of the corpus callosum, Leigh syndrome, decreased white matter, and cortical atrophy are common (311–312).

SDH consists of four nuclear-encoded subunits. It participates in succinate catabolism in the Krebs cycle and the electron transfer in the respiratory chain. Mutations in the four genes, SDHA, B, C and D, have been reported. Interestingly, SDHA mutations have been reported to cause an encephalomyopathy in childhood, resembling a respiratory chain defect (see below), while mutations in the genes encoding the other three subunits have been associated only with tumor formation (313).

Defects in Gluconeogenesis

Gluconeogenic defects involve deficiencies in the four regulatory enzymes of this pathway: PC, phosphoenolpyruvate carboxykinase (PEPCK), fructose-1, 6-diphosphatase (FDP), and glucose-6-phosphatase. Deficiency of the latter affects gluconeogenesis as well as glycogen degradation and is responsible for the glycogen storage disease Type 1. In general, patients with gluconeogenic defects present not only lactic acidosis but also hypoglycemia and hepatomegaly.

PC, a biotin-dependent enzyme responsible for the carboxylation of pyruvate to oxaloacetate (Fig. 4), plays an important role in gluconeogenesis, lipogenesis and energy production. Decreased availability of oxaloacetate also impairs the synthesis of aspartate and glutamate with secondary abnormalities in the urea cycle and the synthesis of glutamine-derived neurotransmitters. Deficiency of the PC can be isolated or as a part of the biotinidase or holocarboxylase synthetase deficiencies (see organic acidemias). Isolated PC deficiency has been described in many patients. Three clinical presentations are differentiated. The most severe form presents in neonates with lactic acidosis, hypotonia, and tachypnea during the first hours of life. Tremors, hypokinesia, and abnormal ocular movements appear to be distinctive, while seizures are infrequent.

A rapid fatal outcome is described for most patients (294,314,315). A less severe phenotype, mainly described in North American Indians, presents in infancy with developmental delay, failure to thrive, and seizures, progressing to severe mental retardation. Mild hepatomegaly is present in both clinical presentations. Macrocephaly and brain abnormalities, such as decreased myelination, ischemia-like lesions, cyst, periventricular leukomalacia, Leigh syndrome, subdural hematomas, and brain atrophy have been described (294,316,317). These abnormalities are thought to be related to the important role of PC in astrocyte metabolism. The third, less common phenotype, is characterized by episodic attacks of lactic acidosis with slight neurological involvement (294).

PEPCK deficiency is very rare. Symptoms appear in the newborn period or early infancy and include failure to thrive, hypotonia, lethargy, and hepatomegaly. Renal tubular acidosis and skeletal and cardiac muscular involvement have been reported (294).

FDP-deficient patients present in the newborn period with symptoms of hypoglycemia, hypotonia, and liver enlargement. Neurological involvement in these patients is only related to the hypoglycemic episodes (318).

Mitochondrial Oxidative Phosphorylation Diseases

The OXPHOS process is mediated by the respiratory chain, which carries electrons through a series of complex reactions to generate ATP. The respiratory chain is located in the mitochondria and is divided into five complexes, I through V. Each complex has several protein components, some encoded by nuclear DNA (nDNA) and others by mitochondrial DNA (mtDNA) (319). The only exception is complex II, which has only nDNA-encoded proteins. Additionally, transport of proteins into the mitochondria and assembly of the different components of the respiratory chain require coordinate regulation of nuclear and mitochondrial genes (319,320).

The mtDNA is a small circular molecule (16,500 base pairs) that encodes for 13 polypeptide subunits of the respiratory chain together with ribosomal and transfer RNAs needed for protein synthesis. Each cell contains hundreds of mitochondria and thousands of mtDNA molecules. In patients with mtDNA abnormalities, normal and abnormal mtDNA may coexist in the same cells (heteroplasmy). During cell division, mitochondria are randomly distributed to the new cells. Therefore, the relative proportions of normal and abnormal mtDNA change as the cells divide (319–321).

The clinical implication of mtDNA biology is that some tissues or organs can exhibit the effects of an mtDNA genetic defect while others are functioning normally, depending on the relative proportion of normal and abnormal mtDNA. Furthermore, normal tissues may be affected over time if the number of abnormal mitochondria reaches a threshold for phenotypical expression (320). For these reasons, genotype–phenotype correlations are difficult, as the same genetic defect can cause different phenotypes even within the same sibship, and phenotypes can change over time (320–323). This also emphasizes the importance of obtaining affected tissues for enzymatic diagnosis, such as liver in patients with acute liver failure or endomyocardial biopsy for patients with cardiomyopathies.

Clinical presentation of patients with OXPHOS defects is extremely broad, ranging from lesions in single tissues (i.e., optic nerve) to multisystemic manifestations, with age of onset ranging from birth to adulthood. An early-onset disease with a chronic and progressive clinical course and unexplained association of symptoms, and involving seemingly unrelated organs (i.e., diabetes and deafness) is characteristic of OXPHOS disorders (322). The most frequent findings are shown in Table 8.

Predominant clinical manifestations in neonates are severe lactic acidosis and encephalopathy, while infants frequently present with hypotonia or dystonia, recurrent vomiting, failure to thrive, developmental delay, pyramidal signs, and seizures. Oculomotor abnormalities and cerebellar signs are common, as well as renal tubular acidosis and cardiac and endocrine abnormalities (mainly diabetes) (322,323).

Almost all organs and systems can be affected in OXPHOS diseases, and even though some well-defined mitochondrial syndromes have been described, overlapping in clinical presentation is common. Table 9 lists the classical syndromes associated with mtDNA

Table 8 Most Frequent Findings Associated with OXPHOS Diseases

Neuromuscular
  Hypotonia
  Muscle weakness, myopathy
  Myalgia, exercise intolerance, myoglobinuria
  Developmental delay
  Progressive encephalopathy, regression
  Dementia
  Peripheral sensory-motor neuropathy
  Seizures, myoclonus
  Migraine headaches
  Stroke-like episodes
Movement disorders
  Recurrent ataxia
  Dystonia
  Parkinsonism
Brain abnormalities
  Absence of corpus callosum
  Porencephalic cysts
  Abnormal signaling of the basal ganglia
  Leukodystrophy
  Cortical atrophy/poliodystrophy
  Leigh's disease
Eye
  Cataracts, corneal opacities
  Retinitis pigmentosa
  Optic neuropathy
Ear
  Sensorineural hearing loss
Heart
  Cardiomyopathy (mainly hypertrophic)
  Cardiac conduction defects
Endocrine
  Diabetes mellitus
  Growth hormone deficiency
  Hypothyroidism, hypoparathyroidism
Gastrointestinal
  Episodic vomiting
  Chronic diarrhea, villous atrophy
  Exocrine pancreatic dysfunction
  Liver failure
  Dysmotility, pseudo-obstruction
Renal
  Renal Fanconi syndrome
  Tubulointerstitial nephritis, renal failure
Miscellaneous
  Sudden infant death
  Failure to thrive, intrauterine growth retardation
  Anemia (sideroblastic), myelodysplasia
  Recurrent hypoglycemia
  Craniofacial dysmorphic features
  Hair abnormalities (dry, thick, brittle hair)
  Skin abnormalities (mottled pigmentation in exposed areas)

Table 9 Most Common Clinical Syndromes Associated with mtDNA Defects

Mainly associated to mtDNA mutations	
MELAS	Mitochondrial encephalomyopathy, lactic acidosis, and stroke-like episodes
MERRF	Myoclonic epilepsy and ragged-red fibers
NARP	Neuropathy, ataxia and retinitis pigmentosa
LHON	Leber's hereditary optic neuropathy
Diabetes mellitus and deafness	
SNHL	Nonsyndromic aminoglucoside-induced hearing loss
Mainly associated with mtDNA deletions/duplications	
Pearson syndrome	Anemia (sideroblastic)/pancytopenia, exocrine pancreatic insufficiency, failure to thrive, liver dysfunction, myopathy, lactic acidosis
Kearns Sayre syndrome	Age before 20 years, progressive external ophthalmoplegia, retinitis pigmentosa, cerebellar ataxia, increased cerebrospinal protein, complete heart block, diabetes mellitus
Wolfram syndrome	Diabetes insipidus, diabetes mellitus, optic atrophy, and deafness
PEO	

common cardiac manifestations are hypertrophic cardiomyopathy (58%), dilated cardiomyopathy (29%), and left ventricular noncompaction (13%) (323). Arrhythmias, being the most common ventricular tachycardia, were detected in 11% of patients.

Another important phenotype that is being increasingly recognized is liver failure associated with neurological manifestations and lactic acidosis (hepatocerebral syndrome) as a presentation of nuclear-encoded mutations that lead to mtDNA depletion (324–326).

Adult patients present more frequently with classical mtDNA-encoded syndromes (Table 9) or a combination of muscle disease (myopathy, muscle weakness, exercise intolerance, rhabdomyolysis, etc.) associated with variable CNS involvement (ataxia, hearing loss, seizures, retinopathy, polyneuropathy, movement disorders) (320,321).

Once a mitochondrial disease is suspected, a complete evaluation of the most frequently affected organs or systems should be performed, which might include MRI and MR spectroscopy of the brain, EKG and echocardiogram, ophthalmological and hearing evaluation, and renal, liver, and endocrine function

defects, while Table 10 shows phenotypes associated with known mutations in nuclear genes.

In a series of 113 pediatric patients, the most common clinical subtypes were cardiomyopathy and myopathy, nonspecific encephalomyopathy, Leigh syndrome (subacute necrotizing encephalomyopathy), classical mitochondrial syndromes, and lethal infantile mitochondrial disease (323). It is important to recognize that OXPHOS defects represent a major cause of cardiomyopathy in children, with a reported incidence ranging from 24% (322) to 40% (323). The most

Table 10 Mitochondrial OXPHOS Diseases Due to Nuclear Mutations

	Phenotype	Disease
Genes controlling the stability of mtDNA		
ANT1	Multiple deletions mtDNA, PEO, muscle weakness, ataxia, depression, hypogonadism, hearing loss, peripheral neuropathy	AD-PEO
Twinkle		
Polymerase gamma1	Infantile hepatocerebral syndrome	Alpers' polidystrophy
Thymidine phosphorylase	Multiple deletion/depletion mtDNA, ophthalmoparesis, peripheral neuropathy, leucoencephalopathy, and gastrointestinal symptoms with intestinal dismotility	MNGIE
Thymidine kinase2	Fatal infantile congenital myopathy with or without a DeToni–Fanconi renal syndrome	MDS
DGUOK	Fatal infantile hepatopathy leading to rapidly progressive liver failure	
Deoxynucleotide carrier	Congenital microcephaly of Amish	
Genes encoding protein respiratory chain components		
Complex I NDUFS1	Leigh syndrome, complex I deficiency	AR mutations
Complex I NDUFS2	Cardiomyopathy–encephalomyopathy	AR mutations
Complex I NDUSFS4	Leigh-like syndrome	AR mutations
Complex I NDUFS7	Leigh syndrome	AR mutations
Complex I NDUFS8	Leigh syndrome	AR mutations
Complex I NDUFV1	Leigh syndrome, leucodystrophy, myoclonus	AR mutations
Complex II SDHA	Leigh syndrome	AR mutations
Complex II SDHB	Phaeochromocytoma, cervical paraganglioma	AD or sporadic
Complex II SDHC and SDHD	Hereditary paraganglioma	AR mutations
Complex III UQCRB gene subunit VII	Hypokalaemia and lactic acidosis	AR homozygous deletion
Defects of nonprotein respiratory chain constituents		
Coenzyme Q deficiency	Ataxia, seizures, myopathy	(?)
Tafazzin (cardiolipin acyltransferase?)	Barth syndrome	X-linked recessive
Genes encoding respiratory chain assembly components		
SURF1	COX_ Leigh syndrome	AR mutations
SCO1	COX_ hepathopathy and ketoacidotic coma	AR mutations
SCO2	COX_ infantile cardiomyopathy	AR mutations
COX10	COX_ leucodystrophy and renal tubulopathy	AR mutations
COX15	COX_ hypertrophic cardiomyopathy	AR mutations
BCS1L	Complex III-deficient encephalopathy, liver failure, renal tubulopathy	AR mutations
LRPPRC (mRNA-binding protein)	COX_ Leigh syndrome	AR mutations
ATP12	Complex V deficiency–encephalopathy	AR mutations

Abbreviations: ANT, adenine nucleotide translocator; AR, autosomal recessive; AD, autosomal dominant; COX: cytochrome C-oxidase; PEO, progressive external ophthalmoplejia; MNGIE, mitochondrial neuro-gastro-intestinal encephalomyopathy; MDS, mitochondrial DNA depletion syndrome.
Source: From Ref. 320.

tests. Common findings in MRI are bilateral and symmetrical hyperintense signals in the basal ganglia and involvement of brain stem (typical of Leigh disease). Different degrees and patterns of demyelination have also been described.

Diagnosis

Initial laboratory work-up is similar for a patient with suspected PLA of any etiology. In patients with intermittent symptoms, it is best to obtain samples during the acute decompensation. Blood levels for chemistry panel, blood gases, lactate (L), pyruvate (P), ammonium and AAs, and urine for organic acids are required. Additional information can be obtained by measuring blood levels of 3-OH-butyrate (3OHB), acetoacetate (AcAc), total and free carnitine, and urine AAs.

Accurate measurement of L and P requires rapid and proper handling of the specimens. Arterial or free-flowing venous samples are preferred. Patients

with acute decompensation usually have severe metabolic acidosis with high anion gap and markedly elevated lactic acid. The lactic/pyruvate (L/P) ratio is low or normal in PDHC and elevated in PC and respiratory chain defects (complex I, III, and IV) (327). Reduced 3OHB/AcAc ratio is expected in PC deficiency (294). Secondary lactic acidosis due to poor perfusion, hypoxia, liver insufficiency, sepsis, or sedation with propofol should be ruled out (327,328). In general, they do not present with ketosis.

In chronic patients, even slight elevations of lactate provide a clue for diagnosis. More severe biochemical abnormalities might only be present during attacks, which are usually triggered by fasting or intercurrent illnesses.

In some patients with PDHC or OXPHOS defects, increased lactic acid levels are only detected one to two hours after a regular or a high-carbohydrate meal. In contrast, elevated fasting levels of lactic acid that decrease after a high CHO meal, with simultaneous increase in ketone bodies, are suggestive of PC deficiency (294). In patients with CNS involvement and normal lactic acid in blood, lactate should be measured in cerebral spinal fluid.

Hypoglycemia is associated with lactic acidemia during fasting in patients with gluconeogenic defects, while hyperglycemia can be found in OXPHOS and PDHC deficiencies (327). Mild hyperammonemia is present in neonates with PC and fumarase deficiencies and increased uric acid and hypophosphatemia are found in FDP deficiency. In the latter, provocative tests with fructose and glycerol, performed under close supervision, are useful for diagnosis. Glucose tolerance tests should be avoided, as they can trigger an acute decompensation in PDHC-deficient patients.

UOA analysis is useful but, with the exception of the TCA cycle defects, cannot determine the site of the metabolic block. Usual findings in OXPHOS defects are elevated lactic, pyruvic, and 2-hydroxybutyric acids, mild elevation of TCA cycle intermediates (succinic, fumaric, malic and α-ketoglutaric acids), and ketonuria. PC presents with increased lactic acid and ketones, while the latter are usually absent in PDHC deficiency. Glycerol and glycerol-3-phosphate can be found in patients with FDP deficiency.

α-Ketoglutaric and lactic acids are increased in α-keto glutarate dehydrogenase, but the former could be increased only intermittently (309). Increased α-ketoglutaric is also found in patients with glycogen storage disease Type I, while in patients with lipoamide dehydrogenase (E_3deficiency), the increased levels of α-keto glutaric is accompanied by metabolites of 2-hydroxy- and 2-ketoacids. Fumarase deficiency is characterized by increased fumaric acid with different degrees of lactic, succinic, and α-ketoglutaric acid (312). Methylglutaconic acid has been reported in several patients with OXPHOS defects, as well as in other diseases (see organic acidemias) and it appears to be a nonspecific marker of mitochondrial dysfunction (327).

Isolated elevations of lactic acid in urine can be found in urinary infections due to Enterobacter cloacae (329) and in patients with short gut or blind loop syndrome, who excrete high amounts of d-lactic acid, which is undistinguishable from the l-isomer (330).

Quantitative plasma AAs typically show an elevation of alanine, while elevated glutamate and glutamine may be present in PDHC, α-KGD, and OXPHOS deficiencies (294,327). A typical AA profile is seen in the neonatal form of PC deficiency, with increased alanine, proline, citrulline, and lysine and decreased levels of aspartate and glutamine (294,314–317). In the E_3 subunit deficiency, mild elevations of BCAAs and alanine are characteristic.

Skeletal muscle biopsy for morphological, histochemical, and biochemical studies is useful for diagnosis of OXPHOS diseases. The most typical abnormality is the presence of "ragged-red fibers," which are caused by accumulation of abnormal mitochondria under the sarcolemmal membrane.

A positive stain for SDH and negative stain for cytochrome C oxidase (COX; complex IV) are also typical. Electron microscopy reveals abnormal mitochondria in size and shape, with paracrystal inclusions (319–322,331,332). Abnormalities in muscle biopsy are more frequently found in adults, while normal results in muscle histology and histochemistry are common in children. Therefore, a normal muscle biopsy does not rule out the diagnosis of an OXPHOS defect.

Measurement of respiratory chain activity in muscle can be performed in experienced laboratories, but inconclusive results are common. Most frequent findings are decreased activity of complex I, combined deficiencies in more than one complex, and isolated complex IV (COX) deficiency (323). Results in different centers may vary due to different diagnostic approaches (e.g., fresh isolated mitochondria vs. frozen muscle) and the different techniques used to measure respiratory chain activity.

Molecular characterization of patients with OXPHOS defects is challenging. Differentiation between diseases caused by gene defects in nDNA or mtDNA is important to characterize the disease, establish genotype–phenotype correlations, and provide prenatal diagnosis and genetic counseling: OXPHOS diseases due to nDNA defects follow a Mendelian inheritance while mtDNA defects are maternally transmitted (320,321). Different panels that screen for the most common mtDNA mutations and deletions are available commercially. Their utility is limited because they only include mutations and deletions associated with frequent classic mitochondrial syndromes such as the 3243A > G mutation for MELAS or 8344A > G for MERRF. Additionally, a negative result in blood does not exclude a possible mutation in other tissues. Many "nonclassical" mutations have been associated with OXPHOS disease in children, which highlights the need for full sequencing of the mitochondrial genome in patients with strong clinical presentation and/or pedigree suggestive of maternal inheritance.

Hundreds of nuclear genes are involved in the respiratory chain activity and are believed to account for the majority of the mitochondrial diseases in children. About 30 of those nuclear genes have been characterized and linked to diseases. Therefore, molecular diagnosis is rarely achieved in children. Some laboratories offer sequencing of genes associated with complex IV and mtDNA depletion.

Enzymatic diagnosis for defects in pyruvate oxidation, the TCA cycle, and gluconeogenesis can be done in blood, fibroblasts, or other tissues (294).

Treatment: The Acute Episode

Treatment of acute neonatal lactic acidemia requires an intensive care unit. Sodium bicarbonate in large amounts is required to control the metabolic acidosis. If hypernatremic acidosis develops, it should be treated with hemodialysis or peritoneal dialysis (solutions should have sodium bicarbonate instead of sodium chloride and should not contain acetate or lactate). A high GIR can severely worsen the lactic acidemia in patients with PDHC deficiency. Therefore, initial IV fluids should be given with D 5%. The GIR can be increased according to clinical and biochemical response. A high GIR is indicated in PC deficiency.

After the appropriate samples for diagnosis have been obtained, pharmacological treatment with one or several drugs can be started in patients with life-threatening lactic acidemia (Table 11).

A wide range of doses have been used. Assessment of the response to vitamin therapy is difficult and well-documented data are rare. The most commonly used are biotin, thiamine, riboflavin, and coenzyme-Q_{10}. These compounds are cofactors involved in the different metabolic pathways. Vitamins C and K have been used as artificial electron acceptors (294,333). Dichloroacetate (DCA) stimulates the activity of the PDHC and is used, in doses of 15 to 200 mg/kg/day, in the treatment of PDHC (294,333). Some reports have documented improvement following treatment with coenzyme Q_{10} or, its synthetic analog, idebenone (334,335). When final diagnosis becomes available, an attempt to withdraw those vitamins not involved in the metabolic block should be done, one at the time, with careful monitoring of the clinical and biochemical response. Carnitine should be used in patients with low carnitine levels (50–100 mg/kg/day).

Long-Term Management

In patients with PDHC deficiencies, thiamine (500–2000 mg/day), lipoic acid (which is bound to the E_2 component), carnitine, and DCA have been tried, with variable results (294,303). Additionally, a high-fat (75–80%), low-CHO (5%) diet has been useful in some patients. The rationale is to provide alternative sources of acetyl-CoA, not derived from pyruvate (294). However, a detailed study showed mild improvement in development but not change in long-term survival of these patients (336). In PDHC deficiency, due to abnormalities in the E_3 component, dietary treatment is more difficult as the affected enzymes impair protein, carbohydrate, and fat metabolism. Restriction of branched chain AAs (as in MSUD) is helpful to reduce blood levels of branched chain AAs and their metabolites in urine (294).

In patients with PC deficiency, treatment with biotin (10–50 mg/day) indicated. Citrate and aspartate have also been tried in this condition, with improvement in blood chemistry but poor long-term neurological outcome (317). A low-fat high-CHO diet with frequent feeds is also indicated in PC deficiency as well as in all the other gluconeogenic defects (294,333). Additionally, restriction of protein intake to reduce production of gluconeogenic substrates has been proposed in PC deficiency. Recently, a patient with neonatal-onset PC had a remarkable biochemical response after treatment with triheptanoate, which has an anaplerotic effect in TCA cycle. However the natural course of the disease could not be changed (315).

In patients with FDP deficiency, mild restriction of sucrose and fructose is indicated.

Long-term treatment for OXPHOS diseases has been disappointing (337–338), except for the above-mentioned responses to CoQ$_{10}$ treatment (334–335). Controlled exercise may be helpful in some patients to enhance the aerobic capacity and decrease lactic acid levels (319). Liver transplantation has been performed in patients with hepatic respiratory chain disorders, but extrahepatic manifestations may appear later, despite successful transplantation (339). Treatment with valproic acid and phenobarbital should be avoided, as they inhibit the respiratory chain (332). Supportive treatment for the different manifestations of OXPHOS diseases (exocrine pancreatic deficiency, anemia, diabetes, renal Fanconi syndrome, etc.), as well as psychological support for patients and family, should be provided.

Table 11 Pharmacological Treatment for Primary Lactic Acidemias

Treatment	Dose (range)	Deficiency
Thiamine (vitamin B$_1$)	500–2000 mg/day	PDHC
	200–300 mg/day	OXPHOS
Lipoic acid	10–50 mg/kg/day	PDHC
Dichloroacetate	15–200 mg/kg/day	PDHC
Biotin	10–50 mg/day	PC
Riboflavin (vitamin B$_2$)	50–300 mg/day	OXPHOS
Coenzyme-Q$_{10}$	100–300 mg/day	OXPHOS
Idebenone	30–90 mg/day	OXPHOS
Ascorbic acid (vitamin C)	500–4000 mg/day	OXPHOS
Vit.K$_3$,menadione/ K$_1$,phylloquinone	50–100 mg/day	OXPHOS
Tocopherol (vitamin E)	50–200 μg/day	OXPHOS

Abbreviations: PDHC, pyruvate dehydrogenase complex; PC, pyruvate carboxylase; OXPHOS, oxidative phosphorylation.

REFERENCES

1. Saudubray JM, Ogier de Baulny H, Charpentier C. Clinical approach to inherited metabolic disorders. In: Fernandes J, Saudubray JM, van den Berghe G, eds. Inborn Metabolic Diseases. 2nd ed. Berlin: Springer-Verlag, 2000:3–42.
2. Wilken B, Wiley V, Hammond J, Carpenter K. Screening newborns for inborn errors of metabolism by tandem mass spectrometry. N Engl J Med 2003; 348:2304–2312.
3. Scriver CR, Beaudet AL, Sly WS, Valle D, eds. The Metabolic and Molecular Bases of Inherited Disease. 8th ed. New York: McGraw-Hill, 2001.
4. Fernandes J, Saudubray JM, van den Berghe G, eds. Inborn Metabolic Diseases. 2d ed. Berlin: Springer-Verlag, 2000.
5. Brusilow SW, Horwich AL. Urea cycle enzymes. In: Scriver CR, Beaudet AL, Sly WS, Valle D, eds. The Metabolic

and Molecular Bases of Inherited Disease. 8th ed. New York: McGraw-Hill, 2001:1909–1963.

6. Leonard JV. Disorders of the urea cycle. In: Fernandes J, Saudubray JM, van den Berghe G, eds. Inborn Metabolic Diseases. 2nd ed. Berlin: Springer-Verlag, 2000: 214–222.

7. Butterworth RF. Effects of hyperammonemia on brain function. J Inherit Metab Dis 1998; 21(suppl 1):6–20.

8. Gropman AL, Batshaw ML. Cognitive outcome in urea cycle disorders. Mol Genet Metab 2004; 81:S58–S62.

9. Connelly A, Cross JH, Gadian DG, et al. Magnetic resonance spectroscopy shows increased brain glutamine in ornithine carbamoyl transferase deficiency. Pediatr Res 1993; 33:77–81.

10. Picker JD, Puga AC, Levy HL, et al. Arginase deficiency with lethal neonatal expression: evidence for the glutamine hypothesis of cerebral edema. J Pediatr 2003; 142:349–352.

11. Guffon N, Schiff M, Cheillan D, Wermuth B, Haberle J, Vianey-Saban C. Neonatal hyperammonemia: the N-carbamoyl-L-glutamic acid test. J Pediatr 2005; 147(2): 260–262.

12. Nassogne MC, Heron B, Touati G, Rabier D, Saudubray JM. Urea cycle defects: management and outcome. J Inherit Metab Dis 2005; 28:407–414.

13. Christodolou J, Qureshi IA, McInnes RR, et al. Ornithine transcarbamylase deficiency presenting with stroke-like episodes. J Pediatr 1993; 122:423–427.

14. Sperl W, Felber S, Skladal D, Wermuth B. Metabolic stroke in carbamyl phosphate synthetase deficiency. Neuropediatrics 1997; 28:229–234.

15. Mattson LR, Lindor NM, Goldman DH, et al. Central pontine myelinolysis as a complication of partial ornithine carbamoyl transferase deficiency. Am J Med Genet 1995; 60:210–213.

16. Rowe PC, Newman SL, Brusilow SW. Natural history of symptomatic partial ornithine transcarbamylase deficiency. N Engl J Med 1986; 314:541–547.

17. Arn PH, Hauser ER, Thomas GH, et al. Hyperammonemia in women with a mutation at the ornithine transcarbamylase locus. New Engl J Med 1990; 322:1652–1655.

18. Crombez EA, Cederbaum SD. Hyperargininemia due to liver arginase deficiency. Mol Genet Metab 2005; 84(3):243–251.

19. Elpeleg O, Shaag A, Ben shalom E, Schmid T, Bachman C. N-acetylglutamate synthase deficiency and the treatment of hyperammonemic encephalopathy. Ann Neurol 2002; 52:845–849.

20. Caldovic L, Morizono H, Daikhin Y, et al. Restoration of ureagenesis in N-acetylglutamate synthase deficiency by N-carbamylglutamate. J Pediatr 2004; 145(4):552–554.

21. Hudak ML, Jones D, Brusilow S. Differentiation of transient hyperammonemia of the newborn and urea cycle enzyme defects by clinical presentation. J Pediatr 1985; 107:712–719.

22. Tuchman, Lichtenstein GR, Rajagopal BS, et al. Hepatic glutamine synthetase deficiency in fatal hyperammonemia after lung transplantation. Ann Intern Med 1997; 127:446–449.

23. Stanley CA, Lieu YK, Hsu BY, et al. Hyperinsulinism and hyperammonemia in infants with regulatory mutations of the glutamate dehydrogenase gene. N Engl J Med 1998; 338:1352–1357.

24. Saheki T, Kobayashi K, Iijima M, et al. Adult-onset type II citrulinemia and idiopatic neonatal hepatitis caused bi citrin deficiency: involvement of the aspartate glutamate carrier for urea synthesis and maintenance of the urea cycle. Mol Genet Metab 2004; 81:S20–S26.

25. Maestri NE, Lord CR, Glynn M, et al. The phenotype of ostensibly healthy women who are carriers for ornithine transcarbamylase deficiency. Medicine 1998; 77:389–397.

26. Bonham JR, Guthrie P, Downing M, et al. The allopurinol load test lacks specificity for primary urea cycle defects but may indicate unrecognized mitochondrial disease. J Inherit Metab Dis 1999; 22:174–184.

27. Tuchman M, Morizono H, Rajagopal BS, et al. The biochemical and molecular spectrum of ornithine transcarbamylase deficiency. J Inherit Metab Dis 1998; 21(suppl 1):40–58.

28. McCullogh BA, Yudkoff M, Batshaw ML, et al. Genotype spectrum of ornithine transcarbamylase deficiency: correlation with the clinical and biochemical phenotype. Am J Med Genet 2000; 93:313–319.

29. Hendricks KM. Estimation of energy needs. In: Hendricks KM, Walker WA, eds. Manual of Pediatric Nutrition. 2nd ed. Philadelphia: B.C. Decker Inc., 1990:59–71.

30. Chen CY, Chen YC, Fang JT, Huang CC. Continuous arteriovenous hemodiafiltration in the acute treatment of hyperammonaemia due to ornithine transcarbamylase deficiency. Ren Fail 2000; 22:823–836.

31. Donn SM, Schwartz RD, Thoene JG. Comparison of exchange transfusion, peritoneal dialysis and hemodialysis for the treatment of hyperammonemia in an anuric newborn infant. J Pediatr 1979; 95:67–70.

32. Feillet F, Leonard JV. Alternative pathway therapy for urea cycle disorders. J Inherit Metab Dis 1998; 21(suppl 1): 101–111.

33. Batshaw M, MacArthur RB, Tuchman M. Alternative pathway for urea cycle disorders: twenty years later. J Pediatr 2001; 138:S46–S55.

34. Summar Marshall. Current strategies for the management of neonatal urea cycle disorders. J Pediatr 2001; 138: S30–S39.

35. UCYCLYD Pharma. 8125 North Hayden RD, Scottsdale, Arizona, U.S.A. 85258.

36. Praphanphoj V, Boyadjiev SA, Waber LJ, et al. Three cases of intravenous sodium benzoate and sodium phenylacatate toxicity occurring in the treatment of severe hyperammonaemia. J Inherit Metab Dis 2000; 23:129–136.

37. Oechsner M, Steen C, Sturenburg HJ, Kohlschutter A. Hiperammonaemic encephalopathy after initiation of valproate theraphy in unrecognised ornithine transcarbamylase deficiency. J Neurol Neurosurg Psychiatry 1998; 64:680–682.

38. Uchino T, Endo F, Matsuda I. Neurodevelopmental outcome of long-term therapy of urea cycle disorders in Japan. J Inherit Metab Dis 1998; 21(suppl 1):151–159.

39. Saudubray JM, Touati G, Delonay P, et al. Liver transplantation in urea cycle disorders. Eur J Pediatr 1999; 158(suppl 2):S55–S59.

40. Maestri NE, Hauser ER, Bartholomew D, Brusilow SW. Prospective treatment of urea cycle disorders. J Pediatr 1991; 119:923–928.

41. The Urea Cycle Disorders Conference Group. Consensus statement from a conference for the management of patients with urea cycle disorders. J pediatr 2001; 138:S1–S5.

42. Whitington PF, Alonso EM, Boyle JT, et al. Liver transplantation for the treatment of urea cycle disorders. J Inherit Metab Dis 1998; 21(suppl 1):112–118.

43. Leonard JV, McKiernan PJ. The role of liver transplantation in urea cycle disorders. Mol Genet Metab 2004; 81:S74–S78.

44. Horslen SP, McCowan TC, Goertzen, et al. Isolated hepatocyte transplantation in an infant with a severe urea cycle disorder. Pediatrics 2003; 111:1262–1267.

45. Lee B, Dennis JA, Healy PJ, et al. Hepatocyte gene therapy in a large animal: a neonatal bovine model of citrullinemia. Proc Natl Acad Sci USA 1999; 96:3981–3986.

46. Ensenauer R, Vockley J, Willard JM, et al. A common mutation is associated with a mild, potentially asymptomatic phenotype in patients with isovaleric acidemia diagnosed by newborn screening. Am J Hum Genet 2004; 75(6):1136–1142.

47. Koeberl DD, Millington DS, Smith WE, et al. Evaluation of 3–methylcrotonyl-CoA carboxylase deficiency detected by tandem mass spectrometry newborn screening. J Inherit Metab Dis 2003; 26(1):25–35.

48. Matern D, He M, Berry SA, et al. Prospective diagnosis of 2–methylbutyryl-CoA dehydrogenase deficiency in the Hmong population by newborn screening using tandem mass spectrometry. Pediatrics 2003; 112:74–78.

49. Ofman R, Ruiter JP, Feenstra M, et al. 2–Methyl-3–hydroxybutyryl-CoA dehydrogenase deficiency is caused by mutations in the HADH2 gene. Am J Hum Genet 2003; 72(5):1300–1307.

50. Morris AA. Disorders of ketogenesis and ketolysis. In: Fernandes J, Saudubray JM, van den Berghe G, eds. Inborn Metabolic Diseases. 2nd ed. Berlin: Springer-Verlag, 2000:151–156.

51. Sass JO, Sander S, Zschocke J. Isobutyryl-CoA dehydrogenase deficiency: isobutyrylglycinuria and ACAD8 gene mutations in two infants. J Inherit Metab Dis 2004; 27(6):741–745.

52. Chambliss KL, Gray RG, Rylance G, Pollitt RJ, Gibson KM. Molecular characterization of methylmalonate semialdehyde dehydrogenase deficiency. J Inherit Metab Dis 2000; 23(5):497–504.

53. Ogier de Baulny H, Saudubray JM. Branched-chain organic acidurias. In: Fernandes J, Saudubray JM, van den Berghe G, eds. Inborn Metabolic Diseases. 2nd ed. Berlin: Springer-Verlag, 2000:195–212.

54. Fenton WA, Gravel RA, Rosenblatt DA. Disorders of propionate and methylmalonate metabolism. In: Scriver CR, Beaudet AL, Sly WS, Valle D, eds. The Metabolic and Molecular Bases of Inherited Disease. 8th ed. New York: McGraw-Hill, 2001:2165–2194.

55. Ieradi-Curto, Kaplan P, Saitta S, Mazur A, Berry GT. The glutamine paradox in a neonate with propionic acidaemia and severe hyperammonaemia. J Inherit Metab Dis 2000; 23(1):85–86.

56. Massoud AF, Leonard JV. Cardiomyopathy in propionic acidaemia. Eur J Pediatr 1993; 152:441–445.

57. D'angio CT, Dilon MJ, Leonard JV. Renal tubular dysfunction in methylmalonic acidemia. Eur J Pediatr 1991; 150:259–263.

58. Dudley J, Allen J, Tizard J, McGraw M. Benign methylmalonic acidemia in a sibship with distal renal tubular acidosis. Pediatr Nephrol 1998; 12:564–566.

59. Rutledge SL, Geraghty M, Mroczek E, et al. Tubulointerstitial nephritis in methylmalonic acidemia. Pediatr Nephrol 1993; 7:81–82.

60. Baumgartner ER, Viardot, et al. Long term follow-up of 77 patients with isolated methylmalonic acidemia. J Inherit Metab Dis 1995; 138–142.

61. Dechaux M, Touati G, Vargas Poussou R, et al. Renal function in children with methylmalonic acidaemia. J Inherit Metab Dis 2000; 23:(suppl 1):97A.

62. Rosenblatt DS. Disorders of cobalamin and folate transport and metabolism. In: Fernandes J, Saudubray JM, van den Berghe G, eds. Inborn Metabolic Diseases. 2nd ed. Berlin: Springer-Verlag, 2000:283–300.

63. Buyukgebiz B, Jakobs C, Scholte HR, Huijmans JG, Kleijer WJ. Fatal neonatal malonic aciduria. J Inherit Metab Dis 1998; 21:76–77.

64. Wolf B. Disorders of biotin metabolism. In: Scriver CR, Beaudet AL, Sly WS, Valle D, eds. The Metabolic and Molecular Bases of Inherited Disease. 8th ed. New York: McGraw-Hill, 2001:3935 3964.

65. Hoffmann GF. Disorders of Lysine catabolism and related cerebral organic-acid disorders. In: Fernandes J, Saudubray JM, van den Berghe G, eds. Inborn Metabolic Diseases. 2nd ed. Berlin: Springer-Verlag, 2000:241–254.

66. Goodman SI, Frerman FE. Organic acidemias due to defects in Lysine oxidation: 2–ketoadipic acidemia and glutaric acidemia. In: Scriver CR, Beaudet AL, Sly WS, Valle D, eds. The Metabolic and Molecular Bases of Inherited Disease. 8th ed. New York: McGraw-Hill, 2001:2195–2205.

67. Strauss KA, Puffenberger EG, Robinson DL, Morton DH. Type I glutaric aciduria, part 1: natural history in 77 patients. Am J Med Genet C Semin Med Genet 2003; 121C:38–52.

68. Gibson KM, Hoffmann GF, Hodson AK, Bottiglieri T, Jacobs C. 4–hydroxybutyric acid and the clinical phenotype of succinic semialdehyde dehydrogenase deficiency, an inborn error of GABA metabolism. Neuropediatrics 1998; 29:14–22.

69. Traeger EC, Rapin I. The clinical course of Canavan disease. Pediatr Neurol 1998; 18:207–212.

70. Topku M, Aydin OF, Yalcinkaya C, et al. L-2–hydroxyglutaric aciduria: a report of 29 patients. Turk J Pediatr 2005; 47(1):1–7.

71. Barth PG, Hoffmann GF, Jaeken J, et al. L-2–hydroxyglutaric acidaemia: clinical and biochemical findings in 12 patients and preliminary report on L–2–hydroxyacid dehydrogenase. J Inherit Metab Dis 1993; 16:753–761.

72. Struys EA, Salomons GS, Achouri Y, et al. Mutations in the D-2–hydroxyglutarate dehydrogenase gene cause D-2–hydroxyglutaric aciduria. Am J Hum Genet 2005; 76(2):358–360.

73. Van der Knaap MS, Jacobs C, Hoffmann GF, et al. D-2–hydroxyglutaric aciduria. Biochemical marker or clinical disease entity? Ann Neurol 1999; 45:111–119.

74. Burlina AB, Dionisi-Vici C, Bennet M, y col. A new syndrome with ethylmalonic aciduria and normal fatty acid oxidation in fibroblasts. J Pediatr 1994; 124:79–86.

75. Tirani V, D'adamo P, Briem E, et al. Ethylmalonic encephalopathy is caused by mutations in ETHE1, a gene encoding a mitochondrial matrix protein. Am J Hum Genet 2004; 74:239–252.

76. McGowan, Nyhan WL, Barshop BA, et al. The role of methionine in ethylmalonic encephalopathy with petechiae. Arch Neurol 2004; 61(4):570–574.

77. Sweetman L, Williams JC. Branched chain organic acidurias. In: Scriver CR, Beaudet AL, Sly WS, Valle D, eds. The Metabolic and Molecular Bases of Inherited Disease. 8th ed. New York: McGraw-Hill, 2001:2125–2164.

78. Hoffmann GF. Organic acid analysis. In: Blau N, Duran M, Blaskovics ME, eds. Physician's Guide to the Laboratory Diagnosis of Metabolic Diseases. 1st ed. London: Chapman and Hall Medical, 1996:32–49.

79. Thompson GN, Walter JH, Bresson JL, et al. Sources of propionate in inborn errors of metabolism. Metabolism 1990; 11:1133–1137.

80. Leonard JV. Stable isotope studies in propionic and methylmalonic acidaemia. Eur J Pediatr 1996; 156(suppl 1): S67–S69.

81. Coude FX, Sweetman L, Nyhan WL. Inhibition by propionyl-coenzyme A of N-acetyglutamate synthtase in rat liver mitochondria. J Clin Invest 1979; 1544–1551.

82. Coude FX, Ogier H, Grimber G, et al. Correlation between blood ammonia concentration and organic acid accumulation

in isovaleric and propionic acidemia. Pediatrics 1982; 69:115–117.

83. Shapira SK, Ledley FD, Rosenblatt DS, Levy HL. Ketoacidotic crisis as a presentation of mild methylmalonic acidemia. J Pediatr 1991; 119:80–84.

84. Sethi KD, Ray R, Roesel RA, et al. Adult onset chorea and dementia with propionic acidemia. Neurology 1989; 39:1343–1345.

85. Nyhan WL, Bay C, Beyer EW, Mazi M. Neurologic nonmetabolic presentation of propionic acidemia. Arch Neurol 1999; 56:1143–1147.

86. Matern D, Seydewitz HH, Lehnert W, Niederhoff H, Leititis J, Brandis M. Primary treatment of propionic acidemia complicated by acute thiamine deficiency. J Pediatr 1996; 129(5):758–760.

87. Tracy E, Arbour L, Chessex P, et al. Glutathione deficiency as a complication of methylmalonic acidemia: response to high doses of ascorbate. J Pediatr 1996; 129:445–448.

88. Griffin TA, Hostoffer RW, Tserng KY, et al. Parathyroid resistance and B cell lymphopenia in propionic acidemia. Acta Paediatr 1996; 85:875–878.

89. Khaler SG, Sherwood WG, Woolf D, et al. Pancreatitis in patients with organic acidemias. J Pediatr 1994; 124:239–243.

90. Fiumara A, Barone R, Nigro F, Ribes A, Pavone L. Pancreatitis in organic acidemias. J Pediatr 1995; 126:852.

91. Burlina AB, Dionisi-Vici, Piovan S, et al. Acute pancreatitis in propionic acidemia. J Inherit Metab Dis 1995; 18:169–172.

92. Boeckx RL, Hicks JM. Methylmalonic acidemia with the unusual complication of severe hyperglycemia. Clin Chem 1982; 28:1801–1803.

93. Attia N, Sakati N, al Ashawal A, et al. Isovaleric acidemia appearing as diabetic ketoacidosis. J Inherit Metab Dis 1996; 19:85–86.

94. Rashed MS, Bucknall MP, Little D, et al. Screening blood spots for inborn errors of metabolism by electrospray tandem mass spectrometry with a microplate batch process and a computer algorithm for automated flagging of abnormal profiles. Clin Chem 1997; 43:1129–1141.

95. Vreken P, van Lint AEM, Bootsma AH, et al. Quantitative plasma acylcarnitine analysis using electrospray tandem mass spectrometry for the diagnosis of organic acidemias and fatty acid oxidation defects. J Inherit Metab Dis 1999; 22:302–306.

96. Rutledge SL, Havens PL, Haymond MW, et al. Neonatal hemodialysis: effective therapy for the encephalopathy of inborn errors of metabolism. J Pediatr 1990; 116:125–128.

97. Zytkovicz TH, Fitzgerald E, Marsden D, et al. Tandem mass spectrometry analysis for amino, organic and fatty acid disorders in newborn dried blood spots: a two year summary from the New England Newborn screening program. Clin Chem 2001; 47:1945–1955.

98. Schenone AB, Abdenur JE, Guinle A, Fuertes A, Chamoles N. Detection of inherited metabolic disorders in cord blood samples by tandem mass spectrometry, SIMD March 07–10, Orlando, Florida, U.S.A., 2004.

99. Osorio JH, Pourfarzam M. Diagnostico temprano de enfermedades neurometabolicas por espectrometria de masas en tandem. Perfil de acilcarnitinas en la sangre del cordon umbilical. Rev Neurol 2004; 38:11–46.

100. Gibson KM, Burlingame TG, Hogema B, et al. 2-methylbutyryl-CoA-dehydrogenase deficiency: a new inborn error of L-Isoleucine metabolism. Pediatr Res 2000; 47:830–833.

101. Abdenur JE, Chamoles NA, Schenone AB, et al. Diagnosis of isovaleric acidemia by tandem mass spectrometry: false positive result due to pivaloylcarnitine in a newborn

screening programme. J Inherit Metab Dis 1998; 21:624–630.

102. Bonafe L, Troxler H, Kuster T, et al. Evaluation of urinary acylglycines by electrospray tandem mass spectrometry in mitochondrial energy metabolism defects and organic acidurias. Mol Genet Metab 2000; 69:302–311.

103. Tuchman M, Yudkoff M. Blood levels of ammonia and nitorgen scavenging aminoacids in patients with inherited hyperammonemia. Mol Genet Metab 1999; 66:10–15.

104. Thompson GN, Chalmers RA. Increased urinary metabolite excretion during fasting in disorders of propionate metabolism. Pediatr Res 1990; 27:413–416.

105. Millington DS, Roe ChR, Maltby DA, Inoue F. Endogenous catabolism is the major source of toxic metabolites in isovaleric acidemia. J Pediatr 1987; 110:56–60.

106. Bodamer OAF, Hoffman GF, Visser GH, et al. Assessment of energy expenditure in metabolic disorders. Eur J Pediatr 1997; 156(suppl 1):S24–S28.

107. Kalloghlian A, Gleispach H, Ozand PT. A patient with propionic acidemia managed with continuous insulin infusion and total parenteral nutrition. J Child Neurol 1992; 7(suppl):S88–S91.

108. Khaler SG, Millington DS, Cederbaum SD, et al. Parenteral nutrition in propionic and methylmalonic acidemia. J Pediatr 1989; 115:235–241.

109. Acosta P, Yannicelli S. The Ross Metabolic Formula System: Nutrition Support Protocols. 4th ed. 2001.

110. Roth B, Younossi A, Skopnik H, Leonard JV, Lehnert W. Haemodialysis for metabolic decompensation in propionic acidemia. J Inherit Metab Dis 1987; 10:147–151.

111. Ogier de Baulny H, Saudubray JM. Emergency treatments. In: Fernandes J, Saudubray JM, van den Berghe G, eds. Inborn Metabolic Diseases. 2nd ed. Berlin: Springer-Verlag:53–61.

112. Praphanphoj V, Brusilow S, Hamosh A, Geraghty MT. The use of intravenous sodium benzoate and sodium phenylacetate in propionic acidemia with hyperammonemia. J Inherit Metab Dis 2000; 23(suppl 1):91A.

113. Levrat V, Blanc S, Schiff M, Vianey-Saban C, Boyer S, Guffon N. N-carbamoyl-L-glutamic acid: a beneficial effect in the treatment of acute decompensation of organic acidurias (methylmalonic and propionic aciduria) with hyperammonemia? J Inherit Metab Dis 2005; 28:81A.

114. Gebhardt B, Vlaho S, Fischer D, Sewell A, Bohles H. N-carbamylglutamate enhances ammonia detoxification in a patient with decompensated methylmalonic aciduria. Mol Genet Metab 2003; 79(4):303–304.

115. Fries MH, Rinaldo P, Schmidt-Sommerfeld E, et al. Isovaleric acidemia: response to a leucine load after three weeks of supplementation with glycine, L-carnitine, and combined glycine-carnitine therapy. J Pediatr 1996; 129:449–452.

116. Al essa M, Rahbeeni Z, Jumaah S, et al. Infectious complications of propionic acidemia in Saudi Arabia. Clin Genet 1998; 54:90–94.

117. Koopman RJJ, Happle R. Cutaneous manifestations of methylmalonic acidemia. Arch Dermatol Res 1990; 282:272–273.

118. Heidenreich R, Natowicz M, Hainline B, et al. Acute extrapyramidal syndrome in methylmalonic acidemia: "metabolic stroke" involving the globus pallidus. J Pediatr 1988; 113:1022–1027.

119. Haas RH, Marsden DL, Capistrano-Estrada S, et al. Acute basal ganglia infarction in propionic acidemia. J Child Neurol 1995; 10:18–22.

120. Bergman AJ, Van der Knaap MS, Smeitink JA, et al. Magnetic resonance imaging and spectroscopy of the brain in

propionic acidemia: clinical and biochemical considerations. J Pediatr 1996; 129:758–760.

121. Brandstetter Y, Weinhouse E, Splaingard M, Tang T. Cor Pulmonale as a complication of methylmalonic acidemia and homocystinuria (Cbl–C type). Am J Med Genet 1990; 36:167–171.

122. Guigonis V, Fremeaux-Bacchi V, Giraudier S, et al. Late onset thrombotic microangiopathy caused by cblC disease: association with factor H mutation. Am J Kidney Dis 2005; 45(3):588–595.

123. Baethmann M, Wendel U, Hoffmann GF, et al. Hydrocephalus internus in two patients with 5–10–methylenetetrahydrofolate reductase deficiency. Neuropediatrics 2000; 31:314–317.

124. Rossi A, Biancheri R, Tortori–Donati P. The patogenesis of hydrocephalus in inborn errors of single carbon transfer pathway. Neuropediatrics 2001; 32:335–336.

125. Feillet F, Bodamer OA, Dixon M, et al. Resting energy expenditure in disorders of propionate metabolism. J Pediatr 2000; 136:659–663.

126. Prasad C, Nurko S, Borovoy J, Korson MS. The importance of gut motility in the metabolic control of propionic acidemia. J Pediatr 2004; 144(4):532–535.

127. Thompson GN, Chalmers RA, Walter JH, et al. The use of metronidazole in management of methylmalonic and propionic acidemias. Eur J Pediatr 1990; 149:792–796.

128. Vockley J, Rogan PK, Anderson BD, et al. Exon skipping in IVD RNA processing in isovaleric acidemia caused by point mutations in the coding region of the IVD gene. Am J Hum Genet 2000; 66:356–367.

129. Ugarte M, Perez Cerda C, Rodriguez Pombo P, et al. Overview of mutations in the PCCA and PCCB genes causing propionic acidemia. Hum Mutat 1999; 14:275–282.

130. Desviat LR, Perez B, Perez Cerda C, et al. Propionic acidemia: mutation update and functional and structural effects of the variant alleles. Mol Genet Metab 2004; 83:28–37.

131. Fuchshuber A, Mucha B, Baumgartner ER, et al. Muto methylmalonic acidemia: eleven novel mutations of the methylmalonyl CoA mutase including a deletion-insertion. Hum Mutat 2000; 16:179.

132. Crane AM, Martin LS, Valle D, Ledley FD. Phenotype of disease in three patients with identical mutations in methylmalonyl CoA mutase. Hum Genet 1992; 89:259–264.

133. Weinberg GL, Laurito CE, Geldner P, et al. Malignant ventricular disrythmias in a patient with isovaleric acidemia receiving general and local anesthesia for suction lipectomy. J Clin Anesth 1997; 9:668–670.

134. Harker HE, Emhardt JD, Hainline BE. Propionic acidemia in a four-month-old male: a case study and anesthetic implications. Anesth Analg 2000; 91:309–311.

135. North KN, Korson MS, Gopal YR, et al. Neonatal onset propionic acidemia: neurologic and developmental profiles and implications for management. J Pediatr 1995; 126:916–922.

136. Van der Meer SB, Poggi F, Spada M, et al. Clinical outcome and long term management of 17 patients with propionic acidemia. J Pediatr 1996; 155:205–210.

137. van der Meer SB, Poggi F, Spada M, et al. Clinical outcome of long term management of patients with vitamin B-12 unresponsive methylmalonic acidemia. J Pediatr 1994; 125:903–908.

138. Varvogli L, Repetto GM, Waisbren SE, Levy HL. High cognitive outcome in an adolescent with mut- methylmalonic acidemia. Am J Med Genet 2000; 96:192–195.

139. Anderson HC, Marble M, Shapira E. Long-term outcome in treated combined methylmalonic acidemia and homocystinemia. Genet Med 1999; 1:146–150.

140. Nicolaides P, Leonard JV, Surtees R. Neurological outcome of methylmalonic acidemia. Arch Dis Child 1998; 78:508–512.

141. Saudubray JM, Touati P, Delonlay P, et al. Liver transplantation in propionic acidaemia. Eur J Pediatr 1999; 158(suppl 2):S65–S69.

142. De Raeve L, Meirleir L, Ramet J, Vandenplas Y, Gerlo E. Acrodermatitis enteropathica-like cutaneous lesions in organic aciduria. J Pediatr 1994; 124:416–420.

143. Yannicelli S, Hambidge KM, Picciano MF. Decreased selenium intake and low plasma selenium concentrations leading to clinical symptoms in a child with propionic acidemia. J Inherit Metab Dis 1992; 15:261–268.

144. Collins J, Kelly D. Cardiomyopathy in propionic acidemia. Eur J Pediatr 1994; 153:53–54.

145. Bhan AK, Brody C. Propionic academia. A rare cause of cardiomyopathy. Congest Heart Fail 2001; 7:218–219.

146. van't Hoff WG, Dixon M, Taylor J, et al. Combined liver-kidney transplantation for methylmalonic acidemia. J Pediatr 1998; 132:1043–1044.

147. van't Hoff WG, McKiernan PJ, Surtees RAH, Leonard JV. Liver transplantation for methylmalonic acidemia. Eur J Pediatr 1999; 158(suppl 2):S70–S74.

148. Packman S, Rosenthal P, Weisiger K, et al. Liver transplantation in Cbl B methylmalonic acidemia. J Inherit Metab Dis 2000; 23(suppl 1):95A.

149. Yorifuji T, Muroi J, Uematsu A, et al. Living-related liver transplantation for neonatal–onset propionic acidemia. J Pediatr 2000; 137:572–574.

150. Chuang DT, Shih V. Maple syrup urine disease (branched–chain ketoaciduria). In: Scriver CR, Beaudet AL, Sly WS, Valle D, eds. The Metabolic and Molecular Bases of Inherited Disease. 8th ed. New York: McGraw-Hill, 2001:1971–2005.

151. Chuang DT, Chuang JL, Wynn RM. Lessons from genetic disorders of branched-chain amino acid metabolism. J Nutr 2006; 136(1):243S–249S.

152. Peinemann, Danner DJ. Maple syrup urine disease 1954 to 1993. J Inherit Metab Dis 1994; 17:3–15.

153. Temudo T, Martins E, Pocas F, Cruz R, Vilarinho L. Maple syrup disease presenting as paroxysmal dystonia. Ann Neurol 2004; 56(5):749–750.

154. Heldt K, Schwahn B, Marquardt I, Grotzke M, Wendel U. Diagnosis of MSUD by newborn screening allows early intervention without extraneous detoxification. Mol Genet Metab 2005; 84(4):313–316.

155. Puffenberger EG. Genetic heritage of the old order Mennonites of southeastern Pennsylvania. Am J Med Genet C Semin Med Genet 2003; 15(121):18–31.

156. Chuang JL, Wynn RM, Moss CC, et al. Structural and biochemical basis for novel mutations in homozygous Israeli maple syrup urine disease patients: a proposed mechanism for the thiamin-responsive phenotype. J Biol Chem 2004; 279(17):17792–17800.

157. Henneke M, Flaschker N, Helbling C, et al. Identification of twelve novel mutations in patients with classic and variant forms of maple syrup urine disease. Hum Mutat 2003; 22(5):417.

158. Jouvet P, Poggi F, Rabier D, et al. Continuous venovenous haemofiltration in the acute phase of neonatal maple syrup urine disease. J Inherit Metab Dis 1997; 20:463–472.

159. Jouvet P, Hubert P, Saudubray JM, Rabier D, Man NK. Kinetic modeling of plasma leucine levels during continuous venovenous extracorporeal removal therapy in neonates with maple syrup urine disease. Pediatr Res 2005; 58(2):278–282.

160. Hmiel SP, Martin RA, Landt M, Levy FH, Grange DK. Amino acid clearance during acute metabolic decompensation

in maple syrup urine disease treated with continuous venovenous hemodialysis with filtration. Pediatr Crit Care Med 2004; 5(3):278–281.

161. Friedrich CA, Marble A, Maher J, et al. Successful control of branched–chain aminoacids in maple syrup urine disease using elemental aminoacids in total parenteral nutrition during acute pancreatitis. Am J Hum Genet 1992; 51:A350.

162. Riviello JJ, Rezvani I, Digeorge AM, et al. Cerebral edema causing death in children with maple syrup urine disease. J Pediatr 1991; 119:42–47.

163. Treacy E, Clow CL, Reade TR, et al. Maple syrup urine disease: interrelations between branched-chain amino-oxo-and hydroxyacids; implications for treatment: associations with CNS dysmyelination. J Inherit Metab Dis 1992; 15:121–135.

164. Brismar J, Aqeel A, Brismar G, et al. Maple syrup urine disease: findings on CT and MRI scans of the brain in 10 infants. Am J Neuroradiol 1990; 11:1219.

165. Sakai M, Inoue Y, Oba H, Ishiguro A, Sekiguchi K, Tsukune Y, et al. Age dependence of diffusion-weighted magnetic resonance imaging findings in maple syrup urine disease encephalopathy. J Comput Assist Tomogr 2005; 29(4):524–527.

166. Di Rocco M, Biancheri R, Rossi A, Allegri AE, Vecchi V, Tortori-Donati P. MRI in acute intermittent maple syrup urine disease. Neurology 2004; 63(6):1078.

167. Schonberger S, Schweiger B, Schwahn B, Schwarz M, Wendel U. Dysmyelination in the brain of adolescents and young adults with maple syrup urine disease. Mol Genet Metab 2004; 82(1):69–75.

168. Jan W, Zimmerman RA, Wang ZJ, Berry GT, Kaplan PB, Kaye EM. MR diffusion imaging and MR spectroscopy of maple syrup urine disease during acute metabolic decompensation. Neuroradiology 2003; 45(6):393–399.

169. Hallam P, Lilburn M, Lee PJ. A new protein substitute for adolescents and adults with maple syrup urine disease (MSUD). J Inherit Metab Dis 2005; 28(5):665–672.

170. Nord A, van Doorninck WJ, Greene C. Developmental profile of patients with maple syrup urine disease. J Inherit Metab Dis 1991; 14:881–889.

171. Hilliges C, Awiszus D, Wendel U. Intellectual performance of children with maple syrup urine disease. Eur J Pediatr 1993; 152:144–147.

172. Hoffmann B, Helbling C, Schadewaldt P, Wendel U. Impact of longitudinal plasma leucine levels on the intellectual outcome in patients with classic MSUD. Pediatr Res 2006; 59(1):17–20.

173. Wendel U, Saudubray JM, Bodner A, Schadewaldt P. Liver transplantation in maple syrup urine disease. Eur J Pediatr 1999; 158(suppl 2):S60–S64.

174. Bodner-Leidecker A, Wendel U, Saudubray JM, Schadewaldt P. Branched-chain L-amino acid metabolism in classical maple syrup urine disease after orthotopic liver transplantation. J Inherit Metab Dis 2000; 23(8):805–818.

175. Roe CRDJ. Mitochondrial Fatty Acid Oxidation Disorders. 8th ed. New York: McGraw Hill, 2001:2297–3327.

176. Brivet M, Boutron A, Slama A, et al. Defects in activation and transport of fatty acids. J Inherit Metab Dis 1999; 22:428–441.

177. Stahl A. A current review of fatty acid transport proteins (SLC27). Pflugers Arch 2004; 447:722–727.

178. Rinaldo P. Fatty acid transport and mitochondrial oxidation disorders. Semin Liver Dis 2001; 21:489–500.

179. Odaib AA, Shneider BL, Bennett MJ, et al. A defect in the transport of long-chain fatty acids associated with acute liver failure. N Engl J Med 1998; 339:1752–1757.

180. Wanders RJ, Vreken P, den Boer ME, et al. Disorders of mitochondrial fatty acyl-CoA beta-oxidation. J Inherit Metab Dis 1999; 22:442–487.

181. Bonnefont JP, Djouadi F, Prip-Buus C, et al. Carnitine palmitoyltransferases 1 and 2: biochemical, molecular and medical aspects. Mol Aspects Med 2004; 25:495–520.

182. Stoler JM, Sabry MA, Hanley C, et al. Successful long-term treatment of hepatic carnitine palmitoyltransferase I deficiency and a novel mutation. J Inherit Metab Dis 2004; 27:679–684.

183. Korman SH, Waterham HR, Gutman A, et al. Novel metabolic and molecular findings in hepatic carnitine palmitoyltransferase I deficiency. Mol Genet Metab 2005; 86:337–343.

184. Wanders RJ, Denis S, Ruiter JP, et al. 2,6–Dimethylheptanoyl-CoA is a specific substrate for long-chain acyl-CoA dehydrogenase (LCAD): evidence for a major role of LCAD in branched-chain fatty acid oxidation. Biochim Biophys Acta 1998; 1393:35–40.

185. Frerman FEGS. Defects of Electron Tranfer Flavoprotein and Elctron Transfer Flavoprotein-Ubiquinone Oxidoreductase: Glutaric Aciduria Type II. 8th ed. New York: McGraw-Hill, 2001:2357–2366.

186. Olpin SE, Clark S, Andresen BS, et al. Biochemical, clinical and molecular findings in LCHAD and general mitochondrial trifunctional protein deficiency. J Inherit Metab Dis 2005; 28:533–544.

187. Spiekerkoetter U, Khuchua Z, Yue Z, et al. General mitochondrial trifunctional protein (TFP) deficiency as a result of either alpha- or beta-subunit mutations exhibits similar phenotypes because mutations in either subunit alter TFP complex expression and subunit turnover. Pediatr Res 2004; 55:190–196.

188. Spiekerkoetter U, Bennett MJ, Ben-Zeev B, et al. Peripheral neuropathy, episodic myoglobinuria, and respiratory failure in deficiency of the mitochondrial trifunctional protein. Muscle Nerve 2004; 29:66–72.

189. Angdisen J, Moore VD, Cline JM, et al. Mitochondrial trifunctional protein defects: molecular basis and novel therapeutic approaches. Curr Drug Targets Immune Endocr Metabol Disord 2005; 5:27–40.

190. Sander J, Sander S, Steuerwald U, et al. Neonatal screening for defects of the mitochondrial trifunctional protein. Mol Genet Metab 2005; 85:108–114.

191. Fukao T, Lopaschuk GD, Mitchell GA. Pathways and control of ketone body metabolism: on the fringe of lipid biochemistry. Prostaglandins Leukot Essent Fatty Acids 2004; 70:243–251.

192. Wolf NI, Rahman S, Clayton PT, et al. Mitochondrial HMG-CoA synthase deficiency: identification of two further patients carrying two novel mutations. Eur J Pediatr 2003; 162:279–280.

193. Morris AA. Cerebral ketone body metabolism. J Inherit Metab Dis 2005; 28:109–121.

194. Pie J, Casals N, Puisac B, et al. Molecular basis of 3–hydroxy-3–methylglutaric aciduria. J Physiol Biochem 2003; 59:311–321.

195. Saudubray JM, Martin D, de Lonlay P, et al. Recognition and management of fatty acid oxidation defects: a series of 107 patients. J Inherit Metab Dis 1999; 22:488–502.

196. Bonnet D, Martin D, Pascale De L, et al. Arrhythmias and conduction defects as presenting symptoms of fatty acid oxidation disorders in children. Circulation 1999; 100:2248–2253.

197. Wilcken B, Carpenter KH, Hammond J. Neonatal symptoms in medium chain acyl coenzyme A dehydrogenase deficiency. Arch Dis Child 1993; 69:292–294.

198. Thiel C, Baudach S, Schnackenberg U, et al. Long-chain 3–hydroxyacyl-CoA dehydrogenase deficiency: neonatal manifestation at the first day of life presenting with tachypnoea. J Inherit Metab Dis 1999; 22:839–840.

199. Iafolla AK, Thompson RJ Jr. Roe CR. Medium-chain acyl-coenzyme A dehydrogenase deficiency: clinical course in 120 affected children. J Pediatr 1994; 124:409–415.

200. Spierkerkoetter U, Khuchua Z, Yue Z, et al. The early-onset phenotype of mitochondrial trifunctional protein deficiency: a lethal disorder with multiple tissue involvement. J Inherit Metab Dis 2004; 27:294–296.

201. Ibdah JA, Dasouki MJ, Strauss AW. Long-chain 3-hydroxyacyl-CoA dehydrogenase deficiency: variable expressivity of maternal illness during pregnancy and unusual presentation with infantile cholestasis and hypocalcaemia. J Inherit Metab Dis 1999; 22:811–814.

202. Tripp M KM, Peters HA et al. Systemic carnitine deficiency presenting as familial endocardial fibroelastosis. New Engl J Med 305:385–390.

203. Tyni T, Paetau A, Strauss AW, et al. Mitochondrial fatty acid beta-oxidation in the human eye and brain: implications for the retinopathy of long-chain 3-hydroxyacyl-CoA dehydrogenase deficiency. Pediatr Res 2004; 56:744–750.

204. Ibdah JA, Yang Z, Bennett MJ. Liver disease in pregnancy and fetal fatty acid oxidation defects. Mol Genet Metab 2000; 71:182–189.

205. Chakrapani A, Olpin S, Cleary M, et al. Trifunctional protein deficiency: three families with significant maternal hepatic dysfunction in pregnancy not associated with E474Q mutation. J Inherit Metab Dis 2000; 23:826–834.

206. Bellig LL. Maternal acute fatty liver of pregnancy and the associated risk for long-chain 3-hydroxyacyl-coenzyme a dehydrogenase (LCHAD) deficiency in infants. Adv Neonatal Care 2004; 4:26–32.

207. Ibdah JA. Role of genetic screening in identifying susceptibility to acute fatty liver of pregnancy. Nat Clin Pract Gastroenterol Hepatol 2005; 2:494–495.

208. Nelson J, Lewis B, Walters B. The HELLP syndrome associated with fetal medium-chain acyl-CoA dehydrogenase deficiency. J Inherit Metab Dis 2000; 23:518–519.

209. Innes AM, Seargeant LE, Balachandra K, et al. Hepatic carnitine palmitoyltransferase I deficiency presenting as maternal illness in pregnancy. Pediatr Res 2000; 47:43–45.

210. Matern D, Hart P, Murtha AP, et al. Acute fatty liver of pregnancy associated with short-chain acyl-coenzyme A dehydrogenase deficiency. J Pediatr 2001; 138:585–588.

211. Boles RG, Buck EA, Blitzer MG, et al. Retrospective biochemical screening of fatty acid oxidation disorders in postmortem livers of 418 cases of sudden death in the first year of life. J Pediatr 1998; 132:924–933.

212. Lundemose JB, Kolvraa S, Gregersen N, et al. Fatty acid oxidation disorders as primary cause of sudden and unexpected death in infants and young children: an investigation performed on cultured fibroblasts from 79 children who died aged between 0–4 years. Mol Pathol 1997; 50:212–217.

213. Treacy EP, Lambert DM, Barnes R, et al. Short-chain hydroxyacyl-coenzyme A dehydrogenase deficiency presenting as unexpected infant death: A family study. J Pediatr 2000; 137:257–259.

214. Nuoffer JM, de Lonlay P, Costa C, et al. Familial neonatal SIDS revealing carnitine-acylcarnitine translocase deficiency. Eur J Pediatr 2000; 159:82–85.

215. Rinaldo P, Stanley CA, Hsu BY, et al. Sudden neonatal death in carnitine transporter deficiency. J Pediatr 1997; 131:304–305.

216. Chalmers RA, Stanley CA, English N, et al. Mitochondrial carnitine-acylcarnitine translocase deficiency presenting as sudden neonatal death. J Pediatr 1997; 131:220–225.

217. Poplawski NK, Ranieri F, Harrison JR, et al. Multiple acyl-coenzyme A dehydrogenase deficiency: diagnosis by acyl-carnitine analysis of a 12-year-old newborn screening card. J Pediatr 1999; 134:764–766.

218. Rashed MS, Ozand PT, Bennett MJ, et al. Inborn errors of metabolism diagnosed in sudden death cases by acylcarnitine analysis of postmortem bile. Clin Chem 1995; 41:1109–1114.

219. Chace DH, DiPerna JC, Mitchell BL, et al. Electrospray tandem mass spectrometry for analysis of acylcarnitines in dried postmortem blood specimens collected at autopsy from infants with unexplained cause of death. Clin Chem 2001; 47:1166–1182.

220. Rinaldo P, Yoon HR, Yu C, et al. Sudden and unexpected neonatal death: a protocol for the postmortem diagnosis of fatty acid oxidation disorders. Semin Perinatol 1999; 23:204–210.

221. el-Schahawi M, Bruno C, Tsujino S, et al. Sudden infant death syndrome (SIDS) in a family with myophosphorylase deficiency. Neuromuscul Disord 1997; 7:81–83.

222. de Klerk JB, Duran M, Huijmans JG, et al. Sudden infant death and lysinuric protein intolerance. Eur J Pediatr 1996; 155:256–257.

223. Dionisi-Vici C, Seneca S, Zeviani M, et al. Fulminant Leigh syndrome and sudden unexpected death in a family with the T9176 mutation of the mitochondrial ATPase 6 gene. J Inherit Metab Dis 1998; 21:2–8.

224. Pastores GM, Santorelli FM, Shanske S, et al. Leigh syndrome and hypertrophic cardiomyopathy in an infant with a mitochondrial DNA point mutation (T8993). Am J Med Genet 1994; 50:265–271.

225. Bennett MJ, Weinberger MJ, Kobori JA, et al. Mitochondrial short-chain L-3-hydroxyacyl-coenzyme A dehydrogenase deficiency: a new defect of fatty acid oxidation. Pediatr Res 1996; 39:185–188.

226. Bennett MJ, Spotswood SD, Ross KF, et al. Fatal hepatic short-chain L-3-hydroxyacyl-coenzyme A dehydrogenase deficiency: clinical, biochemical, and pathological studies on three subjects with this recently identified disorder of mitochondrial beta-oxidation. Pediatr Dev Pathol 1999; 2:337–345.

227. Molven A, Matre GE, Duran M, et al. Familial hyperinsulinemic hypoglycemia caused by a defect in the SCHAD enzyme of mitochondrial fatty acid oxidation. Diabetes 2004; 53:221–227.

228. Eaton S, Chatziandreou I, Krywawych S, et al. Short-chain 3-hydroxyacyl-CoA dehydrogenase deficiency associated with hyperinsulinism: a novel glucose-fatty acid cycle? Biochem Soc Trans 2003; 31:1137–1139.

229. Clayton PT, Eaton S, Aynsley-Green A, et al. Hyperinsulinism in short-chain L-3-hydroxyacyl-CoA dehydrogenase deficiency reveals the importance of beta-oxidation in insulin secretion. J Clin Invest 2001; 108:457–465.

230. Treem WR WC, Picoli DA, et al. Medium chain and long chain acyl CoA dehidrogenase deficiency: clinical, pathologic and ultrastructural differentiation from Reye's Syndrome. Hepatology 1986; 6:1270–1278.

231. Rashed MS. Clinical applications of tandem mass spectrometry: ten years of diagnosis and screening for inherited metabolic diseases. J Chromatogr B Biomed Sci Appl 2001; 758:27–48.

232. Rinaldo P, Matern D, Bennett MJ. Fatty acid oxidation disorders. Annu Rev Physiol 2002; 64:477–502.

233. Bennett MJ, Rinaldo P, Strauss AW. Inborn errors of mitochondrial fatty acid oxidation. Crit Rev Clin Lab Sci 2000; 37:1–44.

234. Wilcken B, Wiley V, Sim KG, et al. Carnitine transporter defect diagnosed by newborn screening with electrospray tandem mass spectrometry. J Pediatr 2001; 138:581–584.

235. Fingerhut R, Roschinger W, Muntau AC, et al. Hepatic carnitine palmitoyltransferase I deficiency: acylcarnitine profiles in blood spots are highly specific. Clin Chem 2001; 47:1763–1768.

236. Sim KG, Wiley V, Carpenter K, et al. Carnitine palmitoyltransferase I deficiency in neonate identified by dried blood spot free carnitine and acylcarnitine profile. J Inherit Metab Dis 2001; 24:51–59.

237. Zschocke J, Penzien JM, Bielen R, et al. The diagnosis of mitochondrial HMG-CoA synthase deficiency. J Pediatr 2002; 140:778–780.

238. Abdenur JE CN, Schenone AB, et al. Supplemental newborn screening of aminoacids and acylcarnitines by electrospray tandem mass spectrometry: experience in Argentina. J Inherit Metab Dis 2000; 23(Suppl 1):13.

239. Bonnefont JP, Demaugre F, Prip-Buus C, et al. Carnitine palmitoyltransferase deficiencies. Mol Genet Metab 1999; 68:424–440.

240. Brivet M, Slama A, Millington DS, et al. Retrospective diagnosis of carnitine-acylcarnitine translocase deficiency by acylcarnitine analysis in the proband Guthrie card and enzymatic studies in the parents. J Inherit Metab Dis 1996; 19:181–184.

241. Wilcken B, Wiley V, Hammond J, et al. Screening newborns for inborn errors of metabolism by tandem mass spectrometry. N Engl J Med 2003; 348:2304–2312.

242. Abdenur JE, Chamoles NA, Schenone AB, et al. Multiple acyl-CoA-dehydrogenase deficiency (MADD): use of acylcarnitines and fatty acids to monitor the response to dietary treatment. Pediatr Res 2001; 50:61–66.

243. Bonafe L, Troxler H, Kuster T, et al. Evaluation of urinary acylglycines by electrospray tandem mass spectrometry in mitochondrial energy metabolism defects and organic acidurias. Mol Genet Metab 2000; 69:302–311.

244. Costa CG, Dorland L, Holwerda U, et al. Simultaneous analysis of plasma free fatty acids and their 3-hydroxy analogs in fatty acid beta-oxidation disorders. Clin Chem 1998; 44:463–471.

245. Jones PM, Burlina AB, Bennett MJ. Quantitative measurement of total and free 3-hydroxy fatty acids in serum or plasma samples: short-chain 3-hydroxy fatty acids are not esterified. J Inherit Metab Dis 2000; 23:745–750.

246. Brivet M, Slama A, Saudubray JM, et al. Rapid diagnosis of long chain and medium chain fatty acid oxidation disorders using lymphocytes. Ann Clin Biochem 1995; 32 (Pt 2): 154–159.

247. Young SP, Matern D, Gregersen N, et al. A comparison of in vitro acylcarnitine profiling methods for the diagnosis of classical and variant short chain acyl-CoA dehydrogenase deficiency. Clin Chim Acta 2003; 337:103–113.

248. Shen JJ, Matern D, Millington DS, et al. Acylcarnitines in fibroblasts of patients with long-chain 3-hydroxyacyl-CoA dehydrogenase deficiency and other fatty acid oxidation disorders. J Inherit Metab Dis 2000; 23:27–44.

249. Sim KG, Hammond J, Wilcken B. Strategies for the diagnosis of mitochondrial fatty acid beta-oxidation disorders. Clin Chim Acta 2002; 323:37–58.

250. Gregersen N, Andresen BS, Bross P. Prevalent mutations in fatty acid oxidation disorders: diagnostic considerations. Eur J Pediatr 2000,159(suppl 3):S213–S218.

251. Andresen BS, Dobrowolski SF, O'Reilly L, et al. Medium-chain acyl-CoA dehydrogenase (MCAD) mutations identified by MS/MS-based prospective screening of newborns differ from those observed in patients with clinical symptoms: identification and characterization of a new, prevalent mutation that results in mild MCAD deficiency. Am J Hum Genet 2001; 68:1408–1418.

252. Tyni T, Pihko H. Long-chain 3-hydroxyacyl-CoA dehydrogenase deficiency. Acta Paediatr 1999; 88:237–245.

253. Gregersen N, Bross P, Andresen BS. Genetic defects in fatty acid beta-oxidation and acyl-CoA dehydrogenases. Molecular pathogenesis and genotype-phenotype relationships. Eur J Biochem 2004; 271:470–482.

254. Njolstad PR, Skjeldal OH, Agsteribbe E, et al. Medium chain acyl-CoA dehydrogenase deficiency and fatal valproate toxicity. Pediatr Neurol 1997; 16:160–162.

255. Abdenur JE, Chamoles NA, Guinle AE, et al. Diagnosis of isovaleric acidaemia by tandem mass spectrometry: false positive result due to pivaloylcarnitine in a newborn screening programme. J Inherit Metab Dis 1998; 21:624–630.

256. Baillet L, Mullur RS, Esser V, et al. Elucidation of the mechanism by which (+)-acylcarnitines inhibit mitochondrial fatty acid transport. J Biol Chem 2000; 275: 36766–36768.

257. Ogier H S-FA. Disorders of Mitochondrial Fatty Acid Oxidation and Ketone Body Metabolism. 1st ed. Berlin: Springer-Verlag, 2006:147–160.

258. Gillingham MB, Weleber RG, Neuringer M, et al. Effect of optimal dietary therapy upon visual function in children with long-chain 3-hydroxyacyl CoA dehydrogenase and trifunctional protein deficiency. Mol Genet Metab 2005; 86:124–133.

259. Harding CO, Gillingham MB, van Calcar SC, et al. Docosahexaenoic acid and retinal function in children with long-chain 3-hydroxyacyl-CoA dehydrogenase deficiency. J Inherit Metab Dis 1999; 22:276–280.

260. Abdenur JE, Chamoles NA, Specola N, et al. MCAD deficiency. Acylcarnitines (AC) by tandem mass spectrometry (MS-MS) are useful to monitor dietary treatment. Adv Exp Med Biol 1999; 466:353–363.

261. Abdenur JE LS, Schenone AB, Guinle A, et al. Complex carbohydrates in the treatment of LCHAD deficiency. Mol Genet Metab 2004; 81:166(A).

262. Roe CR, Sweetman L, Roe DS, et al. Treatment of cardiomyopathy and rhabdomyolysis in long-chain fat oxidation disorders using an anaplerotic odd-chain triglyceride. J Clin Invest 2002; 110:259–269.

263. Van Hove JL, Grunewald S, Jaeken J, et al. D,L-3-hydroxybutyrate treatment of multiple acyl-CoA dehydrogenase deficiency (MADD). Lancet 2003; 361:1433–1435.

264. Djouadi F AF, Schlemmer D, et al. Potential of fibrates in the treatment of fatty acid oxidation defects: revival of classical drugs? J Inherit Metab Dis 2005; 28:115.

265. Marsden D. Expanded newborn screening by tandem mass spectrometry: the Massachusetts and New England experience. Southeast Asian J Trop Med Public Health 2003; 34(suppl 3):111–114.

266. Millington DS. Newborn screening for lysosomal storage disorders. Clin Chem 2005; 51:808–809.

267. Superti-Furga A. Glutaric aciduria type 1 and neonatal screening: time to proceed–with caution. Eur J Pediatr 2003; 162(suppl 1):S17–S20.

268. Chace DH, Sherwin JE, Hillman SL, et al. Use of phenylalanine-to-tyrosine ratio determined by tandem mass spectrometry to improve newborn screening for phenylketonuria of early discharge specimens collected in the first 24 hours. Clin Chem 1998; 44:2405–2409.

269. Meyburg J, Schulze A, Kohlmueller D, et al. Acylcarnitine profiles of preterm infants over the first four weeks of life. Pediatr Res 2002; 52:720–723.

270. Matern D. Tandem mass spectrometry in newborn screening. Endocrinol 2002; 12:50–57.

271. Naylor EW, Chace DH. Automated tandem mass spectrometry for mass newborn screening for disorders in fatty acid, organic acid, and amino acid metabolism. J Child Neurol 1999; 14(suppl) 1:S4–S8.

272. http://genes-r-us.uthscsa.edu/nbsdisorders.pdf.

273. Zytkovicz TH, Fitzgerald EF, Marsden D, et al. Tandem mass spectrometric analysis for amino, organic, and fatty acid disorders in newborn dried blood spots: a two-year summary from the New England Newborn Screening Program. Clin Chem 2001; 47:1945–1955.

274. Insinga RP, Laessig RH, Hoffman GL. Newborn screening with tandem mass spectrometry: examining its cost-effectiveness in the Wisconsin Newborn Screening Panel. J Pediatr 2002; 141:524–531.

275. Chace DH, Kalas TA, Naylor EW. The application of tandem mass spectrometry to neonatal screening for inherited disorders of intermediary metabolism. Annu Rev Genomics Hum Genet 2002; 3:17–45.

276. Schulze A, Lindner M, Kohlmuller D, et al. Expanded newborn screening for inborn errors of metabolism by electrospray ionization-tandem mass spectrometry: results, outcome, and implications. Pediatrics 2003; 111:1399–1406.

277. Gennaccaro M, Waisbren SE, Marsden D. The knowledge gap in expanded newborn screening: Survey results from paediatricians in Massachusetts. J Inherit Metab Dis 2005; 28:819–824.

278. Waisbren SE, Albers S, Amato S, et al. Effect of expanded newborn screening for biochemical genetic disorders on child outcomes and parental stress. JAMA 2003; 290:2564–2572.

279. Schenone A AJ, Guinle A, Fuertes A, Chamoles NA. Detection of inborn metabolic disorders in cord blood samples by tandem mass spectromety. Mol Genet Metab 2004; 81:178-A.

280. http:// www.californiaMsMs.org.

281. Gallagher RC, Cowan TM, Goodman SI, et al. Glutaryl-CoA dehydrogenase deficiency and newborn screening: retrospective analysis of a low excretor provides further evidence that some cases may be missed. Mol Genet Metab 2005; 86:417–420.

282. Smith WE, Millington DS, Koeberl DD, et al. Glutaric acidemia, type I, missed by newborn screening in an infant with dystonia following promethazine administration. Pediatrics 2001; 107:1184–1187.

283. Ly TB, Peters V, Gibson KM, et al. Mutations in the AUH gene cause 3-methylglutaconic aciduria type I. Hum Mutat 2003; 21:401–407.

284. Browning MF, Larson C, Strauss A, et al. Normal acylcarnitine levels during confirmation of abnormal newborn screening in long-chain fatty acid oxidation defects. J Inherit Metab Dis 2005; 28:545–550.

285. Waddell L, Wiley V, Carpenter K, et al. Medium-chain acyl-CoA dehydrogenase deficiency: genotype-biochemical phenotype correlations. Mol Genet Metab 2006; 87:32–39.

286. Dantas MF, Suormala T, Randolph A, et al. 3-Methylcrotonyl-CoA carboxylase deficiency: mutation analysis in 28 probands, 9 symptomatic and 19 detected by newborn screening. Hum Mutat 2005; 26:164.

287. Spiekerkoetter U, Sun B, Zytkovicz T, et al. MS/MS-based newborn and family screening detects asymptomatic patients with very-long-chain acyl-CoA dehydrogenase deficiency. J Pediatr 2003; 143:335–342.

288. Rinaldo P, Tortorelli S, Matern D. Recent developments and new applications of tandem mass spectrometry in newborn screening. Curr Opin Pediatr 2004; 16:427–433.

289. http://www.genes-r-us.uthscsa.edu.

290. http://www.childrenshospital.org/newenglandconsortium/.

291. www.dhs.ca.gov/gdb.

292. http://www.baylorhealth.com/medicalspecialties/metabolic/newbornscreening.htm.

293. http://www.mayoclinic.org/laboratorygenetics-rst/newbornscreening.html.

294. Robinson BH. Lactic acidemia: disorders of pyruvate carboxylase and pyruvate dehydrogenase. In: Scriver CR, Beaudet AL, Sly WS Valle D, eds. The Metabolic and Molecular Bases of Inherited Disease. 8th ed. New York: McGraw-Hill, 2001:2275–2295.

295. De Vivo DC, Di Mauro S. Disorders of pyruvate metabolism, the citric acid cycle and the respiratory chain. In: Fernandes J, Saudubray JM, Tada, eds. Inborn Metabolic Diseases. Diagnosis and management. 1st ed. Springer-Verlag.

296. Cameron JM, Levandovskiy V, Mackay N, Tein I, Robinson B. Deficiency of pyruvate dehydrogenase caused by novel and known mutations in the E1 alpha subunit. Am J Med Genet 2004; 131:59–66.

297. Lissens W, De Meirleir L, Seneca S, et al. Mutations in the X-linked pyruvate dehydrogenase (E1) a subunit gene (PDHA1) in patients with a pyruvate dehydrogenase complex deficiency. Hum Mutat 2000; 15:209–219.

298. Head RA, Brown RM, Zolkipli Z, Shahdadpuri R, King MD, Clayton PT, Brown GK. Clinical and genetics spectrum of pyruvate dehydrogenase deficiency: dihydrolipoamide acetyltransferase (E2) deficiency. Ann Neurol 2005; 58:234–41.

299. Brown RM, Head RA, Boubriak II, Leonard JV, Thomas NH, Brown GK. Mutations in the gene for the E1beta subunit: a novel cause of pyruvate dehydrogenase deficiency. Hum Genet 2004; 115:123–127.

300. Robinson BH, Mac Kay N, Petrova-Benedict R, et al. Defects in the E2 lipoyltransacetylase and the X-lipoyl containing component of the pyruvate dehydrogenase complex in patients with lactic acidemia. J Clin Invest 1990; 85:1821–1824.

301. Ito M, Kobashi H, Naito E, et al. Decrease of pyruvate dehydrogenase phosphatase activity in patients with congenital lactic acidemia. Clin Chim Acta 1992; 209:1–7.

302. Yoshida I, Sweetman L, Kulovich S, Nyhan WL, Robinson B. Effect of lipoic acid in a patient with defective activity of pyruvate dehydrogenase, 2-oxoglutarate dehydrogenase and branched-chain keto acid dehydrogenase. Pediatr Res 1990; 27:75–79.

303. Elpeleg ON, Ruitenbeek W, Jakobs C, et al. Congenital lactic acidemia caused by lipoamide dehydrogenase deficiency with favorable outcome. J Pediatr 1995; 126:72–74.

304. Saada A, Aptowitzer I, Link E, Elpeleg ON. ATP synthesis in lipoamide dehydrogenase deficiency. Biochem Biophys Res Commun 2000; 16:382–386.

305. Makino M, Horai S, Goto Y, Nonaka I. Mitochondrial DNA mutations in Leigh syndrome and their phylogenetic implications. J Hum Genet 2000; 45:69–75.

306. DiMauro S, Bonilla E, De Vivo D. Does the patient have a mitochondrial encephalomyopathy? J Child Neurol 1999; 14(suppl 1):S23–S35.

307. Odievre MH, Chretien D, Munich A, et al. A novel mutation in the dihydrolipoamide dehydrogenase E3 subunit gene resulting in an atypical formo f alpha-keto-glutarate dehydrogenase deficiency. Hum Mutat 2005; 25:323–324.

308. Kohlschutter A, Behbehani A, Langenbeck U, et al. A familial progressive neurodegenerative disease with 2-oxo-glutaric aciduria. Eur J Pediat 1982; 138:32–37.

309. Dunckelmann RJ, Ebinger F, Schulze A, et al. 2-ketoglutarate dehydrogenase deficiency with intermittent 2-ketoglutaric aciduria. Neuropediatrics 2000; 31:35–38.

310. Bourgeron T, Chretien D, Poggi-bach J, et al. Mutation of the fumarase gene in two siblings with progressive encephalopathy and fumarase deficiency. J Clin Invest 1994; 2514–2518.

311. Coughlin EM, Christensen E, Kunz P, et al. Molecular analysis and prenatal diagnosis of human fumarase deficiency. Mol Genet and Metab 1998; 63:254–262.

312. Kerrigan JF, Aleck KA, Tarby TJ, et al. Fumaric aciduria: clinical and imaging features. Ann Neurol 2000; 47: 583–588.

313. Briere JJ, Favier J, Ghouzzi VE, et al. Succinate dehydrogenase deficiency in humans. Cell Mol Life Sci 2005; 62:2317–2324.

314. Garcia-Cazorla A, Rabier D, Touati G, et al. Pyruvate carboxylase deficiency: metabolic characteristics and new neurological aspects. Ann Neurol 2006; 59:121–127.

315. Mochel F, De Lonlay P, Touati F, et al. Pyruvate carboxylase deficiency: clinical and biochemical response to anaplerotic diet therapy. Mol Genet Metab 2005; 84: 305–12.

316. Brun N, Robitaille Y, Grignon A, et al. Pyruvate carboxylase deficiency: prenatal onset of ischemia–like brain lesions in two sibs with acute neonatal form. Am J Med Genet 1999; 84:94–101.

317. Ahmad A, Khaler S, Kishnani PS, et al. Treatment of pyruvate carboxylase deficiency with high doses of citrate and aspartate. Am J Med Genet 1999; 87:331–338.

318. Fructose 1,6-diphosphatase deficiency. In: Nyhan WL, Ozand PT, eds. Atlas of Metabolic Diseases. 1st ed London: Chapman & Hall Medical, 1998:273–277.

319. Shoffner JM. Oxidative phosphorylation diseases. In: Scriver CR, Beaudet AL, Sly WS, Valle D, eds. The Metabolic and Molecular Bases of Inherited Disease. New York: McGraw-Hill, 2000:2367–2423.

320. Zeviani M, Di Donato S. Mitochondrial disorders. Brain 2004; 127:2153–2172.

321. DiMauro S, Schon E. Mitochondrial respiratory-chain diseases. N Engl J Med 2003; 348:2656–2668.

322. Munnich A, Rotig A, Cormier Daire V, Rustin P. Clinical presentation of respiratory chain deficiency. In: Scriver CR, Beaudet AL, Sly WS, Valle D, eds. The Metabolic and Molecular Bases of Inherited Disease. New York: McGraw-Hill, 2001:2261–2274.

323. Scaglia F, Towin JA, Craigen WJ, et al. Clinical spectrum, morbidity and mortality in 113 pediatric patients with mitochondrial disease. Pediatrics 2004; 114:925–931.

324. Rabinowitz S, Gelfond D, Chen CK, et al. Hepatocerebral mitochondrial DNA depletion syndrome: clinical and morphologic features of a nuclear gene mutation. J Pediatr Gastroenterol Nutr 2004; 38:216–220.

325. Ferrari G, Lamantea E, Donati A, et al. Infantile hepatocerebral syndromes associated with mutations in the mitochondrial DNA polymerase-γA. Brain 2005; 128:723–731.

326. Labarthe F, Dobbelaere D, Devisme L, et al. Clinical, biochemical and morphological features of hepatocerebral syndrome with mitochondrial DNA depletion due to deoxiguanosine kinase deficiency. J Hepatol 2005; 43: 333–341.

327. Poggi-Travert F, Martin D, Billette de Villemeur T, et al. Metabolic intermediates in lactic acidosis: compounds samples and interpretation. J Inherit Metab Dis 1996; 19:478–488.

328. Cray SH, Robinson B, Cox PN. Lactic acidemia and bradyarrhythmia in a child sedated with profolol. Crit Care Med 1998; 26:2087–2092.

329. Rogers JG, Wilkinson RG, Skelton I, Danks DM. Tertiary lactic acidosis. J Pediatr 1981; 99:272–273.

330. Bongaerts G, Bakkeren J, Severijen R, et al. Lactobacilli and acidosis in children with short small bowel. J Pediatr Gastroenterol Nutr 2000; 30: 288–293.

331. Romero NB, Lombes A, Touati G, et al. Morphological studies of skeletal muscle in lactic acidosis. J Inher Metab Dis 1996; 19:528–534.

332. Munnich A. Defects of the respiratory chain. In: Fernandes J, Saudubray JM, van den Berghe G, eds. Inborn Metabolic Diseases. 2nd ed. Berlin: Springer-Verlag, 2000:158–168.

333. Morris AAM, Leonard JV. The treatment of congenital lactic acidoses. J Inher Metab Dis 1996; 19:573–580.

334. Lerman-Sagie T, Rustin P, Lev D, et al. Dramatic improvement in mitochondrial cardiomyopathy following treatment with idebenone. J Inher Metab Dis 2001; 24:28–34.

335. Salviati L, Sacconi S, Murer L, et al. Infantile encephalomyopathy and nephropathy with CoQ10 deficiency: a CoQ10-responsive condition. Neurology. 2005; 65(4): 606–608.

336. Wexler ID, Hemalatha SG, McConnell J, et al. Outcome of pyruvate dehydrogenase deficiency treated with ketogenic diets. Studies in patients with identical mutations. Neurology 1997; 49:1655–1661.

337. Chinnery PF, Bindoff LA. 116th ENMC international workshop: the treatment of mitochondrila disorders. Neuromuscul Disord 2003; 13:757–764.

338. Chinnery P, Majamaa K, Turnbull D, Thorburn D. Treatment for mitochondrial disorders. Cochrane Database Syst Rev 2006; 25 (1):CD004426.

339. Sokal EM, Sokol R, Cormier V, et al. Liver transplantation in mitochondrial respiratory chain disorders. Eur J Pediatr 1999; 158 (suppl 2):S81–S84.

18

Private Practice of Pediatric Endocrinology

Richard Mauseth

Woodinville Pediatrics, Woodinville, Washington and Department of Pediatrics,
University of Washington School of Medicine, Seattle, Washington, U.S.A.

INTRODUCTION

Prevalence of private practice endocrinology is rising in the United States, with 30.9% of the applicants for the 2003 pediatric endocrine board certification exam indicating involvement with private practice (1). This is up from 19.3% for those registered for the 1992 exam. Of those taking the 2003 exam, 10.3% were full-time subspecialty physicians in private practice (up from 4.1% in 1992), 7.4% were in a part-time subspecialty and part-time general pediatrics (down from 11.1% in 1992), and 13.2% were full-time subspecialty, partly in private practice and partly in an academic setting (up from 4.1% in 1992). However, these statistics do not account for pediatric endocrinologists who have shifted their time and effort to a full-time practice of the specialty after attaining the board certification, nor do they account for full-time academic colleagues engaged in direct patient care as their principal activity. This chapter attempts to assist and encourage those considering private practice, as well as to offer some guidance from my own experience. Hopefully, some of these factors will benefit those in academic medicine, much of which is changing to become increasingly like private practice with the same concerns about patient issues, reimbursement, and contracting.

PRIVATE AND ACADEMIC PRACTICES

One major factor in a successful practice is putting out a good product that satisfies the patient's needs, as well as fulfills the referring doctor's expectation of your involvement in their patient's care. A private pediatric endocrinologist has the personal satisfaction of developing a patient-care program of one's own making, one that is not subject to as many external forces as university-based physicians have to deal with, such as department heads, hospital administrators, and others giving input in the running of—and reimbursement to—the program. Private practice endocrinologists are required and able to meet directly with insurance companies and negotiate contracts, and to either accept or reject them based on their worth. Conversely, university-based or hospital-based endocrinologists' contracts are often negotiated by surgeons, neonatologists, cardiologists, and cardiac surgeons. These specialists have a major stake in the overall contract and are willing to undersell pediatric endocrinology reimbursements because these are considered a "lost leader" service. Most private pediatric endocrinologists take an active role in the billing and evaluation of their practice and have the right to refuse or accept different insurances, depending on whether the reimbursement for pediatric endocrinology is adequate.

Many university- and hospital-based endocrinology groups have become more like private practices within the university setting. Visible benefits include physicians having more say as to how to run their practices and calculate their reimbursement. The position of the university- or hospital-based physician is generally salaried and includes some incentives, with the majority of income guaranteed. Many aspects of a successful private pediatric endocrinologist practice may be appealing to the academic endocrinologist. Pressure on academic endocrinology departments to improve their reimbursement and to become more streamlined is increasing. Furthermore, academic endocrinologists have teaching and research responsibilities that cause difficulty when also having to attend to the details required to run a successful private practice. These endocrinologists are also somewhat inhibited by the difference in coding for—and reimbursement of—hospital-related visits, which is often different than that of the private practice endocrinologist. This again addresses the subject of private practice endocrinologists' negotiating contracts by themselves, rather than referring to a full hospital or multispeciality clinic scale for reimbursement. On the other hand, independent endocrinologists experience added stress as well as risk in not having the safety net of a department in the event their practice does not succeed.

Pediatric endocrinologists in private practice often participate in clinical research as well as in teaching students, residents, and fellows within their own settings.

A major difference between academic and private practice endocrinologists is flexibility. Generally, private practice physicians can set their own hours. However, an academic institution does not provide that flexibility to the pediatric endocrinologist, and often demands "productivity" in clinical services without consideration to teaching and research activities. Private practice endocrinologists can control their overhead and employ a small or large staff. They also have the ability to develop programs within the office setting, such as diabetes education classes and support groups. While some programs have no direct financial benefit, overall they are seen as beneficial for the clinic or community. In addition, these programs are not subject to the scrutiny of a hospital or academic administrator.

A successful pediatric endocrinology practice must adapt to various fluctuations, such as age of patient, as well as their socioeconomic and educational backgrounds. The practice also needs to be able to adapt to changing insurance coverage and insurance circumstances such as HMOs, private insurance, and welfare. It needs to deal with patients who lose or change their insurance coverage or employment. In addition, the practice must adapt to the doctor's changing age, energy, and personal commitments. A new physician may be able to devote an extensive amount of time to getting established, whereas a more established endocrinologist may be able to afford more time away from the practice. On the other hand, a young physician may also have personal commitments such as young children and, therefore, not be able to work as many hours or weekends/evenings due to family needs. Of course, as the children get older the physician's ability to devote more time to the practice will also evolve.

Building a successful private pediatric endocrinology practice, be it an independent practice or one within an academic or hospital setting, requires a number of things. Primarily, hard work, organization, and a commitment to the practice are critical. Also required are good listening skills and empathy, as well as the ability to adapt and be able to provide a good service at all times. For instance, community outreach programs such as lectures to the general public and participating in health groups help to earn the physician's respect from other physicians and the general public, as well as to establish the physician's reputation as an expert in the field. Continuing medical education through conferences is valuable, as is communication with referring doctors through prompt updates on their patients and answers to medical queries not related to specific consultations. Being available to doctors to deal with their concerns and support their services requires flexible hours, which makes the pediatric endocrinologist more available to deal with emergencies and other urgent matters of physicians and of parents. Adjusting to parents' working hours is often necessary, which indicates that you care enough for patients, their families, other physicians, and the community to make yourself available during nontraditional working hours. The important ability to listen to parents enables you to understand concerns and bring them into a partnership with the care of their child. It is essential to address each patient's needs, both personal and specific to each patient group, such as diabetics. Availing yourself to other physicians and their concerns is key and may enhance your value, not to mention produce for you more timely and appropriate referrals. Also, tune in to the needs of the community and respond with any resources you may be in a position to provide, which are not presently available or are inadequate.

PERSONAL EXPERIENCE

Early in my career, I was a fellow in Seattle. At the end of my fellowship, I decided to stay in the area because my family was there. I became a junior faculty member at the University of Washington. At that time, there was only one academic faculty member in the Division of Endocrinology, and he did no clinical practice. The clinics at Children's Hospital were maintained by me and other local private practice pediatric endocrinologists. Two other private practice endocrinologists and I did most of the inpatient consultations at the hospital.

Feeling frustrated with the university system, I decided to establish an independent private practice. I had been told at the university that the patients were clinic patients, and they were not to be seen by a specific doctor in order to allow more exposure to residents for teaching. It was very difficult for me to let go of that close relationship I had with patients and their families, particularly my diabetic patients. I very much enjoyed the teaching and close contact with the residents, but the time required to attend the various meetings was burdensome. I was concerned, however, about the possible financial ramifications of opening an independent practice because, although private practice brought the potential for higher financial rewards and I was not tenured at the university, the position I had did provide relative security.

I chose a geographic area about 25 minutes from Children's Hospital in the community where I lived. The choice of this area was based on a number of factors: there were several school districts (with a total of 30,000 students) without a pediatrician. One district was increasing in population by two new houses per day. These were all three- to four-bedroom houses indicating an increase of families with children. I set up an office of general pediatrics open six half-days per week, and then spent the other four half-days a week attending clinics at Children's Hospital doing pediatric endocrinology.

Because I was initially practicing general pediatrics, there was a great deal of resistance from local pediatricians to refer their endocrinology patients to me. They were concerned they would lose their patients to me. It took a great deal of time to convince them that I was not recruiting their patients for my general pediatrics practice. I had to be very careful to refer the patients back to their primary-care doctors and not allow patients to transfer over to my practice. After two and half years of solo pediatric practice, I recruited a trained pediatric hematologist–oncologist as a partner, who was also willing to practice general pediatrics with some time committed to hematology–oncology. Because of our affiliation with the local Children's Hospital and the lack of any other pediatrician in the large area around where we had set up our practice, we became a referral service for high-risk pediatrics patients and the practice continued to grow.

Subsequently, more and more pediatricians joined us, thus allowing me to decrease the amount of time I spent in general pediatrics and increase the time I could devote to pediatric endocrinology. After about 10 years of work in private practice, I no longer took new pediatric patients and accepted only new pediatric endocrinology patients. At the present time, I spend about 95% of my time doing pediatric endocrinology and 5% of my time doing general pediatrics. The latter percentage is mainly taking care of children of former patients of mine, most of whom are now adult Type I diabetics. The practice has grown from a staff of 1 (me), to 26 years later, having 14 providers, eight partner pediatrician MDs, three part-time employee MDs (one a pediatric endocrinologist), and three nurse practitioners (one in pediatric endocrinology), and more than 20,000 active patients. We also have a part-time certified diabetes educator nutritionist. A nurse practitioner is able to see and bill patients without a physician seeing the patient. In my case, I usually see most of the patients briefly just for continuity and for the ability to handle phone inquiries about them, should they arise. Nutritionists have recently gained the ability to be reimbursed for their services in my area, but I am not sure this is the case nationwide. Often the reimbursement is better if it is associated with some type of physician contact.

In my opinion, the key to the growth and success of the practice was the selection of an area that was underserved and that had a great potential for growth, along with acquiring high-quality partners to provide the best of care. In many ways, starting a pediatric endocrinology practice without the general pediatrics would be easier, both in terms of less night calls and fewer worries by the referring doctors that their patients would switch to another practice. However, income is generated more quickly with general pediatrics. A possible solution would be to practice pediatric endocrinology without general pediatrics and offer to perform locums tenums for a large general pediatric group to become known to the community and to increase referrals.

After being in practice for 10 years, the university decided to hire a full-time clinical endocrinologist to care for their patients. My time commitment to the Children's Hospital had decreased by then. As the general pediatric portion of my practice decreased, so did the concern of other pediatricians that referrals to me would result in a loss of their patients. Interestingly enough, when there was an emphasis on managed care (which is minimal in our area today) and people were being assigned physicians, there was a large influx into our practice of endocrinology patients selecting us as their primary-care doctors in order to avoid the necessity of eliciting an approved referral every time. In the more recent years, this has become less of a concern. However, being a primary-care physician for endocrinology patients has proven to be a unique challenge, in that it requires a greater involvement in immunizations as well as in addressing general pediatric health-care issues at each visit.

Every doctor entering my practice realizes they need to be familiar with diabetes management, because there are times when they are asked to cover for me when I am out of town. I have had the privilege of having an extremely capable nurse who can handle most of these cases and can aid in the assistance of the other pediatricians handling these cases when I am not available. As the practice matured, the more severe cases of endocrine abnormalities have been directly referred to Children's Hospital, which can provide more intensive care. Mild DKA patients and existing known diabetics within my practice are usually taken care of at the local hospital or as outpatients in our office. A collegial relationship has developed between me and the Children's Hospital staff, and I have participated in working with several of their research patients, and they have assisted me in taking care of my inpatients at the hospital when I am not available.

TYPE OF PRACTICE

The type of practice desired and the location in which to set it up are much intertwined, and both are equally important topics.

Type

There are multiple types of practices: solo, group practice, partnership with adult endocrinologist, and affiliation with a hospital or even being owned by a hospital or a major group. Each of these has pros and cons for the pediatric endocrinologist.

A solo practice allows you to have control over your staff, your hours, and your ability to change your practice as needed. You control your overhead and you make the hiring and firing decisions. But the downside is that you have to be very much involved in the business aspects (which results in time away from the clinical aspect of the practice). There is some degree of isolation and no one to talk to. And, coverage becomes a major issue.

A group practice has the advantage of being kinetic, so the higher volume results in less overhead. Coverage becomes easier. However, you no longer have sole control over decision making; rather, any decisions need to be made by consensus. There can be differences in billing practices, differences in work practices, differences in educational tools (i.e., diabetes educators and diabetes classes) and differences in treatment styles. If one is entering a group practice, or deciding to start one, it is important to get smart people. Trading less on-call for poorer quality physicians usually ends up making things more difficult for you.

Some of the advantages of partnering with an adult endocrinologist include the large volume of patients brought into the practice. These physicians often own many of the laboratory facilities that can increase income. The pediatric endocrinologist can transition patients directly to the adult endocrinologist, making the transition convenient for both the physicians and the family. However, the disadvantage of this partnership is that the pediatric endocrinologist often has more overhead. Pediatric patients, especially young diabetics, demand more of your time along with that of diabetes educators and dietitians. Occasionally, the resources for diabetes education and nutritional advice can be obtained in the community and not at the physician's expense. However, in most instances, these resources are geared for adults. This leaves the pediatric patient and parents having to search elsewhere for information.

Affiliation with a hospital or a university, whether the practice is owned by the hospital or is partially managed by the hospital or university or a large health-care organization, has the advantage of somewhat more secure income, less physician-funded startup costs, most established referral patterns, and immediate recognition for the community of a large number of doctors. Depending on the relationship to the hospital, there would be some concern about who controls the staffing and the contracting, as well as who establishes the work hours, coverage, and on-call schedules. However, this affiliation may also create some restriction on which laboratories, X ray, and magnetic resonance imaging facilities are used, resulting in the possible use of a facility that may not have a lot of pediatric experience.

These are among the various issues facing each type of practice, and each one needs to be anticipated and addressed up front.

Location

A good doctor can make a reasonable living almost anywhere, despite all the current day encumbrances with market healthcare. First and foremost, consider the location in which you would like to live. The United States has an increasing number of pediatric endocrinology patients, particularly the ever-growing number of diabetics and their need to attain better control of their disease. Therefore, the need for pediatric endocrinologists is only going to be increasing over time. The number of qualified caregivers is not increasing as fast as the number of patients. Of the 989 board-certified pediatric endocrinologists, 22.5% of these are over 60 years old and another 16.3% are 56 to 60 years old (1). The median age is 52.9 years old. Only 62 pediatricians passed the 2003 pediatric endocrine certification exam, which is given every two years (1). In many areas, the need for pediatric endocrine services is provided by other specialists and general physicians. However, pediatricians are most often reluctant to care for and participate in the treatment of diabetics. And although adult endocrinologists are often willing to transfer the care of their pediatric patients to a pediatric endocrinologist, this willingness may not be evident with the care of other pediatric endocrine patients, i.e., those with thyroid or growth disorders.

The population required to support a pediatric endocrinology practice varies. In general, a population of 100,000 to 200,000 is needed. But it all depends how on the doctor functions, attracts patients, establishes a referral pattern. The typical pediatric endocrine practice consists of a large proportion of Type 1 diabetic patients (50–60%) (2). In our practice, this is also the case: diabetics account for 54% of visits, growth disorders 27%, pubertal disorders 9%, and other endocrine disorders 10%. There are more than 13,000 new children who develop diabetes every year (Vol. 1; Chap. 3), thus the need for pediatric endocrinology will continue to grow. Moreover, the current epidemic of obesity has also been associated with a higher prevalence of Type 2 diabetes and of insulin resistance in children (Vol. 1; Chap. 3), and because of this, the higher demand for pediatric endocrine services will need to be met. A practice that cares for diabetics will also grow faster, though it requires more personnel and clinical associates. Diabetics need to be seen more frequently and by more individuals.

The distance patients need to or are willing to drive to see a pediatric endocrinologist depends on the presence of other competitive pediatric subspecialists in practice or in academic centers (however, the service that that physician provides to the family and to the referring physician can make all the difference). It is not uncommon for a patient in Montana to drive 400 miles in a day for a clinic visit. Their only other option is to get on an airplane, because as of this date, there are no pediatric endocrinologists in that state. The reverse may also apply, as pediatric endocrinologists may want to serve and cover the need in far distant places. But one needs to exercise caution when doing this, because these areas may be so economically depressed that the number of uninsured or poorly insured patients makes it economically unfeasible for a pediatric endocrinologist to succeed.

In checking location, it would be important to examine the demographics of the insured: the percentage of patients on welfare, the number of uninsured patients, the percentage of patients who have HMOs, and the general reimbursement by the major insurance companies. This information can be obtained through the local medical society and other physicians. Local hospitals would be able to provide information on the percentage of patients who are with each insurance company. Look at the major industries in the area and the type of insurance they provide. It is important to see if an area is growing or declining in population, particularly if families with young children are moving into the area. Oftentimes, poorer patients have higher needs, require more paperwork because of their state-provided insurance, have more social issues, and often create an increased number of no-shows. Patients with a lower level of education may be more difficult to work with, but all of these factors need to be balanced against a personal social conscious level for providing for these patients.

Setting up a practice in a wealthier neighborhood brings its own challenges. Setup costs may be higher. The staff has to be more professional and should have higher technical skills. However, these costs will be balanced against higher collections. Working with well-to-do patients often has its own issues: they are more demanding; they often have achieved a higher level of education, and, as a result, are more up-to-date on the medical issues. They have better access to Internet and, therefore, can demand answers to questions they have researched. One local pediatric neurologist has become so popular that he no longer takes insurance: he requires payment up front. Therefore, he has no billing. He has very few cancellations and has a very full practice, and he meets his social consciousness by giving 10% of his practice as free care. I do not know of a pediatric endocrinologist who has this luxury.

Oftentimes in looking at a location where other pediatric endocrinologists exist, certain things should be considered. You may have the option of joining an existing practice. If you are going to eventually buy the practice, look at the age of the doctor who may be near retirement and may want to slow down. This decrease in overall production will increase the burden of overhead on a younger physician. An older pediatric endocrinologist may have an older group of patients who may not remain in the practice for a long period of time, thus decreasing the value of the older pediatrician's practice; i.e., if the average age of growth hormone–deficient patients in the practice is 14 years old, those patients will most probably move on to an adult practitioner sooner than a growth hormone–deficient patient who is six years old. All of these factors must be taken into consideration when choosing a location.

BUILDING A NEW PRACTICE

Beware of what you wish for. Having more patients does not always mean making more money and often means less free time. You can expect to see two kinds of patients: one is very demanding, has been through three or four other pediatric endocrinologists, requires a lot of time, and has a lot of needs. It is important to listen to these patients and try to meet their needs, but it is also very important to set limits with them. The other type of patient is one who is newly diagnosed and wants to see a doctor right away. This patient has been referred to you by his/her pediatrician because you are new in town and can get them in fast. It is important to spend time with these patients and to also have direct contact with their primary-care physician by phone. Usually when you start a practice, you are going to have plenty of time and, therefore, a good service to the primary-care physician by a letter and personal phone call often can introduce you to them and increase your referral base. It is important to be personable with your referring physicians, but, on the other hand, sooner or later, your privacy is going to become a major issue. I found out the hard way to not give out my pager number, cell phone number, or residential phone number. You have to establish the maximal amount of acceptable intrusion into your life.

Giving talks to the public is a good way to increase your exposure and, in turn, your practice. Some excellent venues are local hospitals, major pediatric groups, JDRF or ADA functions, as well as parent support groups such as the Turner's Group or the Human Growth Foundation groups. Attending the state pediatric society meeting is also helpful, not only to get yourself known, but oftentimes they have very good seminars on topics such as practice management billing, and coding for insurance, which can all be very helpful. As we will discuss later, billing and coding are ever-changing and require constant attention and revision to get the most for your efforts.

In setting the hours of your practice, it is wise, and even advantageous, to provide evening and weekend hours. If you are involved with a pediatric practice, it is often possible to have evening hours or weekend hours when you are on call for some other reason. Making yourself more available can be an initial drawing factor to you. But as your practice matures, you may find that you do not want to maintain these extended hours. Once a precedent is established, however, as time goes by, it may be more difficult to change it. This must be weighed carefully.

Staffing and Office Space

When starting up a practice, two of the biggest costs are staffing and rent. The space needs to be large enough to accommodate your growing practice and your ability to work. However, leases can be negotiated so that the first several months can either be free with an increase over a period of time, or reduced rent or help with the cost of leaseholder improvements. It is a common practice to give several months of free rent with an allowance for tenant improvements. The more free rent and the higher tenant improvements are usually associated with a longer lease commitment. This is all negotiable.

In starting a solo practice, it is not necessary to have a lot of employees. Your initial hire should be a billing person, as this is the lifeblood of your practice. The person needs to be committed to the practice, and is probably the most key employee in the office. The billing person needs to be aggressive in discussing the bills submitted with the insurance companies, needs to be convinced that your services are worthwhile and legitimate, needs to be compassionate in discussing bills with patients and their families and also be able to solve problems. The person needs to be intelligent and have good communication skills, but does not necessarily have to have completed a college degree. This person must keep you informed and be accountable to you. A person who does not have billing experience can receive training through seminars with medical associations, or can attend national seminars that are set up by different corporations on coding, billing, and collecting. In my experience, every penny that has been spent on education has returned itself many times on the investment.

Initially, the billing person will have enough time to check in patients, make sure that the billing codes are accurate, and answer phones. Prescription refills can be a major problem, especially for diabetics. We have developed a form with all the diabetes supplies (insulins, test strips, syringes, pen needles, ketostix, lancets, etc.) with frequency of use, amount used, supply quantity, and duration of prescription (Table 1). My nurse or I fill this out for a year. We then make multiple photocopies (mail-order, local pharmacy, travel, lost prescription, and one for our files), so the receptionist can fax if needed without my involvement. We have also instituted a diabetic prescription line on our phone system, which gives specific instructions on the information needed to fill a prescription. We request that the patient have the pharmacy fax us an order to be signed, which cuts down on workload. Growth hormone is handled differently. After each clinic visit, the note is sent to the distributing company for them to resubmit for insurance approval. As the practice grows, there will be more phone calls and more patients, and more staff will need to be added. I would suggest hiring a nurse with either significant pediatric experience or experience in endocrinology; having both would be ideal. The less experience a nurse has in either field, the more time it is going to require you as the doctor to educate the patient. You can have meetings; they can sit in with patients. They can listen to phone discussions, and how problems are handled. They could attend the Pediatric Endocrine Nurses' Association

and Diabetes Educator Association meetings. There are also local pediatric endocrine programs. They should be encouraged to attend these programs and to discuss unique and interesting patients. This gives them a feeling of responsibility, confidence, and respect, and allows them to feel that they are a worthwhile part of your practice. You can also increase their knowledge of pediatric endocrinology by enrolling them in the Pharmaceutical Growth Hormone Registries, which all have meetings the nurses can attend. Their education is key to the success of the practice.

Eventually, as the practice gets larger and the demand increases, the hiring of a receptionist and/or a medical assistant may become necessary. This depends on the volume of the practice and the desire of the physician for staffing. Again, staff is part of overhead, and more overhead, either in space or in staff, decreases the amount of income to the physician.

Originally starting out, it is possible for the physician to supplement his/her salary by doing locums for other physicians. I would suggest, however, that this be done a distance from the primary pediatric endocrine office in order to avoid a sense of competition from other pediatricians who may, in turn, decrease their referrals. Another source of potential income is covering on call for the university or being partly involved in the university clinic system and receiving reimbursement. This would increase rapport between the academic and private pediatric endocrinologist as well as create collegial relationships with them.

Equipment

A pediatric endocrinologist does not need a lot of equipment to set up an office. A main computer system, depending on whether you want to have scheduling as well as billing, is a good start. An electronic medical record system would be ideal and may be worth the original expense, because it is very difficult to institute later on and it may also be more costly. In-office equipment would include a bone age book, orchidometer, blood pressure cuffs, Lange calipers for skin fat fold thickness and, ideally, an A1c-glycosylated hemoglobin machine. Very little other equipment is necessary, such as DEXA scans and X-ray machines. The value of having these pieces of equipment could be considered at a later time and depends on your association with others who would utilize this expensive equipment.

In considering a laboratory, it is important to have the age-related norms for the various tests. It is also important to have a good turnaround time and results that are presented in a readable manner. Most of the laboratories understand that pediatric endocrinologists have a great deal of testing and are very willing to change their forms and systems around to meet your needs. Very often, there can be competition between different laboratories for your testing, and

Table 1 Prescription Form

Name:_____   Date:____/____/____

Diabetes Supplies Prescriptions:

Insulin Type	Amount	Directions	# days supply	Renewal, length
Humulin R	_____Vials	_____Units/day	30 60 90	6 mo. 1 yr.
Humulin L	_____Vials	_____Units/day	30 60 90	6 mo. 1 yr.
Humulin N	_____Vials	_____Units/day	30 60 90	6 mo. 1 yr.
Humulin U	_____Vials	_____Units/day	30 60 90	6 mo. 1 yr.
Humalog(H)	_____Vials	_____Units/day	30 60 90	6 mo. 1 yr.
Humalog Disposable Pen	_____Boxes; 5/box	_____Units/day	30 60 90	6 mo. 1 yr.
Novolin R	_____Vials	_____Units/day	30 60 90	6 mo. 1 yr.
Novolin N	_____Vials	_____Units/day	30 60 90	6 mo. 1 yr.
Novolin L	_____Vials	_____Units/day	30 60 90	6 mo. 1 yr.
Novolog Dispos. Flex Pen	_____Boxes;5/box	_____Units/day	30 60 90	6 mo. 1 yr.
Novolog	_____Vials	_____Units/day	30 60 90	6 mo. 1 yr.
Lantus (Glargine)	_____Vials	_____Units/day	30 60 90	6 mo. 1 yr.
Novolog 3 cc cartridges	_____Boxes;5/box	_____Units/day	30 60 90	6 mo. 1 yr.
Lantus 3 cc cartridges	_____Boxes; 5/box	_____Units/day	30 60 90	6 mo. 1 yr.
Test Strips				
Freestyle	_____Box/100 ea	Use_____X/day	30 60 90	6 mo. 1 yr.
One Touch (Ultra)	_____Box/100 ea	Use_____X/day	30 60 90	6 mo. 1 yr.
Glucometer	_____Box/100 ea	Use_____X/day	30 60 90	6 mo. 1 yr.
Precision	_____Box/100 ea	Use_____X/day	30 60 90	6 mo. 1 yr.
Advantage or Complete (Comfort Curve)	_____Box/100 ea	Use_____ X/day	30 60 90	6 mo. 1 yr.
Compact (17 strips/drum)	_____Box/2drums	Use_____X/day	30 60 90	6 mo. 1 yr.
Ascensia Autodisk (10 strips/disk)	_____Box/5 disks	Use_____X/day	30 60 90	6 mo. 1 yr.
Ascensia Microfill	_____Box/100 ea	Use_____X/day	30 60 90	6 mo. 1 yr.
True Track	_____Box/100 ea	Use_____X/day	30 60 90	6 mo. 1 yr.
Blood-glucose test strips	_____Box/100 ea	Use_____X/day	30 60 90	6 mo. 1 yr.
Syringes				
B-D Ultrafine .3 cc .5 cc 1.0 cc short needle II-III normal needle	_____Boxes of 100	Use_____X/day	30 60 90	6 mo. 1 yr.
Other syringes	_____Boxes of 100	Use_____X/day	30 60 90	6 mo. 1 yr.
Needles for Pens				
B-D normal short II-III	_____Boxes of 100	Use_____X/day	30 60 90	6 mo. 1 yr.
Novo normal short II-III	_____Boxes of 100	Use_____X/day	30 60 90	6 mo. 1 yr.
Ketone test strip (foil wrap)	_____Box/50 ea	Use as directed	30 60 90	1 yr.
Glucagon Kit	_____Kits	Unconscious	30	1 yr.
Lancets ( )	_____Boxes of 100	Use X/day	30 60 90	6 mo. 1 yr.
Phenergan Supp. mg	pr q6h prn	#	30	1 yr.

Richard S. Mauseth, MD_____

this should be considered when choosing a laboratory. Also to be considered when choosing a laboratory is the volume of blood necessary for each test, handling of specimens, and turnaround time. The willingness of the company to resolve conflicts, such as when mistaken tests are ordered or the wrong test was performed, is important. Resolving billing issues for the patient should also be considered. All of these can be negotiated and you might find that companies are very willing to do so.

Performing stimulation testing in the office can be profitable. It requires good staff, well-organized procedure documentation, and some equipment. Intravenous (IV) equipment is relatively inexpensive. Oxygen and crash carts are necessary, but the necessity of other equipment depends on the test being done, proximity to medical backup, and abilities of the doctor and staff. IV hydration of diabetic patients at times is inconvenient for the doctor, but can also be profitable. Often insurance companies and HMO's will look at the pediatric endocrinologist who performs such services as being a cost savings to them and, therefore, will be more favorable in their reimbursement for not only this procedure but also other billings as well.

Credentialing and Privileges

Private practice pediatric endocrinologists have numerous ways to obtain CME credits. Regional pediatric endocrinology meetings are held annually. In the Seattle area, we have a monthly speaker at our local Children's Hospital. The Adult Endocrine Department has weekly seminars and a quarterly daylong "Endocrine Days" conference, which often has topics of interest to the pediatric endocrinologist. In addition, the National Growth Hormone postmarketing study groups supply updates and, if you are involved in their study, can have the study paid for by the group. The Lawson Wilkins Pediatric

Endocrine Society is a great place to keep up-to-date and also earn CME credits while being able to network with other physicians. I also try to attend either or both the ADA and Endocrine Society's national scientific meetings. These supply the most up-to-date research but also are more clinician oriented. Over the last several years, the American Association of Clinical Endocrinologists meetings has become more pediatric oriented and provide further opportunities for obtaining practice management information as well as clinical information.

I am on the active staff at my local hospital as well as at the local Children's Hospital. As a physician has fewer patients in the hospital, it is becoming harder for the credentialing bodies within these institutions to evaluate physicians performance. Therefore, it is beneficial for a physician to have some involvement with hospitalized patients. If this is not possible, there are methods for gaining credentialing.

BILLING

When establishing a private practice, the physician must be directly involved with the negotiations of the contracts with various insurance companies. Every three months, I sit down with my bookkeeper and we review our billing (number of visits for each code, number of tests, and the reimbursement for each from our major contractual companies). Often there are significant discrepancies between companies. When this happens, we will point this out to the company with the lesser reimbursement and inquire as to how we could bill differently to get the more appropriate reimbursement. In one instance, one company gave us a separate diabetes education code, which reimbursed significantly more than what we were charging. Two years later, they decided not to accept that code. We then had to renegotiate with them the code for that service, upon which they suggested a different method to bill for our services. It pays to be aggressive at getting reimbursement and not merely settle for what they will give you. Again, an aggressive billing person is your lifeblood.

One of the most important functions in a private office is billing appropriately and accurate documentation of your time. If you spend 1 hour and 15 minutes with a patient and you bill an hour for the visit, this bill will be coded as a prolonged visit with extenders. Each requires close documentation of time and decision making. Unless you can meet the criteria for each of the codes as well as the requirement for the extended coding time, the billing will be disallowed and they will downgrade your reimbursement. The amount of time spent with each patient should be noted in their chart. If a bill is contested, you may be requested to provide records as to how much time you had routinely scheduled with the patient. Therefore, the time should not be

exaggerated. Or, if any extenuating circumstances should arise, these should be clearly explained in your notes.

A 99215 code, which is oftentimes used as a follow-up visit charge, requires an interim history, evidence of complex decision making, evidence of review of systems, interim social history, dietary history, and a full physical exam. If the insurance company requests the patient's chart, the claim will oftentimes be rejected if the information denoting the extended service is not satisfactory. In my practice, I have developed a form for each visit, which mandates that I fill in each box (Table 2). The letter generated by the first part of this form is listed in Table 3, while the latter part satisfies the complexity of the billing code. This makes it more convenient and easy for me to remember to complete the forms. It also clearly shows to anyone auditing the visit that each of the criteria for that billing code is satisfied. This also helps in the defense of a bill, stating that you have done what is needed to satisfy a certain billing code and, therefore, deserve to be paid. Oftentimes the nurse checking the patient in can fulfill these forms. The forms can very easily be incorporated into an electronic medical record with a template for each of the major pediatric endocrine diseases. Templates would include Type I diabetes, Type II diabetes, congenital adrenal hyperplasia, polycystic ovarian syndrome, congenital hypothyroidism, thyroiditis, hyperthyroidism, growth disorders, growth hormone deficiency or insufficiency, Turner's syndrome, early puberty, early pubertal disorders (premature adrenarche, premature pubarche, and premature thelarche), precocious puberty, delayed maturation, hypogonadism, panhypopituitarism, and a blank general form that has no specific disease. Each would have general descriptions of the chief complaint, along with height, weight, stats from the physical, as well as a review of systems, social history, dietary history, and interim history—all of which are required for the 99215 coding. If each form is set up correctly, it can automatically provide a letter that can be customized to fulfill a narrative, but sound like a personal dictation. It would include all the information, but would not look like a standard form letter, therefore eliminating much of the need for dictation.

In our experience, coding for a 99214 is less likely to create chart notes requests and requires less documentation, but it also receives less reimbursement. A 99213 is the same code that a general pediatrics office uses for an ear infection. It requires very little documentation or past history. It is unlikely to be audited. Again, this has a lower reimbursement scale. The difference in billing a 99215 versus a 99214 is very important. A 99215 is usually quoted as a 30 to 40-minute visit, where a 99214 is coded as a 20 to 25-minute visit. The criteria of history taking, complexity of decision–making, and physical examination for each of the different billing codes are listed on Charts 1 to 4. The 99215 requires more extensive documentation, which can easily be taken care of by organized

Table 2 History and Physical Examination Form

Short Diabetes VISIT/MDI Date:

Dr. Name:

Pt. Name:

His / Her

A1C_____ / Down From _____ / _____ mo. Ago

Control: Excellent Good Fair Poor

Avg. Blood Sugar _____mg/ dl

Lantus_____Units at _____

Novolog/Humalog _____units/ _____carbs

_____units/ _____mg/dl

Drop _____Desired_____

_____Units/kg/day: Very High High Avg Low Very Low

lows/week: 0, 1, 2, 3, 4, 5, 6 Symptomatic at_____

Rec. of lows: All, Most, Less than half, Only part, None

Concern for lows: A Major Mod Slight No

Height_____cm Weight_____kg

Tanner Stage: I, II, III, IV, V

Recommendations:

a.

b.

c.

d.

PHYSICAL EXAM: B/P _____/ A.P._____

HEENT NI / Abn. _____

Eyes NI / Abn _____

Thyroid NI / Abn _____

Chest NI / Abn_____

Cardia NI / Abn_____

Abd NI / Abn_____

Skin NI / Abn_____

Exrem NI / Abn_____

Neuro NI / Abn_____

Pubic Hair I II III IV V

Breast

Genitalia I II III IV V

ROS_____

General NI / Abn_____

Respiratory NI / Abn_____

Cardiac NI / Abn_____

G.I. NI / Abn_____

Urinary NI / Abn_____

Neuro NI / Abn_____

Reproductive NI / Abn_____

Skin NI / Abn_____

Muscular NI / Abn_____

Social_____

Grade_____ Doing Well, Fair, Poor

Living with Parents, Mom_____ Dad _____

Friends Good, Bad_____

Living in house, Apt _____

Interim/Past Medical History _____

Family History

No Change_____ Divorced

_____

Health Parents ok_____ No change_____

Siblings ok, no change_____

Grandparents ok, no change _____

Comments _____

forms of EMR templates. If you bill for two patients per hour and you compare 99215 versus 99214, the collections, at least in our experience, are 42% more with the 99215, making it worth the increased effort to fulfill the documentation requirements.

Reimbursement for coding can often change and differs greatly from region to region and year to year. Several years ago, a 99244, which is a consultation code with the same documentation criteria as a 99205 (a new patient code), had higher reimbursement. The latter allowed resumption of care for the diagnosis code, whereas the former code had a limit of two visits. More recently, the 99205 has reimbursed better for not only the original visit but also for subsequent visits. This was about a $32 difference per visit. When multiplied by the number of visits per year (1500–3000 visits), a small increase becomes very significant. This is what has happened in my area and, although it may not be representative nationwide, shows the need to pay close attention to coding, reimbursement, and the change in reimbursement by each coding criteria over time.

It is often beneficial to organize your diagnoses according to billing codes. For example, a diagnosis of early puberty is for patients who are being followed for early puberty and is coded as such, whereas the code for precocious puberty is for a patient who is on treatment. This would allow you to retrieve all your patients by specific diagnosis and treatment codes if at some time you wanted to compare these, either for research or for your own knowledge. It also allows you to retrieve your diabetes patients according to coding. These records can be cross-referenced with their last visit to see how many patients are not coming in for routine visits, thereby allowing you to send them reminder notes to schedule an appointment.

An initial physician's visit, which often takes an extended period of time, needs accurate documentation. Making note of time in and time out is often useful. One of the techniques that works best for me in explaining the complexity of the discussion I have had with parents and family is to make sure that I have copies of all documents, particularly drawings I have made during the review of the original disease, different treatment options, pros and cons of treatment, risks, and other topics I have discussed with my patients and their families. In order to prove a prolonged visit of 45 minutes to two hours, a copy of the written documentation can be sent to the insurance company to illustrate the complexity and time spent with the patient. These visits almost always will require clinic notes to be attached. For a new onset diabetic patient who is being treated as an outpatient, we have created a checklist of things that are discussed at each visit. Either the diabetes educator, the nutritionist, or I will sign off on each one of the items that is supposed to be covered. This checklist documentation can be used at any time, to teach injection technique, institute insulin pump therapy, or address other common problems (see Table 4 for example of initial new onset diabetes outpatient education). These will again explain the complexity and necessary time spent on each one of these patients at each one of these visits.

Table 3   Letter Generated by Form Note January 30, 2006

Doctor _____

RE: _____ Birthdate ____/ ___/ ____

Dear:_____

I recently saw _____ for her/his diabetes. Her/His A1c was ____, up/down from _____ _____months ago. This represents excellent/very good/good/poor concerning diabetes control. Her/His average blood sugar was _____. She/He is on _____ units Lantus at __:__ AM/PM and a NovoLog/Humalog__ unit/10 carbs;__ unit/50 mg/dl drop. She/He has __ units in the a.m., __ with snack, __ with lunch, __ with dinner and __ at hs. This represents an insulin dose of _.__ units/kg/day, which is very high/high/average/low for her/his age, weight and stage of puberty.

She/He is having __ low blood sugars per week, with symptoms in the __'s in the AM/PM, and is recognizing these all/most/some/none of the time. These appear to represent a slight/moderate/great concern to the patient and family.

On physical examination her/his height is ____.__ cm, weight __.__ kg. and pubertal stage is Tanner ___. My recommendations are:

1.

2.

3.

Thank you very much for allowing me to see one of your patients. If you have any questions or concerns, please give me a call.

Sincerely,

Richard S. Mauseth, MD, FAAP, PS

RSM:lj

The reimbursement for nutritional visits and diabetes educator visits has improved. It can be done one of two ways: bill for the nutritionist or for the diabetes educator separately, or, incorporate each of these allied health professionals into a physician visit, which can then be coded at a higher level. In many cases, documentation can be done by the nutritionist or diabetes educator who would expand on it with written notes, followed by the physician's acknowledgment of reviewing the notes with the patient. This acknowledgment not only verifies direct patient–physician contact, but also allows the physician to review the visit, discuss future plans with the patient, and arrange for follow-up. If a billing code has been denied or reduced, a letter to the insurance company, or even a phone call to the medical director explaining the bill and explaining the time (even documentation retroactively) will often be successful in gaining a better reimbursement. If this is a persistent problem, either the documentation accompanying the original bill should be reconsidered, or a standard letter of explanation should be adopted to accompany a submitted bill. Oftentimes, the original denial of a claim is made by a nonmedical person looking at records he/she did not recognize as illustrating the complexity of decision-making, physician exam, or history.

Going to the medical director or to a supervisor who has some background will often be successful, as is aggressive follow-up on coding with the insurance company. There are some instances where the insurance company, after having several of these disputed claims, will suggest certain coding which, to

them, justifies your claim and increases your likelihood of receiving more appropriate reimbursement.

It is often worth knowing what each insurance company pays for each one of the billing codes, so you can know what to expect for reimbursement. This is important if you are in a partnership, and one partner is billing 99214s and receiving a higher percentage of reimbursement than another partner who is billing 99215s and receiving a lower percentage of reimbursement. This is particularly important if the distribution of income to each partner is based on total billing.

Often it is beneficial to meet with the medical director and staff of the insurance company, who will be reviewing your bill. This creates rapport and will eventually enable you and your staff to save time, not to mention receive better reimbursement. These do not need to be long talks, and can often occur outside of routine office hours, so you do not lose billable time. It is often best to have your billing person accompany you so that problems can be discussed directly with the staff at the insurance company. The Barbara Davis Center in Colorado has negotiated for bundled care for the first several months of new onset diabetes care with the insurance company, allowing the center to provide excellent, yet more flexible care of these patients while not having to admit them to the hospital. I am not sure of the specifics of how they have worked this out, but it serves as a good example of how someone with a good product can show the contractual payers that it is cost effective and works well.

Stimulation tests and tests in the office are often difficult to get reimbursed. The major factor to improve reimbursement is documentation and more

---

Chart 1   Type of Medical Decision-Making (2 of 3 Factors Must Apply)

Complexity of Medical Decision Making	Number of Possible Diagnoses/ Management Options	Amount and/or Complexity of Data Reviewed	Risk of Complication, Morbidity, or Mortality
Low Complexity	Limited	Limited	Low
Moderate Complexity	Multiple	Moderate	Moderate
High Complexity	Extensive	Extensive	High

Chart 2   Type of Examination

Expanded	An examination of the affected body area to organ system and other symptomatic or related organs
Detailed	An extended examination of the affected body area and other symptomatic or related organ systems
Comprehensive	A complete single system specialty examination or a complete multi-system examination

documentation. Often the drugs that are used for these tests are more expensive than the insurance will cover. One method of dealing with this is to have the patient pick up the drug at the pharmacy and bring it to the office for the test. Protocols must be firmly established, and it helps to have a flow sheet to document every step. The flow sheet should have all medicines given, all blood draw times and quantity, and tests to be run. It should include any IV starts, description of procedure, and discontinuation of procedure in order to establish length of IV therapy. Documentation of the physician's visits with the patient firmly establishes that the test is being done under the physician's supervision and that he or she is directly or indirectly observing the patient during the entire length of the test. This information should be readily available for billing as well as malpractice purposes.

Because of the continuous changing nature of reimbursements, physicians should frequently review them with their billing staff and think of creative ways to improve outcomes. At times, it is worth doing such things as a bone age or a glycosylated hemoglobin for very little reimbursement because it takes more time and effort to find the results and then to recontact the patient. One alternative to this is if the lab or X-ray facility is in proximity to the practice, have a diabetes patient come in and have glycosylated hemoglobin measurement an hour prior to the clinic visit at the external lab. An X ray, if requested from the previous physicians' note, can be done similarly if X-ray facilities are available nearby. Considerations include the close proximity and availability of facilities versus the time spent having to hunt them down. By reevaluating your billing and reimbursement, oftentimes you can decide what is your most efficient practice visit, and that may, to some extent, influence your scheduling of patients. It may be better

Chart 3   Type of History

Expanded	Chief complaint: brief history of present illness; problem persistent system review
Detailed	Chief complaint: extended history of present illness; extended system review; present, past, family, and/or social history
Comprehensive	Chief complaint: extended history of present illness; complete system review, complete past, family and/or social history

to see a patient two or three times in a row for a 99215 visit, rather than trying to do everything at one visit, requiring extended time. Some insurances reimburse fairly well for prolonged visits as long as good documentation of time and content is made. However, other insurances do not cover prolonged codes at all. Patient travel time and compliance must be taken into consideration when making this decision.

Successful billing/coding is an ever-changing phenomenon that requires time, vigilance, imagination, persistence, communication with other doctors, and reeducation of staff and doctor. It is different in various regions of the country and often differs from one insurance company to the next. Just when you think you have it figured out, it changes.

ELECTRONIC MEDICAL RECORDS

Record keeping by charts has been standard in the past, but with the institution of electronic medical records, a new practice has a great opportunity to set up their office with systems that will allow much better utilization of time and staff. Not only will a physician be able to access patients' records at home when returning a phone call, he or she will also be able to document that phone call. At some time in the future, these phone calls may be reimbursable, particularly when related to insulin adjustment. Not only can medical records be set up with templates that would allow documentation of clinic visits, they could also present the data for fulfillment of billing codes in a clear and easily readable manner to the reviewer.

The other issue of record keeping concerns space. Electronic medical records do not require a large amount of square footage in the office like file cabinets do, which can increase the cost of rent. They make retrieval of records and laboratory tests much easier.

This technology is still in its infancy and changes every few months. When determining what type of system to purchase for your practice, consideration must be given to its ability to be updated and serviced, as well as to whether or not it is compatible with the local hospital's system, the local lab's system, and any other outside entity with which your practice has a relationship.

OUTREACH CLINICS

Outreach clinics can be very helpful. Not only do they build your practice by getting you known by the doctors in the community, they can provide a service to local areas that are often underserved and create relationships with people in the communities that are long lasting. They can be used to enhance local education to the primary care doctors, their staff, and the community through lectures. They often provide a quiet, less-stressed environment that is devoid of

Chart 4 Outpatient Evaluation and Management Codes

	Key Components			Contributory Factor	
	Complexity of Medical Decision Making	Type of Examination Performed	Type of History Taken	Nature of Presenting Problem	Face to Face Minutes
New Patient Visit (All 3 Factors Must Apply)					
99203	Low	Detailed	Detailed	Moderate	30
99204	Moderate	Comprehensive	Comprehensive	Moderate to high	45
99205	High	Comprehensive	Comprehensive	Moderate to high	60
Established Patient Visit (2 of 3 Factors Must Apply)					
99213	Low	Expanded	Expanded	Low to Moderate	15
99214	Moderate	Detailed	Detailed	Moderate to High	20–25
99215	High	Comprehensive	Comprehensive	Moderate to High	30–40
Outpatient Consultation (All 3 Factors Must Apply)					
99243	Low	Detailed	Detailed	Moderate	40
99244	Moderate	Comprehensive	Comprehensive	Moderate to High	60
99245	High	Comprehensive	Comprehensive	Moderate to High	80

interruptions a physician in a primary office may experience. They can provide the opportunity for a physician to practice with low overhead: ie, the cost of being at an outreach clinic is often very low to non-existent, depending on the space that is utilized, and often local hospitals or clinics see the clinic as a benefit. However, Stark Laws have to be considered. These are laws designed to prevent a clinic or hospital from enticing physicians to provide services through their institution by providing the physician unduly cheap rent or services. Outreach clinics are ideal for a physician who is at a primary office only two to three days a week, because sharing their primary office with another physician would greatly reduce overhead costs. Of course, there is a downside of working at an outreach clinic. You must consider the need for travel, difficulties with follow-up, and difficulties with obtaining lab results. However, electronic record keeping makes this less of a problem. Maintaining the involvement of the patient's primary care doctor helps to cut down on your need for evening and weekend phone calls, as well as your involvement in medication refills.

PARTICIPATING IN RESEARCH

National studies such as the Diabetes Control and Complications Trial (DCCT) or the Diabetes Prevention Trial are among those in which a private pediatric endocrinologist can become involved, geographic distance notwithstanding. This not only keeps the physician at the cutting edge of research, but also allows great collaboration with our academic partners. The academic pediatric endocrinologists in general are always looking for patients for different kinds of research proposals, and having an open collegial relationship with academic physicians increases the likelihood of exposure to interesting and unusual patients. Attendance at national meetings such as the Lawson and Wilkins Pediatric Endocrine Society, the American Diabetes

Table 4 New Onset Outpatient Diabetes Education Checklist Initial Outpatient Management of New Onset Type 1 Diabetes: Institution of Insulin Therapy

Date	Initials	Topic
_____	_____	1. Understanding of why they are in clinic
_____	_____	2. Review signs and symptoms which have been occurring
_____	_____	3. Review differential diagnosis of hyperglycemia
_____	_____	4. Integrate these to establish why this is purely Type 1 D.M.
_____	_____	5. Review glucose metabolism (pancreas, islets, insulin, cells, ketones, polyuria, polydypsia)
_____	_____	6. Describe difference between Type 1 versus Type 2 diabetes (age onset, etiology, treatment)
_____	_____	7. Further discuss etiology of Type 1 (genetics, siblings, predisposition, viral, exposures, prevention trials, prior diet-sugar did not cause)
_____	_____	8. Discuss past and present treatment plans
_____	_____	9. Discuss how new treatment plans and improved control
_____	_____	10. Discuss outcomes of DCCT
_____	_____	11. Discuss complications and how they relate to present treatment
_____	_____	12. Discuss new onset management (hospital versus outpatient)
_____	_____	13. Physical examination, complex history
_____	_____	14. Review management of diabetes at present time and near future
_____	_____	15. Discuss diabetes education plan
_____	_____	16. Discuss psychological adjustments within family

Association, and/or the Endocrine Society, not only increases your knowledge of the specialty, but also allows you to network with pediatric endocrinologists around the country. The pharmaceutical-sponsored growth hormone registries offer meetings that provide education for the physician, nurses, and diabetes educators, as well as the ability to collaborate with nationally recognized basic science pediatric endocrinologists. These registries can provide income that can offset the cost of staff time to fill out growth hormone insurance forms, which take a great deal of time and expense. We are involved in four pharmaceutical company registries. We also collaborated on several diabetes studies (Search, Trigger, Trial Net, and, in the past, the DCCT and Diabetes Prevention Trial). I have been very involved with bone marrow transplant patients and am currently involved with several projects with the Fred Hutchison Cancer Research Center. Furthermore, we have requested and received several research grants. I believe that our low overhead helps counterbalance the financial disadvantage of not being in a university setting, as long as the project is within our capabilities.

FINAL CONSIDERATIONS

Private practice pediatric endocrinology has been a wonderful and rewarding experience. I have met many wonderful people, learned a lot, and have had very meaningful relationships with my patients, although at times I have felt isolated and desired to be able to discuss a case with university colleagues. As the practice has grown, the isolation decreased, but the trade-off is in the increased complexity of a larger group. Ultimately, diligence, hard work, and being responsive to the needs of those in your practice are a recipe for success.

REFERENCES

1. Annual Report of the American Board of Pediatrics to the Pediatric Endocrine Program Directors. American Board of Pediatrics; September 21, 2005: Lyon, France.
2. Rosenbloom AL et al. Characteristics of pediatric endocrinology practice: a work force study. Endocrinologist 1998; 8:213–218.

19

Clinical Research in Children

Phillip D. K. Lee

*Reproductive Medicine and Metabolism, Clinical Development, Serono, Inc.,
Rockland, Massachusetts, U.S.A.*

INTRODUCTION

Clinical research is the crucial process that provides justification for the translation of practical experience and related scientific knowledge into clinical practice standards. In recent decades, increased understanding of physiology and disease processes, improved technologies for diagnostic tools, and a wider range of potential treatment modalities has led to an increased need for credible clinical research. However, a lack of commensurate increases in clinical research funding and training coupled with increased regulation of clinical research activities, largely warranted in the interest of protecting human rights, has worked against fulfillment of this need. Nonetheless, there has been a near-exponential growth in citations related to clinical trials and randomized clinical trials over the past four decades, as shown in Figure 1.

Despite a long and colorful history of experimentation in children (1), modern clinical research specific to the pediatric age group is relatively lacking in quantity and quality (2,3). This may not seem particularly surprising because the detailed study of childhood physiology and the organized recognition of pediatrics as a practice specialty have occurred only within the past approximately 125 years, beginning in the United States with the creation of the American Medical Association (AMA) Section on Diseases of Children in 1880 and the American Pediatric Society in 1888 (4,5). Prior to and for many years following these events, the medical care of children was often considered an extension of the medical care of adults and many academic clinical services continue to include pediatrics as a subdivision of general medicine. In the United States, it was not until 1912 that a federal agency, the Children's Bureau, was established to represent and lobby for the interests of child health. In 1930, the American Academy of Pediatrics (AAP) was founded by several members of the AMA Section on Diseases of Children, partly in protest against the AMA opposition to the 1921 Congressional Maternity and Infants Act, "aka" the Sheppard-Towner Act, which had been supported by the Children's Bureau to reduce infant mortality rates by providing states with federal matching grants to improve health education and diagnosis.

Since the mid-1960s, the number of clinical research publications related to pediatrics has increased dramatically, with a particular upswing in the past 15 years (Fig. 1), perhaps due to focused attention by government regulatory agencies. However, as shown in Figure 2, the proportion of publications related to pediatric clinical trials or randomized clinical trials has decreased over the past four decades. Possible contributory factors include the relative emphasis on development of pharmaceutical agents for adults and, perhaps, the wider range of treatable disorders affecting the adult population. However, it is also evident that a large proportion of medications prescribed to children have not been specifically tested in this population and may lack appropriate safety and efficacy testing (6,7).

Coordinated, comprehensive, multicenter clinical research has been a standard in pediatric and adult oncology for five decades, and has led to major advances in cancer diagnosis and treatment (8). For example, the treatment of childhood leukemia has been revolutionized by this approach (9). A recent review of the National Institutes of Health (NIH) clinical trials database (www.clinicaltrials.gov) reveals that 25% of 12,000 current trials involve cancer research. In the United States and elsewhere, most children with cancer enroll in a clinical research study as part of their treatment protocol (10). Data is compiled into common databases (e.g., www.seer.cancer.gov), and analyzed for treatment safety, efficacy, and other clinical end points. A major exception is thyroid cancer, which is traditionally treated by pediatric and adult endocrinologists rather than oncologists and for which comprehensive multicenter natural history and treatment efficacy data are notably lacking. The usual barriers for recruitment of patients for clinical research, including allowance for third-party reimbursement of nonstandard, "unapproved" therapies, have evidently been overcome for pediatric and adult oncology, but not to the same degree for pediatric endocrinology.

Nonetheless, the subspecialty of pediatric endocrinology has played a leading and ongoing role in the development of pediatric clinical research. Early examples include clinical studies by Wilkins and coworkers beginning in the 1930s, which began to define

All Clinical Trials

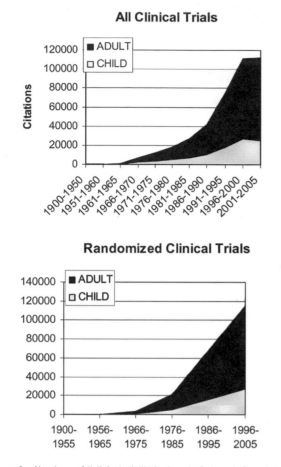

Randomized Clinical Trials

Figure 1 Numbers of "clinical trial" citations in Pubmed. Search limits: child, 0 to 18 years; adult, 19+ years.

Pediatric Clinical Research Citations
(% of Total Citations)

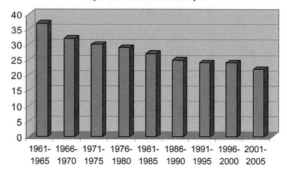

Pediatric RCT Citations
(% of Total Citations)

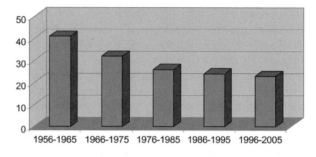

Figure 2 Ratio (×100) of pediatric to total clinical research and RCT citations in Pubmed. Search limits: pediatric, 0 to 18 years; adult 19+ years. *Abbreviation*: RCT, randomized controlled trial.

the etiology and treatment of congenital adrenal hyperplasia (11). Food and Drug Administration (FDA) labeling of recombinant-DNA–derived insulin and growth hormone (GH), in 1982 and 1985, respectively, were the first successful pharmaceutical applications of this technology (12). Pediatric endocrinology has also played an integral role in the establishment of postmarketing surveillance studies, as discussed in a later section. However, even for GH, a drug which was initially intended to specifically target a childhood disorder, the proportion of citations favors adult clinical research (Fig. 3).

The material presented in this chapter focuses primarily on pediatric clinical research in the United States, with an emphasis on pediatric endocrine research. Regulatory guidelines are similar, but not identical, in other industrialized countries. The field of pediatric clinical research is still in a formative period and information is somewhat inconstant. Therefore, only basic points and guidelines will be reviewed.

DEFINITIONS

Clinical research could refer to a wide range of scientific endeavor involving human or nonhuman

materials that indirectly or directly affect clinical care. However, broad definitions have limited utility in the formulation of public policy and funding priorities.

In 1997, the U.S. NIH Director's Panel on Clinical Research proposed a three-part consensus definition

Randomized Endocrine Trials

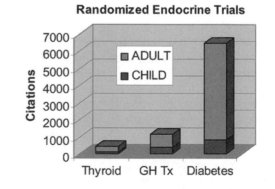

Figure 3 Numbers of randomized, controlled trials relating to thyroid-growth hormone and diabetes as cited in Pubmed. Search limits: child, 0–18 years; adult, 19 + years.

of clinical research "...particularly for tracking and monitoring funding activities," as follows (13):

1. Patient-oriented research. Research conducted with human subjects (or on material of human origin such as tissues, specimens, and cognitive phenomena) for which an investigator (or colleague) directly interacts with human subjects. This area of research includes the following:

   - Mechanisms of human disease
   - Therapeutic interventions
   - Clinical trials
   - Development of new technologies

2. Epidemiologic and behavioral studies
3. Outcomes research and health services research

Specifically excluded are studies using human tissues but for which the identity of the source is unknown and unnecessary.

In 2005, the Medical Research Council of the United Kingdom issued a similar definition (14): "...research defined as clinical should encompass at least one of the following categories:

1. Human participation: ...face-to-face contact with patients and/or healthy human participants...
2. Records based studies: ...require access to personal data on health or lifestyle without involving face-to-face contact, e.g., epidemiological studies, health economic studies, public health interventions, health services research and meta-analyses...
3. Clinical samples: ...involve laboratory studies on human material, which are specifically designed to understand or treat a diseases/disorder.
4. Technology development for clinical use..."

A clinical trial is defined by the U.S. NIH (http://grants2.nih.gov/grants) as "prospective biomedical or behavioral research study of human subjects that is designed to answer questions about biomedical or behavioral interventions...used to determine whether new...interventions are safe, efficacious and effective." In 2004, the International Committee of Medical Journal Editors (ICMJE) offered this definition of a clinical trial: "Any research project that prospectively assigns human subjects to intervention and comparison groups to study the cause-and-effect relationship between a medical intervention and health outcome" (15). For the purposes of trial registration (*vide infra*), this definition was further updated to require a control or comparison group(s) (16). In accordance with these guidelines, clinical "trial" in this chapter will refer specifically to clinical research that is concerned with testing therapeutic interventions.

PEDIATRIC CONSIDERATIONS

Pediatric clinical research usually refers to research involving human subjects within the pediatric age range, i.e., in utero to 21 years of age, as is specified in the NIH

Policy on Inclusion of Children (17) and a previous statement from the AAP (18). U.S. federal guidance further subdivides the pediatric population into age-related subgroups: (i) newborn or neonate: birth to one month, (ii) infant: greater than one month to two years, (iii) child: more than 2 to 12 years, (iv) more than 12 to 21 years (19). Clinical investigations in pediatric centers often involve subjects above the age of 21 and fetal/maternal studies, e.g., in relation to prenatal maternal care, genetics, and congenital disorders; arguably, some or these studies should also be classified as "pediatric."

On the other hand, the definition of pediatric research is sometimes limited to subjects younger than the legal age of consent. In a 1995 statement regarding conduct of drug research in children, the AAP defined children as "persons who have not attained the legal age for independent consent to treatments or procedures involved in research, under the applicable law of the jurisdictions in which the research is conducted" (20). This AAP definition is utilized in the U.S. Department of Health and Human Services (DHHS) Regulation 45 CFR Part 46, Subpart D, pertaining to protection of children involved as research subjects. The popular medical information search engine, PubMed (www.pubmed.gov) sets the "all child" search limit at 0 to 18 years old, and adult as 19+.

Justification for separate attention to the pediatric population may seem intuitive and scientifically obvious to pediatric specialists; but is not as well understood by others. The two major life tasks that distinguish the pediatric population from adults are physical growth and intellectual development. These tasks encompass a wide range of physiologic, mental, and behavioral processes that are not observed in adults. Because of these processes, there are special considerations in pediatrics related to definition of normal physiology, diagnostic criteria, drug pharmacokinetics, treatment effects, and adverse reactions. In relation to adverse effects, effects on body growth and intellectual development are particularly unique to the pediatric population.

Pediatric-specific clinical research can be subcategorized as follows:

1. Normal physiology: e.g., studies of infant development, normal growth patterns, normal hormone levels, physiologic reference ranges.
2. Diagnostic: delineation of abnormal and potentially treatable disturbances of growth and development, e.g. derivation of diagnostic criteria and validation of diagnostic testing.
3. Therapeutic (clinical trial): treatment efficacy and adverse effects.
4. Monitoring: ongoing clinical monitoring of individual patients or populations with a particular diagnosis and/or undergoing a specific treatment.
5. Outcomes: evaluation of therapeutic outcomes and cost-benefit.

Although the bulk of recent interest in pediatric clinical research is related to therapy and outcomes, there are substantial deficits in our understanding of basic physiology and definition of normal/abnormal boundaries. As an example, although there are multiple pediatric treatment indications for GH therapy and extensive therapeutic monitoring databases, there are continuing controversies over the appropriate assessment of the GH axis and the criteria used to define an abnormality of GH secretion (21).

Pediatric clinical research is most often conducted in those venues where groups of children and adolescents are usually located. Pediatric endocrinology clinical services historically evolved as academic practices; in the United States and many other countries, the majority of pediatric endocrinology patients are cared for in institutionally based or affiliated clinics rather than in solo private practice settings. Therefore, it is not surprising that the majority of clinical research in pediatric endocrinology originates from academic centers. In the United States, the quality of academic pediatric clinical research has been enhanced by the creation of government-supported, academic inpatient and outpatient clinical research facilities such as the U.S. Department of Agriculture (USDA)/Agricultural Research Service Children's Nutrition Research Center (www.kidsnutrition.org) and the NIH Clinical Research Centers (www.ncrr.hihi.gov/clinical/cr-gcrc.asp).

Clinical research in private practice and in non-medical settings, such as summer camp programs and schools, has become increasingly difficult due in part to regulatory requirements and costs. In addition, many childhood conditions are somewhat uncommon and the pediatric population tends to be mobile with respect to both geographic location and health-care provision, which creates difficulties with recruitment and longitudinal follow-up, respectively.

In 1986, the AAP established the Pediatric Research in Office Settings (PROS) (www.aap.org/pros), which currently includes approximately 2000 practitioners at more than 700 private practice sites (22). Although primarily concerned with topics related to general pediatrics, PROS conducted a landmark investigation on female pubertal development (23,24); a similar study regarding male puberty is currently in progress.

The U.S. National Children's Study, authorized by the Children's Health Act 2000 of the U.S. Congress, is expected to enroll 100,000 children beginning in 2007. Study subjects will be monitored from birth until 21 years, using a variety of physical and biochemical parameters, to analyze environmental influences on childhood health and development. This is a multi–hypothesis-driven effort, for which specific hypotheses have not been finalized at the time of this writing.

In 2005, the Lawson Wilkins Pediatric Endocrine Society (www.lwpes.org) established the pediatric endocrinology research network to facilitate recruitment of subjects. As of this writing, only one protocol is listed on this site. However, it is hoped that these and other efforts will facilitate future clinical research in pediatrics and pediatric endocrinology.

PROTOCOL DESIGN

In the early days of pediatrics, simple observational reports, frequently limited to only a few patients from a single clinic, were often adequate to provide new information and wider application of new therapies. For instance, early experimentation with insulin therapy in individual patients beginning in the 1920s led to the global therapeutic use of this hormone for children and young adults with Type I diabetes mellitus (25). Patients involved in this early research were clinically observed during treatment but not enrolled in a clinical trial as we might envision one today.

Over the past few decades, the body of medical knowledge, including new laboratory techniques, statistical methodologies, and therapeutic options has increased dramatically. Clinical research leading to new methods of diagnosis and/or therapy is now judged primarily on the basis of protocol design and statistical credibility. Therefore, it is incumbent upon each researcher and clinician conducting or making use of clinical research to be appropriately knowledgeable in these areas.

A full discussion of clinical research protocol design and statistical analysis is beyond the scope of this chapter, and only basic considerations will be mentioned. The reader is referred to a number of excellent publications for additional information (19,26–29). In addition, academic institutions, research organizations, and government agencies frequently hold seminars and courses on clinical research. Presented here is a selected list of components in clinical research protocol design.

Hypothesis

The study hypothesis should be formulated prior to designing a protocol and clearly stated in one or two sentences in a manner that is amenable to being tested using the proposed procedures. As a general rule, if the hypothesis cannot be concisely stated, then it probably cannot be concisely proven. Common misconceptions are that the answer to the hypothesis should be known prior to study or that it must always be proven correct. The hypothesis basically states a testable unknown; the possibility of proving the hypothesis incorrect should exist within the study design.

The terms "purpose" or "objectives" are sometimes used interchangeably with "hypothesis"; however, they are not necessarily equivalent. For instance, the stated purpose of a study might be "to determine whether GH therapy is beneficial in children with Noonan Syndrome." The testable hypothesis might then be stated as "one year of GH therapy given in standard doses will increase height velocity by +1 SD in prepubertal children with Noonan Syndrome."

Background and Significance

What work has been previously done to address the question(s) posed in the hypothesis? What new information will be obtained from the current protocol? Is the current work justified based on previous knowledge, or the lack of it? This portion of the protocol design provides the basis for investing in the effort. It should be carefully researched, focused, and logically presented, with attention to all sides of the topic to be investigated.

End Points

The end points for the study are the measured parameters that will be the focus of the data analysis. As such, the end points should be closely tied to the hypothesis. For instance, in a study with a hypothesis that GH therapy will increase height by $+1SD$ in Noonan syndrome, the primary end point measure would be height. All other aspects of the study design should focus on optimizing assessment of the primary end point measure(s). Secondary end points (e.g., weight, educational outcomes, and psychosocial adjustment in the example given) can also be defined, but do not provide the primary focus for the study design and data analyses.

General Design Elements

Retrospective or Prospective Design

A retrospective study examines previously collected data, usually recorded for reasons unrelated to the current hypothesis and without forethought regarding systematic analysis. In a prospective study, the purpose for the data collection and the methodology is defined prior to commencing the study, with specific attention given to eventual systematic analysis against the hypothesis and end points. In general, prospective study design is preferable whenever feasible, because the elements of the data collection relevant to later analysis can be predetermined and applied.

Systematic collection of data alone does not define data as being prospective. For instance, a pediatric endocrinologist has over many years examined all GH treated patients every three months. After 10 years, the data for patients with Noonan syndrome are analyzed. Although the data collection was systematic and reliable, the purpose of the collection, enrollment criteria, and plans for analysis were not defined "a priori." Therefore, the data would be considered retrospective.

Randomized, Controlled Design

Randomized, controlled study design is considered to be the "sine qua non" of clinical research, and is particularly valued in relation to clinical trials, i.e., clinical research relating to therapeutic efficacy. However, this study design can be problematic for pediatric clinical research.

For many pediatric therapeutic trials, the ethics of including a no-treatment or placebo arm is questionable because there may be preceding efficacy data in adult populations and/or off-label pediatric

experience. Typical pediatric endocrine study end points, such as height and pubertal development, are unlikely to be subject to a placebo effect in a nutritionally healthy population. In addition, because some childhood disorders have a time-limited window for effective treatment, prolonged assignment to no-treatment could be detrimental. For instance, randomized, controlled study of GH treatment of GH deficiency to final height could be problematic for the untreated group. In some cases, the use of a placebo group can be avoided by randomization to different treatment levels, without inclusion of a no-treatment arm. A placebo-controlled trial of zidovudine treatment of HIV-infected pregnant women and similar studies have raised ethical questions regarding the relative rights of the individual patient as opposed to the value to society of a well-designed study (30,31).

Another important consideration is that many childhood disorders are relatively uncommon. Therefore, accumulating sufficient numbers of subjects for a randomized, controlled or a concurrent nonrandomized control group study is often not feasible. In these situations, comparison to well-characterized historical controls or predefined reference ranges may be sufficient. For instance, studies of GH effects in uncommon genetic conditions rely on comparisons to growth charts derived from the unaffected population and/or an affected, untreated population (32).

Regardless of the method chosen, all clinical studies involving definition of diagnostic criteria or treatment effect must have an appropriate comparison population. More complete discussions of ethical and statistical considerations related to randomization and selection of appropriate control groups are available, including a useful 2001 Guidance for Industry from the U.S. FDA (33). Recommendations for reporting of randomized control trial data, generated by the international Consolidated Standards of Reporting Trial (CONSORT) group and adopted by several major journals, are regularly updated online (www.consort-group.org) and can provide useful guidance for planning a simple randomized, controlled trial (34–36).

An important consideration for all clinical trials is whether provisions are needed for interval analysis and possible trial termination. Particularly in the case of randomized, controlled trials, if significant treatment effects or adverse events, either for individual subjects or for the group(s), are identified during the study course, early termination or redirection of the trial may be ethically and/or legally necessary. However, implementation of an interval-analysis process can be problematic, especially for blinded trials, where special procedures may be required to break the code. In addition, premature termination of a trial can lead to inappropriate analyses and conclusions. For instance, early termination for a positive treatment effect could cause the investigators to miss a serious adverse effect occurring later in the course of treatment. Decisions about whether to provide for and implement interval analysis and early termination should be carefully considered on the basis of ethical boundaries to protect both the patient from harm and the society from erroneous data and conclusions regarding a therapy. Whenever possible, the conditions and procedures for interval data analysis and trial termination should be included in the planning of the study protocol.

Sites and Personnel

Due to the uncommon nature and complexity of many pediatric conditions, multisite, multinational, and multidisciplinary collaborations are often the best options for obtaining adequate numbers of study subjects. However, in the case of multiple sites, the protocol design may need to take into account geographic, regulatory/legal, ethnic, and cultural differences that could impact on the study end point(s). For example, a multinational study of the incidence of precocious puberty in girls may need to consider known ethnic and regional differences in "normal" pubertal onset.

In studies involving multiple researchers at one or more sites, the role of each individual and eventual data access, presentation, and authorship rights should be decided prior to commencing the study.

Sample Size Calculation

An integral part of planning a study protocol is an a priori assessment of the study sample size requirement (37). Selection of an inappropriate target sample size can severely limit the data analysis and decrease the value of the study in proving or disproving the hypothesis.

For a simple parallel design, randomized controlled trial, this calculation can be easily made using a number of commercial statistical software programs or online resources. In a power analysis or power calculation, the investigator specifies the expected effect size and required Type I and II errors; the required sample size is then calculated. In some cases, the investigator may choose to approach this in the opposite direction, calculating the statistical power of an effect at different levels of sample size.

Data Handling and Adverse Events

The methods for data collection and tabulation should be decided before commencing a clinical research project, based on the selected end points and projected analytical methods. Without this preplanning, a project may end up collecting data that is difficult or impossible to analyze. Preconsultation with an experienced statistician can lead to immense downstream savings of time and effort (38). In addition to the collection of data related to the study hypothesis and end points, rigorous attention should be paid to monitoring of adverse events.

In the United States, all clinical trials (research related to assessment of therapeutic efficacy) require an Institutional Review Board (IRB)-approved data and safety monitoring plan (or board, in the case of multisite studies) to insure data integrity and the safety of study participants. All adverse events should be recorded and scored according to the likelihood of being related to the study intervention or procedures. A similar process should be considered for other types of clinical research that involves human contact. Detailed recommendations for reporting of safety data from randomized clinical trials have been recently published by the international CONSORT group (39).

Protection of Human Subjects

Early clinical practice and research in the Western world was guided primarily by the Hippocratic Oath, on which a physician swears to act in the best interests of the patient. In 1938, the United States took a first step toward formalizing this protection by instituting the FDA, requiring demonstration of drug safety prior to marketing. An international recommendation for informed consent and risk-benefit considerations for clinical research resulted from the Nuremberg Code of 1947. However, the first U.S. law requiring informed consent for clinical research was not passed until 1962, followed by adoption of international clinical research guidelines, the Helsinki Declaration, in 1964. The IRB system was mandated by the U.S. Surgeon General in 1966, with further strengthening of associated regulations over the subsequent years. In 1983, special protections for children involved in clinical research were adopted under Health and Human Services regulation 45 CFR 46 Part D.

Currently, all clinical research studies in the industrialized world are required to be preapproved by an appropriate IRB, with reapprovals as mandated by the IRB. A statement of IRB approval and supervision, with appropriate consent procedures, is required by all legitimate scientific journals.

While human rights protection and informed consent procedures are essential, application to pediatric clinical research has been the subject of considerable ethical and legal debate (40–42). It is generally accepted that prior to the legally defined age of majority, the parent(s) or legally designated guardian(s) serve a surrogate role for the child in approving participation in clinical research. In the United States, the federally defined age of majority, 18 years, is generally accepted, but this can be complicated by regional differences in the definition of an emancipated minor, e.g., a teenager who is legally considered an adult by virtue of motherhood and/or marriage. Furthermore, the types of research that can be consented to on behalf of a child have been called into question. In one case, a Maryland court ruled that parents may not give consent to nontherapeutic research on behalf of their child if there is risk involved (43). Other studies have shown that parents have relatively poor understanding of research procedures described during the consent process, relying heavily on physician input and perceived individual benefit to their child for their decision (40,44,45).

The requirement for a surrogate consent process coupled with the facts that (i) research subjects cannot be completely protected from risk and (ii) new, beneficial treatments for children cannot be definitely proven without research in children have led to considerable ethical debate over the process by which children become involved in clinical research.

Although children are not legally able to give consent, IRBs require adherence to the U.S. federal guidance that older children be informed and give assent as part of the consent process (46). However, the legal validity of assent procedures is relatively untested and it is apparent that children often have little understanding of what they are assenting to. Many pediatric study subjects probably base their decision largely on the opinions of their parent(s)/guardian(s) and the clinical researcher and, in some cases, based on their perceptions of the procedures involved such as fear of phlebotomy (47) or other study procedures. In some cases, financial or other incentives may provide motivation for child (or parent approval for) participation, raising ethical questions about the consent process (48).

In addition, there is the question of parental consent given on behalf of infants, young children, or handicapped children who may not be able to adequately comprehend the procedures involved. This becomes particularly problematic for dependent handicapped children over the age of 18. In many cases involving these "adult children," guardianship has not been legally extended and the consent process could be questioned.

These and other concerns have contributed to ongoing discussion and debate regarding legal and ethical protection of children's rights in clinical research (49). For all clinical trials, the appropriate and acceptable risk to benefit must be addressed. Interpretation of federal guidelines has led to a requirement of grading of risk for potential harm or discomfort, e.g., "minimal risk" and "minor increase over minimal risk," with both IRB and DHHS approval needed for higher-risk research (20,50). These and similar terms should be carefully explained to the parent and child, if feasible, during the consent process using comparisons to daily life situations or familiar medical procedures.

It is imperative that pediatric clinical researchers participate in the process and be aware of changes in regulatory, ethical, and legal guidance (19,20). Starting in 2000, the NIH has required that all U.S. clinical investigators complete a course in protection of human research participants (51). In addition, many IRBs require investigator certification in patient/subject confidentiality and privacy protection, and ethics courses are required by some IRBs and state medical licensing boards.

SPECIAL CONSIDERATIONS

Reference Ranges and Diagnostic Testing

The pediatric age range is unique in the large age- and sex-related variability in normal biological and physiological parameters. Failure to compare individual biological measures against normal age- and sex-related variability can lead to major errors in diagnosis and treatment. For instance, normal children can be expected to have an abnormally low T-score for bone mineral density (BMD), consistent with the definition for osteoporosis, before mid-puberty (52). Similar problems are encountered for hormone levels. This author has seen many patients referred inappropriately based on comparison of pediatric patient results to adult reference ranges for BMD, testosterone and gonadotropins, and other measures. Even in the relatively well-established area of thyroid testing, it is not clear whether controversies over low TSH levels apply to pediatric populations. Moreover, the higher upper-normal variability for pediatric thyroid hormone levels, coupled with inclusion of thyroid hormone tests on routine panels, has led to many inappropriate referrals for hyperthyroidism.

The need for pediatric reference intervals for biochemical testing has been admirably addressed by several standard texts; a particularly useful, regularly updated text is published by the American Association for Clinical Chemistry (AACC) (53). However, there is general acknowledgment that the methodologies for derivation of reference ranges and, specifically, pediatric ranges are not always well defined, and published ranges for a particular analyte may not be applicable for different assay methods, laboratories, or populations.

Key problems in establishing reference ranges are the selection of an appropriate "normal" reference population and the numbers of subjects needed to establish the age- and sex-related ranges. For instance, in establishing reference ranges for insulin-like growth factor-I (IGF-I), does one select only those healthy subjects with "normal" heights, as has been done in some studies (54), or should the reference population be selected from the general healthy population regardless of height? Because IGF-I levels show a general correlation with height, inclusion of shorter individuals, even if otherwise healthy, may tend to blur the distinction between GHD and normal populations. Some biochemical parameters, such as IGF-I and testosterone, change dramatically during puberty; should the reference ranges be corrected for age or for pubertal stage?

After selecting the reference population, the numbers of samples needed and the distribution by age and sex need to be determined. However, for analytes where the natural variability is wide, it is often impossible to know whether an adequate number has been selected. As quoted in a recent article, one expert has estimated that a typical pediatric reference range may require, on average, 1200 to 1400 samples (55), representing a considerable cost in time and effort.

Analysis of reference range data can also be complex (56). A common manipulation in pediatrics is to use standard deviations or conversion of values to standard deviation, or z-scores. These conversions require that the data be normally distributed about the mean at any given age. This criterion is often not met by endocrine measures, necessitating the use of log-normalization or other adjustments.

Closely linked to the reference range discussion is the topic of diagnostic accuracy of a test; i.e., "the ability of a test to identify a condition of interest." An initial international effort to address deficiencies in reporting of tests of diagnostic accuracy is the Standards for Reporting of Diagnostic Accuracy (STARD) Statement (57,58). As stated by the STARD group: "Exaggerated results from poorly designed studies can trigger premature adoption of diagnostic tests and can mislead physicians to incorrect decisions about the care for individual patients" (57).

A full discussion of the controversies surrounding reference ranges and diagnostic testing for biochemical and physical parameters is beyond the scope of this chapter, and is more fully discussed in other publications (53,59). It is incumbent upon pediatric clinical researchers to be cognizant of developments in these fields and to properly apply accepted analytical methods whenever feasible. Furthermore, it is important for researchers to educate laboratory directors and practicing physicians regarding the limitations of pediatric reference ranges for biochemical and physical parameters, and the need to include basic knowledge and clinical judgment before applying test results to individual patients.

Clinical Trials

As mentioned above, clinical trials are defined by the U.S. FDA as a category of clinical research concerned with determining the efficacy, safety, and effectiveness of therapeutic interventions. A clinical trial is the typical mechanism required for regulatory approval of new pharmaceuticals and medical treatment devices. The need for premarket safety, efficacy testing, and federal regulation of clinical trials in the United States was recognized following the disastrous marketing of liquid elixir sulfanilamide in 1937, in which more than 100 patients died from ingestion of the diethylene glycol diluent (60). In 1938, the U.S. Food, Drug and Cosmetic Act essentially established the role of the FDA as a regulatory body.

Until the mid-1970s, clinical trials specific to pediatrics were scarce (2). In 1968, this situation prompted Shirkey to describe children as "therapeutic or pharmaceutical orphans" (61). In 1977, the AAP formed a Committee on Drugs, which subsequently addressed the lack of pediatric drug labeling (20). In 1985, human GH became the first recombinant-DNA–derived medication marketed solely for pediatric use. However, it was not until the FDA Modernization Act (FDAMA) in 1997 that a requirement for pediatric labeling was considered at the federal level in the U.S. after the failure of several voluntary programs. FDAMA provided an incentive to manufacturers of six months market exclusivity in

return for studies resulting in pediatric labeling. In 1998, this was extended to require pediatric studies for certain drugs. The FDAMA exclusivity provision expired in January 2002 and was essentially replaced by the Best Pharmaceuticals for Children Act, which further required that the NIH and FDA collaborate in efforts to perform necessary pediatric studies not initiated by industry. In 2003, the Pediatric Research Equity Act (PREA) formalized a requirement for pediatric studies of certain drugs retroactive to 1999, including new drugs and previously approved drugs with new dose form(s), regimen(s), administration, and ingredient(s) (62). In addition, PREA included a mandate for pediatric expertise on advisory panels when appropriate (63). As a result of these government initiatives, the numbers of drugs obtaining pediatric labeling have increased dramatically.

A similar process mandating pediatric clinical drug trials was initiated by the European Commission in 1997, but implementation has been somewhat more gradual than in the United States. In 2005, the European Parliament voted to adopt a panel recommendation to extend manufacturers patent protection for six months in return for investment in pediatric clinical drug trials (64,65).

A full FDA clinical trial is usually preceded by laboratory research and preclinical animal testing. The subsequent trial is divided into phases as follows (www.fda.gov/edu/):

1. Phase 1: Initial testing, usually conducted in a small group of healthy people (e.g., 20–80), although patients may also be involved. The purpose of this phase is to evaluate safety, including safe dosage and side effects. Drug pharmacokinetics and metabolism are also studied.
2. Phase 2: Controlled study in a group of patients with the relevant target condition. This phase typically involves several hundred subjects and is intended to further define efficacy, as well as common short-term risks and adverse effects.
3. Phase 3: Controlled studies in a larger group (100s–1000s) to evaluate efficacy in comparison to other interventions, to monitor for adverse effects, and to collect additional safety data.

All phases are closely monitored, with regular interactions between the sponsor, usually but not always a manufacturer, and the Center for Drug Evaluation and Research (CDER), a branch of the FDA, which regulates clinical trials. At any stage, the CDER can place a hold on a trial based on safety or efficacy concerns.

Phase 1 studies are preceded by sponsor submission and FDA consideration and approval of an investigational new drug (IND) application. At the end of Phase 3, a new drug or device application (NDA) is submitted by the sponsor to the FDA. An Advisory Committee is convened by the FDA to review the application and recommend approval or denial of the application to market the product. Final decision, however, rests with the FDA. For pediatric research, clinical trial, product labeling, and other issues, the FDA is mandated to seek the advice of pediatric consultants. To satisfy this latter goal, a 13-member pediatric advisory committee has been chartered by the FDA (66). In some cases, the approval process may be followed by a required or voluntary postmarketing surveillance study, sometimes called a Phase 4 study, as described below.

In addition to this standard drug development process, the FDA currently provides three alternative tracks, which allow the use of a new drug.

1. The Treatment IND program, established in 1987, makes investigational drugs available to a seriously ill patient if there is no comparable alternative therapy and the patient does not qualify for an ongoing clinical trial. Investigational drugs must usually be in Phase 3 trials before being considered for use in a Treatment IND. Treatment IND applications are usually submitted by the pharmaceutical manufacturer upon consideration and approval of a request from the patient's physician. If approved by the FDA, the drug is then distributed to the physician for subsequent administration to the patient. Treatment INDs are carefully monitored and the data is added to the collective experience with the drug.
2. The parallel track program, established in 1990, allows access of investigational drugs to individuals with HIV-related disorders who do not qualify for participation in the clinical trial process. Requests to participate in a parallel track treatment program can be initiated by the patient. Parallel track drug use is monitored and added to the collective experience with the drug.
3. Accelerated approval (accelerated development and review): In 1992, the FDA established a process for rapid approval of new drugs to treat serious, life-threatening conditions. This process essentially eliminates the need to follow the three-phase process. The sponsor must show that the drug provides benefit over currently available therapy and that a surrogate end point (e.g., a laboratory or radiological marker) reasonably predicts clinical benefit. In addition, accelerated approval requires a subsequent postmarketing study commitment.

Of special interest to pediatric clinical researchers is the Orphan Drug Act of 1983, which supports the development and approval of medications to treat rare diseases (www.fda.gov/orphan/). Included is the Humanitarian Use Device Program, established in 1996, to encourage development of treatment devices and diagnostic products for use in rare disorders. Prior to the Orphan Drug Act, rare disorders were often ignored by drug development companies, which is not surprising given the limited market potential. Incentives to manufacturers include tax benefits, marketing exclusivity, eligibility for grants (through the Orphan Products Grant program), and flexibility regarding the approval process. Although drugs in the Orphan Drug Development program are still required to go through the FDA approval process, many qualify for accelerated approval, while others may have a limited data collection requirement due to the rarity of the condition. As of this writing, approximately 200 drugs and products have been marketed through the Orphan Products Development Program.

Postmarketing Safety and Efficacy Studies

Treatment-monitoring studies are an integral element of modern medical research. However, it is only within the past two decades that such studies have become accepted as part of the new drug approval process, and pediatric endocrinology has played a key role in this process.

In the U.S., human cadaver-donor–derived human GH was distributed "gratis" to patients (via their physician) beginning in the 1960s, by a government agency, the National Hormone and Pituitary Program (67). Similar programs were subsequently established in other countries. Commercial marketing of a similar preparation began in the 1970s. Supplies were limited and sporadic, and comprehensive monitoring of safety and efficacy was not routine. In 1985, following a report of Creutzfeldt disease in a patient previously treated with cadaver-derived pituitary GH (68), biosynthetic GH was quickly moved through the FDA approval process, prior to completion of the usual safety and efficacy trials. A unique system for comprehensive postmarketing surveillance was established by agreement between the GH manufacturers and the FDA, due in large part to continuing concerns that GH itself rather than the then-mysterious "slow virus" may have contributed to the cases of Creutzfeldt disease. Several dozen additional cases of this condition in patients treated with pituitary GH have been identified (69), many with symptomatic onset prior to the 1985 case, further emphasizing the unfortunate lack of systematic monitoring for adverse events. In 1987, Genentech Inc. established the National Cooperative Growth Study in the United States and Kabi Pharmaceuticals (now Pfizer) established the Kabi International Growth Database. Although the original regulatory mandates for GH surveillance studies have long since expired, manufacturers have continued these efforts, collecting valuable information regarding the safety and efficacy of GH therapy (70).

A formal process for postmarketing surveillance studies, or Phase 4 commitments, was established by the FDA in 2000 (71,72). Phase 4 commitments are mandated for any drug approved through the accelerated approval program and may be required under the PREA. As of October 31, 2005, 155 Phase 4 commitments are listed as being required under the PREA.

In the United States, drug safety and medication errors have been monitored by The Office of Drug Safety within the CDER branch of the FDA. In 2005, a separate Drug Safety Oversight Board was established (73), and a new program was established by the FDA to facilitate reporting of drug safety information to consumers. In addition, as part of the adverse event reporting system established in 1969, the FDA maintains a medical product safety information program (MedWatch; www.fda.gov/medwatch/) with avenues for voluntary and mandatory reporting of adverse events for consumers, physicians, and industry. However, especially for medical products which do not have a mandated postmarketing reporting requirement, underreporting and other issues remain problematic (74).

Outcomes Research

Health outcome, an essential element in evidence-based medical practice, is a relatively new area of pediatric clinical research. Such research includes assessment of clinical benefits of therapeutic interventions (e.g., the Diabetes Control and Complications Trial), cost benefit studies (e.g., for newborn screening and managed care programs), and systematic reviews of health-care done, such as those performed by the Cochrane Collaboration (75). In the future, it is likely that for better or worse, health outcomes research will become a primary guide for reimbursement for clinical care services.

Medical Device Trials

Many nonindustry clinical researchers may not be aware that clinical trials are required for a host of non-pharmaceutical medical devices. In the United States, medical device regulation is handled by the FDA Center for Devices and Radiological Health (CDRH). In vitro diagnostic devices, such as laboratory reagents and assays, are the responsibility of The Office of In Vitro Diagnostic Device Evaluation and Safety within the CDRH. A variety of programs are applicable to medical devices. Although some devices are waived and can be marketed without a formal approval process, others need to show substantial equivalence to a predicate device (510 K application) or may require a more extensive process, a premarket approval application (PMA), which is similar to the new drug application (NDA) for pharmaceutical products. Diagnostic or treatment devices intended for rare conditions may qualify under the humanitarian use device exemption, while an investigational device exemption may be applicable if a device is used clinically during collection of data to support a PMA. Similar to the Phase 4 commitments for drugs, device manufacturers may be required to conduct ongoing postmarketing surveillance studies. Devices that have no known or accepted use in human clinical diagnosis or treatment may be marketed under a research use only designation.

The process of performing laboratory testing is regulated by the Clinical Laboratory Improvements Amendments (CLIAs), first implemented in 1988. Tests, which are simple, accurate, and not substantially subject to user error may be CLIA-waived, as are many tests performed in physician offices and in home testing.

Medical device regulations are designed to protect the public against faulty or ineffective diagnostic procedures and device-dependent therapies and, as such usually require submission of data in humans. Clinical research needed to satisfy CDRH, CLIA, and other regulatory guidelines is usually handled by the device manufacturer. However, nonindustry clinical researchers may participate directly or indirectly in this process. At the stage of regulatory review, CDRH is required to include pediatric advisors when appropriate (76). Further information on device regulation in the United States may be found on the CDRH website (www.fda.gov/edits/). Similar guidelines are in place for the European Union (www.europa.eu.int) and most industrialized countries.

Registration

In 2004, the ICMJE issued an update to the Uniform Requirements for Manuscripts Submitted to Medical Journals standardizing reporting of clinical trial data and requiring that all clinical trials considered for publication be fully registered on a searchable public database (18). Such registration had been federally mandated by section 113 of the FDAMA of 1997, leading to establishment of the FDA-sponsored Protocol Registration System (PRS). The process and requirements for trial registration are detailed and regularly updated on the PRS (10) and ICMJE (www.icmje.org) websites. In addition, the World Health Organization in May 2005 initiated a process to establish international standards for clinical trials registration and reporting (www.who.int).

Registration is required for trials that are "clinically-directive," i.e., intended to test a hypothesis regarding the relationship between an intervention and health outcome. The study design must include a concurrent, prospective control or comparison group. For new drug trials, this would be equivalent to an FDA Phase 3 trial. Investigators conducting or planning to conduct clinical trials should consult recent updated information on trial registration as part of the protocol planning process.

Funding and Conflicts of Interest

In the United States, funding for clinical research originates from multiple sources, with the largest contribution coming from government agencies (NIH, USDA, and NSF). However, the majority of funding for clinical drug trials comes from pharmaceutical companies, as might be expected. Clinical research is also supported by private foundations, including innovative programs such as The Glaser Pediatric Research Network (www.gprn.org). Links between public and private interests are evidenced by the proliferation of science and biotechnology parks and incubators, encouraging marketable and clinically beneficial research.

As most physicians are aware, the close links between the interests of patients, the public, researchers/physicians, and commercial entities can create potential and actual conflicts of interest. In the best of worlds, all clinical research would be conducted only in the interests of the patient and public. However, in the real world, financial support and future financial gain are major factors contributing to the purpose and goals of conducting clinical research and, in particular, clinical trials. Many clinical researchers hold investments in or receive research or consultancy funds directly from industry (77). In addition, financial reimbursement and/or incentives may be offered to enhance recruitment of subjects for clinical trials (78). Nonfinancial personal interests, such as academic reputation and promotion, are often involved for all types of clinical research (79). To address concerns that these external interests might compromise the integrity of clinical research, regulatory restrictions and guidance have been imposed at multiple levels, including pharmaceutical company self-regulation, governmental regulations, and institutional restrictions, with variable levels of agreement between regulatory bodies (80). Investigator disclosure of financial support and interests is now considered routine for scientific publication and presentation.

In some cases, it can appear that the regulations to prevent external influence on conduct of research may be inhibiting the exercise of academic and personal freedoms on the part of the investigator(s) despite their beneficial intent (81). For instance, publication requirements for industry-sponsored research recently implemented by JAMA were deemed "unfair" and "absurd" in an editorial in BMJ (82). Similar arguments have been made against restrictions placed on intramural NIH investigators limiting interactions with both industry and academia (83).

The ethical conduct of clinical research is a constantly evolving area in which we are likely to see further standardization of regulations. Input from experienced clinical researchers in industry, universities, and other settings will be needed to make certain that a balance is reached between regulatory requirements and necessary progress in clinical science.

Training

Given the rapidly growing need for credible clinical research and the increasing emphasis on evidence-based medical practice, one might assume that physician training in clinical research would be a highly structured training requirement. In 1997, the NIH Director's panel on clinical research made four specific recommendations for improvement of clinical research training and support (13). Current programs administered by the NIH to encourage clinical scientist training include the intramural NIH clinical research training program for individuals, the extramural Mentored Clinical Scientists Development Program Award (K-12 Award) to institutions, and both intramural and extramural loan repayment programs for clinical scientists.

However, as of this writing, specific standards for such training are limited, particularly for those medical programs and trainees not supported by one of the NIH clinical scientist initiatives. In the United States, training programs in pediatrics and pediatric subspecialties are regulated by the Accreditation Council for Graduate Medical Education (ACGME) (www.acgme.org). Clinical research training is not specified in the current ACGME pediatric program requirements (updated 7/2003), nor is it detailed in the pediatric endocrinology program requirements (7/2000).

The American Board of Pediatric (www.abp.org), which is responsible for post-training certification, specifies in the general Eligibility Criteria Certification in the Pediatric Subspecialties (11/2005) that for those starting their training before 7/1/2004: "Subspecialty residents must be instructed in the scientific and ethical bases of clinical research, including study design, modeling and methodology, statistical concepts, and data collection and analysis. The institution must provide the support necessary for a subspecialty resident to participate in such scholarly activities."

In addition, the criteria specify that such training in clinical research must start in year one and continue for the duration of training.

Surprisingly, the requirement for clinical research training appears to be less stringently detailed for those beginning their training after 7/1/2004, for whom the above criteria are substituted by the following: "In addition to participating in a core curriculum in scholarly activities, all fellows will be expected to engage in projects in which they develop hypotheses or in projects of substantive scholarly exploration and analysis that require critical thinking. Areas in which scholarly activity may be pursued include but are not limited to basic, clinical, or translational biomedicine; health services; quality improvement; bioethics; education; and public policy."

In the opinion of this author, the lack of required clinical research training for physicians is a serious oversight that will hopefully be addressed within the near future. As perhaps a first step in that direction, the American Association of Clinical Endocrinologists White Paper on Endocrine Clinical Research (84) commits the AACE to "educate the practicing endocrinologist on clinical research" and "bring a clinical research curriculum to endocrinology training programs."

CLINICAL RESEARCH AND EVIDENCE-BASED MEDICINE

A goal of modern medicine is the development of evidence-based clinical practice standards and guidelines. While knowledgeable physician judgment should take precedence in caring for individual patients, a recommended approach to a particular problem, evidenced by credible research, can provide considerable benefit. Examples of such guidelines are those generated by expert panels on behalf of the American Diabetes Association (www.diabetes.org) and the American Association of Clinical Endocrinologist (www.aace.com). In addition, schemes for analyzing evidence for clinical recommendations have been described (85,86).

Despite these goals and efforts, it is readily apparent that subspecialty care is still largely guided by anecdotal experience and opinion (87,88). For instance, clinical trials have clearly shown that GH improves height velocity for a variety of conditions; however, evidence for improvement in final adult height, psychosocial benefit, and favorable cost-benefit is less clear. Even for a more traditional condition, adrenal insufficiency, there is ongoing controversy over appropriate evidence-based diagnosis and therapy. Full attainment of the goals of evidence-based medicine will depend on proper training of researchers coupled with regulatory, institutional, and financial support of clinical research.

CONCLUSIONS

Clinical research is considered to be the necessary backbone of modern clinical medicine. Few physicians would deny the potential value of basing all patient assessment, diagnosis, and treatment on scientifically sound research studies. Rapid, ongoing technological advances have greatly increased diagnosis and treatment possibilities. However, for pediatrics and its subspecialties, support for necessary clinical research studies and training of competent clinical researchers have been inadequate (89,90). It is only within the past decade, starting with FDAMA and the Pediatric Rule, that there has been a continued forward momentum of regulatory support for pediatric clinical research, particularly clinical trials, in the United States. In Europe and elsewhere, the process has only just started. Clinical research training remains inadequate and very unlikely to generate the needed quantity and quality of independent investigators.

Coupled with increased attention to pediatric research has been controversy over ethical and legal boundaries, and imposition of regulatory guidelines and requirements that many researchers find increasingly onerous and limiting. To generate the necessary data to test interventions, incentivizing potential subjects, their parents and investigators to participate in the clinical trial process has become routine. Clinical research related to normal physiology has become increasingly difficult, even as the need for normal childhood data has escalated.

Especially within the pediatric subspecialties, including pediatric endocrinology, many of the important conditions are relatively uncommon, further complicating the conduct of relevant clinical research regarding pathogenesis and treatment. For many disorders, individual research centers may not have sufficient patients to generate statistically sound data. Postmarketing studies, such as those conducted for GH, provide a limited solution, but are limited on many levels, including the lack of hypothesis-driven primary design, lack of no-treatment control or comparison groups, limitations on the extent of data that can be collected, and an industry-oriented focus. Looking forward, pediatric clinical researchers and non–industry funding sources should explore avenues for collaborative projects, perhaps along the lines of the cancer registries (10), the completed Diabetes Prevention Trial-1 (91) and the currently ongoing multinational T1DM-related studies, TRIGR (www.trigr.org) and TrialNet (www.diabetestrialnet.org).

If the dilemmas facing clinical research are not addressed in a way that will facilitate free scientific inquiry and good clinical research, it is unlikely that the goal of universal evidence-based medicine will be achieved. Physicians and other clinical researchers have a duty to direct the evolution of the process whether via individual actions or through involvement in professional organizations.

REFERENCES

1. Lederer SE. Children as guinea pigs: historical perspectives. Account Res 2003; 10:1–16.
2. Murphy D. Pediatric trials: the impact of U.S. legislative and regulatory efforts. Appl Clin Trials 2005:1–4. (www.actmagazine.com/appliedclinicaltrials).
3. Steinbrook R. Testing medications in children. N Engl J Med 2002; 347:1462–1463.
4. Faber HK. History of the American Pediatric Society, 1887–1965. New York: McGraw-Hill, 1996.
5. Baker JP, Pearson HA. Dedicated to the Health of All Children: 75 Years of Caring, 1930–2005. Elk Grove Village: American Academy of Pediatrics, 2005.
6. Conroy S, Choonara I, Impicciatore P, et al. Survey of unlicensed and off label drug use in the paediatric wards in European countries. BMJ 2000; 320:79–82.
7. 't Jong GW, Vulto AG, de Hoog M, et al. Unapproved and off-label use of drugs in a children's hospital. N Engl J Med 2000; 343:1125.
8. Reaman GH. Pediatric cancer research from past successes through collaboration to future transdisciplinary research. J Pediatr Oncol Nurs 2004; 21:123–127.
9. Ziegler DS, Dalla Pozza L, Waters KD, Marshall GM. Advances in childhood leukaemia: successful clinical-trials research leads to individualised therapy. Med J Aust 2005; 182:78–81.
10. Sateren W, Trimble EL, Abrams J, et al. How sociodemographics, presence of oncology specialists and hospital cancer programs affect accrual to cancer treatment trials. J Clin Oncol 2002; 20:2109–2117.
11. Fisher DA. A short history of pediatric endocrinology in North America. Pediatr Res 2004; 55:1–11.
12. Steinberg FM, Raso J. Biotech pharmaceuticals and biotherapy: an overview. J Pharm Pharm Sci 1998; 1:48–59.
13. Executive summary. NIH director's panel on clinical research Bethesda: National Institutes of Health, 1997. (www.nih.gov/news/crp/97 report/execsum.htm).
14. Medical Research Council. MRC definition of clinical research, 2005. (www.mrc.ac.uk).
15. DeAngelis C, Drazen HM, Frizelle FA, et al. Clinical trial registration: a statement from the international committee of medical journal editors. N Engl J Med 2004; 351:1250–1251.
16. DeAngelis CD, Drazen JM, Frizelle FA, et al. Is this clinical trial fully registered? A statement from the international committee of medical journal editors. N Engl J Med 2004; 352:2436–2438.
17. NIH Policy and Guidelines on the Inclusion of Children as Participants in Research Involving Human Subjects. Bethesda: National Institutes of Health, 1998. (http://grants.nih.gov/grants/guide/notice-files/not 98-024.html).
18. Council on Child Health, American Academy of Pediatrics. Age limits of pediatrics. Pediatrics 1972; 49:463.
19. Kodish E. Ethics and Research with Children: A Case-Based Approach. Oxford: Oxford University Press, 2005.

20. Committee on Drugs, American Academy of Pediatrics. Guidelines for the ethical conduct of studies to evaluate drugs in pediatric populations. Pediatrics 1995; 95:286–294; reaffirmed: Pediatrics 2005; 116:796.

21. Cianfarani S, Liguori A, Germani D. IGF-I and IGFBP-3 assessment in the management of childhood onset growth hormone deficiency. Endocr Dev 2005; 9:66–75.

22. Wasserman RC, Slora EJ, Bocian AB, et al. Pediatric research in office settings (PROS): a national practice-based research network to improve children's health care. Pediatrics 1998; 102:1350–1357.

23. Herman-Giddens ME, Bourdony CJ. Assessment of sexual maturity stages in girls. Elk GroveVillage: American Academy of Pediatrics, 1995.

24. Herman-Giddens ME, Slora EJ, Wasserman RC, et al. Secondary sexual characteristics and menses in young girls seen in office practice: a study from the pediatric research in office settings network. Pediatrics 1997; 99:505–512.

25. Bliss M. The Discovery of Insulin. Chicago: University of Chicago Press, 1982.

26. DeRenzo EG, Moss J. Writing Clinical Research Protocols: Ethical Considerations. Amsterdam: Elsevier, 2006.

27. Haynes RB. Clinical Epidemiology: How to do Clinical Practice Research. Philadelphia: Lippincott Williams & Wilkins, 2006.

28. Machin D, Campbell MJ. Design of Studies for Medical Research. Hoboken: Wiley, 2005.

29. Schuster DP, Powers WJ. Translation and Experimental Clinical Research. Philadelphia: Lippincott Williams & Wilkins, 2005.

30. Hellman D. Trials on trial. Rep Inst Philo Public Policy 1998; 18:13–18.

31. Hellman S, Hellman D. Of mice, but not men: problems of the randomized clinical trial. N Engl J Med 1991; 324:1585–1589.

32. De Sanctis V. Manual of Growth Charts and Body Measurements. Pisa: Pacini, 2001:1–119.

33. Guidance for Industry. E 10 choice of control group and related issues in clinical trials. Rockville: U.S. Food and Drug Administration, 2001:1–33. (www.fda.gov/cder/guidance/4155fnl.htm).

34. Moher D, Sampson M, Campbell K, et al. Assessing the quality of reports of randomized trials in pediatric complementary and alternative medicine. BMC Pediatr 2002; 2:2.

35. Moher D, Schulz KF, Altman DG. The CONSORT statement: revised recommendations for improving the quality of reports of parallel-group randomized trials. Lancet 2001; 357:1191–1194.

36. Nuovo J, Melnikow J, Chang D. Reporting number needed to treat and absolute risk reduction in randomized controlled trials. JAMA 2002; 287:2813–2814.

37. Hsieh FY, Lavori PW, Cohen HJ, Feussner JR. An overview of variance inflation factors for sample-size calculation. Eval Health Prof 2003; 26:239–257.

38. Sprent P. Statistics in medical research. Swiss Med Wkly 2003; 133:522–529.

39. Ioannidis JPA, Evans SJW, Gøtzsche PC. Better reporting of harms in randomized trials: An extension of the CONSORT statement. Ann Intern Med 2004; 141:781–788.

40. Barfield RC, Church C. Informed consent in pediatric clinical trials. Curr Opin Pediatr 2005; 17:20–24.

41. Field MJ, Behrman RE. Ethical Conduct of Clinical Research Involving Children. Washington, D.C., National Academies Press, 2004.

42. Gill D, Kurz R. Practical and ethical issues in pediatric clinical trials. Appl Clin Trials 2003:1–4. (www.actmagazine.com/appliedclinicaltrials).

43. Spriggs M. Canaries in the mines: children, risk, non-therapeutic research and justice. J Med Ethics 2004; 30:176–181.

44. Chappuy H, Doz F, Blanche S, et al. Parental consent in pediatric clinical research. Arch Dis Child 2005.

45. Rothmeier JD, Lasley MV, Shapiro GG. Factors influencing parental consent in pediatric clinical research. Pediatrics 2003; 111:1037–1041.

46. Whittle A, Shah S, Wilfond B, Gensler F, Wendler D. Institutional review board practices regarding assent in pediatric research. Pediatrics 2004; 113:1747–1752.

47. Dlugos DJ, Scatterfood TM, Ferraro TN, et al. Recruitment rates and fear of phlebotomy in pediatric patients in a genetic study of epilepsy. Epilepsy Behav 2005; 4:444–446.

48. Weise KL, Smith ML, Maschke KJ, Copeland HL. National practices regarding payment to research subjects for participating in pediatric research. Pediatrics 2002; 110:577–582.

49. Hampton T. Experts ponder pediatric research ethics. JAMA 2005; 294:2148–2151.

50. Kopelman LM, Murphy TF. Ethical concerns about federal approval of risky pediatric studies. Pediatrics 2004; 113:1783–1789.

51. Required education in the protection of human research participation (NIH Notice OD-00–039). Bethesda: National Institutes of Health, 2000.

52. Ellis K, Shypailo RJ, Hardin DS, et al. Z score prediction model for assessment of bone mineral content in pediatric diseases. J Bone Miner Res 2001; 16:1658–1664.

53. Soldin SJ, Brugnara C, Wong EC. Pediatric Reference Intervals. 5th ed. Washington, D.C., American Association for Clinical Chemistry, 2005.

54. Rosenfeld RG, Wilson DM, Lee PD, Hintz RL. Insulin-like growth factors I and II in evaluation of growth retardation. J Pediatr 1986; 109:428–433.

55. Pizzi R. Pediatric reference intervals, a big need for little patients. Clin Lab News 2005; 31:1, 5–6.

56. Barry PL, Westgard JO. Method validation—reference interval transference (Lesson of the month #30). Westgard Quality Corp, 1999. (www.westgard.com).

57. Bossuyt PM, Reitsma JB, Bruns DE, et al. The STARD statement for reporting studies of diagnostic accuracy: explanation and elaboration. Clin Chem 2003; 49:7–18.

58. Bossuyt PM, Reitsma JB, Bruns DE, et al. Towards complete and accurate reporting of studies of diagnostic accuracy: the STARD initiative. Clin Chem 2003; 49:1–6.

59. Hytltoft Petersen P, Henny J. Special issue on reference values and reference intervals. Clin Chem Lab Med 2004; 42:685–867.

60. Wax PM. Elixirs, diluents, and the passage of the 1938 Federal Food. Drug and Cosmetic Act Ann Intern Med 1995; 122:456–461.

61. Shirkey H. Therapeutic orphans. J Pediatr 1968; 72:119–120.

62. Guidance for industry (draft guidance). How to comply with the Pediatric Research Equity Act. Rockville: U.S. Department of Health and Human Services, Food and Drug Administration, 2005.

63. Guidance for industry and FDA staff. Pediatric expertise for advisory panels. Rockville: U.S. Department of Health and Human Services, Food and Drug Administration, 2003. (www.fda.gov/cdrh/ode/guidance/1208.pdf).

64. Oortwijn WJ, Horlings E, Anton S, et al. Extended impact assessment of a draft EC regulation on medicinal products for paediatric use. Santa Monica: RAND Corp, 2004.

65. Grosstête F. Report on the proposal for a regulation of the European Parliament and of the Council on medical products for paediatric use and amending Regulation (EEC) No 1768/92, Directive 2001/83/EC and Regulation (EC) No 726/2004 (Document A6-0247/2005). Brussels: European Parliament, 2005. (www.europarl.eu.int).

66. Charter. Pediatric Advisory Committee. Rockville: U.S. Food and Drug Administration, 2004. (www.fda.gov/oc/advisory/OCPedsChapter.html).

67. Frasier SD. The not-so-good old days: working with pituitary growth hormone in North America, 1956 to 1985. J Pediatr 1997; 131:S1–S4.

68. Hintz RL. Eternal vigilance—mortality in children with growth hormone deficiency. J Clin Endocrinol Metab 1996; 81:1691–1692.

69. Will RG. Acquired prion disease: iatrogenic CJD, variant CJD, kuru. Brit Med Bull 2003; 66:255–265.

70. Hintz RL. The prismatic case of Creutzfeldt-Jakob disease associated with pituitary growth hormone treatment. J Clin Endocrinol Metab 1995; 80:2298–2301.

71. Department of Health and Human Services, Food and Drug Administration. 21 CFR Parts 314 and 620 Postmarketing studies for approved human drug and licensed biological products: status reports. Fed Reg 2000; 65:64607–64619.

72. Report to Congress. Reports on postmarketing studies (FDAMA 130). Rockville: U.S. Food and Drug Administration, 2002.

73. Okie S. Safety in numbers—monitoring risk in approved drugs. N Engl J Med 2005; 352:1173–1176.

74. Wysowki DK, Swartz L. Adverse drug event surveillance and drug withdrawals in the United States, 1969–2002: the importance of reporting suspected reactions. Arch Intern Med 2005; 165:1363–1369.

75. Richter B, Clar C. Systematic reviews in endocrinology. The Cochrane metabolism and endocrine disorders review group. Endocrinol Metab Clin North Am 2002; 31:613–617.

76. Guidance for Industry and FDA Staff. Premarket assessment of pediatric medical devices. Rockville: U.S. Food and Drug Administration, 2004:1–22.

77. Topol EF, Blumenthal D. Physicians and the investment industry. JAMA 2005; 293:2654–2657.

78. Bryant J, Powell J. Payment to healthcare professionals for patient recruitment to trials: a systematic review. BMJ 2005; 331:1377–1378.

79. Levinsky NG. Nonfinancial conflicts of interest in research. New Engl J Med 2002; 347:759–761.

80. Mello MM, Clarridge BR, Studdert MD. Academic medical centers' standards for clinical-trial agreements with industry. N Engl J Med 2005; 352:2202–2210.

81. Nathan D, Weatherall DJ. Academic freedom in clinical research. N Engl J Med 2002; 347:1368–1371.

82. Rothman KJ, Evans S. Extra scrutiny for industry funded trials. BMJ 2005; 331:1350–1351.

83. Hampton T. NIH eases ethics rules on employees: consulting ban to remain. JAMA 2005; 294:1749–1750.

84. AACE Clinical Research Committee. American association of clinical endocrinologists white paper on endocrine clinical research. First Messenger 2004; 13:12–13.

85. Harbour R, Miller J for the Scottish Intercollegiate Guidelines Network Grading Review Group. A new system for grading recommendations in evidence-based guidelines. BMJ 2001; 323:334–336.

86. Moher D, Soeken K, Sampson M, et al. Assessing the quality of reports of systematic reviews in pediatric complementary and alternative medicine. BMC Pediatr 2002; 2:3.

87. Gipson D, Trachtman H. The clinical trial imperative. Pediatr Nephrol 2005; 20:5–9.

88. Montori VM. Evidence-based endocrinology: how far have we come? Treat Endocrinol 2004; 3:1–10.

89. Beitins IZ. Opportunities and challenges in pediatric clinical research. J Clin Endocrinol Metab 1999; 84:4302–4306.

90. Feigin RD. Prospects for the future of child health through research. JAMA 2005; 294:1373–1379.

91. Pozzilli P. The DPT-1 trial: a negative result with lessons for future type 1 diabetes prevention. Diab Metab Res Rev 2002; 18:257–259.

20

Reference Charts and Tables Frequently Used by Endocrinologists

Adriana A. Carrillo

*Department of Pediatric Endocrinology, Mailman Center for Child Development and
Department of Pediatrics, Miller Medical School, University of Miami, Miami, Florida, U.S.A.*

Fima Lifshitz

*Pediatric Sunshine Academics Inc. and Sansum Medical Research Institute,
Santa Barbara, California, and Department of Pediatrics, University of Miami,
Miami, Florida, and Department of Pediatrics, Health Science Center,
State University of New York, Brooklyn, New York, U.S.A.*

■ **GROWTH CHARTS FOR CHILDREN WITH GENETIC CONDITIONS**

STANDARDS OF GROWTH
Neonates

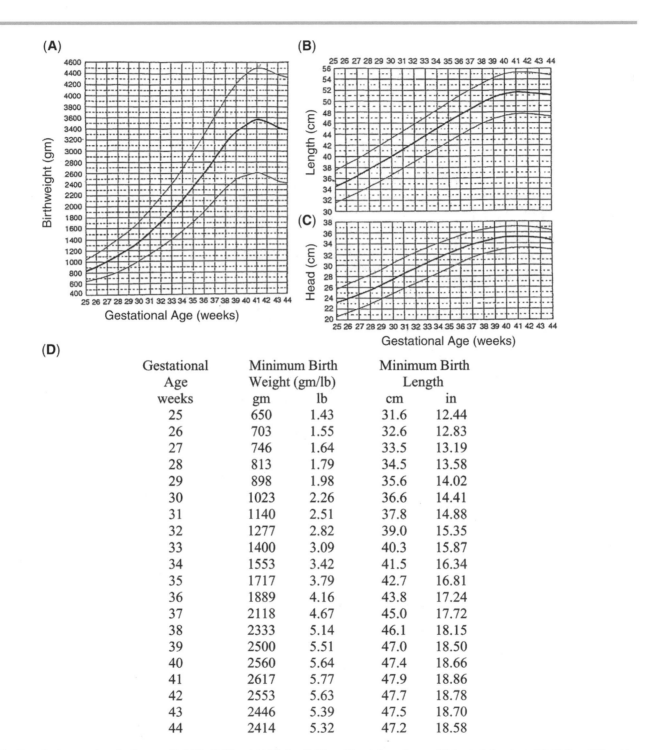

(A)

(B)

(C)

(D)

Gestational Age weeks	Minimum Birth Weight (gm/lb)		Minimum Birth Length	
	gm	lb	cm	in
25	650	1.43	31.6	12.44
26	703	1.55	32.6	12.83
27	746	1.64	33.5	13.19
28	813	1.79	34.5	13.58
29	898	1.98	35.6	14.02
30	1023	2.26	36.6	14.41
31	1140	2.51	37.8	14.88
32	1277	2.82	39.0	15.35
33	1400	3.09	40.3	15.87
34	1553	3.42	41.5	16.34
35	1717	3.79	42.7	16.81
36	1889	4.16	43.8	17.24
37	2118	4.67	45.0	17.72
38	2333	5.14	46.1	18.15
39	2500	5.51	47.0	18.50
40	2560	5.64	47.4	18.66
41	2617	5.77	47.9	18.86
42	2553	5.63	47.7	18.78
43	2446	5.39	47.5	18.70
44	2414	5.32	47.2	18.58

Figure 1 Smoothed curve values for the mean± 2 SD of birth weight (**A**), length (**B**), and head circumference (**C**) for gestational age (**D**). Birth weight and/or length 2 SD below the mean, adjusted for gestational age. *Source*: From Usher R, McLean F. Intrauterine growth of live-born Caucasians infants at sea level: standards obtained from measurements in 7 dimensions of infants born between 25 and 44 weeks of gestation. J Pediatr 1969; 74:901–910; with permission from Elsevier.

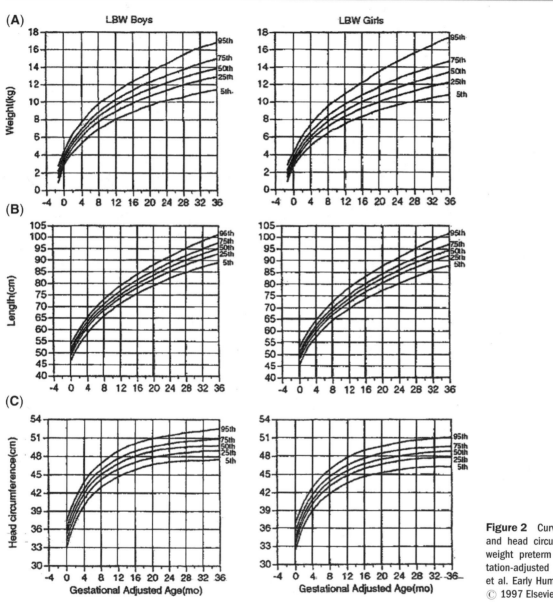

Figure 2 Curves for weight (**A**), length (**B**), and head circumference (**C**) for low birth-weight preterm infants in relation to gestation-adjusted ages. *Source*: From Guo SS et al. Early Human Dev 1997; 47:305–325; © 1997 Elsevier Ireland Ltd., by permission.

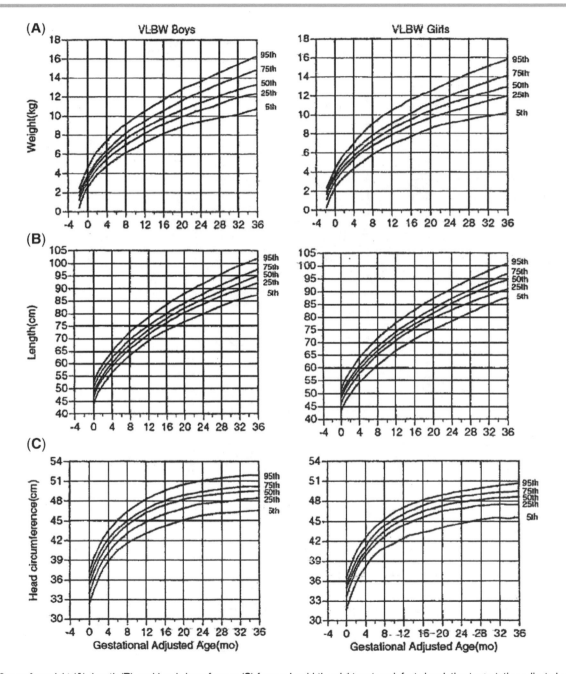

Figure 3 Curves for weight (**A**), length (**B**), and head circumference (**C**) for very low birth-weight preterm infants in relation to gestation-adjusted ages. *Source*: From Guo SS et al. Early Human Dev 1997; 47:305–325; © 1997 Elsevier Ireland Ltd., by permission.

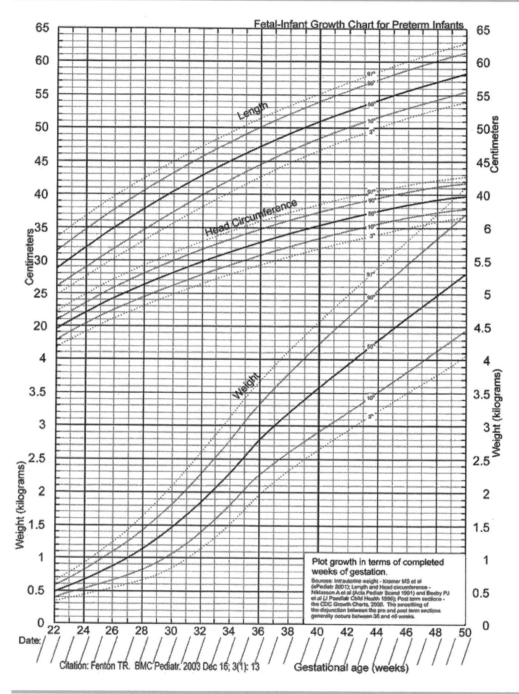

Figure 4 Fetal infant growth chart for preterm infants from a meta-analysis. *Source*: From Fenton TR. BMC Pediatrics 2003; 3:13 (open access).

Infants

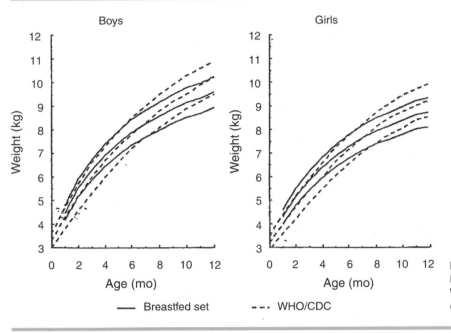

Figure 5 Weight quartiles of infants breast-fed at least 12 months (*n* = 226) in comparison with the WHO/CDC reference (1986). *Source:* From Dewey KG et al. Pediatrics 1995; 96:495; by permission of AAP.

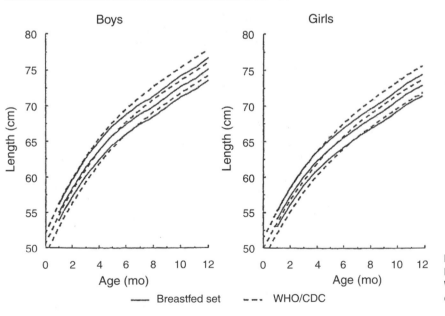

Figure 6 Length quartiles of breast-fed infants at least 12 months (*n* = 226) in comparison with the WHO/CDC reference (1986). *Source:* From Dewey KG et al. Pediatrics 1995; 96:495; by permission of AAP.

Females

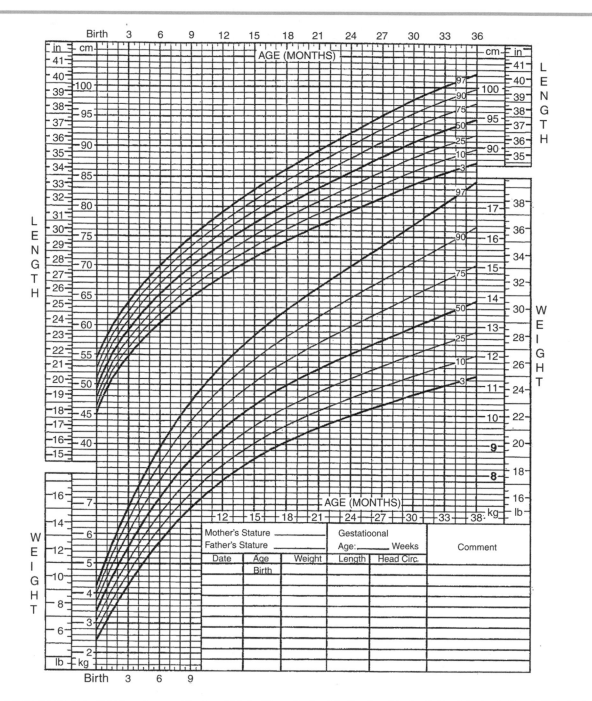

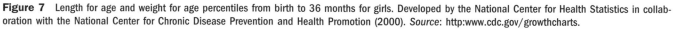

Figure 7 Length for age and weight for age percentiles from birth to 36 months for girls. Developed by the National Center for Health Statistics in collaboration with the National Center for Chronic Disease Prevention and Health Promotion (2000). *Source*: http:www.cdc.gov/growthcharts.

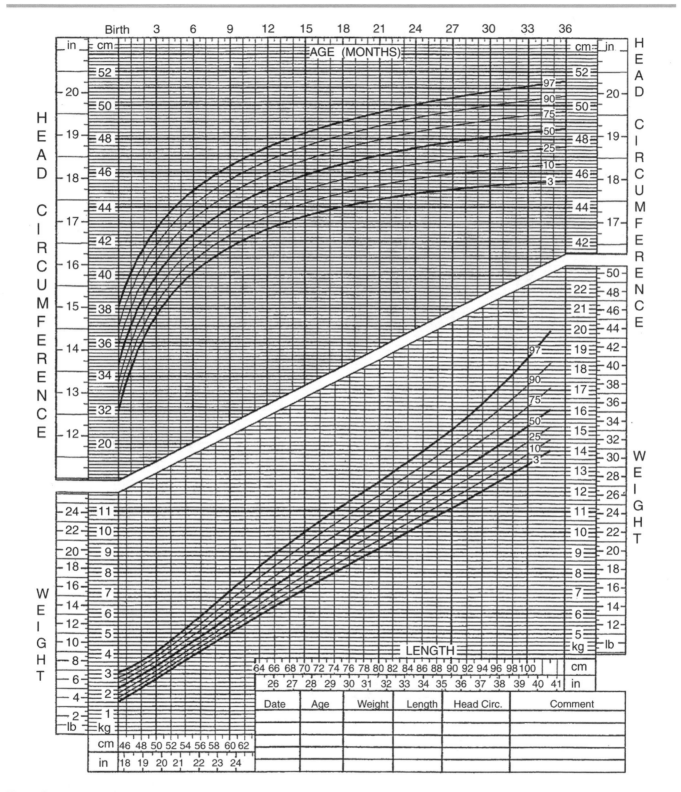

Figure 8 Head circumference for age and weight for length percentiles. Developed by the National Center for Health Statistics in collaboration with the National Center for Chronic Disease Prevention and Health Promotion (2000). *Source*: http:www.cdc.gov/growthcharts.

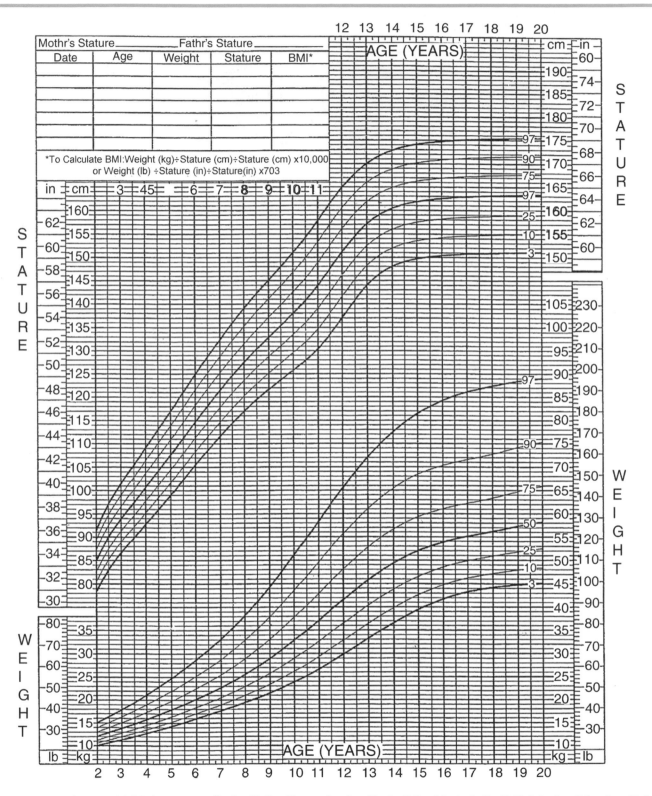

Figure 9 Stature for age and weight for age percentiles for girls 2 to 20 years. Developed by the National Center for Health Statistics in collaboration with the National Center for Chronic Disease Prevention and Health Promotion (2000). *Source*: http:www.cdc.gov/growthcharts.

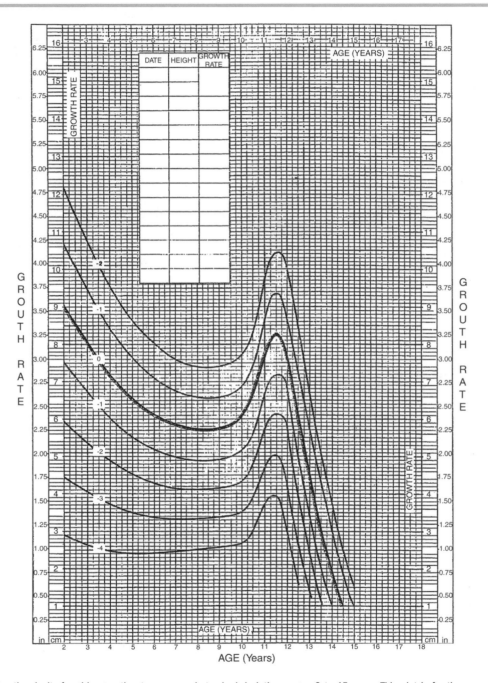

Figure 10 Yearly growth velocity for girls; growth rate, mean and standard deviations; ages 2 to 15 years. This plot is for the average-maturing children. Developed by the National Center for Chronic Disease Prevention and Health Promotion (2000). *Source:* http:www.cdc.gov/growthcharts.

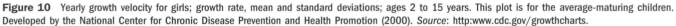

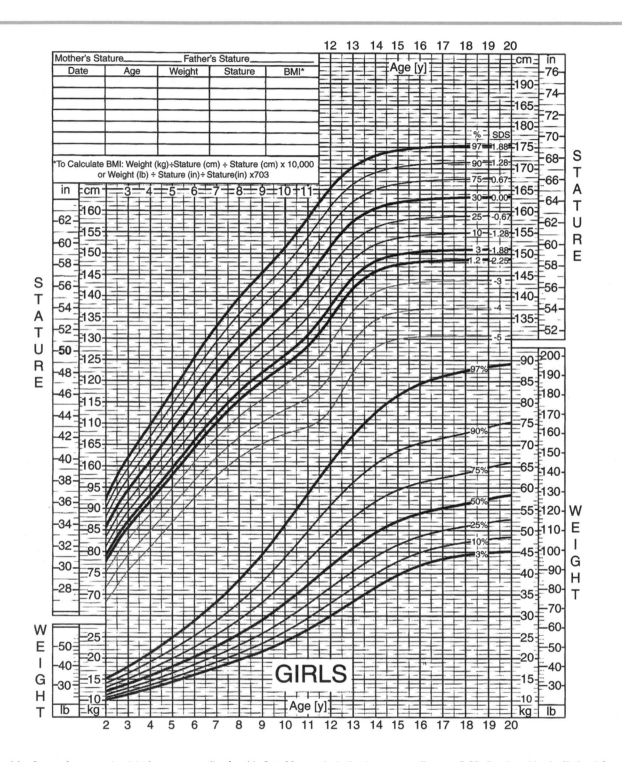

Figure 11   Stature for age and weight for age percentiles for girls 2 to 20 years including lower percentiles to −5 SD. Developed by the National Center for Health Statistics in collaboration with the National Center for Chronic Disease Prevention and Health Promotion (2000). *Source*: http:www.cdc.gov/growthcharts.

Males

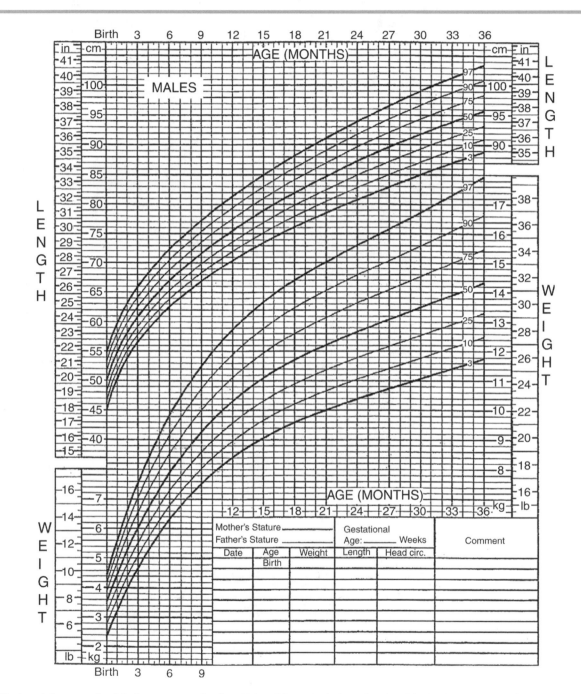

Figure 12 Length for age and weight for age percentiles from birth to 36 months for boys. Developed by the National Center for Health Statistics in collaboration with the National Center for Chronic Disease Prevention and Health Promotion (2000). *Source*: http:www.cdc.gov/growthcharts.

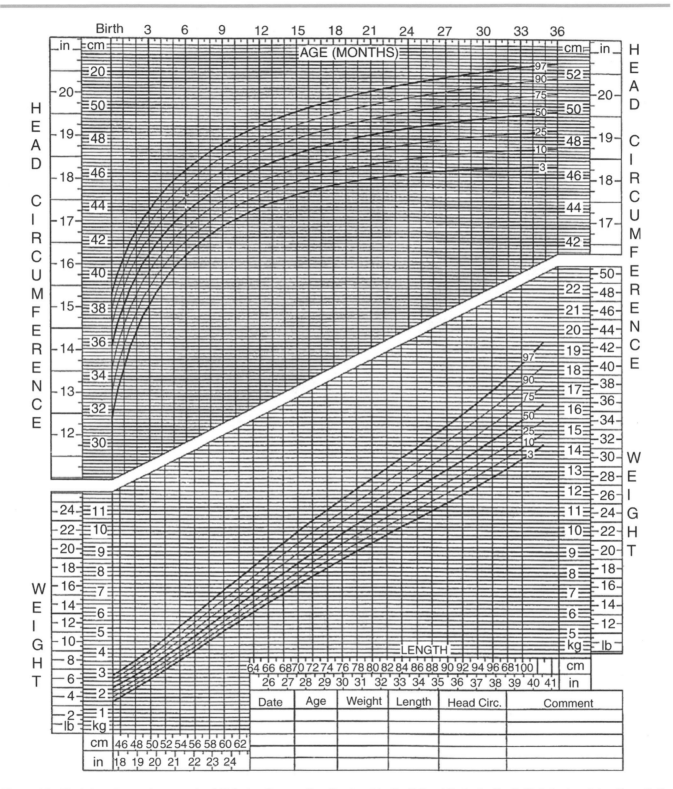

Figure 13 Head circumference for age and weight for length percentiles. Developed by the National Center for Health Statistics in collaboration with the National Center for Chronic Disease Prevention and Health Promotion (2000). *Source:* http:www.cdc.gov/growthcharts.

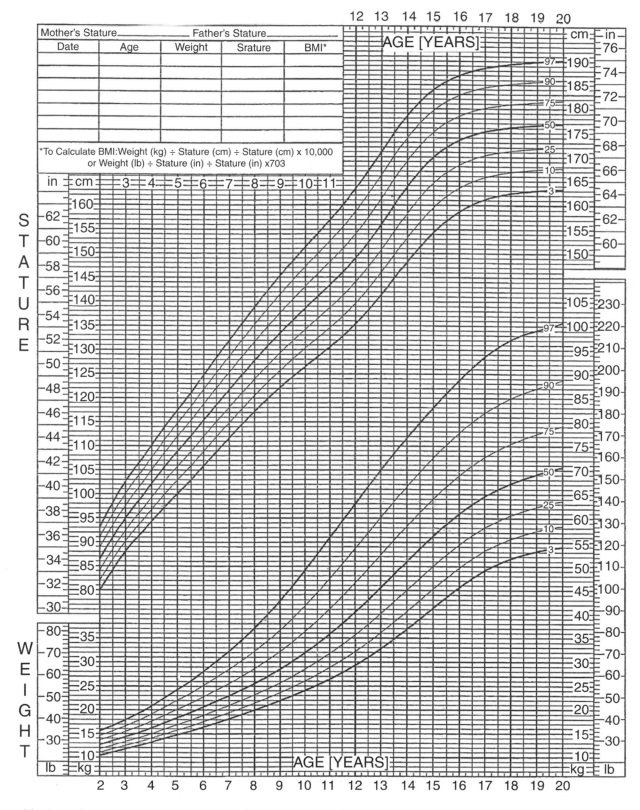

Figure 14 Stature for age and weight for age percentiles for boys 2 to 20 years. Developed by the National Center for Health Statistics in collaboration with the National Center for Chronic Disease Prevention and Health Promotion (2000). *Source*: http:www.cdc.gov/growthcharts.

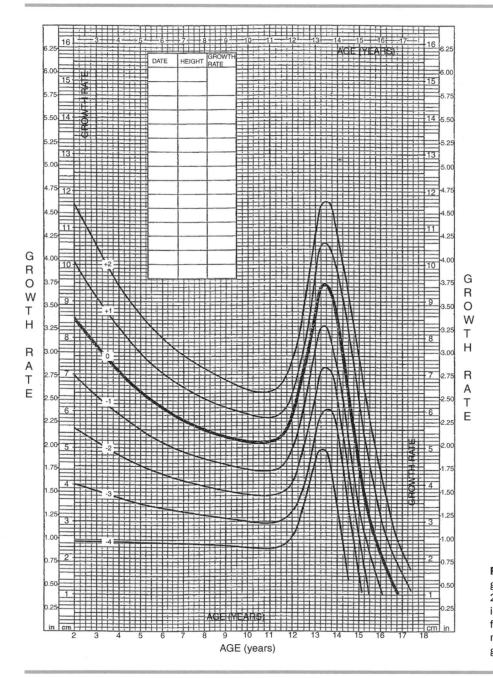

Figure 15 Yearly growth velocity for boys; growth rate, mean and standard deviations; ages 2 to 15 years. This plot is for the average-maturing children. Developed by the National Center for Chronic Disease Prevention and Health Promotion (2000). *Source*: http:www.cdc.gov/growthcharts.

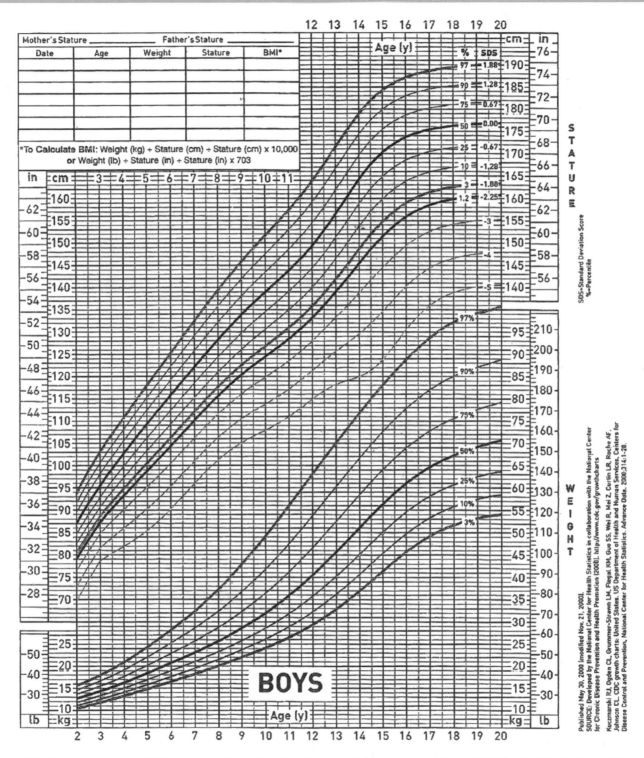

Figure 16 Stature for age and weight for age percentiles for boys 2 to 20 years including lower percentiles to -5 SD. Developed by the National Center for Health Statistics in collaboration with the National Center for Chronic Disease Prevention and Health Promotion (2000). *Source*: http:www.cdc.gov/growthcharts.

MISCELLANEOUS MEASUREMENTS AND STANDARDS

| | HEIGHT (In.) | | SPAN | | | |
| | | | Absolute | | Relative | |
AGE	M	F	M	F	M	F
Birth	20.2	19.9	19.3	18.9	95.7	95.2
1 Mo.	21.9	21.5	21.0	20.5	95.7	95.2
2 Mos.	23.1	22.7	22.1	21.6	95.7	95.2
3 Mos.	24.1	23.7	23.1	22.6	95.8	95.3
4 Mos.	25.0	24.6	24.0	3.4	95.8	95.3
5 Mos.	25.7	25.3	24.6	24.1	95.8	95.3
6 Mos.	26.4	26.0	25.3	24.8	95.8	95.3
7 Mos.	27.1	26.6	26.0	25.4	95.9	95.4
8 Mos.	27.6	27.1	26.5	25.9	95.9	95.4
9 Mos.	28.1	27.6	26.9	26.3	95.9	95.4
10 Mos.	28.6	28.1	27.4	26.8	95.9	95.9
1I Mos.	29.1	28.6	27.9	27.3	96.0	95.5
12 Mos.	29.5	29.0	28.3	27.7	96.0	95.5
15 Mos.	30.7	30.2	29.5	28.9	96.1	95.6
18 Mos.	31.9	31.4	30.7	30.0	96.2	95.7
21 Mos.	32.9	32.4	31.7	31.0	96.3	95.7
24 Mos.	33.9	33.4	32.6	32.0	96.3	96.8
30 Mos.	35.7	32.1	34.4	33.7	96.4	96.0
36 Mos.	37.3	30.7	30.0	35.0	96.6	96.2
42 Mos.	38.8	38.2	37.5	36.5	96.8	96.4
48 Mos.	40.2	39.6	39.0	38.2	97.0	96.6
54 Mos.	41.5	40.9	40.3	39.6	97.2	96.8
60 Mos.	42.7	42.2	41.6	40.9	97.4	97.0
5-1/2 Yrs.	43.9	43.4	42.8	42.2	97.6	97.2
6 Yrs.	45.0	44.6	44.0	43.4	97.8	97.4
6-1/2 Yrs.	46.1	45.7	45.2	44.6	98.1	97.6
7 Yrs.	47.2	46.8	46.4	48.9	98.4	97.8
7-1/2 Yrs.	48.2	47.9	47.6	47.0	98.7	98.1
8 Yrs.	49.2	48.9	48.8	48.1	99.1	98.3
8-1/2 Yrs.	50.2	49.9	50.0	49.2	99.6	98.6
9 Yrs.	51.2	50.9	51.2	50.3	100.0	98.8
9-1/2 Yrs.	52.2	51.9	52.4	51.4	100.4	99.0
10 Yrs.	53.2	53.0	53.6	52.6	100.7	99.2
10-1/2 Yrs.	54.2	54.1	54.7	53.8	100.9	99.4
11 Yrs.	55.2	55.3	55.8	55.1	101.2	99.6
11-1/2 Yrs.	56.2	56.5	56.9	56.3	101.4	99.8
12 Yrs.	57.1	57.6	58.0	57.6	101.6	100.0
12-1/2 Yrs.	58.0	58.7	59.1	58.7	101.8	100.1
13 Yrs.	58.9	59.7	60.1	59.9	102.0	100.3
13-1/2 Yrs.	59.8	60.6	61.1	60.9	102.2	100.4
14 Yrs.	60.7	61.4	62.1	61.7	102.3	100.6
14-1/2 Yrs.	61.6	62.0	63.1	62.4	102.5	100.7
15 Yrs.	62.4	62.5	64.0	63.0	102.6	100.8
15-1/2 Yrs.	63.2	62.9	64.9	63.5	102.7	100.9
16 Yrs.	64.0	63.2	65.8	63.0	102.8	101.0
16-1/2 Yrs.	64.7	63.5	66.6	64.2	102.9	101.0
17 Yrs.	65.4	63.7	67.4	64.4	103.0	101.2
17-1/2 Yrs.	66.0	63.9	68.1	64.6	103.1	101.2
18 Yrs.	66.6	64.0	68.7	64.8	103.2	101.3
18-1/2 Yrs.	67.1	64.0	69.3	64.8	103.3	101.3
19 Yrs.	67.5	64.0	69.8	64.8	103.4	101.3
19-1/2 Yrs.	67.8	64.0	70.1	64.8	103.4	101.3
20 Yrs.	68.0	64.0	70.4	64.8	103.5	101.3

Figure 17   Span in relation to age and standing height. *Source*: From Tanner JM, et al. 1985; 107:317–327.

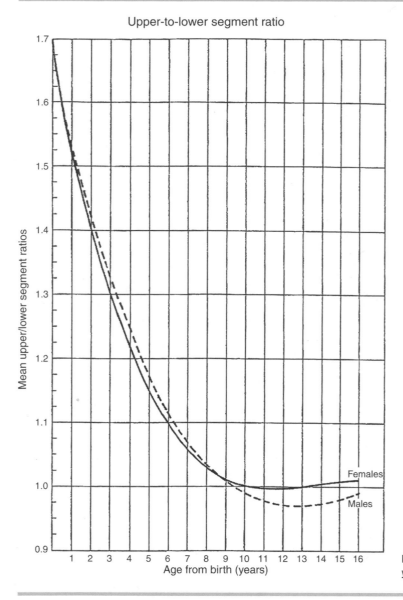

Figure 18 Upper-to-lower segment ratio, both sexes, birth to 16 years. *Source*: From Harriet Lane Handbook, 1975.

AGE:	STANDING HEIGHT (In.)		SITTING HEIGHT, ABSOLUTE		SITTING HEIGHT, RELATIVE	
	M	F	M	F	M	F
Birth	20.2	19.9	13.6	13.4	67.3	67.3
1 Month	21.9	21.5	14.6	14.4	66.7	66.8
2 Months	23.1	22.7	15.3	15.1	66.2	66.3
3 Months	24.1	23.7	15.8	15.6	65.6	65.7
4 Months	25.0	24.6	16.3	16.1	65.1	65.2
5 Months	25.7	25.3	16.6	16.4	64.6	64.7
6 Months	26.4	26.0	16.9	16.7	64.1	64.2
7 Months	27.1	26.6	17.3	17.0	63.8	63.9
8 Months	27.6	27.1	17.5	17.2	63.4	63.5
9 Months	28.1	27.6	17.7	17.4	63.1	63.2
10 Months	28.6	28.1	18.0	17.7	62.8	62.9
11 Months	29.1	28.6	18.2	17.9	62.6	62.7
12 Months (1 yr)	29.5	29.0	18.4	18.1	62.3	62.4
15 Months	30.7	30.2	18.9	18.6	61.6	61.7
18 Months	31.9	31.4	19.4	19.1	60.9	61.0
21 Months	32.9	32.4	19.8	19.5	60.3	60.4
24 Months (2 yrs)	33.9	33.4	20.3	20.0	59.8	59.9
30 Months	35.7	35.1	21.0	20.7	58.9	59.0
36 Months (3 yrs)	37.3	36.7	21.7	21.4	58.2	58.3
42 Months	38.8	38.2	22.3	22.0	57.6	57.6
48 Months (4 yrs)	40.2	39.6	22.9	22.5	57.0	56.9
54 Months	41.5	40.9	23.4	23.1	56.5	56.4
60 Months (5 yrs)	42.7	42.2	23.9	23.6	56.0	55.9
5½ Years	43.9	43.4	24.4	24.1	55.6	55.5
6 Years	45.0	44.6	24.9	24.6	55.2	55.2
6½ Years	46.1	45.7	25.3	25.1	54.9	54.9
7 Years	47.2	46.8	25.8	25.5	54.6	54.5
7½ Years	48.2	47.9	26.2	26.0	54.3	54.2
8 Years	49.2	48.9	26.6	26.4	54.1	54.0
8½ Years	50.2	49.9	27.1	26.9	53.9	53.8
9 Years	51.2	50.9	27.5	27.3	53.7	53.6
9½ Years	52.2	51.9	27.9	27.7	53.4	53.3
10 Years	53.2	53.0	28.3	28.1	53.2	53.0
10½ Years	54.2	54.1	28.8	28.6	53.0	52.8
11 Years	55.2	55.3	29.2	29.1	52.9	52.6
11½ Years	56.2	56.5	29.6	29.7	52.7	52.6
12 Years	57.1	57.6	30.0	30.3	52.6	52.6
12½ Years	58.0	58.7	30.4	30.9	52.5	52.7
13 Years	58.9	59.7	30.9	31.5	52.4	52.8
13½ Years	59.8	60.6	31.3	32.0	52.3	52.8
14 Years	60.7	61.4	31.7	32.5	52.3	52.9
14½ Years	61.6	62.0	32.2	32.8	52.4	52.9
15 Years	62.4	62.5	32.8	33.0	52.5	52.9
15½ Years	63.2	62.9	33.3	33.2	52.6	52.9
16 Years	64.0	63.2	33.7	33.4	52.7	52.9
16½ Years	64.7	63.5	34.1	33.5	52.8	52.9
17 Years	65.4	63.7	34.5	33.6	52.8	52.8
17½ Years	66.0	63.9	34.8	33.7	52.8	52.8
18 Years	66.6	64.0	35.1	33.8	52.7	52.8
18½ Years	67.1	64.0	35.3	33.8	52.6	52.8
19 Years	67.5	64.0	35.5	33.8	52.6	52.8
19½ Years	67.8	64.0	35.6	33.8	52.5	52.8
20 Years	68.0	64.0	35.7	33.8	52.5	52.8

Figure 19 Sitting height in relation to age and standing height—birth to 20 years. (From Engelbach W Endocrine) Medicine. *Source*: Courtesy of Charles C. Thomas, Springfield: Illinois, 1932.

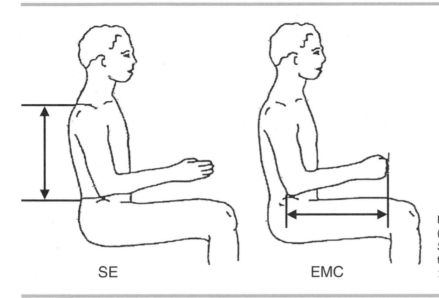

Figure 20   Measurement of the shoulder-to-elbow length (SE) and elbow-to-end-of-third metacarpal length (EMC). *Source*: From Cervantes C, Lifshitz F. Tubular bone alterations in familial short stature. Human Biol 1988; 60: 151–165.

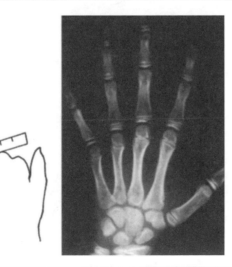

Figure 21   Clinical assessment of brachymetacarpia. A straight ruler is applied against the distal end of the third, fourth, and fifth metacarpals of a tightly closed fist. The clinical observation of brachymetacarpia V was confirmed radiologically when the fifth metacarpal bone failed to intercept a straight line connecting the distal ends of the third and fourth metacarpal bones by more then 2 mm. *Source*: From Cervantes C, Lifshitz F, Levenbrown J. Radiologic anthropometry of the hand in patients with familial short stature. Pediat Radiol 1988; 18:210–214.

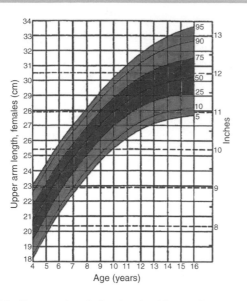

Figure 22   Upper arm length, females, 4 to 16 years. *Source*: From Manila RM, Hamill PVV, Lemeshow S. Manual of Physical Performance in Childhood. Vol 1B. New York: Plenum Press, 1973:1048.

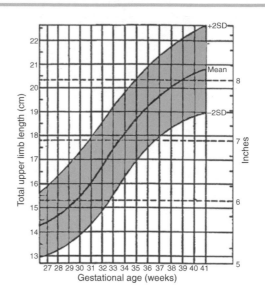

Figure 24   Total upper limb lengths at birth by gestational age. *Source*: From Sivan Y, Merlob P, Reisner SH. Am J Dis Child 1983; 137: 829.

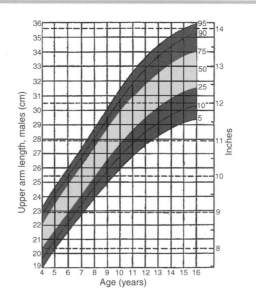

Figure 23   Upper arm length, males, 4 to 16 years. *Source*: From Manila RM, Hamill PVV, Lemeshow S. Manual of Physical Performance in Childhood. Vol 1B. New York: Plenum Press, 1973:1048.

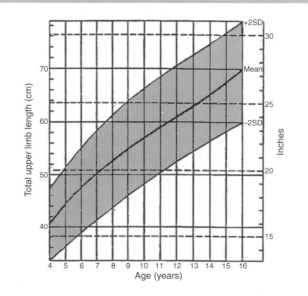

Figure 25   Total upper limb lengths, both sexes, 4 to 16 years. *Source*: From Martin and Saller. Lehrbuch der Antropologie, Gustave Fische, Stuttgart.

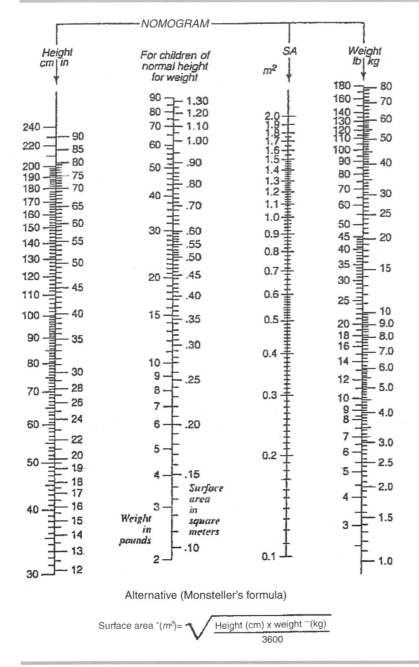

Alternative (Monsteller's formula)

$$\text{Surface area }^-(m^2)= \sqrt{\frac{\text{Height (cm) x weight }^-\text{(kg)}}{3600}}$$

Figure 26 Body surface area nomogram. *Source:* From Arch Dis Child 1994; 70:246.

Bone Development Standards

PRIMARY (DECIDUOUS) TEETH

Designation	Calcification (fetal month)	Eruption (months)	Shedding (years)
central incisor	5	6–8	7–8
lateral incisor	5	8–11	8–9
cuspid	6	16–20	11–12
first primary molar	5	10–16	10–11
second primary molar	6	20–30	10–12

MAXILLARY

MANDIBULAR

Designation	Calcification (fetal month)	Eruption (months)	Shedding (years)
second primary molar	6	20–30	11–13
first primary molar	5	10–16	10–12
cuspid	6	16–20	9–11
lateral incisor	5	7–10	7–8
central incisor	5	5–7	6–7

DESIGNATION OF TEETH

$$\frac{211111 \mid 101112}{211110 \mid 11111}$$

Deciduous teeth designated by 1; permanent teeth by 2, missing teeth by O. Upper row indicates maxillary teeth, lower row of numbers indicates mandibular teeth. Vertical line locates the midline.

SECONDARY (PERMANENT) TEETH

Designation	Calcification begins	Eruption
central incisor	3–4 mo.	7–8 yr.
lateral incisor	10–12 mo.	8–9 yr.
cuspid	4–5 mo.	11–12 yr.
first bicuspid	18–21 mo.	10–11 yr.
second bicuspid	24–30 mo.	10–12 yr.
first molar	birth	6–7 yr.
second molar	30–36 mo.	12–13 yr.
third molar (wisdom)	7–9 mo.	17–22 yr.

MAXILLARY

MANDIBULAR

Designation	Calcification begins	Eruption
third molar (wisdom)	8–10 mo.	17–22 yr.
second molar	30–36 mo.	12–13 yr.
first molar	birth	6–7 yr.
second bicuspid	24–30 mo.	11–13 yr.
first bicuspid	18–21 mo.	10–12 yr.
cuspid	4–5 mo.	9–11 yr.
lateral incisor	3–4 mo.	7–8 yr.
central incisor	3–4 mo.	6–7 yr.

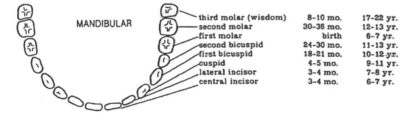

Figure 27 Development of dentition. *Source*: From Simon FA, Stevenson RE. Pediatric Patient Care. University of Texas Press, 1975.

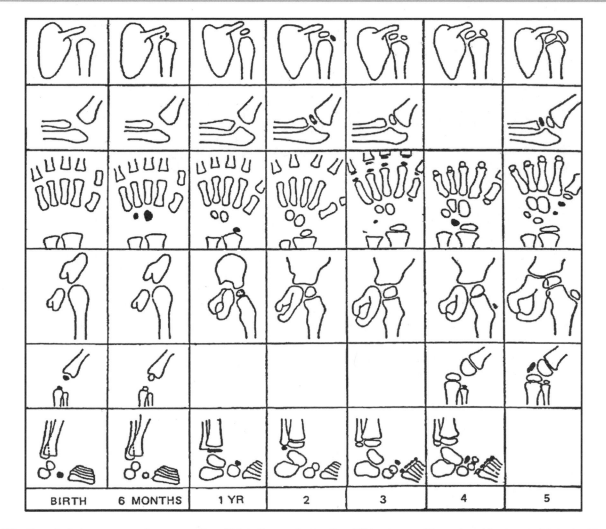

Figure 28 Chronological appearance of osseous centers—birth to 5 years. *Source*: From Wilkins, Lawson. Diagnosis and Treatment of Endocrine Disorders in Childhood and Adolescence. Springfield: Illinois, 1966. Courtesy of Charles C. Thomas.

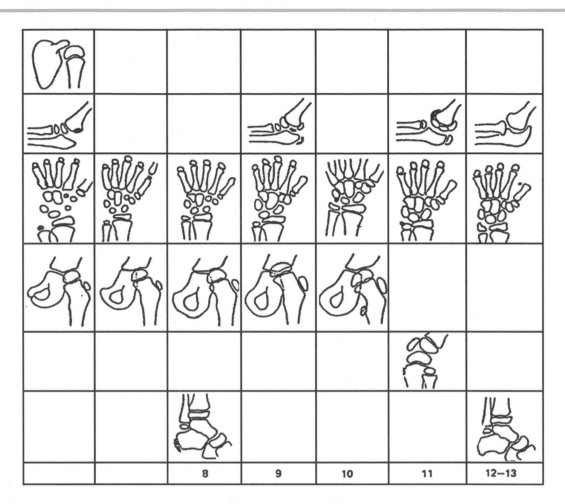

Figure 29 Chronological appearance of osseous centers—6 to 13 years. *Source*: From Wilkins, Lawson. Diagnosis and Treatment of Endocrine Disorders in Childhood and Adolescence. Springfield: Illinois, 1966. Courtesy of Charles C. Thomas.

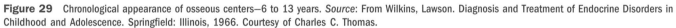

	12 Yrs	13 Yrs	14 Yrs	15 Yrs	16 Yrs	17 Yrs	18 Yrs
Shoulder							Head of humerus Great tuberosity
Elbow	Trochlen & capitelium	Olecranon	Ext. epicondyle Head of radious				
Hand		Styloid of ulna		Ep. metacarpals & phalanges			Ep. radious & ulna
Hip				Head of femur Trochanters			
Knee							Ep. femur, tibia % fibula
Foot	Ep. os raleis			Ep. metatarsals & phalanges		Ep. tibia & fibula	

Figure 30 Chronological order of union of epiphysis with diaphysis. *Source*: From Wilkins, Lawson. Diagnosis and Treatment of Endocrine Disorders in Childhood and Adolescence. Springfield: Illinois, 1966. Courtesy of Charles C. Thomas.

Fatness Standards

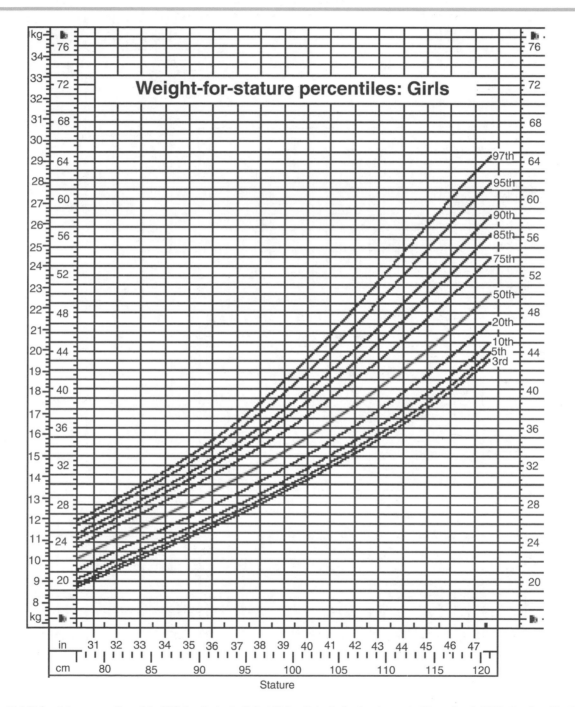

Figure 31 Weight-for-stature percentiles, girls, CDC growth charts: United States. *Note*: Revised and corrected December 4, 2000. Developed by the National Center for Health Statistics in collaboration with the National Center for Disease Prevention and Health Promotion (2000). *Source*: www.CDC.gov/growthcharts.

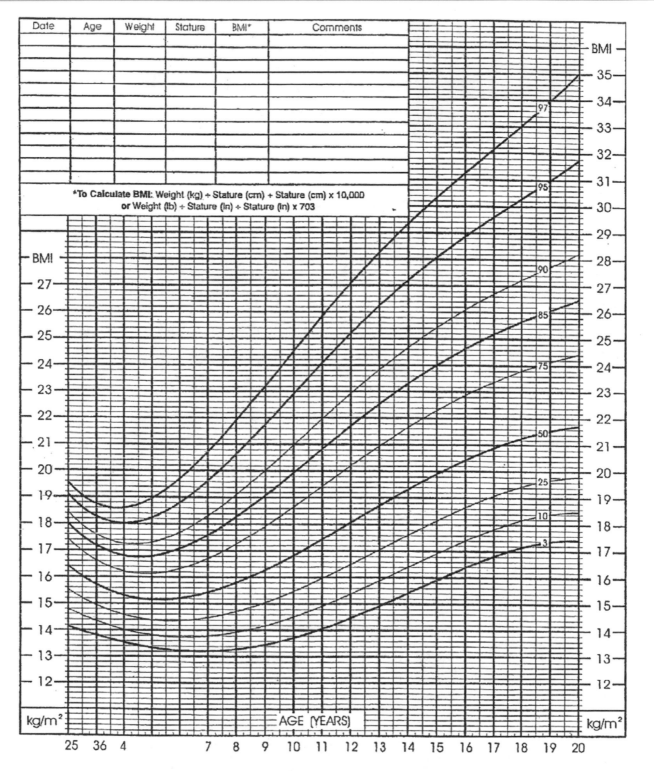

Figure 32 Body mass index for age percentiles, females. Developed by the National Center for Health Statistics in collaboration with the National Center for Chronic Disease Prevention and Health Promotion (2000). *Source*: http:www.cdc.gov/growthcharts.

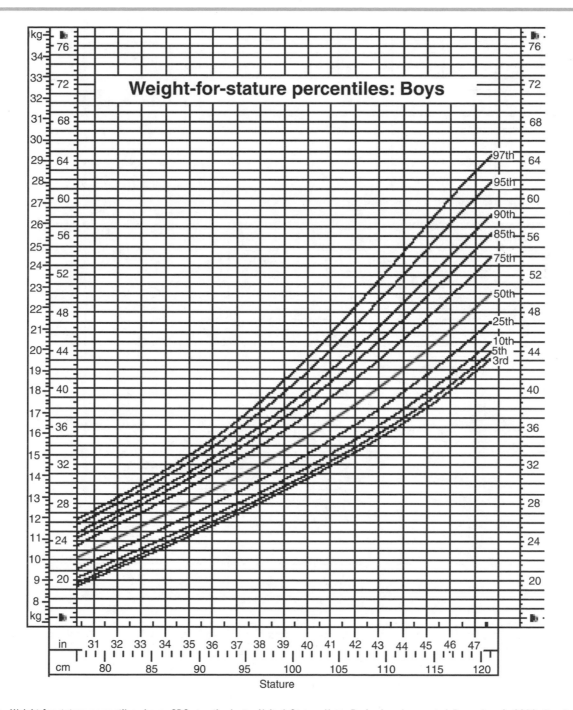

Figure 33 Weight-for-stature percentiles, boys, CDC growth charts: United States. *Note*: Revised and corrected December 4, 2000. Developed by the National Center for Health Statistics in collaboration with the National Center for Disease Prevention and Health Promotion (2000). *Source*: www.CDC.gov/growthcharts.

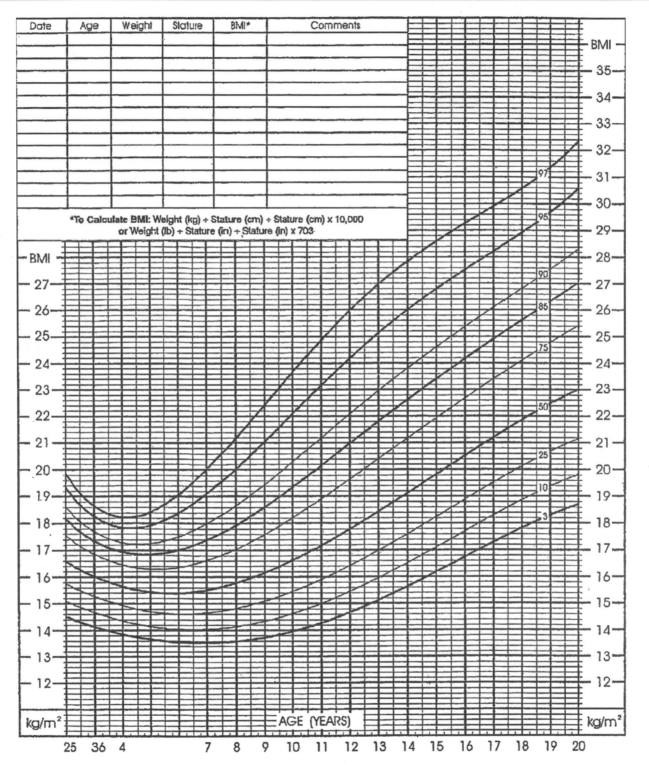

*To Calculate BMI: Weight (kg) ÷ Stature (cm) ÷ Stature (cm) x 10,000
or Weight (lb) ÷ Stature (in) ÷ Stature (in) x 703

Figure 34 Body mass index for age percentiles, males. Developed by the National Center for Health Statistics in collaboration with the National Center for Chronic Disease Prevention and Health Promotion (2000). *Source*: http:www.cdc.gov/growthcharts.

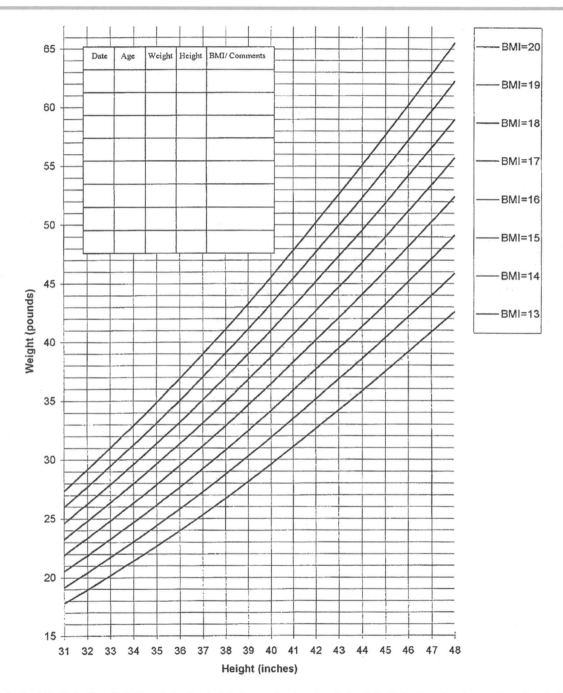

Figure 35 Portland Health Institute Body Mass Index Graph, 2 to 5 years. Developed by Portland Health Institute, Inc. *Source*: Reproduced with permission from Pediatrics 2004; 113:425–426; © 2004 by AAP.

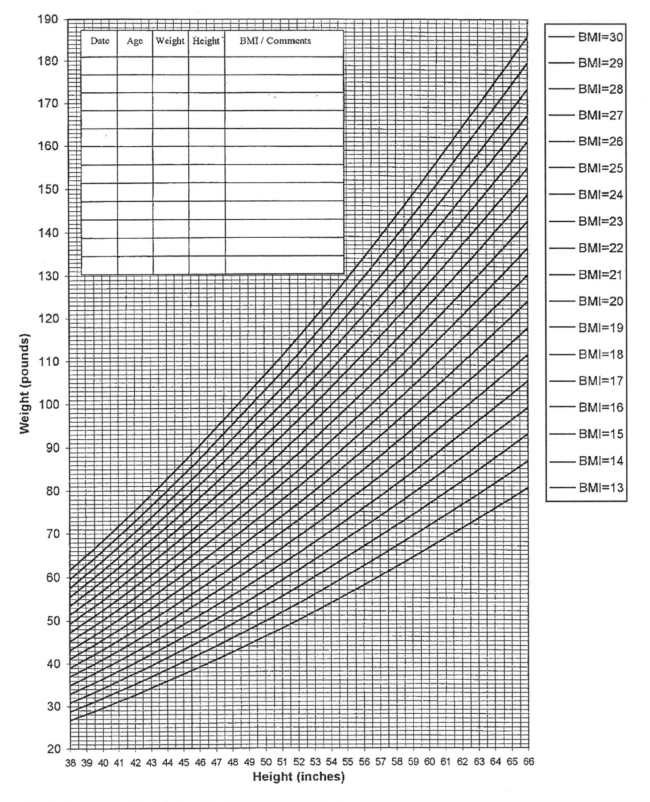

Figure 36 Portland Health Institute Body Mass Index Graph, 5 to 12 years. Developed by Portland Health Institute, Inc. *Source:* Reproduced with permission of Pediatrics 2004; 113:425–426; © 2004 by AAP.

Estimated value for percentile regression for European-American children and adolescents, according to sex

	Percentile for boys					Percentile for girls				
	10th	25th	50th	75th	90th	10th	25th	50th	75th	90th
Intercept	39.3	43.2	42.9	43.3	43.8	39.5	41.3	43.6	45.0	46.8
Slope	1.8	1.9	2.1	2.6	3.4	1.6	1.7	1.9	2.3	2.9
Age (y)										
2	42.9	46.9	47.1	48.6	50.6	43.1	45.1	47.4	49.6	52.5
3	44.7	48.8	49.2	51.2	54.0	44.7	46.8	49.3	51.9	55.4
4	46.5	50.6	51.3	53.8	57.4	46.3	48.5	51.2	54.2	58.2
5	48.3	52.5	53.3	56.5	60.8	47.9	50.2	53.1	56.5	61.1
6	50.1	54.3	55.4	59.1	64.2	49.5	51.8	55.0	58.8	64.0
7	51.9	56.2	57.5	61.7	67.6	51.1	53.5	56.9	61.1	66.8
8	53.7	58.1	59.6	64.3	71.0	52.7	55.2	58.8	63.4	69.7
9	55.5	59.9	61.7	67.0	74.3	54.3	56.9	60.7	65.7	72.6
10	57.3	61.8	63.7	69.6	77.7	55.9	58.6	62.5	68.0	75.5
11	59.1	63.6	65.8	72.2	81.1	57.5	60.2	64.4	70.3	78.3
12	60.9	65.5	67.9	74.9	84.5	59.1	61.9	66.3	72.6	81.2
13	62.7	67.4	70.0	77.5	87.9	60.7	63.6	68.2	74.9	84.1
14	64.5	69.2	72.1	80.1	91.3	62.3	65.3	70.1	77.2	86.9
15	66.3	71.1	74.1	82.8	94.7	63.9	67.0	72.0	79.5	89.8
16	68.1	72.9	76.2	85.4	98.1	65.5	68.6	73.9	81.8	92.7
17	69.9	74.8	78.3	88.0	101.5	67.1	70.3	75.8	84.1	95.5
18	71.7	76.7	80.4	90.6	104.9	68.7	72.0	77.7	86.4	98.4

Figure 37 **(A)**   Waist circumference percentiles for European-American children and adolescents according to sex. *Source*: Fernandez JR, Redden DT, Pietrobelli A, Allison DB. Waist circumference percentiles in nationally representative samples of African–American, European–American, and Mexican–American children and adolescents. J Pediatr 2004; 145:439–444. © 2004 Mosby, with permission from Elsevier.

Estimated value for percentile regression for African-American children and adolescents, according to sex

	Percentile for boys					Percentile for girls				
	10th	25th	50th	75th	90th	10th	25th	50th	75th	90th
Intercept	40.1	41.2	42.7	44.1	43.6	39.9	41.2	41.7	42.1	42.8
Slope	1.6	1.7	1.9	2.2	3.2	1.6	1.7	2.1	2.8	3.7
Age (y)										
2	43.2	44.6	46.4	48.5	50.0	43.0	44.6	46.0	47.7	50.1
3	44.8	46.3	48.3	50.7	53.2	44.6	46.3	48.1	50.6	53.8
4	46.3	48.0	50.1	52.9	56.4	46.1	48.0	50.2	53.4	57.5
5	47.9	49.7	52.0	55.1	59.6	47.7	49.7	52.3	56.2	61.1
6	49.4	51.4	53.9	57.3	62.8	49.2	51.4	54.5	59.0	64.8
7	51.0	53.1	55.7	59.5	66.1	50.8	53.2	56.6	61.8	68.5
8	52.5	54.8	57.6	61.7	69.3	52.4	54.9	58.7	64.7	72.2
9	54.1	56.4	59.4	63.9	72.5	53.9	56.6	60.9	67.5	75.8
10	55.6	58.1	61.3	66.1	75.7	55.5	58.3	63.0	70.3	79.5
11	57.2	59.8	63.2	68.3	78.9	57.0	60.0	65.1	73.1	83.2
12	58.7	61.5	65.0	70.5	82.1	58.6	61.7	67.3	75.9	86.9
13	60.3	63.2	66.9	72.7	85.3	60.2	63.4	69.4	78.8	90.5
14	61.8	64.9	68.7	74.9	88.5	61.7	65.1	71.5	81.6	94.2
15	63.4	66.6	70.6	77.1	91.7	63.3	66.8	73.6	84.4	97.9
16	64.9	68.3	72.5	79.3	94.9	64.8	68.5	75.8	87.2	101.6
17	66.5	70.0	74.3	81.5	98.2	66.4	70.3	77.9	90.0	105.2
18	68.0	71.7	76.2	83.7	101.4	68.0	72.0	80.0	92.9	108.9

Figure 37   **(B)** Waist circumference percentiles for African-American children and adolescents according to sex. *Source*: Fernandez JR, Redden DT, Pietrobelli A, Allison DB. Waist circumference percentiles in nationally representative samples of African–American, European–American, and Mexican–American children and adolescents. J Pediatr 2004; 145:439–444. © 2004 Mosby, with permission from Elsevier.

Estimated value for percentile regression for Mexican-American children and adolescents, according to sex

	Percentile for boys					Percentile for girls				
	10th	25th	50th	75th	90th	10th	25th	50th	75th	90th
Intercept	41.0	41.8	43.3	44.3	46.2	41.4	42.1	43.9	44.8	47.1
Slope	1.7	1.9	2.2	2.7	3.5	1.5	1.8	2.1	2.6	3.2
Age (y)										
2	44.4	45.6	47.6	49.8	53.2	44.5	45.7	48.0	50.0	53.5
3	46.1	47.5	49.8	52.5	56.7	46.0	47.4	50.1	52.6	56.7
4	47.8	49.4	52.0	55.3	60.2	47.5	49.2	52.2	55.2	59.9
5	49.5	51.3	54.2	58.0	63.6	49.0	51.0	54.2	57.8	63.0
6	51.2	53.2	56.3	60.7	67.1	50.5	52.7	56.3	60.4	66.2
7	52.9	55.1	58.5	63.4	70.6	52.0	54.5	58.4	63.0	69.4
8	54.6	57.0	60.7	66.2	74.1	53.5	56.3	60.4	65.6	72.6
9	56.3	58.9	62.9	68.9	77.6	55.0	58.0	62.5	68.2	75.8
10	58.0	60.8	65.1	71.6	81.0	56.5	59.8	64.6	70.8	78.9
11	59.7	62.7	67.2	74.4	84.5	58.1	61.6	66.6	73.4	82.1
12	61.4	64.6	69.4	77.1	88.0	59.6	63.4	68.7	76.0	85.3
13	63.1	66.5	71.6	79.8	91.5	61.1	65.1	70.8	78.6	88.5
14	64.8	68.4	73.8	82.6	95.0	62.6	66.9	72.9	81.2	91.7
15	66.5	70.3	76.0	85.3	98.4	64.1	68.7	74.9	83.8	94.8
16	68.2	72.2	78.1	88.0	101.9	65.6	70.4	77.0	86.4	98.0
17	69.9	74.1	80.3	90.7	105.4	67.1	72.2	79.1	89.0	101.2
18	71.6	76.0	82.5	93.5	108.9	68.6	74.0	81.1	91.6	104.4

Figure 37 **(C)** Waist circumference percentiles for Mexican-American children and adolescents according to sex. *Source*: Fernandez JR, Redden DT, Pietrobelli A, Allison DB. Waist circumference percentiles in nationally representative samples of African–American, European–American, and Mexican–American children and adolescents. J Pediatr 2004; 145:439–444. © 2004 Mosby, with permission from Elsevier.

Estimated value for percentile regression for all children and adolescents combined, according to sex

	Percentile for boys					Percentile for girls				
	10th	25th	50th	75th	90th	10th	25th	50th	75th	90th
Intercept	39.7	41.3	43.0	43.6	44.0	40.7	41.7	43.2	44.7	46.1
Slope	1.7	1.9	2.0	2.6	3.4	1.6	1.7	2.0	2.4	3.1
Age (y)										
2	43.2	45.0	47.1	48.8	50.8	43.8	45.0	47.1	49.5	52.2
3	44.9	46.9	49.1	51.3	54.2	45.4	46.7	49.1	51.9	55.3
4	46.6	48.7	51.1	53.9	57.6	46.9	48.4	51.1	54.3	58.3
5	48.4	50.6	53.2	56.4	61.0	48.5	50.1	53.0	56.7	61.4
6	50.1	52.4	55.2	59.0	64.4	50.1	51.8	55.0	59.1	64.4
7	51.8	54.3	57.2	61.5	67.8	51.6	53.5	56.9	61.5	67.5
8	53.5	56.1	59.3	64.1	71.2	53.2	55.2	58.9	63.9	70.5
9	55.3	58.0	61.3	66.6	74.6	54.8	56.9	60.8	66.3	73.6
10	57.0	59.8	63.3	69.2	78.0	56.3	58.6	62.8	68.7	76.6
11	58.7	61.7	65.4	71.7	81.4	57.9	60.3	64.8	71.1	79.7
12	60.5	63.5	67.4	74.3	84.8	59.5	62.0	66.7	73.5	82.7
13	62.2	65.4	69.5	76.8	88.2	61.0	63.7	68.7	75.9	85.8
14	63.9	67.2	71.5	79.4	91.6	62.6	65.4	70.6	78.3	88.8
15	65.6	69.1	73.5	81.9	95.0	64.2	67.1	72.6	80.7	91.9
16	67.4	70.9	75.6	84.5	98.4	65.7	68.8	74.6	83.1	94.9
17	69.1	72.8	77.6	87.0	101.8	67.3	70.5	76.5	85.5	98.0
18	70.8	74.6	79.6	89.6	105.2	68.9	72.2	78.5	87.9	101.0

Figure 37 **(D)** Waist circumference percentiles for all children and adolescents according to sex. *Source*: Fernandez JR, Redden DT, Pietrobelli A, Allison DB. Waist circumference percentiles in nationally representative samples of African–American, European–American, and Mexican–American children and adolescents. J Pediatr 2004; 145:439–444. © 2004 Mosby, with permission from Elsevier.

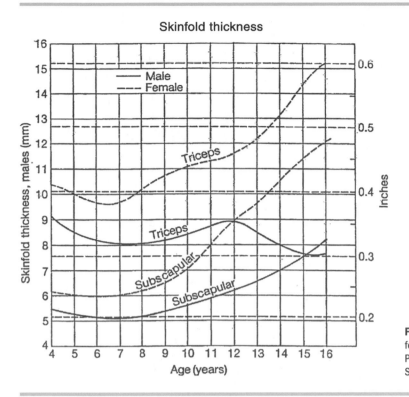

Figure 38 Triceps and subscapular skinfolds, males and females, 4 to 16 years. *Source*: From Schulueter K, Funfack W, Pachalay J, Weber B. Eur J Pediatr 1976; 123:255; courtesy of Springer Science and Business Media.

Age	% fat males		% fat females	
	AAP[1]	Formula[2]	AAP[1]	Formula[2]
Birth	14	--	15	--
6 months	25	--	26	--
12 months	22	--	24	--
2 years	20	22	20	26
4 years	16	20	18	23
6 years	14	18	16	22
8 years	13	17	17	21
10 years	14	17	20	21
12 years	19	17	24	23
14 years	18	17	25	23
16 years	14	18	24	21
18 years	13	18	23	21
20 years	13	19	25	20

Figure 39 Ideal body fat percentages. *Source*: (*1*) from American Academy of Pediatrics, 1895; (*2*) from Jackson AS, Stanforth PR, Gagnon J, et al. The effect of sex, age, and race on estimating percentage body fat from body mass index: the Heritage Family Study. Int J Obes Relat Metab Disord 2002; 26:789–796; courtesy of Elsevier.

Genitalia and Puberty Stages

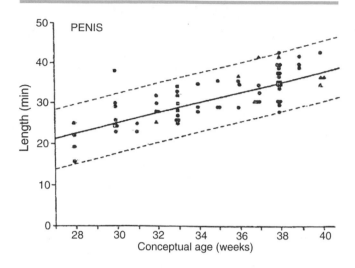

Figure 40   Phallic lengths of premature and full-term infants. Stretched phallic length of 63 normal premature and full-term infants (), showing lines of mean 2 SD. Correlation coefficient is 0.8. Superimposed are data for two small-for-gestational-age infants (), seven large for gestational age infants (), and four twins (), all of which are in the normal range. *Source*: From Feldman KW, Smith DW. Fetal phallic growth and penile standards for newborn male infants. J Pediatr 1975; 86(3):395–398; courtesy of Elsevier.

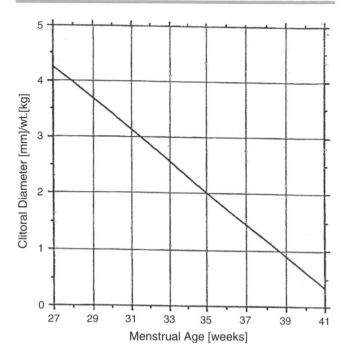

Figure 42   Ratio of clitoral diameter to infant's weight plotted against menstrual age. Measurements were made with calipers on 69 premature and 90 term infants in the first three days of life. There were no differences in measurements between black and white infants. *Source*: From Riley WS, et al. J Pediatr 1980; 96:918.

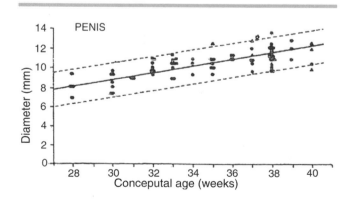

Figure 41   Phallic diameters of premature and full-term infants. *Source*: From Feldman KW, Smith DW. Fetal phallic growth and penile standards for newborn male infants. J Pediatr 1975; 86(3):395–398; courtesy of Elsevier.

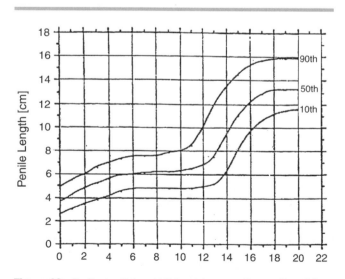

Figure 43   Penile growth from birth to adolescence. *Source*: From Schonfield WA. Am J Dis Child 1943; 65:535.

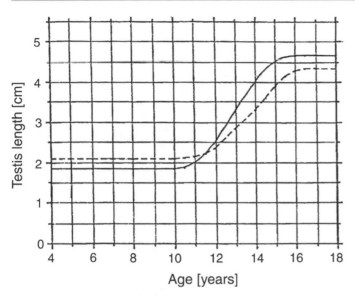

Figure 44 Testicular growth from ages 4 to 18 years. *Source:* From Laron A, Zilka E. J Clin Endocrinol Metab 1969; 29:1409; Adapted from data of Praeder A. Recognizable Patterns of Human Malformation. 3rd ed. Philadelphia: WB Saunders, 1982.

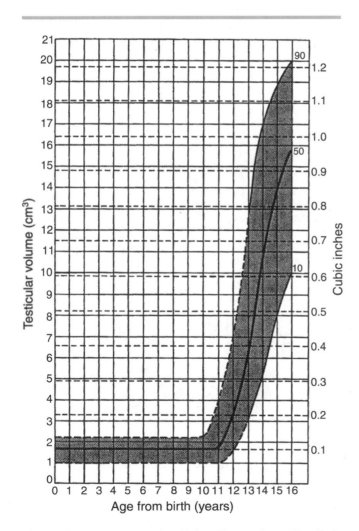

Figure 45 Testicular volume from birth to 16 years. *Source:* From Zachman et al. (1974) and Goodman and Gorlin (1983).

Progression of puberty stages of breasts in females.

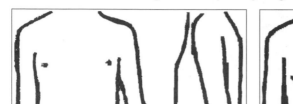 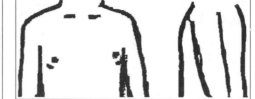

Stage 1. The breasts are preadolescent. There is elevation of the papilla only. No palpable glandular tissue. Areola not pigmented. Breast does not project from the chest wall.

Stage 2. Breast bud stage. A small mound is formed by the elevation of the breast and papilla. The areolar diameter enlarges. Glandular tissue is palpable, continuous to the areola.

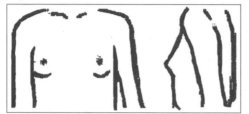 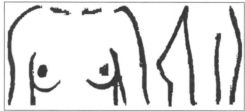

Stage 3. There is further enlargement of breasts and areola with no separation of their contours. Glandular tissue beyond the areola. Nipple enlarged and becoming pigmented.

Stage 4. There is a projection of the areola and papilla to form a secondary mound above the level of the breast. Increased areola pigmentation.

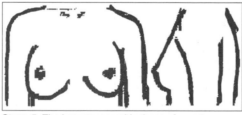

Stage 5. The breasts resemble those of a mature female as the areola has recessed to the general contour of the breast.

Progression of puberty stages of female pubic hair.

Stage 1. There is no pubic hair.

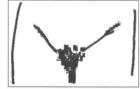 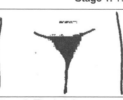 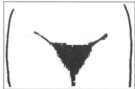 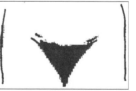

Stage 2. There is sparse growth of long slightly pigmented downy hair, straight or only slightly curled, primarily along the labia.

Stage 3. The hair is considerably darker and more curled.The hair spreads sparsely over the junction of the pubis.

Stage 4. The hair is now adult in type, covering mons pubi pattern, but not extending to thighs.

Stage 5. The hair is adult in quantity and type with extension onto the thighs.

Figure 46   Progression of puberty stages of breast and pubic hair.

Progression of puberty stages of male genitalia.

Stage 1. The penis, testicle (< 2.4 cm and volume < 3.0 mL), and scrotum are of childhood size and there is no pubic hair.

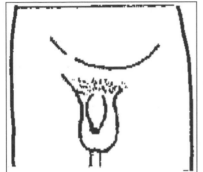

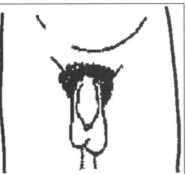

Stage 2. There is enlargement of the scrotum and testes but the penis usually does not enlarge. The scrotal skin reddens. The testicle size is < 2.5 cm and volume < 3.0 mL. There is sparse growth of pubic hair at the base of the penis, slightly pigmented, downy, and straight.

Stage 3. There is further growth of the testes and scrotum and enlargement in the penis, mainly in length. The testicle size is > 2.5–3.0 cm and volume > 6.0–10 mL. There is darker coarse curly hair that spreads over the junction of the pubis.

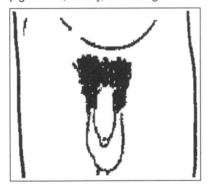

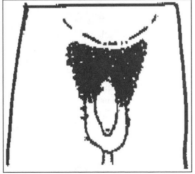

Stage 4. There is further growth of the testes and scrotum and further growth in the the penis, especially in breadth. Length > 3.5–4.0 cm and volume > 10–15 mL. The hair is now adult in type covering a smaller area than in the adult without extending onto the thighs.

Stage 5. The genitalia are adult in size and shape. Length > 4.0 cm and volume > 15 mL. Adult quantity and type in an inverse triangle with extension to the linea alba and lower abdomen.

Figure 47 Progression of puberty stages of male genitalia and pubic hair.

Site	Grade	Definition
1. Upper lip	1	A few hairs at outer margin.
	2	A small moustache at outer margin.
	3	A moustache extending halfway from outer margin.
	4	A moustache extending to midline.
2. Chin	1	A few scattered hairs.
	2	Scattered hairs with small concentrations.
	3 and 4	Complete cover, light and heavy.
3. Chest	1	Circumareolar hairs.
	2	With midline hair in addition.
	3	Fusion of these areas, with three-quarter cover.
	4	Complete cover.
4. Upper back	1	A few scattered hairs.
	2	Rather more, still scattered.
	3 and 4	Complete cover, light and heavy.
5. Lower back	1	A sacral tuft of hair.
	2	With some lateral extension.
	3	Three-quarter cover.
	4	Complete cover.
6. Upper abdomen	1	A few midline hairs.
	2	Rather more, still midline.
	3 and 4	Half and full cover.
7. Lower abdomen	1	A few midline hairs.
	2	A midline streak of hair.
	3	A midline band of hair.
	4	An inverted V-shaped growth.
8. Arm	1	Sparse growth affecting not more than a quarter of the limb surface.
	2	More than this: cover still incomplete.
	3 and 4	Complete cover, light and heavy.
9. Forearm	1,2,3,4	Complete cover of dorsal surface; 2 grades of light and 2 of heavy growth.
10. Thigh	1,2,3,4	As for arm.
11. Leg	1,2,3,4	As for arm.

Figure 48 Hair grading system Hirsutism. *Source:* From Ferriman D, Gallwey JD. J Clin Endocrinol Metab 1961:1440–1447.

GROWTH CHARTS FOR CHILDREN WITH GENETIC CONDITIONS

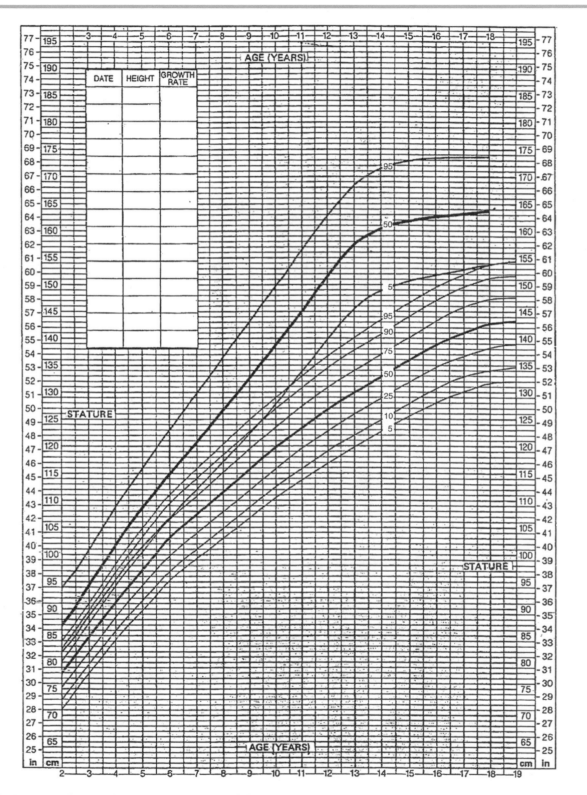

Figure 49 Growth chart for Turner Syndrome compared to normal female growth. The broken line shows growth in untreated Turner syndrome grils. *Source*: Percentiles derived from Lyon AJ, Precee MA, Grant DB. Arch Dis Child 1985; 60:932–935.

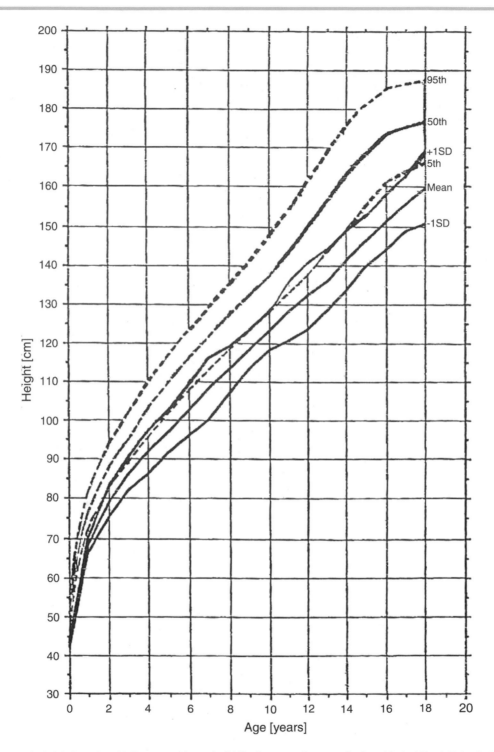

Figure 50 Growth curve for height in males with Noonan syndrome (*solid lines*) compared to normal values (*dashed lines*). Data obtained from 64 Noonan syndrome males from a collaborative retrospective review. *Source*: From Witt DR et al. Clin Genet 1986; 30:150.

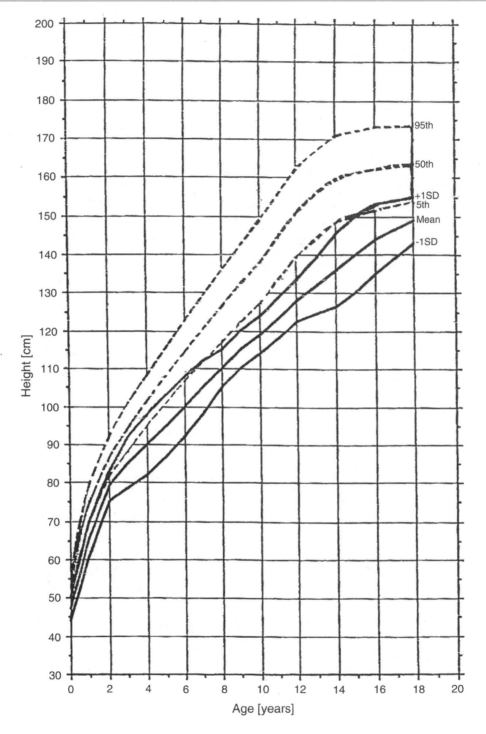

Figure 51 Growth curve for height in females with Noonan syndrome (*solid lines*) compared to normal values (*dashed lines*). Data obtained from 48 Noonan syndrome females from a collaborative retrospective review. *Source*: From Witt DR et al. Clin Genet 1986; 30:150.

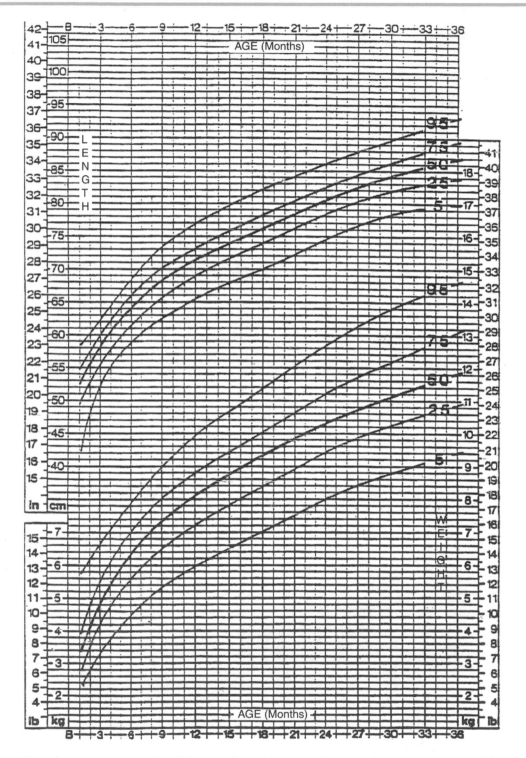

Figure 52 Length and weight for males with Down syndrome from birth to 36 months. *Source*: From Pediatrics 1988; 81:102.

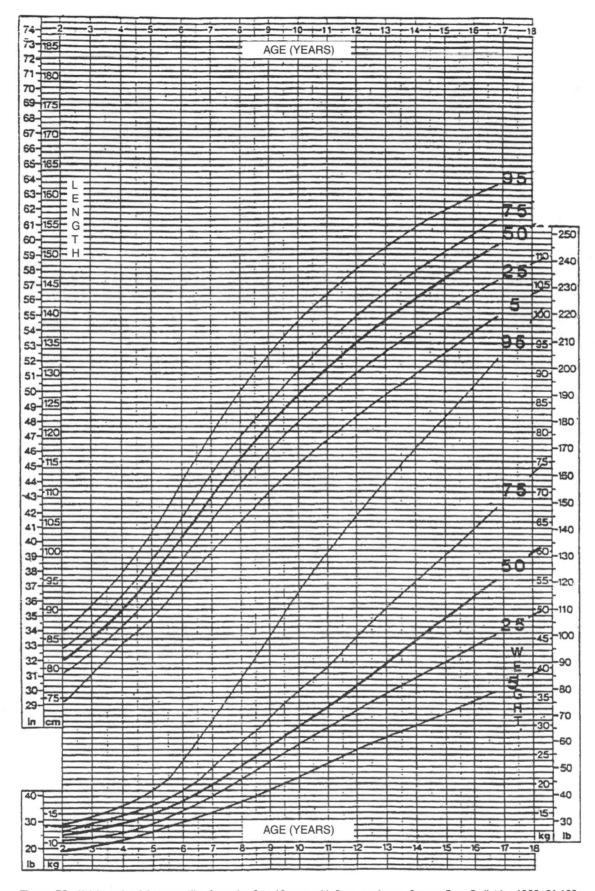

Figure 53 Height and weight percentiles for males 2 to 18 years with Down syndrome. *Source:* From Pediatrics 1988; 81:102.

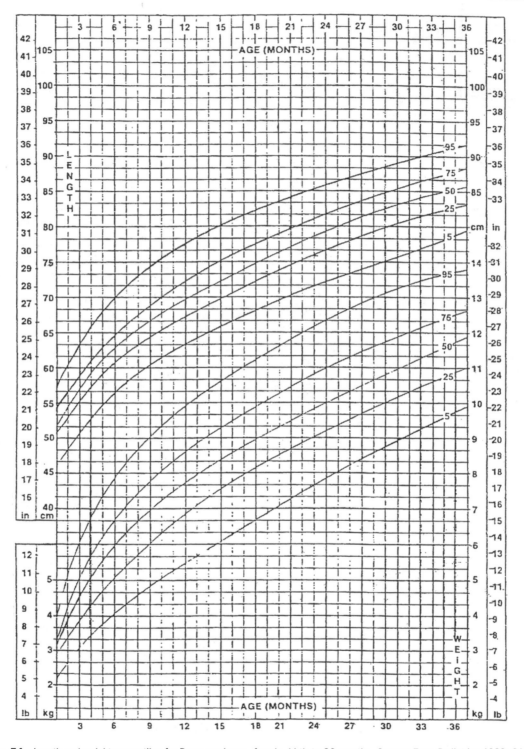

Figure 54 Length and weight percentiles for Down syndrome—female, birth to 36 months. *Source:* From Pediatrics 1988; 81:102.

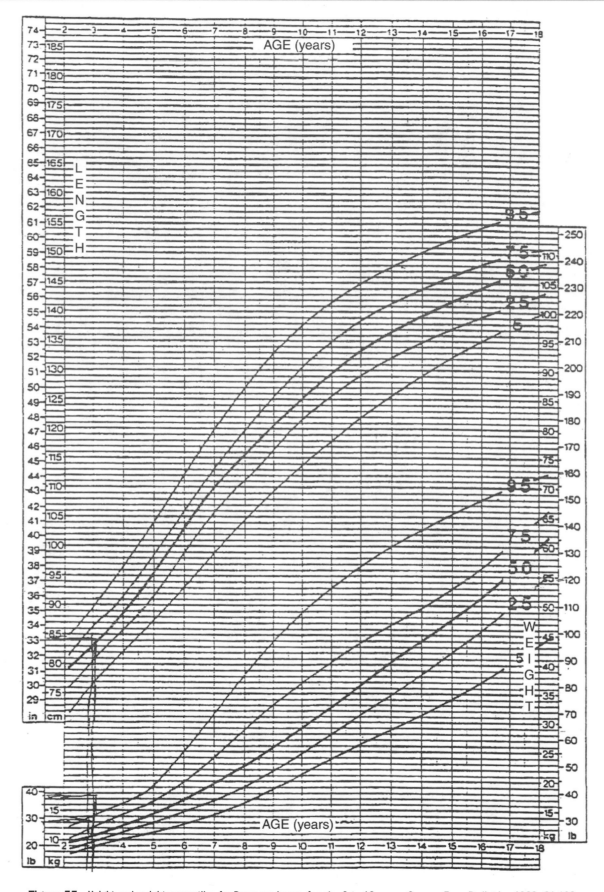

Figure 55 Height and weight percentiles for Down syndrome—female, 2 to 18 years. *Source:* From Pediatrics 1988; 81:102.

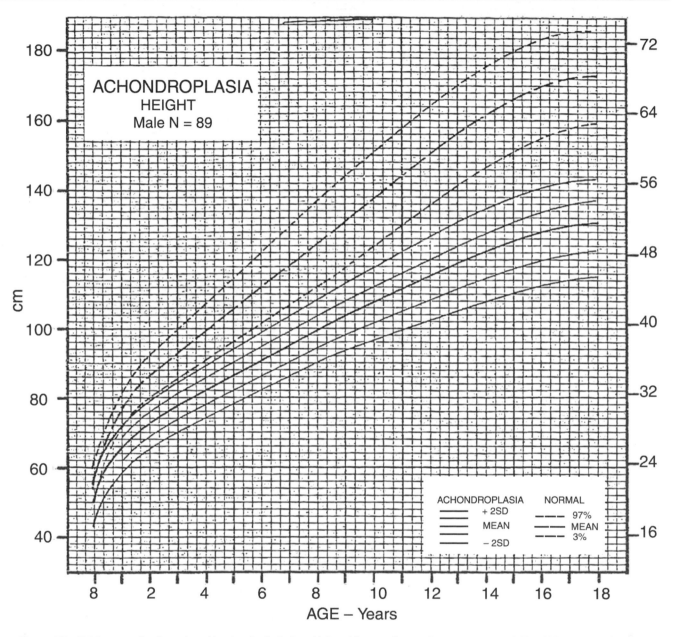

Figure 56   Height percentiles for males with achondroplasia from birth to 18 years. *Source*: From J Pediatr 1978:435–438; courtesy of Elsevier.

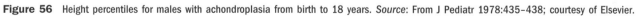

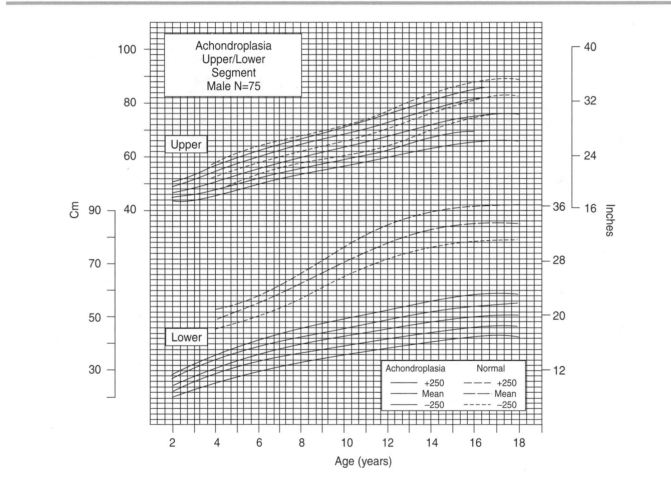

Figure 57 Upper and lower segments for achondroplasia–males, birth to 18 years. *Source*: From J Pediatr 1978:435–438; courtesy of Elsevier.

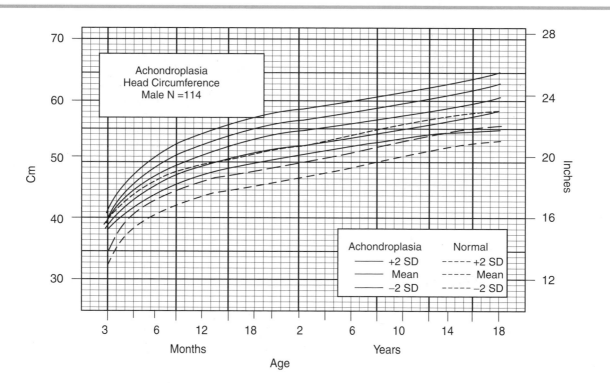

Figure 58   Head circumference for males with achondroplasia. *Source*: From J Pediatr 1978:435–438; courtesy of Elsevier.

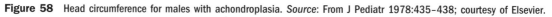

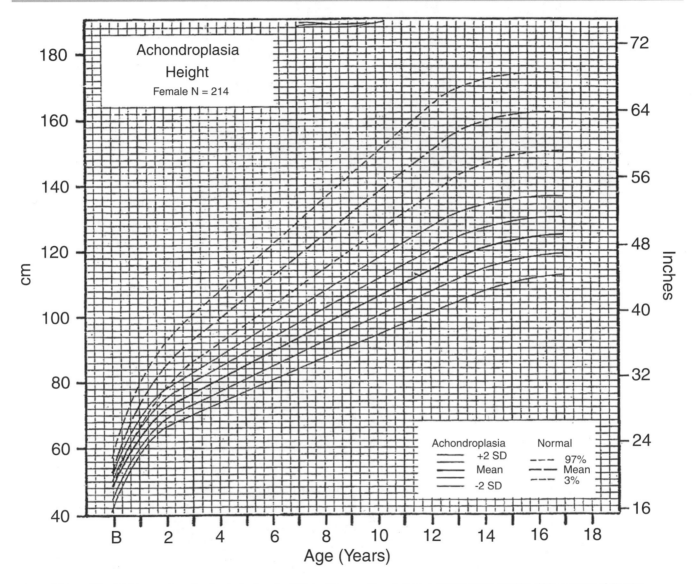

Figure 59   Height curve for achondroplasia—female, birth to 18 years. *Source*: From J Pediatr 1978; 93:435–438; courtesy of Elsevier.

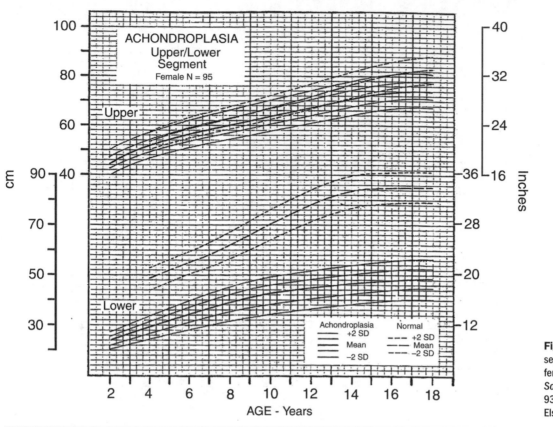

Figure 60 Upper and lower segments for achondroplasia—females, birth to 18 years. *Source*: From J Pediatr 1978; 93:435–438; courtesy of Elsevier.

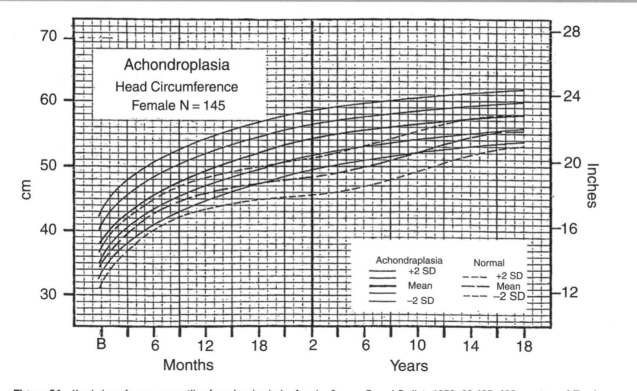

Figure 61 Head circumference percentiles for achondroplasia—female. *Source*: From J Pediatr 1978; 93:435–438; courtesy of Elsevier.

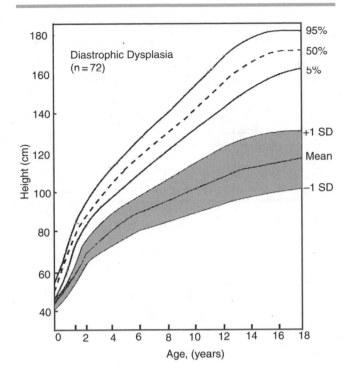

Figure 62 Growth percentiles for diastrophic dysplasia—birth to 18 years (no gender specified). *Source*: From Am J Dis Child 1983; 136:316–319.

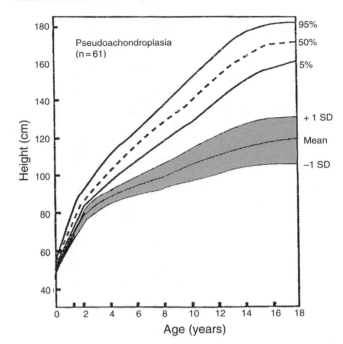

Figure 64 Growth percentiles for pseudoachondroplasia—birth to 18 years (no gender specified). *Source*: From Am J Dis Child 1983; 136:316–319.

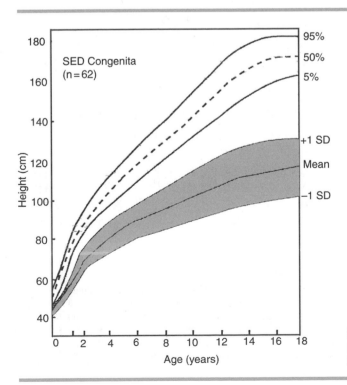

Figure 63 Growth percentiles for spondyloepiphyseal dysplasia congenital—birth to 18 years (no gender specified). *Source*: From Am J Dis Child 1983; 136:316–319.

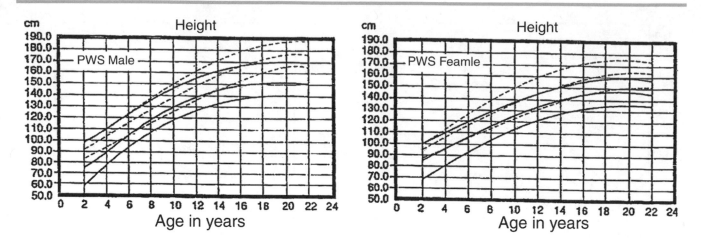

Figure 65   Height percentiles for males and females with Prader-Willi syndrome (*solid lines*) and healthy individuals (*broken lines*). *Source*: From Pediatrics 1991; 88:853.

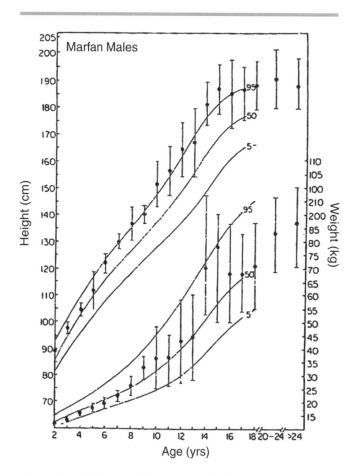

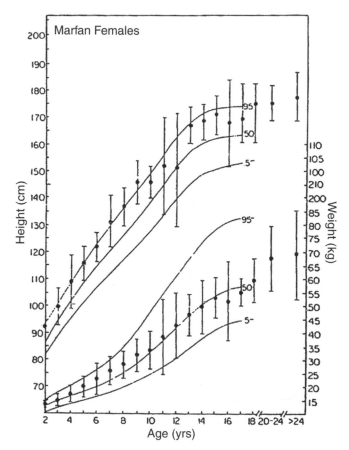

Figure 66   Height and weight percentiles for Marfan syndrome—male, 2 to 24 years, superimposed in normal growth curves (5th, 50th, and 95th percentiles). Cross-sectional and longitudinal data from 200 Caucasian patients with Marfan syndrome were included. Bars shown ± one standard deviation. *Source*: From Pyeritz RE. Marfan Syndrome. Principles and Practice of Medical genetics. New York: Churchill Livingstone, 1983.

Figure 67   Height and weight percentiles for Marfan syndrome—female, 2 to 24 years, superimposed in normal growth curves (5th, 50th, and 95th percentiles). Cross-sectional and longitudinal data from 200 Caucasian patients with Marfan syndrome were included. Bars shown ± one standard deviation. *Source*: From Pyeritz RE. Marfan Syndrome. Principles and Practice of Medical genetics. New York: Churchill Livingstone, 1983.

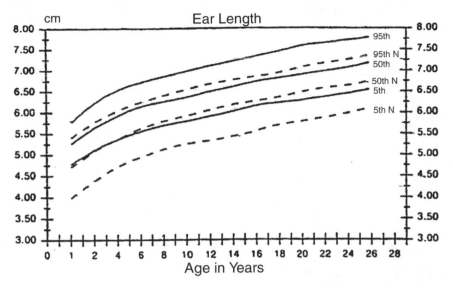

Figure 68 Curve of ear length for males with fragile X syndrome (*solid lines*) and normal individuals (*dotted lines*). *Source*: From Butler MG, Brunschwig A, Miller LK, et al. Pediatrics 1992; 89:1059–1062.

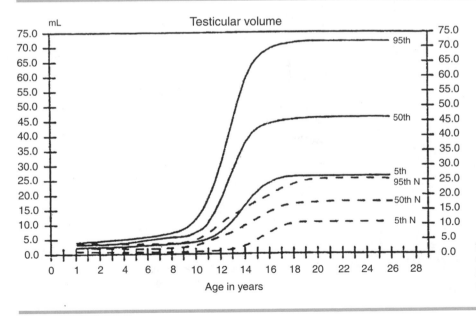

Figure 69 Curves for testes volume for males with fragile X syndrome—birth to 28 years. *Source*: From Butler MG, Brunschwig A, Miller LK, et al. Pediatrics 1992; 89:1059–1062.

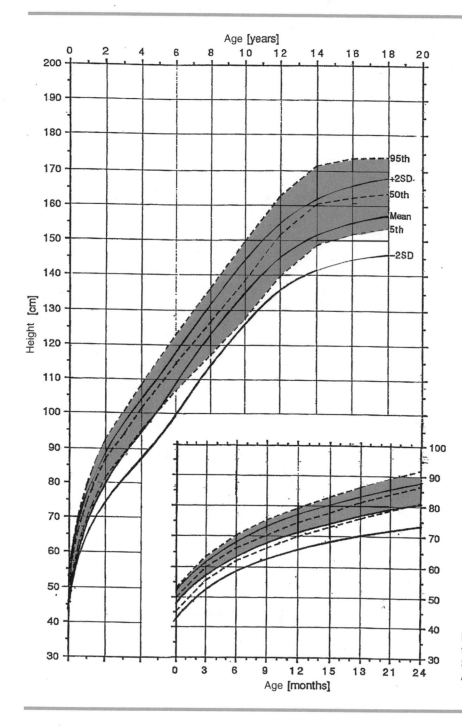

Figure 70 Height percentiles for William syndrome females, 0 to 20 years. *Source*: From Saul RA, Geer Js, Seaver LH, et al. Growth References: Third Trimester to Adulthood. Greenwood, SC: Greenwood Genetic Center, 1998.

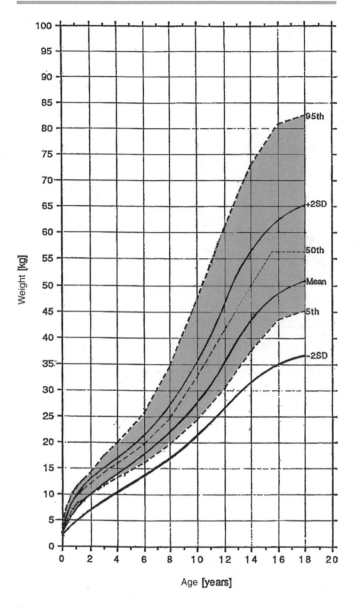

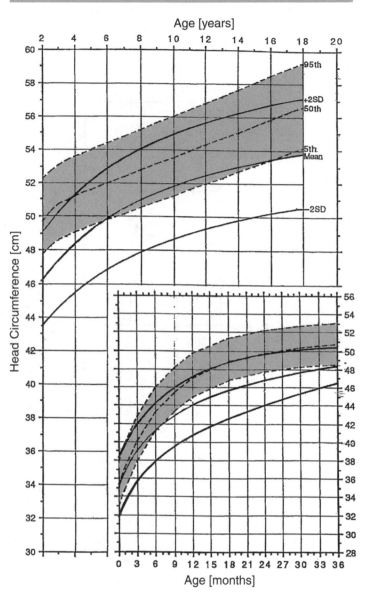

Figure 71 Weight percentiles for William syndrome females, 0 to 20 years. *Source*: From Saul RA, Geer Js, Seaver LH, et al. Growth References: Third Trimester to Adulthood. Greenwood, SC: Greenwood Genetic Center, 1998.

Figure 72 Head circumference percentiles for William syndrome females, 0 to 20 years. *Source*: From Saul RA, Geer Js, Seaver LH, et al. Growth References: Third Trimester to Adulthood. Greenwood, SC: Greenwood Genetic Center, 1998.

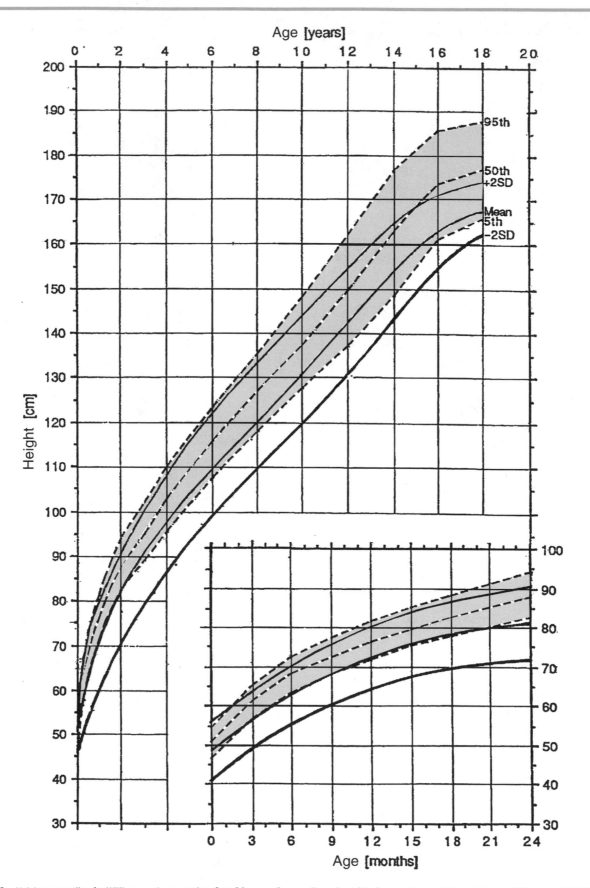

Figure 73 Height percentiles for William syndrome males, 0 to 20 years. *Source*: From Saul RA, Geer Js, Seaver LH, et al. Growth References: Third Trimester to Adulthood. Greenwood, SC: Greenwood Genetic Center; 1998.

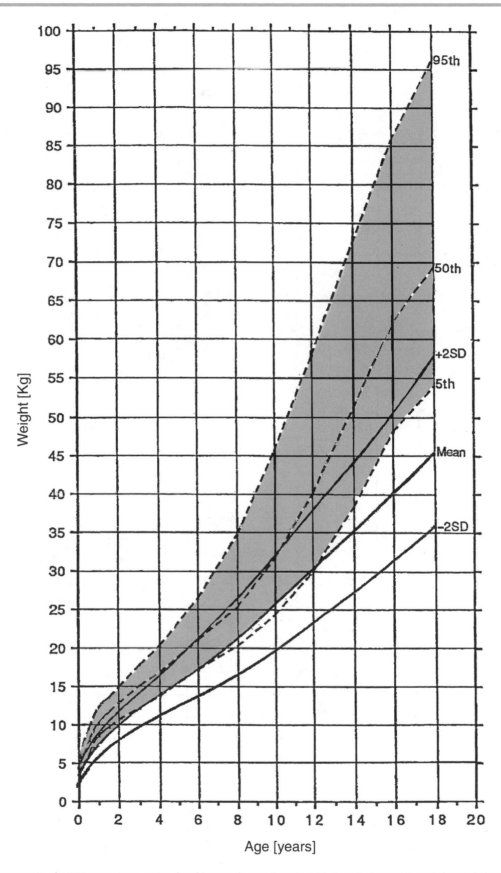

Figure 74 Weight percentiles for William syndrome males, 0 to 20 years. *Source:* From Saul RA, Geer Js, Seaver LH, et al. Growth References: Third Trimester to Adulthood. Greenwood, SC: Greenwood Genetic Center, 1998.

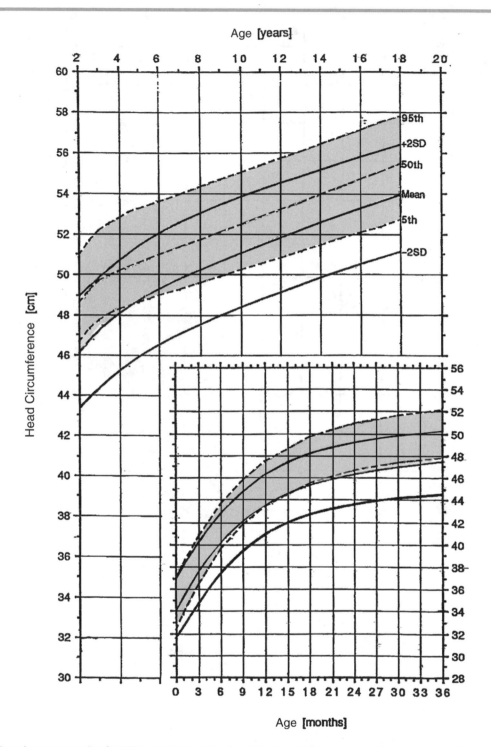

Figure 75 Head circumference percentiles for William syndrome males, 0 to 20 years. *Source*: From Saul RA, Geer Js, Seaver LH, et al. Growth References: Third Trimester to Adulthood. Greenwood, SC: Greenwood Genetic Center, 1998.

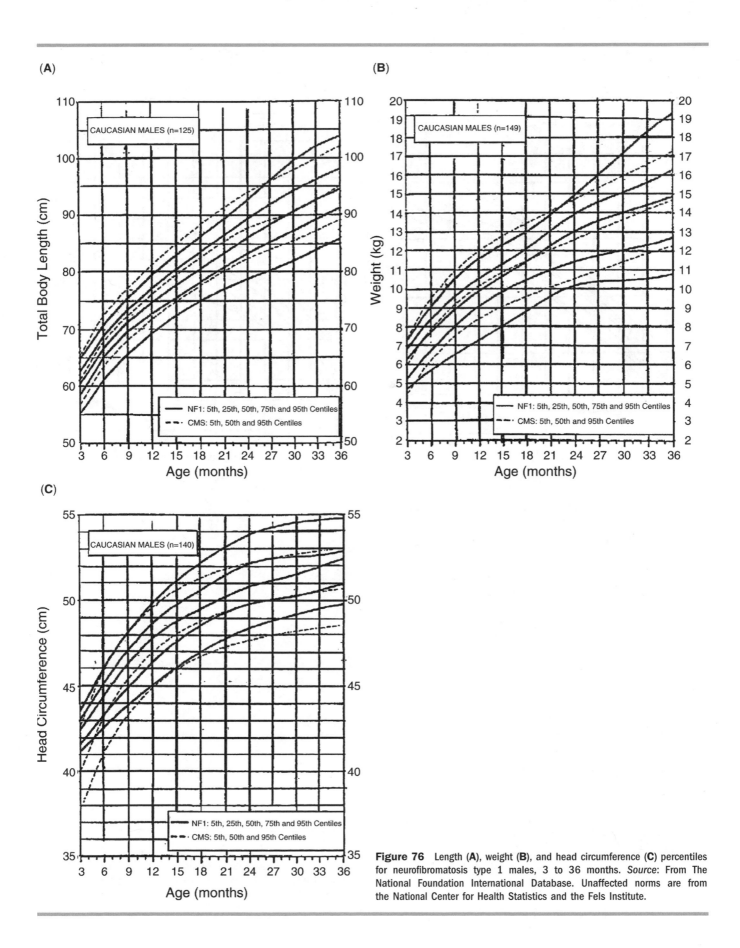

Figure 76 Length (**A**), weight (**B**), and head circumference (**C**) percentiles for neurofibromatosis type 1 males, 3 to 36 months. *Source:* From The National Foundation International Database. Unaffected norms are from the National Center for Health Statistics and the Fels Institute.

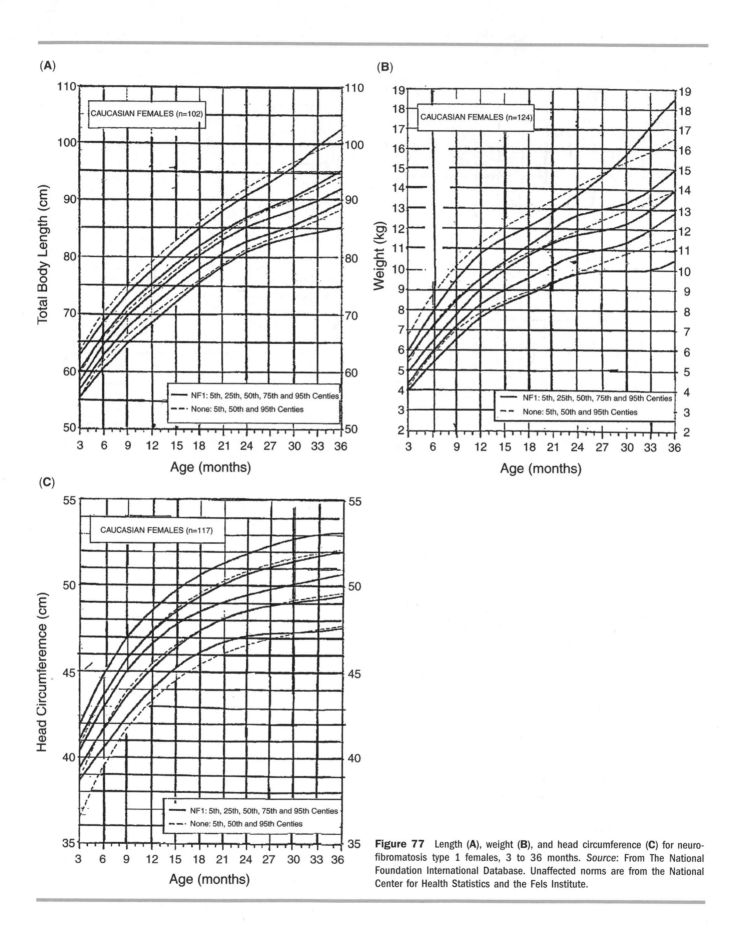

(A)

(B)

(C)

Figure 77 Length (**A**), weight (**B**), and head circumference (**C**) for neurofibromatosis type 1 females, 3 to 36 months. *Source*: From The National Foundation International Database. Unaffected norms are from the National Center for Health Statistics and the Fels Institute.

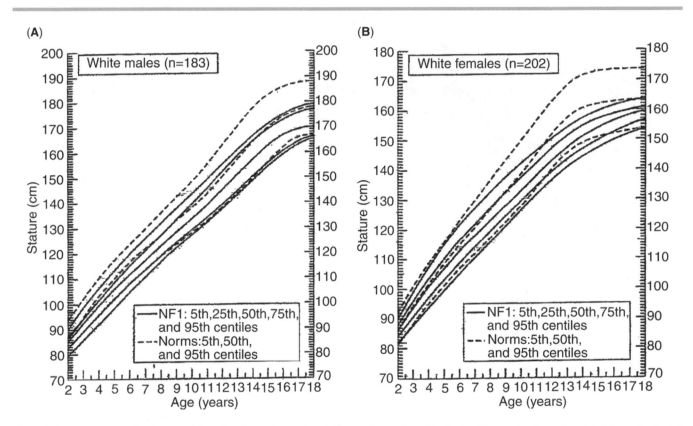

Figure 78 Height percentiles for NF1 males (**A**) and females (**B**) 2 to 18 years. *Source*: From The National Foundation International Database. Unaffected norms are from the National Center for Health Statistics and the Fels Institute; Szudek J, Birch P, Friedman JM. J Med Genet 2000; 37:933–938; courtesy of BMJ Publishing Group LTd, 2000.

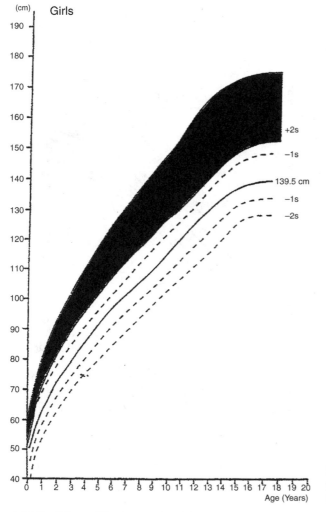

Figure 79 Height percentiles for Russell–Silver syndrome girls from 0 to 20 years. *Source*: From Wollman HA et al. Eur J Pediatr 1995; 154:958; courtesy of Springer Science and Business Media.

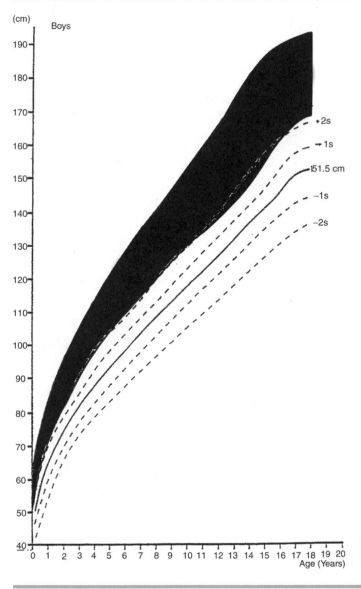

Figure 80 Height percentiles for Russell–Silver syndrome males from 0 to 20 years. *Source*: From Wollman HA et al. Eur J Pediatr 1995; 154:958; courtesy of Springer Science and Business Media.

Miscellaneous Data

Table 1 Eating Attitudes Score

	Always	Very often	Often	Sometimes	Rarely	Never
Am terrified about being overweight	( )	( )	( )	( )	( )	( )
Avoid eating when I am hungry	( )	( )	( )	( )	( )	( )
Find myself preoccupied with food	( )	( )	( )	( )	( )	( )
Have gone on eating binges where I feel that I may not be able to stop	( )	( )	( )	( )	( )	( )
Cut my food into small pieces	( )	( )	( )	( )	( )	( )
Aware of the calorie content of foods I eat	( )	( )	( )	( )	( )	( )
Particularly avoid foods with high carbohydrate content (e.g., bread, potatoes, rice)	( )	( )	( )	( )	( )	( )
Feel that others would prefer if I ate more	( )	( )	( )	( )	( )	( )
Vomit after I have eaten	( )	( )	( )	( )	( )	( )
Feel extremely guilty after eating	( )	( )	( )	( )	( )	( )
Am preoccupied with a desire to be thinner	( )	( )	( )	( )	( )	( )
Think about burning up calories when I exercise	( )	( )	( )	( )	( )	( )
Other people think that I am too thin	( )	( )	( )	( )	( )	( )
Am preoccupied with the thought of having fat on my body	( )	( )	( )	( )	( )	( )
Take longer than others to eat my meals	( )	( )	( )	( )	( )	( )
Avoid foods with sugar in them	( )	( )	( )	( )	( )	( )
Eat diet foods	( )	( )	( )	( )	( )	( )
Feel that food controls my life	( )	( )	( )	( )	( )	( )
Display self-control around food	( )	( )	( )	( )	( )	( )
Feel that others pressure me to eat	( )	( )	( )	( )	( )	( )
Give too much time and thought to food	( )	( )	( )	( )	( )	( )
Feel uncomfortable after eating sweets	( )	( )	( )	( )	( )	( )
Engage in dieting behavior	( )	( )	( )	( )	( )	( )
Like my stomach to be empty	( )	( )	( )	( )	( )	( )
Enjoy trying new rich foods	( )	( )	( )	( )	( )	( )
Have the impulse to vomit after meals	( )	( )	( )	( )	( )	( )

Note: Scores are derived as follows: a mark on "always" yields 3 points, "very often" 2 points, "often" 1 point, and "others" 0 point. The only exception is number 25, which is reversed scoring. Any patient who scores above 20 points may have a severe eating disorder
Source: From Gardner MP, Bohr Y, Garfinkel PE. The Eating Attitude Test: psychometric features & clinical correlates. Psych Med 1982; 12:871–878.

Table 2 Serum Total Cholesterol Levels for Children and Adolescents by Sex, Age, and Race NHANES III

Population group	N	Mean (SE)*	Percentiles						
			5	10	25	50	75	90	95
Age[a] (years)									
4–5	1,707	162 (0.9)	124	132	144	161	177	194	204
6–8	1,367	168 (1.0)	126	134	149	165	282	197	209
8–11	1,488	171 (1.0)	131	139	151	168	187	206	222
12–15	1,502	161 (1.2)	118	126	141	158	178	197	209
16–19	1,435	165 (1.6)	118	124	141	158	182	207	222
12–19	2,937	163 (1.0)	518	125	141	158	180	201	217
Total (4–19)	7,499	165 (0.6)	121	130	145	162	181	200	216
Sex and age[b] (years)									
Male									
4–5		161 (1.5)	122	132	143	159	175	191	202
8–8		160 (1.7)	126	134	146	164	183	202	212
9–11		173 (2.0)	135	140	153	170	188	208	226
12–15		158 (1.6)	116	124	140	157	174	192	203
16–19		158 (1.8)	116	122	138	155	174	199	213
12–19		158 (1.2)	116	123	139	156	174	195	206
Total (4–19)		163 (1.0)	119	127	143	161	179	198	212
Female									
4–5		164 (1.3)	125	133	145	182	178	196	206
6–8		166 (1.4)	126	138	149	165	180	596	203
9–11		169 (1.5)	130	137	148	166	185	204	218
12–15		164 (1.9)	122	129	142	159	181	201	218
16–19		171 (2.3)	118	128	145	163	189	217	237
12–19		167 (1.3)	119	128	144	181	185	209	225
Total (4–19)		167 (0.8)	124	132	147	163	184	202	220
Race/ethnicity and sex									
Non-Hispanic black									
Male		168 (1.0)	122	132	148	165	186	304	219
Female		171 (1.2)	122	134	149	167	189	213	226
Non-Hispanic white									
Male		162 (1.2)	118	126	143	160	178	195	207
Female		166 (1.1)	123	132	146	163	182	200	217
Mexican American									
Male		183 (1.0)	121	129	143	159	180	202	213
Female		165 (1.1)	121	128	144	161	183	201	216
Race/ethnicity and age (years)									
Non-Hispanic black									
4–5		166 (1.3)	121	128	147	164	182	200	214
6–8		172 (1.7)	128	138	150	168	190	210	219
9–11		173 (1.8)	131	138	152	168	191	212	228
12–15		168 (1.2)	119	127	147	168	186	208	222
16–19		168 (1.7)	120	131	147	163	186	214	226
12–19		168 (1.1)	119	130	147	164	186	211	224
Total (4–19)		170 (0.9)	122	133	148	168	187	209	223
Non-Hispanic white									
4–5		162 (1.5)	128	134	144	160	175	188	202
6–8		166 (1.3)	125	133	149	165	181	196	204
9–11		170 (1.1)	131	140	151	168	186	201	219
12–15		159 (1.4)	117	126	140	157	176	193	203
16–19		163 (2.1)	117	123	139	157	182	205	221
12–19		161 (1.4)	117	124	139	157	179	199	215
Total (4–19)		164 (0.8)	119	129	144	162	180	198	212
Mexican American									
4–5		161 (1.7)	120	127	143	159	177	197	204
6–8		164 (1.8)	126	134	145	162	179	192	208
9–11		168 (1.2)	126	135	147	163	186	206	216
12–15		160 (1.7)	118	123	139	155	176	198	212
16–19		168 (2.3)	121	129	145	162	186	211	227
12–19		163 (1.6)	119	126	141	157	181	204	218
Total (4–19)		164 (0.9)	121	129	144	160	182	201	214

Source: From Hickman TB, Briefel RR, Carroll MD, et al. Distributions and trends of serum lipid levels among United States children and adolescents ages 4–19 years: data from the Third National Health and Nutrition Examination Survey. Prev Med 1998; 27:879–890.

Table 3 Serum HDL-C Levels for Children and Adolescents by Sex, Age, and Race NHANES III

Population group	N	Mean (SE)*	Percentiles						
			5	10	25	50	75	90	95
Age (years)									
4-5	1,697	49 (0.5)	30	35	40	47	55	64	70
6-8	1,362	52 (0.6)	33	37	43	50	59	67	71
9-11	1,479	52 (0.6)	35	38	43	51	59	68	74
12-15	1,494	50 (0.6)	33	35	41	48	57	64	69
16-19	1,426	49 (0.5)	31	34	40	48	56	64	70
12-19	2,920	49 (0.4)	32	35	40	48	56	64	69
Total (4-19)	7,458	50 (0.3)	32	36	41	49	57	65	71
Sex and age* (years)									
Male									
4-5		50 (0.7)	31	35	41	49	56	65	71
6-8		53 (0.6)	33	37	43	51	60	68	73
9-11		534(0.6)	37	39	44	52	61	71	76
12-15		48 (0.7)	32	35	39	46	55	62	67
16-19		46 (0.9)	30	33	38	45	51	61	67
12-19		47 (0.6)	31	34	38	46	53	62	67
Total (4-19)		50 (0.4)	32	35	40	48	57	65	71
Female									
4-5		48 (0.6)	30	34	39	46	55	62	68
6-8		50 (0.9)	33	37	43	49	57	64	70
9-11		51 (0.7)	33	38	42	50	57	65	69
12-15		51 (0.8)	33	36	42	50	58	66	70
16-19		52 (0.7)	33	37	43	52	59	66	72
12-19		52 (0.5)	33	37	43	51	59	66	71
Total (4-19)		51 (0.4)	33	36	42	50	58	65	70
Race/ethnicity and sex									
Non-Hispanic black									
Male		55 (0.5)	37	39	46	53	63	72	77
Female		56 (0.4)	36	40	46	54	63	72	78
Non-Hispanic white									
Male		48 (0.5)	31	35	39	47	55	63	68
Female		50 (0.5)	32	36	41	49	56	63	68
Mexican American									
Male		51 (0.5)	31	35	41	49	58	66	72
Female		52 (0.4)	34	37	43	50	58	57	73
Race/ethnicity and age (years)									
Non-Hispanic black									
4-5		53 (0.7)	35	38	45	52	59	68	75
6-8		58 (0.7)	39	42	49	57	66	73	80
9-11		58 (0.7)	35	41	47	57	56	76	83
12-15		55 (0.8)	36	39	46	54	63	72	77
16-19		53 (0.5)	36	38	45	51	59	69	74
12-19		54 (0.5)	36	39	45	52	61	71	76
Total (4-19)		55 (0.4)	36	40	46	54	63	72	78
Non-Hispanic white									
4-5		47 (0.8)	29	34	39	46	53	63	67
6-8		50 (0.8)	32	36	42	49	56	65	69
9-11		51 (0.8)	35	38	42	50	58	66	71
12-15		48 (0.7)	32	35	40	47	54	61	65
16-19		48 (0.6)	30	33	39	47	54	61	67
12-19		48 (0.5)	31	34	40	47	54	61	66
Total (4-19)		49 (0.4)	32	35	41	48	55	63	68
Mexican American									
4-5		50 (0.6)	29	35	41	49	57	64	69
6-8		53 (0.6)	35	38	44	52	59	66	72
9-11		52 (0.0)	33	37	42	51	60	70	76
12-15		50 (0.7)	32	35	42	49	57	65	70
16-19		50 (0.6)	32	36	42	48	57	65	72
12-19		50 (0.6)	32	36	42	49	57	65	71
Total (4-19)		51 (0.4)	32	36	42	50	58	66	72

Source: From Hickman TB, Briefel RR, Carroll MD, et al. Distributions and trends of serum lipid levels among United States children and adolescents ages 4-19 years: data from the Third National Health and Nutrition Examination Survey. Prev Med 1998; 27:879-890.

Table 4   Serum LDL-C Levels for Children and Adolescents by Sex, Age, and Race NHANES III

Population group	N	Mean (SE)*	Percentiles						
			5	10	25	50	75	90	95
Age (years)									
12–15	551	91 (2.0)	51	56	73	88	106	125	135
16–19	544	99 (2.8)	56	63	78	90	113	146	162
Total (12–19)	1,095	95 (1.6)	53	61	76	89	109	132	152
Sex and age* (years)									
Male									
12–15		88 (2.4)	50[d]	54[d]	68	83	103	119[d]	131[d]
16–19		94 (3.8)	54[d]	64[d]	76	89	103	132[d]	153[d]
Total (12–19)		91 (2.1)	52	60	73	88	103	126	149
Female									
12–15		94 (2.8)	54[d]	59	77	90	110	127	145[d]
16–19		103 (4.4)	59[d]	63	79	94	123	147	167[d]
Total (12–19)		99 (2.4)	54	62	78	92	115	139	161
Race/ethnicity and sex									
Non-Hispanic black									
Male		99 (2.4)	60	68	80	98	115	127	138
Female		102 (1.9)	58	71	81	96	123	142	154
Non-Hispanic white									
Male		91 (3.2)	48[d]	58	72	87	102	131	152[d]
Female		100 (3.4)	54[d]	60	76	90	115	145	161[d]
Mexican American									
Male		93 (2.2)	56[d]	63[d]	74	93	107	123	135[d]
Female		92 (3.1)	52[d]	57	74	88	108	124	139[d]
Race/ethnicity and age (years)									
Non-Hispanic black									
12–15		101 (2.1)	57	70	81	99	119	133	142
16–19		100 (2.0)	60	69	80	96	116	134	156
Total (12–19)		101 (1.4)	59	69	81	97	119	134	146
Non-Hispanic white									
12–15		89 (2.7)	46[d]	53	70	86	105	122	133[d]
16–19		101 (3.9)	58[d]	65	78	90	113	151	163[d]
Total (12–19)		95 (2.6)	51	59	75	88	107	135	155
Mexican American									
12–15		91 (3.0)	53[d]	57	73	90	106	123	130[d]
16–19		95 (2.1)	57[d]	63	76	91	109	126	140[d]
Total (12–19)		93 (2.1)	54	61	74	91	107	123	136

Source: From Hickman TB, Briefel RR, Carroll MD, et al. Distributions and trends of serum lipid levels among United States children and adolescents ages 4–19 years: data from the Third National Health and Nutrition Examination Survey. Prev Med 1998; 27:879–890.

Table 5 Serum Triglycerides Levels for Children and Adolescents by Sex, Age, and Race NHANES III

Population group	N	Mean (SE)[b]	Percentiles						
			5	10	25	50	75	90	95
Age[c] (years)									
12–15	554	91 (4.4)	38	44	56	74	108	147	208
16–19	545	95 (3.7)	39	45	58	78	119	173	207
Total (12–19)	1,099	93 (2.4)	38	45	57	76	110	160	207
Sex and age[c] (years)									
Male									
12–15		87 (7.0)	35[d]	41[d]	54	72	101	135[d]	178[d]
16–19		94 (6.1)	36[d]	45[d]	58	79	119	165[d]	200[d]
Total (12–19)		91 (4.0)	36	42	55	74	107	150	196
Female									
12–15		96 (5.6)	41[d]	48	59	81	110	170	213[d]
16–19		96 (5.9)	43[d]	46	60	76	118	168	207[d]
Total (12–19)		96 (3.9)	43	47	60	77	115	171	208
Race/ethnicity and sex									
Non-Hispanic black									
Male		72 (4.5)	35[d]	39	48	63	84	99	117[d]
Female		72 (3.2)	36[d]	40	50	63	81	110	144[d]
Non-Hispanic white									
Male		95 (6.5)	37[d]	43	56	76	109	164	205[d]
Female		99 (5.0)	41[d]	47	60	80	118	172	218[d]
Mexican American									
Male		95 (5.5)	37[d]	44	55	79	109	146	203[d]
Female		98 (4.6)	45[d]	53	62	85	111	156	202[d]
Race/ethnicity and age (years)									
Non-Hispanic black									
12–15		74 (5.2)	35[d]	39	49	64	82	103	151[d]
16–19		70 (2.7)	35[d]	41	48	63	83	100	120[d]
Total (12–19)		72 (3.0)	35	39	49	63	82	101	126
Non-Hispanic white									
12–15		94 (6.7)	38[d]	43	57	74	108	168	211[d]
16–19		99 (4.6)	39[d]	48	59	81	123	173	223d
Total (12–19)		97 (3.4)	39	35	57	78	115	171	216
Mexican American									
12–15		95 (4.0)	43[d]	48	60	83	109	144	191[d]
16–19		98 (6.2)	38[d]	46	60	82	112	158	210[d]
Total (12–19)		96 (3.7)	42	47	60	83	111	150	205

Source: From Hickman TB, Briefel RR, Carroll MD, et al. Distributions and trends of serum lipid levels among United States children and adolescents ages 4–19 years: data from the Third National Health and Nutrition Examination Survey. Prev Med 1998; 27(6):879–890.